Special Operations Forces Medical Handbook

Second Edition

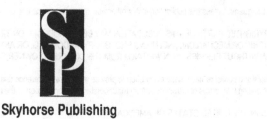

Skyhorse Publishing

Chief Editor:	COL Warner Dahlgren "Rocky" Farr, MC, US Army
Senior Medical Editor:	CDR Leslie H. Fenton, MC, US Navy (Ret)
Project Manager:	Robert Clayton, SF, US Army (Ret)
Managing Editor:	Gay Dews Thompson, BSN, MPH
Style Editor:	Holly Hardison Pavliscsak, BS, MHSA
Production Manger:	Jeanette D. Rasche, BS, MS
Medical Illustrators:	Jordan Mastrodonato, MS, CMI
	Brad Sullivan, BFA, MS
Network Administrator:	Rick Wise

Dosage Selection: The authors and the Department of Defense have made every effort to ensure the accuracy of dosages cited herein. However, it is the responsibility of every practitioner to consult appropriate information sources to ascertain correct dosages for each clinical situation, especially for new or unfamiliar drugs and procedures. The authors, editors, publisher, and the Department of Defense cannot be held responsible for any errors found in this book.

Use of Trade or Brand Names: Use of trade or brand names in this publication is for illustrative purposes only and does not imply endorsement by the Department of Defense.

Neutral Language: Unless this publication states otherwise, masculine nouns and pronouns do not refer exclusively to men.

The authors and publisher have made every effort to provide an accurate reference text. However, they shall not be held responsible for problems arising from errors or omission, or from misunderstandings on the part of the reader.

PRINTED IN THE UNITED STATES OF AMERICA

First Skyhorse Publishing Edition © 2011 for additional material only.

Library of Congress Cataloging-in-Publication Data is available on file.

ISBN: 978-1-61608-278-9

Second Edition Authors and Contributors:

LTC John Albano, MC, US Army
MAJ Abel Alfonso, MC, US Army
COL Shannon Allison, DC, US Army Reserve
COL Warner Anderson, MC, US Army Reserve
MAJ Richard Angel, MC, US Army
COL Frank Anders, MC, US Army
CPT Steven Ballard, MC, US Army
LTC Scott Barnes, MC, US Army
MAJ Steven Batty, VC, US Army
Col Charles Beadling, US Air Force, MC
Alexander Bertelsen, PA-C
MSG Samuel Blazier, US Army
CPT Kristin S. Bloink, VC, US Army
LTC William Bosworth, VC, US Army
MAJ Adam Buchanan, MC, US Amy
COL Chester Buckenmaier, III, MC, US Army
CDR Timothy Burgess, MC, US Navy
CPT Samuel Burkett, MC, US Army
COL David Burris, MC, US Army
COL Leopoldo C. Cancio, MC, US Army
LTC Marc Caouette, MS, US Army
BG Joseph Caravalho, Jr., MC, US Army
Lt Col George Christopher, US Air Force, MC
COL Ted Cieslak, MC, US Army
COL Robert Cinatl, DC, US Army
COL Clifford Cloonan, MC, US Army (Ret)
CPT Christopher Cole, SP, US Army
Maj Nicholas Conger, US Air Force, MC
CAPT Joseph Cosentino, Jr., NC, US Navy
Phillip Coule, MD
MAJ John Croushorn, MC, MSARNG
MSgt G. Steven Cum, US Air Force
Lt Col Gregory Deye, US Air Force, MC
LTC Prospero Donan, Jr., AN, US Army
LTC Michael Doyle, MC, US Army
COL Edward Eitzen, MC, US Army (Ret)
LTC Ethan Emmons, MC, US Army
LTC Raymond Enzenauer, MC, US Army (Ret)
LTC Robert Enzenauer, MC, US Army (Ret)
LTC Kathleen Dunn Farr, MC, US Army
COL Warner Farr, MC, US Army
CDR Leslie H. Fenton, MC, US Navy (Ret)
CAPT Scott Flinn, MC, US Navy
LTC Robert Forsten, MC, US Army
CDR Raymond A. Fritz, MSC, US Navy Reserve (Ret)
COL Michael Fuenfer, MC, US Army Reserve
SFC Dominique Greydanus, US Army (Ret)
MAJ Leonard Gruppo, SP, US Army
COL Henry Hacker, MC, US Army
CDR John Hammes, MC, US Navy
COL Karla Hansen, MC, US Army
COL Jackie Hayes, MC, US Army
Katherine Helmick, RN, CNRN, CRNP
Mary Ellen Hoehn, MD
Maryann Hoftiezer, MSN, FNP-C
COL John Holcomb, MC, US Army
COL Duane Hospenthal, MC, US Army
MAJ (P) Daniel Hsu, MC, US Army
LT John Hyatt, MC, US Navy Reserve
LTC Michael Jaffee, MC, US Army
CDR Christopher Jankosky, MC, US Navy
Lt Col W. Scott Jones, US Air Force, MC
LT Traci Johnson, NC, US Navy
COL Ismail Jatoi, MC, US Army
LTC Sean Keenan, MC, US Army
COL Kenneth R. Kemp, MC, US Army

LCDR Steven Kriss, MC, US Navy
MAJ Paul Kwon, MC, US Army
MAJ William Lefkowitz, MC, US Army
COL Martha Lenhart, MC, US Army
Brooke Lerner, Ph.D.
MAJ Christopher J. Lettieri, MC, US Army
CAPT D. Mark Llewellyn, MC, US Navy
LTC Douglas Lougee, MC, US Army
LCDR Robert Lueken, MC, US Navy
LTC Robert Lutz, MC, US Army
MAJ Robert Malsby III, MC, USA
COL Kurt Maggio, MC, US Army
COL Peter McNally, MC, US Army (Ret)
COL John Mercier, MS, US Army
COL Charles Middleton, DC, US Army Reserve
MAJ Charles Moon, MC, US Army
MAJ L. Bradley Morgans, AN, US Army
COL Michael Morris, MC, US Army (Ret)
LTC (P) Robert Mott, Jr., MC, US Army
LTC Clinton Murray, MC, US Army
LTC Jeffery Nelson, MC, US Army
MAJ Karin Nicholson, MC, US Army
LTC Ric Ong, MC, US Army
CPT Carl Pavel, MC, US Army
COL Ronald Poropatich, MC, US Army
MAJ Timothy Pellini, MC, US Army
LTC Andre Pennardt, MC, US Army
CPT Michael Perkins, MC, US Army
MAJ Robert Price, MC, US Army
LCDR Timothy Quast, MC, US Navy
MAJ James Reed, AN, US Army
Col Glen Reeves, US Air Force, MC (Ret)
Capt Dara Regn, US Air Force, MC
COL Glenn Reside, DC, US Army (Ret)
CPT Jesse Reynolds, MS, US Army
COL Paul Rock, MC, US Army (Ret)
COL Michael Roy, MC, US Army
CDR John Sanders, MC, US Navy
LTC E. Glenn Sanford, MC, US Army
CPT Jeffrey Savage, MC, US Army
LTC (P) Daniel Schissel, MC, US Army
LT Susan Schmidt, NC, US Navy Reserve
Richard Schwartz, MD
Maj Ricky Sexton, US Air Force, NC
Capt Joshua Sill, US Air Force, MC
LTC (P) Douglas Soderdahl, MC, US Army
COL Richard Tenglin, MC, US Army (Ret)
Steven J. Thomas, MD
Gay Dews Thompson, RN, MPH
LTC Gwendolyn Thompson, MS, US Army
LT Frank Tratchel, NC, US Navy
COL Robert Vigersky, MC, US Army
Lt Col Jeff Vista, US Air Force, MC
CDR Robert Wall, MC, US Navy
COL Winston J. Warme, MC, US Army (Ret)
LTC Steve Waxman, MC, US Army
LCDR Timothy Whitman, MC, US Navy Reserve
Col John Wightman, US Air Force, MC
LTC Joseph Wilde, MC, US Army
MSG Lennox Wildman, US Army
LTC Marvin Williams, MC, US Army
LTC Joseph Williamson, VC, US Army
CPT James Woodrow, MC, US Army
COL Glenn Wortmann, MC, US Army
MAJ Victor Yu, SP, US Army (Ret)
MAJ Thomas B. Zanders, MC, US Army

Table of Contents

PART 4: ORGAN SYSTEMS

Chapter 1: Cardiac/Circulatory

Chapter 2: Blood

Chapter 3: Respiratory

Chapter 4: Endocrine

Introduction

The Office of the Surgeon, John F. Kennedy Center for Military Assistance published the first *Special Forces Medical Specialist Handbook* in January 1969. It has a red cover and I have the only copy that I have seen in years. In 1982, the John F. Kennedy Special Warfare Center published the second edition. It was green covered and titled *ST 31-91B US Army Special Forces Medical Handbook*. This office, the Command Surgeon, United States Special Operations Command, under Colonel Steve Yevich, a Special Forces qualified Army medical officer, published the first edition of the familiar black covered *Special Operations Forces Medical Handbook* 1 June 2001. This "single-source" reference provided many nontraditional approaches to accessing medical information, such as a treatment hierarchy based on available resources and mission parameters commonly facing Special Operations Forces (SOF) Medics. Our handbook continues to be an innovation in military medicine, organized into a problem-oriented template for reference to diagnoses and treatments with contributions by over 130 authors, 57 reviewers, and 4 editors.

As a Special Forces medic in Vietnam with the Studies and Observations Group, I used the "red book" to do my utmost to care for our wounded and sick. Current Global War On Terror SOF medics, called "Doc" by the men they serve, rely on the medical resources at their disposal-what supplies they brought on their backs to the war along with ingenuity, and courage. I am profoundly grateful for the time and effort put forth by the authors, editors, and production staff of the Special Operations Forces Medical Handbook's second edition, especially, Mr. Bob Clayton, USSF(Ret.); CDR Les Fenton, USN (Ret), and Mrs. Gay Thompson, RN. I recognize with heartfelt appreciation the time sacrificed by all contributors from their busy schedules, deployments, families and friends, in order to meet our requirements. The rules of employment were stringent, the template a struggle, and the salary was none. They are listed in this introductory section.

Thirteen years passed between the first and second SF Medic handbooks and a further nineteen years before the first SOF Medic handbook. It has been only eight years to this second SOF edition. The world has changed dramatically; we are at war and we have new weapons, enemies, friends and threats. New diseases and new types of injuries have emerged, and as always in war, new treatments and therapies have been developed. Advancing technology and an explosive proliferation of medical information on the Internet have revolutionized medicine. The mission of SOF medics has not changed; unaided, medics provide care with limited resources in austere, hostile, stressful, and isolated environments, without the capability of timely patient evacuation. The scope and standards of SOF medical missions are radically different from those found in a fixed, fully equipped, and staffed hospital in a peaceful America. Few in civilian (or even conventional military) medicine ever are challenged with the conditions in which SOF medics practice daily. Despite the proliferation of medical information, no other single reference source has emerged addressing the varied and complicated needs of SOF Medics. Prior to the last edition, conflicting information and even misinformation had created confusion over the most basic medical questions, possibly endangering the lives of those we are committed to help. The SOF medical community mitigated this danger by creating the SOF Medical Handbook. This Handbook is part of an evolving system, taking advantage of new information technology. I deliberately limited the printed version in size. The system includes an electronic version that is in exhaustive detail. It provides guidance to medics in our special environment, answering the hard diagnostic and treatment questions as best as possible. These answers are based on the best possible knowledge and tailored to the austere mission — in plain, straightforward language, without excuses, conditions, or academic musings. This is not a trauma manual; this is a primary care medicine manual. We developed the Tactical Combat Casualty Care (TCCC) guidelines under Captain Frank Butler, a SEAL qualified medical officer and my predecessor, and it has its own manual. Some will view the advice in this handbook as dangerous, outrageous in traditional, conservative, hospital-based medical settings. Only someone struggling with life and death decisions in the difficult environment of SOF medics can appreciate the need for this advice. Some will view it as inappropriate, possibly even bordering on malpractice.

Be well advised that the Handbook has limited application outside of SOF and we did not intend it for anything other than use by highly trained SOF medics in deployed situations.

All the authors have experience with SOF and its environment. We charged all with the same question: *"How would you diagnose and treat this patient if it was your wife, child, or parent and you were alone, with no assistance, evacuation, or consultation, in an isolated environment, armed only with the most basic of medical tools?"* These authors struggled answering this difficult question, knowing they had to break with the conservative paradigms of medicine, possibly facing the censure of their peers in doing so. The SOF community and I salute their efforts. We offer this handbook in remembrance of noble deeds and honorable intentions of all SOF medic warriors and all those who have served so ably and well since inception, from World War II OSS to GWOT USSOCOM, so that those SOF medics who follow can serve at an even higher level of medical skill and knowledge.

"Unconventional Warfare - Unconventional Medicine!"

Colonel Warner D. ("Rocky") Farr, M.D., M.P.H.
USSOCOM Command Surgeon

Chief Editor
Special Operations Forces Medical Handbook
Second Edition 2008

Tactical Combat Casualty Care
Col Charles Beadling, USAF, MC

Introduction: Combat mortality has been steadily reduced by improvements in equipment, tactics and training. However, preventable deaths still occur on the battlefield. To determine which deaths may have been prevented, a thorough analysis of the causes of death for combat fatalities has been conducted. TCCC focuses on the most common causes of preventable combat death. Controllable hemorrhage is by far the leading cause of death in this category, followed by tension pneumothorax and loss of airway. TCCC describes the appropriate level of care during 3 phases of the tactical environment. During Care Under Fire, the casualty and rescuer are still under effective hostile fire. If there is no longer effective enemy fire, then it is the Tactical Field Care phase. This may apply to injuries sustained when there has been no hostile fire. The final phase, Combat Casualty Evacuation Care, is rendered during transport to a higher level of care. Additional medical resources may be available during this phase.

Subjective: Symptoms
Focused History: The purpose of questions is to identify immediate life-threatening injuries and determine functional status. Remote assessment: *Are you bleeding badly?* (Identify exsanguinating hemorrhage) *Can you move to cover and return fire?* (Determine functional capacity) Attending casualty: *Are you having trouble breathing?* (Identify airway or breathing problem) *Where do you hurt?* (Identify other injuries)

Objective: Signs
Using Basic Tools:
General: Altered mental status may indicate open or closed head injury, hypovolemic shock, or inadequate oxygenation/ventilation. Inspection: Identify uncontrolled bleeding immediately. Observe depth and rate of respirations (breathing >30 times per minute indicates significant respiratory distress), asymmetric chest wall movement (flail chest) and gross deformity of extremities. Tracheal deviation or jugular venous distention may indicate tension pneumothorax. Auscultation: Unnecessary during Care Under Fire and you may not be able to hear during other phases. Absent or decreased breath sounds on one side suggest pneumothorax. Palpation: Presence (absent radial), rate (rapid) and quality (weak) of pulses suggest hypovolemia. Crepitus on chest wall can indicate pneumothorax or flail chest. Abdominal rigidity, tenderness or rebound suggests internal injury. Quickly palpate extremities and spine to locate injuries. Pulse oximetry: <95% saturation indicates an airway or breathing problem. Consider tension pneumothorax if airway is open.

Using Advanced Tools:
It is unlikely that advanced tools will be available for TCCC. If they are available, keep in mind that the hemoglobin and hematocrit will not immediately reflect the degree of blood loss from an acute hemorrhage.

Assessment:
During the Care Under Fire phase, you may be limited to remotely assessing a casualty and directing him to move to cover or administer self-aid. Additional personnel should not be put at risk to recover a casualty that appears dead or with un-survivable injuries. Initial assessment is based on XABC: eXsanguinating hemorrhage, Airway, Breathing, Circulation.

Differential Diagnosis
Loss of consciousness/altered mental status: Open or closed head injury, inadequate cerebral perfusion (due to hypovolemic shock) or inadequate ventilation
Respiratory distress: Tension pneumothorax, flail chest, hemo/pneumothorax

Plan: If capable, casualty should move to cover and return fire.
Primary Treatment
Care Under Fire: Hemorrhage is controlled by tourniquet. Airway management is limited to nasopharyngeal airway. Suspected tension pneumothorax should be treated with needle decompression.
Tactical Field Care: Definitive airway can be secured with endotracheal intubation or cricothyrotomy as needed. Open chest wounds should be covered with occlusive dressing. Consider converting tourniquets to pressure dressings (Combat Gauze) and hemostatic agents (WoundStat). Intravenous or intraosseous access should be obtained and converted to saline lock. Shock, evidenced by poor mentation/absent radial pulse, is managed by bolus of 500mL hetastarch (Hextend). Repeat bolus once if needed. Remember that administration of fluids with uncontrollable internal hemorrhage (thoracic, abdominal or pelvic) can exacerbate bleeding and worsen outcomes. Pain and antibiotic medications are administered if appropriate. Open wounds should be covered with dressings and fractures splinted. Documentation of treatment should be initiated.
Tactical Evacuation Care: Additional medical assets may be available. Hypothermia, especially with aeromedical evacuation, must be prevented to avoid acidosis and coagulopathy. If available, Blizzard Wrap or Readi-Heat blanket and cap can be used. Patient must be carefully monitored for decompensation during transport.

Counter-insurgency Medical Operations
LTC Sean Keenan, MC, USA & MSG Samuel J. Blazier, 18Z, USA

Counter-insurgency (COIN) operations are characterized by decentralized, independent, intelligence-driven tactical operations with both kinetic (typical military force use) and non-kinetic (humanitarian aid, civil-military affairs, and information operations) components. The decentralized focus must center around sometimes geographically remote areas and ultimately supports a fledgling or immature government. With this in mind, medical operations should be tailored to reflect the operational conditions and tactical effects required.

Evacuation and Hospitalization: Medical service organization and procedures will require adaptation to the type of operations envisioned. Medical support is complicated by: (1) distances between the installations where support must be provided; (2) use of small mobile units in independent or semi-independent combat operations in areas where ground evacuation may be impossible or from areas where aerial evacuation of patients cannot be accomplished or will be significantly delayed; (3) vulnerability of ground evacuation routes to guerrilla ambush.

There are several factors and measures that may be utilized to overcome the complicating factors. The following are examples of such measures: Establish aid stations with a treatment and holding capacity at lower echelons, including static security posts and combat bases. Patients to be evacuated by ground transport may be held until movement by secure means is possible. Use forward-stationed surgical teams for area medical support of both US and host nation (HN) patients. Provide sufficient air or ground transportation to move medical elements rapidly to establish or reinforce existing treatment and holding installations where patients have been unexpectedly numerous (ie, mass casualty situations). Maximize use of air evacuation, both casualty evacuation and medical evacuation, to include both scheduled and on-call evacuation support of static installations and combat elements in the field. Provide small medical elements to augment extended combat patrols. Assign specially trained enlisted medical personnel (Special Forces medical sergeants, independent duty corpsmen, etc.) who are capable of operating medical treatment facilities for short periods of time with a minimum of immediate supervision. Use HN medical assistance for supervised work and formation of indigenous litter bearer teams. Strictly supervise sanitation measures, maintenance of individual medical equipment (both individual first aid kits and combat lifesaver/vehicle kits), and advanced first aid training (combat lifesavers or equivalent) throughout the command. Increase emphasis on basic combat training of medical service personnel, arming medical service personnel, and using armored carriers for ground evacuation where feasible. Use indigenous medical resources and capabilities when available and professionally acceptable. Establish medical clinics at each firebase. Establishing and running medical clinics at each firebase affords trauma-level treatment to stabilize wounded until medical evacuation can occur. Additionally, clinics can serve to assist the local populace in areas where there is no medical support or affordable care. This service to the local populace is a major non-kinetic strategy tool that is highly effective.

Local National Medical Care as a Non-kinetic Strategic Tool: The utilization of host nation medical care and clinics are a valid and integral part of a non-kinetic strategy of fighting a COIN operation. Through the use of inherent SOF medical talents, each firebase can utilize medical care of local nationals to help achieve the overall goal of peace and stability in their respective areas of operation (AO). There are some key tenants and tasks that an individual medic should consider which are outlined in this section.

In order to fully take advantage of this non-kinetic experience, the individual SOF medic should consider establishing, operating, and managing a local medical clinic designed to address (or augment) medical care for the local populace. The rapport gained by providing a local medical clinic is forefront for a Special Operations team in their AO. Looking back on the stories of Vietnam and the "G-Hospitals," a recurring theme is the provision of more sophisticated medical care to an underserved population.

The SOF medic should first conduct an assessment of the area to determine the local medical capabilities, and availability of medical personnel – both host nation and friendly force or foreign assets. The assessment should include HN medical supplies and pharmacy services available. This will vary widely depending on the operating base location, but some undeveloped areas will have complete lack of some basic services and adequate medical or pharmacy supply. The SOF medic should establish and build rapport with any local medical personnel, and determine if they have the resources needed to carry out their responsibilities. There may be an opportunity to assist local clinics or hospitals, by physically assisting and advising, or with the procurement of local supplies and medications.

There may be numerous "established" programs that a team may be able to utilize, and Civil Affairs (CA) specialists will be an invaluable resource. There may be national or regional programs that can be promoted by the Special Operations teams in remote areas that are not being serviced as intended. Especially with a fledgling government in a primitive environment, outreach by the central governmental organizations may be sporadic to the rural areas. An example of this may be national vaccination programs which seek to vaccinate all children in a host nation. By supporting and enabling the local medical clinic, it is legitimizing the local clinic and its personnel, which furthers the rapport process.

The Special Operations team can conduct "mini-MEDCAPs" locally to introduce themselves into the area and to show support for the local populace. These visits are usually in conjunction with tactical operations into formally denied areas. As for medical care, it is far from definitive and should serve more as an advertisement for the firebase clinic or local national establishments of which remote towns may be unaware until these planned encounters. Medics should consider carrying small boxes or kit bags to take advantage of medical targets of opportunity while out on patrols. Medical interactions with the local populace are a very safe and valuable non-threatening encounter that should be considered as an augmentation to many tactical scenarios. These can sometimes be planned in conjunction with tactical CA assessments and project nomination site surveys.

Establishing and Running a Firebase Medical Clinic: When considering the permanent structure for a firebase local national clinic, the location should be planned carefully. The SOF medic should establish a clinic in a safe area and the clinic should be run purely by the team. An ideal location is outside the inner perimeter but still attached to the firebase. The firebase clinic should be accessible to indigenous personnel, yet have adequate security. Firebase clinics need a controlled access point, and the personnel entering the control point should be scanned with a metal detector or be searched physically by a host nation soldier or security. This is necessary to protect both the local civilians as well as the Special Operations team personnel. From this controlled access point they should go into a waiting area that is over-watched by the HN soldiers or security personnel. This holding area provides an excellent opportunity for interaction with the waiting patients; whether it is for patient education, PSYOP presentations, or CA interaction. The clinic itself, however, is the main effort.

Many operating bases choose to have the local national clinic (the outer clinic) and the "American" clinic (the inner clinic). The local national clinic is rudimentary, has basic exam tables and screening equipment, and the bulk of its medications can be local national medications supplied by CERP funding. The inner or "American" clinic contains the traditional Class VIII supplies, monitors and everything needed for procedures and more complicated patients. A technique is to screen the vast majority of patients at the local national clinic, and bring the sickest patients or those needing more advanced care to the inner clinic.

The SOF medic working in this clinical setting finds a tremendous opportunity to train team members, HN military medics and interpreters to assist in medical procedures, taking vital signs, and the operational procedures of the clinic. This not only helps the medic with his daily duties, but provides vital hands-on training to first responders. Simple duties such as wound care and IV practice are a daily occurrence. This on-the-job training is a vital supplement to classroom or pre-deployment medical training for our own operators. The confidence derived from this training pays enormous dividends during tactical combat casualty care.

Scope of Practice: What we are seeing in these clinics is that the SOF medic has historically in our operations been the most medically qualified person in the majority of the remote operating areas. Medics must be cautious not to overstep their bounds in terms of scope of practice. SOF medics should practice within their medical training and comfort level of the Unit Surgeons and pass the patients to a higher medical level when appropriate and available.

An understanding of the medical operational environment is essential. Each medic should be thoroughly familiar with both military and civilian evacuation chains, understanding full well that there may be a very non-permissive (military) or non-existent (civilian) evacuation situation system in place. This is a continual problem that should be considered early in the treatment of medical problems, and the medics will soon get an understanding of not only their capabilities, but necessary limitations. In other words, there must be an appreciation for not "biting off more than they can chew." After working in the environment, a medic quickly realizes there are some problems best left not addressed, especially chronic problems or problems so overwhelming that intervention will only delay inevitable deterioration or death. Every provider in this austere environment goes through a period of adjustment from the way they were taught to the way they will practice, effectively modifying the "standard of care." A provider should always remember the axiom: "First, do no harm."

At times the SOF medic has so many people that come for treatment that he cannot physically screen, assess and treat them all. The medics must develop a system to triage patients and refer to the local HN clinic as appropriate. This legitimizes the local clinic and local medical personnel, which serves to increase the rapport in the AO, while dissuading the local populace from an over-reliance on the medical care provided by the "temporary" firebase, eroding the incentive for local national health care development.

Medical Supplies: The established local national clinic should maximize the use of locally purchased medications. CA units may have access to local development money allocated for medical projects. The use of these types of funds is encouraged to purchase local national medications. This will serve a number of purposes: it bolsters the economy by the spending of money in the community, it discourages an over-reliance on American products and medications, and it legitimizes the local medications provided on the economy. It also gives the local military or civilian medical personnel the necessary training and practice in supply and logistics, which is an often under-developed skill set in other nations.

Patient Population and Treatment Challenges: Patient demographics tend to be greater than 50% pediatric, with many of those pediatric cases being less than 2 years of age. This necessitates Broselow Kits (or similar weight-based treatment aids), pediatric references, pediatric medications, and good lines of communications with pediatric and higher medical consultation. In colder or primitive societies, burns can be a prominent injury presenting to operating bases. Each medic should be familiar with burn care and procedural sedation since much of the wound care will necessarily be handled at the operating base clinic.

Caution needs to be exercised in medications and treatment plans. Our experience is that local national patients seldom take the medication as directed, may sell the medications you have given them, or may take dangerously large doses despite what you consider to be adequate education. Also, follow-up is sometimes non-existent, so common treatments such as daily wound dressing changes actually become weekly. The medic should prepare for this contingency and frequently modify treatment plans. The KISS (keep it simple, stupid) principle should be foremost in every treatment and follow-up plan provided.

Unconventional Warfare and Guerrilla Hospitals
COL Warner Farr, MC, USA

UW medical organization and procedures tend to be unique to the partisan situation and will require adaptation to the types of operations conducted by the resistance force. In general, UW medical support is complicated by:

- Distances between battle sites and secure locations under resistance control where care can be provided. This results in long evacuation times and increased mortality due to delays in addressing non-compressible (truncal) hemorrhage. A good example of this was the first Afghan war where the Afghan forces fighting the Russians sent casualties to hospitals in Pakistan. This resulted in a preponderance of extremity wounds that could survive this long evacuation path. In contrast to this, the use of small mobile units with limited surgical and holding capabilities placed near areas of combat operations was done in Yugoslavia in World War II. The Allies inserted two Forward Surgical Teams (FST) into Tito's forces to serve in areas where ground evacuation to partisan hospitals was difficult and aerial evacuation of patients could not be accomplished or would be significantly delayed. US doctrine still calls for FST insertion and limited indigenous wounded evacuation.

- Vulnerability of ground evacuation routes to counter-guerrilla forces. The literature on all guerrilla forces mentions the difficulties of moving a guerrilla force encumbered with casualties. It also always mentions that guerrilla forces must spend the manpower and considerable efforts to have a medical force to inspire their fighters. This dichotomy led some guerrilla forces to cache casualties in friendly homes rather than develop a hospital system. This was particularly done by the French Marquis. They at first used French hospitals until they realized that the Gestapo swept up their wounded and then transitioned to a system of cached patients and "circuit rider" medics. Recruitment of local national fighters may require promises of both health care, to include family care, burial services, and death benefits (life insurance).

- Personnel availability of trained medical soldiers is always a problem for guerrilla forces. Some resistance forces in fairly developed countries attract enough local national medical personnel to serve as guerrilla force medical officers and as members of the auxiliary and underground. A robust auxiliary and underground is imperative to manage casualties, especially in a disbursed system of care (rather than in guerrilla hospitals in remote secure areas). Many larger guerrilla forces in WW II (the Ukrainians, the Yugoslavs) trained their own medical personnel. Current US doctrine (FM 8-43/FM 4-02.43) dictates medical support to indigenous forces by US personnel when the indigenous forces cannot attract sufficient numbers of medical personnel.

- Equipment is always short in a resistance movement. Some larger ones do significant manufacturing in denied areas but the most common source of supply is from external sources of support or from capturing medical supplies from the enemy. Many guerrilla forces have mounted operations solely to capture medical supplies. More recent partisan organizations have attempted to obtain medical supplies from nongovernmental organizations, private voluntary organizations and other non-state actors on the modern battlefield. Guerrilla forces in developed countries may be able to tap the nation's (the enemy's) hospitalization, workman's compensation, and other social welfare systems.

Triage in MASCAL
Richard Schwartz, MD & E. Brooke Lerner, PhD

Introduction: The term triage means to sort or select and on the modern battlefield involves the dynamic process of sorting casualties to provide the greatest good for the greatest number of casualties. It is important that casualties be re-triaged at each phase and level of care and whenever clinically and tactically allowable because the initial triage category may change as the clinical status changes. Additionally, it is important to remember that triage categories are different than MEDEVAC priority criteria and when using air evacuation appropriate evacuation priority categories should be assigned.

When: Triage occurs when there is more than 1 casualty and a decision is made to provide care to 1 patient over another. In situations where there are larger numbers of casualties or fewer resources to respond, the importance of accurate triage increases. In this setting, having an organized standard approach to the triage of casualties assumes an increasing importance. Additionally, the tactical environment presents unique challenges to the medic performing triage on the battlefield. Triage will vary depending on the phase of care (Care Under Fire, Tactical Field Care, Tactical Evacuation Care).

What You Need: In some instances, triage tags will be available for tagging individual casualties with their triage category. The tags should allow for changes in triage category as the patients' clinical condition changes. Use a marker to indentify the first letter of the assigned triage category on the casualties' forehead if tags are unavailable. Alternatively, casualties can simply be separated into groups based upon their triage category.

What To Do:

    Triage Categories: Casualties will be divided into 5 categories: Immediate, Delayed, Minimal, Expectant, and Dead. These categories can be remembered by the mnemonic ID-MED.

        Immediate casualties are designated by the color **red** and are those who need immediate medical attention due to obvious threat to life or limb. Patients under this group include: unresponsive, altered mental status, respiratory distress, uncontrolled hemorrhage, amputations proximal to the elbow or knee, sucking chest wounds, unilateral absent breath sounds, cyanotic patient, and rapid weak pulses.

        Delayed casualties are designated by the color **yellow** and are those who are in need of definitive medical care, but should not decompensate rapidly if care is delayed initially. Examples of this group include: deep lacerations with bleeding controlled and good distal circulation, open fractures, abdominal injuries with stable vital signs, amputated fingers, or hemodynamically stable head injuries with an intact airway.

        Minimal casualties are designated by the color **green** and are assigned to the "walking wounded." These patients are those who have minor injuries such as: abrasions, contusions, and minor lacerations. Their vital signs will be stable and while they require medical attention, it can be delayed for days if necessary without an adverse effect.

        Expectant casualties are designated by the color **gray** and are patients that have little or no chance for survival despite maximum therapy. Initially, resources should not be directed towards this group other than comfort care as they will be needed to care for the other patients. As the event progresses and resources become available, then resources will be dedicated to these casualties and efforts may be directed to resuscitation.

        Dead casualties are designated by the color **black**.

    Triage in the Phases of Care:

        Care Under Fire: During this phase of care, triage and care is limited to identifying and treating those casualties that may need a Life Saving Intervention (LSI) when the tactical environment allows. The focus needs to be on completing the objective and getting the casualty to a more secure situation where greater care can be provided.

        Tactical Field Care: During this phase of care, triage is completed and casualties are placed into the triage categories and are prioritized for evacuation. The casualties are provided a higher level of care after immediate LSIs have been performed. The initial medical care will focus upon the immediate casualty group. After the immediate casualties' have been cared for, the other categories should be re-triaged as the casualties clinical status may have changed.

        Tactical Evacuation Care: During this phase of care, the casualties must be re-triaged at each level of evacuation. As the casualties are transported and greater resources are available, all groups need to be re-triaged and the expectant group should be evaluated. If excess resources exist, then consideration for resuscitation should be considered even though there is little chance of a successful resuscitation.

Mass Casualty Triage:

SALT Triage: This triage system (a proposed national standard) should be used when sorting large numbers of injured patients during a multi-casualty incident. The acronym SALT can be used to remember this process: Sort, Assess, Life Saving Interventions, Transport/Treatment.

Step 1: Global Sorting of Patient

Start by globally sorting patients into groups based on voice commands. The first command is "If you can walk, please move over here." Victims who move to the designated area should be prioritized as last for individual assessment. The rescuer should then say "If you can, please wave your hand or leg and I will come to you in a few minutes to help you." The victims who remain still or have obvious life-threatening conditions should then be assessed first as they may need immediate life saving interventions. Those who can follow your command to wave or are making purposeful movements should be assessed second, followed by those who moved out of the area.

- Priority 1: Still/obvious life threat
- Priority 2: Wave/purposeful movement
- Priority 3: Walk

Figure 1-1. Step 1 - Global Sorting of Patients

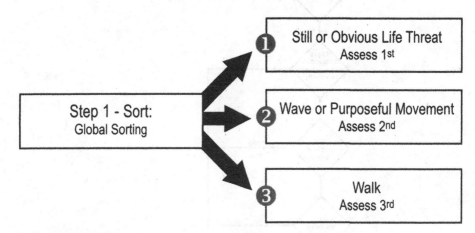

Step 2: Individual Assessment

Individual assessment should be initiated once victims have been prioritized for assessment based on their ability to follow your commands. Individual assessment begins by providing limited rapid lifesaving interventions. These include:

1. Controlling major hemorrhage through the use of tourniquets or direct pressure provided by other patients or other devices
2. Opening the airway through positioning or basic airway adjuncts (if the patient is a child, consider giving 2 rescue breaths)
3. Chest decompression
4. Auto-injector antidotes

These should only be performed within the responder's scope of practice and only if the equipment is immediately available. Further, these procedures should be time limited and the medics must move quickly to next patient and not spend large amounts of time with any one patient. Next, assess if the victim is breathing, obeys commands, has a peripheral pulse, is in respiratory distress, or has major hemorrhage that is not controlled. The medic must also assess whether the victim is likely to survive given their observed injuries and the available resources or if the victim's injuries appear to be minor injuries for which a delay in care will not increase mortality. Patients should be prioritized for treatment and/or transport by assigning them to 1 of 5 triage categories:

1. Immediate
2. Delayed
3. Minimal
4. Expectant
5. Dead

Patients who do not obey commands, or do not have a peripheral pulse, or are in respiratory distress, or have uncontrolled major hemorrhage should be triaged as immediate and should be designated with the color red. The patients triaged as delayed are stable patients that need definitive care and should be designated with the color yellow. Patients who have mild injuries that are self-limited and if not treated can tolerate a delay in care without increased risk of mortality should be triaged as minimal and should be designated with the color green. Providers should consider if these patients have injuries that are likely to be incompatible with life given the currently available resources; if they are, then the provider should triage these patients as expectant and they should be designated with the color gray. Patients who are not breathing even after life-saving interventions are attempted should be triaged as dead and should be designated with the color black.

Figure 1-2. Step 2 - Individual Assessment

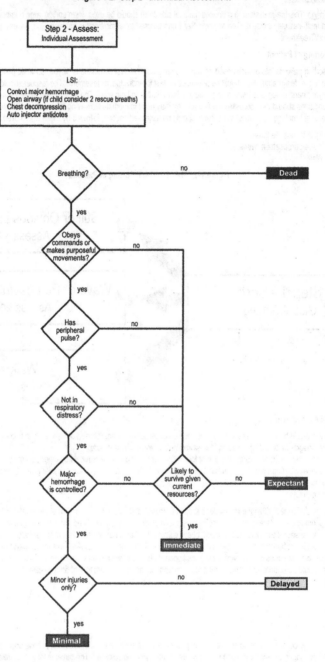

Reassessment

The SALT triage process is rapid and uses a minimum number of resources and rescuers. Individual assessment is dependent on the provider's skill level. Prioritization for treatment and/or transport is dynamic and may be effected by changing patient conditions, resources, and scene safety. As more resources become available, including more highly trained medical personnel, patients should be reassessed. Reassessment is important since patients' conditions may change and rapid initial evaluations may miss important and life-threatening injuries. Unfortunately in a mass casualty incident, the goal has to be to do the most good for the most people and this may mean that some individuals will not receive the treatment that they need in the time that they need it. Further, efficient use of assets may require the mixing of patients designated with different priorities rather than transporting them strictly in their priority order.

Air Evacuation Priorities: For patients that need to be transported by MEDEVAC the patients should be further subdivided into evacuation priorities. The following is an overview of the MEDEVAC priorities:

Priority I: URGENT is assigned to emergency cases that should be evacuated as soon as possible and within a maximum of 2 hours in order to save life, limb, or eyesight, to prevent complications of serious illness, or to avoid permanent disability.

Priority IA: URGENT-SURG is assigned to patients who must receive far forward surgical intervention to save life and stabilize for further evacuation.

Priority II: PRIORITY is assigned to sick and wounded personnel requiring prompt medical care. This precedence is used when the individual should be evacuated within 4 hours or his medical condition could deteriorate to such a degree that he will become an URGENT precedence, or whose requirements for special treatment are not available locally, or who will suffer unnecessary pain or disability.

Priority III: ROUTINE is assigned to sick and wounded personnel requiring evacuation but whose condition is not expected to deteriorate significantly. The sick and wounded in this category should be evacuated within 24 hours.

Priority IV: CONVENIENCE is assigned to patients for whom evacuation by medical vehicle is a matter of medical convenience rather than necessity.

What Not To Do:

1. Do not consider triage complete after initial triage. Re-triage is as important as initial triage. Patients' clinical status will change and the provider must re-triage patients at each phase and level of care and as often as tactically and clinically possible. Triage is not complete until all patients are cared for.

2. Do not ignore the expectants. The expectant category is a subjective category that includes patients that in the best estimate by the triage officer will not survive their injuries. These patients should receive comfort care and be re-triaged like the other casualties. An expectant casualty may improve and become an immediate. When resources become available the expectant casualties should be provided medical treatment.

3. Do not provide complex medical care during the triage process. Treatment during the triage process should be limited to life-saving interventions and complex medical procedures such as intubation, chest tube insertion, and traction splinting should be delayed until after the initial round of triage so all patients who may benefit from LSI are identified and treated.

Prepare a Patient for Evacuation Using Special Equipment

COL Warner Anderson, MC, USA

When: You must prepare a patient for transport insuring that the patient's airway is secure, all hemorrhage is controlled, IV infusions are secure, all fractures and dislocations are splinted, patient care and condition are documented and the patient is safely secured in the extraction device.

What You Need: Jungle penetrator, Stokes litter, 3 A7-A cargo straps, 2 sling ropes, 2 snap links, a STABO suspension rope, or SKED

What To Do:

1. Insure the patient has a secure airway.
2. Reinforce all pressure bandages.
3. Secure splinted arms to the body trunk.
4. Secure splinted legs together if fractured or dislocated. **Note:** If using the jungle penetrator, do not secure the casualty's legs together.
5. Reinforce IV sites by wrapping the catheter site and a 4-6 inch loop of tubing with an Ace wrap. If fluid administration can be interrupted, change to saline locks. Wrap the site and the tubing with gauze in a spiral to prevent ripping out the IV.
6. Just prior to pickup, clamp off the IV infusion set and secure the IV bag.
7. Document the patient's injuries and condition to include vital signs on card and attach to the patient.
8. Prepare the casualty for transport using one of the following methods (**Note:** Follow steps 1-7 above for all casualties regardless of the extraction equipment being used.):

   A. Jungle penetrator:
   (1) Select a proper site for extraction.
      a) The capabilities and limitations of the mission aircraft are primary factors in site selection
      b) Consider site altitude and temperature, as hot or thin air reduces the helicopter payload
      c) Extremely dense overhead foliage prevents lowering the jungle penetrator. Select a spot that provides some overhead clearing to allow safe lowering and retrieval
   (2) Allow the penetrator to touch the ground in order to discharge static electricity. Do not touch the hoist cable or rescue seat until after ground contact, because static electricity may cause severe electrical shock. In swamp or open water, the shock may effect persons at some distance.
      • For one man rescue, do the following:
         a) Assume a kneeling position to make holding and mounting the jungle penetrator easier
         b) Hold the jungle penetrator upright in front of you
         c) Pull the seat blade down until the retaining hook engages and locks the seat blade in the extended position
         d) Mount and straddle the seat while facing the shank
         e) Open the safety strap cover and remove the safety strap

f) Position the safety strap around the body under the armpits and pull it tight

g) Attach the snap fastener to the bar located at the top of the safety strap

h) When ready for retrieval, signal the helicopter by one of the following means:
- Give "thumbs up" signal
- Radio
- Vigorously shake hoist cable from side to side
- Hold on with both arms around the shank

i) Keep the crotch close to the jungle penetrator with the head and shoulders close to the cable. **Caution:** The hoist hook swivel will spin rapidly as tension is placed on the cable. Do not hold the swivel.

j) Upon reaching a position level with the helicopter door, the crewman will turn you to face away from the door and pull you inside. **Note:** Do not attempt to help him or to dismount the rescue seat until instructed to do so. The crewman will disconnect you from the jungle penetrator when you are safely inside.

k) While in flight, do not cross your legs because of possible injury when you enter the aircraft.

l) Make certain the hoist cable does not become entangled with the safety straps or with any part of the body.

- For a two man rescue do the following:

a) Place least injured individual (#1) on one seat and secure the safety strap.

b) Place the more severely injured individual (#2) on the two remaining seats with his legs over #1 man's legs. Secure the safety strap.

c) Instruct the men to hold on to each other.

d) Signal the helicopter for retrieval (as above).

e) Hoist operator will unload #2 man into aircraft first, followed by #1 man. **Note:** For rescue of wounded or injured personnel, or rescue under emergency conditions, the rescuer always dons and tightens the safety strap. Personnel can be safely retrieved without being mounted on the seat. The same jungle penetrator, equipped with a flotation collar, can be used for water rescue.

B. Stokes litter: Place the casualty into the basket using one of the following methods:
- 3-4 man lift
- Log roll
- Secure the casualty with the straps provided:
  (1) One strap below the knee
  (2) One strap above the knee
  (3) One strap at waist level
  (4) One strap at chest level; ensure that the chest strap is not so tight that it interferes with respiration.

Warning: Never attempt to "ride up" by standing or hanging on to a Stokes litter. This will cause the litter to become unbalanced and spin, making it impossible to retrieve into the aircraft and possibly endangering the aircraft.

C. Horse collar (Note: The horse collar rescue device is a padded strap that is lowered on the end of the hoist to extract one soldier at a time.):

(1) Extend one arm through the loop

(2) Slip it over your head and shoulders

(3) Put your other arm through the loop

(4) Place the collar behind your back

(5) Connect the chest strap

(6) Give the ready signal to the aircraft

Note: The horse collar cannot be used to extract severely injured or unconscious patients.

D. Hansen rig (Note: The Hansen rig is constructed from an A-7A strap with a D-ring and snap link.):

(1) Thread the strap through the D-ring

(2) Hold the D-ring so that it is pointing in the opposite direction of the thick-lip floating bar of the friction adapter

(3) Remove any twists in the strap and thread the end through the friction adapter. Note: The device is now ready to be donned

(4) Place the D-ring and the friction adapter on the casualty's left shoulder with the running end strap to the casualty's front.

(5) Stand on the strap with the left foot and pull the running end tight

(6) Hold the hardware on top of the casualty's left shoulder with your left hand. Reach behind the casualty with your right hand and pull the strap around to the front.

(7) With your left hand, grasp and hold both left and right straps.

(8) Reach between the casualty's legs and pull up the third section, forming a diaper.

(9) Connect all three sections with a snap link and retighten the strap.

(10) Hook up to the extraction rope (the extraction rope is the STABO suspension rope) by connecting the snap link at the end of the extraction rope to the D-ring on the A7A strap.

(11) Give the ready signal to the aircraft.

Note: If time permits, the suspension rope hook can be passed through the D-ring and run down to the snap link holding the A-7A strap together.

E. Palmer rig:

(1) Form a standard rappel seat

(2) Make the extraction rope by using a standard 120 rappel rope and connecting a snap link to the end or using a STABO suspension rope.

(3) With either rope, tie a second rope (about 6-8 feet long) near the end to form a loop. Use a Prusik knot to attach the loop so that it can be slid up or down.

(4) When the extraction line is lowered, connect the snap link at the end of the rope through the single wrap around the waist and through the ropes that form the overhand knot at the waist.

(5) Slide the Prusik knot down to the patient's chest level.

(6) Pass the loop over the patient's shoulder and give the thumbs-up signal.

(7) With a conscious patient, instruct him to adjust the Prusik knot up or down as he is lifted so that he is in the seated position.

Note: The SPIES, FRIES, and STABO rigs can all be used in their normal configuration for casualty extraction. For information on the use of the Fulton STAR system, refer to TC 31-24.

What Not To Do:

1. Do not send an "expectant" patient by aircraft if it will present a danger to the A/C or ground party, or divert resources from other needs.

2. Do not hand an unstable patient off to a lower level of care. The A/C may be a lower level of care than the ground party or facility. In CONUS, such a hand-off may be a violation of Federal law. In general, dysbaric patients require special arrangements and care on the A/C, and any casualty who has dived within 24 hours must receive special attention.

3. Do not fail to sedate psychiatric patients or casualties.

4. A patient with significant chest trauma, including blast injury should, when possible, have chest tubes inserted prior to transfer.

5. A patient with facial burns involving the oropharynx or nasal vibrissae should, when possible, be intubated (or LMA) and sedated for the flight.

6. When protocols permit, the patient's C-spine should be clinically cleared prior to flight, to avoid the encumbrance of backboard or KED.

7. Do not assume others team members are familiar with these procedures; identify opportunities to include use of special equipment in unit medical training.

SKEDCO Personnel Placement for Evacuation Using Special Equipment

Skedco, Inc.

When: The purpose of a tag line is to prevent dangerous litter spin, which occurs when hoisting a litter by helicopter. This kit is designed prevent spin while preventing other problems normally associated with tag lines, such as tangled rope, deployment difficulties, and storage problems. The Skedco Helitag Kit contains 250 feet of 7mm water rescue rope. It has a polypropylene core with a nylon sheath, which allows it to float in the water and have good abrasion resistance. Both ends have a figure 8 knot on a bight that is backed up with a double overhand knot for safety. The rope is placed in a throw bag, which has a closed cell foam disc in the bottom for extra flotation when used for water applications. The carry handle of the bag is an adjustable strap with a side release buckle to allow securing the kit in an aircraft. The bottom end of the bag has a grommetted hole through which one end of the rope protrudes. This provides a hand loop for a victim in the water to grasp when a litter is not used, so that he or she can be towed to a safe area. The other end of the rope has a loop with a screw link attached to allow a weak link to be utilized. Another screw link is then passed through the nylon weak link to secure the tag line to a V strap, which is attached to the two side grommets at the foot end of the Sked litter, or to the corners at the foot end of a Stokes basket litter, for safe hoisting.

What You Need: **SK-1010 SKEDCO HELITAG KIT (NSN 6545013810654)**

Table 1-1. Helicopter Tag Line Kit Contents

1 250' x 7MM PMI Water Rescue Rope	1 V Strap	1 rope maintenance card
2 locking aluminum carabiners	1 Package of 10 weak links	1 rope history card
2 screw links 1 Helitag throw bag	1 instruction sheet	

What To Do:

Hoisting. Loosen the drawstring of the Helitag bag and pull out the end of the rope with a screw link, weak link, screw link, V strap and carabiners attached. Attach the ends of the V strap to the two side grommets at the foot end of the Sked stretcher or to the corners of a basket litter at the foot end (*see Figure 1-3*). It is not necessary to pull extra rope from the bag. As the litter is hoisted, it is only necessary to maintain enough tension on the rope to keep the litter from spinning. As the litter is hoisted, allow the rope to slide through your hand. When the litter is secured into the helicopter, the tag line is released and dropped to the ground. The person on the ground should then stuff the rope back into the bag and close the drawstring. The tag line is now ready for the next use.

Deployment from the Helicopter Loosen the drawstring on the bag and pull out 2-3 feet of rope. While holding on to the end of the rope, throw the bag down (not out or upward) from the aircraft. A person in the water can place his hand through or simply hold onto the loop protruding from the bag and be towed to safety or kept afloat while the rescue effort progresses. If a litter is to be lowered, attach the tag line kit to the appropriate point on the litter and throw the tag line bag down to a person on the ground. The person on the ground will then maintain enough tension on the rope to prevent litter spin during the lowering process. Please read the rope care instructions and maintain a rope use log to keep your tag line in top and useful condition.

Warning: A new weak link must be used each time a human load is hoisted!

What Not To Do:

1. No personnel should perform a helicopter hoist of a patient without understanding the dangers of stretcher spin and the proper utilization of a tag line.

2. Do not perform a second lift on the same link.

Stretcher Spin. Skedco believes that there is a degree of risk involved any time a person is packaged in a stretcher and hoisted to a helicopter. There is risk not only to the patient in the stretcher, but to the helicopter and crew as well. All stretchers, including the sked stretcher, have an inherent potential to spin when being hoisted by a helicopter. A spinning stretcher presents a variety of dangers to the patient, and cases have been recorded where an improperly packaged patient has been discharged from a stretcher and fallen to the ground. Skedco Inc. was asked for a tag line with a weak link and responded immediately with the **Skedco Helitag Kit** (NSN 6545-01-381-0654).

Figure 1-3. Recommended Personnel Placement for Helicopter Hoisting of a Stretcher

Preferred Placement

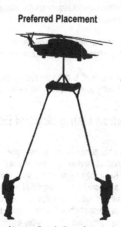

Ideal placement. Use of two tag lines is the safest way to prevent any litter from spinning. Two tag lines should always be used in training and non-hostile situations for best litter control. Maximum visibility for pilot and crew.

Good Placement

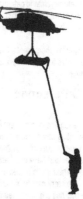

Good placement to prevent stretcher spin with minimum tension applied to tag line. Maximum visibility for pilot and ground crew.

Improper Placement

While better than no tag line at all, this placement of personnel and equipment tilts the stretcher, increasing the likelihood of spin, and requires greater tension on the tag line to prevent the spin, creating an increased possibility of weak link separation.

Causes of Stretcher Spin. The rotor wash from a helicopter creates a natural wind force that can cause a stretcher to spin. Other factors that increase the tendency of a stretcher to spin include:

- Improper loading: Uneven loading will exacerbate the tendency of the stretcher to spin.
- Weather conditions: The stronger the winds, the higher the risk of spin!
- Improper attachment of the tag line. Skedco recommends that the tag line be attached to the center grommet at the foot end of the stretcher.
- Improper placement and performance of personnel. Personnel should not be located directly below the helicopter.

Pulling the tag line tight while below the helicopter will tilt the stretcher, creating a natural air foil, and resulting spin. Skedco Inc. recommends that the tag line handler should (if at all possible) be positioned forward of the aircraft and visible to the pilot and crew, rather than directly below the aircraft. *See Figure 1-3* which diagrams proper personnel placement.

Use and Risks of a Tag Line. The utilization of a tag line can prevent the stretcher from spinning. Attaching the line to the stretcher have having ground personnel maintain tension while the stretcher is being lifted will provide the best available protection against stretcher spin However, the presence of an attached line to the ground presents a potential danger to the aircraft and its crew, particularly in a combat environment.

Should the tag line become entangled on the ground the helicopter crew could be placed in a position of having to release the patient to save the aircraft. Some organizations involved in helicopter hoists choose to utilize a tag line, which does not incorporate a weak link. These organizations recognize that, in the event the aircraft is in jeopardy, the patient must be released from the hoist.

SK-1011 Weak Links (NSN 6530-01-445-7291). The utilization of the "weak link" in a tag line represents a compromise, providing the best level of protection for the patient and the minimum risk to the aircraft. The weak link is designed to separate at a tension point at which the aircraft is jeopardized.

After extensive consultation with military and civilian rescue personnel, Skedco included a weak link in the Helitag kit, which is made to break at 265 to 310 pounds. Recommendations from US Army Aeromedical Research Laboratories is between 265 to 310 pounds.

Weak links that break at the higher poundage not only present a risk to the aircraft, but also would allow ground personnel to be inadvertently lifted from the ground by the aircraft. Weak links provided with the Skedco Helitag Kit are made of line rated to break at 135 pounds. Laboratory tests indicate that, when tied in a loop and pulled from both ends, Skedco weak links break at from 275 to 310 pounds.

Personnel utilizing the Skedco Helitag Kit should recognize that when a weak link breaks it is doing its job. However, the separation of a weak link places renewed risk on the patient. Skedco believes that a spinning litter is preferable to a falling litter. In the case of weak link failure, the litter should be lowered back to the ground, and the conditions that led to the failure analyzed, to determine if further hoisting could be done safely.

Patient Evacuation Considerations
Col Charles Beadling, USAF, MC

Introduction: Patient movement, or evacuation, usually occurs from the point-of-injury to initial stabilization, then by intra-theater movement to an aeromedical staging facility, and finally by inter-theater evacuation to definitive care or CONUS. Movement by non-medical air or ground vehicles is called CASEVAC. Evacuation by vehicles equipped for patient movement is called MEDEVAC.

While each service has the capability for intra-theater patient movement, the Air Force performs strategic, inter-theater aeromedical evacuation for the entire DoD. Patients are placed in the AF evacuation system by a Patient Movement Control Center (PMCC). The Global Patient Movement Requirements Center (GPMRC) at Scott AFB, IL regulates the movement of all military patients.

A Theater Patient Movement Requirements Center (TPMRC) acts at the AOR level. The following are patient considerations and classifications that should be used to inform the Patient Movement Control Center (PMCC) the patient's status. The AF uses several codes to make communication easier and they should be used when requesting patient evacuation.

Patient Classifications/Category:

1=Psychiatric	2=Litter Inpatient	3=Ambulatory Inpatient
4=Infant	5=Outpatient	6=Attendant

Note: When contacting the PMCC, use the numerical code.

Patient Movement Precedence: (Joint Pub 4-02.2)

Rotary-wing (All Services):

Urgent/Urgent Surgical: Immediate movement to save life, limb, eyesight, or far forward surgical intervention is required (ASAP – maximum 2 hours).

Priority: Sick or wounded requiring prompt medical care (maximum 4 hours).

Routine: Sick or wounded requiring care within 24 hours; psychiatric patients (maximum 24 hours).

Convenience: Patients for whom air evacuation is a matter of convenience rather than medical necessity.

Fixed-wing (Air Force):

Urgent: Immediate movement to save life, limb or eyesight (ASAP).

Priority: Patients requiring prompt medical care not available locally, used when the medical condition could deteriorate and the patient cannot wait for routine evacuation, (movement within 24 hours).

Routine: Patient requires medical evacuation, but their condition is not expected to deteriorate significantly (movement within 72 hours).

Table 1-2. Timing by Category and Fixed-Wing Patient Movement

Category	Rotary-wing	Fixed-wing
Urgent	Within 2 hours	ASAP
Priority	Within 4 hours	Within 4 hours
Routine	Within 24 hours	Within 72 hours

Note: Ensure that the PMCC understands you are with a SOF unit and your request is not an everyday request. Relay any unusual circumstances or need to send this patient to a particular destination. They will respond accordingly.

Patient Information: You should be prepared to provide patient information to the PMCC. Information should include why the patient is being evacuated (ie, What is medically wrong with the patient?), a brief synopsis of current history and past significant medical history, allergies and current medications, if known. The following information sheet will help you organize the information:

Figure 1-4. Patient Movement Information Sheet

Patient Identification: _____   Organization: _____

Name: _____   Nationality: _____

Rank: _____

SSN: _____

HPI: _____   Significant PMH: _____

Allergies: _____   Medications: _____

Patient Classification: _____   Evacuation Precedence: _____

Date: _____   Destination: _____

Special Medical Considerations: _____   Special Equipment: _____
(eg, chest tube)   (eg, ventilator)

Note: The PMCC can assist you in finding an accepting physician, if needed.

Patient Preparation/Documentation: Document on one of the following forms, if available:

- DD Form 1380 (US Medical Card)
- DD Form 600 (Chronological Record of Medical Care)
- DD Form 602 (Patient Evacuation Tag)
- AF Form 3899 (AE Patient Record)

If the forms above are not on hand, please provide the PMCC with any concise clinical documentation that is available.

9 Line MEDEVAC Request

LINE	ITEM	EXPLANATION	REASON
1	Location of pickup site	Encrypt the grid coordinates of the pickup site. When using the DRYAD Numeral Cipher, the same "SET" line will be used to encrypt the grid zone letters and coordinates. To preclude misunderstanding, a statement is made that grid zone letters are included in the message (unless unit SOP specifies its use at all times).	Required so evacuation vehicle knows where to pickup patient. Also, so the unit coordinating the evacuation mission can plan the route for the evac vehicle (if the evac vehicle must pick up from more than one location).
2	Radio frequency, call	Encrypt the frequency of the radio at the pickup site, not a relay frequency. The call sign (and suffix if used) of person to be contacted at the pickup site may be transmitted in the clear.	Required so evac vehicle can contact requesting unit en route (obtain additional information or change in situation or directions).
3	Number of patients by precedence	Report only applicable information and encrypt the brevity codes. A - Urgent D - Routine B - Urgent-Surg E - Convenience C - Priority If two or more categories must be reported in the same request, insert the word "BREAK" between each category.	Required by unit controlling the evac vehicles to assist in prioritizing missions
4	Special equipment required	Encrypt the applicable brevity codes. A - None C - Extraction equipment B - Hoist D - Ventilator	Required so that the equipment can be placed on board the evac vehicle prior to the start of the mission
5	Number of patients by type	Report only applicable information and encrypt the brevity code. If requesting medical evacuation for both types, insert the word "BREAK" between litter entry and ambulatory entry. L+# of PNT – Litter A+# of PNT – Ambulatory (sitting)	Required so that the appropriate number evac vehicles may be dispatched to the pickup site. They should be configured to carry the patients requiring evac.
6a	Security of pickup site (wartime)	N - No enemy troops in area P - Possible enemy troops in area (approach with caution) E - Enemy troops in the area (approach with caution) X - Enemy troops in area (armed escort required)	Required to assist the evac crew in assessing the situation and determining if assistance is required. More definitive guidance can be provided to the evac vehicle while en route (specific location of enemy to assist aircraft in planning its approach).
6b	Number and type of wound, injury, or illness (peacetime)	Specific information regarding patient wounds by type (gunshot or shrapnel) Report serious bleeding with patient blood type, (if known)	Required to assist evac personnel in determining treatment and special equipment needed.
7	Method of marking pickup site	Encrypt the brevity codes. A - Panels D - None B - Pyrotechnic signal E - Other C - Smoke	Required to assist the evacuation crew in identifying the specific location of the pickup. Note that the color of panels or smoke should not be transmitted until the evac vehicle contacts the unit (just prior to its arrival). For security, the crew should identify the color and the unit verifies it.
8	Patient nationality and status	The number of patients in each category need not be transmitted. Encrypt only the applicable brevity codes. A - US military D - Non-US civilian B - US civilian E - Enemy prisoner of C - Non-US military war (EPW)	Required to assist in planning for destination facilities and need for guards. Unit requesting support should ensure that there is English speaking representative at the pickup site.
9a	CBRN contamination (wartime)	Include this line only when applicable. Encrypt the applicable brevity codes. C - Chemical R - Radiological B - Biological N - Nuclear	Required to assist in planning for the mission (determines which evac vehicle will accomplish the mission and when it will be accomplished)
9b	Terrain Description (peacetime)	Include details of terrain features in and around proposed landing site. If possible, describe relationship of site to prominent terrain features (eg, mountain, lake, tower).	Required to allow evac personnel to assess route/avenue of approach into area. Of particular importance if hoist operation is required.

Helicopter Landing Zones
Col Charles Beadling, USAF, MC

Responsibility: The unit requesting aeromedical evacuation support is responsible for selecting and properly marking the helicopter landing zones (LZs).

Criteria for Landing Sites: The helicopter LZ and the approach zones to the area should be free of obstructions. Sufficient space must be provided for the hovering and maneuvering of the helicopter during landing and takeoff. The approach zones should permit the helicopter to land and take off into the prevailing wind whenever possible. It is desirable that landing sites afford helicopter pilots the opportunity to make shallow approaches. Definite measurements for LZs cannot be prescribed since they vary with temperature, altitude, wind, terrain, loading conditions, and individual helicopter characteristics. The minimum requirement for light helicopters is a cleared area of 30 meters in diameter with an approach and departure zone clear of obstructions.

Figure 1-5. Semi-Fixed Base Operations (Day)

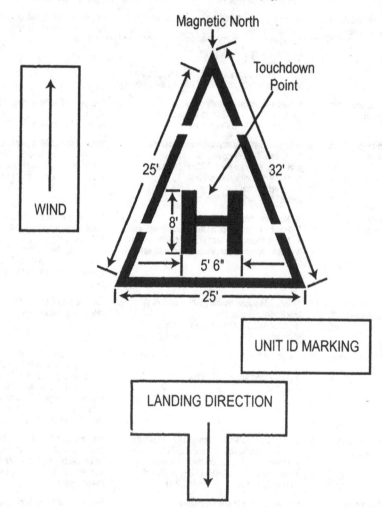

Removing or Marking Obstructions: Any objects (paper, cartons, ponchos, blankets, tentage, or parachutes) likely to be blown about by the wind from the rotor should be removed from the landing area. Obstacles, such as cables, wires, or antennas at or near LZs, which cannot be removed and may not be readily seen by a pilot, must be clearly marked. Red lights are normally used at night to mark all obstacles that cannot be easily eliminated within a LZ. In most combat situations, it is impractical for security reasons to mark the tops of obstacles at the approach and departure end of a LZ. If obstacles or other hazards cannot be marked, pilots should be advised of existing conditions by radio.

Identifying the Landing Site: When the tactical situation permits, a landing site should be marked with the letter "H" or "Y", using identification panels or other appropriate marking material. Special care must be taken to secure panels to the ground to prevent them from being blown about by the rotor wash. Firmly driven stakes will secure the panels tautly; rocks piled on the corners are not adequate.

If the tactical situation permits, the wind direction may be indicated by:

- Small windsock or rag tied to the end of a stick at the edge of the LZ.
- Man standing at the upwind edge of the site with his back to the wind and his arm extended forward.
- Smoke grenades, which emit colored smoke as soon as the helicopter is sighted. Smoke color should be identified by the aircrew and confirmed by ground personnel.

Figure 1-6. Semi-Fixed Base Operations (Night)

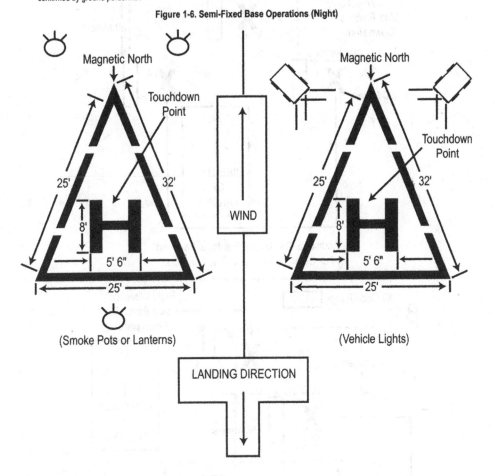

(Smoke Pots or Lanterns)   (Vehicle Lights)

In night operations, the following factors should be considered: One of the many ways to mark a landing site is to place a light, such as a chemical light, at each of the four corners of the usable LZ. These lights should be colored to distinguish them from other lights that may appear in the vicinity. A particular color can also serve as one element in identifying the LZ. Flare pots or other types of open lights should only be used as a last resort as they are usually blown out by the rotor downwash. Further, they often create a hazardous glare or reflection on the aircraft's windshield. The site can be further identified using a coded signal flash to the pilot from a ground operator. This signal can be given with the directed beam of a signal lamp, flashlight, vehicle lights, or other means. When using open flames, ground personnel should advise the pilot before he lands. Burning material must be secured in such a way that it will not blow over and start a fire in the LZ. Precautions should be taken to ensure that open flames are not placed in a position where the pilot must hover over or be within 3 meters of them. The coded signal is continuously flashed to the pilot until recognition is assured. After recognition, the signal operator, from his position on the upwind side of the LZ, directs the beam of light downwind along the ground to bisect the landing area. The pilot makes his approach for landing in the line with the beam of light and toward its source, landing at the center of the marked area. All lights are displayed for only a minimum time before arrival of the helicopter. The lights are turned off immediately after the aircraft lands. When standard lighting methods are not possible, pocket-sized white (for day) or blue (for night) strobe lights are excellent means to aid the pilot in identifying the LZ.

Figure 1-7. Field Expedient Landing Zone (Day)

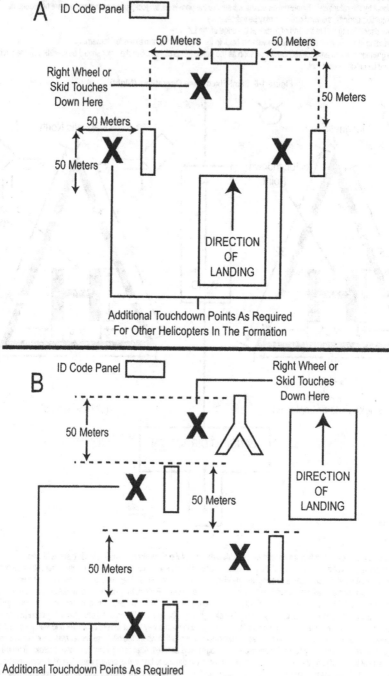

Additional Touchdown Points As Required
For Other Helicopters In The Formation

Figure 1-8. Field Expedient Landing Zone (Night)

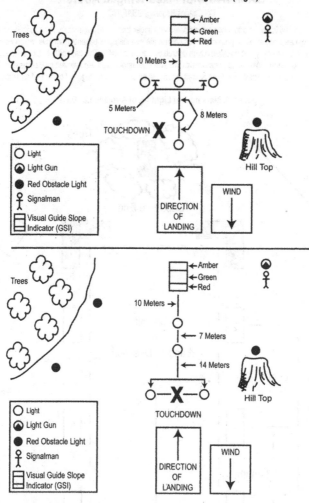

During takeoff, only those lights requested by the pilot are displayed; they are turned off immediately after the aircraft's departure. When the helicopter approaches the LZ, the ground contact team can ask the pilot to turn on his rotating beacon briefly. This enables the ground personnel to identify the aircraft and confirm its position in relation to the LZ (north, south, east, or west). The rotating beacon can be turned off as soon as the ground contact team has located and identified the aircraft. The ground contact team helps the pilot by informing him of his location in relation to the LZ, observing the aircraft's silhouette, and guiding the aircraft toward the LZ. While the aircraft is maneuvering toward the LZ, two-way radio contact is maintained and the type of lighting or signal being displayed is described by the pilot and verified by ground personnel via radio. The signal should be continued until the aircraft touches down in the LZ.

The use of FM homing procedures can prove to be a valuable asset, especially to troops in the field under adverse conditions. Through the use of FM homing, the pilot can more accurately locate the ground personnel. The success of a homing operation depends upon the actions of the ground personnel. First, ground personnel must be operating an FM radio, which is capable of transmitting within the frequency range of 30.0 to 69.95 megahertz; then they must be able to gain maximum performance from the radio (refer to appropriate technical manual for procedure). The range of FM radio communications is limited to line of sight; therefore, personnel should remain as clear as possible of obstructions and obstacles that could interfere with or totally block the radio signals. Ground personnel must have knowledge of the FM homing procedures. For example, when the pilot asks the radio operator to "key the microphone," he is simply asking that the transmit button be depressed for a period of 10-15 seconds. This gives the pilot an opportunity to determine the direction to the person using the radio.

Note: When using FM homing electronic countermeasures, the possible site detection of LZs by means of electronic triangulation presents a serious threat and must be considered.

CASEVAC with Fixed Winged Aircraft

Col Charles Beadling, USAF, MC

Small fixed-wing aircraft are limited in speed and range as compared with larger transport-type aircraft. The capability of small fixed-wing aircraft to land or take off from selected small, unprepared areas permits the evacuation of patients from AOs, which would be inaccessible to larger aircraft. These aircraft can fly slowly and maintain a high degree of maneuverability. This capability further enhances their value in forward areas under combat conditions. When adequate airfields are available, larger fixed-wing aircraft may be used in forward areas for patient evacuation. This is a secondary mission for these aircraft, which will be used only to augment dedicated air ambulance capabilities.

Figure 1-9. Marking and Lighting of Airplane LZ (Day)

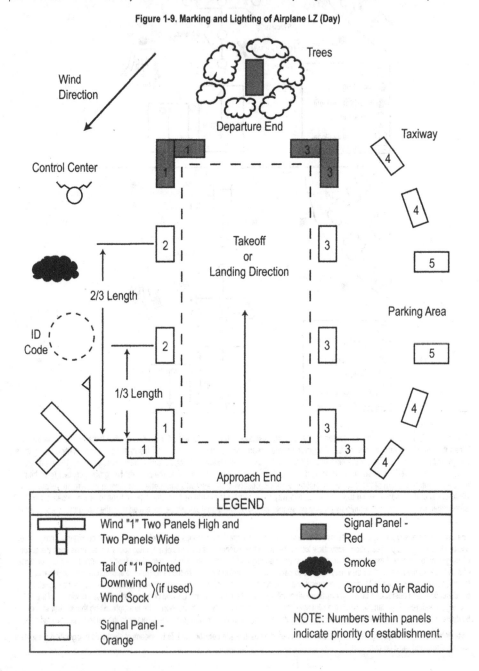

Figure 1-10. Marking and Lighting of Airplane LZ (Night)

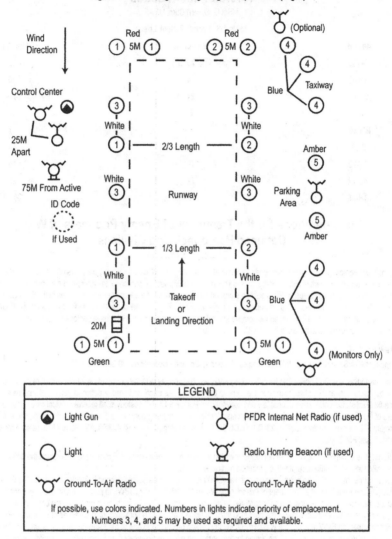

LEGEND

⬤ Light Gun		☿ PFDR Internal Net Radio (if used)
◯ Light		☿ Radio Homing Beacon (if used)
☿ Ground-To-Air Radio		▤ Ground-To-Air Radio

If possible, use colors indicated. Numbers in lights indicate priority of emplacement.
Numbers 3, 4, and 5 may be used as required and available.

Air Evacuation Phone List
MSgt G. Steven Cum, USAF

Global Patient Movement Requirement Center (GPMRC)
AE Intertheater and CONUS: 1-800-303-9301, DSN 779-4200
AE Support EUCOM: 011-49-6371-47-8040, DSN 314-480-8040
AE Support PACOM: 011-81-3117-55-4700, DSN 315-448-1602
AE Support SWA: DSN 318-436-4417/4418

Air Force Recovery Coordination Center (AFRCC)
CONUS Tyndall AFB 1-800-851-3051

Joint Recovery Coordination Center (JRCC)
PACOM Hickam AFB, HI: 1-808-535-3333
EUCOM Ramstein AB, GE: DSN 314-478-6885/4552/4547
SWA Al Udied Doha, Qatar: DSN 318-436-4215
South and Central America, Key West, FL: 305-295-5415, DSN 483-5835
Gulf of Mexico/Caribbean, San Juan, PR: DSN 894-1490

Aircraft Patient Loads
MSgt G. Steven Cum, USAF

Table 1-3. Aircraft Patient Loads

Aircraft	Max Litter	Max Amb
C-130	70	92
MH-5	14	20
Ch-47	24	33-44
UH-1	6	12
MH-60	4	11
C-17	36	54
CV-22	12	15
MV-22	22	28
CH-46	22	30-40

Considerations for the Treatment of Enemy Prisoners of War, Detained Personnel, and Civilians
LTC Robert Lutz, MC, USA

Introduction: SOF medical personnel will frequently be required to provide medical care for enemy prisoners of war (EPWs), detained personnel, and civilians on the battlefield. In doing so, it is important for SOF medical personnel to understand the basis of the rules and regulations that they are required to follow. This section starts with an explanation of the legal basis for the rules that US military medical personnel must follow, and concludes with some operational considerations. The majority of the text includes excerpts from HQDA ST 4-02.46. The operational considerations section is compiled from feedback from personnel who have deployed in support of the War on Terrorism, in addition to excerpted guidance from HQDA ST 4-02.46.

Part I – Legal Aspects

1. **Reference:** HQDA Special Text No. 4-02.46 "Medical Support to Detainee Operations" 30 September 2005

2. **General Guidance:** It is DoD policy that the US military services shall comply with the principles, spirit, and intent of the international law of war, both customary and codified, to include the Geneva Conventions. As such, captured or detained personnel shall be accorded an appropriate legal status under international law and conventions. Personnel in US custody shall receive medical care consistent with the standard of medical care that applies for US military personnel in the same geographic area. For additional information refer to Department of Defense Directive (DoDD) 2310.1, DoDD 5100.77, Army Regulation (AR) 40-400, AR 190-8, FM 3-19.40, FMs 4-02- and 8-10-series, and FM 27-10.

3. **Definitions:** It is essential for all medical personnel involved in the care of personnel in US custody to understand the differences between categories of captured, retained, or detained personnel.
   A. Enemy Prisoner of War: An enemy prisoner of war (EPW) is a detained person as defined in Articles 4 and 5 of the Geneva Convention Relative to the Treatment of Prisoners of War of August 12, 1949 (GPW). In particular, one that is engaged in combat under orders of his government, who is captured by an enemy armed force. As such, he is entitled to the combatant's privilege of immunity from the municipal law of the capturing state for warlike acts that do not amount to breaches of the law of land warfare. For example, an EPW may be, but is not limited to, any person belonging to one of the following categories who has fallen into the power of the enemy: a member of the armed forces, organized militia or volunteer corps; a person who accompanies the armed forces without actually being a member thereof; a member of a merchant marine or civilian aircraft crew not qualifying for more favorable treatment; or individuals who, on the approach of the enemy, spontaneously take up arms to resist the invading forces. These personnel may also be referred to as prisoners of war (POW).
   B. Retained Personnel: Enemy personnel who come within any of these categories below are eligible to be certified as retained personnel (RP):
      1. Medical personnel exclusively engaged in the:
         • Search, collection, transport, or treatment of the wounded or sick
         • Prevention of disease
         • Staff administration of medical units and establishments exclusively
         • Chaplains attached to enemy armed forces
         • Staff of national Red Cross societies and other voluntary aid societies
   C. Civilian Internees: A civilian internee is a person that is interned during armed conflict, occupation for security reasons, for protection or because he has committed an offense against the detaining power. This term is used to refer to persons interned and protected in accordance with the Geneva Convention Relative to the Protection of Civilian Persons in Time of War, 12 August 1949 (GC).

D. Other Detainees: Persons in the custody of the US Armed Forces that have not been classified as an EPW (Articles 4, GPW), a retained person (Article 33, GPW), or civilian internee (Article 78, GC), shall be treated as an EPW until a legal status is ascertained by competent authority.

It is possible that other detainees may be designated additional classifications according to the policies promulgated by the President of the US or the DOD. Such additional classifications do not impact the planning and execution of detainee operations. Instead, these additional classifications impact issues such as possible criminal charges for engaging in unprivileged military activities.

The designation of enemy combatant (EC), established in relation to the global war on terrorism (GWOT) to designate individuals that engage in unprivileged hostilities against the US, is an example of such additional classification. Individuals designated as ECs under the provisions of Executive Order (EO) 13224 are subject to potential criminal sanctions for their activities. However, for the purposes of detainee operations such individuals are simply regarded as other detainees because they do not fall into a specific category of detainee according to the Geneva Conventions.

4. **Law of Land Warfare:**
   A. The conduct of armed hostilities on land is regulated by the Law of Land Warfare. This body of law is inspired by the desire to diminish the evils of war by:
      * Protecting both combatants and noncombatants from unnecessary suffering
      * Safeguarding certain fundamental human rights of persons that fall into the hands of the enemy, particularly POWs, the wounded and sick, and civilians
      * Facilitating the restoration of peace

   B. The Law of Land Warfare places limits on the exercise of a belligerent's power in the interest of furthering that desire (diminishing the evils of war) and it requires that belligerents:
      * Refrain from employing any kind or degree of violence that is not actually necessary for military purposes
      * Conduct hostilities with regard for the principles of humanity and chivalry

5. **Sources of the Law of Land Warfare:**
   A. The Law of Land Warfare is derived from two principal sources:
      * Lawmaking treaties or conventions (such as the Hague and Geneva Conventions)
      * Custom (practices which by common consent and long-established uniform adherence have taken on the force of law)
   B. Under the US Constitution, treaties constitute part of the Supreme Law of the Land, and thus must be observed by both military and civilian personnel. The unwritten or customary Law of Land Warfare is also part of the US law. It is binding upon the US, citizens of the US, and other persons serving this country. For additional information on the Law of Land Warfare, refer to Department of the Army Pamphlet (DA Pam) 27-1 and FM 27-10.

6. **Geneva Conventions:** The US is a party to numerous conventions and treaties pertinent to warfare on land. Collectively, these treaties are often referred to as The Hague and Geneva Conventions. Whereas the Hague Conventions concern the methods and means of warfare, the Geneva Conventions concern the victims of war or armed conflict. The Geneva Conventions are four separate international treaties, signed in 1949.

The Conventions are very detailed and contain many provisions, which are tied directly to the FHP mission. These Conventions are entitled:
   * Geneva Convention for the Amelioration of the Condition of the Wounded and Sick in Armed Forces in the Field (GWS)
   * Geneva Convention for the Amelioration of the Condition of Wounded, Sick, and Shipwrecked Members of Armed Forces at Sea
   * Geneva Convention Relative to the Treatment of Prisoners of War (GPW)
   * Geneva Convention Relative to the Protection of Civilian Persons in Time of War

7. **Protection of the Sick and Wounded:** The essential and dominant idea of the GWS is that the soldier who has been wounded or is sick, and for that reason is out of the combat in a disabled condition, is from that moment protected. Friend or foe must be tended with the same care. From this principle, numerous obligations are imposed upon parties to a conflict.

8. **Protection and Care:** Article 12 of the GWS imposes several specific obligations regarding the protection and care of the wounded and sick.
   A. The first paragraph of Article 12, GWS, states "Members of the armed forces and other persons mentioned in the following Article, who are wounded or sick, shall be respected and protected in all circumstances."
      * The word respect means "to spare, not to attack," and protect means "to come to someone's defense, to lend help and support." These words make it unlawful to attack, kill, ill-treat, or in any way harm a fallen and unarmed enemy soldier. At the same time, these words impose an obligation to come to his aid and give him such care as his condition requires. This obligation is applicable in all circumstances. The wounded and sick are to be respected just as much when they are with their own army or in no man's land, as well as when they have fallen into the hands of the enemy.
      * Combatants, as well as noncombatants, are required to respect the wounded. The obligation also applies to civilians; Article 18, GWS, specifically states: "The civilian population shall respect those wounded and sick, and in particular abstain from offering them violence." The GWS does not define what "wounded or sick" means, nor has there ever been any definition of the degree of severity of a wound or a sickness entitling the wounded or sick combatant to respect. Any definition would necessarily be restrictive in character and would thereby open the door to misinterpretation and abuse. The meaning of the words "wounded and sick" is thus a matter of common sense and good faith. It is the act of

falling or lying down of arms because of a wound or sickness that constitutes a claim to protection. Only the soldier that is himself seeking to kill may be killed.

- The benefits afforded the wounded and sick extend not only to members of the armed forces, but to other categories of persons as well, classes of whom are specified in Article 13, GWS. Even though a wounded person is not in one of the categories enumerated in the Article, we must still respect and protect that person. There is a universal principle which says that any wounded or sick person is entitled to respect and humane treatment and the care that his condition requires. Wounded and sick civilians have the benefit of the safeguards of the GC.

B. The second paragraph of Article 12, GWS, provides that the wounded and sick "...shall be treated humanely and cared for by the party to the conflict in whose power they may be, without any adverse distinction founded on sex, race, nationality, religion, political opinions, or other similar criteria...."

- All adverse distinctions are prohibited. Nothing can justify a belligerent in making any adverse distinction between wounded or sick that require his attention, whether they be friend or foe. Both are on equal footing in the matter of their claims to protection, respect, and care. The foregoing is not intended to prohibit concessions, particularly with respect to food, clothing, and shelter, which take into account the different national habits and backgrounds of the wounded and sick. The wounded and sick shall not be made the subjects of biological, scientific, or medical experiments of any kind that are not justified on medical grounds and dictated by a desire to improve their condition.
- The wounded and sick shall not willfully be left without medical assistance nor shall conditions exposing them to contagion or infection be created.
- The only reasons that can justify priority in the order of treatment are reasons of medical urgency.
- Paragraph 5 of Article 12, GWS, provides that if we must abandon wounded or sick, we have a moral obligation to, "as far as military considerations permit," leave medical supplies and personnel to assist in their care. This provision is in no way bound up with the absolute obligation imposed by paragraph 2 of Article 12 to care for the wounded. A belligerent can never refuse to care for enemy wounded on the pretext that his adversary has abandoned them without medical personnel and equipment.

9. **Enemy Wounded and Sick:** The protections accorded the wounded and sick apply to friend and foe alike without distinction. Certain provisions of the GWS, however, specifically concern enemy wounded and sick. There are also provisions in the GPW which, because they apply to POWs generally, also apply to enemy wounded or sick.

- Article 14 of the GWS states that persons who are wounded and then captured have the status of POWs. However, that wounded soldier is also a person who needs treatment. Therefore, a wounded soldier who falls into the hands of an enemy who is a Party to the GWS and the GPW, such as the US, will enjoy protection under both Conventions until his recovery. The GWS will take precedence over the GPW where the two overlap.
- Article 16 of the GWS requires the recording and forwarding of information regarding enemy wounded, sick, or dead. See AR 190-8 for disposition of an EPW after hospital care.
- When intelligence indicates that large numbers of EPWs may result from an operation, medical units may require reinforcement to support the anticipated additional EPW patient workload. Procedures for estimating the medical workload involved in the treatment and care of EPW patients are described in FM 8-55.

10. **Search for and Collection of Casualties:** Article 15 of the GWS imposes a duty on combatants to search for and collect the dead, wounded, and sick as soon as circumstances permit. It is left to the tactical commander to judge what is possible and to decide to commit his medical personnel to this effort. If circumstances permit, an armistice or suspension of fire should be arranged to permit this effort.

11. **Assistance for the Civilian Population:** Article 18, GWS, addresses the civilian population. It allows a belligerent to ask civilians to collect and care for wounded or sick of whatever nationality. This provision does not relieve the military authorities of their responsibility to give both physical and moral care to the wounded and sick. The GWS also reminds the civilian population that they must respect the wounded and sick, and in particular, must not injure them.

12. **Enemy Civilian Wounded and Sick:**
    A. Certain provisions of the GC are relevant to the FHP mission. Article 16 of the GC provides that enemy civilians who are "wounded and sick, as well as the infirm, and expectant mothers shall be the object of particular protection and respect." The Article also requires that, "as far as military considerations allow, each Party to the conflict shall *facilitate* the steps taken to search for the killed and wounded (civilians), to assist...other persons exposed to grave danger, and to protect them against pillage and ill-treatment (emphasis added)."
    - The "protection and respect" to which wounded and sick enemy civilians are entitled is the same as that accorded to wounded and sick enemy military personnel.
    - While Article 15 of the GWS requires Parties to a conflict to search for and collect the dead, wounded, and sick members of the armed forces, Article 16 of the GC states that the Parties must "facilitate the steps taken" in regard to civilians. This recognizes the fact that saving civilians is the responsibility of the civilian authorities rather than of the military. The military is not required to provide injured civilians with medical care in a combat zone (CZ). However, if we start providing treatment, we are bound by the provisions of the GWS. Provisions for treating civilians (enemy or friendly) will be addressed in division, corps, and theater regulations.
    B. In occupied territories, the Occupying Power must accord the inhabitants numerous protections as required by the GC. Provisions relevant to medical care include the:
    - Requirement to bring in medical supplies for the population if the resources of the occupied territory are inadequate.
    - Prohibition on requisitioning medical supplies unless the requirements of the civilian population have been taken into account.

- Duty of ensuring and maintaining, with the cooperation of national and local authorities, the medical and hospital establishments and services, public health, and hygiene in the occupied territory.
- Prohibition on requisitioning civilian hospitals on other than a temporary basis and then only in cases of urgent necessity for the care of military wounded and sick and after suitable arrangements have been made for the civilian patients.
- Requirement to provide adequate medical treatment to detained persons.
- Requirement to provide adequate medical care in internment camps.

13. Protection and Identification of Medical Personnel:

A. Article 24 of the GWS provides special protection for "Medical personnel *exclusively engaged* in the search for, or the collection, transport, or treatment of the wounded or sick, or in the prevention of disease, and staff exclusively engaged in the administration of medical units and establishments…(emphasis added)." Article 25 provides limited protection for "Members of the armed forces specially trained for employment, should the need arise, as hospital orderlies, nurses, or auxiliary stretcher-bearers, in the search for or the collection, transport, or treatment of the wounded and sick…*if they are carrying out those duties at the time when they come into contact with the enemy or fall into his hands* (emphasis added)."

B. There are two separate and distinct forms of protection.

- The first is protection from intentional attack if medical personnel are identifiable as such by an enemy in a combat environment. Normally this is facilitated by medical personnel wearing an armband bearing the distinctive emblem (a Red Cross or Red Crescent on a white background), or by their employment in a medical unit, establishment, or vehicle (including medical aircraft and hospital ships) that displays the distinctive emblem. Persons protected by Article 25 may wear an armband bearing a miniature distinctive emblem only while executing medical duties.
- The second protection provided by the GWS pertains to medical personnel who fall into the hands of the enemy. Article 24 personnel are entitled to "retained person" status. They are not deemed to be POWs, but otherwise benefit from the protections of the GPW. They are authorized to carry out medical duties only, and "shall be retained only in so far as the state of health…and the number of POWs require." Article 25 personnel are POWs, but shall be employed to perform medical duties in so far as the need arises. They may be required to perform other duties or labor, and they may be held until a general repatriation of POWs is accomplished upon the cessation of hostilities.

Part II – Operational Considerations

1. **Emergency Care and Treatment:** Wounded EPWs and detained personnel in US custody shall receive medical care consistent with the standard of medical care that applies for US military personnel in the same geographic area. At the SOF Advanced Tactical Provider (ATP) level this means that personnel in these categories will receive the same standard of medical care that they provide to the personnel in their unit.

2. **Medical Screening of EPWs and Detained Personnel:** Unit medics should provide the initial screening of EPWs and detained personnel as soon as practical after capture. If at all possible, a brief screen should be done after the objective is secure and any medications the detainee is currently taking should be recovered. Because of the differences in medication names and dosages for foreign medications, it will provide a starting point to work from if the detainee is on chronic medications. SOF Medics should become familiar with higher HQ policy on the time frames within which after capture EPW and detained personnel are required to have a medical screening examination. It should be as soon as practical after capture and should be part of the EPW/detainee processing. In addition, it is particularly important to medically screen detainees before and after transfer to a host nation facility, as it will provide documentation of the detainee's health status and it will serve to protect your command from potential allegations of abuse.

A. Detainees will be examined in an environment appropriate for the preservation of individual dignity and safety. Graduated levels of privacy will be used, appropriate to the type of examination. The detainee will be asked only to expose as much body surface as medically necessary for a complete examination. Every effort will made to provide an examiner of the same gender as the detainee.

B. During the initial screening of detainees any preexisting medical conditions, wounds, fractures, and bruises should be noted. Documentation of these injuries/conditions will provide a baseline for each detainee. Thorough written documentation and/or photographs of wounds/bruises present at the time of capture serve two purposes:

- Careful documentation of injuries present at the time of capture prevents the EPW/detained person from claiming that their injury was received in the internment facility.
- Careful documentation of injuries present at the time of capture will facilitate the identification of any injuries received in the internment facility.

3. Release of Medical Information:

A. Detained personnel must have access to the same standard of medical care as the US and coalition forces to include respect for their dignity and privacy. In general, the security of detainees' medical records and confidentiality of medical information will be managed the same way as for the US and coalition forces. During detainee operations, the Patient Administration Division (PAD), the Criminal Investigation Division (CID), the International Committee of the Red Cross (ICRC), and medical chain of command can have access to detainee medical records besides the treating medical personnel. At no time, the military police (MP) or other detention facility personnel will have access to medical records and at no time will detainee's medical information be used during interrogation.

B. The obligation to safeguard patient confidences is subject to certain exceptions which are ethically and legally justified because of overriding social considerations. Where a patient threatens to inflict serious bodily harm to another person or to him or herself and there is a reasonable probability that the patient may carry out the threat, the medical provider should take reasonable precautions for the protection of the intended victim, including notification of the chain of command.

C. Because the chain of command is ultimately responsible for the care and treatment of detainees, the internment facility chain of command requires some medical information. For example, detainees suspected of having infectious diseases such as tuberculosis (TB) should be separated from other detainees. Guards and other personnel who come into contact with such patients should be informed about their health risks and how to mitigate those risks.

D. Releasable medical information on internees includes that which is necessary to supervise the general state of health, nutrition, and cleanliness of internees, and to detect contagious diseases. Such information should be used to provide health care; to ensure health and safety of internees, Soldiers, employees, or others at the facility; to ensure law enforcement on the premises; and ensure the administration and maintenance of the safety, security, and good order of the facility.

4. **Protection of Medical Personnel:** Articles 24 and 25 of the GWS provide special protection for medical personnel exclusively involved in medical activities. Given that SOF medical personnel are often integrated into the assault force, and in some cases are part of the assault team, it is not appropriate for them to claim the special protections afforded by the GWS. These special protections can only be claimed if the SOF medical provider is "exclusively engaged" in providing medical care.

5. **Prohibited Acts:** The GPW describes acts that are prohibited under the Conventions and specifies that all detainees will receive humane treatment.

A. Prohibited acts include killing, torture, medical/scientific experimentation, physical mutilation, removal of tissues/organs for transplantation, and causing serious injury, pain, and suffering.

B. Torture can take many guises in wartime situations. Historically, it has been used to extract tactical information from an uncooperative EPW. However, it has also been applied for the sake of punishment and/or to inflict pain and suffering. Regardless of the rationale, the torture of EPWs is prohibited. Medical personnel do not participate in the interrogation of prisoners; however, some actions can be construed as prohibited acts. Medical personnel, who administer drugs to facilitate interrogation or advise interrogators on the ability of an individual to withstand torture, can be considered complicit in that torture.

C. Under current DoD policy, medical personnel cannot certify a detainee for interrogation and cannot provide consultation to interrogators if they are detainee medical providers.

D. Physical Abuse: Slapping, hitting, bruising, beating, or any other intentional act that causes someone physical pain, injury, or suffering. The use of painful physical restraints or the use of restraints for purely punitive action rather than safety reasons may be considered abuse.

E. Emotional Abuse: Threatening, humiliating, causing emotional pain, distress, or anguish. Emotional abuse can be verbal or nonverbal; it includes insults and threats of harm.

F. Sexual Abuse: Any sexual activity to which the individual does not consent or is incapable of consenting; any sexual activity between detainees and internment facility personnel is without question abusive because it cannot be truly "consensual." Nonconsensual sexual activity includes everything from exhibitionism to inappropriate touching to sexual intercourse.

6. **Potential Pitfalls:**

A. EPW/Detainee transport: When enemy personnel have been captured on an objective and are being returned to the FOB for processing and internment, there is potential for injury. These personnel frequently are restrained and placed in a vehicle or aircraft for transport. They are generally only allowed limited movement and limited communication. There is a high risk for injury during transport and the detained personnel should be frequently checked to ensure their restraints are not too tight or that they have not been placed against an exhaust pipe or on a hot surface. There have been cases of injuries from decreased circulation from restraints that are too tight in transport and cases of burns from placement next to a hot surface.

B. Delayed diagnosis and/or recognition of a medical problem: A medical screening exam should be done as soon as practical after capture and preferably before internment into a holding facility.

C. Scope of practice and standard of care: If a detainee has a medical complaint that would prompt the medic to refer US personnel to a higher level of care, then the detainee should be referred to a higher level of care. Detainees are entitled to the same standard of care as US personnel in the same geographic area. It can be logistically challenging to move detained personnel to a Combat Support Hospital or other higher level of care, however the medic must work with the chain of command to ensure that this is safely done in order to maintain standards of care.

7. **Reporting Requirements:**

A. Medical personnel are obligated to report any suspected abuse or torture through the chain command. Reports may be made through other channels such as the MP, the Staff Judge Advocate, or the IG.

B. Failure to report abuse or mistreatment can be cause for UCMJ action.

Part III – Conclusion

Proper care and treatment of EPWs, Detained Personnel, and civilians on the battlefield is not only required by policy, law, and treaties, it is our obligation as citizens of the United States. Mistreatment of ill, wounded, or injured personnel under US control can have an adverse impact at the strategic level in our fight to reign in terrorism. It is the duty of all medical personnel, to include those in US Special Operations Command, to ensure that appropriate medical aid is rendered to both enemy and US injured and wounded on the battlefield.

Medical History and Physical Examination

LTC Andre Pennardt, MC, USA

Efficient, focused, problem-oriented medical care is the goal of the Special Operations Forces medic. The S-O-A-P note format is a primary tool used to efficiently organize a concise, focused, problem-oriented medical examination and treatment plan.

The same SOAP format has been consistently used throughout the handbook to present medical information about diseases and conditions seen by the SOF medic. The goal is to provide the essential medical information for the most common diseases seen by the SOF medic using the same SOAP format that SOF medics use to collect information, define problems and develop treatment plans.

> *Subjective* complaints (to include pertinent positives and negatives of patient's history and focused review of systems)
>
> *Objective* findings (from physical examination and tests)
>
> *Assessment* defined and prioritized list of problems
>
> *Plan* of management and treatment (for each problem)

The focused medical examination is the most frequently used tool of the SOF medic. The comprehensive medical examination follows the same SOAP format and includes details for each organ system. Although the Subjective and Objective sections of the comprehensive medical examination include more detail, the basics of the diagnostic and therapeutic process are the same for both the focused and the comprehensive medical examination. The goal is to accurately define and efficiently solve the patient's medical problems.

The Focused Medical Examination:

Subjective: (Chief Complaint & Pertinent HPI)

Symptoms:	Acute:	Sub-acute:	Chronic:
Constitutional:			
CNS:			
Skin:			
HEENT:			
Chest:			
Back:			
GU:			
Abdominal:			
Extremity:			
Hand:			
Foot:			
Other:			

Pertinent History (PMH, FH, SH, ROS) including allergies:

Objective:

Signs:	Acute:	Sub-acute:	Chronic:
Inspection (see):			
Palpation (feel):			
Percussion (tap):			
Auscultation (listen):			

Diagnostic Tests and Procedures (essential [eg, vital signs], recommended):

Assessment

Prioritized List of Problems: 1.   2.   3.   etc.

Plan (for each problem)

Treatment:
   Primary:
   Alternative:
   Primitive:
   Empiric:

Patient Education:
   General:
   Diet:
   Activity:
   Medications:
   Prevention and Hygiene:
   Wound Care:

Follow-up Actions:
   Return Evaluation:
   Evacuation/Consultation Criteria:

The Comprehensive Medical Examination is an organized hierarchy for all medical history and physical findings noted in the Subjective and Objective portions of the SOAP format. These sections of the SOAP note contain all findings, including tests and laboratory studies, to provide the basis that all "clinical" diagnoses (the prioritized problem list) are made. The final assessment of information and plan to confirm the diagnosis of an illness or injury, begin treatment, educate the patient, and form any follow up plans is contained in the Assessment and Plan portion of the SOAP format. The SOAP problem-oriented approach is a universal standard in medical education, recording medical information, and communicating medical information to other health care providers.

Subjective: A necessary part of all medical histories is collecting the patient's basic information: name, rank, social security number, unit, gender, and date of birth. The medical history may be divided into four parts: the chief complaint (CC), history of present illness (HPI), review of systems (ROS), and past, family, and or social history (PFSH).

Chief Complaint (CC): This consists of a concise statement describing the symptom, problem, condition, diagnosis, or other factors that is the reason the patient is seeking treatment. It is usually stated in the patient's own words.

History of Present Illness (HPI): This consists of a chronological description of the patient's illness or injury. There are 8 elements associated with the HPI:

LOCATION:	Specific area of body involved; radiation; bilateral, anterior, distal, etc.
QUALITY:	Specific patterns and descriptions: dull, sharp, throbbing, stabbing, constant, intermittent, worsening, etc.
SEVERITY:	Degree of severity or intensity (scale of 1-10): "feels like when...", severe, mild, etc.
DURATION:	Onset of problem or symptom: started 3 days ago, 1 hour ago; since yesterday; until this morning; for about 2 months, etc.
TIMING:	Indicates frequency and progression, how long it lasts, how often it occurs, etc.
CONTEXT:	Setting in which it occurs: what was patient doing when signs/symptoms started; occurs after meals, etc.
MODIFYING FACTORS:	What has patient done to relieve signs/symptoms: type of medications taken, how it relieved or made worse; rest makes it better; movement makes it worse, etc.
ASSOCIATED SIGNS AND SYMPTOMS:	Other signs and symptoms patient has experienced or has at presentation: Medic should ask direct questions (eg, nausea/vomiting, blurred vision, change in bowel habits).

Review of Systems (ROS): This is an inventory of body systems obtained through a series of questions seeking to identify any signs/symptoms the patient may be experiencing. There are 14 elements to the ROS.

CONSTITUTIONAL:	Weight changes, fever, fatigue, weakness, etc.
EYES:	Pain, redness, blurring, photophobia, decreased visual acuity, diplopia, etc.
ENT:	Decreased hearing, pain, vertigo, tinnitus, epistaxis, sore throat, etc.
CARDIOVASCULAR:	Palpitations, fainting, tachycardia, orthopnea, ECG results, etc.
RESPIRATORY:	Wheezing, cough, sputum (color and quantity), dyspnea, pleuritic pain, etc.
GASTROINTESTINAL:	Nausea, vomiting, diarrhea, bloody stools, constipation, abdominal pain, anorexia, etc.
GENITOURINARY:	Frequency, painful urination, hematuria, testicular pain, incontinence, penile discharge, last menstrual period, etc.
MUSCULOSKELETAL:	Joint pain or stiffness, muscle pain, decreased range of motion, swelling, etc.
SKIN/BREAST:	Dryness, rashes, itching, jaundice, lumps, sores, changes in hair or skin, nipple discharge, etc.
NEUROLOGICAL:	Seizures, focal weakness, slurred speech, tremors, difficulty walking, paralysis, numbness, headaches, etc.
PSYCHIATRIC:	Nervousness, depression, mood changes, insomnia, etc.
ENDOCRINE:	Excessive thirst and polyuria (eg, diabetes), cold/heat intolerance (eg, thyroid dysfunction), sweating, etc.
HEMATOLOGIC / LYMPHATIC:	Anemia, easy bruising or bleeding, adenopathy, past transfusions, etc.
ALLERGIC / IMMUNOLOGIC:	Allergies, prior immunizations, HIV test results, etc.

Past, Family, and Social History (PFSH):

PAST MEDICAL HISTORY:	This includes the patient's significant prior medical problems, past surgeries, current medications, food and medication allergies, and immunization history.
FAMILY HISTORY:	This consists of a review of medical events in the patient's family that may be hereditary, or place patient at increased risk (eg, colon cancer, father had heart attack at age 40)
SOCIAL HISTORY:	This is an age-appropriate review of past and current activities that may affect the illness/injury. It includes employment, marital status, alcohol, drug and tobacco use, living arrangements, etc.

Objective:
Physical Examination
Constitutional:

VITAL SIGNS:	Height, weight, blood pressure, pulse rate, respiratory rate, temperature and level of pain
GENERAL APPEARANCE:	Development, nutrition, growth, body habitus, attention to grooming, etc.

Eyes: Pupils (equal, round, react to light, accommodate), move in all directions to command, no spontaneous abnormal movement (nystagmus), sclerae clear, conjunctivae without inflammation. Document visual acuity for each eye (with/without glasses).

Ears, Nose, Mouth, and Throat:

EARS:	Overall appearance of auricles, auditory canals (swelling, drainage, etc.), tympanic membranes (erythema, blood, mobility, etc.), and assessment of hearing acuity.
NOSE:	Examination of external nose, nasal mucosa, sinuses, septum, and turbinates for swelling, redness, polyps, blood, rhinorrhea, deviation, perforation, etc.
MOUTH:	Examination of lips, teeth, tongue, gums, etc. for dental caries, gingivitis, periodontal disease, tooth loss, loose teeth, cyanosis, etc.
THROAT:	Examination of oropharynx for lesions, symmetry, erythema, tonsillitis, etc.

Respiratory: Examination should include inspection of chest (shape, symmetry, expansion, use of accessory muscles, and intercostal retractions), percussion of chest (dullness, hyperresonance), palpation of chest (tenderness, masses, tactile fremitus), and auscultation of lungs (equality of breath sounds, rubs, rales, rhonchi, and wheezes).

Cardiovascular: Examination should include palpation of heart (location, forcefulness of the point of maximal impact, thrills, etc.), auscultation of heart (murmurs, abnormal sounds), assessment of pulse amplitude and presence of bruits in various arteries (carotid, femoral, popliteal, etc.), assessment of jugular veins (distention, A, V, or cannon A waves), palpation of pedal and other pulses, and measurement of ankle-brachial index.

Breasts (Chest): The breasts may be inspected for contour, symmetry, nipple discharge, gynecomastia, and palpated for lumps/masses and tenderness. Remember that breast tissue extends from the clavicles to the "bra-line" and from the mid-sternum to the mid-axillary line.

Gastrointestinal: The abdomen should be inspected for obesity, distention, and scarring, followed by auscultation in all four quadrants for bowel sounds. Percussion may be performed to detect abdominal tenderness, ascites, or tympani. Palpation is performed to assess for tenderness, guarding, rebound, and other signs of peritoneal irritation, enlargement of the spleen or liver, masses, and pulsatile enlargement of the aorta (abdominal aortic aneurysm). Digital examination of the rectum may be performed to detect hemorrhoids or rectal masses, assess rectal tone, obtain stool for Hemoccult determination, and examine the prostate.

Genitourinary (Male): External examination of the penis may be performed to detect lesions or discharge. The testicles may be examined for symmetry, tenderness, masses, hydrocele, or varicocele. The prostate may be assessed for enlargement, tenderness, or masses during digital rectal examination. The bladder may be palpated to assess for distention or tenderness.

Genitourinary (Female): The external genitalia and vagina may be examined for general appearance, estrogen effect, lesions, or discharge. The cervix may be inspected for lesions or discharge using a speculum, at which time specimens may be obtained for microscopy and culture. Bimanual examination of the internal GU organs is performed to detect cervical motion tenderness, as well as uterine and/or ovarian enlargement, tenderness, or masses. The bladder may be palpated to assess for distention or tenderness.

Musculoskeletal: The spine may be examined for tenderness, range of motion, step-offs, scoliosis, or other deformity. Muscles may be examined for strength, tenderness, swelling, or spasm. Joints may be examined for range of motion, tenderness, warmth, discoloration (erythema/ecchymosis), swelling, and instability. Other bones should be palpated for tenderness, deformity, and crepitus as appropriate.

Neurologic: The patient should have his mental status assessed (mini-mental status exam) for higher cognitive function (including level of consciousness). The Glasgow Coma Scale (GCS) is a useful adjunct to assess the current mental status and progression of trauma victims. Cranial nerves (CN) II through XII are routinely assessed as part of the neurologic examination:

CN I	Olfactory is difficult to assess in the field since this requires testing of smell.
CN II	Visual acuity and fields
CN III, IV, and VI	Extraocular movements, pupillary reflex (III)
CN V	Facial sensation and corneal reflex
CN VII	Facial symmetry and strength
CN VIII	Hearing
CN IX	Gag reflex and reflex palatal movement
CN X	Voluntary movement of soft palate or vocal cord function
CN XI	Shoulder shrug strength
CN XII	Tongue protrusion (midline)

Cerebellar function is tested by having the patient perform actions requiring coordination such as finger/nose or rapid alternating movements. Motor assessment includes strength and symmetry of major muscle groups. Standard deep tendon reflexes tested include the knee, ankle, and biceps. Sensation testing may include light touch, pinprick, vibration, and proprioception. Gait testing is another good measure of central nervous system function.

Psychiatric: If psychiatric examination is indicated, it should include a number of elements, including a description of speech (rate, volume, pressured, etc.), assessment of thought process (rate and content), association (loose, tangential, intact, etc.), abnormal or psychotic thoughts (hallucinations, delusions, suicidal or homicidal ideation, etc.), and mood/affect (depression, anxiety, agitation, etc.). Other psychiatric components that may be assessed as part of overall examination include orientation, memory, concentration, and attention span. SOF medical personnel must identify, support (and refer as required) team members who are at increased risk for PTSD and other mental health issues (eg, depression/mania, anxiety disorders, psychosis, substance abuse).

Lymphatic: Evaluation may include palpation for enlarged nodes in the neck, groin, and axillae.

Skin: Examination may include quantity, texture, and distribution of hair, as well as assessment of skin for rashes, lesions, moles, birthmarks, hyperhidrosis, etc.

Results of labs and tests:

Assessment: Prioritized Problem List: Keep it as simple, accurate, complete and consistent with what you know. Example: It is perfectly correct to list **SEVERE CHEST PAIN** (suspect myocardial infarction) and **SEVERE SHORTNESS OF BREATH** (suspect pulmonary edema) as problem #1. Then you may execute a diagnostic and therapeutic plan (that might include oxygen, aspirin and monitored medical evacuation) that will eventually tell you whether patient's complaints are the result of a heart attack, pulmonary embolism, pneumonia, esophageal spasm, anxiety attack or other (the differential diagnosis). The goal is to define the problem in the terms that you are most certain of and move forward to more accurately diagnose and subsequently treat the patient.

Plan: Specific plans for each problem (may include any or all of the following as required):
a. Diagnostic (specific tests, labs or other action required to choose between a list of possible diagnoses/the differential diagnoses)
b. Therapeutic
c. Rehabilitation
d. Patient/family education

Acute Abdominal Pain

COL Peter McNally, MC, USA (Ret)

Introduction: Acute abdominal pain is an internal response to a mechanical or chemical stimulus. The pain can be separated into three categories: visceral (dull and poorly characterized), somatoparietal (more intense and precisely localized) and referred (pain felt remote from the origin). The most important elements in the evaluation of acute abdominal pain are the history and physical examination. Attention to the chronology and description of the pain can often suggest the origin of acute abdominal pain. Determining whether the underlying cause of the abdominal pain requires early surgical intervention is a primary consideration.

Subjective: Symptoms

Listed in Table 3-1 below are some of the most common causes of acute abdominal pain and their associated symptoms. Some patients will voluntarily provide a typical description of the details about the onset, location, and character of the pain. For others, the medic will have to ask pertinent questions (eg, *Where does it hurt? How would you describe the pain?*) to obtain the necessary information. Integrate past medical and surgical history, family history and medications into the search for the origin of acute abdominal pain. If the patient also has jaundice, constipation, diarrhea and vomiting, *see Part 3: General Symptoms: Jaundice; Part 3: General Symptoms: Constipation & Part 3: General Symptoms: Diarrhea, Acute.* GU and GYN illnesses may present as abdominal pain, although they typically present as flank pain or pelvic pain respectively. For additional information *see Part 4: Organ Systems: Chapter 8 & Part 3: General Symptoms: Gynecologic Problems.*

Table 3-1. Common Causes of Acute Abdominal Pain and their Associated Symptoms

Descriptor	Onset/Intensity	Location/Radiation	Character	Key History	Etiology
Burning, Knifelike	Sudden/severe	Epigastric/back	Localized early, diffuse late	Aspirin or NSAID ingestion. Chronic alcohol use	Perforated ulcer
Agonizing	Sudden/severe	Periumbilical/none	Diffuse	Arteriosclerotic heart disease, diabetes mellitus, high cholesterol, smoker	Intestinal ischemia/ infarction
Tearing	Sudden/severe	Abdomen/back & flank	Diffuse	Pulsatile abdomen	Ruptured aneurysm
Excruciating	Sudden/severe	Periumbilical	Diffuse	African or Mediterranean heritage	Sickle cell crisis
Orthostatic	Sudden/severe	Either adnexal (pelvic) area/none	Localized	Missed menses, nipple discharge, & AM nausea	Ruptured ectopic pregnancy
Constricting, bandlike	Rapid/moderate	Right upper quadrant/scapula	Localized	Family history of gallstones, rapid weight reduction. Postprandial, possibly recurrent	Cholelithiasis if intermittent/recurring Cholecystitis
Burning/sticking	Postprandial	Epigastric/back	Localized	Postprandial, recurrent	Reflux
Boring/drilling	Rapid/severe	Epigastric/back	Localized	History of gallstones, high triglycerides, abdominal trauma, alcohol abuse.	Pancreatitis
Ache	Slow/moderate	Periumbilical-early, Right lower quadrant-late/none	Diffuse early, localized late	Unless prior appendectomy, it is always a potential cause	M/F– Appendicitis, F– ovulation, tubo-ovarian abscess, ectopic pregnancy
Ache	Slow/mild to moderate	Left lower quadrant/ none	Localized	Often onset after straining at defecation	Diverticulitis F– ovulation, ectopic, tubo-ovarian abscess
Crampy	Slow/moderate	Periumbilical/none	Diffuse	Previous abdominal surgery & vomiting	Small bowel obstruction
Spastic	Slow/mild to moderate	Periumbilical	Diffuse	Nausea, vomiting and diarrhea	Gastroenteritis
Ache	Slow/moderate	Either adnexal (pelvic) area/none	Localized	Sexual promiscuity, vaginal discharge	Pelvic inflammatory disease

Objective: **Signs**

Using Basic Tools: Temperature: Fever suggests infection or inflammation, ie, appendicitis, cholecystitis, pancreatitis, diverticulitis, gastroenteritis or pelvic inflammatory disease. BP and pulse: Pain typically causes a reflex increase in heart rate and BP. If the BP <90, consider causes of blood or vascular fluid loss, ie, bleeding ulcer, pancreatitis (fluid third spacing), gastroenteritis (diarrheal losses). Signs of shock suggest rapid loss of blood, eg, ruptured ectopic pregnancy, hemorrhaging ulcer or ruptured abdominal aneurysm. Inspection: Surgical scars may suggest small bowel obstruction. Assumption of the fetal or knee-chest position by the patient may suggest pancreatitis or sickle cell crisis. Palpation: The abdominal examination should start gently away from the site of discomfort. Localization of pain in the RLQ suggests appendicitis or pelvic inflammatory disease. Sudden inspiratory arrest during steady palpation of the RUQ (Murphy's sign) suggests cholecystitis. Rebound tenderness and involuntary guarding highly suggest peritonitis from bowel perforation. Pelvic Examination: Severe cervical motion tenderness or a tender adnexal mass, coupled with fever, suggests pelvic inflammatory disease. Extremities: Loss of lower extremity pulse(s) suggests abdominal aneurysm. Rectal: Tarry, sticky, foul-smelling stool (melena suggests bleeding ulcer. Large volume of bright red blood on rectal exam with hypotension can indicate massive bleeding from an ulcer. Recurrent moderate bright red blood on rectal examination, but no hypotension may suggest hemorrhoids, or if associated with diarrhea, inflammatory bowel disease, infectious or ischemic colitis. Small volume of blood adherent to stool, dripping into the toilet or found on toilet paper suggests anorectal source. Recurrent rectal bleeding with "tenesmus" (uncontrollable urgency to have a bowel movement) suggests ulcerative proctitis. For further objective signs, *see Table 3-2.*

Table 3-2. Abdominal Pain: Objective Signs

Basic Tools:	Clinical Findings:	Interpretations:
Vital Signs	• Pulse >100 beats per minute	• Probable hypovolemia
	• Systolic BP <90 (loss of radial pulse in an uninjured extremity indicates severe hypovolemia)	• Probable hypovolemia
	• Orthostatic change in VS (systolic BP drop of 20mmHg or pulse rise 20 beats per minute)	• Significant hypovolemia
	• Temperature (above 101.5°F)	• Suggests infection or inflammation
Appearance	• Pallor of anemia, diaphoresis	• Suggests significant blood loss
Gastric Contents [examine if (+) history of melena or hematemesis]	NG aspirate: • Bile; no blood or coffee grounds • Coffee ground • Bright red blood	 • No active bleeding • Recent bleeding • Active bleeding
Abdomen	• Rigid abdomen with guarding	• Peritonitis
	• Abdominal distention without bowel sounds	• Ileus
	• Abdominal distention with high pitched and tinkling bowel sounds	• Small bowel obstruction
	• Disproportionate pain to abdominal distention	• Intestinal ischemia, infarction, sickle cell crisis, or abdominal aneurysm
Rectal Exam	• Melena (black, sticky, and tar-like stool)	• Recent UGI bleeding

Using Advanced Tools: Labs: CBC for infection and anemia, and UA for infection, stones, etc.

Assessment: **Differential Diagnosis**

Self-limiting causes of abdominal pain are usually milder in severity and remit either spontaneously within 24 hrs, or after administration of antacids, H-2 blockers, proton pump inhibitors, laxatives, etc. Examples of common self-limiting causes of abdominal pain would include gastroesophageal reflux, gastritis, intestinal gas, constipation, etc. *See discussion and Table 3-1 in Subjective for other diagnoses to consider.* Also include OB (labor), GYN, GU causes of abdominal pain. *See Part 3: General Symptoms: Gynecologic Problems & Part 4: Organ Systems: Chapter 8.*

Plan:

Treatment

Goals for field management: Diagnose underlying etiology and treat appropriately. Determine whether condition is a surgical emergency. Manage primary airway, breathing circulation issues (maintain intravascular volume), treat infection, manage pain. Follow clinical condition with repeat examinations. Persistent or worsening abdominal pain with duration >4 hours, fever, signs of hypovolemia, intestinal bleeding, shock or peritonitis are indications for medical evacuation.

1. Place 1 large IV (>18 gauge). If hypotensive or bleeding, then place 2 IVs.
2. Use lactated Ringers or normal saline to replace fluid loss and maintain intravascular volume.
3. Insert NG tube for gastric decompression for significant abdominal distention or vomiting.
4. Use pain control medications as required (with consideration of effect of pain medications on subsequent physical examination). See Part 8: Procedures: Chapter 30: Pain Assessment and Control
5. Use antiemetic of choice (eg, **prochlorperazine** 5-10mg IM q3-4h, max 40mg/day).
6. Acid suppression for patients thought to have GI ulceration able to take oral medications, **famotidine** 20mg po daily or **omeprazole** 20-40mg po daily. For all patients on prolonged NPO: **famotidine** 20mg per NG tube q6h, or **famotidine** 20mg (10mg/mL) IV over 2 minutes q12h or **esomeprazole** IV 20-40mg IV (mix with 5cc D5W or LR and give over no less than 3 minutes) or infusion (mix with 50cc D5W or LR and give over 30 minutes) daily.

7. If moderately to severely ill with fever and/or peritoneal signs present, initiate empiric IV antibiotic management for presumed intra-abdominal infection and continue antibiotic through medical evacuation. **Note:** As is the case for "field use" of antibiotics for combat wounds, the "field use" of antibiotics for a presumed intra-abdominal infection is an attempt to mitigate the risk of life-threatening infection while patient is en route to definitive medical care.
   a. Give **ceftriaxone** 2g IV daily or **cefotaxime** 2g IV q8h plus **metronidazole** 500mg IV q6h or
   b. Give **ciprofloxacin** 400mg IV q12h or **levofloxacin** 750mg IV q24h plus **metronidazole** 500mg IV q6h or
   c. Give **ertapenem** 1g IV daily or **moxifloxacin** 400mg po daily (when IV access is not possible and patient able to tolerate po meds)

Patient Education:
Maintain hydration, healthy diet with high fiber, low fat content. Exercise daily.

Follow-up Actions:
Evacuation/Consultant Criteria: Evacuate urgently for continuing pain or unstable condition. Consult general surgery early and other appropriate specialties as needed.

Anxiety
LTC Michael Doyle, MC, USA

Introduction: Anxiety is a vague feeling of apprehension due to the anticipation of danger. It is a common, normal reaction to any internal or external threat, is usually transient, and does not tend to recur frequently. Some situations, like jumping out of an airplane, are inherently anxiety provoking. When the symptoms of anxiety begin to interfere with duty or with social/occupational functioning, the medic may need to intervene. Anxiety, as a symptom, is often associated with most mental disorders and combat and operational stress reactions. In the deployed setting, service members may experience a wide variety of anxiety symptoms that are normal responses to the unusual stress of combat, but are not in and of themselves evidence of a disorder. This section identifies those specific conditions in which anxiety is the disorder and not just a symptom of a condition.

Subjective: **Symptoms**
Free-floating anxiety not attached to any particular idea or notion, fear, agitation, tension, panic. Patients may then complain of sleep, appetite or activity disturbances.
Focused History: *When did you start feeling this way? Have you ever felt this way before?* (identify precipitating events) *Are these feelings constant or do they come and go? How long do the spells last?* (Panic attacks come and go and are usually brief; anxiety due to an underlying medical condition or from post traumatic stress disorder [PTSD] or other chronic anxiety conditions usually is always present.) *Does the anxiety keep you from sleeping or wake you up? How is your appetite?* (If there are significant appetite and sleep problems, then a mood disorder may be the culprit.) *Can you do your job?* (Occupational impairment is important to document and monitor.) *Do you have thoughts of hurting yourself or anyone else?* (Always consider safety.) *What helps you feel better?* (Incorporate the patient in treatment plans)

Objective: **Signs**
Using Basic Tools: Distracted, jittery, skittish, easily startled, and often confused.
   Mental Status Exam: Alert and oriented in all spheres; may appear easily distracted or startled
      Activity: Restless, hyper vigilant, easily startled
      Speech: May be rapid, breathless, but also can be slowed with hesitancy or stuttering
      Thought content: Not delusional, may have hopelessness and dread that gives rise to suicidal ideation. Obsessions (recurring irresistible thoughts or feelings that cannot be eliminated by logical effort) may be present.
      Thought processes: Usually logical, linear and goal directed; may perseverate (go over and over) on one idea or theme
      Mood: Generally miserable, worried, or sad
      Affect: Often anxious, but if describing panic attacks, may appear normal.
      Cognition: Intact, though present anxiety may slow cognition or responsiveness
      Insight: Variable; may be poor to good

Assessment:
Differential Diagnosis: Always maintain a high index of suspicion for a physical or CNS injury!
   Occult injury: Hypotensive or hypoxic service member will appear anxious! DO NOT MISS THIS!
   Substance withdrawal: Patients in early alcohol withdrawal look anxious. *See Part 5: Specialty Areas: Chapter 18: Substance Abuse*
   Intoxication: Caffeine, nicotine, amphetamine are common substances associated with development of anxiety symptoms
   Medications: Medications commonly associated with anxiety include steroids (prednisone), mefloquine.
   Hyperthyroidism: *See Part 4: Organ Systems: Chapter 4: Thyroid Disorders*
   Combat or Operational Stress Reaction: *See Part 5: Specialty Areas: Chapter 18: Operational Stress*
   Battle Fatigue: *See Part 5: Specialty Areas: Chapter 18: Operational Stress*
   Mental disorders associated with anxiety:
      Panic Disorder: Discrete recurring episodes of sudden onset panic attacks
      Phobias: Specific fears, triggered by environmental stimuli, that are unreasonable under the circumstances.
      Generalized Anxiety Disorder: A pervasive, nearly constant and impairing sense of free-floating anxiety.
      Acute Stress Disorder: Circumscribed period lasting 2+ days of anxious symptoms and unpleasant, intrusive recollections of a recent unusual or traumatic event; occurring within 4 weeks of the event and resolving within 4 weeks of onset.
      Post Traumatic Stress Disorder: Chronic symptoms of anxiety with recurring, unpleasant, intrusive recollections of a past unusual or traumatic event, beginning anywhere from immediately following the event to years later.

Plan:

Primary Treatment - Basic

Symptomatic relief through rest and reassurance. Where possible, remove or minimize potential cause (eg, situation, caffeine, medication).

Benzodiazepines (**lorazepam** 1-2mg po q6-8h or **diazepam** 2-5mg po q8-12h as needed)

Relaxation exercise:

- Slow deep breathing: Use a paper bag or simply work with patient to take slow deep breaths.
- Progressive muscle relaxation: Focus on separate muscle groups (such as the balls of the feet); contract them, then relax slowly on the count of 5, move on to next muscle group.
- Visualization: Encourage patient to visualize a relaxing setting like sitting on a beach or fishing by a cool stream.

Primary Treatment - Advanced

Consider initiation of definitive treatment with a Selective Serotonin Reuptake Inhibitor (SSRI), starting with a low dose (1/2 therapeutic dose). *See Part 3: General Symptoms: Depression and Mania.* Patients should be referred for evaluation and treatment as operations permit.

Patient Education

General: Reassure patient that this condition is not life-threatening, and he is not going "crazy", which is often a fear of patients suffering from acute anxiety.

Activity: Normal. Try to keep on duty.

Diet: Avoid caffeine or other stimulants.

Prevention and Hygiene: Sleep, relaxation, stress management

Follow-up Actions

Return Evaluation: Frequent, scheduled follow-ups as opposed to "come in as needed"; support and assist patients with management of their anxiety.

Evacuation/Consultation Criteria: Most anxiety disorders do not need to be evacuated. Consult when there is evidence of mild impairment in function that has not been responsive to rest and reassurance.

Back Pain, Low

CAPT Scott Flinn, MC, USN

Introduction: Low back pain is an extremely common affliction. Most low back pain results from strain or mechanical stress, is self-limited and resolves in 4-6 weeks. Identification of worrisome signs or symptoms (ie, pain over 6-8 weeks, night pain, weight loss, progressive neurological injury including loss of bowel and bladder control) will determine which patients require additional testing or treatment. Evaluate trauma causing low back pain for the presence of a fracture and/or neurologic injury. Immobilize properly if trauma suspected to prevent possible permanent neurologic injury. Although very common in adults, low back pain is unusual in children and adolescents and warrants investigation.

Subjective: Symptoms

Constitutional: Worrisome symptoms include persistent fever, night pain, weight loss and progressive neurological symptoms such as progressing weakness or saddle anesthesia. Loss of bowel or bladder control in a nontrauma patient suggests cauda equina syndrome, a rare condition that is a surgical emergency to prevent permanent neurologic damage.

Location: Low back pain may be midline, one-sided, radiate into the hip or buttock. Numbness or tingling radiating past the knee, and/or lower extremity weakness suggests a herniated nucleus pulposus (HNP) pushing on a nerve.

Focused History: *Was there any trauma?* (suspect a fracture) *Are there neurological symptoms such as numbness, tingling or weakness?* (If acute from trauma, suspect fracture, otherwise suspect a nerve impingement from a herniated disc or other cause.) *Are there warning signs that pain is due to a serious condition?* (Night pain, unexplained weight loss of a large amount [eg, 20 lbs], progressive neurologic deficit, or loss of bowel/bladder control.) *Is the pain chronic?* (if >2-3 months induration, may need evaluation for worrisome/surgical cause like herniated disc, tumor) *Is there a persistent fever (>2 weeks) and/or fatigue malaise?* (suggests infection, eg, tuberculosis, brucellosis or other pathogens, or other cause)

Objective: Signs

Using Basic Tools: Acute traumatic low back pain – screen for signs of fracture. Inspection: Obvious deformities: acute trauma (think fracture) or chronic pain (look for scoliosis). Any mass: tumor. Skin erythema: Infection or tumor. Palpation: Step-off on spinous processes: sign of fracture. Palpable spasm: sign of trauma. Palpable mass: tumor. Abnormal neuro exam indicates a possible HNP or other nerve root injury: L4 motor: tibialis ant - pull foot up, reflex - quadriceps, sensation - medial malleolus; L5 motor: extensor hallucis longus - great toe pulled up, no reflex, sensation - first dorsal toe web space; S1 motor: peroneals - feet held up and out/everted, reflex -Achilles tendon, sensation - lateral malleolus. If there is loss of sensation in the anal area, check the anal sphincter tone. Loss of sphincter tone and sensation about the anus suggests neurologic damage to the sacral nerves, such as in cauda equina syndrome or serious damage to the spinal cord. Unless other red flags are present, initial evaluation of low back pain does not require x-rays. Manual muscle test scale is 0-5 with 0 being absent and 5 normal. Deep tendon reflexes are 0-4 scale, with 0 being absent, 2 normal, and 4 being hyperactive with clonus.

Assessment: Differential Diagnosis

The differential diagnosis of low back pain is extensive and includes mechanical low back pain, sciatica, herniated disc with or without nerve impingement, spondylolysis with or without spondylolisthesis, scoliosis, sacroiliac joint dysfunction, infection, ankylosing spondylitis, spinal stenosis, abdominal aortic aneurysm in elderly patients, various benign and malignant tumors, fracture, and cauda equina syndrome. *See Part 3: General Symptoms: Joint Problems: Joint Pain* and other related topics in this book. Urological conditions such as stone disease and pyelonephritis may present as back pain (*see Part 4: Organ Systems: Chapter 8*). Other problems may be referred to the back from the abdomen, including labor (*see Part 3: General Symptoms: Obstetric Problems*) and pancreatitis (*see Part 4: Organ Systems: Chapter 7: Acute Pancreatitis*).

Plan:

Treatment

Primary: Usual treatment of mechanical low back pain includes ice, anti-inflammatories such as **ibuprofen** 800mg po tid with food and progressive range of motion exercises and trunk strengthening. In patients who can tolerate the side effects (dizziness, somnolence), short term (7 days) use of **cyclobenzaprine** 10mg po tid may be used with or without NSAIDs. Bed rest is not indicated unless absolutely essential, as it merely causes deconditioning. Epidural steroids are sometimes used; oral steroids are not recommended. Cauda equina syndrome, a rare complication where there is compression of the cauda equina in the spinal column causing neurological impairment, may become permanent if not surgically repaired in 12-24 hours. Suspected fractures should be immobilized on a spine board or the nearest field equivalent and evacuated to the nearest appropriate facility that can perform appropriate radiological studies and surgery if necessary.

Patient Education

General: Most low back pain is self-limited and will resolve in 4-6 weeks.

Activity: Gradually resume activity. Avoid bed rest if possible as it only weakens the back muscles.

Diet: Normal

Medications: Anti-inflammatory medicine may cause bleeding ulcers, kidney and liver problems with chronic use.

Prevention and Hygiene: Use proper mechanics when lifting; bend at the knees, not the waist. Core strengthening helps prevent injury

No Improvement/Deterioration: Loss of bowel or bladder control warrants immediate referral.

Follow-up Actions

Return Evaluation: Worrisome signs for further referral for imaging (such as x-ray and MRI) and evaluation include fever, night pain, unexplained weight loss, persistent pain (greater than 4-6 weeks), progressive neurological deficit.

Evacuation/Consultation Criteria: Loss of bowel or bladder control, and/or urinary retention warrants immediate evacuation. Obtain delayed evacuation for imaging and evaluation, if fever, night pain, unexplained weight loss, persistent pain (greater than 4-6 weeks), and progressive neurologic deficit.

Breast Problems: Clinical Breast Examination
COL Ismail Jatoi, MC, USA

The three most common breast complaints for which women seek medical attention are breast pain, nipple discharge, and a breast mass ("lump"). Although mammography and/or ultrasound are frequently required to make a definitive diagnosis, there are several things that SOF medics can provide in the field setting that may assist in ruling out serious problems.

Perform a clinical breast exam: Have the patient disrobe from the waist up, and ask her to sit with her arms at her side. Observe patient from the front and from both sides then have the woman lift her arms over her head to exposes the lateral aspects and inferior portions of the breast, making it possible to examine all parts of the breast. Again, examine from the front and sides of the patient. Consequently, if there is a tumor involving Cooper's ligaments, contracting the pectoralis major muscle by having the patient push in on her hips will cause an indentation of the skin or skin retraction. With the patient in a sitting position; palpate the axillary, supraclavicular, and infraclavicular lymph nodes and the supraclavicular and infraclavicular nodes. Next support the woman's arm at the elbow so that the arm is relaxed, passively abducting the arm so the examining hand can palpate the axilla and the lymph nodes.

Have the patient lie down and ask her to put her one arm above her head. If the woman has large breasts, placing a towel underneath her back and shoulders will help the breast fall medially against the chest wall to facilitate the exam. When the patient lies down, the breast tissue will move toward the clavicles. The area to be examined is not just the breast mound, but also tissue from the clavicle to the bra line, and from the lateral sternum to the midline of the lateral chest. When palpating the breast, assess the degree of nodularity and whether there is a dominant mass or thickening. Use the pads of the first three fingers, covering an area about the size of a dime for each examining finger. Palpation should be done using a light touch, then a medium touch, and then a deep touch. Be sure to also palpate the nipple and areola. It is the second most likely place for cancer to occur. It is not necessary to try to elicit nipple discharge in a woman who is not complaining of spontaneous discharge. Now have the woman put her raised arm by her side, raise her other arm, and repeat the exam on the other breast.

Breast Problems: Breast Pain
COL Ismail Jatoi, MC, USA

Introduction: Common complaint, frequently encountered in the primary care setting and most often of little clinical significance. It is important to allay the patient's anxiety.

Subjective: **Symptoms**

Focused History: *Where is the pain?* (If it diffuse or localized, have the woman point to the area of pain with one finger.) *Is it in both breasts, or just one? When did you first notice the pain? Does it change with your menstrual cycle?* (*See Differential Diagnosis: Cyclic Mastalgia*). Reassure patient that many women experience breast pain, and that this is generally not a symptom associated with a life-threatening condition (eg, cancer which generally presents as a painless mass).

Objective: **Signs**

Using Basic Tools: Perform a thorough examination of the breasts (*see Part 3: General Symptoms: Breast Problems: Clinical Breast Examination*). A breast cyst may present as a discrete tender breast mass, however, most patients with breast pain will not present with a discrete, palpable cyst.

Using Advanced Tools: Ultrasound can be used to distinguish between a breast cyst and a solid breast mass. Although aspiration of mass may provide immediate relief from her breast pain, cyst aspiration should only be done by individuals who have experience with this procedure. If you have no experience aspirating a cyst, it is better to leave it alone. Most cysts will resolve spontaneously over time.

Assessment: **Differential Diagnosis**

Mastalgia: Fibrocystic changes in the breast. The intensity of the pain might vary according to the menstrual cycle (cyclical mastalgia), or the pain might have no correlation with the menstrual cycle at all (acyclical mastalgia).
Mastitis: *See Part 3: General Symptoms: Breast Problems: Mastitis*

Plan:

Treatment

Have patient restrict caffeine intake (coffee, tea, chocolates, etc.), which may reduce breast pain. If the patient smokes, she should be told to stop. Eliminating nicotine may resolve the breast pain. Reassure the patient that her symptoms do not represent a life-threatening condition and will most likely resolve on their own.

Patient Education

General: Reassure the patient to reduce her anxiety. Breast pain is generally not associated with malignancy, and patients find this information reassuring.

Diet: Restrict caffeine and nicotine (*see Plan: Treatment*)

No Improvement/Deterioration: The use of evening primrose oil 1.5-3g po daily (found in many health food stores in the USA) may help relieve symptoms of breast pain. There are also prescription medications that can be used to relieve breast pain, but these should generally not be used in the field setting.

Follow-up Actions

Return Evaluation: See the patient in about 2-3 weeks after telling her to restrict use of caffeine and (if applicable) to stop smoking.
Evacuation/Consultation Criteria: Most breast pain resolves with the simple measures discussed. Evacuation and further consultation is generally not required.

Breast Problems: Nipple Discharge
COL Ismail Jatoi, MC, USA

Introduction: Nipple discharge may prompt a visit to a health care provider and has been reported to occur in up to 7% of women. Although it is usually due to a benign process, it could be the sole sign of cancer (1% of all breast cancer patients). **Note:** The nipple has between 5 and 10 milk ducts, which open to the surface and it is important to note whether the discharge is from a single duct or multiple ducts.

Subjective: **Symptoms**

Focused History: *Is the discharge spontaneous?* (A discharge that appears only when the nipple is stimulated or compressed is generally physiologic. Most physiologic, non-spontaneous discharge is bilateral and involves multiple ducts.) *Does the discharge stain your underclothes or bedding?* (This indicates a true spontaneous nipple discharge, and must be evaluated.) *Is it coming out of one breast or both?* (Unilateral spontaneous persistent nipple discharge may suggest underlying breast pathology.) If the discharge is bilateral, it should be classified as galactorrhea [milky]. Galactorrhea is generally not a symptom of breast cancer or primary breast pathology. The most likely cause of galactorrhea in a premenopausal woman is pregnancy. However, pituitary adenomas may also produce galactorrhea.) *Is the discharge coming out of one duct or multiple ducts?* (The patient may not be able to tell you this.) *Are you taking any new medications?* (Oral contraceptives, antihypertensive drugs, phenothiazines, and many tranquilizers may cause galactorrhea.) *If the discharge is not milky, what color is the discharge?* (Although bloody nipple discharge is the more common, watery discharge is more likely to represent carcinoma. Among women who had spontaneous discharge because of cancer, 45% had watery discharge, 25% had bloody discharge, 12% had serosanguineous discharge, and 6% had a serous discharge. Milky, green, gray or black discharge expressed from several ducts [especially bilaterally] is generally not suspicious for cancer.)

Pearls:
1. Nipple discharge, particularly if bilateral or multi-ductal, or milky, green, gray, or black, is generally due to a benign process. If milky discharge is profuse, the patient should be referred for a medical work-up.
2. A woman with any kind of nipple discharge <u>and</u> a palpable mass should be referred to a surgeon.
3. If discharge is suspicious for neoplasm (spontaneous; unilateral; confined to a single duct; occurring in older patient; clear, bloody, serous, or serosanguineous), refer the woman to a surgeon.
4. Bloody nipple discharge may indicate carcinoma, depending on the age group, with older women much more likely to have cancer, and younger women more likely to have an intraductal papilloma.
5. Spontaneous nipple discharge generally requires surgical referral.

Objective: **Signs**

Using Basic Tools: Inspection: Observe breasts for evidence of spontaneous discharge. Assess color of discharge. Palpation: Physical examination of nipple discharge consists of a "milking" type of motion, exerting deep pressure on the breast tissue from the periphery toward the nipple. Pressure should be distributed evenly as the duct system is milked for each number on the clock. Observe carefully to see if discharge comes out of one or more ducts. Document location as on a clock's face.
Using Advanced Tools: Labs: In the field setting, there might be few tools available to further evaluate nipple discharge. Cytology is sometimes helpful, but may not be available. If you suspect a pituitary adenoma (in a young woman with bilateral spontaneous milky discharge who is not pregnant), then a prolactin level might be useful. If the prolactin level is elevated, an MRI might be needed to assess for a pituitary adenoma. However, this technology will not be available in the field setting.

Assessment: **Differential Diagnosis**

Bilateral, spontaneous milky discharge in younger women might be due to pregnancy. In women who are not pregnant, it might be due to a pituitary adenoma. A unilateral nipple discharge might occasionally be associated with a malignancy. It should be noted that, in younger women, the most common etiology of a unilateral bloody nipple discharge is an intraductal papilloma. In most instances, nipple discharge is due to benign conditions.

Plan: A detailed history and meticulous physical examination should be obtained.
Treatment
In a hospital setting, some instances of nipple discharge might be further evaluated with a mammogram, ductogram, and even MRI to rule out a pituitary adenoma. This sort of evaluation is generally not possible in the field setting. If there are any concerns, patients should be referred to a surgeon for further evaluation. However, as noted previously, nipple discharge is, in most instances, attributable to benign conditions.
Patient Education
General: As noted, most nipple discharge is attributable to benign conditions.
No Improvement/Deterioration: Patients may need to be referred to a surgeon for further evaluation.
Follow-up Actions
Return Evaluation: Persistent nipple discharge in non-pregnant women may require surgical evaluation.
Evacuation/Consultation Criteria: A women with nipple discharge should generally be referred for further evaluation.

Breast Problems: Breast Lump
COL Ismail Jatoi, MC, USA

Introduction: Patients may seek medical attention for either nodularity of the breast or a discrete lump (or mass) in the breast. It is important to distinguish between the two. Diffuse nodularity of the breasts is common, and often attributable to fibrocystic changes. Diffuse nodularity (fibrocystic changes) might also be associated with breast pain (*see Part 3: General Symptoms: Breast Problems: Breast Pain*). Generally, no further work-up is required, other than that for the management of breast pain. In contrast, there are 3 common etiologies for a discrete breast mass: fibroadenoma, cyst, or cancer. These can occur in women of any age group. However, fibroadenomas tend to occur in younger women (often women in their late teens or twenties) and cancers tend to occur in older women. As mentioned previously, a discrete, palpable breast cyst might be associated with pain.

Subjective: **Symptoms**
Focused History: *How old are you?* (Fibroadenomas tend to occur in younger women [often women in their late teens or twenties] and cancers tend to occur in older women.) *How long has the lump been present?* (If a patient tells you that a large breast lump appeared suddenly, it might be a cyst. This is especially true if the lump is tender.) *Do you have a family history of breast-related problems (particularly breast cancer)?*

Objective: **Signs**
Using Basic Tools: Inspection: Skin retraction over a breast lump suggests cancer. Palpation: A firm, mobile lump may indicate a fibroadenoma (marble rolling under your finger). In contrast, a hard, fixed mass may suggest cancer. A breast cyst may feel firm, and is sometimes tender to palpation.
Using Advanced Tools: Mammogram and/or ultrasound with histology/cytology are required for definitive diagnosis.

Assessment: **Differential Diagnosis**
As mentioned previously, it is important to determine whether the patient is complaining of diffuse nodularity or a discrete breast lump.
Diffuse nodularity: Most often attributable to fibrocystic changes and no further work-up is generally required. A screening mammogram is recommended especially for patients >40 years.
Discrete breast mass: Could be a fibroadenoma, cyst, or cancer.

Plan:
Treatment
Mammography/ultrasound and cytological or histological assessment are required for definitive diagnosis of a discrete breast mass. Patient should be referred to a surgeon for diagnosis and management.
Patient Education
General: Two large randomized prospective trials have shown that there is no benefit to breast self-examination (in reducing breast cancer mortality). Thus, there is no proven value to teaching breast self-examination.
No Improvement/Deterioration: In general, most patients with a discrete breast mass should be referred to a surgeon for further evaluation.
Follow-up Actions
Return Evaluation: A woman with a breast mass should be referred for surgical evaluation.
Evacuation/Consultation Criteria: If possible, any woman who presents with a breast mass should be referred for surgical evaluation.

Breast Problems: Mastitis
COL Ismail Jatoi, MC. USA

Introduction: Mastitis most commonly presents as a cellulitis in a lactating breast (1-3% of breastfeeding women). The causative organisms, *S. Aureus, E. Coli and streptococcus* (rarely), are easily treated with antibiotics. Tuberculosis mastitis is very rare (1% of cases) even where TB is endemic. One of the risk factors for mastitis is plugging or obstruction of one of the milk ducts which drain to the nipple. Obstruction can be secondary to delayed infant feedings, which can lead to engorgement, and tight clothing (poorly fitting brassieres). Other risk factors include cracked nipples, maternal stress and fatigue.

Do not let mastitis interrupt breastfeeding. The infected breast will worsen if the baby does not empty it, and the infection cannot be transmitted to the infant through the milk.

Untreated or delayed and inappropriate treatment can lead to breast abscesses. If an abscess occurs, it is necessary to stop lactation in the affected breast, which deprives the infant of its food source. This may be devastating, particularly in developing countries.

Subjective: Symptoms

Localized pain, redness, swelling, warmth in one breast; fever; chills; body aches; fatigue; headache; occasionally nausea and vomiting.
Focused History: *Have you recently given birth? If nursing; are you having any problems with breast feeding?* (Mastitis is most common in lactating women and generally presents several weeks to a month after giving birth.)

Objective: Signs

Using Basic Tools: Fever - often greater than 101°F. Inspection: Pink, wedge-shaped area on the breast. Patient appears in mild to moderate distress. Palpation: Tender, occasionally indurated, warm area. There SHOULD NOT be a palpable, fluctuant mass; that is a sign of abscess.

Assessment: Differential Diagnosis

Plugged duct: Tender lump in the breast of a mother who is otherwise well. Caused by partial obstruction of a duct. Infection is not present but MAY RESULT if the duct remains blocked. *See Plan: Treatment for Plugged Duct*

Breast engorgement: Gradual onset in the immediate postpartum period (peak on days 2-4) of bilateral breast swelling and warmth. Pain is generalized. Fever may occur but is rarely over 101°F. The breasts feel better after they are emptied. Caused by inadequate emptying of the breasts. A risk factor for mastitis. *See Plan: Treatment for Engorgement.*

Breast abscess: Painful, fluctuant mass. 10-15% of women who delay treatment of mastitis will develop a breast abscess. Should be suspected if a patient on antibiotics for mastitis does not improve after 72 hours of antibiotic therapy. *See Part 3: General Symptoms: Breast Problems: Breast Abscess Incision and Drainage Procedure*

Breast cancer: In rare instances, breast cancer will present with erythema and resemble cellulitis. This type of breast cancer is referred to as inflammatory breast cancer, and has a poor prognosis. Thus, persistent mastitis must be evaluated urgently by appropriate radiological and surgical approaches. Patients with persistent mastitis should therefore be referred immediately for surgical evaluation.

Plan:

Treatment for Mastitis

Primary:
1. Ensure infant nurses on both breasts, starting on the unaffected side. Even after feeding, the affected breast may need to be more thoroughly emptied by manual expression or pumping.
2. Ensure mother completes full course of antibiotic therapy:
   a. **Dicloxacillin** or **cephalexin** 500mg po q6h x 10 days
   b. Patients allergic to penicillin: **clindamycin** 300mg po q6h x 10 days or **erythromycin** 500mg po q6h x 10 days
   c. If patient does not improve after 48 hours of rest and therapy, switch to **amoxicillin/clavulanate** 875/125mg po bid or 500/125mg po tid
3. Apply ice packs or warm packs to the breast (whichever the mother prefers). Hot packs provide drainage and pain relief.
4. Ensure mother drinks plenty of fluids.
5. Advise mother to wear a support bra or other supportive clothing that does not cause painful pressure on the breast.

Alternate:
Some patients with severe mastitis may need IV therapy. Use **nafcillin** or **oxacillin** 2.0g IV q4h or **cefazolin** 1.0g IV q8h until systemic signs of infection have resolved and patient is showing clinical improvement at which time po medications (in Primary Treatment) should be given. Penicillin allergic patients can be given **clindamycin** 300mg IV q6h.

Primitive:
If antibiotics are not available, initiate rest, hydration and MOST IMPORTANTLY, drainage (nursing) of the affected breast. Mastitis will recur in at least 50% of women not treated with antibiotics, and the breast abscess rate will be high.

Patient Education

General: Counsel family to assist the mother.
Activity: The patient should be instructed to limit her daily activities (rest as much as possible). If patient is improving, she may gradually increase her activity level after 72 hours.
Diet: Fluids and well-balanced diet
No Improvement/Deterioration: Improvement in systemic symptoms is expected in 24-48 hours. The focal breast tenderness should be significantly improved in 72 hours then gradually resolve in 7-10 days.

Follow-up Actions

Return Evaluation: 48-72 hours Reassess vital signs and perform breast examination for mass or fluctuance (evaluate for abscess). Reemphasize compliance with antibiotic therapy and rest.
Assess breastfeeding frequency and nutritional status of the infant. Be sure the mother is emptying the infected breast. If the patient is not improving, consider changing antibiotics to amoxicillin/clavulanate.

If the patient remains febrile after 72 hours:
1. If possible, transfer the patient immediately. If not, continue to item #2.
2. If non-compliant, administer **ceftriaxone** 1g IM. See if the patient would also take **azithromycin** 1g po. Follow-up in 24 hours and repeat the **ceftriaxone**.
3. If compliant, add **clindamycin** IV.
4. Find an experienced person in the community who can stay with the patient and assist with breastfeeding and manual expression.

Evacuation/Consultation Criteria: Suspicion of breast abscess, continued fever after 72 hours of antibiotics. Breast abscess requires incision and drainage, which should be done by a trained physician if possible.

Treatment for Plugged Duct:
Massage the area, gently pressing toward the nipple. Warm compresses help. The most important intervention is frequent feeding on the affected side. Consecutive feedings should be started on the affected side to facilitate flow from the obstruction. Because different lobes of the breast are drained better with different nursing positions, place the infant with its chin pointing toward the blocked duct. If the mother is separated from her infant for any reason, the breast should be emptied by hand-expression or by using an effective breast pump. Be sure to follow the mother closely as mastitis can occur. **Note:** Plugged ducts will last only for short periods of time (a few days). Any lump that persists for many days must be evaluated for malignancy.

Treatment for Engorgement:
Frequent breastfeeding is the most effective treatment. If the nipples are engorged, it may be difficult for the baby to latch on. Relieve nipple engorgement by applying warm compresses before the feeding, gently express some milk to soften the breast, or lean the breasts into a large bowl of warm water (or take a warm shower) just before the feeding to facilitate milk release and soften the nipples. After the feeding, apply cold compresses, or cool cabbage leaves to the breast for 20 minutes leaving the nipple exposed. Use standard doses of **acetaminophen** and/or **ibuprofen** for pain relief. Use mild narcotics (**acetaminophen** with **codeine #3**) in severe cases. Support the breasts with a good-fitting brassiere. Do not bind the breasts as this will increase the engorgement.

Breast Problems: Breast Abscess Incision and Drainage Procedure

COL Ismail Jatoi, MC. USA

When: A breast abscess may present as a fluctuant mass, and might be related to non-resolving or worsening mastitis (*see Part 3: General Symptoms: Breast Problems: Mastitis*). In some instances, an abscess can be treated with needle aspiration and antibiotics. However, in most cases, incision and drainage is required to adequately treat an abscess. Thus, any patient suspected of having a breast abscess should generally be referred to a surgeon as soon as possible. Aspiration and/or incision and drainage of a breast abscess should generally only be done by individuals who have experience with these procedures.

What You Need: Sterile prep and drape, 18 and 24-26 gauge needles, 5cc and 10cc syringes, alcohol prep pads, local anesthetic agent such as 1% **lidocaine** with **epinephrine**, 2x2 and 4x4 dressings, scalpel with #15 blade (but any blade will work), sterile irrigation if available, gloves, and a small Penrose drain.

What To Do:

Needle Aspiration: Anesthetize skin and subcutaneous tissues over fluctuant area using 5cc syringe and 24-26 gauge needle. Insert 18 gauge needle attached to 10cc syringe into the abscess, aspirating as you advance the needle. Drain as much pus as possible once the cavity is entered. Then remove needle and cover puncture site with a small dressing.

Incision and Drainage of Abscess: Anesthetize the skin and subcutaneous tissues over the fluctuant mass. If possible, choose your incision point close to but not in the areola (allow room for an infant to nurse without contacting the incision). Make the incision parallel to the edge of the areola and over the fluctuant area. Try not to make transverse incisions as they leave an unacceptable scar. Circumareolar incisions will heal with a better cosmetic result. Keep the incision small, only large enough to allow entrance of your 5th digit. Do not cut deeply into the breast tissue, but start superficially and advance carefully. Make your incision deeper until the cavity is just reached and pus begins to drain. Insert your 5th digit into the wound to break up any loculations and to ensure complete drainage. Irrigate the wound, and pack the wound open with gauze.

Follow-up care: The patient will require dressing changes bid. These should be wet to dry dressing changes (moist dressing is applied on the wound, and it is generally dry and adherent to the underlying tissue when it is removed several hours later, thereby debriding the infected tissue). Once an abscess is adequately drained, oral antibiotics (*see Part 3: General Symptoms: Breast Problems: Mastitis*) should be given to resolve associated cellulitis. After that, continue with the wet to dry dressing changes alone, without the antibiotics. Engorgement of the breast will interfere with healing. Feed infant or empty the affected breast on a regular basis, every 2-2½ hours. The milk is clean as long as the abscess drains to the outside (through the skin). Nursing can continue when the abscess is surgically drained as long as the incision is away from the areola. Milk may drain from the incision during breastfeeding. Apply pressure over the incision while breastfeeding to minimize leakage. If the patient cannot do this herself, her spouse or another person may hold light pressure over the incision.

Follow-up Exam: 24 hours and as needed thereafter. The patient and family members can be taught how to do wet to dry dressing changes on the open wound, until granulation tissue forms and the wound heals. Evidence of healing of the wound from the inside out should be evident within 3-5 days.

Referral Criteria: Persistent fever despite treatment; worsening pain; increased size of abscess.

What Not To Do:
1. Do not make incision any deeper than necessary.
2. Do not make the incision too close to the areola to avoid compromising breastfeeding.
3. Do not allow the skin to close until the wound has healed from the inside out to the surface.

Chest Pain

BG Joseph Caravalho, Jr., MC, USA

Introduction: The primary goal in the evaluation of chest pain is to determine whether or not this relatively common symptom is the presentation of a life-threatening condition or is symptomatic of another non life-threatening condition. It is not uncommon for patients to have more than one component of chest pain, each of which needs to be assessed separately, as noncardiac pain can mask angina pectoris (ie, chest pain associated with underlying coronary artery disease). Acute, single episodes more likely to be related to life-threatening conditions: Acute Coronary Syndrome (myocardial ischemia), aortic dissection, pulmonary embolism (PE), tension pneumothorax, pericardial tamponade, mediastinitis (rupture of esophagus or stomach) or gas embolism (*see Part 6: Operational Environment: Chapter 20: Decompression Injuries: Pulmonary Over Inflation Syndrome [including Arterial Gas Embolism]*). You should also consider the possibility of drug related coronary artery spasm and in an athlete (eg, young Soldier), the possibility of hypertrophic cardiomyopathy, which is the leading cause of sudden death in athletes younger than 30 years of age. Possibility of an effect of specific occupational exposures (eg, gas embolism or decompression sickness following diving or HALO parachuting) should be evaluated and managed appropriately (*see Part 6: Operational Environment: Chapter 20 & Chapter 22*). A prior history of any of these conditions should lead to a presumptive diagnosis in favor of recurrence. Most myocardial infarction victims who are going to die do so in the first 1-4 hours due to ventricular fibrillation, asystole, myocardial rupture or cardiogenic shock. In the field, the full capability to immediately respond may be limited; additionally, certain medications, such as heparin, may be beneficial in some settings (eg, acute coronary syndrome and PE), but detrimental and contraindicated in others (eg, esophageal rupture, hemothorax, cardiac tamponade, and aortic dissection). Chronic, recurring chest pain that typically represents a non life-threatening condition involve the heart (eg, stable angina, pericarditis, mitral valve prolapse); lungs/pleura (eg, pneumonia, tracheitis, bronchitis); GI tract (eg, dyspepsia, hiatal hernia, gastroesophageal reflux, gall stones, pancreatitis); musculoskeletal system (costochondritis [painful inflammation at the cartilage-bone junctions], intercostal muscle strains, rib fractures or contusions); or other (eg, decompression sickness, herpes zoster [shingles], subacromial bursitis, mastitis). See appropriate sections for detailed discussions of these conditions.

Subjective: Symptoms

(**"PQRS&T":** Obtain the patient's history by asking questions in a logical order, but use this mnemonic to ensure you can fully characterize the symptoms).

Provocation/Palliation: *What brings on the chest pain or makes it worse? What makes it better? Do activities such as walking uphill, hurrying, exposure to cold, emotional stress or the postprandial state bring on the pain? Is pain influenced by motion, position, or respiration? Does the supine position influence the pain? Does pain come on without any precipitating factor or during sleep? Have you been diving or HALO jumping?* (Angina pectoris is brought on by exertion [eg, walking uphill] and relieved by rest or sublingual nitroglycerin which may also relieve lower esophageal sphincter spasm, gall bladder disease or intestinal angina. Nothing relieves the pain of aortic dissection, perforated peptic ulcer or pneumothorax except narcotics; pleuritic pain [occasionally associated with PE, pneumonia] is worsened by deep breaths; drinking cold liquids can bring on esophageal spasm; dyspepsia comes on after eating is worsened by lying down and relieved by antacids. Gallstone pain is brought on by fatty foods. Musculoskeletal pain [eg, costochondritis] is brought on by movement of the arms or chest and can be decreased limiting motion, ASA or NSAIDS, or by digital pressure to the area of pain on the chest wall. Movement of the neck aggravates cervical disk pain. Eating or antacids relieve peptic ulcer disease pain.)

Quality: *What does the chest pain feel like?* (Myocardial ischemia [ACS or routine angina] can be described as a pressure, fullness, deep ache, squeezing, burning, sharp, gas, heartburn, indigestion, a need to belch, numbing or prickly. Some cardiac pain may be felt in the epigastrium only. Aortic dissection is an intense, tearing pain. Esophageal rupture is worsened by eating or drinking and relieved only by narcotics. Shingles pain is burning and worsened by clothing touching the area. Determine the consistency of the pain over time. Distinguish between pinpoint or sharply localized pain from more diffuse and generalized pain.) *Does the pain remain steady or wax and wane* (like a roller coaster) *during an episode? How rapidly does the pain subside?* (Pneumothorax pain is sharp like a knife located within the chest [ie, cannot be touched with a finger]. GI pain is an aching discomfort located centrally substernally or in the upper abdomen. Musculoskeletal pain is dull pain localized to a finger point area.) **Pearl:** Anxiety and psychogenic chest pain can be sharp and last for seconds or be dull and last for days.

Radiation: *Where else does the sensation travel?* (Cardiac pain commonly radiates to shoulders, arm, back, neck, throat, jaw or the interscapular area. Upper extremity numbness or tingling may represent referred pain. Aortic dissection and peptic ulcer pains typically radiates from the chest or epigastrium straight to the back. Pain moving to the right shoulder blade may be due to gallbladder disease. Pain moving to the top of the shoulder is likely to be from pneumonia, pneumothorax or subacromial bursitis. Splenic pain may be referred to the left shoulder.)

Severity: *How strong/devastating are the symptoms? How much does it hurt on a scale of 1 to 10?* (Use a 1-10 scale to characterize severity. I find the semi-quantitative severity scale more useful than descriptive words, as most patients cannot easily describe minor changes in discomfort. The self-reported severity scale also allows the patient to be his/her own barometer over time. Do not let the patient give you a number greater than 10.) Associated symptoms: *What appears whenever the palpitations occur?* (Breathlessness, marked fatigue, diaphoresis, pre-syncope, syncope, apprehension and sense of impending doom may occur with cardiac etiologies. Sweating, nausea, vomiting and palpitations may be nonspecific. An acid taste in the mouth [water brash] suggests esophageal reflux. Pneumonia is associated with fever and a productive cough.)

Time: *How do the episodes start and stop? How long do the episodes last? How frequently do they recur? Does the pain begin abruptly at full intensity or does it build up gradually? Does the pain last for seconds, minutes or hours? Are there quick jabs or stabs or does the pain last for hours at a time? Is there lingering pain after the worst of the episode has cleared?* (Angina is usually relieved over 5 minutes while myocardial infarction pain may last for 30 minutes to an hour. Musculoskeletal pain may come and go. Pneumothorax pain lasts until relieved by an intervention. Aortic dissection pain continues for hours. Dyspepsia resolves in minutes with treatment.)

Coronary Risk Factors: The presence of three or more coronary risk factors increases the likelihood of the disease presence: smoking, hypertension, family history of premature coronary artery disease (ie, myocardial infarction before age 55 for men or before 65 for women), diabetes, abnormal lipid profile (ie, high total cholesterol, high LDL or low HDL), or obesity. Peripheral artery disease also places an individual at increased risk for coronary artery disease.

Pearls:
1. Pain that lasts seconds is not serious.
2. Pain that moves from the chest into arms and then legs is not myocardial ischemia.
3. Pain relieved by sublingual **nitroglycerin** suggests a smooth muscle origin of the pain: heart, esophagus, gall bladder, intestinal.
4. Chest pain with collapse and shock is due to one of the life-threatening causes of chest pain.
5. Anxiety and psychiatric chest pain can be sharp and last for seconds or dull and last for days. Although it may be unresponsive to all empiric therapies, psychogenic chest pain is a diagnosis of exclusion. It is NOT the diagnosis until other causes have been ruled out!

Objective: Signs
Using Basic Tools:
General: Pale, sweaty, cool clammy skin suggests decreased cardiac output; cyanosis suggests PE. Vital signs: Fever suggests infectious cause such as pneumonia or bronchitis. Irregular pulse suggests cardiac cause. Absent pulses in the left arm or a blood pressure >10 mmHg lower than the right suggest an aortic dissection. SBP <100mmHg with HR >120 bpm suggest decreased cardiac output (eg, cardiac tamponade, myocardial infarction, others). Respirations >30 rpm suggests decreased cardiac output or hypoxemia.

Neck Veins: Elevated suggests right heart failure (with or without left heart failure) or cardiac tamponade.

Chest Wall: Point tenderness over the costochondral junction or the intercostal muscles suggests a non-cardiac musculoskeletal etiology (eg, costochondritis or muscle strain). Numbness in a subcostal nerve distribution suggests nerve injury from trauma. Lateral compression of the chest cage will accentuate pain from a rib fracture. Tenderness and warmth of the breast suggests mastitis. Exquisite pain in a dermatomal distribution (ie, does not cross midline) suggests shingles.

Lungs: Absence of breath sounds or increased resonance to percussion suggests pneumothorax. A shift in the trachea supports a tension pneumothorax. Rales (fine crackling sounds heard on auscultation) may suggest pulmonary edema associated with cardiac cause. Rhonchi (coarse crackling sounds) suggest pneumonia or bronchitis. Egophony ("E->A" changes heard on auscultation) suggests pneumonia.

Heart: Muffled heart sounds suggest cardiac tamponade or pneumothorax. A "rubbing leather" sound with each heart beat suggests pericarditis.

Abdomen: Right upper quadrant tenderness suggests gall bladder. Peritoneal findings suggest ruptured peptic ulcer or pancreatitis

Extremities: A pulse deficit between upper and lower extremities suggests aortic dissection. Swelling and tenderness of the calf or thigh suggests a deep venous thrombosis and a possible source for PE.

Using Advanced Tools: O_2 saturation <85% suggests PE, but may be present with pneumothorax or MI with pulmonary edema. WBC for infection (pneumonia). ECG: ST elevation (1mm or more) may indicate an acute myocardial infarction. ST depression of 1mm suggests ischemia. ST elevation, along with PR depression suggests pericarditis, and one should then rule out cardiac tamponade

Assessment: Determine whether the patient has a life-threatening condition. An acute, single episode of symptom (eg, chest pain, SOB) is more likely to be related to a life-threatening condition. *See Part 3: General Symptoms: Chest Pain & Part 3: General Symptoms: Shortness of Breath (Dyspnea)*

Life-Threatening
Acute coronary syndrome (AMI or unstable angina): *See Part 4: Organ Systems: Chapter 1: Acute Coronary Syndrome (Acute Myocardial Infarction and Unstable Angina)*

Aortic dissection: Classically acute onset with excruciating "tearing" type of pain and severe cardiovascular compromise. History of blunt trauma or deceleration injury. (eg, hard parachute or aircraft landing)

Pulmonary embolism: *See Part 4: Organ Systems: Chapter 3: Deep Vein Thrombosis and Pulmonary Embolism & Part 6: Operational Environment: Chapter 20: Decompression Injuries: Pulmonary Over Inflation Syndrome (Including Arterial Gas Embolism)*

Tension pneumothorax: *See Part 4: Organ Systems: Chapter 3: Pneumothorax*

Pericardial tamponade: *See Part 4: Organ Systems: Chapter 1: Pericarditis*

Mediastinitis (ruptured esophagus or stomach): May have history of peptic ulcer disease or recent, severe vomiting. *See Part 4: Organ Systems: Chapter 3: Pneumomediastinum*

Diving/Aerospace injuries: History of exposure to changes in atmospheric pressure. *See Part 6: Operational Environment: Chapter 20 & Chapter 21*

Non-life-threatening
Cardiac: Pericarditis: *See Part 4: Organ Systems: Chapter 1: Pericarditis*

Pulmonary: *See Part 4: Organ Systems: Chapter 3: Pneumonia*

GI cause (reflux, dyspepsia): *See Part 4: Organ Systems: Chapter 7: Acute Gastritis & Part 4: Organ Systems: Chapter 7: Acute Peptic Ulcer*

Musculoskeletal: Pain with movement of the trunk or arms, point tenderness over the ribs or costochondral joint areas. *See Objective Signs: Chest Wall.*

Other (eg, shingles, decompression sickness): *See Part 4: Organ Systems: Chapter 6: Viral Infections: Herpes Zoster (Shingles) & Part 6: Operational Environment: Chapter 20: Decompression Injuries: Pulmonary Over Inflation Syndrome (Including Arterial Gas Embolism)*

Plan:

Primary Treatment for Life-Threatening Chest Pain

Basic:

Stabilize and identify specific life-threatening condition. Have patient lie down (rest to decrease O_2 consumption), provide O_2 to maintain saturation >95%. Give **aspirin** (non-enteric coated) 325mg chewed; start IV of normal saline at 100cc/hr. If needed, bolus 1000cc of NS to bring the systolic blood pressure (SBP) over 100mmHg.

Advanced:

Acute Coronary Syndrome (AMI or unstable angina): Defibrillator, ECG, ACLS capability (*see Part 4: Organ Systems: Chapter 1: Acute Coronary Syndrome [Acute Myocardial Infarction and Unstable Angina]*)

Aortic dissection: You must slow the heart rate before (or in conjunction with) lowering SBP: Give **propranolol** 40-80mg po qid and **diazepam** 5mg po qid. NO HEPARIN!

PE: *See Part 4: Organ Systems: Chapter 3: Deep Vein Thrombosis and Pulmonary Embolism & Part 6: Operational Environment: Chapter 20: Decompression Injuries: Pulmonary Over Inflation Syndrome (Including Arterial Gas Embolism)*

Tension pneumothorax: *See Part 4: Organ Systems: Chapter 3: Pneumothorax & Part 8: Procedures: Chapter 30: Thoracostomy, Needle and Chest Tube*

Pericardial tamponade: If SBP is falling, perform pericardiocentesis. *See Part 8: Procedures: Chapter 30: Pericardiocentesis*

Mediastinitis (ruptured esophagus or stomach): NPO, IV of normal saline at 100cc/hr. If needed, bolus 1000cc of NS to bring the systolic blood pressure (SBP) over 100mmHg.

Diving Injuries: *See Part 6: Operational Environment: Chapter 20: Decompression Injuries: Pulmonary Over Inflation Syndrome (Including Arterial Gas Embolism) & Decompression Sickness (Caisson Disease, the "Bends")*

Evacuation/Consultation: Stabilize and evacuate all patients suspected of having life-threatening condition as soon as possible.

Primary Treatment for Non Life-Threatening Chest Pain:

Basic:

Monitor to confirm non-life threatening, baseline ECG, follow up (See sections pertaining to specific diagnosis)

Advanced:

Cardiac: *See Part 4: Organ Systems: Chapter 1: Pericarditis*

Pulmonary: *See Part 4: Organ Systems: Chapter 3:* Pneumonia

GI cause (reflux, dyspepsia): Liquid antacid, 1 tablespoon q2-4h. **Cimetidine** 400mg po tid or **famotidine** 20mg po bid.

Musculoskeletal: Ibuprofen 400-600mg po tid with food.

Other (eg, shingles): *See Part 4: Organ Systems: Chapter 6: Viral Infections: Herpes Zoster (Shingles)*; Decompression sickness (*see Part 6: Operational Environment: Chapter 20: Decompression Injuries: Decompression Sickness [Caisson Disease, the "Bends"]*)

Patient Education

General: Healthy lifestyle

Activity: Do not restrict physical exertion if medical condition is not life threatening.

Diet: High fiber, low cholesterol, low fat

Medications: Take exactly as prescribed. Beta-blockers cause tiredness and slow HR.

Prevention: Discontinue smoking; obtain treatment for hypertension and hyperlipidemia.

Follow Up Actions

Reevaluate all patients prn to confirm diagnosis and determine cost/benefit of field management vs evacuation based on operational considerations.

Evacuation/Consultation: If pain is unresolved following treatment.

Constipation

COL Peter McNally, MC, USA (Ret)

Introduction: Constipation is a conscious, unpleasant, and subjective sensation of deviating from the "normal" defecation pattern. Most will feel uncomfortably distended and "backed up." Risk Factors: Healthy and active persons may become acutely constipated after a change in lifestyle, decrease in dietary bulk (fruits, vegetables, whole grains), dehydration, or inactivity. When the urge to defecate is repeatedly repressed or ignored, constipation may result. A preceding history of inactivity (eg, prolonged confinement in a vehicle, airplane, or ship) and decreased food and fluid intake is typical for acute constipation.

Subjective: **Symptoms**

The definition of constipation varies person to person, but a reasonable definition is as follows: Two or fewer bowel movements per week, straining >25% of the time, hard stools >25% of the time, incomplete evacuation >25% of the time. Constipation is much more common among women than men, and the young and aged persons are especially prone. Common causes of constipation include inadequate fiber & food intake, repression or ignoring the urge to defecate, and immobility. Medications such as opiates, anticholinergics and antidepressants can slow intestinal transit and promote constipation.

Focused History: Get a personal history of bowel habits. *How often do you usually have a BM when you are stateside?* (Ascertains "norm" for this patient) *How has your pattern changed since you have been deployed? When was your last bowel movement? Has your constipation been alternating with diarrhea? Does it hurt to have a BM?* (This suggests possible anal fissure or hemorrhoids.)

Objective: **Signs**

Using Basic Tools: Should have normal vital signs. Increased pulse and decreased BP may indicate dehydration. Inspection: May look uncomfortable and restless; distended abdomen. Always look for signs of hypothyroidism: fatigue, feeling cold, loss of hair. Check skin turgor and mucous membranes for signs of dehydration. Auscultation: Bowel sounds present. Absent bowel sounds suggest peritonitis or bowel obstruction, not simple constipation. Palpation: Stool-filled loops may be palpable but abdominal tenderness is uncommon. If constipation is long-standing, perform DRE to check for impaction. Percussion: Tympany over distended loops of bowel is common.

Using Advanced Tools: Labs: CBC should be normal. Elevated WBC suggests infection, low HCT suggests obstruction or neoplasm. Abnormally high HCT suggests dehydration.

Assessment:

For acute constipation temporally associated with change in diet and activity, no testing is necessary. For chronic constipation, tests to exclude structural and systemic disease are necessary.

Plan:

Treatment

Primary: Increase fluid intake. Give mild laxative: **docusate** 50-400mg po per day in 1-4 divided doses, take each tablet with 8oz of water.

Alternate: Magnesium citrate 12oz po (effective in 6-8 hrs); **bisacodyl** 5-15mg po as a single dose with 8oz of water; **senna** or **psyllium granules** 1-2 teaspoons in 8oz of water po, 1-4 times a day

Primitive: Perform a digital rectal examination and remove fecal impaction if present. THIS SHOULD BE A PRIORITY, AS IT IS OFTEN DIAGNOSTIC AND THERAPEUTIC. If hard stool is present, **glycerin** or **bisacodyl** suppositories may be helpful. Position the suppository directly against the rectal wall.

Patient Education

General: Promote healthy, high fiber diet, stress the importance of increased fluid consumption and daily exercise. Answer the urge to defecate. Develop a regular bowel habit. Return to medic if you have relapse in constipation, anal pain or rectal bleeding, fever or nausea or vomiting. MREs are excellent sources of nutrition, but may be constipating when insufficient fluids are consumed. Extreme heat may dehydrate and predispose to abdominal cramps and constipation. Extreme cold, stress and lack of privacy often lead to aversion to pass a bowel movement, perpetuating the cycle of constipation. With appropriate caution, always answer the urge to defecate.

Follow-up Actions

Evacuation/Consultation Criteria: Evacuation is not usually necessary. Consult as needed.

Cough
LCDR Timothy M. Quast, MC, USN & MAJ Christopher J. Lettieri, MC, USA

Introduction: Cough is an extremely common condition and is the 5th most prevalent symptom among patients evaluated in the primary care setting. Cough is a normal physiologic function of the respiratory system, and is the only mechanism that clears secretions, mucus, and foreign bodies from the lung. Conditions that cause coughing include primary pulmonary causes such as airway obstruction from increased secretions or foreign body aspiration, airway irritation (infectious, chemical or thermal injury), or chronic lung disease (emphysema). Non-pulmonary causes include cardiac (congestive heart failure [CHF] or pericardial disease), gastroesophageal reflux disease (GERD), rhinitis with post-nasal drip or medication side effects (eg, ACE inhibitors or beta-blockers). Receptors for cough are multiple and include the larynx, trachea, bronchi, ear canal, pleura, stomach, nasal and sinus passages, pericardium and diaphragm. The causes of cough range from the benign (post-nasal drip) to the malignant (bronchogenic carcinoma).

Subjective: Symptoms

This information, in addition to taking a complete medical history, can guide effective therapy in nearly all cases of cough. Key pieces of information such as whether the patient is an active smoker, takes ACE inhibitors, suffers from symptoms consistent with GERD, or has a recent history of upper respiratory tract infection (RTI) are crucial in determining how to proceed. Be aware of more atypical causes of cough, such as CHF, lung cancer, or TB; the history obtained from the patient may guide the work-up in these cases.

Focused History: *How long have you had this cough?* (Viral upper respiratory tract infections [RTI]or viral bronchitis usually lasts 7-10 days; if >14 days, consider underlying lung disease or a more serious type of infection, such as atypical pneumonia. Use the following guide for acute, subacute, or chronic cough to guide in decision-making. Acute cough is <3 weeks. Most common causes of acute cough are infectious in origin, specifically the common cold, allergic rhinitis, acute bacterial sinusitis, COPD exacerbations, and *Bordetella pertussis* infections. Sub-acute cough is 3-8 weeks and most common causes are post-infectious [ie, upper or lower RTI], *Bordetella pertussis* infections, subacute bacterial sinusitis, or asthma. Chronic cough is >8 weeks. Most common causes for chronic cough are postnasal drip syndromes, nonallergic rhinitis, allergic rhinitis, vasomotor rhinitis, chronic bacterial sinusitis, asthma, GERD, chronic bronchitis [smokers], ACE inhibitors, or eosinophilic bronchitis. Among non-smoker, chronic rhinitis and GERD are, by far, the most common causes of chronic cough and empiric therapy for both are almost universally effective.) *Does anything come up when you cough?* (indicates secretions and inflammation in the airway, which are common in infections) *What color is the sputum that you cough up, and is there blood admixed with your sputum (or frank blood)?* (Green sputum is associated with bacterial infection; blood is generally associated with infection or underlying lung disease; clear or white sputum or non-productive cough is associated with asthma or pneumonia from mycoplasma. While helpful, it should be noted that the color and consistency of sputum is unreliable and should not be solely relied upon as a diagnostic criteria.) *Do you cough at night?* (CHF, asthma, GERD)...*or while lying flat?* (GERD)..*during or after exercise?* (asthma) *Have you had a cough that changed? How?* (COPD may have a chronic cough that increases and becomes productive with an infection.) *Do you have a violent cough or cough associated with vomiting?* (*Bordetella pertussis*) *What makes the cough better, and what makes it worse?* (Cough that worsens with talking is usually due to infection or allergy; cough that improves by sitting up, gets worse after eating or when lying down suggests GERD; cough that only occurs after exercise, and is worse in cold weather [the airway is devoid of moisture below 32°F] is highly suggestive of asthma; cough that improves with cold medications suggests allergy and post-nasal drip.) *Do you smoke?* (Morning cough is common, due to chronic bronchitis.) *Did you stop smoking recently?* (After stopping, the clearance mechanisms of the lung begin to recover and mobilize secretions from the lower airways. This type of cough is beneficial to the lungs and improves over several months if they do not resume smoking). *Have you recently started a new medication such as an ACE inhibitor or beta-blocker? Did you recently have a RTI which you felt resolved?* (Post infectious cough is a common cause of cough for those in the subacute category.)

Pearls:

1. Cough associated with eating suggests a mechanical swallowing problem causing aspiration, or a tracheoesophageal fistula (connection between trachea and esophagus), or gastroesophageal reflux (associated with heartburn or a sour taste).
2. Persistent morning cough that improves after expectorating sputum is typical of chronic bronchitis.
3. Nighttime cough associated with SOB may suggest CHF (especially in elderly patients) or asthma (if wheezing).
4. Nighttime cough without SOB indicates a sinus infection or an allergic origin such as post-nasal drip.

Objective: Signs

Using Basic Tools: Vital signs: Low-grade fever (99–100.5°F) may mean viral or mycoplasma infection. High-grade fever (>102°F) may mean bacterial infection. <14 breath/min most likely allergies, post-nasal drip, bronchitis, GE reflux. If >14 breaths/min, think asthma, pneumonia, acute exacerbation of chronic bronchitis. Inspection: Barrel chested may mean COPD/chronic bronchitis. If splinting respiration, think pleurisy or pneumonia. Auscultate Lungs: If sound is resonant and normal, think upper airway cause (eg, sinusitis.). If wheezes heard, think asthma or emphysema (or rarely foreign body aspiration). If rhonchi heard, think secretions in the airway, eg, bronchitis or pneumonia. If rales heard, think inflammation or fluid in the alveoli, eg, pneumonia. If dull sound, think parapneumonia effusion, pneumonia or collapsed lung.

Using Advanced Tools: Labs: Gram's stain and culture of sputum: >15 white cells/high power field indicates bacterial infection CXR: If clear, think asthma or upper airway cause. If infiltrate, think pneumonia. If a cavity, think lung cancer or TB. Confirm PPD negative for TB.

Assessment: Differential Diagnosis

Infections: Bronchitis (acute or chronic), pneumonia (viral, bacterial, fungal, mycoplasma including TB), sinusitis, pharyngitis, laryngitis. Rule out all of the previous by observing lack of fever, lack of productive cough with dark yellow to green sputum, with or without mixed blood; rule out pneumonia by observing a normal radiograph; rule out sinusitis by observing non-boggy sinuses with an absence of sinus tenderness +/- sinus CT if felt to be indicated under ambiguous physical exam findings. Rule out pharyngitis by observing a normal appearing oropharynx without redness or exudates. PPD negative.

Aspiration: Foreign body, gastric contents. Rule out with a normal auscultation of the throat and lungs, ie, lack of high pitched breath sounds or stridor. Rule out aspiration of gastric contents with a finding of a normal chest radiograph.

Allergic or sensitization response: Asthma, pneumonitis (chemical, biological), allergic rhinitis. Rule out asthma by observing a lack of wheeze on auscultation of the thorax. Formally rule out asthma with a normal pulmonary function testing (no signs of obstruction; this should be done with pulmonary consult if available.) Formal allergy testing may be indicated to rule out allergy as a cause for chronic cough.

Chronic lung disease: Emphysema, COPD, chronic bronchitis, smoking, cancer. To rule this out, observe on clinical exam a prolonged expiratory to inspiratory breathing ratio (eg, 1 to 3) as well as pursed lip breathing in the case of advanced emphysema. Formal pulmonary function testing via a pulmonary consult is indicated to rule out COPD/emphysema, if these assets are available.
Lung cancer is initially evaluated with a chest radiograph; a follow on chest CT is indicated if clinical suspicion is high enough for cancer or if abnormalities are seen on plain radiograph, eg, a pulmonary nodule or mass.

Other lung disease: Pulmonary embolism, pneumothorax, pleurisy. To evaluate, note whether the patient has tachypnea or respiratory distress (for pulmonary embolus or pneumothorax). A chest CT specifically designed to evaluate for pulmonary embolus is indicated if clinical suspicion warrants this. For pneumothorax, a plain film chest radiograph is adequate to diagnose. Pleurisy is diagnosed by symptoms alone, ie, evidence of pain with breathing, or obvious splinting with breathing. Atelectasis may be seen on plain chest radiograph in this setting.

Other non-pulmonary disease: Congestive heart failure, irritant rhinitis, gastroesophageal (GE) reflux, medication effect.
Congestive heart failure would be ruled out with a chest radiograph that does not show pulmonary vascular congestion, and/or the lack of symptoms of orthopnea and paroxysmal nocturnal dyspnea, in addition to the lack of evidence on exam of lower extremity edema.

Plan:

Treatment

1. *See Part 4: Organ Systems: Chapter 3* for treatment for asthma, pneumonia, pleurisy, pneumothorax, allergic pneumonitis, emphysema, COPD, pulmonary embolism.
2. Antibiotics are only indicated in patients with evidence of a bacterial infection, or at high risk due to a chronic underlying pulmonary disease, particularly COPD (empirically treat for both gram-positive and negative organisms). For *Bordetella pertussis*, give **erythromycin** 500mg po q4h x 14 days, or if allergic to same, **trimethoprim-sulfamethoxazole DS** (160mg-800mg) po bid x 14 days.
3. Treat symptomatically when the findings on history and physical examination do not warrant antibiotics. A good first strategy when post-nasal drip is strongly suspected is to treat with a combined antihistamine/decongestant (eg, **chlorpheniramine/ pseudoephedrine** sustained action (8mg/120mg) 1 cap po bid x 7-14 days) Addition of nasal steroids (eg, **fluticasone propionate** 50mcg/spray 2 sprays per nostril q day x one month trial initially) should be strongly considered in this case, and a short course (3 days) of nasal **oxymetolazone** may help alleviate symptoms more rapidly. Only prescribe this medication for short courses to prevent addiction. A combination of nasal steroids, nasal saline rinses, nasal antihistamines and systemic antihistamine decongestants is typically extremely effective as either an initial approach or in patients who fail to respond to other therapies. Once symptoms have improved, these medications should be weaned consecutively with nasal steroids and saline remaining for long-term therapy. Do not suppress a productive cough unless it interferes with obtaining adequate rest/sleep or jeopardizes concealment.
   Dextromethorphan in tablet or liquid form (children over age 2:2.5mg, to age 12:10mg, Adults: 30-60mg, q hs or q4h) or combined with expectorants like **guaifenesin** are often used. Expectorants have not been proven to be effective.
   Codeine (children over age 6:5mg; age 12, 10mg; adults: 30-60mg, po q hs or q4h) for severe cough. QHS is preferred for severe cough that interferes with the ability to rest and will not impair the ability to clear secretions during the daytime. Use no more than 3 nights.

4. If you cannot determine a clear etiology for the cough, treat empirically for allergy, since this is one of the most common causes in otherwise healthy individuals and treatment is well tolerated. One should also consider empiric treatment for GERD with PPIs or H2 blockers if other modalities have been employed empirically, without success.

5. Have a low threshold to order ancillary tests such as pulmonary function tests, chest radiograph, or sinus CT series if specific diagnoses are being considered (eg, asthma, bronchogenic carcinoma, or chronic sinusitis, respectively). Any cough that does not resolve with therapy deserves further evaluation with a chest radiograph, pulmonary function tests and referral to a pulmonologist.

Patient Education

Follow-up Actions: Return if cough persists for more than 2 weeks or worsens. Determine history of PPD and confirm non reactive status.

Note: Cough can be associated with psychological symptoms. However, "psychogenic cough" is a diagnosis of exclusion, but can be associated with severe anxiety or becomes part of a conversion reaction.

Depression and Mania
LTC Michael Doyle, MC, USA

Introduction: Everyone experiences happiness and sadness. However, command and medical personnel should be concerned when service members' variations in mood begin to impair duty performance. 20% of the general population will at some point experience depression outside of the level of sadness expected in daily life. Another 2-5% will experience sustained mood elevation, called mania or hypomania. Both depression and mania appear in all cultures. SOF medics may be called upon to evaluate host nation civilian and military personnel.

Subjective: Symptoms

Depression: Loss of pleasure in activities, social isolation and withdrawal, subjective cognitive impairments, anxiety, worry, excessive guilt, preoccupation with thoughts of death or suicide, insomnia or hypersomnia, changes in appetite and weight, loss of energy and feelings of helplessness, hopelessness, and worthlessness.

Mania: Mood elevation, grandiosity, increased seeking of pleasurable stimuli (hyper-sexuality, spending money, etc.), intrusiveness, belief in special powers, skills or relationships.

Focused History: *When did you start feeling this way, and have you ever felt this way before?* (Many people with depression have had it before.) *Are these feelings constant or do they come and go?* (Severe depression is usually ever-present; mood swings are related to personality; mania rarely switches rapidly enough to seem to "come and go.") *How is your sleep?* (Depressed patients complain of poor sleep or too much sleep, but never feeling rested; manic patients insist they feel fine on very little sleep.) *How is your appetite?* (Often decreased in depression, but some patients complain of cravings or eating too much in order to feel better) *Can you do your job?* (Hypo-manic patients appear to do their job very well [and try to do everyone else's]; manic and depressed patients have obvious impairment in work functioning.) *Do you have thoughts of hurting yourself or anyone else?* (Always, always ask!) *What helps you feel better?* (Manic patients feel even better with sex, alcohol or spending money; depressed patients find that little interests them or helps them feel better.)

Objective: Signs

Let a patient talk for a few minutes uninterrupted and try to sit quietly and follow where the train of thought goes.

* What themes are present? Depressed themes? Grand themes?
* Are the thoughts connected? Are there delusions?
* How severe is the depression? On a scale of 1-10, where 5 is normal, 0 is "the worst I've ever felt" and 10 is "the best I've ever felt".

Using Basic Tools: Normal vitals; manic patients may have slightly elevated pulse and BP.

Mental Status Exam:

Depressed persons appear sad or sometimes worried. They move slowly but may also be agitated, unable to sit still. Look for hand wringing. A depressed person will often avoid eye contact, preferring to gaze downward.

Depressed persons may have difficulty concentrating or completing thoughts. Mental processes are generally slowed.

Manic persons are happy or irritable. They talk profusely -that is, with pressured speech. Interrupting them is like trying to stop a freight train. Manic persons can be grandiose -believing they are God, or simply have grand ideas about how to solve the world's problems. They are energetic and intrusive. Sometimes ideas are very loosely connected or hard to follow. Always ask about suicidal and homicidal ideations, intents, or plans. Both depressed and manic patients may develop fixed false beliefs called delusions. This represents more severe illness.

Assessment:

Differential Diagnosis. Always maintain a high index of suspicion for a physical or CNS injury to explain a change in mood.

Table 3-3. Differential Diagnosis for Depression and Mania

Condition	Manic Symptoms	Depressive Symptoms
Substance Intoxication	PCP, LSD, amphetamines, cocaine	Barbiturates, benzodiazepines, alcohol, marijuana
Trauma or Mass Lesion	Head injury, tumor Hypoxia (from any source)	Head injury, tumor Hypoxia (from any source)
Endocrine	Hyperthyroidism Diabetes	Hypothyroidism Diabetes

Table 3-3. Differential Diagnosis for Depression and Mania, continued

Condition	Manic Symptoms	Depressive Symptoms
Mental Disorder	Bipolar Disorder: A severe illness in which there is a prominent and distinct period of significant mood elevation that impairs the affected individual's social and occupational functioning.	Major Depressive Disorder: A severe illness of 2 or more weeks duration with most of the symptoms and signs described.
	Cyclothymia: Periods of low mood alternating with periods of elevated mood; distinct from elevated mood; "mood swings" in response to social cues or irritability. Low or elevated mood or the swings between interfere with social or occupational functioning.	Dysthymia: A longstanding pattern of low mood more days than not, for more than 2 years, but not as severe as Major Depression Adjustment Disorders (MDAD).
	Schizophrenia: A disturbance in the perception of reality, evidenced by hallucinations, delusions, or thought disorganization with manic behavior	MDAD: As the name indicates, there is some difficulty adjusting to a new stressor that results in functional impairment. Of these listed, adjustment disorders are the most common conditions causing depressive symptoms.
		Schizophrenia: A disturbance in the perception of reality, evidenced by hallucinations, delusions, or thought disorganization with depressive behavior.
Post Traumatic Stress Disorder	A disorder characterized by complex somatic, cognitive, affective and behavioral effects of psychological trauma with symptoms of agitation, irritability and poor sleep or insomnia.	A disorder characterized by complex somatic, cognitive, affective and behavioral effects of psychological trauma with associated symptoms of sense of foreshortened future, sadness, anxiety and worry, and suicidal ideation.

Plan:
Treatment
Primary
1. Ensure safety of the patient (suicide risk) through physical or chemical restraint, 1 on 1 watch or merely increased supervision (as the situation dictates) until definitive care is available.
2. Treat patient appropriately:
   A. **Mania:** Manage the behavioral disturbance through benzodiazepines or neuroleptics.
      1. Benzodiazepines (**diazepam** 5-10mg po or IM q8-12h prn agitation or **lorazepam** 2mg po, IM or IV q-6-8h prn agitation.)
      2. Neuroleptics (**haloperidol** 2-5mg IM or po or **chlorpromazine** 50-100mg po or IM q6-8h prn agitation). Consider **diphenhydramine**, 25-50mg po or IM coincident with the neuroleptic for reduction of risk of adverse reactions (dystonia).
      3. If these fail to settle down an agitated patient, consider restraints. If leather restraints are unavailable, consider physical restraint with sheets wrapped around patient on litter.
   B. **Depression:** Selective Serotonin Re-uptake Inhibitors (SSRIs) such as **fluoxetine, sertraline, paroxetine,** and **citalopram** are mainstays of therapy, but take 1-2 weeks before becoming effective. In an uncomplicated patient without other medical problems, starting an anti-depressant medicine like an SSRI sooner (rather than later) can be very helpful. Starting dose is ½ the therapeutic dose and held at this dose for 1-2 weeks depending on side effects. This tends to minimize side-effects and may improve compliance. In most patients, **fluoxetine** and **sertraline** are best taken in the morning with food; **paroxetine** and **citalopram** tend to be sedating and may be taken at bedtime.

Table 3-4. Primary Treatment Drugs for Depression

Drug Name	Starting Dose (mg/day)	Therapeutic Dose (mg/day)
fluoxetine	10mg	20mg
sertraline	50mg	100mg
paroxetine	10mg	20mg
citalopram	20mg	40mg

3. Refer to local civilian or military health authorities as soon as possible. This may not be immediate.
4. Treat side effects that may emerge with use of SSRIs (nausea, loose stools and headache) symptomatically. Evaluate other physical symptoms (severe headache, diarrhea) as a separate condition and rule out distinct causes.
5. Implement weapons access restrictions.
6. Educate commanders to provide time, opportunity, and conditions for sleep.
7. As with any impairing condition—physical or behavioral—command must be apprised of what limitations, if any, the condition places on the service member's ability to conduct his or her mission.

Patient Education
General: Get adequate rest. Go to bed and arise on same schedule daily. Avoid tobacco, alcohol, and caffeine in the evenings.
Medications: Take SSRIs with food. They may cause headache, diarrhea and nausea.
Follow-up Actions
Return Evaluation: Follow frequently with scheduled and prn visits.
Evacuation/Consultation Criteria: Evacuate urgently, particularly if functionally impaired, suicidal or a danger to others.

Diarrhea, Acute
CDR John Sanders, MC, USA

Introduction: Diarrhea is usually defined as 3 or more loose or liquid stools in 24 hours. Diarrhea can be characterized by days of illness: acute (1-14 days), persistent (14-30 days), or chronic (>30 days), and by symptoms; watery diarrhea (voluminous liquid stools); dysentery (stools mixed with blood and mucus), and "gastroenteritis," (predominance of vomiting). Acute diarrhea is one of the most common illnesses seen in deployed military forces and can cause a significant decrease in unit readiness. It is the 3rd leading cause of death of children in developing countries. Although there are numerous causes of diarrhea, most cases occurring in deployed personnel are caused by an infectious agent; bacteria (~85%), viruses (5-10%) or parasites (5-10%). Other causes; food poisoning (pre-formed toxin), exposure to chemical agent, chronic disease and malabsorption syndromes must also be considered. **Geographic Associations:** Most common in developing countries with poor sanitary conditions. **Seasonal Variation:** The incidence of diarrhea tends to increase in warmer and rainy seasons, but it can occur at any time of the year. **Risk Factors:** Ingestion of contaminated food or water is the primary risk factor. Poorly maintained latrine facilities, lack of hand washing, and large numbers of flies likely also increases risk. The use of medicines to block stomach acid production increases the risk of infection.

Subjective: **Symptoms**
Diarrhea may be accompanied by abdominal cramps, nausea, vomiting, fever, blood, and/or pus/mucus in stool, and tenesmus (rectal pain on defecation). The presence of these symptoms is dependent on both the patient and the cause of illness (ie, certain pathogens are more likely to cause some of these symptoms than other pathogens). The patient can present with a broad range of symptoms (thirsty, lightheadedness, delirium, decreased level of consciousness) caused by dehydration.
Focused History: *How many loose stools have you had in the last 24 hours? How many loose stools since the illness started?* (Change in the consistency of stools without a change in frequency is not diarrhea and more likely caused by stress or change in diet.) *Are you dizzy when you stand up?* (Orthostatic hypotension suggests the patient needs rehydration.) *How are these symptoms impacting your ability to work/recreate?* (measure of severity of condition; treatment is warranted if readiness is affected.) *How long have you had diarrhea?* (symptoms <7 days, most likely due to bacteria or virus; >7 days, the likelihood of parasitic infection increases [eg, *Entamoeba histolytica*]; if >30 days, the likelihood of a non-infectious process increases [eg, inflammatory bowel disease]). *Have you had blood in your stool?* (Bloody diarrhea [dysentery] is suggests an invasive organism, such as *Shigella* or *Campylobacter*; loperamide is contraindicated.) *Have you had numerous large volume, watery stools (voluminous diarrhea, >1 liter of stool/hr?)* (seen with toxin producing bacteria, such as *Vibrio cholerae* [cholera], enterotoxigenic *E. coli*.) *Have you had lots of vomiting with minimal diarrhea?* (Typical of viral gastroenteritis, [eg, norovirus or food poisoning due to pre-formed toxin], and treatment with an antibiotic and loperamide are not indicated.) *Have you been taking antibiotics?* (increases risk pseudomembranous colitis [*C. difficile*] - toxic megacolon) *Does anyone else in your unit have similar symptoms?* (important to define and mitigate risk to mission readiness; may suggest etiology)

Objective: **Signs**
Using Basic Tools: Vital signs: Fever, hypotension, tachycardia, orthostatic changes in heart rate and blood pressure. Inspection: May appear dehydrated, weak and disoriented. Urine concentrated. Auscultation: Usually rapid bowel sounds are evident. Absent bowel sounds with abdominal distention and tympani suggest megacolon or perforation. Percussion: Tympani and distention suggest dilated loops of bowel. Palpation: Mild diffuse tenderness is common. Poor skin turgor (the skin tents when pinched).
Using Advanced Tools: For acute diarrhea (symptoms <14 days), diagnostic testing is not usually required until after empiric treatment has been tried. If symptoms are severe or persistent, examine stool for blood & fecal leukocytes (suggests invasive organism); O & P (to identify organism).

Assessment: **Differential Diagnosis**
Malaria: Can present as fever and diarrhea. If in a malarious area, this should be ruled out by blood smear in any patient presenting with fever and diarrhea. *See Part 5: Specialty Areas: Chapter 12: Parasitic Infections: Malaria*
Typhoid fever: Can present with fever and diarrhea. Usually associated with increasing "stepladder" fever, abdominal pain, and splenomegaly (by second week). Distinguish by culture of stool or blood. *See Part 5: Specialty Areas: Chapter 12: Bacterial Infections: Typhoid Fever*
Bacillary dysentery: Fever, abdominal pain, urgency/pain (tenesmus), stool contains blood, mucus, and pus. This is typically due to *Shigella, Campylobacter,* or *Salmonella.* Distinguish with stool culture. Fecal leukocytes suggestive.
Amebic dysentery: Chronic bloody diarrhea. Distinguish with O & P (stool microscopy).
Cholera: Voluminous diarrhea with "ricewater" stools" (clear watery stools with flecks of mucus). Can lead to hypovolemic shock and death within 1-2 days. Usually occurs in outbreak settings. Distinguish with culture. *See Part 5: Specialty Areas: Chapter 12: Bacterial Infections: Cholera*
Inflammatory bowel disease: Chronic or intermittent diarrhea associated with abdominal pain and often associated with bloody stools. Requires work-up by specialist for diagnosis.
Giardiasis: Chronic diarrhea, cramping, increased flatulence, weight loss, pale and greasy stools. Distinguished by stool O & P (microscopy).
Other parasites: *Cryptosporidium, Cyclospora, Isospora,* etc. Suggested by symptoms persisting more than a week. Distinguished by stool O & P (microscopy); *see Part 5: Specialty Areas: Chapter 12: Parasitic Infections* for specific parasite.
Viral gastroenteritis (stomach flu): Usually presents in "outbreak settings" (ie, the whole camp is getting sick). Norovirus is most

common in military outbreaks and is typically initially foodborne and then often spread person-to-person. Classically presents with significant vomiting.

Food poisoning (pre-formed toxin): Usually presents with severe vomiting and some diarrhea 4-12 hours after ingesting meal. Symptoms usually resolve in <24 hours. *See Part 4: Organ Systems: Chapter 7: Acute Bacterial Food Poisoning*

Plan:
Treatment
Primary: Rehydration; all patients should receive oral or IV fluids (eg, lactated Ringers), until signs and symptoms of dehydration have resolved. For mild symptoms that are not interfering with ability to work, rehydration and observation may be adequate.
Loperamide 4mg po initially (followed by 2mg after each loose stool, up to 16mg in 24 hours) may be used as required to meet operational requirements. For moderate to severe symptoms, **ciprofloxacin** 500mg po bid x 3 days (less if symptoms resolve; many people only need one dose) can be added. Loperamide is contraindicated in patients who appear septic or whose symptoms include fever, severe abdominal pain or bloody stools.
Alternative: Azithromycin 1000mg po once or 500mg po daily x 3 days (or until symptoms resolve; many patients only require one dose) combined with **loperamide**.
Empiric: Empiric therapy for acute diarrhea during deployment (travelers' diarrhea) is the combination of an appropriate antibiotic (**ciprofloxacin** or **azithromycin**) with **loperamide**. Empiric therapy may be required for acute diarrhea during deployment to minimize symptoms and reduce the potential impact on the mission. If empiric therapy fails, further work-up can be conducted.
Primitive: If antibiotics and loperamide are not available, Oral Rehydration Solution (ORS) may provide some symptomatic relief and will help to maintain hydration status. The World Health Organization ORS recipe is 1L of purified water + 20g glucose + 3.5g salt + 5g sodium bicarbonate + 1.5g potassium chloride. If ingredients not available, basic ORS can be made by mixing 8 level teaspoons of sugar and 1 level teaspoon of salt in 1L of clean water.

Patient Education
General: Most patients recover very quickly with appropriate therapy. The most important aspect of therapy is maintaining hydration. Empiric therapy with antibiotics and loperamide will usually cut duration of symptoms from approximately 4 days to <1 day.
Activity: As tolerated, but should be restricted from food preparation or handling until symptoms have fully resolved.
Diet: As tolerated.
Medications: Loperamide can cause constipation and is rarely associated with drowsiness. Ciprofloxacin can be associated with nausea/vomiting, headache, and difficulty sleeping, but these side effects are rare (especially if they only need one dose). Azithromycin (especially at the 1000mg dose) may be associated with nausea and vomiting.
Prevention and Hygiene: Encourage good hand washing; avoid consumption of local food and water. If local food must be consumed; "peel it, boil it, cook it, or forget it."
No Improvement/Deterioration: Should return if symptoms do not improve or worsen.
Follow-up Actions
Return Evaluation: As needed.
Evacuation/Consultation Criteria: If the patient does not respond to empiric therapy or if symptoms are chronic (especially if associated with bloody stool), the patient should be referred for more intensive evaluation.
Note: Travelers' diarrhea appears to be associated with the subsequent development of irritable bowel syndrome (IBS) within a year of the initial infection in some patients.

Dizziness
CDR Christopher Jankosky, MC, USN

Introduction: Dizziness is a common complaint but often difficult for a patient to describe. Is the person describing an alteration of consciousness (*see Part 3: General Symptoms: Syncope [Fainting]*), an alteration of balance, or a feeling of lightheadedness that accompanies standing up?
Do they have a perceived (false) sense of motion, ie, the patient feels they or the surroundings are moving (vertigo)? One should attempt to localize the pathology to the inner ear, the central nervous system or a systemic disorder.

Subjective: **Symptoms**
Focused History: *Does the patient have a prior history that can account for recurrent dizziness such as Ménière's disease?*
Duration: *How long has the patient had symptoms?* (Acute symptoms may represent a self-limited illness such as otitis media or labyrinthitis. Chronic symptoms may suggest an anatomic abnormality, such as acoustic neuroma.)
Illness: *Has the patient been ill, especially any upper respiratory illnesses?* (Recent URI can lead to vertigo through otitis media or labyrinthitis.) *Any vomiting and/or diarrhea?* (dizziness caused by volume depletion)
Fullness: *Has the patient been experiencing ear pain fullness?* (This can be associated with otitis media.)
Trauma: *Has the patient been exposed to any direct trauma to the ear or barotrauma?* (This can result in serous otitis media.) *Has the patient been flying or diving recently? See Part 6: Operational Environment: Chapter 20: Decompression Injuries: Decompression Sickness (Caisson Disease, the "Blends")*
Hearing/Ringing: *Does the patient have a persistent ringing (tinnitus) in their ears? If so, do they also have a hearing loss?* (The combination makes Ménière's more likely.)
Spinning: *Does the patient have a sensation of motion/spinning? If so, does head movement bring it on?* (Consider benign paroxysmal vertigo, which may be accompanied by vomiting.)
Walking: *Does the patient have difficulty walking? If so, do they feel dizzy when this happens?* (Abnormal gait without dizziness is most likely ataxia [difficulty walking], a motor control problem.)
Falling: *Does the patient constantly fall toward the same direction?* (An anatomic abnormality [ie, tumor] in the middle ear will classically cause the patient to fall toward the affected side.)

Objective: Signs

Using Basic Tools:

Vital signs: Low blood pressure (or a change with standing of >20mmHg systolic) suggests volume depletion caused by dehydration.

Fever: Possible ear infection.

Ear exam: Tympanic membrane (TM) injected, loss of light reflex, +/- purulent fluid in middle ear - purulent otitis media can cause vertigo by stimulating of the vestibular apparatus. TM bulging, clear fluid in middle ear suggests serous otitis media. Perform Rinne and Weber test to evaluate for an associated hearing loss. The Rinne test is performed by placing a vibrating 512Hz tuning fork initially on the mastoid, then next to the ear. If a conductive hearing loss is present, then bone conduction from the mastoid is louder to the patient than air conduction through the ear. The Weber test is performed by placing the vibrating tuning fork in the middle of the forehead, equal distance from each ear. If a conductive hearing loss is present in one ear, then the sound appears louder in the affected ear. If a sensorineural hearing loss is present in one ear, the sound appears louder in the unaffected ear.

Neurologic: Assess for Benign Paroxysmal Positional Vertigo (BPPV) using the Dix-Hallpike Maneuver: Have patient sit so that when lying supine, the head extends over the end of the table. Instruct the patient to keep his eyes open and to stare at the examiner's nose during the test. To test the left posterior canal, have the patient turn his head 45° to the left. Keeping the head in this position, lie the patient down rapidly until the head is dependent and extended below the table. In each position, observe the eyes closely for up to 40 seconds for development of a rotational nystagmus (eyes beat upward and torsionally, with the upper poles of the eyes beating toward the ground). Return the patient to the upright position and nystagmus will recur but in the opposite direction. To test the right posterior canal, repeat maneuver with the head turned 45° to the right side. With each repetition, the intensity and duration of nystagmus will typically diminish. If patient has other neurological symptoms or specific focal neurologic signs, consider evacuation for a definitive diagnosis of underlying etiology.

Assessment: Differential Diagnosis

Systemic disorders: Medications or toxins, hypotension, infectious diseases, endocrine (diabetes, hypothyroid).

Ménière's Disease: A chronic disorder resulting in decreased hearing acuity over long duration, accompanied by multiple exacerbations of vertigo and tinnitus.

Labyrinthitis: Causes dizziness and a decrease in hearing acuity. This can be due to bacterial or viral infection.

Benign Paroxysmal Positional Vertigo (BPPV): The cause is a displaced otolith (debris) in a vestibular organ. An acute spinning sensation brought on with head movement that generally lasts less than a minute, and is associated with a rotatory nystagmus on physical exam. There is no change in the patient's hearing.

Plan:

Treatment

BPPV: Treat using the modified Epley maneuver. Through a series of particle repositioning maneuvers, the goal is to move debris in the posterior vestibular canals away from the hair cells that directly influence balance. The modified Epley maneuver is performed as follows: Have the patient lie involved ear down with head dependent (as in Dix-Hallpike maneuver) until the observed nystagmus has fatigued. Then turn the head with the neck extended until the noninvolved ear is facing downward. Nystagmus may recur at this point (if so, it should be in the same direction as it was when initially). Hold this position until the nystagmus fatigues or for approximately 30-60 seconds. Then roll the patient onto their side into a lateral decubitus body position, with the nose pointed downward, for another 30-60 seconds. Finally, the chin is tucked toward the chest and the patient is helped up into the seated position. Because sitting up will sometimes elicit a vestibular response, maintain contact with the patient at this point to prevent a fall from the table.

Ménière's Disease: Consider evacuation or consultation to confirm diagnosis and management plan. For milder symptoms, consider **meclizine** 25mg po qid. For severe symptoms, use **meclizine** 25mg po q6h or **prochlorperazine** 25mg per rectum q12h. **Diazepam** 5mg po qid may also provide benefit. The duration of drug treatment depends on response and individual situation; there is not a set number of treatment days for symptomatic treatment of dizziness.

Purulent Otitis Media: Analgesics, decongestants, and antibiotics (often **amoxicillin** 250mg po tid for 7-10 days). *See Part 3: General Symptoms: ENT Problems: Ear Pain*

Serous Otitis Media: Analgesics, antihistamines and decongestants. *See Part 3: General Symptoms: ENT Problems: Ear Pain*

Labyrinthitis: May provide symptomatic treatment with medications noted for Ménière's disease. The symptoms of labyrinthitis often resolve in less than a week, but may persist longer.

Patient Education

General: Patient should be aware that dizziness can arise from many different conditions, and should communicate changes to his medic. If severe vertigo limits oral intake, then IV hydration should be initiated.

Follow-up Actions

Close follow-up required if dizziness or medication side effects potentially limit occupational functioning. Follow up will vary depending on suspected etiology of dizziness. Rapid follow up if symptoms worsen, if new symptoms occur, or if patient is not responding as expected to treatment.

Evacuation/Consultation Criteria: Evacuate patients with persistent or recurrent symptoms of vertigo or dizziness when an etiology for the symptoms cannot be readily determined in the field. Some neurological conditions, such as cerebellar hemorrhage, may be difficult to diagnose accurately in the field and will require specialty evaluation.

ENT Problems: Ear Pain

COL Karla Hansen, MC, USA

Introduction: Ear pain may be felt on the outer ear, in the canal, or deep in the ear. Pain may be from the ear itself or referred from areas innervated by cranial nerves V, VII, IX or X, or by cervical nerves C2 or C3. A complete head and neck exam may be necessary to identify the source of pain.

Subjective: Symptoms

Focused History: *Where is the pain: outer ear (pinna), external ear canal, or deep inside the ear?* If outer ear: *Have you noticed a loss of hearing?* (There may be swelling or blockage of external auditory canal [EAC], or fluid behind the tympanic membrane [TM].) *Is there drainage from the ear?* (otitis externa or otitis media with perforated TM) *Does your ear itch?* (acute or chronic otitis externa) *Have you been in a very cold environment?* (frostbite) *If external ear canal: Is it tender when you pull on your ear?* (helps to differentiate ear canal from inner ear problem) *Does chewing cause or increase pain?* (External ear canal problems tend to cause pain with chewing.) *Have you been in the water?* (common cause of otitis externa – swimmer's ear) *Have you stuck anything in your ear?* (Attempting to scratch can traumatize the skin and lead to infection.) *If deep inside the ear: Have you noticed a loss of hearing?* (causes may include upper respiratory infection, otitis media) *Have you had a head cold recently?* (Edema from upper respiratory infection may occlude the eustachian tube, leading to otitis media, hearing loss.)

Objective: Signs

Using Basic Tools: Vital signs: Elevated temperature suggests infection. Inspection: Redness, exudate or swelling of pinna and canal. Check adjacent skin of face or neck and post-auricular region. Foul smelling drainage from EAC may be from otitis externa or cholesteatoma. Use otoscope to identify foreign bodies, exudate, swelling of canal walls, inflamed or perforated TM, or blood, mass, fluid in the middle ear space behind the TM. Assess hearing with whisper test or tuning fork; *see Part 3: General Symptoms: ENT Problems: Hearing Loss.* Examine the oropharynx; pharyngitis, peritonsillar abscess or GERD can cause referred pain to the ear. Palpation: Manipulate pinna and tragus (pointy part just anterior to EAC meatus) to localize pain. Swelling or "doughiness" of the mastoid process behind the ear suggests mastoiditis.

Using Advanced Tools: Labs: Culture any discharge from EAC or any wound near ear before initiating treatment.

Assessment: Differential Diagnosis

External Ear Pain

Trauma: Swelling, ecchymosis, lacerations. Severe swelling (subcutaneous hematoma) may cause "cauliflower ear" and loss of cartilage.

Perichondritis: Infection of the cartilage of the pinna with sparing of the flesh lobule. Severe pain out of proportion to the physical exam. Red, swollen pinna. Slow to resolve even with appropriate antibiotic therapy.

Frostbite: Pallor and numbness of pinna secondary to cold; thawing causes redness and swelling; vesicles are seen with second degree and necrotic tissue occurs with third degree injury; initial numbness replaced with constant pain. *See Part 6: Operational Environment: Chapter 23: Freezing Injury (Frostbite)*

Mastoiditis: Cancer, psoriasis and other skin conditions. *See Differential Diagnosis: Internal or Middle Ear Conditions (Beyond TM): Mastoiditis*

Pain and Abnormalities of the EAC and TM

Foreign body: Canal may be swollen from inflammation; object (commonly cerumen) usually seen with otoscope

Otitis externa (bacterial): Infection of the ear canal, usually due to retained moisture; pinna usually normal but retraction causes ear pain; canal is swollen, red, moist and has debris. Hearing is usually decreased due to obstruction of the canal.

Otitis externa (otomycosis): Fungal infection of the canal, occasionally extending to the TM; usually very itchy. Fungus may appear as fine coal dust or cotton-like white patches.

Furunculosis: Staph infection secondary to microtrauma (often caused by cleaning) of the canal causes furuncle; occurs only in the external, hair-bearing portion of the canal; tragal tenderness; red, swelling of the canal limited to hair-bearing portion.

Bullous myringitis: Normal EAC; sudden onset of severe pain; multiple, isolated vesicles or hemorrhagic bullae on TM (may be associated with *Mycoplasma pneumoniae* upper respiratory infection)

Malignant external otitis: Osteomyelitis of the temporal bone and skull base; usually in diabetic patient or immune compromised patient; life-threatening infection; increasing pain; debris and granulation tissue in canal at junction of cartilaginous and bony canal. *Pseudomonas aeruginosa* is the causative organism; may be associated with cranial nerve palsies (especially facial nerve); slowly progressive to soft tissue

TM perforation: May be small or quite large; very severe pain at the time or moment of injury, gradually diminishing thereafter; ringing in ear; hole in TM is usually visible, although area may have blood around it; may have conductive hearing loss if hole is large

Internal or Middle Ear Conditions (Beyond TM)

Acute otitis media (OM): Effusion (fluid) of middle ear space with infection; marked ear pain or throbbing; hearing loss; tinnitus; may have fever; purulent ear drainage if TM ruptures. TM is usually red, bulging, but sometimes opaque, or white with loss of landmarks.

Chronic OM: Mild symptoms; prolonged course; TM has pale, thickened appearance; may have chronic drainage if TM is perforated

Mastoiditis: Surgical emergency, large amount of pain or discomfort, "doughy" swelling and redness over post auricular region; fevers/chills. The ear canal may frequently become swollen, particularly the posterior canal wall, and have debris or discharge. It may occur in the late phases of a resolving OM.

Cholesteatoma (skin cyst of middle ear): Frequently painless; recurrent, foul smelling drainage from ear; TM perforation or retraction pocket; white, fluffy, cotton-like debris that is the cholesteatoma; conductive hearing loss

Eustachian tube dysfunction: Loss of ability to equilibrate external air (or water pressure with submersion) with air pressure in the middle ear space, resulting in negative pressure in the middle ear space; feeling of pressure or fullness in ear or "water in the ear"; occasional bout of lancinating or shooting pain within ear or extending down into neck. Ear may crackle or pop; TM may be retracted.

Barotrauma: Blood behind TM or injected TM with history of exposure to change in pressure. *See Part 6: Operational Environment: Chapter 20: Barotrauma: Barotrauma to Ears*

Blast trauma: Causes over pressure, frequently causing a combination injury of TM rupture with pain and hearing loss from sensorineural damage.

Other causes of ear pain to consider other than the ear

Dental: (eg, temporomandibular joint pain): Pain radiates to ear; exacerbated by biting or chewing; tenderness to pressure over joint; clicking or grinding of joint

Salivary gland: Swelling over salivary gland; may worsen just after eating; may have pus from duct into mouth

Lesions or tumors of oral cavity, larynx or pharynx may also cause pain that is referred to the ear.

Plan:

Treatment

Trauma: Treat lacerations as described for other wounds. Do not suture cartilage. Prevent swelling and "cauliflower ear" by applying ice to pinna and bacitracin-soaked supportive dressings in cavities of pinna. Fresh subcutaneous hemorrhage may be aspirated under sterile conditions. Recurrent, resistant or prolonged hemorrhage requires evacuation. Evaluate for TM rupture and fractures as appropriate.

Perichondritis: Treat with hot packs and systemic antibiotics, initially **nafcillin** or **oxacillin** 2g IV q6h until clearly improved, usually 4-5 days. If not responsive by 48 hours, change to **vancomycin** 1g IV q12h until improved, usually 4-5 days and evacuate.

Frostbite: Re-warm pinna rapidly without rubbing. Use **silver nitrate** soak (.05%) for superficial infections. *See Part 6: Operational Environment: Cold Related Illnesses and Injuries: Freezing Injury (Frostbite)*

Mastoiditis: Use **ceftriaxone** 1.5g IVPB q day or **vancomycin** 500mg IV q6, or for pediatric patients, start at 10mg/kg q6h. Install topical drops: **(hydrocortisone/neomycin/polymyxin B otic [Cortisporin]** 5-6 drops tid or **gentamicin ophthalmic** drops 5-6 tid). Continue treatment for 5-7 days after response is initially seen. Evacuate when possible.

Foreign body:

Basic: Ensure the TM is intact. Gently irrigate the canal using syringe and water, followed by rubbing alcohol to dry the ear. Avoid water or saline if the object is a bean or other vegetable matter that can swell when wet. If the object is a live insect, flood the canal with **lidocaine** to stop the motion of the insect before removal.

Advanced: Gently remove object under visualization with otoscope. Batteries in ear need to be removed immediately secondary to possible acid or alkaloid leakage that can result in scarring and stenosis of the canal.

Otitis externa: Bacterial:

Primary: Clean canal of debris with ear loop. If ear is severely swollen, place a wick made of cotton into canal and apply topical medications or drops to wick: **Cortisporin otic** suspension or **gentamicin** ophthalmic drops 5-6 drops tid x 5-7 days. Oral antibiotics may be indicated for severe cases: **amoxicillin** 250mg tid x 7-10 days , or if penicillin allergic, use **erythromycin** 250mg qid or **ciprofloxacin** 250mg or 500mg po bid x 7-10 days.

Primitive: Acidify canal with white vinegar and dry with rubbing alcohol (mix half and half) bid/tid x 7 days.

Otitis externa: Otomycosis:

Primary: Clean canal of debris with ear loop. Use **Cortisporin otic drops** 5-6 drops tid x 5-7 days. Rarely, an oral antifungal may be needed **(ketoconazole** 200-400mg q day x 5-7 days).

Alternate: Apply **Gentian violet** in the canal.

Primitive: Acidify canal with white vinegar and dry with rubbing alcohol (mix half and half) tid x 7-10 days.

Furunculosis:

Primary: Clean ear if possible with white vinegar and rubbing alcohol (50/50 mix) as above. Use anti-staphylococcal antibiotic like **amoxicillin/clavulanate** 500mg po bid x 7 days.

Alternate: Incise lesion with needle after anesthetizing the area with **lidocaine**.

Primitive: Warm soaks with saline may cause spontaneous drainage.

Bullous myringitis: Use topical antibiotic and anesthetic drops like **Cortisporin otic** (5-6 drops tid x 7 days) and **antipyrine/ benzocaine** (5-6 drops bid x few days), as well as a broad-spectrum antibiotic like **amoxicillin/clavulanate** 500mg po bid x 7-10 days.

Malignant external otitis:

Primary: Clean canal of debris with ear loop. Install anti-*Pseudomonas* drops, **gentamicin** ophthalmic 5-6 drops tid long term, usually requires weeks (6 weeks) and evacuate.

Alternate: If unresponsive, add IV antibiotics such as **gentamicin** 1mg/kg IVPB q8h, **tobramycin** 1mg/kg IVPB q8h or **amikacin** 15mg/kg up to 1500 mg/d IVPB divided q8h and evacuate. If the patient truly has malignant otitis externa, IV therapy for 6 weeks to 6 months may be necessary.

TM perforation:

Primary: Keep ear dry. Apply **ofloxacin otic** 5-6 drops bid x 5-7 days. Other drops may damage nerves. TM perforation followed by contamination (ie, dirty water, sea water) should receive a prophylactic course of oral antibiotics: **amoxicillin** 250mg po tid x 7 days or **erythromycin** 250mg po qid x 7 days

Primitive: Most heal spontaneously. Keep ear dry of water by placing a cotton ball impregnated with a generous amount of petroleum jelly in EAC.

Acute OM:

Primary: Treat febrile patients or those in severe pain with **amoxicillin** 250mg po tid x 7-10 days or **amoxicillin/clavulanate** 500mg po bid x 7-10 days or, if penicillin allergic, **erythromycin** 250mg po qid x 7-10 days.

Primitive: Most cases resolve spontaneously.

Chronic OM:

Primary: 1-2 courses of oral antibiotic (same regimen as for acute OM) for minimum of 2 weeks each and decongestants like **pseudoephedrine** 30mg po tid/qid.

Primitive: May resolve without antibiotic treatment although time course may be prolonged (8-12 weeks).

Cholesteatoma: Keep ear dry of water while awaiting evacuation. Treat secondary infection with topical drops like **Cortisporin otic** or

gentamicin ophthalmic 5-6 drops tid x 7-10 days. **Amoxicillin/clavulanate** 500mg po bid x 7-10 days may be used for severe symptoms.

Eustachian tube dysfunction:

Primary: Use decongestant like **pseudoephedrine** 30mg po tid/qid, or **chlorpheniramine maleate** and **pseudoephedrine HCl** one tablet po tid. May need to treat upper respiratory infection or rhinitis (*see Part 4: Organ Systems: Chapter 3: Common Cold [Upper Respiratory Infections] & Part 3: General Symptoms: ENT Problems: Rhinitis/Rhinorrhea*).

Primitive: Gently try to equalize pressure with Valsalva maneuver to prevent further ear trauma.

Dental, Salivary Gland and Other Conditions: *See Part 5: Specialty Areas: Chapter 10: Oral and Dental Problems & Part 3: General Symptoms: ENT Problems: Salivary Gland Disease*

Patient Education

General: Keeping the ear dry prevents numerous ear problems. Water in an ear with a perforation will likely lead to infection and pain.

Activity: Avoid water in the ears, particularly with a TM perforation. Keep ear dry by placing a cotton ball impregnated with a generous amount of petroleum jelly in EAC, and do not go underwater.

Diet: Regular

Medications: Antibiotics may cause GI upset or yeast infections.

Prevention and Hygiene: Avoid the use of Q-tips or other objects in the ear canal as they may cause extensive injury and infection. Clean ear by placing drops of white vinegar with rubbing alcohol (50/50 mix) into the canal to rinse the whole canal surface. Do not do this if there is a hole in the eardrum.

Follow-up Actions

Return Evaluation: If symptoms persist or increase following therapeutic trial of appropriate medications, consider changing antibiotics or referring for specialty care.

Evaluation/Consultation Criteria: Patients should respond to therapy within 24 hours of starting IV antibiotics (up to 48 hours for oral antibiotics). If pain, fever, and, headache persist after >24 hours of IV antibiotic therapy, consider urgent medical evacuation.

ENT Problems: Hearing Loss

COL Karla Hansen, MC, USA

Introduction: Hearing loss (HL) can be classified by type: conductive (involving external ear, canal, tympanic membrane [TM] and middle ear contents), sensorineural (involving cochlea and acoustic nerve), mixed (a combination of conductive and sensorineural hearing loss), or central (brain processing). Onset can be slow or sudden, and may be an isolated problem or associated with other symptoms such as ear infection, dizziness or vision changes. If recognized early, sudden hearing loss can be improved greatly with intervention. **Risk Factors:** A family history of hearing loss, particularly in any family member before age 40, is associated with increased risk of hearing loss. A recent head cold (more common in winter) causing eustachian tube dysfunction increases the risk of temporary conductive hearing loss secondary to fluid in the middle ear. Prolonged periods of loud noise exposure are a very common cause for hearing loss among service members. Sudden extreme loud noise or blast injuries, ie, Improvised Explosive Device (IED) explosions, are high risk factors for sudden decrease in hearing from both conductive losses secondary to tympanic membrane rupture and from acoustic damage to the sensorineural mechanism.

Subjective: **Symptoms**

Acute (within 72 hours): Sudden loss of hearing (one side), +/- vertigo, ear fullness

Sub-Acute (>72 hours, <1 month): Decreased hearing, ear fullness

Chronic (>1 month): Decreased hearing, ear congestion

Focused History: *Do you have a head cold?* (HL may be conductive secondary to fluid behind the eardrum or perceived loss secondary to eustachian tube dysfunction.) *Do you have any ear drainage?* (may indicate a TM perforation or infection) *Have you had any ear trauma?* (suggests TM perforation) *Did the hearing loss occur within the last few hours?* (Sudden HL secondary to a viral nerve insult will occur quickly.) *Are you dizzy or is the room spinning?* (Viral labyrinthitis or Ménière's Disease will have vertigo and possible hearing loss associated with it.) *Have you been exposed to loud noise, and if so for how long?* (Very loud sounds may cause hearing threshold shifts, both temporary and permanent.) *Have you had a blast trauma?* (Sudden blast cause both TM rupture and sensorineural hearing loss.) *Have you had ear surgery? If so, what was done?* (may indicate repeat hole in eardrum or ossicular [hearing bone] problem) *What medications do you take, and how long have you taken them?* (Medications like aminoglycosides, erythromycin, vancomycin and tetracycline are associated with HL.) *Have you been diving in the past 48 hours?* (especially with 100% oxygen rebreather)

Objective: **Signs**

Using Basic Tools: Inspection: Look for external signs of redness, tenderness or swelling in the ear canal, and drainage (bloody or purulent) or inflammation that suggest an external auditory canal infection or obstruction. Debris may block the ear canal. Gently clean the canal with water or vinegar/water mix, if available, with a syringe. Do not use excessive force, which can rupture TM. Look for other signs such as nystagmus, ataxia, and imbalance. Palpation: Feel behind the ear for any swelling or tenderness suggesting external otitis and mastoiditis. Hearing tests: Do tuning fork exams with 512Hz fork. Weber Test: For lateralization of hearing, strike the forked end, and then place the stem on the midline of the patient's skull or the incisor teeth. Have the patient report in which ear the tone seems louder. Patients with normal hearing or equal loss in both ears report the sound in the midline or in both ears. Patients with a unilateral sensorineural loss will perceive the tone louder in their better ear. Patients with a unilateral conductive loss will perceive the tone louder in the poorer ear. Rinne Test: Compares a patient's air and bone conduction hearing. Strike the tuning fork at the forked end, and then place the stem on the mastoid process. Then hold the fork off the patient's head approximately two inches from the opening of the external auditory canal with the tines of the fork in a line with the opening of the external ear canal. Have the patient report which position was louder, on the mastoid or next to the external ear canal. Patients with normal hearing or sensorineural hearing loss will perceive the tone of the fork held off the ear being louder. Patients with conductive hearing losses of greater than 25-30dB will perceive the sound behind the ear as louder.

Using Advanced Tools: Otoscope to examine the ear canals for obstruction or debris, and examine the TMs for perforations or fluid behind the drum.

Assessment: Differential Diagnosis

Serous otitis media: A fluid collection behind the eardrum will decrease the mobility of the TM, pain, pressure, fullness, and causing conductive hearing loss. This is associated with viral respiratory illness, head colds, and allergy problems.

Sudden sensorineural hearing loss: The hearing in one ear can acutely (<72 hours) decrease. This may be accompanied by tinnitus (ringing) in the affected ear. Sometimes there can be an associated short period of vertigo. This problem can occur at any age. The patient may have a history of a viral illness in the past several weeks. The origin of the disease is usually a viral insult to the hearing nerve itself.

Acute threshold shift: Noise-induced trauma to the ear that causes a decrease in hearing. The patient will have a history of significant loud noise exposure, such as a concert or explosions. Most threshold shifts are temporary. IED and loud explosions are high risk for permanent loss of hearing.

TM perforation: Patient has a history of ear trauma, usually associated with pain. There may be bloody drainage from the ear. A hole may be seen in the TM; the bigger the hole, the greater the conductive hearing loss. Many times with blast trauma, the patient has a mixed conductive and sensorineural hearing loss.

Inner ear barotrauma: Exposure to sudden, large changes in ambient pressure from diving or flying. Causes tinnitus, vertigo, and hearing loss.

Basilar skull fracture: A significant head trauma causing a basilar skull fracture can produce either a conductive or a sensorineural hearing loss.

Lateral skull fractures: Tend to cause TM rupture or ossicular disruptions.

Frontal/occipital fracture: Tend to cause sensorineural hearing loss due to cochlear injury. Associated signs may include hemotympanum, cerebrospinal fluid otorrhea or bruising behind the ears (Battle's sign).

Plan:

Treatment

Serous otitis media: Most effusions will slowly resolve over 4-6 weeks. If the patient has pain or fever, a course of antibiotics such as **azithromycin** 500mg po on day 1, then 250mg po days 2-5 or **amoxicillin** 250mg po tid x 7-10 days may help to resolve the fluid buildup.

Sudden sensorineural hearing loss: Many patients will have a spontaneous recovery of their hearing. The prognosis can be improved by treatment with a short course of high dose steroid with taper: **prednisone** 80mg/day po x 3 days, then 60mg/day po x 3 days, then 40mg/ day po x 3 days, then 20mg/day po x 3 days.

Acute threshold shift: Withdrawal from the noise and additional hearing protection may help recovery of full hearing. Not all patients will recover completely.

Blast trauma: Withdrawal from the noise and additional hearing protection may help recovery of full hearing. Trial of short course of high dose steroid with taper may help: **prednisone** 80mg/day po x 3 days, then 60mg/day po x 3 days, then 40mg/day po x 3 days, then 20mg/day po x 3 days. Early evidence from ongoing research shows a positive impact of steroids on the overall recovery of sensorineural hearing after an acoustic trauma. Unless there is a contraindication, a therapeutic trial of steroids post injury may benefit the patient and improve hearing. Optimal timing for steroids is within 72 hours of injury.

Patient Education

General: Sudden hearing changes need to be evaluated for possible treatment to improve the outcome. Many people will gradually have a decrease in hearing as they age but significant hearing loss before age 40 should be evaluated.

Prevention and Hygiene: Avoid excessive noise. Use hearing protection!

No Improvement/Deterioration: Should the hearing continue to decline in a short period of time (1 week); the patient must be evaluated with a hearing test and examination by an otolaryngologist.

Follow-up Actions

Return Evaluation: Re-examine the patient to check for restoration or deterioration of hearing.

Evaluation/Consultation Criteria: Patients with significant head trauma (including basal skull fracture), or trauma associated with vertigo lasting greater than one day, should be evacuated.

ENT Problems: Hoarseness

COL Karla Hansen, MC, USA

Introduction: Aside from habitual throat clearing, hoarseness is the most common symptom of laryngeal disease. Most cases of hoarseness will be secondary to an irritating process such as a viral illness, post-nasal drip or gastroesophageal reflux. The other structures of the upper aerodigestive tract (nose, sinuses, esophagus) may be actively involved in the same disease process or even be the cause of hoarseness. Be alert for serious disease processes that may involve potential for airway compromise. Never refer patients with unstable airways before first securing the airway by either endotracheal intubation or a surgical airway. **Risk Factors:** A large portion of the population will experience hoarseness with over usage of the voice. Working in a loud environment fosters loud speech and significant additional vocal abuse. A history of tobacco and/or alcohol use increases the risk of larynx cancer. Chemical or smoke exposure may also cause hoarseness.

Subjective: Symptoms

Acute (less than 3 weeks): Suggestive of viral illness. Pain, dry cough, URI symptoms

Sub-Acute (>3 weeks): Suggestive of benign process. No pain, cough, +/- Gastroesophageal Reflux Disease (GERD)

Chronic (>6 weeks): If symptom comes and goes, then something irritating is occurring such as post-nasal drip or GERD or vocal abuse. A constant coarse or breathy/weak voice is suggestive of malignancy or mass. Pain, +/- cough, hemoptysis, painful or difficult swallowing also suggests malignancy in long-term hoarseness.

Focused History: *How long have you been hoarse?* (Acute processes should resolve within 3 weeks.) *Have you been yelling, instructing, or working in a loud environment recently?* (suggestive of vocal abuse) *Does it hurt to swallow?* (Acute pain supports infection, but chronic pain supports cancer.) *Is it difficult to swallow?* (Suggests serious infection, or in chronic case, suggests cancer.) *Have you noticed any lumps or masses in your neck?* (Possible metastatic lymph nodes especially if very hard or fixed; neck lumps/masses could also be lymphadenopathy in acute infection and tend to be tender and firm but not hard or fixed.) *Have you had any recent neck trauma?* (Coughing up blood suggests significant larynx injury.) *Do you have allergies or post-nasal drip?* (Hoarseness is frequently caused by drainage from the nose.) *Do you have heartburn or indigestion?* (GERD may cause hoarseness.)

Objective: Signs

Using Basic Tools: Listen to voice quality. Constant course, rough, gravelly or husky voice may all indicate a true vocal cord lesion. A weak or breathy voice may indicate a paralysis of one of the vocal cords. Loss of range of pitch indicates excessive strain or tension dysphonia. An intermittent whisper or complete aphonia suggests a psychogenic origin. Inspection: Thoroughly inspect the oral cavity and posterior pharynx, looking for any evidence of irritation, inflammation or drainage. Look into the nasal cavity for rhinorrhea. Palpation: Thoroughly palpate the neck, paying attention to any enlarged lymph nodes, tenderness, or swelling. The normal larynx will have palpable crepitus when the larynx is rocked back and forth between the hands as the thyroid cartilage and cricoid cartilage rub against each other. Loss of this crepitus may suggest a mass lesion is present and should increase the suspicion for cancer.

Using Advanced Tools: X-ray: Soft tissue x-ray of the anterior neck may reveal fracture of hyoid bone or cartilage of the larynx in trauma.

Assessment: Differential Diagnosis

Acute laryngitis: Ascending or descending viral infection (with risk of bacterial superinfection) characterized by pain, dryness or "rough" feeling in larynx brought on by dry cough and/or habitual throat clearing. Hoarseness may progress to painful inability to speak (aphonia). Noninfectious causes include dry and dusty air, gases and caustic vapors, and repeated coughing attacks. Recovery should be within 3 weeks of onset.

Vocal abuse: Hoarseness (from vocal exertion) that is most pronounced in the evening and is accompanied by frequent throat clearing. Can lead to abnormal speech patterns. Frequently found in drill sergeants, teachers, workers in loud environments, mothers, and little boys.

Vocal nodules: Benign, painless growths on vocal cords secondary to chronic vocal cord abuse (yelling, loud singing, singing or speaking outside normal frequency range). Symptoms include hoarseness, habitual throat clearing and foreign body sensation. Limits ability to sing softly or reach high tones.

Trauma: The larynx may be injured by external trauma (vehicle accident, gunshot, stab wound, sports injury) or by damage to internal surfaces (physical or chemical agents such as endotracheal tube, foreign body, caustic substance). Pain and hoarseness are typical symptoms, and patient may develop hemoptysis. Watch for impending loss of airway.

Tumors: Benign tumors: Produce a uniform symptom complex consisting of foreign body sensation, habitual throat clearing, cough, hoarseness (occasionally progressing to aphonia) and possible dyspnea (depending on size and location). These tumors include papillomas, polyps, and granulomas. Cancers: The most common warning signs, in order of frequency, are hoarseness, throat clearing, cough, hemoptysis, dyspnea, pain and difficulty swallowing. Pain is generally a late symptom signifying perichondritis (infection of membrane surrounding cartilage). Depending on the tumor location, metastasis to lymph nodes may occur early, late or not at all.

GERD: Very common cause of hoarseness usually, but not always, accompanied with signs of heartburn, indigestion, foreign body sensation in the throat and occasional sour taste. Usually worse in AM.

Chronic rhinitis: Chronic drainage, clear or purulent, can lead to chronic throat irritation and hoarseness. May be accompanied by sneezing, nasal congestion, facial pain, or pressure.

Plan:

Treatment

Acute laryngitis: Supportive measures, including hydration, humidity, throat lozenges and vocal rest, are appropriate. When bacterial superinfection is suspected (fever, purulent discharge), use **amoxicillin** 250–500mg po tid x 7-10 days or **erythromycin** 250mg po qid (for PCN allergic patients) x 7-10 days. All cases should improve greatly within 3 weeks. Use steroids if there is airway swelling with risk of possible loss of airway (or speaker must use voice for pressing engagement). **Prednisone** 60mg po qd x 5 days is tolerable for most patients without withdrawal effects.

Chronic laryngitis: Try to remove irritants, fumes, alcohol, resolve sinusitis, and possibly empirically treat for GERD

Vocal abuse: Vocal rest is essential. Greatly limit speech and ban whispering, which is a greater strain than plain speech. Soldiers may need varying amounts of rest with a minimum of 24-48 hours. Some may need to be reassigned, eg, drill instructors.

Vocal nodule: Vocal rest may be helpful, pending referral to a speech therapist for retraining.

Trauma: Hoarseness after laryngeal trauma requires a thorough evaluation and examination. Look for signs of impending airway loss such as stridor, drooling, anxiety, and sitting with a forward lean to maximize the airway patency. Never force the patient to lie down since this may precipitate airway compromise. Never send a patient out without first securing the airway, by either endotracheal intubation or a surgical airway (cricothyroidotomy or tracheostomy). If the trauma is significant, it may be safer to start with a surgical airway rather than risk the loss of airway with a difficult intubation complicated by swelling and blood.

Tumors: Refer to ENT surgeon quickly. Tumors can cause sudden loss of airway when they occlude the larynx.

GERD: Use **aluminum hydroxide gel** 30cc po q hs and/or **ranitidine** 150mg po bid or **famotidine** 20mg po q PM and elevate the head of the bed at night to keep acid in stomach.

Chronic rhinitis: See Part 3: General Symptoms: ENT Problems: Rhinitis/Rhinorrhea

Patient Education

General: Hoarseness is a common complication of upper respiratory viral illness. It should resolve within 3 weeks.

Activity: Vocal rest during acute phase of illness and avoid additional vocal abuse.

No Improvement/Deterioration: Return to clinic if symptoms fail to resolve after 3 weeks. Increasing pain, difficulty swallowing or shortness of breath need to be reported immediately.

Follow-up Actions

Evacuation/Consultation Criteria: Evacuate any patient with a strong suspicion of a tumor, malignancy, or worsening airway. Be careful not to send out unstable airway patients; always secure the airway first in patients with signs of impending airway loss or compromise. The airway may be secured with either endotracheal intubation or a surgical airway like cricothyroidotomy.

ENT Problems: Neck Masses
COL Karla Hansen, MC, USA

Introduction: Neck masses may be congenital, or the result of an infection or neoplastic disease (benign or malignant). Neoplastic disease should be suspected if the mass has been slowly increasing in size, especially if associated with symptoms of painful or difficulty swallowing, hoarseness, weight loss or night sweats. The possibility of airway obstruction must always be considered especially if acute onset of stridor, noisy breathing, dyspnea, swallowing difficulties (such as drooling) or obvious expansion is noted. **Geographic Associations:** Certain causes of lymph node enlargement (adenopathy) are more common in specific geographical areas (eg, tuberculosis and HIV are more common in Asia and Africa). **Risk Factors:** Exposure to individuals with TB or exposure to animals such as cats, rodents or birds may increase risk of contracting zoonoses that can cause lymphadenopathy of the neck. Smoking and alcohol consumption are risk factors for the development of upper aerodigestive tract cancers, including cancer of the mouth, throat, tongue, and esophagus. Patients under the age of 40 tend to have infectious disease processes, while patients over the age of 40 should be strongly suspected to have cancer as a cause for their neck mass. Most neck masses will require referral for definitive diagnosis. Patients with neck masses that do not resolve after 2 weeks, increasing in size or are associated with malignancy need to be evacuated.

Subjective: **Symptoms**

Acute (1 day - 1 week): Suggests infection: pain, sore throat, fever/chills, painful or difficulty swallowing, tenderness.

Sub-Acute (1 week - 1 month): Suggests chronic infection: +/- fevers/chills, +/- pain.

Chronic (>1 month): Suggests neoplasm: night sweats, +/- pain, weight loss, painful or difficulty swallowing, hoarseness.

Focused History: *How long has the mass been present?* (Recent onset of days to a few weeks suggests infectious origin.) *Have you had an upper respiratory tract infection recently?* (Congenital, cystic masses can fill with fluid in association with a viral infection or RUI. Reactive lymph nodes may be present after a URI.) *Do you have fevers or chills?* (suggests infection) *Does the mass hurt?* (suggests infection) *Do you have night sweats?* (suggestive of cancer, especially lymphoma) *Have you lost weight? How much?* (Significant weight loss tends to occur with cancer.) *Do you have painful and/or difficulty swallowing?* (suggests infection or neoplasm) *Can you swallow your own spit?* (If not, there is a strong potential for airway compromise.) *Are you short of breath?* (increased potential for airway obstruction) *Are you able to drink?* (Poor oral intake may lead to dehydration.)

Objective: **Signs**

Using Basic Tools: Inspection: Inspect the neck for evidence of trauma, swelling, redness, and compare to the other side for symmetry. Do a complete head and neck exam, evaluating the structures of the mouth, scalp, nose, skin, and throat. Note any lesions or ulcerations, as well as location and symmetry of structures. Look for signs of drainage. See Objective: Signs: Location: Lymph Node Region: Area Drained. Palpation: Gently palpate the mass to determine if it is a single mass, single node, multiple nodes or generalized inflammation. Check the mobility of the mass to determine whether it is solid or cystic. Check the consistency (hard, firm, soft, fluctuant). Note any tenderness or pain with palpation. Be sure to measure the diameter (use a ruler for precision) of the mass to monitor changes in the size of the mass during the clinical course.

Location: Lymph Node Region: Area Drained

Mandibular angle: Mouth, tonsils, teeth, tongue, pharynx

Retroauricular: External ear canal, ear temporal scalp

Preauricular: Anterior scalp, external ear, lateral eyelid, upper face, parotid gland

Submaxillary/submental: Lower half of face, lips, teeth, nose, salivary glands

Nuchal: Skin of head and occiput

Superior cervical chain: Entire head and upper neck region

Inferior cervical chain: Lower neck, axilla, arm, chest

Posterior cervical: Nasopharynx

Assessment: **Differential Diagnosis**

Thyroglossal duct cyst: A tense, painless cystic mass with smooth contour located in the midline at the level of the hyoid (may occur as low as the jugular fossa), caused by persistent remnant of the embryonic thyroglossal duct. The cyst is often not noticed until it distends with debris after an upper respiratory infection or head cold. Noting that the mass follows the movements of the hyoid bone on swallowing and tongue protrusion can make the diagnosis. Lymph nodes will not move with swallowing or protrusion of the tongue.

Branchial cleft cyst: This congenital cyst usually presents in early childhood or early adulthood because of inflammatory reaction after an upper respiratory infection. Most are located laterally, anterior to the sternocleidomastoid muscle at the level of the hyoid or anterior to the tragus, but they can be at any level in the neck. They tend to be soft, cystic and non-tender. They may rarely become secondarily infected and demonstrate tenderness, redness or purulent drainage.

Tumor (neoplasm): Soft tissue neoplasms are rare in the neck, but neck nodes may frequently enlarge from tumor metastasis or lymphomas.

a. **Metastatic disease:** Upper aerodigestive tract cancers of the mouth, throat, pharynx, larynx and esophagus frequently present as neck masses (metastatic nodes). There is usually a strong history of tobacco and alcohol use in the patient. Patients may have other symptoms specific to the location of their disease (pain on swallowing, difficulty swallowing, and hoarseness, spitting or coughing up blood). The nodes can be single or multiple, are usually firm, nodular, non-tender and initially mobile (but become fixed).

b. **Lymphoma:** Single or multiple nodes that are usually enlarged, non-tender, painless and firm or rubbery feeling. The patient is usually between ages 10-35 or older than 50. Nonspecific systemic signs include fatigue, an undulant fever that rises slowly to moderate levels with afebrile intervals, night sweats, weight loss, and pruritus. Later there is significant malaise. The patient may also have axillary or groin lymph node enlargement.

Goiter: Enlarged thyroid is a common condition throughout the world and can be severe in 3rd world countries where medical care may not be readily available. Slow growth can lead to insidious development of symptoms; usually very visible unless goiter is completely substernal; dyspnea with position change or lying down; rare from wheezing; 10-30% cough, few dysphagia, and hoarseness.

Infectious adenopathy: Many infectious diseases cause enlargement of the lymph nodes. Only a few of the more common ones are listed.

a. **Viral upper respiratory tract infection:** Common cause of cervical node enlargement. Symptoms should subside in 7-10 days. Enlarged nodes should resolve in no more than 3 weeks from a cold.

b. **Bacterial cervical adenitis:** Most commonly associated with infection by Group A Beta-hemolytic *Streptococcus* or *Staphylococcus aureus*. The node feels firm to fluctuant and very tender. The skin over it may be inflamed and red. The patient may have fevers and elevated white cell count. The node enlargement should resolve within 2-3 weeks of treatment.

c. **HIV:** AIDS affects the whole body with frequent (40%) manifestations in the head and neck. Symptoms may be very diverse. Adenopathy is usually painless in single, or numerous nodes (more common) that slowly increase in size. There are generalized symptoms of fever, anorexia, muscle/joint pain, diarrhea and weight loss.

d. **Tuberculous lymphadenopathy:** Painless swelling of groups of cervical nodes. Most prevalent in children and adolescents, but increasingly common in the 20-50 age range. The lesions can be solitary or multiple, may be bilateral, small or large, firm or fluctuant and may be associated with fistula formation. If a fistula forms or an I&D procedure is attempted, the patient will develop unrelenting chronic drainage. The adenopathy can be associated with pulmonary TB infection, consuming unpasteurized milk, traveling in Asia or Africa, living among Alaskan natives and recent immigration. Intradermal tuberculin test (PPD) is usually positive.

e. **Other diseases** that may be associated with enlarged lymph nodes:

  Toxoplasmosis: Protozoan parasite usually ingested from inadequately cooked contaminated animal meat or contact with infected cat feces. 50-90% are asymptomatic; cervical adenopathy, sore throat, myalgia, malaise and fevers; decrease over many months; usually resolves spontaneously.

  Cat-Scratch fever: Most common cause of chronic localized adenopathy in children in the US; 90% inoculated into skin or onto mucous membrane by cat scratch or bite. Kittens more likely to transmit; adenopathy near inoculated site with skin inflammation; about 3-12 days after injury; 80% single node; significant number will have oculoglandular syndrome with conjunctivitis, ipsilateral preauricular node; enlarges over 3-4 weeks; 30% are warm, tender, red fevers; usually self limited.

  Tularemia: Regional or generalized adenopathy; most from bite of infected tick, some from deer flies or infected animals or under cooked contaminated animal meat; pharyngeal tularemia has painful exudative tonsillitis and cervical adenopathy, oculoglandular disease; skin may become erythematous; enlarged nodes are tender over months and may suppurate.

  Brucellosis: History of ingestion of non-pasteurized milk or milk product or contact with cattle; nontender adenopathy, fevers, sore throat, arthralgia or arthritis and abdominal pain; 10-20% hepatomegaly.

  Cytomegalovirus (CMV): Commonly seen in babies 1-3 months and toddlers; mononucleosis-like sydrome with malaise, fevers, adenopathy; rarely produces pharyngitis or tonsillitis; splenomegaly may occur; usually self-limited and uncomplicated.

  Mucocutaneous lymph node syndrome (Kawasaki): Exclusively in children, usually under 4 years old; non-purulent conjunctivitis, erythema of the lips, tongue, oral cavity, polymorphous erythematous rash, indurative edema and erythema of hands and feet; unilateral or bilateral cervical adenopathy; diagnosis most include 5 or more days of significant fevers and at least 4 other findings; cervical node in only 50-70%; vasculitic syndrome involving medium size coronary vessels; 1% mortality.

  Epstein-Barr virus: Common cause of acute to chronic adenopathy throughout childhood; mononucleosis; fever, malaise, fatigue, worsening sore throat, enlarged discrete, painless to moderately tender anterior and posterior cervical nodes, 1-3 cm; exudative tonsillitis in 60%; 50-80% enlarged spleen.

  Other possibilities: Leishmaniasis, actinomycosis, sarcoid, mumps, measles, cytomegalovirus

Deep neck infection: The neck has several potential spaces that can become infected, causing pain or difficulty swallowing, fevers, chills and potential airway compromise secondary to swelling. These patients tend to be very ill on presentation

a. **Ludwig's angina:** A cellulitis process involving the oral floor above the hyoid. The submental area is hard, bulging and extremely tender with tense, reddened skin. The condition may progress at any time to a deep compartment abscess or descending cervical cellulitis. The patient can have severe airway compromise secondary to swelling, with the tongue being pushed backward to occlude the airway. This condition is frequently associated with dental work or dental infection. This is an airway emergency with pending airway collapse.

b. **Compartment abscess:** This infection is an abscess in one of the fascial compartments of the neck, usually originating in the mouth or pharynx (tonsillitis, dental abscess, or injury) or can result from lymphadenitis. The patient often holds the head and neck in a guarded position and trismus (inability to open the mouth > ~3cm) may occur. There is constant and severe pain, painful swallowing, swelling of the floor and/or one side of the neck with exquisite tenderness, and possible circumscribed redness and tension of the overlying skin. High fever and pronounced left shift in the WBC are also typical. In later stages, there may be chills, septic fever and rapid deterioration reflecting thrombophlebitis or general sepsis.

c. **Others:** Benign and malignant masses of the salivary glands, parathyroid or thyroid glands; expanding hematomas (traumatic); epidermal inclusion cysts; lipomas; calcified carotid bodies (junction of internal and external carotid arteries).

Plan:

Treatment: Patients may be sitting up and leaning forward to maximize their airway. Do not force the patient to lie back down as this may occlude the airway.

1. Thyroglossal duct cyst: If inflamed and infected, treat with oral antibiotic such as **amoxicillin/clavulanate** 500mg po bid x 7-10 days. When possible, refer for surgical removal.

2. Branchial cleft cyst: If infected, treat with antibiotics like **amoxicillin/clavulanate** 500-875mg po bid x 10 days or **clindamycin** 300mg po qid x 7-10 days. If cyst is painfully swollen, decompress it with a 20-22 gauge needle until the patient can be referred for surgery. Avoid incision as this may lead to scarring and potential damage to underlying structures.

3. Tumors - metastatic disease or lymphoma: evacuate ASAP.

4. Infections
   a. Viral: Supportive care, keep well hydrated.
   b. Bacterial: **Amoxicillin/clavulanate** 500-875mg po bid x 10 days or **clindamycin** 900mg IV q8h until tolerating po, then change to oral regimen. If node becomes very fluctuant, it may need to be drained with an 18-20 gauge needle. If the neck mass persists after a complete course of antibiotics, make a referral for further evaluation.
   c. HIV: *See Part 5: Specialty Areas: Chapter 12: Viral Infections: Human Immunodeficiency Virus*
   d. Others: *See Part 5: Specialty Areas: Chapter 12* for treatment of toxoplasmosis, tularemia, brucellosis, cytomegalovirus, cat scratch disease (Bartonellosis). Kawasaki's: usually self limited but may need IV immune globulin therapy; refer out.

5. Deep neck infection: When this diagnosis is suspected, the patient is usually very ill. Start IV access. The patient will need high dose antibiotics like **clindamycin** 900mg IV q8h or **cefuroxime** 1.5g, and **metronidazole** 1g IV Piggy Back (IVPB) loading dose followed by 500mg q6h x 5-7 days or until improved and can change over to po antibiotics to complete 10 day regimen. Consider given **dexamethasone** 10mg IV (over 1 min or less) q8h x 3 doses. The patient may need to have the airway secured by either endotracheal intubation or by a surgical airway if showing signs of drooling or stridor. If the patient has severe swelling, it is safer to do a surgical airway under local anesthesia while the patient is maintaining his own airway. These patients will need further evaluation for potential surgical drainage of their infection.

6. Others: See appropriate topic on the electronic version.

Patient Education

General: No neck mass is routine. They always need medical evaluation. Neck masses associated with head colds should completely resolve within two weeks.

Activity: Light if acutely ill

Medications: Antibiotics can cause GI upset. Complete all medication unless directed otherwise. Report any severe side effects or diarrhea

No Improvement/Deterioration: Return to the clinic immediately for any signs of difficulty breathing, difficulty swallowing, drooling of secretions, stridor or noisy breathing, or appearance of air hunger or distress.

Follow-up Actions

Return Evaluation: All neck masses need to be re-evaluated. For non-acute, smaller masses, a time interval of 2 weeks is appropriate. If no improvement, refer to a surgeon. If the mass has started to decrease in size, it may be followed for another 2 weeks.

Evacuation/Consultation Criteria: Patients with neck masses that do not resolve after 2 weeks, are increasing in size or are associated with malignancy need to be evacuated. Make timely referral for masses that increase in size or associated with symptoms suggestive of malignancy. Patients with possible airway obstructions should have a secure airway either by intubation or surgical airway prior to evacuation.

ENT Problems: Control of Persistent Nosebleed (Epistaxis)

COL Karla Hansen, MC, USA

What: Control of severe and/or persistent bleeding from the nose using various techniques, including cautery and packing. Most cases of nosebleed (epistaxis) in young patients are from trauma or spontaneous rupture of superficial blood vessels located in the anterior portion of the septum. Bleeding disorders are rare but may present as recurrent bouts of epistaxis. Older patients may have epistaxis during periods of hypertension or from breathing dry air. The septum must be examined for a hematoma after trauma as a hematoma in nasal septum can cause necrosis and destruction of nasal cartilage. Use an otoscope to examine the anterior septum for any swollen, soft (palpate with Q-tip), compressible mass consistent with a hematoma (*see What To Do: Step 6: Drain a hematoma*). Posterior bleeding originates from the junction of the hard and soft palate, from beneath the inferior turbinate, from the nasopharynx or from the orifice of the posterior choana. These sources cannot be reached from an anterior approach.

When: If a nosebleed persists for more than 10-15 minutes (or fills a teacup) despite adequate compression.

What You Need: A nasal speculum (or otoscope with large speculum), cotton-tipped applicators (Q-tips) if available, bayonet forceps (if available), silver nitrate sticks, ½" by 72" petroleum gauze (two) or alternates: Surgicel (oxidized regenerated cellulose), or Oxycel (oxidized cellulose) or Merocel (commercially made nasal sponge), Foley catheter (16 or 18 Fr) with 30cc balloon, or tonsil sponges (large size), umbilical clamp or other small clip, suction (if available), scalpel. A simple feminine hygiene product (tampon) can also be used. While this is larger than optimal, it can be an adequate substitute. The tampon may be cut down in size to fit.

What To Do:

1. Attempt direct pressure control:
   a. Have the patient blow his nose to remove all old clots.
   b. Pinch the nasal soft tissues between thumb and index finger to compress the lateral nasal walls to the septum. (Most anterior nosebleeds arise from the anterior septum.)
   c. Hold pressure for at least 5 minutes.
   d. After releasing pressure, do not blow nose or traumatize with manipulation.
   e. If nose continues to bleed, compress for an additional 10 minutes.
   f. If nose continues to bleed, *see nasal packing (Steps 3, 4, & 5) or cautery (Step 2)*.
2. Cauterize (if the bleeding site is visible):
   a. Have patient vigorously blow his nose to remove all old clots.
   b. Have patient breathe through his mouth during the procedure.
   c. Use light source and nasal speculum (or otoscope with large speculum) and suction if available to maximize visibility.
   d. Apply silver nitrate stick to the site, holding pressure for several seconds. Gently roll the stick at the site. The silver nitrate should be applied for approximately 20 seconds. Only apply silver nitrate to one side of the septal mucosa. Application of silver nitrate to both sides will devascularize the septum, causing a perforation.
3. Apply anterior packing (if the bleeding site CANNOT be seen):
   a. Use a ½ Vaseline gauze impregnated with antibiotic ointment. Alternatively, a small pledget of oxidized cellulose wedged in the bleeding site or commercially made nasal sponge such as Merocel may control epistaxis.
   b. Start by unraveling approximately 8cm of gauze. Keep the very end of the gauze out of the nose, next to the cheek. If placed into the nose, it can become dislodged and the patient may swallow it or choke on it.
   c. Use bayonet forceps to pack the space between the floor of the nose and the inferior turbinate first. Be sure to place packing completely back into the nasal cavity, approximately 6cm. If the packing is just anterior, it may act as a wick and promote bleeding. This packing should be moderately tight. Remember that the nasal cavity should be packed by placing gauze straight back, parallel to the ground, along the nasal floor and not up toward the skull base.
   d. Pack the space between the middle turbinate and the inferior turbinate (which are both lateral structures) and the space between the septum and turbinates.
   e. Leave packing intact for 3-5 days to allow development of mature thrombosis.
   f. Antibiotics (*see step 7*) to mitigate risk of infection.
4. Insert posterior packing with a Foley catheter
   a. Use a Foley catheter with a 30cc balloon to occlude the nasopharynx. Place the catheter along the floor of the nose until the tip is visible in the back of the mouth. Inflate the balloon fully with air, not water, unless air evacuation or flight may occur since balloon would be affected by altitude changes.
   b. Set the catheter by putting traction on it until it is against the posterior choana or posterior part of the nose and wedged in the nasopharynx.
   c. Hold the catheter firmly in place and pack ½ inch gauze into the anterior nose bilaterally as described for an anterior nose bleed.
   d. Clamp the Foley catheter in place by applying the umbilical clamp or other clamp at the level of the nostril. Be sure to provide padding between the clamp and the nose to prevent a pressure sore.
   e. Have patient breathe through mouth.
   f. Packing should be left intact for 72 hours or up to 5 days to allow development of mature thrombosis.
   g. Give prophylactic antibiotics; *see step 7*
   h. Remove packing by deflating Foley catheter and withdrawing through nose.
5. Apply posterior packing with tonsil sponges or gauze
   a. If a Foley catheter is not available, use a pack made of tonsil sponges or gauze large enough to occlude the nasopharynx but not interfere with swallowing.
   b. Attach two heavy silk sutures to the sponge or gauze.
   c. Place a catheter (or other flexible tube) through the nose, grasp it and pull it out the mouth.
   d. Attach one of the sutures to the catheter tip. Keep the other suture outside the mouth.
   e. Pull the catheter and suture back out the nose, then seat the pack firmly into the posterior end of the nasal cavity by pulling the suture. Use a finger or a clamp to get the packing around the soft palate into the nasopharynx.
   f. Secure the one silk suture through the nose by tying it around a small gauze or dental roll in front of the nose.
   g. Tape the other silk suture from the oral cavity next to the cheek.
   h. Pack the anterior nose as described *in step 3*.
   i. Have patient breathe through mouth.
   j. Leave packing intact for 5 days to allow development of mature thrombosis.
   k. Prescribe prophylactic antibiotics; *see step 7*
   l. Remove packing by pulling on the suture through the oral cavity.
6. Drain a hematoma (nasal septum):
   a. First, determine that a hematoma is present (obvious mass in the nasal septum).
   b. Inject approximately 1cc of **lidocaine** (1% with 1:100,000 **epinephrine**) into the septum mucosa on one side of the hematoma.
   c. Make a shallow incision through the septum mucosa approximately 1cc in length. This is easy to do since the hematoma is usually pushing the mucosa out away from the underlying cartilage. Be sure to not incise through the whole septum since this may lead to a perforation.
   d. Now milk the blood clot out by gently applying pressure on both sides of the septum with cotton tip applicators or other soft instruments.

    e. After thoroughly evacuating the clot, pack both sides of the nose using the previous guidelines for anterior packing to prevent reaccumulation of the hematoma.

    f. Remove the packing after 72 hours.

    g. Give patient an oral antibiotic to decrease chances of infection.

7. Antibiotics (to mitigate risk of infection): **Amoxicillin/clavulanate** 875mg po bid or **erythromycin** 250mg po bid or **cephalexin** 250mg po qid for the duration of the packing and a few days after will help prevent nasal and sinus infections. Use of antibiotic may mitigate risk of bacterial infection but is not a treatment for the rare complication of toxic shock syndrome. If the patient demonstrates fever, nausea, vomiting, or diarrhea usually within 24-48 hours of nasal packing, remove the packing and treat for toxic shock syndrome.
See Part 5: Specialty Areas: Chapter 12: Bacterial Infections: Streptococcal Infections, Life-Threatening

What Not To Do:

1. Do not fail to provide adequate pressure by squeezing or packing to control epistaxis.
2. Do not allow the patient to reinjure (pick, scratch, Valsalva, hard blowing) the clotted area and cause recurrent epistaxis. Instruct him to avoid cleaning the nose aggressively, sneeze with his mouth open, not to blow his nose for several days and avoid "clearing the ears" by mouth closing with increased pressure.
3. Do not fail to use antibiotics for those with nasal packing.

ENT Problems: Pharyngitis, Adult

COL Karla Hansen, MC, USA

Introduction: Trauma, viral or bacterial infections, including sinusitis, mononucleosis and peritonsillar abscess can all present with pharyngitis, or sore throat. Viral infection is the most common cause. Supportive care is usually the only treatment necessary. Several potential causes, including life-threatening ones, are discussed in this section. Pharyngitis may be associated with other upper respiratory symptoms. **Seasonal Variation:** Increased incidence during winter or cold season. **Risk Factors:** Prior history of pharyngitis may precipitate recurrent attacks. Lack of immunizations, particularly MMR, diphtheria and HIB, increases risk for serious causes of pharyngitis. For diagnosis and management of pharyngitis in children, *See Part 5: Specialty Areas: Chapter: 15: Most Common Pediatric Diseases: Throat Problems: Pharyngitis.*

Subjective: **Symptoms**

Sore throat, difficult and/or painful swallowing, fevers/chills, cough or malaise. Pain may be referred to the ears.

Focused History: *How long have you had a sore throat?* (tells if this is an acute problem or a chronic one. Acute tends to be infectious/ trauma vs. chronic, especially with other symptoms such as weight loss may indicate a serious condition such as throat cancer.) *Do you have a fever/chills?* (suggests infection) *Have you been around anyone else who is sick?* (suggests contagious infection) *Did your symptoms start after eating/drinking something? What was it?* (rule out caustic ingestion or foreign body) *Are you having difficulty swallowing?* (look for signs of dehydration) *How is your breathing?* (look for signs of impending airway obstruction such as drooling, anxiety, air hunger, or leaning forward)

Objective: **Signs**

Using Basic Tools: Inspection: Look at the oral and pharyngeal mucosa, noting any raw areas, dryness, redness, ulcerations, areas of swelling, pustules, foreign bodies and asymmetry of structures, particularly the tonsils. Inspect the neck for symmetry and midline trachea. Palpation: Identify lymph nodes that may be enlarged or tender. Perform bimanual examination of the oral cavity (1 finger in the mouth and 1 on the skin) to examine the parotid and submandibular glands and floor of the mouth for enlargement and tenderness.

Using Advanced Tools: Labs: CBC/WBC to differentiate viral from bacterial infection (elevated segmented lymphocytes); Mono spot test to rule out mononucleosis (can initially be negative and may need to be repeated a few days later); Rapid Strep Antigen Test; throat culture.

Assessment: **Differential Diagnosis**

Viral pharyngitis: Typical symptoms are raw, dry, burning sensation in throat, frequently with concomitant involvement of the nose, larynx, trachea and bronchi (cough, clear sputum, and temporary hoarseness). Pain may radiate to the ear. The pharynx may be coated with mucus or purulent exudates. Children usually have fevers and frequent anterior and posterior cervical adenopathy. The blood count can show a relative lymphocytosis. Adults usually run a milder course with little malaise but significant throat pain. Tonsils and surrounding tissue are usually involved. Causative agents include influenza and adenoviruses. Respiratory syncytial virus (RSV) is common in young children. Bacterial superinfection may follow.

Acute tonsillitis/strep throat: Acute, burning throat pain and pain on swallowing become severe and usually radiate to the ear. Other symptoms include fever, chills, severe malaise. Tonsils and surrounding areas appear red with yellow stipples or spots typically visible on the tonsils. Cervical lymph nodes at the mandibular angle are swollen and painful. Airway distress and obstruction may be an issue if swelling of the tonsils is severe. Usual cause is group A beta-hemolytic *Streptococcus pyogenes*. *Neisseria gonorrhea* is less frequently seen.

Peritonsillar abscess: Rapidly increasing, typically unilateral throat pain that can become quite severe and usually radiates to the ear. Other symptoms: high fever, malaise, anorexia, eating difficulties, muffled voice, trismus (difficulty opening the mouth), "hot potato voice", drooling and fetid breath. The tonsil and surrounding tissue will be red and bulging on one side. The uvula may be pushed to the unaffected side, with swollen lymph nodes on the affected side. The soft palate will appear full or bulging on the side of the abscess. Peak occurrence is second and fourth decades. *See Part 3: General Symptoms: ENT Problems: Peritonsillar Abscess Needle Aspiration*

Influenza: Important to recognize because it is a treatable pathogen, is readily transmitted, and is important epidemiologically. Distinguishing features of the sore throat, which can accompany influenza compared to viral pharyngitis caused by other viruses, are associated cases in the community (epidemic), fever, and myalgias. *See Part 4: Organ Systems: Chapter 3: Influenza*

Mononucleosis: *See Part 5: Specialty Areas: Chapter 12: Viral Infections: Infectious Mononucleosis*

Epiglottitis: Less frequently in children were HiB vaccinations are given, but increasingly seen in adults. Fulminate clinical course usually develops over 1-6 hours. Symptoms include severe pain on swallowing, fever and rapid deterioration. Some patients develop increasing dyspnea (stridor) due to massive swelling of the epiglottis and must sit upright. Patient may use accessory muscles to breathe and will appear restless. There is no cough, usually little to no change in voice, excessive salivation and possible drooling. Usually caused by *Haemophilus influenzae*. There is great potential for loss of airway, so the patient needs immediate attention. *See Part 4: Organ Systems: Chapter 3: Epiglottitis & Part 5: Specialty Areas: Chapter 15: Serious Pediatric Diseases: Epiglottitis*

Diphtheria: Usually begins with relatively mild sore throat, slight pain on swallowing and moderate fevers (<102°F). The tonsils and pharyngeal mucosa are moderately red and swollen and coated with a thick, grayish-white, adherent membrane that later turns dusky. The extra-tonsillar extent of the confluent membrane distinguishes it from a simple acute tonsillitis. Cervical nodes are markedly swollen, hard and tender. Pulse is rapid. Airway obstruction can occur. Diphtheria is rare but is still endemic in some regions. Cause is infection with *Corynebacterium diphtheriae* transmitted via droplets or contact.

Trauma: Sore throat and difficulty swallowing correlate with an exogenous insult (foreign body or indigestion of toxic, scalding and/or caustic substance). There may be bleeding from the mouth or blood-tinged saliva. Small foreign objects (fish bone fragments, etc.) tend to lodge near the tonsil.

Deep neck infection: *See Part 3: General Symptoms: ENT Problems: Neck Masses*

Plan:

Treatment

1. **Viral pharyngitis:** Supportive measures including hydration, pain management and fever control with **acetaminophen**. Patients with a severe sore throat that limits oral intake may benefit from a one-time dose of **dexamethasone** 10mg IM.

2. **Acute tonsillitis/Strep:** Treatment decreases risk of rheumatic fever, development of peritonsillar abscesses and transmission of disease. Supportive measures, **penicillin V** 500mg po bid x 10 days or **erythromycin** (for penicillin allergic) 250mg po qid x 10 days. Approximately 10% will fail penicillin secondary to beta lactamase production. Use **amoxicillin/clavulanate** 500mg po bid x 10 days for those cases. If suspected gonorrhea, *see Part 5: Specialty Areas: Chapter 11: Urethral Discharge* for treatment guidelines.

3. **Peritonsillar abscess:** Drain abscess (*see Part 3: General Symptoms: ENT Problems: Peritonsillar Abscess Needle Aspiration*) and administer antibiotics as follows: Mildly ill patient and uncomplicated procedure: **amoxicillin/clavulanate potassium** 875mg po bid or 500mg po tid x 10 days or **clindamycin hydrochloride** 150-450mg po q6h x 10 days. Severely ill patient: **clindamycin phosphate** 600-900 mg IV q8h or **penicillin G** 24 million units per day IV by continuous infusion or divided q4-6h + **metronidazole** 1g IV q12h or 1 g IV load, then 0.5g IV q6h. Continue IV until patient afebrile and follow with full 10 day course of either **amoxicillin/clavulanate** po or **clindamycin** po (as above).

4. **Mononucleosis:** *See Part 5: Specialty Areas: Chapter 12: Viral Infections: Infectious Mononucleosis*

5. **Epiglottitis:** *See Part 4: Organ Systems: Chapter 3: Epiglottis & Part 5: Specialty Areas: Chapter 15: Epiglottitis*

6. **Diphtheria:** The treatment of respiratory diphtheria includes administration of diphtheria antitoxin with antibiotic therapy. Adults with known diphtheria or high clinical suspicion of diphtheria should receive **penicillin G** 600,000 units IM q12h (maximum 1.2 million units/day) x 14 days. May switch to **penicillin V potassium** 250mg po qid when patient able to swallow. **Erythromycin** 20 to 25 mg/kg IV q12h x 7-14 days may be used in patients allergic to penicillin. Plus **Diphtheria antitoxin:** Pharyngeal or laryngeal disease of less than 48 hours duration: **Diphtheria antitoxin** 20,000 to 40,000 units IM or IV. Nasopharyngeal lesions: **Diphtheria antitoxin** 40,000 to 60,000 units IM or IV. Extensive disease, disease of greater than 3 days duration, or diffuse neck swelling: **Diphtheria antitoxin** 80,000 to 120,000 units IM or IV. **Note:** Diphtheria antitoxin hyperimmune antiserum, produced in horses, binds and inactivates the diphtheria toxin. Only effective before toxin enters the cell and must be administered early. Is not commercially available in the US. May be obtained from the CDC that also provides telephone consultation for diagnosis and treatment questions; call 1-404-639-2889 and ask to have the person responsible for diphtheria paged. Approximately 10% risk of hypersensitivity and/or serum sickness, so give a scratch test dose of 1:100 dilution. The test dose may be followed by 0.02mL of 1:1000 dilution of antitoxin and then the therapeutic dose. **Epinephrine** should be immediately available to treat anaphylaxis. **Isolation and follow-up:** Respiratory droplet isolation and contact precautions for cutaneous disease. Where available, cultures should be taken at 24-48 hours and 2 weeks following infection to document clearance. Continue isolation until 2 consecutive cultures taken at least 24 hours apart are negative. Natural infection does not induce immunity and patients require diphtheria toxoid immunization during their convalescence. **Close Contacts:** After cultures have been taken, give **penicillin G** 600,000 units IM x 1 dose or **erythromycin** 250mg po qid x 10 days.

7. **Trauma:** If a foreign body (FB) like a small fishbone is visible, attempt to gently remove the object. Grasp and pull the tongue out over the teeth with a gauze pad to improve access, and then remove the FB with forceps or similar instrument. If the object is lodged in the lateral aspect of the oral pharynx, from the tonsil area posterior, it should be left in place. Objects deeply imbedded may damage blood vessels and nerves, so removal may cause significant bleeding or aspiration. Treat with antibiotics as in acute tonsillitis and evacuate the patient. Objects that are piercing the cheek may safely be removed without fear of significant hemorrhage.

8. **Deep neck infection:** *See Part 3: General Symptoms: ENT Problems: Neck Masses.*

Patient Education

General: Most sore throats are simple viral illnesses that need supportive care only. Significant breathing or swallowing problems should be reported ASAP.

Activity: Light activity during acute phase of illness. Patients with mononucleosis need to rest and avoid strenuous activities or contact sports for 6 weeks.

Diet: Consume clear liquids or a soft diet depending on the patient's comfort level.

Medications: Complete all antibiotics to avoid complications such as rheumatic fever (3%) and acute glomerulonephritis (10-15%).

Patients with mononucleosis who are given penicillin, yet have no history of allergy may develop a rash. This is not an allergy.

Prevention and Hygiene: Do not cough/sneeze on others, and wash your hands before visiting to avoid spreading these illnesses.

No Improvement/Deterioration: Report any worsening swallowing difficulties, increased pain or airway problems immediately. Otherwise, return if no improvement after 48 hours.

Wound Care: Apply cold or frozen foods and drinks to peritonsillar abscess area.

Follow-up Actions

Return Evaluation: Ensure airway is patent and secure. Consider alternate antibiotic regimen or evacuation.

Evacuation/Consultation Criteria: If clinical condition suggests risk of obstruction of airway, stabilize airway (endotracheal intubation or cricothyroidotomy) and evacuate.

ENT Problems: Peritonsillar Abscess Needle Aspiration

COL Karla Hansen, MC, USA

What: A method of evacuating a peritonsillar abscess (PTA) to hasten healing and prevent extension of infection.

When: The diagnosis of PTA is reasonably certain (*see Part 3: General Symptoms: ENT Problems:* Pharyngitis, Adult) and the abscess needs to be drained. The simplest, low-risk method to drain the abscess is a needle aspiration (success rate is approximately 90% for one-time aspirations). Procedure is used on cooperative and reliable adults who have the ability to protect their airway, but is not a good choice for children or patients unable to protect their airway. Procedure may need to be repeated (10-20% of patients).

What You Need: A stable bright light source and reliable (not using the medic's hands) means of directing light into the mouth, tongue blades or a flat stick to move tongue out of the way, an assistant to direct light and manipulate tongue blade, topical **lidocaine** or **Hurricane** spray, 1% **lidocaine** with 1:100,000 **epinephrine** (5cc), 22 or other small gauge needle for injection, 18 gauge needle for aspiration (you may use a needle with a catheter tip that has been shortened to help prevent deep neck penetration), suction, basin, or bowl for patient to spit into.

Figure 3-1. Aspiration of Peritonsillar Abscess

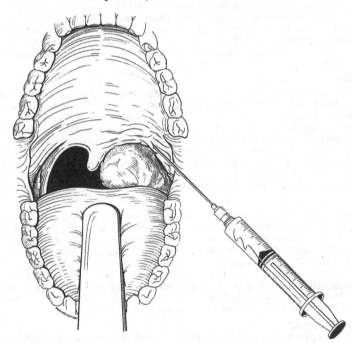

What To Do:
1. The patient will most likely have a significant degree of trismus (inability to open the mouth). To assist with opening, have the patient work at increasing his mouth opening by placing increasing numbers of tongue depressors or other objects between his teeth. This will allow better visibility and room for reaching the posterior oral cavity.
2. Spray the posterior oral cavity and bulging peritonsillar area with topical anesthetic.
3. Wait a few minutes, start by injecting at the superior pole of the tonsillar junction with the soft palate, 2-3cc of local is usually sufficient. This area is usually edematous, since approximately 90% of abscesses occur at this location. Be sure to aspirate back on the syringe prior to injecting the local anesthetic. If blood is aspirated, do not inject the local anesthetic! Withdraw the needle and insert it in a new location. (Injecting local anesthetic into a vein can cause cardiovascular collapse). Patients will usually still have some discomfort because local anesthetic is not as effective in infected tissue.

4. Allow a few minutes for the local anesthetic to work. Slowly advance the 18 gauge needle into the suspected area of abscess. (Again, 80-90% of the abscesses will be located at the superior pole where the tonsil meets the soft palate.) Be sure to aspirate back on the needle as it is advanced. When you see purulence in the syringe, stop advancing the needle and continue to aspirate until no more drainage comes out.

5. If no purulence is aspirated at the superior pole, the abscess may be located at the mid-pole or the inferior pole of the tonsil. Using similar technique as step 4, insert the needle at the mid-pole region between the tonsil (not into it) and the lateral tissue, which is the superior constrictor muscle. Aspirate back on the syringe until purulence is obtained. Make sure that the needle is directed posteriorly and not laterally since the carotid artery and jugular vein are located posterior laterally to the tonsillar fossa.

6. If no purulence is aspirated, follow the same technique inserting the needle at the inferior pole of the tonsil. The abscess must be adequately drained to avoid complications that include extension to the retropharyngeal, deep neck, and posterior mediastinal spaces.

7. Be sure to re-examine the area the next day, (and daily until resolution of infection/symptoms) because a small percentage of abscesses will re-accumulate and need repeat aspiration.

8. Give antibiotics (see Part 3: General Symptoms: ENT Problems: Pharyngitis, Adult) and provide pain control. See Part 8: Procedures: Chapter 30: Pain Assessment and Control

What Not To Do:

1. Do not overuse the topical anesthetic since it may cause seizures if overdosed. One or two sprays per tonsil are usually sufficient.
2. Do not inject the local anesthetic if blood is aspirated back into the syringe. A vascular injection may cause cardiopulmonary collapse.
3. Once the aspiration needle is placed, do not move it excessively or direct it laterally in order to avoid potentially lacerating nearby vessels.

ENT Problems: Rhinitis/Rhinorrhea

COL Karla Hansen, MC, USA

Introduction: Normal mucus drainage is important for maintaining the protective functions of the nasal mucosa. Rhinitis is an inflammation of the nasal mucosa that can be caused by numerous stimuli (upper respiratory infections, immune responses, hormones, drugs, structural problems, metabolic and vascular conditions) resulting in anterior and posterior rhinorrhea (nasal drainage) and obstruction. Pathologic drainage can be unilateral or bilateral, acute, chronic or intermittent and have a quality, consistency, color or odor that differs from normal nasal drainage. It may be characterized as watery or purulent; blood-tinged or fetid. **Seasonal Variation:** More colds with rhinorrhea are seen in wintertime. Seasonal allergies are worse in spring and fall. **Risk Factors:** A history of allergies or sinusitis increases the chance of recurrent rhinitis symptoms.

Subjective: Symptoms

Acute (4-8 days): Acute rhinitis/common cold: Sneezing, nasal congestion, mild fever, marked decrease in sense of smell.
Sub-Acute (seasonal/ months): Allergic rhinitis: Itching of nose/eyes, nasal obstruction, head fullness, decrease in sense of smell.
Chronic (>2 months): Vasomotor rhinitis: Profuse, watery discharge; little discomfort; no pain; normal smell sense.
Focused History: How long have you had a runny nose? (acute versus subacute versus chronic problem) Is the drainage thick and yellow or green? (suggests sinus infection or nasal foreign body) Do you have any pain in your face or in your sinuses? (suggests sinus infection) Do you have environmental allergies? Do your eyes or nose itch? (suggests allergic rhinitis) Are you pregnant? (possible rhinitis secondary to pregnancy or hormone usage) Are you using any nasal sprays or medications? (Overuse of oxymetazoline can cause irritation or rebound symptoms of worsening congestion.) Have you recently had any significant head or nose trauma? (possible fracture with cerebrospinal fluid leak) Is there any possibility of a foreign body?

Objective: Signs

Using Basic Tools: Inspection: Examine the anterior and posterior nasal cavity with an otoscope for any obstruction or foreign body, characteristics of any drainage and appearance of the turbinates. The turbinates can be unremarkable, inflamed, bluish or pale depending on the cause. Check the posterior oral pharynx for drainage, which can be clear, purulent, bloody, thick or thin depending on the cause. Color of discharge may suggest diagnosis (rhinitis may be mixed): Clear watery mucus-like fluid: Allergic rhinitis, vasomotor rhinitis, hormonal rhinitis, rebound rhinitis due to decongestant abuse (rhinitis medicamentosa), cerebrospinal fluid leak. Yellow/green thick mucus: Infectious rhinitis with sinusitis, nasal foreign body (usually unilateral and associated with a foul odor), other upper respiratory infection Blood/blood-tinged mucus: (Usually unilateral): Nosebleed, nasal fracture, nasal foreign body, tumor, cerebrospinal fluid leak. Palpation: Palpate over the sinuses, examining the maxillary sinuses above the cheekbones, the ethmoid sinuses between the eyes and the frontal sinus above the eyebrows. Note if the areas are tender or swollen.

Assessment: Differential Diagnosis

Allergic rhinitis: Seasonal or perennial manifestations after exposure to causative allergens (Type I antigen-antibody reaction). Symptoms include itching and tickling in the nose with a profuse, bilateral, watery discharge that may lead to nasal obstruction. Conjunctivitis/itchy eyes, pharyngitis and malaise may be associated with it. Exam reveals pale or bluish, swollen nasal mucosa (or red during acute attack), profuse watery drainage and possible "allergic shiners" or dark circles under the eyes.
Infectious rhinitis: Yellow discharge is usually associated with the "common cold" or a viral infection, whereas green discharge is more likely due to bacterial infection of the sinuses or around a foreign body. Secondary symptoms such as sore throat may be seen. See Part 4: Organ Systems: Chapter 3: Common Cold (Upper Respiratory Tract Infections); Influenza; Part 3: General Symptoms: ENT Problems: Sinusitis; Pharyngitis, Adult & Part 5: Specialty Areas: Chapter 12: Viral Infections: Adenoviruses.
Vasomotor rhinitis: Profuse, bilateral, watery rhinorrhea without allergic itching. Attacks are usually sudden and can be associated with exposure to triggering agents such as pollution, perfume, and smoke. Sometimes associated with pressure headaches over the sinus areas.

Cerebrospinal fluid (CSF) leak: Leakage of CSF can occur through the nose after a significant head injury or after surgery. The fluid is usually clear, watery or mixed with some blood. The drainage is usually one-sided. The leak is frequently but not always provoked or aggravated by bending or straining, and certain head positions. This dural defect poses a risk of meningitis, so signs of meningeal irritation (headache, light photophobia, and neck stiffness) may be seen.

Hormonal rhinitis: A frequent side effect of pregnancy, but can be seen in puberty and with use of oral contraceptives.

Rhinitis medicamentosa (oxymetazoline abuse): Caused by excessive use of topical nasal decongestants, with profuse rhinitis seen as a rebound phenomenon after stopping medication.

Nasal foreign body (FB): Typically, a unilateral discharge that is initially clear or bloody, but may become purulent if the FB remains over several days.

Plan:

Treatment

Allergic rhinitis: Avoid the antigen, if known. Treat with antihistamines: **diphenhydramine** 25-50mg po tid or low-sedating loratidine 10mg po q day. Combination drugs like **chlorpheniramine maleate/pseudoephedrine** po tid will treat the congestion also. In severe cases, consider steroid burst (prednisone 60mg po q day x 5 days) or taper (burst + 40mg po q day x 5 days, 20mg po q day x 5 days).

Infectious rhinitis: *See Part 4: Organ Systems: Chapter 3: Common Cold (Upper Respiratory Tract Infections); Influenza; Part 3: General Symptoms: ENT Problems: Sinusitis; Pharyngitis, Adult & Part 5: Specialty Areas: Chapter 12: Viral Infections: Adenoviruses*

Vasomotor rhinitis: Avoid irritants. Use steroid nasal sprays such as **beclomethasone** 2 sprays per nostril bid.

Cerebrospinal fluid leak: Elevate the patient's head. Avoid strenuous activity, nose blowing and flying or sudden changes in altitude. Gove stool softener like **docusate sodium** po bid. Give prophylactic **ceftriaxone** 1-2g IV q24h and evacuate.

Hormonal rhinitis: Symptoms will resolve upon delivery, resolution of puberty or change in oral contraception.

Rhinitis medicamentosa (oxymetazoline abuse): Discontinue use in one nostril, then 1-2 weeks later discontinue use in the other nostril while supporting patient with systemic decongestants like **pseudoephedrine** 30mg po tid if no hypertension, or non-addictive steroid: **beclomethasone** 2 sprays in nostril bid. Can use steroid burst such as **prednisone** 60mg/d po x 5 days for severely dependent cases.

Nasal foreign body: Locate FB with otoscope and remove (with bayonet forceps if available). May need decongestant spray (**oxymetazoline**) to reduce inflammation of nasal mucosa and/or control rhinorrhea or bleeding before trying again.

Patient Education

General: Seek treatment for severe or persistent symptoms that interfere with job performance.

Activity: Remain indoors if allergic to pollen or other outdoor allergens.

Medications: Many antihistamines have a sedating side effect. Avoid operation of heavy equipment or other activities that may require full alertness for safe usage decongestants, particularly in older males, may cause urinary retention and inability to void. Decongestants may increase blood pressure.

Prevention and Hygiene: Avoid allergens to help prevent attacks.

No Improvement/Deterioration: Return immediately if other symptoms such as shortness of breath arise.

Follow-up Actions

Return Evaluation: Re-evaluate for severe symptoms. Readjust therapy regimen as necessary.

Evacuation/Consultation Criteria: Evacuate patients with severe symptoms (ie, life-threatening symptoms of SOB or wheezing) that do not response to therapy. Evacuate any patient with a suspicion of a CSF leak, especially in light of a history of trauma or recent surgery to the head, nose or cranium.

ENT Problems: Salivary Gland Disease
COL Karla Hansen, MC, USA

Introduction: Disease processes affecting the salivary gland(s) include bacterial or viral infection, stones, obstruction, tumors (benign and malignant) and numerous systemic diseases such as autoimmune diseases, sarcoidosis, diabetes, allergic reaction, or hypothyroidism. They may cause pain, swelling or disturbances in saliva production, and may be associated with medication. The disease may affect an isolated single gland, all glands or be related to other body systems. The parotid gland is located in front of the ear and blends with facial contour. The submandibular gland is located under the mandible in the submandibular trigone. The sublingual glands lie between the tongue and the oral floor musculature. Most salivary gland diseases cause visible swelling.

Subjective: **Symptoms**

Acute (>1 week): Suggests infection or gland obstruction: pain, swelling, +/- purulent drainage, fevers/chills

Sub-Acute (1 week to 1 month): Suggests obstruction: pain after eating, swelling worse after eating, +/- drainage

Chronic (>one month): Suggests tumor or chronic systemic disease: rarely painful, swelling unchanged w/ eating, no drainage

Focused History: *Have you had this condition before?* (suggests recurrent obstruction) *Is there any drainage or a sour taste in your mouth?* (possible bacterial infection) *Does the swelling come up after eating? Does it slowly go down?* (suggests obstruction pattern) *Are your immunizations up to date?* (possible mumps if no MMR shot) *Do you have any chronic medical conditions like diabetes or hypertension?* (Many medications can cause painless enlargement of the glands over time.) *How long have you had this mass?* (>1 month without infection means neoplasm, either benign or malignant)

Objective: **Signs:**

Using Basic Tools: Inspection: Compare potentially enlarged parotid to the opposite gland by viewing both glands from the posterior aspect. The parotid gland empties into the mouth via Stensen's duct (opposite the second upper molar), while the submandibular gland empties via Wharton's duct on the floor of the mouth just lateral to the frenulum and behind the lower incisors. Examine the oral cavity for any drainage or purulence by gently pushing on the parotid or submandibular gland while examining the duct region. Check for motion and symmetry between the sides of the face. Weakness of the facial nerve (runs through parotid) is a very worrisome sign for malignant tumor. Look at the skin over the glands for redness. Palpation: Perform bimanual palpation of gland tissue (1 finger in the oral cavity and 1 on the skin). Check for gland enlargement, tenderness, mobility or masses. Evaluate whether any mass is solid like a tumor or fluctuant like infection or abscess. Note any stone.

Assessment:
Differential Diagnosis
Acute bacterial sialadenitis (salivary gland inflammation): The parotid is most commonly affected but submandibular gland may have recurrent episodes of infection. Pain is very severe and occurs in waves. The gland is hard, swollen, and warm and the overlying skin may be erythematous. The earlobe may protrude on the affected side. A discharge, usually purulent, cloudy, viscous can be expressed from the punctum of the duct. The patient may have fever. This is a common condition among patients who are debilitated and dehydrated, especially following trauma or surgery. The organism is usually *Staphylococcus aureus*.

Chronic recurrent sialadenitis: Symptoms of recurrent, slightly painful enlargement of the gland, especially after eating. Decreased salivary flow, stone formation, stasis and alteration in composition of saliva usually cause the condition.

Viral sialadenitis (mumps): A common viral disease affecting mostly children from ages 4-10 years. The infection period is 14-21 days and the duration of symptoms is 7-10 days. Bilateral parotid swelling, malaise and trismus characterize the infection. Other organs systems may be affected. Look for symptoms of orchitis, pancreatitis, meningitis or encephalitis.

Sialolithiasis (salivary gland stone): 80% of all salivary gland stones are found in the submandibular glands. The calculi are often composed of hydroxyapatite and are multiple in 25% of cases. About 65% of parotid calculi are radiolucent while 65% of submandibular ones are radiopaque. This condition is most common in middle-aged men and is characterized by pain and swelling of the affected area which worsens during mealtime.

Xerostomia (severe dry mouth): Numerous causes including medications, working in a hot, dusty environment and autoimmune disorders. Dry mouth associated with dry eyes may be Sjogren's syndrome.

Tumors: Salivary tissue can manifest both benign and malignant tumors. They occur equally in men and women. The parotid gland is the most common site (73%) for all salivary tumors, followed by the minor salivary tissue (14%) and the submandibular gland (11%). The incidence of malignancy or cancer in those tumors is roughly 20% of parotid tumors, 45% of submandibular gland tumors and 75-80% of minor salivary tumors.

Submandibular odontogenic (tooth-related infection): *See Part 5: Specialty Areas: Chapter 10: Oral and Dental Problems*

Plan:
Treatment
Acute bacterial sialadenitis: Rehydration, warm compresses, antibiotics such as **amoxicillin/clavulanate** 500mg or 875mg po bid x 7-10 days or **clindamycin** 900mg IV q8h initially until patient is able to tolerate oral antibiotics. Sucking on sour candies or lemons will help stimulate saliva formation to expel infection from the gland.

Chronic recurrent sialadenitis: Massage, warm compresses and lemon drops will help drain the gland. Treat with antibiotics (*See Acute bacterial sialadenitis*) if associated with purulent drainage, fever, or chills. The gland may need removal for persistent problems.

Viral sialadenitis: Usually self-limited. Treat supportively. Adults who have not had mumps should be vaccinated.

Sialolithiasis: Massage gland toward duct to mobilize and expel stone. Refer those with persistent or recurrent symptoms.

Xerostomia: Treatment is largely supportive. Drink non-caffeinated beverages. Increase oral hygiene to prevent tooth decay. Avoid sugar candies or gums.

Tumors: All salivary lesions, tumors or persistent masses must be referred for specialty evaluation. Never attempt to biopsy nodules or masses that are pre-auricular (parotid) or beneath the level of the platysma muscle, the broad, thin muscle that runs from the fascia of both sides of the neck up to the jaw.

Patient Education
General: Most salivary gland infections will resolve with antibiotics, warm compresses and massage.
Activity: Rest for several days as needed during severe phase of infection.
Diet: Sour food and candies will help move saliva through the gland but may cause some discomfort during usage.
Drink lots of liquids to increase saliva production. Avoid caffeine since it dehydrates the body.
Medications: Any antibiotic can cause some GI upset. Notify a health care provider of severe diarrhea if it occurs.
Prevention and Hygiene: Continue to do good basic oral hygiene, and stay well hydrated.
No Improvement/Deterioration: Return if not improving in 24-48 hours, or for worsening fevers, pain or difficulty swallowing.

Follow-up Actions
Return Evaluation: Repeat exam looking for stone, tumor, or occult obstruction. Consider alternate antibiotic.
Evacuation/Consultation Criteria: Refer patients with significant swallowing difficulty and those who, after initial management, have increasing pain, worsening swallowing, or persistent fevers.

ENT Problems: Sinusitis
COL Karla Hansen, MC, USA

Introduction: Sinusitis is a symptomatic upper respiratory tract infection (RTI) usually caused by bacteria. It is associated with symptoms lasting longer than 10 days, including purulent nasal drainage, nasal congestion, fever, headache, facial pain or pressure, pain between the eyes or dental pain. The patient will frequently complain of sore throat or cough secondary to post-nasal drip. Patient may develop respiratory complications or asthma exacerbation with wheezing, shortness of breath, or coughing. **Seasonal Variation:** May see a seasonal increase in wintertime secondary to a viral illness (such as a cold) progressing into sinusitis, or a slight increase in springtime due to high levels of plant allergens. **Risk Factors:** Patients with other respiratory tract diseases, such as asthma or cystic fibrosis, are predisposed to sinus infection. Allergies may increase risk of sinusitis secondary to inflammation in the nasal passage and sinuses. Smoking may increase risk secondary to impaired ciliary action in the sinuses.

Subjective: Symptoms

Acute (10-21 days): Tooth pain, fever, sore throat, nasal discharge, facial/sinus pain, persistent ear infection

Sub-Acute (3 weeks to 12 weeks): Tooth pain, sore throat, nasal discharge, facial/ sinus pain or pressure

Chronic (>12 weeks): Similar symptoms, +/- nasal discharge

All Stages: Nasal congestion, headache, cough, face pain and fatigue

Focused History: *Are your symptoms worse than your usual head cold?* (Severe symptoms or fever may need to be treated before 10 days.) *Have you had this same illness recently?* (may indicate a recurrent problem and need for prolonged medical therapy) *Do you have pain in the mid-face?* (may indicate maxillary sinus disease) *Do you have pain behind your eyes?* (consistent with ethmoid sinus disease) *Do you have any double vision?* (may indicate a complicated sinusitis that requires immediate surgical attention) *Do you have any photophobia, severe headache or stiff neck?* (may indicate central nervous system complications indicating immediate surgical referral)

Objective: Signs

Using Basic Tools: Inspection: **Acute:** Purulent nasal drainage in nose or posterior oral cavity, inflamed turbinates in nose, foul odor to breath. **Sub-Acute:** Same as acute signs **Chronic:** Same as acute signs. Palpation: **Acute:** Facial tenderness, maxilla tender to palpation **Sub-Acute:** Same as acute signs.

Assessment:

Differential Diagnosis

Viral upper RTI or common cold: Similar symptoms but short duration; very common; no sinus tenderness. *See Part 4: Organ Systems: Chapter 3: Common Cold (Upper Respiratory Tract Infections)*

Pharyngitis: Similar symptoms, including marked pain in throat but no sinus tenderness. *See Part 3: General Symptoms: ENT Problems: Sinusitis & Pharyngitis, Adult*

Sinus barotrauma from flight, dive, or altitude change: Sudden, lancinating pain in sinus region during or after exposure to pressure gradient. Mainly effects fliers, divers and parachutists. Patient will have a history of recent flight or dive or altitude change. *See Part 6: Operational Environment: Chapter 20: Barotrauma: Other (Dental, Sinus, GI, Skin and Face Mask) & Part 6: Operational Environment: Chapter 21: Barosinusitis*

Trauma: Severe pain with recent history of trauma. Patient will have external soft tissue swelling, bruising and possible fracture.

Dental decay (cavity) or infection: Nerves from the upper teeth run through the floor of the maxillary sinus, so inflammation of either teeth or sinus is often confused as pain in the other. Swelling over the cheek is usually secondary to a dental abscess and not sinusitis. *See Part 5: Specialty Areas: Chapter 10: Oral and Dental Problems*

Trigeminal neuralgia: Severe, transient pain in distribution of any branch of cranial nerve V, which may include cheek or forehead (rare). No discharge, fever or other infectious symptoms are present. *See Part 4: Organ Systems: Chapter 5: Trigeminal Neuralgia*

Rhinitis: Nasal discharge that may not be purulent and typically not associated with sinus tenderness. May be secondary to allergies, hormone, medications, irritants, metabolic disease, or pregnancy. *See Part 3: General Symptoms: ENT Problems: Rhinitis/Rhinorrhea*

Plan:

Treatment: More than 60% of sinus infections will resolve even without antibiotic treatment

1. Give antibiotics for 10-14 days for acute or sub-acute cases: **amoxicillin** 250mg po tid or **amoxicillin/clavulanate** 500mg po bid, or **trimethoprim/sulfamethoxazole DS** po bid. If penicillin allergic, use **erythromycin** 250mg po qid, or **trimethoprim/ sulfamethoxazole DS** one tablet po bid.
2. Oral decongestants like **pseudoephedrine** 30-60mg tid to qid provide relief from pressure symptoms, but may thicken mucus and slow clearance of the infection. Avoid in older adults (can cause urinary retention) and in hypertensives (can raise blood pressure).
3. Simple remedies may help to clear thick secretions, shrink mucosa and relive pressure: rinse out nose with salt-water solution of 1-teaspoon salt in a liter of water with a pinch of baking soda; or breathe warm steam in shower or over a tea kettle.
4. Chronic cases or those that recur shortly after treatment need re-treatment for 21-30 days: **amoxicillin/clavulanate** 500mg po bid or **cefuroxime** 250-500mg po bid or **trimethoprim/sulfamethoxazole DS** 1 po bid. A short course of **prednisone** 60mg po q day x 5 days will decrease mucosal swelling, allowing sinus drainage.

Patient Education

General: Most infections will resolve without treatment. Severe symptoms may indicate a serious infection. Report them ASAP.

Activity: Light activity for a few days may help with recovery

Medications: Prolonged antibiotic use may cause diarrhea, especially life threatening pseudomembranous colitis from Clostridium difficile overgrowth. Severe, crampy diarrhea should be reported to the healthcare provider ASAP.

No Improvement/Deterioration: Return for persistent or worsening symptoms, including headache or severe pain despite appropriate antibiotic treatment, mental status changes, persistent high fever, signs of orbital complications such as edema around the eye, inability to move eye, or sudden changes in vision.

Follow-up Actions

Return Evaluation: Examine for recurrent or chronic sinusitis.

Evacuation/Consultation Criteria: Rapidly evacuate all cases with complications of infection, including mental status changes, signs of meningitis, or changes in eye movement or vision (*see Part 4: Organ Systems: Chapter 5: Meningitis*) and start treatment if evacuation is delayed

Note: Complications are rare in this day of effective antibiotics, but when they do occur, patients can have a poor outcome. Therefore, when a patient deteriorates or a severe complication begins to develop, initiate either **ceftriaxone** 1-2g IV/IM q8h or **cefuroxime** 1.5g IV q8h. If no significant improvement after 24 hours, evacuate immediately.

Eye Problems: Acute Red Eye Without Trauma
LTC Scott D. Barnes, MC, USA

Introduction: The complaint of "red eye" is common and the differential diagnosis is large. If vision is unaffected, there is no corneal opacity, no photophobia, no evidence of pus (hypopyon) or blood (hyphema) in the anterior chamber, the condition will likely be able to be managed in the field. Unilateral red eye with nausea and vomiting suggests acute angle-closure glaucoma; severe ocular pain, visual deficit, photophobia, hypopyon, or hyphema suggests uveitis/iritis. Suspicion of herpes is an indication for expedited referral to an ophthalmologist. True laser eye injuries (almost always only from looking directly into "friendly" range finders rather than offensive weapons) rarely give any redness. If red eye is associated with trauma, *see Part 3: General Symptoms: Eye Problems:* Eye Injury.

Subjective: Symptoms
Redness, discharge, foreign-body sensation (especially in chemical injuries), eye pain, dry eye, photophobia (including sensitivity to light), loss of vision, nausea and vomiting (if the intraocular pressure [IOP] rises suddenly), possibly fever.

Focused History: *Has your vision changed?* (suggests abnormality in anterior segment) Quality of pain: *Is the pain sharp or dull?* (sharp often cornea etiology; dull more iritis, scleritis, glaucoma) *Is your eye sensitive to light?* (Photophobia points toward iritis/uveitis, less likely cornea.) *Is there any discharge?* (Stringy mucus suggests viral conjunctivitis; purulent suggests bacterial.) Duration of pain: *Was the onset of symptoms sudden, or over hours/days?* (Sudden onset is typically corneal; gradual onset indicates inflammatory processes such as iritis.)

Pearl: *Does the patient notice a relief with one drop of topical anesthesia?* (If so, this generally indicates corneal or conjunctival disease.) *Does the patient notice pain in the affected eye when light is shined in the unaffected eye (consensual photophobia)?* (This is a main sign of ocular inflammation, especially uveitis.)

Objective: Signs
Using Basic Tools: Vital signs: Fever may indicate systemic infection. Pupil exam: Irregular pupil may indicate scarring from iritis; consensual photophobia-uveitis. Mid-dilated, fixed pupil may indicate acute glaucoma. Flashlight: Look for injected conjunctival vessels: perilimbal (cornea-sclera junction) injection indicates uveitis/iritis; diffuse injection indicates infection or corneal disease. Look for discharge: mucoid discharge-viral, purulent-bacterial. Snellen chart (if available): Decreased visual acuity to between 20/40 and 20/100. Decreased vision indicates abnormality in anterior segment (cornea, crystalline lens or iris). If a Snellen chart is not available, reading the print in a book or other printed material will provide a rough measure of visual acuity.

Using Advanced Tools: Fluorescein strip and UV light: Disrupted epithelium (abrasion, infection, chemical injury) allows bright fluorescence in affected area.

Assessment: Differential Diagnosis
Acute angle-closure glaucoma: Age over 40; decrease in visual acuity; history of previous episodes of eye pain; nausea/vomiting usually present; fixed, mid-dilated pupil.

Scleritis: Inflammation of the sclera (white of the eye) may appear similar to episcleritis but more severe; centered on "wall" of the eye. History of previous episodes; significant discomfort; associated systemic disorders.

Uveitis/iritis (linings inside eye): Consensual photophobia usually present; deep, dull pain not relieved by tetracaine; often associated with systemic inflammatory disorders

Herpes simplex keratitis: Unilateral viral process; dendritic (branching line) figure on fluorescein staining; no trauma; often a history of previous episodes or "cold sores."

Dry eye: Usually bilateral and may result in secondary tearing; history of previous episodes; occurs in dry environments.

Subconjunctival hemorrhage: Painless bleeding around the "white" of the eye, often seen with coughing, vomiting, or Valsalva; "bruise" of the eye. Needs no treatment.

Conjunctivitis (pink eye): Acute onset; 95% are viral usually starting unilateral but quickly moving to both eyes; watery, mucoid discharge in viral cases, purulent in the rare bacterial cases.

Blepharitis (inflamed lid margin): Chronic recurrent eyelid inflammation; more common in older patients; usually bilateral, but one eye may be worse.

Corneal abrasion: Stain on fluorescein exam; underlying cornea is clear; history of foreign object falling or blowing into eye; pain relieved with topical tetracaine.

Corneal ulcer: Stain on fluorescein exam with underlying opaque spot on cornea; leading diagnosis of contact lens wearers with painful red eye; pain relieved with topical tetracaine.

Recurrent corneal erosion: Chronic, repeat abrasions; often upon daily awakening after laser vision correction or after a history of previous corneal trauma; pain relieved with tetracaine.

Ultraviolet keratitis: Bilateral eye pain; sunburned face; maximum intensity several hours or longer after exposure; fluorescein staining typically reveals numerous small dots called superficial punctate keratitis (SPK).

Episcleritis: Benign and self-limited inflammation of the episclera (the lining of the eye between the conjunctiva and the sclera); identified by sectors of redness, no discharge and often a history of previous episodes; discomfort is typically mild or absent.

Conjunctival or corneal foreign body: Identification of the foreign material by penlight

Contact lens overwear syndrome: Increased tearing and discharge, mild pain and decreased vision; consensual photophobia; symptoms are magnified by the presence of contact lenses; may show SPK in fluorescein staining.

Plan:
Treatment
Acute angle-closure glaucoma: Acetazolamide 250mg po qid; emergently evacuate since such elevated IOP may result in permanent damage to the optic nerve in 24 hours.

Scleritis or uveitis/iritis: Prednisolone 1% 1 drop q1h continuously until expedited evacuation; **scopolamine** 0.25% 1 drop bid; if no improvement in 24-48 hours and not yet evacuated, start **prednisone** 80mg po q day until evacuated.

Herpes simplex keratitis: Expedited evacuation; do not use steroids, consider antibiotic ointment qid; patch eye for pain relief.

Dry eye: Artificial tears prn to relieve symptoms; rehydration; sunglasses/goggles for protection.

Subconjunctival hemorrhage: May spread to edge of cornea but will resolve over 1-3 weeks.

Conjunctivitis: 95% are viral and need no treatment other than aggressive handwashing to prevent spread; if uncertain, consider **ciprofloxacin** or **moxifloxacin** ophthalmic 1 drop qid x 7 days.

Blepharitis: Erythromycin or **bacitracin** ophthalmic ointment applied to the lid margins q hs x 3-4 weeks; apply qid for 1 week in more severe cases; warm compresses for 10 minutes bid-qid. Follow by gently wiping away of the inflammatory material on the eyelashes.

Corneal abrasion: Erythromycin or **bacitracin** ophthalmic ointment applied qid for 4 days or until eye is back to normal or ointment with eye patching if pain is significant. If use of an ointment adversely affects mission, you may use any antibiotic drop qid until symptoms resolve. Check eye daily.

Corneal ulcer: Any topical fluoroquinolone (**ciprofloxacin, moxifloxacin**, etc) q hour; if unavailable, any ophthalmic antibiotic applied hourly. Do not patch or use bandage contact lens (BCL). If related to contact lens use (most common), stop wearing and dispose of all opened contacts/solutions and all contact lens cases.

Recurrent corneal erosion: If sure of diagnosis by history, pain is increasing, and unable to evacuate, consider a BCL (not standard of care for medics) to allow completion of mission; otherwise manage with artificial tears (every few hours until symptoms resolve) and erythromycin or bacitracin ophthalmic ointment q3-4h if needed symptoms resolve).

Ultraviolet keratitis: Bacitracin ophthalmic ointment qid until resolution; sunglasses; patch severely affected eyes for comfort; **scopolamine** 1 drop bid and/or systemic analgesia may be required for pain relief; monitor daily until staining resolves to ensure no infection develops.

Episcleritis: Usually resolves without treatment over several weeks; may improve with **ibuprofen** 600-800mg tid-qid; use **prednisolone** 1% drops qid x 3 days if persistent.

Foreign body: (*see Part 3: General Symptoms: Eye Problems: Eye Injury*) May be able to remove with Q-tip after topical **tetracaine** (1-2 drops). Use **erythromycin** or **bacitracin** ophthalmic ointment qid for 1-3 days after removal.

Overwear syndrome: Re-wet contact lens and use sunglasses; if ineffective, remove the contact lenses and use glasses; if significant SPK are present on fluorescein staining, use **ciprofloxacin** or **ofloxacin** 1 drop qid until the SPK have resolved. Do not replace contact lenses until the eye is symptom-free.

Primitive Treatment only for completion of the mission: A mission may be compromised due to the pain of a corneal defect and the elimination of vision from patching the eye. A low power soft contact lens (-0.50 or so) may be used as a bandage to allow vision while the eyelid is kept from rubbing over the damaged cornea. Any ophthalmic antibiotic drop can be used, but must be continued qid while the contact lens is in place for the sake of the mission.

Patient Education

General: Discuss the level of injury with the patient but do not give prognosis in diseases that should be managed at a higher level of care.

Activity: As tolerated

Diet: As tolerated

Prevention and Hygiene: Keep eyes clean. Avoid spreading conjunctivitis to the other eye or other individuals (aggressive handwashing). Contact lens wearers in the wilderness should always carry a pair of glasses that can be worn if contact lens problems arise.

Follow-up Actions

Return Evaluation: Follow patients closely on daily basis for signs of improvement or worsening

Evacuation/Consultation Criteria: Consult with an ophthalmologist if possible prior to using steroids in the eye. Evacuate as indicated in the treatment section. Evacuate any patient not showing improvement within 24-48 hours.

Eye Problems: Acute Vision Loss without Trauma

LTC Scott D. Barnes, MC, USA

Introduction: Many disorders may cause acute visual loss in a non-traumatized eye: migraine, optic neuritis, uveitis (aka iritis), posterior vitreous detachment (PVD), retinal detachment (RD), vitreous hemorrhage, significant high-altitude retinal hemorrhage, central retinal artery occlusion (CRAO), central retinal vein occlusion (CRVO), giant cell arteritis (GCA), and anterior ischemic optic neuropathy. These disorders are difficult to diagnose and treat while deployed. In most cases, all that can be done is to arrange for an expedited evacuation. Initial treatment for uveitis, GCA, and CRAO can begin in the field. Vision loss in one eye, if due to GCA, is often rapidly followed by loss in the other eye if untreated. In addition, GCA has a significant mortality. If vision loss is associated with trauma, *see Part 3: General Symptoms: Eye Problems: Eye Injury*.

Subjective: Symptoms

Sudden versus gradual loss of vision, eye pain, seeing bright spots or "floating" spots, fever, headache, foreign-body sensation, increased sensitivity to light (photophobia), dry eye, jaw pain

Focused History: *Have you lost your central or peripheral vision or noticed a blind spot?* (Blind spots represent areas not receiving visual information due to disease.) *Do you have a history of migraine headache or family history of migraine?* (Migraine is the most frequent cause of transient biocular visual loss (TBVL) in young adults.) *Has the sharpness of your vision decreased?* (optic nerve disease such as optic neuritis or inflammation such as uveitis) *Do you have pain in or behind your eye?* (deep, dull ache often due to inflammatory uveitis or scleritis; pain increasing with movement may be optic neuritis) *Do you notice floating spots, "cobwebs," or "bugs" in your periphery?* (PVDs present this way.) *Do you see "flashing" lights?* (retinal detachments) *Do you feel you have something in your eye?* (irritation or trauma of the cornea or conjunctiva) *Did you have sudden or gradual loss of vision?* (Gradual decreases typically indicate a non-emergent process such as cataract or diabetic retinopathy.) *What makes your vision better?* (Dry eyes will improve with blinking; improvement with squinting suggests a refractive [glasses] problem.) **Pearl:** Any flashing lights or floating spots/cobwebs present for days-weeks must be treated as a possible RD; if present for many weeks/months, a RD is much less likely.

Objective: Signs
Partial or total loss of vision, fever, jaw tenderness, conjunctivitis, photophobia
Using Basic Tools: Handheld visual acuity card (if available): Loss of visual acuity may be seen in any of the conditions. Provides baseline to work from. Reading print in a book can approximate function if no card is available. Flashlight: Look for possible residual metallic foreign body; pupil exam may show afferent papillary defect (optic neuritis) and/or significant pain with light (uveitis). Visual Fields: Defects seen in optic neuropathies, retinal detachment, GCA, others. Color Vision: When comparing something of bright color (red cap of eye drops), optic neuritis often shows a moderate to profound decrease in "brightness" in the affected eye.
Using Advanced Tools: Ophthalmoscope/fundus exam: "Cherry red" spot for CRAO; "blood and thunder" for CRVO. Fluorescein strip and UV/blue light: Observe for stained tissue indicating corneal abrasion

Assessment: Differential Diagnosis
Migraine: Transient biocular visual loss for this classic migraine aura typically lasts 20-30 minutes rarely as long as an hour. *See Part 3: General Symptoms: Headache*
Optic neuritis: Central decrease in vision and a color vision deficit, peripheral neurologic signs of history of such may be present. Mild vision loss may progress to severe loss over several days.
Uveitis (aka iritis): Inflammation of the iris or inner lining of the eye (uvea). It presents with extreme photophobia, various degrees of visual loss, dull/boring pain, and redness surrounding the cornea. Generally associated with systemic disease (rheumatoid arthritis, inflammatory bowel conditions, ankylosing spondylitis)
Posterior vitreous detachment (PVD): Common finding which increases with age. Patient notices floating spots, "cobwebs," or "bugs" in the peripheral vision. Does not usually include loss of vision. These compacted vitreous strands are non-pathologic effects of aging but can occur sooner with some head trauma. Generally of no consequence if present for more than some weeks/months, but can be associated with a retinal detachment if present for only days or weeks.
Vitreous hemorrhage: "Shower" of floaters accompanied by significant loss of vision; floaters represent blood cells casting shadows on the retina after a blood vessel ruptures; occurs in older diabetics, but can occur after significant trauma, Valsalva, and time spent at high altitudes.
Retinal detachment (RD): Painless, gradual loss of vision like a "shade", "veil" or "curtain" being pulled over the eyes. Earlier signs include the above floating spots, especially when accompanied with "flashes" of light.
Central retinal artery occlusion (CRAO): Painless, sudden, generally profound vision loss in one eye often due to a "clot"; can range from a subtle to a more common complete loss; fundus may show a "cherry red spot" due to massive, whitish swelling of the entire retina except for a small red spot in the direct center (macula). Typical patient is over 60 though risk factors of smoking, diabetes, birth control pills, and cardiac disease can affect all ages.
Central retinal vein occlusion (CRVO): Sudden, less profound loss of vision than in CRAO; the massive numbers of retinal hemorrhages mixed with creamy-white edematous retina has been called "blood and thunder."
Giant cell arteritis (GCA; aka temporal arteritis): Gradual to sudden onset of decreased vision with associated temporal headaches, weight loss, jaw pain while chewing, fever, and/or joint pain; should be ruled out in any patient over 55 years of age with any combination of the above symptoms. Patients are very sick as this represents an inflammation of all the body's vessels.
Anterior ischemic optic neuropathy (AION): Sudden decrease in vision affecting the lower half of the visual field in patients up to age 55 years; disruption of the blood flow to the optic nerve
Laser eye injury: The vast majority of laser eye injuries come from directly looking into "friendly" range finders. Fortunately, there are very few offensive lasers used on the battlefield and true "offensive" eye injuries are extremely rare. *See Part 3: General Symptoms: Eye Problems: Laser Injuries*

Plan:
Treatment
Primary:
1. For patients with transient biocular visual loss with well documented history of **migraine**, *see Part 3: General Symptoms: Headache*. A **PVD** does not require immediate treatment. Most of the other diagnoses require fairly urgent evacuation when possible.
2. There is no agreed upon successful treatment for **CRAO** but a field expedient treatment would include a trial of oxygen at the highest inspired fraction achievable combined with digitally massaging the eye to dislodge any potential embolus (**CRAO, CRVO**) as soon as possible; stop measures if no change is noted after several minutes. Lower IOP in CRAO, CRVO, and vitreous hemorrhage with **acetazolamide** 500mg po initially, then 250mg po q6h may help.
3. **Uveitis/Iritis** may be helped with 1% **prednisolone** drops every hour and either homatropine or scopolamine ophthalmic drops bid.
4. If **GCA** is suspected, give **prednisone** 80mg po a day (divided dose) and expedite evacuation.

Patient Education
General: Patient has severe visual dysfunction and needs immediate care to have the best chance for vision recovery.
No Improvement/Deterioration: Return ASAP for evaluation.

Follow-up Actions
Return Evaluation: Evacuate ASAP since the greatest potential to improve symptoms exists within the first 90 minutes after onset and significantly decreases after 24 hours.
Evacuation/Consultation Criteria: Immediate consultation if possible. Evacuate as above.

Eye Problems: Eye Injury

LTC E. Glenn Sanford, MC, USA & MAJ Adam Buchanan, MC, USA

Introduction: Ocular trauma is an important cause of ocular disability. The differential diagnosis is broad and includes blunt, penetrating and perforating injuries to the globe and all contiguous orbital/ocular structures. A disciplined and systematic approach to the evaluation of the ocular trauma patient will help identify injuries. Remember the **ABCs of Ocular Trauma:**

A – Visual **Acuity**
B – **Best** exam of **Both** eyes
C – **Contiguous** Structures
D – **Diagnostic** Imaging
E – **Evaluation** and Management (everything else)

Always treat life-threatening injuries and follow appropriate trauma protocols before addressing ocular injuries.

Subjective: Symptoms

Loss or decreased vision, pain, foreign-body sensation (especially in chemical injuries), sensitivity to light or photophobia (corneal injury or iris injury), double vision, increased tearing or ocular discharge, nausea and vomiting (if the intraocular pressure rises suddenly), red eye, proptotic eye ("bug" eye due to hemorrhage).

Focused History: *Is there a change in your vision? Did something hit you in the eye? Was there an explosion? Were you or someone near you hammering or grinding metal?* (High or even low velocity projectiles can penetrate the eye.) *Were you wearing combat eye protection, glasses or other types of safety glasses? If so, are there any broken fragments, etc?* (Look for "missing pieces" which may have become intraocular foreign bodies.) *Can you move your eyes?* (possible blow out fracture with muscle entrapment) *Were you using chemicals? Did you or someone else flush your eyes?* (can decrease extent of injury) *Are you sickle cell positive?* (can have significant impact on intraocular bleeding and pressure after trauma)

Objective: Signs

Using Basic Tools: Do not palpate a potentially ruptured globe! Vital signs: Ensure the patient is stable first. Visual Acuity: This is the most important "vital sign" for the eye. Check using a near card if available, otherwise determine using field expedient means, (ie, count fingers at 3 feet, able to see light, etc.) Vision decreases with hemorrhage inside the eye, damage to the lens, cornea or retina. Normal vision gives reassurance that there are no major injuries, but significant injury may still be present. External: Look for any obvious signs of injury, laceration or penetration (even small wounds may indicate projectiles which have penetrated the eye.) Lid lacerations (do not forget the possibility of laceration of the underlying eye.) Check for proptosis ("bug eye"); also check the inability to open or close lids, inability to move eye, loss of normal pupillary reaction to light, orbit feels abnormally firm when palpated. Eye: Obvious ruptured globe, massive conjunctival hemorrhage, non-circular (irregular) pupil (the iris will "plug" small holes), deviated (dysconjugate) gaze, inability to move eyes normally, eye drainage, tangential light exam may reveal blood in anterior chamber (hyphema) or infection (pus or hypopyon), internal contents of the eye located outside the eye such as the lens or iris.

Using Advanced Tools: Ophthalmoscope: Retinal (red) reflex, blood in anterior (hyphema) or posterior chamber (inability to see into the back of the eye suggests hemorrhage), visible foreign body; fluorescein strips (only if globe intact), ophthalmic anesthetic (1 drop) if available and UV light: look for corneal abrasion or ulcer. Do not use ultrasound for eyes. Ultrasound machines for general body examinations do not have the higher frequency required to image the shallow structures of the globe. Performing the ultrasound may contaminate an open globe or cause expulsion of intra-ocular contents.

Assessment: Differential Diagnosis

Hyphema: Blood seen in anterior chamber

Orbital fracture: Detected by new onset of double vision or difficulty moving eye. (most commonly restricts up gaze)

Orbital hemorrhage: Suspect with proptosis, loss of eye movement, loss of pupil function, loss of vision, firm/hard orbit. This is a medical emergency!

Occult ruptured globe: Suspect with history of blunt, blast or impaling injury; dark brown tissue exposed at junction of cornea and sclera, distorted pupil, decreased vision, massive conjunctival hemorrhage

Traumatic iritis: Pain, redness and photophobia

Subconjunctival hemorrhage: Bright red area of blood overlying the sclera without bulging

Eyelid laceration: Partial or full-thickness, lid margin or medial/ lateral canthus involved yes or no. Also consider **corneal abrasion** (epithelial defect), **corneal ulcer** (epithelial defect with white around defect and the base of the lesion), **foreign body, obvious ruptured globe**.

Plan:

Treatment

1. Cover all injured eyes with a metal shield or other device to prevent further injury. Do not apply a pressure patch.
2. Do not attempt to remove any impaled foreign objects.
3. Orbital hemorrhage: Immediate treatment is necessary to try and save vision. Perform lateral canthotomy and inferior cantholysis. *See Part 3: General Symptoms: Eye Problems: Lateral Canthotomy and Cantholysis.* Consult ophthalmologist and transport emergently.
4. Obvious or suspected penetration or rupture of the globe: Give **moxifloxacin** 400mg po tablet from combat pill pack if available. Alternative is **cephazolin** 1g IV q8h plus **levofloxacin** 500mg IV daily (or **ciprofloxacin** 200-400mg IV q12h or **moxifloxacin** 400mg po q24h) and evacuate immediately!

5. **Corneal abrasion:**
   a. **Moxifloxacin** 0.5% solution 1 drop qid and **bacitracin** or **erythromycin** ophthalmic ointment at night. Other available fluoroquinolone drops may be substituted (**gatifloxacin, ofloxacin** or **levofloxacin**).
   b. **Scopolamine** 0.25% or **homatropine** eye drops 1 drop 1-2 x a day x 1-2 days prn pain relief.
   c. **Ketorolac** 0.4% drops qid or systemic analgesics for pain control.
   d. Sunglasses to reduce irritation from light.
   e. Examine daily or more often as necessary looking for possible infection or development of corneal ulcer. The abrasion should heal within 1-3 days.
   f. If abrasion is related to contact lens wear, there is a higher incidence of gram-negative infection, and the eye should NOT be patched.
6. **Corneal ulcer:** Topical **moxifloxacin** or **gatifloxacin** as follows: 1 drop q5 minutes x 3 doses; 1 drop q15 minutes for 6 hours, then 1 drop q30 minutes. **Scopolamine** 0.25% 1 drop bid, or systemic analgesics may be added for pain control if needed. A corneal ulcer is a vision-threatening disorder that may progress rapidly despite therapy, so evacuate emergently if pain and inflammation continue to increase or expedite evacuation even if the ulcer is responding to therapy.
7. **Subconjunctival hemorrhage** requires no treatment, but carefully inspect the eye for associated injuries. If the subconjunctival hemorrhage is massive and causes outward bulging of the conjunctiva (called chemosis), then suspect an occult ruptured globe and manage as described previously.
8. **Hyphema:** The primary concerns in this disorder are associated globe rupture, increased pressure in the eye and permanent damage to vision. Expedite evacuation. Restrict activity to walking only; no lifting. Use **atropine** 1%, 1 drop tid and **prednisolone acetate** 1% 1 drop qid. Keep patient upright if possible to allow blood to settle in the bottom of the anterior chamber. Do not let these individuals read. Do not treat them with NSAIDs or aspirin. There is a high risk of re-bleed in 3 to 5 days post injury.
9. **Traumatic iritis** typically resolves without treatment, can use 1 drop of **scopolamine** 0.25%. Severe cases may be treated with topical **prednisolone acetate** 1% drops qid x 3 days if evacuation is not available and no lesion is noted on fluorescein exam.
10. **Lid laceration:** Any laceration that is full-thickness, involves the lid edge, located in the medial or lateral corners should be repaired by an ophthalmologist. Suspect other trauma beneath the laceration. Clean wounds with sterile saline. Cover wounds with moistened gauze for transport and keep moist with saline. Repair partial lacerations that are not in the areas previously mentioned with simple 6-0 Prolene sutures, sterile technique, and limited 2% lidocaine in the lid. Do not expose the eye to surgical scrub or preparation solutions. Do not puncture underlying globe! Clean wound and apply **bacitracin** or **erythromycin** ointment bid. Remove sutures in 5-7 days.
11. **Foreign body:** Apply topical anesthesia (1 drop 0.5% **proparacaine** or **tetracaine**). Locate and remove foreign body using enhanced lighting and magnification if available. Evert upper eyelid with a cotton-tipped applicator to identify foreign bodies there and remove them with a cotton-tipped applicator moistened with **tetracaine**. Stain eye with **fluorescein** to check for a corneal abrasion. If symptoms persist, irrigate vigorously with artificial tears or sweep conjunctival corners with a moistened cotton-tipped applicator after applying topical anesthesia.
12. Although topical steroids should not be given except by ophthalmologists, **prednisolone acetate** 1% drops will probably not cause any significant adverse effects in an individual whose eye does not stain with **fluorescein** if used no longer than 3 days. Discontinue immediately if symptoms become worse and consult with an ophthalmologist.

Patient Education

General: Discuss the level of injury with the patient but do not give prognosis in diseases that should be managed at a higher level of care.
Activity: Tailor activity level to severity of injury.
Diet: Keep patient NPO for obvious and occult globe ruptures and lid lacerations that will be evacuated.
Prevention and Hygiene: All eye patients should maintain a high level of hygiene while recovering from the injury.
Wound Care: Keep all suspected open globes protected with an eye shield or other field expedient method. Treat external lacerations. Eye injuries are not generally patched, but they may be covered to keep them clean in a dirty environment. Check frequently (q12-24h at a minimum.) Change dressings daily.

Follow-up Actions

Return Evaluation: Follow patients closely on daily basis for signs of improvement or worsening.
Evacuation/Consultation Criteria: Evacuate patients as indicated in the Treatment section and any patient who does not show improvement within 24-48 hours. Consult with an ophthalmologist if available prior to using steroids in the eye.

Eye Problems: Pain and Poor Vision After Refractive Surgery
LTC Scott D. Barnes, MC, USA

Introduction: Laser Assisted in Situ Keratomileusis (LASIK) and Photorefractive Keratectomy (PRK) are the two main areas of laser refractive surgery or laser vision correction (LVC). PRK is part of a category now called advanced surface ablation (ASA) which includes Laser Assisted Sub-Epithelial Keratomileusis (LASEK) and epi-LASIK; ASA only involves removing the surface epithelium compared to standard LASIK which physically cuts a permanent partial thickness flap in the deeper stroma of the cornea. Although very rare (1 in 500 in Ft. Bragg report), flap dislocations with ocular trauma have been reported as far out as 7 years after LASIK. The differential diagnosis of pain and poor vision specifically after LVC includes dry eye, corneal abrasion, recurrent erosion, corneal haze, and LASIK flap dislocation.

Subjective: **Symptoms**

Mild to significant eye pain, redness, foreign-body sensation, dry eye, and decreased vision
Focused History: *Did you have LASIK or did you have an ASA procedure (PRK/LASEK/epi-LASIK)?* (Flap dislocation is greatest problem after LASIK; there is no flap dislocation with ASA.) *Do you have decreased vision without any pain or redness?* (Corneal haze gives no pain or redness.) *Is the discomfort primarily upon awakening and does it resolve in some minutes/hours?* (If after ASA, this suggests recurrent corneal erosion.) *Did something strike your eye?* (Finger, dog's paw, rifle butt, edge of paper, tree branch have all

caused corneal abrasions and LASIK flap dislocations.) *Does vision improve with blinking or squinting?* (Blinking – dry eyes; squinting – residual refractive error; corrects with glasses.) *Was the onset of symptoms sudden or gradual?* (All diagnoses except corneal haze after ASA are sudden in onset.)

Objective: Signs

Using Basic Tools: Flashlight: May see a "wrinkled" LASIK flap if the dislocation is severe (could look like a folded contact lens in the eye), but generally cannot see anything as the flap is the thickness of a hair. Snellen chart (if available): Decreased visual acuity without pain points to corneal haze.

Using Advanced Tools: Fluorescein strip and UV light: Disrupted epithelium (abrasion, erosion, flap dislocation) allows bright fluorescence in affected area. A LASIK flap dislocation may look exactly like a corneal abrasion.

Assessment: Differential Diagnosis

Dry eye: Usually bilateral and may result in secondary tearing; history of previous episodes; occurs in dry environments. It is more frequent in LASIK than ASA.

Corneal abrasion: Stain on fluorescein exam; underlying cornea is clear; general history of trauma or foreign object into eye. Pain is relieved with topical tetracaine.

Recurrent corneal erosion: Chronic, repeat abrasions; not associated with trauma; often upon daily awakening; pain relieved with tetracaine. It is more common after ASA than LASIK.

Corneal haze: Gradual blurring or decrease in vision, often presenting some months after ASA; may increase in dry environments with increased UV exposure. It is not associated with LASIK.

LASIK flap dislocation: Very rare sliding, folding, or slipping of corneal flap; associated with "trauma" from eye rubbing to IED blasts; cannot be seen with most field tools unless dislocation is so severe as to look like dislocated/folded contact lens. It appears similar to abrasion.

Plan:

Treatment

Dry eye: Artificial tears prn to relieve symptoms; rehydration; sunglasses/goggles for protection

Corneal abrasion: Erythromycin or **bacitracin** ophthalmic ointment applied qid x 4 days or until eye is back to normal or ointment with eye patching if pain in significant. Check eye daily. *See Part 3: General Symptoms: Eye Problems: Acute Red Eye without Trauma*

Recurrent corneal erosion: If sure of diagnosis by history, increasing pain, and unable to evacuate, consider a bandage contact lens (BCL) (not standard of care for medics) to allow completion of mission; otherwise manage with artificial tears and **erythromycin** or **bacitracin** ophthalmic ointment. *See Part 3: General Symptoms: Eye Problems: Acute Red Eye without Trauma*

Corneal haze: No diagnosis generally possible in the field (needs slit lamp exam); if decreased vision is noticed by patient, treatment will often require surgery but prednisolone acetate 1% 1 drop qid is only non-surgical treatment; no urgent evacuation is needed as this is very slow in onset and quite stable but will need close follow up by an eye care specialist.

LASIK flap dislocation: Very rare; the appearance in the field is often identical to a corneal abrasion; treatment includes topical **tetracaine** to only to allow for gentle irrigation with saline and eye patching; placement of a BCL only in event of urgent mission and no possible evacuation. This is an ocular emergency requiring urgent repair by qualified eye surgeon.

Pearl (non-standard treatment): An urgent mission may be compromised due to the pain of a corneal defect or flap dislocation. A low power soft contact lens (-0.50 or so) may be used as a BCL to allow vision while the eyelid is kept from rubbing over the damaged cornea. Any ophthalmic antibiotic drop can be used, but **must** be continued qid while the contact lens is in place. Ophthalmic ointment can cause the lens to slide out.

Patient Education

General: All but LASIK flap dislocation can be managed in the field; most have an excellent return of vision if treated with eye care involvement or directions

Activity: As tolerated

Diet: As tolerated

Prevention and Hygiene: Continue using eye protection in field; do not stop using post-operative steroid eye drops until instructed by eye care professional. Haze in ASA is often caused by failure to complete course of steroids.

Follow-up Actions

Return Evaluation: Follow patients closely on daily basis for signs of improvement or worsening

Evacuation/Consultation Criteria: Consult with an ophthalmologist if possible prior to using steroids in the eye. Evacuate as indicated above in treatment. Evacuate any patient not showing improvement within 24-48 hours. LASIK patients must be evacuated to ensure flap integrity even though most injuries may not actually cause a dislocation.

Eye Problems: Laser Injuries
COL Henry D. Hacker, MC, USA

Introduction: Even low levels of laser energy can burn the cornea or retina of the eye. The retina is particularly vulnerable because the optics of the eye focuses the damaging energy of laser light on the retina. The severity of injury depends on duration of exposure, laser wavelength, area of retina damaged and type of lenses or personal protection used. Due to the importance of vision for mission execution and success, as well as the need to protect others from similar burns, laser injuries must be promptly identified, personnel must be quickly moved from the threat environment and the command (and intelligence personnel) must be immediately notified. It is desirable for medical personnel to introduce themselves to intelligence officials early on in order to enhance communication both ways about the potential for directed energy threats to vision in the theater of operations.

Subjective: Symptoms

Immediate partial or complete loss of vision (may be temporary), or loss of peripheral vision, absent to mild eye irritation to extreme pain and photophobia.

Focused History: *What was the source of the laser?* (Laser is a line of sight hazard typically from any one of a number of laser sources, eg, rangefinders and target designators.) *What color and type of laser was it?*

Objective: Signs

Using Basic Tools: Loss of visual acuity-assess with newsprint, or if available, a Snellen chart or Vision Screener. Loss of visual fields-assess peripheral vision in all quadrants (confrontation test with fingers). If available, use Amsler grid chart. Corneal or periorbital burn-corneal ulcer or inflammation (fluorescein exam), skin burns. Unequal, non-reactive or abnormal pupils.

Using Advanced Tools: Ophthalmoscope: Hemorrhagic debris in the vitreous humor from retinal damage (inability to focus on the retina); disrupted macula.

Figure 3-2a. Amsler Grid

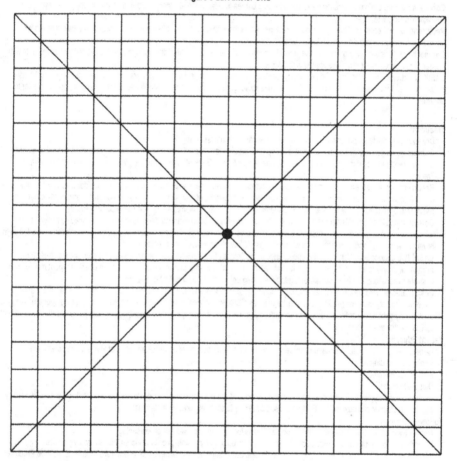

Assessment: Diagnose based on clinical signs and symptoms, environment and probability.

Differential Diagnosis

Traumatic eye injury: Abrasion, blunt trauma, penetrating trauma, etc.

Infection or acquired inflammatory condition: Conjunctivitis, blepharitis, vitritis, retinitis, etc.

Assessment of Macular Damage (*See Figure 3-2a*)

Instructions. Provide Amsler Record Chart pad for solider to draw any irregularities. Test each eye separately in good light, reading the following:

1. Cover your left [right] eye.
2. Hold the card about 40cm or two-card lengths from your eye.
3. Focus on the dot in the center of the grid.
4. While continuing to focus on the center dot, do you notice any dark or hazy areas anywhere on the grid? [If the answer is YES, provide a pen or pencil and say: Please draw in the areas that appear dark or hazy to you.]

5. While still looking at the center dot, do you see all of the horizontal lines? Do these all appear straight? [If the answer is NO, provide a pen or pencil and say: Draw the straight lines where you think they should be.]
6. While still looking at the center dot, do you see all the vertical lines? Do they appear straight? [If the answer to either question is NO, provide a pen or pencil and say: Draw the straight lines where you think they should be.]

Interpreting the Results:

Normal: No dark or hazy area seen. All lines are seen and are straight.

Minor defect: Dark or hazy area (or abnormal lines) which is less than 4 boxes long.

Major defect: Dark of hazy area (or abnormal lines) which is 4 or more boxes long or the affected area includes the center dot.

Plan:

Treatment

Corneal Injury: Treat as an ultraviolet keratitis. **Pain:** Topical anesthetic drops (eg, **tetracaine** or **proparacaine** 0.5% 2-3 drops in affected eye q15-20 minutes during initial examination; do not give bottle to patient). NSAID (eg, **ibuprofen** 600mg po tid–qid). Short acting cycloplegic medication: (eg, 1% **cyclopentolate**, 1 drop to induce cycloplegia.) Repeat in 5-10 min prn to relieve pain of ciliary spasm. Topical ophthalmic antibiotic: (eg, **erythromycin** 0.5% ointment, apply 0.5 inch ribbon tid - qid, or **neosporin** ophthalmic ointment, apply 0.5 inch ribbon bid-tid) Patch: up to 24 hrs (**Note:** May be useful for pain relief but may prolong re-epithelialization; decrease in visual acuity and depth perception may be more of an issue than the pain itself, especially during operational conditions.) Evacuate: When medically or operationally indicated.

Vitreoretinal Injury: Maintain at bedrest if possible, with head elevated and eye(s) patched to facilitate blood settling down and away from the macula. Immediate evacuation is recommended. Seek physician consultation as to steroid or parenteral non-steroidal anti-inflammatory drug (eg, **ketorolac**) use to reduce intraocular inflammation if macular involvement is suspected.

Patient Education: Patient should return for evaluation and management of continued pain and / or changes in vision. Emphasize awareness of laser risk and use of protective gear.

Medication: Do not give bottle of ophthalmic pain medication to patient to prevent overuse leading to delay of epithelialization/healing.

Activity: Bedrest if operationally possible.

Prevention and Hygiene: Use laser protective eyewear in recognized threat environment.

Follow-up Actions

Wound Care: Maintain eye patch for 24 hours for corneal injury, and for the duration of evacuation in the case of vitreoretinal injury.

Evacuation/Consultation Criteria: Evacuate when medically or operationally indicated. *See Table 3-5* for additional guidance. Consult ophthalmology or emergency medicine specialist for all cases of laser eye injuries.

Table 3-5. Laser Exposure Evacuation Criteria

Best Visual Acuity (with correction)	Normal	Minor Defect	Major Defect
20/63 or worse in one/both eyes	Evacuate	Evacuate	Evacuate
20/50 or better in both eyes	Return to duty	Reevaluate in 15 min	Evacuate

If using newsprint or equivalent text and no improvement in vision at 15 & 30 minutes examination, consider evacuation.

Eye Problems: Orbital/Periorbital Inflammation

LTC E. Glenn Sanford, MC, USA & MAJ Adam Buchanan, MC, USA

Introduction: Inflammation of the orbit and surrounding structures may result from infections (bacterial or viral), trauma, allergic reactions or immunologic conditions, and are sometimes idiopathic. Most of these conditions are self-limiting and respond to simple treatments, but they may also represent a severe underlying systemic disorder which, if untreated, can be life or vision-threatening.

Subjective: **Symptoms**

Decrease or change in normal vision, sharp pain, dull or achy pain, increased pain with movement (extra-ocular muscle or lacrimal gland inflammation), photophobia (superficial eye injury or intraocular inflammation), swelling, redness, loss of function (unable to open, close or move eye is very suggestive of orbital inflammation), foreign body sensation (superficial injury, foreign body or dry eye), discharge from the eye. **Focused History:** *Has the sharpness of your vision decreased?* (possible orbital involvement) *Do you have pain in your eye or around your eye?* (Deep achy pain may result from orbital inflammation.) *Where does it hurt? Do you have sharp pain or feel you have something in your eye?* (superficial injury or corneal foreign body) *Do you have any discharge and if so, what kind?* (Watery tears suggest foreign body or virus; muco-purulent discharge suggests bacterial infection or chalazion.) *Is your eye stuck shut when you awaken?* (conjunctivitis or blepharitis) *How is your general health at this time? Has an insect bitten you? Have you had any recent infections in your teeth or sinuses?* (may signify infection adjacent to orbit) *Have you had any recent trauma to this eye? Do you wear contact lenses?* (look for corneal infection)

Objective: **Signs**

Using Basic Tools: Vital signs: Fever may be present with infectious cellulitis and some rheumatologic conditions. Visual acuity: This is the most important "vital sign" for the eye. Use a near card if available, otherwise determine using field expedient means (ie, count fingers at 3 feet, able to see light, etc.). Vision may decrease with inflammation in the orbit. Orbital edema can push on the optic nerve and change the vision. Changes in the tear film or increased discharge may also reduce visual acuity. Normal vision gives reassurance that there are no emergent conditions present at that time. External: Examine the eye for any signs of swelling or erythema. Does the eye protrude forward? (proptosis) Note any signs of superficial skin injuries, insect bites, etc. Look closely at the lid margins for an external or internal hordeolum or crusting. Examine the conjunctiva for foreign bodies and discharge. Pay close attention to see if lid erythema extends beyond the bony orbital rim. Orbital cellulitis frequently does not extend beyond the orbital rim, while pre-septal cellulitis is not bound by this structure. Determine if the patient can open their lids normally and if there is any defect in eye movement. Orbital cellulitis will affect the opening of the eye as well as movement, (ie, frozen globe). Gently palpate the orbit with your finger. The orbit should be soft with the eye "floating" in the orbital fat. A firm orbit suggests inflammation and/or infection of the orbital fat.

Eye: Check pupil function with a flashlight. Abnormal function is a serious sign suggesting involvement of the optic nerve or more distant neural pathways and requires an emergent evacuation.

Using Advanced Tools: Use the ophthalmoscope to examine the visible portions of the eye. Look for signs of infection inside the eye. Also check for corneal abrasion with fluorescein strips and **tetracaine.**

Assessment: Differential Diagnosis

Orbital cellulitis: Associated with a history of sinusitis or upper respiratory tract infection, proptosis (protrusion of the eye), restricted extra ocular muscle motility, abnormal pupil, decreased visual acuity and/or fever. It can progress to meningitis.

Preseptal cellulitis: Associated with a history of periocular trauma or hordeolum (stye), no proptosis (protrusion of the eye), no restriction or pain with eye movement and no change in visual acuity.

Periocular insect bite: May have a papular or vesicular lesion at the site of the bite.

Chalazion: Inflammation isolated to one lid secondary to the rupture of a meibomian gland. Secondary findings include blurry vision, pain, +/- mucopurulent discharge, crusting, eyelid stuck shut in the morning.

Dacryocystitis: A specific type of preseptal cellulitis in which the source of the infection is an obstructed nasolacrimal duct. The erythema and inflammation are localized to the area overlying the lacrimal sac at the inferior nasal aspect of the lower lid. Spontaneous draining may occur. Patient may have a history of recurrent bouts of conjunctivitis or trauma to the lower lid.

Plan:

Treatment

1. **Orbital cellulitis:** Life-threatening disorder requiring emergent evacuation. Give **nafcillin or oxacillin** 2g IV q4h (or **cephazolin** 2g IV q8h) plus **ceftriaxone** 1g IV q day and continue antibiotic through medical evacuation. Give nasal decongestants such as **oxymetazoline** bid prn.
2. **Preseptal cellulitis: Levofloxacin** 500mg po q day x 7-10 days; expedite evacuation if no improvement in 24-48 hours. A second option is **amoxicillin/clavulanate** 875mg po bid.
3. **Periocular insect bite:** Cool compresses and **diphenhydramine** 25–50mg po tid-qid; give **levofloxacin** 500mg po q day x 7-10 days if superficial secondary infection is suspected based on increasing pain, redness, or swelling.
4. **Chalazion:** Hot compresses for 5 minutes qid (long-term for prevention as well), **bacitracin** or **erythromycin** ophthalmic ointment to lashes following hot compresses and in eyes at night x 14 days.
5. **Dacryocystitis:** As for preseptal cellulitis. Use warm compresses on the inflamed eye for 5 minutes qid.

Patient Education

General: Discuss severity of the condition with the patient

Activity: Limited with IV antibiotics.

Diet: Regular as tolerated

Prevention: Good personal hygiene. Early treatment of superficial lesions.

Wound Care: Warm or cool compresses, depending on diagnosis.

Follow-up Actions

Return Evaluation: Return every 12-24 hours.

Evacuation/Consultation Criteria: Immediate evacuation for acute proptosis and/or decreased eye motility or abnormal pupil function.

Eye Problems: Lateral Canthotomy and Cantholysis
LTC Scott Barnes, MC, USA

Introduction: Retrobulbar hemorrhage (bleeding behind the eye) is an ocular emergency whose prompt diagnosis and treatment are essential to prevent blindness. A small amount of bleeding into the orbit, which is a relatively closed compartment, can cause a marked pressure elevation in the orbit (area behind the eye). This is essentially a "compartment syndrome" of the eye/orbit. Retrobulbar hemorrhage most often results from trauma, recent retrobulbar anesthesia, or eyelid surgery. This is exceedingly rare even in significant facial trauma, but must be considered, especially if evacuation is not easily available.

Patients with increased orbital pressure present with pain, decreased vision, diplopia, limited extraocular movements, proptosis, ecchymosis around the eye, bloody chemosis, increased intraocular pressure (IOP), resistance to retropulsion, and an afferent pupillary defect. Untreated, orbital compartment syndrome develops with resultant ischemia of the optic nerve. Orbital pressure can be relieved with an emergent lateral canthotomy. Without decompression, irreversible vision loss due to increasing orbital pressure may occur in as little as 90-120 minutes.

When: Absolute indications for lateral canthotomy include retrobulbar hemorrhage resulting in acute loss of visual acuity, increased IOP, and proptosis (eye "bulging" forward). In the unconscious or uncooperative patient, an IOP greater than 40mmHg (if you have a tonometer or other way to measure eye pressure) is an indication for lateral canthotomy (normal IOP is 10-21mmHg). Lateral canthotomy may also be considered in patients with retrobulbar hemorrhage along with any of the following: afferent pupillary defect, ophthalmoplegia, cherry-red macula, optic nerve head pallor, and severe eye pain. However, these findings are subjective, less reliable, and nonspecific. A CT scan of the orbit may help to clarify the diagnosis. The procedures should NOT be done because of swollen, ecchymotic eyelids which are difficult to open. The procedure is done to relieve the pressure that retrobulbar bleeding causes when the tendons around the eyelids do not allow for forward movement. If the pressure is from bleeding into the eyelids, this will not cause a problem with compression of the globe back into the "socket."

What You Need: Sterile gloves, face shield, gown (if desired), **lidocaine 1-2% with epinephrine,** syringe with 25 gauge needle, sterile drapes, normal saline for irrigation, straight hemostat, sterile iris or suture scissors, forceps

What To Do:

1. Provide adequate anesthesia by injecting 1mL of **lidocaine 1-2% with epinephrine** into the lateral canthus. The combination of lidocaine with epinephrine assists with hemostasis and local anesthesia.

Figure 3-2b. Anesthesia for Lateral Canthotomy

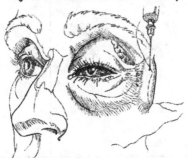

Image Source: Emergency War Surgery 3rd Revision, Borden Institute, 2004, p. 14.9

2. Irrigate the eye with normal saline to clear away debris that may enter the eye or interfere with the procedure.
3. Use a straight hemostat to crimp the skin at the lateral corner of the patient's eye for 30-60 seconds. This crimp functions to achieve hemostasis and to mark the location where the incision is to be made.

Figure 3-3. Lateral Canthotomy, Crimping

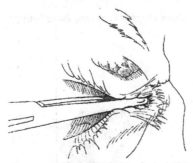

Image Source: Emergency War Surgery 3rd Revision, Borden Institute, 2004, p.14.9

4. Perform the lateral canthotomy by carefully cutting through the crushed, demarcated line to the orbital rim/lateral fornix to avoid traumatizing the orbit.

Figure 3-4. Lateral Canthotomy, Cutting to the Orbital Rim/Lateral Fornix

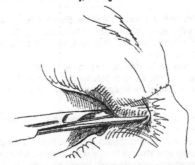

Image Source: Emergency War Surgery 3rd Revision, Borden Institute, 2004, p.14.9

5. This incision decreases some pressure but is often insufficient alone; therefore, proceed to cantholysis by one of the following methods:
    a. **Traditional approach:** Grasp lower eyelid with forceps and pull out/downward away from eye. Identify the canthal ligament by either inspection or palpation. Incise the inferior crus of the lateral canthal ligament with scissors to avoid traumatizing the

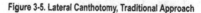

orbit. The canthotomy splits the ligament into two portions, the superior crus and the inferior crus. By cutting the lower portion in half, it allows the lid to "swing" away from the eyeball, thus lowering the pressure.

Figure 3-5. Lateral Canthotomy, Traditional Approach

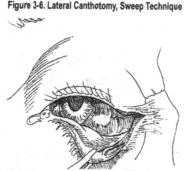

Image Source: Emergency War Surgery 3rd Revision, Borden Institute, 2004, p.14.9

b. **Sweep technique:** Grasp the lower eyelid with forceps and pull out/downward away from eye. Carefully place the lateral side of an opened pair of curved scissors against the conjunctiva of the lateral eyelid. Slowly sweep laterally toward the canthotomy incision. When the inferior crus of the lateral canthal ligament is encountered impeding continued lateral sweeping, carefully move the other scissor blade into position and incise to avoid traumatizing the orbit. The sweep technique may be particularly useful in cases when massive edema makes canthal ligament identification difficult.

Figure 3-6. Lateral Canthotomy, Sweep Technique

Image Source: Emergency War Surgery 3rd Revision, Borden Institute, 2004, p.14.9

What Not To Do:

1. Do not perform a lateral orbital canthotomy if you suspect globe rupture. Signs of globe rupture include hyphema; a peaked, teardrop-shaped, or otherwise irregularly shaped pupil; exposed uveal tissue, which appears reddish-brown; and extraocular movement restriction that is greatest in the direction of the rupture. Subtle signs of globe rupture include subconjunctival hemorrhage, enophthalmos ("sunken" eye), or a conjunctival laceration.
2. Do not injure globe with forceps or scissor tips. Less common complications include bleeding and infection. Unexpected patient head movement can result in iatrogenic injury, including accidental globe puncture. To prevent this, the patient may need to be restrained, undergo conscious sedation, or even be intubated and paralyzed, depending on the situation.

Notes:

- Early and repeat evaluation/documentation of visual acuity in the conscious patient may assist in knowing when to do this procedure (if the vision is decreasing and the patient's pain is increasing, it may be indicated).
- Lateral retraction of the tissue by an assistant during manipulation decreases the chance of a globe injury.
- Despite high intraorbital pressures, only a small amount of blood is usually expressed with the release of the hematoma.
- Tonometry and globe palpation are contraindicated in patients with an open globe injury.
- A successful procedure is marked by improved visual acuity, resolution of a previously detected afferent pupillary defect, and decrease in IOP to below 40mmHg.
- The incision of the inferior crus should result in a very loose or floppy lower eyelid; if not, you generally have not actually transected the lower portion of the ligament.
- Salvaging vision is what is important, don't worry about the cosmetic effect, an eye surgeon can repair the skin/ligament damage at a later time.

- Always seek emergent consultation with an ophthalmologist when this procedure is performed.
- The afferent pupillary defect, or Marcus Gunn pupil, is tested using the swinging flashlight test. The test is positive when the affected pupil dilates in response to light (the other normal pupil also dilates when light is shone in the affected eye). Both pupils constrict when the light is shone in the normal eye.

Unconventional/Field Expedient Tip: An estimate of IOP can be crudely done by gentle palpation of the unaffected globe through closed lids and then comparing this with palpation of the affected globe. The affected eye will feel more firm and resistant to gentle palpation than the "normal" globe; think of a tire with high pressure harder to indent than tire with low pressure. Again, absolute contraindication if suspected globe rupture.

Fatigue

COL Warner D. Farr, MC, USA

Introduction: Active duty military members generally require between 7-9 hours of sleep a night to maintain optimal levels of function. Acute sleep deprivation (>24hrs without sleep) can lead to impairment that resembles or exceeds the level of impairment seen in individuals who meet the legal definition of alcohol intoxication. Minimal effects on performance will be noticed following relatively mild sleep deprivation (ie, 5 hours/night for up to 2 weeks). Chronic sleep deprivation (>2 weeks) can cause more serious side effects with prolonged impairment. Loss of resiliency to acute sleep deprivation, and loss of the ability to recognize impairment are seen relatively early in the course of chronic sleep deprivation. Confusion, poor attention, carelessness, loss of coordination, short-term memory loss, decreased stamina, delusions, and hallucinations are serious effects of severe acute or chronic sleep deprivation. Short naps, power naps, combat naps, cat naps (less than 1/2 hour), especially in early afternoon, are effective in replacing lost sleep. Sleep inertia is a zombie-like state that can occur when a person is awoken from deep sleep occurring after first half hour of sleep and during the following 1-3 hours. A detailed description of the patient's fatigue and thorough review of systems may point to an underlying endocrine disorder, systemic illness, sleep disorder, drug side effect (recreational or prescribed), or psychiatric disorder. If the patient's history does not yield a specific etiology, a careful psychiatric history should be taken to rule out depression. Psychiatric illness (usually depression) can present as a primary complaint of fatigue when seen with a clustering of other symptoms. Attention should be directed toward identifying an underlying organic disease. Never rule out psychogenic causes.

Subjective: **Symptoms**
   Focused History:
     Sleeping: *Have you had trouble with sleeping or had a change in your sleep pattern?* (Fatigue may be a presenting symptom for undiagnosed COPD.) *Early awakening/difficulty getting to sleep?* (often seen with depression.) *Snoring?* (may indicate Obstructive Sleep Apnea [OSA] if coupled with Chronic Fatigue. *See Part 4: Organ Systems: Chapter 3: Chronic Obstructive Sleep Apnea) Told they stop and start breathing when they sleep?* (hallmark sign of OSA) *Wake up with headache on most days?* (secondary symptom of OSA due to nocturnal hypoxemia) *Shift work?* (disordered circadian rhythm) *Do you fall asleep during the day?* (may be seen in OSA or other cause of sleep deprivation)
     Medication: *Do you take any medications or supplements?* (Starting or stopping many medications can cause fatigue. Starting an antihypertensive drug or stopping thyroid replacement are common causes.)
     Drugs/Alcohol: *Do you drink alcohol, use tobacco or use any other type of recreational drugs?* (Alcohol, drugs can alter normal sleep patterns. Although a popular self-treatment; this usually worsens rather than improves the problem. Alcohol has an initial sedative effect, but provides poor sleep quality and paradoxical excitation once it wears off [early awakening]. Caffeine can improve functioning for several hours, but it can cause difficulty falling asleep or maintaining sleep 8-12 hours after consumption. Caffeine has a recognized withdrawal phenomenon.)
     Weight: *Have you lost weight?* (occult malignancy or systemic illness)
     Duration: *How long have you had fatigue?* (6 months to be Chronic Fatigue)
     Night sweats: *Do you have night sweats?* (tuberculosis, lymphoma, malaria, others)
     Exposure: *Have you had any known exposure to HIV, hepatitis, or mononucleosis?* (All can have fatigue as presenting complaint.) *Have you been flying or diving recently?* (possible decompression sickness, *See Part 6: Operational Environment: Chapter 20: Decompression Injuries: Decompression Sickness [Caisson Disease, the "Bends"])*
     Muscle/Joint pain: *Do you have muscle or joint pain?* (connective tissue disorders, eg, rheumatoid arthritis and lupus)
     Depression: *Does the patient have any symptoms related to depression? Difficulty with getting to sleep or early awakening? Lost interest in activities that he/she used to enjoy? Does patient feel guilty about things that they could not control? Decreased energy? Does the patient have difficulty with concentration? Loss of appetite? Does the patient feel like their thoughts are slower than usual, or seem to be fleeting? Has the patient had a decrease in libido? Has the patient contemplated suicide?* (The more symptoms, the more likely the patient has clinical depression. Any time the diagnosis of depression is entertained, patient must be screened for suicidal or homicidal ideation. The possibility of acute combat stress reaction, mild to moderate post traumatic brain injury and post traumatic stress disorder should be considered, documented and if present, managed appropriately.)

Objective: Signs

Table 3-6. Fatigue: Objective Signs

Using Basic Tools	Clinical Findings:	Interpretations:
General	• Assess interaction and general appearance	• Depressed patient will be less likely to engage the clinician and may have decreased personal hygiene.
Vital Signs	• Check pulse ox - if available • Hypotension/Bradycardia-hypothyroid	• Hypoxemia may cause isolated fatigue rather than dyspnea. Hypoxemia may also be a marker of underlying sleep apnea.
HEENT	• Jugular venous distention • Pallor of the mucous membranes • Pharynx erythematous exudate • Thyroid goiter	• Associated with congestive heart failure (CHF) • May suggest anemia • Mononucleosis can cause severe pharyngitis and persistent fatigue.
Cardiovascular	• Systolic ejection murmur • S3/S4 Gallop	• Hypothyroidism is a classic etiology of fatigue. • Anemia will often have a soft ejection murmur. • These abnormal heart sounds will be heard in CHF.
Pulmonary	• Increased AP diameter of chest • Rhonchi/rales/pleural rub	• Possible underlying pulmonary disease (emphysema/COPD) • Possible bronchitis/pneumonia
Abdomen	• Splenomegaly	• Possible mononucleosis
Neurologic	• Sluggish relaxation phase of DTRs • Abnormal muscle tone/muscle girth	• Common finding in hypothyroidism • Possible neuromuscular disorder
Lymphatic	• Lymphadenopathy	• Possible lymphoma, mononucleosis or chronic infection
Rheumatic	• Inflamed joints	• Possible lupus, rheumatoid arthritis, or Lyme disease

Using Advanced Tools: Labs: CBC, rule out anemia, hematologic malignancy, or chronic infection. With a negative history and a normal physical exam, labs are not likely to help with diagnosis. However, a routine set of basic labs should be drawn prior to initiation of treatment of depression or other psychiatric illness.

Plan: Attention to proper sleep/rest, hydration, nutrition, exercise and time management are key to prevention and treatment strategies.
Treatment
  Altered sleep patterns
    Primary: Zolpidem or zaleplon 5-10mg po at bedtime
    Alternate: Antihistamines (more side effects) such as **diphenhydramine** or **hydroxyzine** 25mg po hs
    or **melatonin** 0.3–0.5mg po hs x 4 days may help to restore normal circadian rhythms upset by shift work or jet lag.
    Primitive: Sunglasses that block UA/UVB; blackout curtains in sleeping quarters.
  Snoring and/or Obstructive Sleep Apnea
    Primary: Over-the-counter decongestants or **oxymetazoline** spray or Breathe Right nasal strips (OTC)
    Alternate: Fluticasone 1-2 sprays each nostril q hs
    Primitive: Use a sleep wedge to prevent sleeping on the back
  Depression
    Primary: Specific Serotonin re-uptake inhibitors (SSRI), such as **fluoxetine** or **bupropion** may be useful whereas other
    SSRIs such as **sertraline, paroxetine,** or tri-cyclic antidepressants should be avoided as these often have the side effect
    of fatigue. *See Part 3: General Symptoms: Depression and Mania*
    Alternate: Optimize physical condition (food, sleep, exercise); minimize psychological stressors (sleep deprivation, direct
    combat operations) as operational tempo permits.
Patient Education
  General: Symptom reduction- help the patient to learn to cope with their symptoms and maintain their highest possible
  functioning level. This requires a good medic-patient alliance and a mutual understanding of the diagnosis and treatment goals.
Follow-up Actions
  Follow patient on a routine schedule to assess for improvement of symptoms with treatment interventions. Change therapy, if
  symptoms continue. **Note:** The symptom reduction in depression may take 4-6 weeks; therefore, until the patient has taken therapeutic
  doses of a drug for at least 2 months, therapy should not be discontinued.
  Evacuation/Consultation Criteria: Acute evacuation is not usually necessary, unless the patient is unstable or non-mission capable.
  If labs remain unrevealing and the patient has persistent symptoms of fatigue for greater than 6 months, then a diagnosis of chronic
  fatigue or other (eg, PTSD) may be entertained and the patient referred. Note that chronic fatigue is NOT the same as chronic fatigue
  syndrome, which has specific diagnostic criteria.

Circadian Rhythm Synchronizers and "Go Pills": Use of prescription medications continuously over 14 days can lead to decreased effectiveness and dependence. Herbal and natural products are not recommended. Various military services have adopted policies on the use of "go pills." **Note:** Policies are strenuous, usually requiring home station test dosing, high-level command approval, and close medical supervision.

Dextroamphetamine. The military experience is extensive but use to mitigate the effects of fatigue is an off-label use of this drug that requires informed consent. The recommended dosing for Army aviators is 5-10mg po q4h. This and other aspects of sustained operations can be found in "Leader's Guide to Crew Endurance" published by the US Army Aeromedical Research Laboratory. The USAF has authorized "Go Pills" in specific circumstances for pilots in certain commands. (See "AIRCREW FATIGUE MANAGEMENT PROGRAM" policy on electronic version.) Dextroamphetamine has a high abuse potential and additional adverse side effects include elevated heart rate and elevated blood pressure.

Modafinil is a promising new drug approved by the FDA for the on label use of "shift work sleep disorder." The dosing of **modafinil** is 100-200mg at start of a shift (8 hrs), with a recommendation to not exceed 400mg/day. Modafinil has a much lower potential for abuse and frequently the patient's request for the higher dose (which may cause nausea) is usually a result of the patient not recognizing a perceived stimulant effect of the lower (100mg) dose. Side effects include allergic reactions, serious rashes requiring hospitalization, cardiac dysrhythmias, and ataxia. Do not use with amphetamines.

Guidance for all stimulant use (including caffeine): All personnel should be pretested to identify idiosyncratic adverse reactions under conditions simulating operations but a controlled environment. Follow all service regulations, and administer only under physician supervision, and full knowledge of commanders. Administer at least 1 hour before critical performance times to get peak effect; lower doses are required during daytime; expect the development of tolerance. Give the last dose far enough in advance of scheduled sleep periods to allow drug effects to dissipate. Avoid using hypnotics to induce sleep after these drugs if possible. Emphasis must be placed on the fact that these drugs are, at best, a temporary solution to extreme challenges related to the combat environment. Sleep cannot be postponed indefinitely without significant adverse effects on individual and unit readiness.

Fever

COL Duane Hospenthal, MC, USA

Introduction: Fever (body temperature >101°F) is a common symptom of infection. Fever can be seen in the absence of infection in persons with heat injuries, drug reactions, malignancies, and rheumatologic conditions. Exposure history can be essential to the diagnosis of the cause of febrile illness. Travel history, arthropod exposure, and sexual history are often imperative to arriving at the correct diagnosis or in guiding diagnostic testing. Country specific information on infectious disease threats may be obtained from many official and public sources. Key considerations in the assessment and initial treatment of the febrile patient:

1. All patients need initial assessment for the possibility that they have an infection which could be rapidly life-threatening (prolonged or recurrent fever, exposure history, concerning signs/symptoms (includes hemorrhage/petechiae/purpura, hypotension, altered level of consciousness, or other rashes)
2. Empiric antimicrobial therapy that covers the most likely pathogen(s) should be started promptly in the moderate-severely ill patient.
3. Empiric antimalarial therapy should be promptly started in patients in malarious areas or in travelers from malarious areas unless an alternate diagnosis is obvious or proven.
4. Prompt consideration and initiation of infection control measures for potentially contagious infections.
5. IV fluids are recommended for hypotensive febrile patients.

Subjective: **Symptoms**
   Fever: Temperature of >101°F
   Incubation period of selected febrile diseases:
      Acute (<2 weeks):
         Undifferentiated fever: Malaria, rickettsioses (eg, typhus), dengue, Chikungunya, acute HIV, leptospirosis, relapsing fever, influenza or yellow fever
         Fever with coagulopathy (bleeding, petechiae, purpura): Meningococcemia, viral hemorrhagic fevers, entero viruses, leptospirosis or malaria
         Fever with central nervous system (CNS) symptoms: Malaria, typhoid fever, rickettsioses, encephalitis or meningitis
         Fever with pulmonary symptoms: Influenza, pneumonia (due to typical pathogens, legionellosis, histoplasmosis, coccidioidomycosis, Q fever, SARS, etc.)
         Fever with rash: Rickettsioses, dengue, Chikungunya, typhoid fever, viral exanthems (rubella, measles, varicella, mumps, herpes simplex-6, enteroviruses, parvovirus, etc.)
      Sub-acute (2-6 weeks): Malaria, typhoid fever, viral hepatitis, acute HIV, infectious mononucleosis, schistosomiasis, tuberculosis, visceral leishmaniasis, amebic liver abscess, leptospirosis, viral hemorrhagic fevers or Q fever
      Chronic (>6 weeks): Tuberculosis, visceral leishmaniasis, amebic liver abscess, brucellosis, bartonellosis, deep fungal infections, filariasis, Q fever or malaria
   Focused History: How high is your temperature? (Fever is temperature >101°F.) Is the fever constant? (recurrent fever with some malaria, relapsing fever, leptospirosis) Have you noticed [select: rash, headache, diarrhea, swollen lymph nodes, localized pain, stiff neck, cough]? (identify affected systems) Do you know other persons with similar symptoms? (suggests contagious illness or point source outbreak) Are you taking any medications? (Antimalarials may decrease your ability to diagnose malaria. Use of doxycycline for malaria prophylaxis makes rickettsioses and leptospirosis very unlikely. Fever may be sign of an allergic reaction to medication.)

Figure 3-7. Fever Algorithm

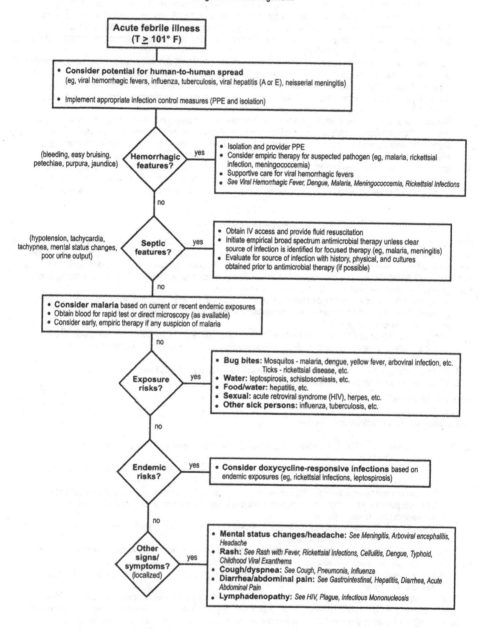

Objective: Signs

Using Basic Tools: Vital signs: Temperature >101°F (also look for relapsing pattern or pulse-temperature dissociation as hints to specific types of infection), respiratory rate over 14 breaths/minute, heart rate over 100 beats/minute, systolic BP <100. Inspection: Evaluate for pallor, diaphoresis, rigors, mental status changes, rash (especially any petechiae or purpura), jaundice, unwillingness to move body parts (stiff neck, limb, back, etc.); evaluate for pharyngitis. Palpation: Feel for inflammatory changes (warmth, tenderness) in areas of symptoms; test range of motion in areas where patient voluntarily restricts movement to see if pain is elicited; check for enlarged lymph nodes and assess if fluctuant, tender or draining; evaluate abdomen for hepatosplenomegaly, peritoneal signs, tenderness. Auscultation: Listen for rales in lungs (egophony or dullness suggest pneumonia); listen for heart murmurs, S3 that could suggest carditis (such as rheumatic fever) or endocarditis; evaluate for abnormal bowel sounds (hyperactive in gastroenteritis, hypoactive in ileus/intra-abdominal abscess)

Using Advanced Tools: Labs: Thick and thin blood smears (malaria, filaria, *Babesia* and other parasites); WBC with differential; urinalysis; Gram's stain of any pus or sputum; stool for fecal leukocytes and O&P if diarrhea. X-Ray: CXR if available (PA and lateral)

Assessment:

Clinical Questions

1. Does patient need outpatient treatment or evacuation/hospitalization for intravenous therapy, resuscitation, possible end organ support (ventilator, dialysis), if available?
2. Does patient need isolation to prevent infecting others (meningococcal meningitis, hemorrhagic fever, plague, pulmonary tuberculosis)?
3. Should the patient receive empiric treatment for several conditions simultaneously (eg, bacterial infection) or should he be treated more specifically (eg, for malaria)?
4. Is the patient at increased risk: elderly, young child, immunocompromised, wounded, concurrent or chronic illness (eg, sickle cell disease, HIV, diabetes, cancer, malnourished)? If so, he will likely require evacuation and/or more resources.
5. Does the patient have signs of sepsis syndrome (fever or hypothermia, heart rate >90 beats/minute, respirations >20 breaths minute and at least one sign of end organ dysfunction; mental status changes, pulse oximetry <90%, urine output less than 30 ml hr)? If so, he will probably require IV fluids, IV antibiotics, evacuation and/or more resources.

Differential Diagnosis: Listed by categories (acute, sub-acute, chronic), associated findings and focused questions under Subjective: Symptoms

Plan:

Treatment

See individual sections of this book for appropriate treatment. Always check for medication allergies and pregnancy before selecting medication for treatment.

Patient Education

General: If fever does not respond to treatment in 72 hours or symptoms progress, seek further medical care.

Activity: As tolerated unless patient requires isolation.

Diet: Regular; avoid alcohol.

Medications: Acetaminophen is preferred for symptom control but avoid if patient has history of alcohol abuse or is jaundiced (history or signs to suggest liver dysfunction).

Gynecologic Problems: Female Pelvic Examination

MAJ Timothy Pellini, MC, USA

When: As indicated per differential diagnosis, which primarily is for abdominal and pelvic complaints. The Pap smear, normally a part of this exam, provides cellular material to screen for pre-cancerous changes of the cervix. However, the Pap smear is not normally done in the field and will not be discussed here. Rectal evaluation may or may not be a part of each examination. Rectovaginal or rectal exam can aid in assessing the posterior aspect of the uterus, the uterosacral ligaments, and posterior cul-de-sac. A stool sample can be obtained and tested for occult blood and lower rectal masses can be palpated. Current recommendations include yearly patient-collected fecal occult blood testing beginning at age 50. Since patient-collected sampling is not very practical in field settings, fecal samples for blood testing will be most often provider collected (during a rectal or rectovaginal exam). For the field medic who will only be performing problem-based pelvic examinations, the exam may be tailored to the specific problem and need not always include bimanual, rectovaginal, and rectal exam. For example, if the patient complains only of abnormal vaginal discharge without pelvic pain, then a vaginal exam, KOH, and wet prep may be all that is necessary. Pelvic exams can cause anxiety for many women regardless of their age. The anxiety can be more pronounced when factors such as the examiner's gender, cultural background, appearance, etc. are considered. Discuss before and after the exam what will happen and what was found. It is necessary to discuss each part of the exam prior to its performance. Before touching or moving any structure the examiner should say, for example, "I am going to touch the right side of the labia now" or "Now I will move the cervix." The exam should be performed expeditiously yet thoroughly. A female chaperone is absolutely necessary for male examiners in the United States. In field situations, a trusted female friend of the patient, her partner, or spouse, and a female assistant to hand you equipment could be an acceptable alternative. Keep the patient as covered as possible. If the examination targets the vulva, ask the patient to undress only from the waist down. Cover the abdomen with a sheet or drape. As soon as the exam is done, allow the patient to dress.

What You Need: For all exams: Good light source (preferably a mobile light), non-sterile gloves, water-soluble lubricant, vaginal speculum of the correct size (small for patients who are virginal, medium Graves are appropriate for most sexually active females and for parous women. Obesity may necessitate a large Graves due to redundant tissue in the vagina). A speculum may be improvised out of two spoons joined by a rubber band, or two bent spoons.

Figure 3-8. Improvised Speculum

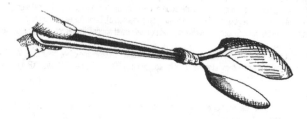

On certain exams: Culture medium for gonorrhea and *chlamydia* testing, large cotton-tipped swabs, pH paper, screening test for fecal occult blood, set-up for wet mount and KOH prep (*see Part 8: Procedures: Chapter 32: Wet Mount and KOH Prep*).

What To Do: The exam described in this section will be appropriate for triage screening and diagnosis. Position the patient in low lithotomy. The head may be elevated 30-60° to allow the patient visual access to the exam. If a lithotomy table with stirrups is not available, the patient may flex her knees to her chest or an exam table can be improvised with a litter, litter stands, IV poles, and small battle dressings. Elevating the patient's buttocks while supine with an emesis basin may also work.

Figure 3-9. Improvised Examination Table

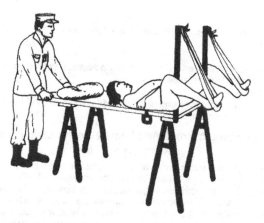

External Genitalia Examination: Prior to touching the perineum, inspect it visually. Observe for symmetry, bulges, rashes, or lesions. If asymmetry or mass is noted, these areas should be palpated to confirm mass, induration, or other abnormality.

Vaginal Examination: Select the appropriate sized speculum. Speculum may be lubricated with warm water prior to insertion. Remember to discuss the examination with the patient. Ask the patient to consciously relax the muscles at the opening of the vagina. Gentle downward pressure with the tip of the speculum or with the finger may help the patient relax, although many times this is not necessary. Place the speculum at the opening of the vagina and gently push it in and downwards until the vaginal apex is reached. Insert the speculum obliquely through the introitus and then rotated to the horizontal plane. Always control the speculum blades, holding them shut with one hand until the blades are opened as the vaginal apex is reached. Observe the vaginal side walls and the cervix. Inspect vaginal discharge for quantity, color, consistency and odor. Evaluate the cervix for erosion, lesion, infection, laceration, polyps, ulceration and tumors. To perform cervical cultures for gonorrhea and chlamydia, place each swab into the cervical os and allow to sit for 20-30 seconds. Replace in culture tube. Assess vaginal pH by obtaining a sample of vaginal discharge from the side wall or from any pooled discharge in the posterior fornix using a small cotton swab. Touch the cotton swab to the pH paper and look for color change. Obtain discharge samples for KOH and wet mount with a similar technique. Blood or cervical mucus will be basic (high pH) and will give false readings, so avoid these while sampling. Bulging of the bladder and/or rectum into the vagina may be seen in patients with pelvic relaxation. Women who have had children vaginally may have some pelvic relaxation. The cervix may descend into the vagina with Valsalva maneuver.

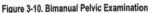

Figure 3-10. Bimanual Pelvic Examination

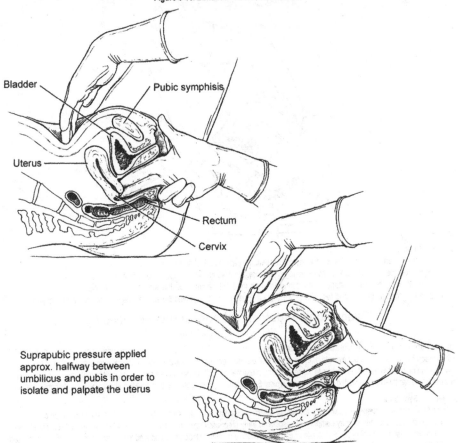

Bladder

Pubic symphisis

Uterus

Rectum

Cervix

Suprapubic pressure applied approx. halfway between umbilicus and pubis in order to isolate and palpate the uterus

Bimanual Examination: With a gloved hand, lubricated with water or gel, insert the index and middle fingers of the dominant hand along the posterior wall of the vagina (*See Figure 3-10*). Place the other hand on the patient's abdomen in the midline above the symphysis pubis. The vaginal fingers should encounter the cervix, which should feel firm and circular. Push the cervix upward in the cervical canal. This will move the body of the uterus. If the uterus is anteverted or midline, it will be palpable with the abdominal hand. If the uterus is retroverted, it will move toward the rectum and the abdominal and vaginal hands will meet in the midline as they come together. If possible, feel the body of the uterus for shape, symmetry and mass. A nulliparous (has never given birth) uterus will be quite small (pear-sized). A parous (has given birth) uterus can be the size of a small grapefruit. Assess the uterus for mobility by moving it side to side by grasping the cervix between the 2 examining fingers. The ovaries may be palpated by moving the vaginal hand to the right or left and reaching upward to the side of the uterus. Sweep the abdominal hand down to meet the vaginal hand along the uterus. Feel the tissue to the side of the uterus. The ovary will normally be pulled down in to the vaginal hand by sweeping along the side of the uterus. Premenopausal ovaries are 3-5cm in length and 2-4cm in width. The ovaries are normally tender to palpation. This tenderness is localized to the time of exam and is usually described as an aching sensation. As a general rule, "normal" ovaries should not be palpated during the exam of a premenarchal (before first menses) or postmenopausal female. A palpable pelvic mass in these age groups needs further evaluation. Ovaries may be palpated about 50% of the time for reproductive-aged women.

Rectovaginal Examination: (*See Figure 3-11*) Always change gloves (so no blood is carried to the rectum) and obtain a large dollop of lubricant prior to rectovaginal examination. Ask the patient to relax the anal sphincter. The middle finger is inserted into the rectum and the index finger into the vagina. It is helpful to have the patient bear down as the rectal finger is inserted slowly. The rectovaginal septum can be felt between the index and middle finger. Palpate the posterior aspect of the uterus, uterosacral ligaments, and posterior cul-de-sac along with the anorectal area. Note masses, nodularity, and pain. A simple rectal examination is the only way to assess the pelvis in an infant or child. Test a sample of fecal material for occult blood.

Figure 3-11. Rectovaginal Examination

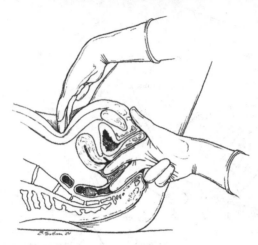

What Not To Do:
1. Do not be insensitive, unprofessional or humorous with the patient during the exam.
2. Do not **routinely** perform pelvic exams during pregnancy. Most women will not require such exams.
3. Do not perform the exam in stages. Do a complete exam the first time and allow the patient to get dressed.
4. Do not perform an occult blood test with gloves that have been used to examine the vagina. The test may be falsely positive.

Gynecologic Problems: Abnormal Uterine Bleeding
MAJ Timothy Pellini, MC, USA

Introduction: The normal menstrual interval is 28 days with a range of 21-35 days. The normal duration (period) of menstrual flow is 2-7 days with average blood loss <80cc per menstrual cycle. Abnormal uterine bleeding (AUB) is a change in the interval and duration of menstrual flow and can range from a relatively minor to life-threatening presentation. AUB presenting as profuse vaginal hemorrhage is the primary focus of this section. Given the limited resources in a typical SOF scenario, stabilization and evacuation should be an early consideration.

Subjective: Symptoms
Significant change in menstrual pattern or amount of bleeding. Excessive blood loss may be described as "gushing"; large clots may be passed; pregnant patients may complain of associated early pregnancy symptoms such as nausea and vomiting, breast tenderness and missing last menstrual cycle. Sub-acute or chronic excessive menstrual blood loss can lead to symptomatic anemia with complaints of fatigue, orthostatic changes, and heart palpitations.
Focused History: *When did your bleeding start?* (with onset of menses, unrelated to period, after/during intercourse) *Are you using any birth control? Are you pregnant? Is there any chance you could be pregnant? Are you having any pain with your bleeding? Are you having any shortness of breath, dizziness, etc?* (A patient's quantification of menstrual bleeding ["passing clots", frequency of tampon changes, etc.] can be difficult to objectively measure. Physical findings [BP, HR, physical exam] and laboratory data [HCT]) are more useful.)

Objective: Signs
Using Basic Tools: Inspection: May have obvious bleeding from the vagina; the cervix may be obscured with blood. Palpation: Uterus may be misshapen by a uterine fibroid (common cause of heavy menses); patients with acute anemia will have heart rate and blood pressure changes based on the volume of blood loss.
Using Advanced Tools: Labs: Assess for anemia via hematocrit; perform pregnancy test

Assessment:
Differential Diagnosis: Physical findings may be minimal and limited to abnormalities found on the pelvic examination. The frequency of each etiology varies according to the patient's age group:
ADOLESCENTS: Pregnancy (always rule out first); anovulation (results in absent followed by irregular/heavy menses); infection (of cervix, uterus, or pelvic inflammatory disease); coagulopathy/bleeding disorders (suspect in a young, newly menstruating female with abnormally heavy flow).
PREMENOPAUSAL WOMAN: Pregnancy (always rule out first); anatomic abnormalities (uterine fibroids, uterine or cervical polyps, cancer of the cervix, uterus, or less common the ovary); anovulation (results in absent followed by irregular/heavy menses); infection (of cervix, uterus, or pelvic inflammatory disease); endocrine disorders (prolactin secretion, hyper or hypothyroidism, adrenal dysfunction all will commonly result in anovulation).
PERIMENOPAUSAL (considered here >45 yrs old): Anovulation (results in absent followed by irregular/heavy menses); anatomic abnormalities (uterine fibroids, uterine or cervical polyps, cancer of the cervix, uterus, or less common the ovary); pregnancy (still consider).
POSTMENOPAUSAL (considered here >51 yrs old): Atrophy of uterine lining; anatomic abnormalities (cancer of uterus > cervix, uterine or cervical polyps). After menopause, most fibroids become asymptomatic. A postmenopausal woman with AUB and an enlarged irregular uterus has cancer until proven otherwise.

Plan:
Treatment
Significant vaginal hemorrhage:
Basic:
1. Stabilize patient (ABCs, etc.), monitor vital signs closely; give IV fluids; transfuse if necessary.
2. Give antibiotics (see *Antibiotic regimens*) liberally for: febrile patient (start immediately); tender uterus (suspect infection of the uterine lining); foul-smelling discharge.
   Antibiotic regimens: With IV regimens, treat until patient has been afebrile for 48hrs.
   Primary: Ampicillin/sulbactam 3g IV q4-6h.
   Alternate: Cefotetan 1-2g IV q12h or **piperacillin** 3-4g IV q4h, or **ticarcillin/clavulanate** 3.1g IV q6h. If patient remains febrile after 48 hours, add **ampicillin** 2g IV q6h.
   Empiric: If IV therapy is not available, treat the patient as per oral PID protocol with **ceftriaxone** 250mg IM x 1 and **azithromycin** 1g po x or **doxycycline** 100mg po bid x 14 days.
3. Medical evacuation

Advanced:
1. If pregnancy ruled out, place a Foley catheter with a 30cc balloon transcervically into uterus. Once inflated, this will tamponade the uterine lining. Leave inflated during evacuation. If unable to evacuate/delayed, deflate the Foley bulb 50% at 12 hrs. If no bleeding, deflate completely and remove. If bleeding apparent (prior to removal), inflate balloon to 30cc again.
2. If evacuation delayed and medicine available, give oral contraceptive (OC) pill (**ethinyl estradiol** 35 micrograms) qid, as estrogen can stabilize the uterine lining. Anticipate nausea and treat with antiemetic like **promethazine** 25mg po/pr/IV/IM q4-6h prn. Acute bleeding will often subside within 48hrs of treatment. A cascading regimen is also reasonable (eg, 5 pills on day 1, 4 pills on day 2, 3 pills on day 3, 2 pills on day 4, and 1 pill on day 5). After day 5, begin a new pill packet and instruct the patient to begin on day 1. If significant anemia is suspected, instruct the patient to take the OC pill (monophasic combination, ie, **Ovral**) in a continuous fashion (do not discontinue medication for 7 day placebo or no pill regime) to prevent a withdrawal bleed and allow for the patient's HCT to recover. Also provide the patient with **elemental iron** 60mg po daily (prenatal vitamin or a multiple vitamin). This regimen may be continued until follow-up with a GYN specialist can be obtained.

Minor menstrual irregularities:
1. If HCG negative, and HCT and physical examination are normal, treatment may be delayed until appropriate consultative services are available.
2. NSAIDs: **Ibuprofen** 800mg po tid or **naproxen** 500mg po bid may reduce blood flow.
3. If available, oral contraceptive pills are the most effective way to control menstrual irregularities. Treatment of other AUB is dependent on appropriate diagnosis that will not be obtainable in the field.

Patient Education
Use of scheduled NSAIDS prior to anticipated menstrual cycle and continued throughout period can decrease the amount of menstrual flow as well as relieve pain associated with period. A greater effect can be seen using oral contraception, either combination birth control or progesterone only pills.

Follow-up Actions
Evacuation/Consultation Criteria: Evacuate after initial stabilization for significant hemorrhage. Consult OB/GYN expert as needed for continued or recurrent symptoms.

Gynecologic Problems: Pelvic Pain, Acute
MAJ Timothy Pellini, MC, USA

Introduction: Internal gynecologic pathology is a common cause of pelvic and abdominal pain. The major causes of acute gynecologic pain are: ovarian pathology (mass, torsion or rupture), pelvic inflammatory disease (PID), ectopic pregnancy, uterine pathology (infection, fibroid degeneration or infarction). Other etiologies include painful menses (dysmenorrhea), intrauterine pregnancy complications (miscarriage), and non-gynecologic issues (gastrointestinal, urologic, neurologic, etc.). Only common gynecologic causes of acute pain will be discussed here. All of these situations require close observation for possible surgical intervention or transfer to an acute care facility.

Subjective: **Symptoms**
Abrupt onset of abdominal/pelvic pain. The duration of the pain by definition (acute) is less than 2 weeks. Character of pain and other symptoms vary depending on the cause.
Ruptured ovarian cyst: Acute lower pelvic pain, often mid-cycle (day 12-16); occasional postcoital onset of pain due to disruption of cyst during intercourse; may have associated nausea; should not have associated fever; may present acutely and improve over 8-12 hours.
Torsion of the ovary: Sudden onset of severe pain (unilateral) with accompanying nausea and vomiting; not initially associated with fever but fever can be present if care is delayed; pain often radiates down inner thigh on affected side; hematologically stable. Torsion most commonly occurs with an ovarian mass, but can occur without a mass, ie, normal ovary.
Pelvic Infection: Pelvic Infection: See Part 3: General Symptoms: Gynecologic Problems: Pelvic Inflammatory Disease
Ectopic pregnancy (aka tubal pregnancy): Classic triad of missed menstrual cycle, vaginal spotting, and lower pelvic pain (not always present); pain will often be increasing prior to rupture of fallopian tube; with ruptured tube a patient may present with circulatory collapse due to hemorrhagic shock; referred shoulder pain, especially while supine, is caused by blood irritating the diaphragm (internal bleeding). History of PID, prior fallopian tube surgery, or previous ectopic pregnancy increase risk.
Focused History: What was the first day of your last menstrual cycle? (Enlarged ovarian follicles often occur during the luteal phase [>2 weeks after first day of last period]. Consider cyst rupture or torsion). *Do you use any contraception?* (Reliable forms of birth control decrease the likelihood of pregnancy and thus ectopic pregnancy. Certain methods like condoms will also decrease infectious etiologies.) *Have you had any fever, vomiting, vaginal discharge?* (can occur with infectious etiologies such as PID. Vomiting and fever may also occur with torsion).

Objective: Signs
Using Basic Tools:

Ruptured ovarian cyst: Tender adnexa (fallopian tubes and ovaries), normal ovaries after rupture. Fullness in posterior cul-de-sac may suggest blood in pelvis. Localized guarding but no rebound until rupture, no abnormal vaginal discharge, normal uterine exam, afebrile or normal vitals.

Torsion of the ovary: Very tender mass in right or left lower quadrant; rebound and guarding; afebrile early with normal WBC, but both elevated later; tachycardia often secondary to pain; delay in diagnosis can result in sepsis (may present with sepsis) due to ovarian necrosis.

Pelvic infection: Lower abdominal tenderness, adnexal tenderness, cervical motion tenderness. *See Part 3: General Symptoms: Gynecologic Problems: Pelvic Inflammatory Disease*

Ectopic pregnancy: If fallopian tube is ruptured: acute abdomen with peritonitis; nausea and vomiting; hemodynamically unstable with tachycardia, hypotension and anxiety; slightly enlarged, tender uterus with severe cervical motion tenderness. If fallopian tube not ruptured: unilateral, palpable, tender mass without peritonitis; early ectopic will not be palpable and may have intermittent, severe, cramping pain; mild vaginal spotting through a closed cervical os (open os with significant vaginal bleeding is a miscarriage).

Note: Perform rectal examination with Hemoccult for blood. Change gloves before rectal exam if the patient is having vaginal bleeding. Positive Hemoccult does not occur with the above diagnoses without co-existing GI disease.

Using Advanced Tools: Labs: WBC count (elevated in later torsion and in PID), urine HCG (ectopic), CBC (anemia due to hemorrhage from ruptured cyst or ruptured fallopian tube), stool Hemoccult (guaiac), cervical cultures for gonorrhea and chlamydia, type blood (pending transfusion if needed)

Assessment: Differential Diagnosis *(see Part 3: General Symptoms: Acute Abdominal Pain)*

Appendicitis: Frequently confused with gynecological acute pathology. Appendicitis begins in the epigastrium, migrates to the periumbilical region and then settles in the right lower quadrant (RLQ) after 6-8 hours, with rebound tenderness and RLQ tenderness to palpation (most common finding). Anorexia, nausea and vomiting are common. Prodromal symptoms include indigestion and irregularity of the bowels. The WBC count is often NOT elevated until the patient has had symptoms for over 24 hours. *See Part 4: Organ Systems: Chapter 7: Appendicitis*

Diverticulitis: Pain due to infected diverticulum is usually left lower quadrant. Past history includes diarrhea and bloody stools, low-grade fever, elevated WBC counts and age over 40.

Severe constipation: Acute cramping pain; anorexia and nausea or vomiting; common in the second and third trimesters of pregnancy; treatment with fluids and fiber will be sufficient for many women. Acute constipation can indicate underlying disease. *See Part 3: General Symptoms: Constipation*

Inflammatory bowel disease or irritable bowel syndrome: Abdominal pain rarely sudden in onset; will have a past history of intermittent symptoms including diarrhea and bloody stools.

Plan:
Treatment
Primary:
1. Stabilize patient (airway, breathing, circulation, etc).
2. Start 2 large bore IVs and initiate fluid resuscitation for unstable patients. *See Part 7: Trauma: Chapter 27: Hypovolemic Shock*
3. If PID, then treat per PID section. *See Part 3: General Symptoms: Gynecologic Problems: Pelvic Inflammatory Disease.* If other abdominal suspected, *see Part 3: General Symptoms: Acute Abdominal Pain*
4. Initiate transfer/evacuation if patient has: <u>possible ovarian torsion, ectopic pregnancy or is hemodynamically unstable</u>. These conditions cannot be managed safely in the field and surgical management can be life-saving.
5. If the patient's diagnosis is consistent with ruptured ovarian cyst and she is hemodynamically stable, she can be placed on bed rest. Repeat vital signs and physical examination q4h. She should improve and be ambulatory in 6-12 hours. NSAIDs may be given, as well as mild narcotics (should only be necessary for the 1st 12-24 hours, if at all. If a significant narcotic need exists beyond 12 hours, the patient should be evacuated).

Primitive: If you are unable to evacuate the patient immediately, institute bed rest and fluid resuscitation with lactated Ringer's or normal saline. Blood transfusion may be life-saving and should be given if patient has failed resuscitation with crystalloid or is otherwise showing signs of inadequate tissue perfusion.

Patient Education
General: Reassure patient and discuss treatment plan even in emergency situations.
Activity: Bed rest
Diet: NPO initially if surgery is a consideration and available.
Medications: Give adequate narcotics to patients whose care is delayed or who must be transferred. Do not over-sedate.
No Improvement/Deterioration: Return for evacuation.

Follow-up Actions
Return Evaluation: Start a patient with recurrent ovarian cysts (*see Mittelschmerz in Part 3: General Symptoms: Gynecologic Problems: Pelvic Pain, Chronic*) on oral contraceptive pills to suppress ovulation. A good pill to start would be **Ortho-Novum** 1/35 if available.

Evacuation/Consultation Criteria: Acute pelvic pain can only be observed if the facility has the capability to intervene surgically. If not, the patient must be transferred. These patients often need abdominal ultrasound or CT, which is not available in primitive areas.

Gynecologic Problems: Pelvic Pain, Chronic
MAJ Timothy Pellini, MC, USA

Introduction: Although no generally excepted definition exists, chronic pelvic pain (CPP) is commonly defined as non-cyclic pelvic pain of at least 6 months duration. There are numerous causes of CPP; determining a source can be very challenging and beyond the scope of this section. In addition to GYN causes, gastrointestinal, urologic, musculoskeletal, neurologic, psychiatric, endocrine, and infectious etiologies are known causes of CPP. For the SOF medic, chronic pelvic pain cannot be cured, but simple, helpful treatments can be initiated. In non-western countries where routine medical care is not available, female patients with chronic pelvic pain may have more serious disease such as cancer (gynecologic, gastrointestinal, urologic) or pelvic tuberculosis. These women are more likely to have weight loss, fatigue, anorexia, night sweats, bloating, bowel/bladder complaints, and abnormal vaginal bleeding. Four commonly seen causes of CPP are discussed in Table 3-7. For further information, *see* http://emedicine.medscape.com/article/258334

Table 3-7. Differential Diagnosis of Chronic Pelvic Pain

	Endometriosis	Dysmenorrhea	Mittelschmerz	IBS
Age of onset	Early 30s-40 but may be seen as early as late teens.	With first menstrual cycles, usually age 12-14.	May occur at any time after the start of menses	May occur at any time in the life cycle
***Subjective:* Symptoms**	New or gradual onset of menstrual pain. May start 7-10 days prior to menstrual cycle, deep pain during intercourse, sacral backache with menses. Pain often radiates to inner thighs. Menses may be heavier. History of infertility.	Pain (cramps), mild to severe start and end with menstruation, radiate to sacrum, vagina and inner thigh area.	Mid-cycle pain days 12-16 of menstrual cycle (count the first day of bleeding as day #1). Gradual onset of crampy lower pelvic pain which peaks in 24-36 hours. Often unilateral. Occasionally sudden onset. Light vaginal bleeding may occur.	Symptoms wax and wane. Pain cycles lasting weeks to months. Colicky pain associated with a feeling of rectal fullness. Pain improves with BM and flatus. Alternating constipation and diarrhea. "Bloating" frequent complaint.
***Objective:* Signs**	Abd exam may elicit mild tenderness. Palpation of uterus and ovaries often very painful. Occasionally may feel nodules behind the uterus, will not have fever or elevated WBC count.	Physical exam will be WNL unless patient is menstruating. Patient will have significant discomfort with exam during menses but no abnormalities of uterus or ovaries should be found. Afebrile, nml WBC.	May have diffuse mild abd tenderness. Enlarged, tender ovary may be present or ovaries may be WNL. Afebrile, WBC count WNL.	Diffuse tenderness on abd exam, greater in LLQ. Often note excessive discomfort with rectal exam. Exam otherwise nonspecific.

Assessment

Endometriosis: Caused by the presence of functional ectopic endometrial glands, which may be located in the ovaries, uterus, uterosacral ligaments or any area within the pelvis. Essentially small bits of the uterine lining are growing in areas where they should not be; the body reacts to these implants causing tissue damage.

Symptoms: Dysmenorrhea (pain with menstruation) will occur in most women with endometriosis. This is usually a change for them with worsening from the normal minor menstrual discomfort; it will often start at least a week prior to the onset of menstruation and may last a few days after blood flow stops. This pain often radiates to the rectum and inner thighs. Pain with intercourse (dyspareunia) is common and sometimes the only complaint; it becomes worse during menses. Patients are often reluctant to engage in sexual activity because of this pain. It is not uncommon for women with endometriosis to have daily pelvic pain. There also appears to be a certain genetic component with 5-10% having a family history positive for the disease.

Focused History: *Does the pain worsen with menstruation? Does the pain occur at times other than during menses? Have you had problems getting pregnant (infertility)? Do you have pain with intercourse?* (Painful intercourse [dyspareunia] caused by endometriosis is described as "deep inside" or high in the vagina. Pain with initial penetration that occurs at the entrance to the vagina is of other origin.)

Pelvic Examination: Palpating the uterus and ovaries often reproduces the pain. The pain may be reproduced with deep abdominal palpation but this is not a reliable finding. As endometriosis can cause scarring in the pelvis, one can find that the uterus and ovaries are immobile due to adhesions. Endometriosis can also cause ovarian cysts known as endometriomas.

Treatment: As endometriosis is a common cause of pelvic pain, it is best keep this disease high in the differential diagnosis. Many women are not diagnosed for years and so treatment is delayed. In a patient with any history consistent with the previous review, it is best to start NSAIDs, birth control pills and refer to gynecology as surgery (laparoscopy) gives the definitive diagnosis and often alleviates symptoms. **Ibuprofen** 800mg po tid or **naproxen** 500mg po bid should be helpful. Birth control pills suppress ovulation, which will decrease the activity of the endometriosis implants. Occasional narcotic OK (eg, **acetaminophen/codeine** #3, 2 tabs po q4-6h prn pain.)

Primary Dysmenorrhea: Dysmenorrhea (painful menstruation) is classified as primary when there is no underlying organic cause other than prostaglandin release from the uterus itself during the time of menstruation.

Symptoms: Once a woman's cycles become ovulatory, anywhere from 6 months to 2 years after the start of her periods, she can experience dysmenorrhea and most do. Age of onset is therefore 6-24 months after the start of menstruation. The pain ranges from very mild to quite severe. It is described as cramping in nature and is felt in the sacral area, low pelvis and inner thigh area. It usually starts and ends with menstruation. The patient feels well throughout the remainder of her cycle. Some will have 1-2 days of premenstrual pain. Many young women will "grow out of" their primary dysmenorrhea. Women may have associated nausea, vomiting and diarrhea (due to excessive prostaglandin release from the uterus). Some may be severely fatigued, pale and ill appearing. Occasionally vasovagal loss of consciousness may occur, but usually with the early years of menstruation only. Fever is not present; anorexia is rare other than with the first day of a severe menstrual cycle.

Focused History: *Is the pain only present during your menstrual cycle?* (*See Table 3-7*)

Diagnosis: Based on history. Physical examination including pelvic should be normal. If the patient is examined during her menstrual cycle, her bimanual examination may be notable for a tender uterus that is of normal shape and size.

Treatment: Involves prostaglandin release suppression with NSAIDs and/or hormonal suppression of ovulation with birth control pills. Any available NSAID (eg, **ibuprofen** 800mg po tid or **naproxen** 500mg po bid) is appropriate; it is important to prescribe at the maximal level and to have the patient take them regularly either once the pain starts or 1-3 days prior to the onset of her periods. Birth control pills are very effective at decreasing menstrual pain and should be prescribed to all who fail NSAIDs. Regular exercise also decreases menstrual pain and premenstrual tension. Patients who do not respond to the previous treatments should be referred to a gynecologist.

Mittelschmerz: Ovulatory pain. Some women have midcycle pain due to either distension of the ovarian capsule or spillage of the ovarian contents at the time of ovulation. This pain usually coincides with the 12th-16th day of the menstrual cycle (count the first day of bleeding as day #1). Women will sometimes have a small amount of vaginal bleeding during this time.

Symptoms: Gradual or rapid onset of pelvic pain that will usually peak in 24 hours and then remit. Occasionally the pain will be acute in onset and more painful then usual. This may be a ruptured ovarian cyst. The most significant piece of history is the timing of the pain-Mittelschmerz will usually be on the 12th-16th day. In women with irregular and/or infrequent periods, the diagnosis will be more difficult.

Focused History: *When does the pain occur in relation to your period and is the pain cyclic?* (This pain should be mid-cycle, approx 12-14 days after the period and be unilateral.)

Pelvic Examination: Often the exam is only significant for generalized lower pelvic discomfort that is mild to moderate in nature. The ovary will sometimes be enlarged. A woman ovulates from only one side each month, so the pain is often lateralizing and changes sides month-to-month.

Diagnosis: A menstrual diary and pain scale are very helpful. The patient can mark the first day of her cycle and then each day that she has pain. If the pain occurs only during midcycle, it is Mittelschmerz. Pain that occurs frequently throughout the month will fall into another category.

Treatment: NSAIDs such as **ibuprofen** 800mg po tid will help to alleviate discomfort. For acute pain, give **ketorolac** 30-60mg IM. Primary treatment is ovulatory suppression with birth control pills.

Irritable Bowel Syndrome (IBS): may be the source of chronic pelvic pain or may occur in conjunction with diseases such as endometriosis. IBS is a disease of abnormal bowel motility triggered by situational stress and certain substances (lactose). Studies show that patients with IBS have increased colonic contractions particularly in response to meals. IBS is often worse the week prior to and during menses and may cause dyspareunia. The discomfort that occurs is often left lower quadrant and lower abdominal, causing many women to interpret their symptoms as related to the uterus and/or ovaries.

Symptoms: Colicky abdominal pain with a sensation of rectal fullness and bloating. Pain is often relieved with bowel movement and exacerbated by meals. The symptoms wax and wane in a cyclic fashion, sometimes lasting for months. The cycles often parallel physical or emotional stress. Abdominal pain is usually accompanied by diarrhea and/or constipation but occasionally may be the only complaint.

Focused History: *Does a specific food or other event trigger your symptoms?* (refer to the symptoms directly)

Physical Examination: In patients with IBS, the uterus and ovaries should be WNL unless a coexisting gynecological problem exists. It is best not to examine these patients in the week prior to and during menses as they may have increased sensitivity to examination. A patient in the midst of an IBS attack may have slight abdominal distension due to gas and mild discomfort to palpation.

Treatment: Involves behavior and dietary modifications. Patients often respond to increased dietary fiber (**psyllium powder**). Fluid intake is often inadequate and should be increased; caffeine should be minimized. Patients should identify and avoid food triggers. Common food triggers include fried and other excessively fatty foods, milk products, rice and beans (in patients not used to a primarily vegetarian diet). Increased aerobic activity may be helpful. Warm baths or heating pads to the abdomen are often helpful during acute exacerbations. *See Part 3: General Symptoms: Acute Abdominal Pain.*

Plan:

Diagnostic Tests

1. Urine culture, cervical cultures to rule out gonorrhea and chlamydia.
2. A pain diary is extremely helpful and diagnostic in many cases. The patient should chart the days of menstruation. She should note pain on a scale of 1-10 and any other accompanying symptoms, including physical and psychological symptoms. If she did something that made the pain better or worse, it should also be noted. Episodes of intercourse are important to mark down. Women with significant pelvic pain will often limit their intercourse.
3. If available, radiographs of the pelvis and lumbar-sacral spine can identify other potential explanations of chronic pelvic pain.

Treatment: *See Treatment sections.*

Patient Education

General: Most chronic pain can be successfully treated in a systematic fashion. There is no quick fix or "magic bullet" for chronic pelvic pain. Comply with therapeutic suggestions. Warm compresses, rest and warm baths can be helpful for many types of chronic pain. Relaxation and meditation have helped many women deal with and decrease pain.

Activity: As tolerated. Maintain a normal lifestyle.

Diet: As tolerated. For patients with constipation, recommend high-fiber with adequate fluids.

Medications: A three-month trial of OCPs is necessary to initiate pain suppression. They will not work immediately.

No Improvement Deterioration: Referral to gynecologist.

Follow-up Actions

Return Evaluation: 3 months if placed on OCPs

Evacuation/Consultation Criteria: Evacuate as needed for acute pain, unclear diagnosis, unresolved pain

Gynecologic Problems: Bacterial Vaginosis

MAJ Timothy Pellini, MC, USA

Introduction: Bacterial vaginosis (BV) is the most common cause of vaginal discharge in women of child-bearing age. BV is caused by a vaginal overgrowth of several indigenous bacterial species. Risk factors for acquisition of BV include multiple or new sexual partners, douching, and smoking. Treatment of male sexual partners has not been shown to prevent recurrence.

Subjective: Symptoms
Vaginal discharge. Symptoms are localized to the vagina rather than throughout the pelvis. Pain with urination and intercourse are rare.
Focused History: *What does the discharge look like? Does it have an odor?* (Most commonly, women present with an off-white, thin vaginal discharge with a foul-fishy odor made worse after intercourse.)

Objective: Signs
Using Basic Tools: Pelvic exam: Thin, off-white discharge adherent to side walls of the vagina; pooled fluid in the posterior vaginal cul-de-sac; amine (fishy) odor to discharge after adding 10% potassium hydroxide (*see Assessment section*).
Using Advanced Tools: Labs: Examine discharge, prepare wet mount (normal saline)/KOH slides (*see Part 8: Procedures: Chapter 32: Wet Mount and KOH Prep*), test pH with urine dipstick. Consider STD and pregnancy evaluation.

Assessment:
Diagnosis based on the discharge having 3 out of these 4 characteristics: pH greater than 4.5; homogenous, thin appearance; fishy odor with the addition of 10% KOH; presence of clue cells (vaginal epithelial cells with their cell borders obscured by bacteria). For a diagnosis of BV, at least 20% of epithelial cells should be clue cells. The presence of clue cells is the most reliable predictor of BV.
Differential Diagnosis
Candida vaginitis or trichomonas: *See Table 3-8*
Gonorrhea/chlamydia: *See Part 5: Specialty Areas: Chapter 11: Urethral Discharge*
PID: May have fever, chills, abdominal/pelvic pain as well as vaginitis complaints. *See Part 3: General Symptoms: Gynecologic Problems: Pelvic Inflammatory Disease*

Plan:
Treatment
Primary: Metronidazole 500mg po bid x 7 days
Alternative: Clindamycin 300mg po bid x 7 days
Primitive: No treatment as BV resolves spontaneously in up to 33% of pregnant and non-pregnant women.
Note: If patient is breastfeeding or in 1st trimester of pregnancy, give **clindamycin**. It is not necessary to treat sexual partners of affected females.
Patient Education
General: Take medications as prescribed and abstain from intercourse during treatment period.
Activity: Regular
Diet: As tolerated Medications: No alcohol consumption (including mouthwash or topical alcohol-containing products) during treatment with metronidazole due to Antabuse-like effect (extreme fatigue, vomiting, anxiety, etc.)
No Improvement/Deterioration: Return immediately
Follow-up Actions
Return Evaluation: If symptoms do not resolve, the most likely cause of persistent disease is noncompliance with medical therapy. If patient has been compliant, may re-treat with the previously mentioned regimes for 14 days. A treatment regimen different from the initial or previous treatment can be considered (eg, if previously treated with metronidazole, try clindamycin and vice-versa). Must also consider other etiologies if treatment fails (trichomonas, gonorrhea, chlamydia, atrophic vaginitis, etc). If the patient has any suggestion of STD/PID, treat immediately.
Consultation Criteria: Worsening; possible PID

Gynecologic Problems: *Candida* Vaginitis/Vulvitis

MAJ Timothy Pellini, MC, USA

Introduction: *Candida* vaginitis and vulvitis (aka "yeast infections") are inflammatory conditions caused by *Candida* yeast. Yeast infections account for 33% of vaginitis cases. Other than the localized symptoms, there are no long-term or immediate sequelae of vaginal/vulvar candidiasis although a small percentage of females will have frequent recurrence requiring prolonged treatment. **Risk Factors:** Pregnancy, diabetes, immunosuppression (includes HIV) and antibiotic use. Yeast infections are not considered sexually transmitted and treatment of partners of affected women is not recommended.

Subjective: Symptoms
Vulvar and vaginal itching are the most common complaints. Women may also complain of painful urination, vaginal/vulvar soreness, and painful intercourse. There is often little or no discharge; if present, typically white and curd-like (cottage cheese). Symptoms will be localized to the vulva and vagina.
Focused History: *Have you had this before?* (may be "exactly like" her last infection) *Do you have a new partner?* (Increased intercourse can change vaginal pH and predispose to *Candida* vaginitis and bacterial vaginosis. Consider STD screening. *See Part 3: General Symptoms: Gynecologic Problems: Pelvic Inflammatory Disease*)

Objective:
Perform physical exam if possible as self-diagnosis can be inaccurate. Incorrect diagnosis and treatment can lead to vulvar dermatitis and delay in appropriate diagnosis/treatment. *See Part 3: General Symptoms: Gynecologic Problems: Female Pelvic Examination &*

Part 8: Procedures: Chapter 32: Wet Mount and KOH Prep

Using Basic Tools: Physical exam shows erythema and edema of the vulva (especially the labia) and vagina. Discharge is classically described as thick, white, curdy discharge, which may look like cottage cheese, adherent to side walls of the vagina. Fissures of the vulva; self-inflicted scratches of the vulva.

Using Advanced Tools: Labs: KOH (potassium hydroxide) wet-mount examination yields yeast hyphae in 50-80% of patients. Test vaginal pH with a urine dipstick. It will be 4-4.5 in patient with *Candida*.

Assessment: Differential Diagnosis

Bacterial vaginosis: *See Part 3: General Symptoms: Gynecologic Problems: Bacterial Vaginosis*
Trichomonas infection: *See Part 3: General Symptoms: Gynecologic Problems: Vaginal Trichomonas*
Gonorrhea: *See Part 5: Specialty Areas: Sexually Transmitted Diseases: Urethral Discharges*
Chlamydia infection: *See Part 5: Specialty Areas: Sexually Transmitted Diseases: Urethral Discharges*

Plan:

Treatment
Primary: Fluconazole 150mg po x1 (preferred if available due to oral route and single dose).
Alternative: Clotrimazole 1% vaginal cream q day x 7 days or **miconazole** 2% vaginal cream q day x 7 days.
Note: Intravaginal antifungals may be used throughout pregnancy. Avoid oral fluconazole. Both intravaginal and oral therapies are safe during breastfeeding.

Patient Education
General: Complete all medication as prescribed since incomplete treatment is a reason for recurrence.
Activity: Normal
Medications: Burning and erythema (sensitivity to meds) may accompany topical treatment; discontinue and treat with oral fluconazole.
Prevention and Hygiene: Wipe urethra/vagina from front to back. Wear cotton underpants and loose clothing. Wash underwear in hot water.
No Improvement/Deterioration: Return immediately for reevaluation.

Table 3-8. Gynecologic Problems: Vaginitis Chart

Infection	Signs/Symptoms	Diagnosis	Treatment	Notes
Candidal Vaginitis	• Vulvar/vaginal itching • Swelling and redness of the vulva with irritation • If discharge present will be odorless, clumpy, white (cottage cheese like) • Dyspareunia may be present because of vaginal irritation. No pelvic pain	• Vaginal pH <4.5 • Discharge visualized either on external genitalia or in the vagina is consistent with diagnosis • KOH prep will show hyphae	*See Part 3: General Symptoms: Gynecologic Problems: Candida Vaginitis/ Vulvitis*	• While not ideal, a patient with complaints consistent with *Candida* may be treated empirically without examination if resources are limited. Follow-up if discharge worsens despite treatment. • Treat with **metronidazole** if patient fails anti-fungal and has a foul smelling discharge. Also consider STD testing.
Bacterial Vaginosis	• Malodorous, off-white vaginal discharge • Vaginal and perineal irritation • Patient will not have pelvic pain or fever. • Dyspareunia usually absent.	• Vaginal pH >4.5 • Odor should be apparent at time of exam (fishy smelling discharge after adding 10% KOH to slide) • Thin, grey discharge present on vulva and vagina • Wet prep reveals clue cells	*See Part 3: General Symptoms: Gynecologic Problems: Bacterial Vaginosis*	• If unable to perform speculum exam and microscopic exam of discharge, the diagnosis can be suggested based on the type of discharge, the patient's symptoms and the abdominal exam. • A bimanual exam is necessary if patient complains of pelvic pain.
Trichomonas	• Malodorous, purulent discharge which may cause significant irritation of the vulva and vagina. • Patients often have dyspareunia and dysuria. • No pelvic pain or fever	• Vaginal pH >4.5 (5-6) • Vulva may appear red and swollen. • Discharge present on vulva with or without odor • Cervix may appear red. • Wet prep reveals motile, flagellated organisms.	*See Part 3: General Symptoms: Gynecologic Problems: Vaginal Trichomonas & Part 5: Specialty Areas: Chapter 11: Urethral Discharge*	• As Trich is virtually always sexually transmitted, partners must be treated and intercourse should be stopped until treatment is complete. • Patients should be tested for STDs if possible.

Gynecologic Problems: Vaginal Trichomonas

MAJ Timothy Pellini, MC, USA

Introduction: *Trichomonas* vaginalis, a flagellated protozoan, is the causative agent of trichomoniasis. *Trichomonas* is virtually always sexually transmitted and is associated with a high prevalence of co-infection with other sexually transmitted diseases (STDs).

Subjective: Symptoms

Purulent, malodorous, thin discharge (green-yellow, frothy); vulvovaginal burning; pruritus; painful urination; painful intercourse

Focused History: *Is there any particular color/odor to the discharge? Any associated vulvar/vaginal pain, burning, itching? Any associated urinary symptoms (burning, frequency, etc)? Any history of sexually transmitted diseases?*

Objective: Signs

Using Basic Tools: Pelvic Exam: Characteristic discharge not always present (10-30%); vulva may be erythematous; redness of the cervix ("strawberry cervix").

Using Advanced Tools: Labs: Vaginal pH should be >4.5 (test with urine dipstick); motile, flagellated trichomonads on wet prep. *See Part 8: Procedures: Chapter 32: Wet Mount and KOH Prep*

Assessment: Differential Diagnosis

Bacterial vaginosis: *See Part 3: General Symptoms: Gynecologic Problems: Bacterial Vaginosis*

Candida vaginitis: *See Part 3: General Symptoms: Gynecologic Problems: Candida Vaginitis/Vulvitis*

Gonorrhea or chlamydial infection: *See Part 5: Specialty Areas: Sexually Transmitted Diseases: Urethral Discharges*

Atrophic vaginitis

Plan:

Treatment

Primary: Metronidazole 2g po x 1 or **metronidazole** 500mg po bid x 7 days (95% cure rate).

Empiric: Treatment of sexual partner reasonable plan while in a deployed setting. Can use oral **metronidazole** during pregnancy. Treatment of asymptomatic pregnant patients is controversial.

Patient Education:

General: Taking medication as directed is essential for cure. Partner must be treated with same regimen. Partner often asymptomatically carries *Trichomonas* in the urethra.

Activity: Refrain from intercourse until treatment complete.

Diet: As tolerated

Medications: Refrain from alcohol and use of alcohol-containing products during treatment because of Antabuse-like effect (vomiting, anxiety, myalgia, etc) with metronidazole

Prevention and Hygiene: Recommend condom use. Discuss STD risks and prevention.

No Improvement/Deterioration: Return for re-evaluation.

Follow-up Actions:

Return Evaluation: Full STD workup is required for both the patient and sexual partner as soon as possible.

Consultation Criteria: No improvement after first course of medication

Notes: If symptoms suggest PID, treat as PID. Partner should receive treatment for trichomonas.

Gynecologic Problems: Pelvic Inflammatory Disease

MAJ Timothy Pellini, MC, USA

Introduction: Pelvic inflammatory disease (PID) refers to an ascending infection (cervical-->upper genital tract) involving any or all of the uterus, fallopian tubes, or ovaries. PID more commonly results from a sexually transmitted agent (gonorrhea, chlamydia, etc) and less commonly from medical procedures, pregnancy, or primary abdominal process (appendicitis, diverticular disease, etc). **Risk factors:** Multiple sex partners, exposure to gonorrhea or chlamydia, patient age (15-25 years old), prior history of PID, and birth control choice. No one diagnostic test has superior sensitivity or specificity. The diagnosis of PID should be based on physical exam findings with available lab tests serving to support the diagnosis, not refute the diagnosis. SOF medics must have a low threshold for considering the diagnosis of PID and initiate empiric antibiotics promptly.

Subjective: Symptoms

Bilateral lower abdominal pain is the usual cardinal presenting symptom. The pain may increase with movement or intercourse. Abnormal vaginal bleeding is present in 1/3 of cases of PID. Fever occurs less than 50% of the time. The onset of symptoms is often within 7 days of the start of menses.

Focused History: *Do you have a history of pelvic inflammatory disease or STD?* (indicates increased risk) *Does your sexual partner have symptoms of a STD?* (increases risk) *Do you have sexual intercourse during menses?* (increased risk of PID) *Have you noticed recent onset of pain during intercourse?* (may be presenting complaint)

Objective: Signs

Using Basic Tools: Physical exam findings of diffuse abdominal tenderness increased in the lower quadrants, bilateral adnexal tenderness, and cervical motion tenderness are diagnostic. Also fever >101°F and/or mucopurulent cervical discharge.

Using Advanced Tools: Labs: Test results positive for gonorrhea or chlamydia, WBC count >10,500; Gram's stain of cervical discharge with gram-negative intracellular diplococci, and presence of white blood cells on saline microscopy of cervical discharge.

Assessment:

Minimum criteria for clinical diagnosis of PID: Lower abdominal tenderness, bilateral adnexal tenderness, cervical motion tenderness. Always rule out pregnancy.

Differential Diagnosis:

GI: Appendicitis, cholecystitis, constipation, gastroenteritis, inflammatory bowel disease (**Note:** Pain limited to RUQ does not exclude PID, which may include symptoms of peri-hepatitis.) Predominance of symptoms related to GI tract suggests a GI diagnosis.

Renal: Urinary tract infection, kidney stone/infection. Predominance of symptoms related to the urinary tract (eg, frequency, urgency, dysuria) suggest a urinary tract diagnosis.

GYN: Ovarian torsion, ruptured ovarian cyst, ectopic pregnancy, painful menses (dysmenorrhea).

Plan:

Treatment

1. **Ceftriaxone** 250mg IM x 1 plus **doxycycline** 100mg po q12h x 14 days. If you have any doubt regarding compliance, substitute **azithromycin** 1g po x 1 for the doxycycline and repeat **azithromycin** 1gm po in 1 week. Doxycycline is contraindicated in pregnancy.
2. If pelvic abscess, bacterial vaginosis, trichomonas suspected, or recent instrumentation of uterus (abortion, etc.), add **metronidazole** 500mg po q12h x 14 days.
3. Bed rest with pelvic rest (no intercourse) is mandatory during the first 72 hours of therapy. Follow-up is mandatory after 48-72 hours. Family members should facilitate patient compliance.
4. Treat partners after patient provides identity.
5. If patient is pregnant and or critically ill, start antibiotic while awaiting transfer. *See Part 4: Organ Systems: Chapter 7: Acute Peritonitis*

Patient Education

General: Comply with follow-up care. Discuss STD prevention and condom use.

Activity: Rest

Diet: As tolerated

Medications: As mentioned previously. If patient develops GI intolerance, pre-medicate with any oral anti-emetic before antibiotic dose.

Prevention: Patient must not have intercourse with untreated partner even if he is asymptomatic. Avoid high-risk sexual behaviors. Use barrier methods to prevent STD transmission.

No Improvement/Deterioration: Return for re-evaluation and management.

Follow-up Actions

Return Evaluation: 48-72 hours

Evacuation/Consultation Criteria: Patients whose diagnosis is unclear or whose pain is worsening despite treatment will require immediate evacuation for management (ie, laparoscopy, pelvic ultrasound, CT scan, cervical cultures for gonorrhea and chlamydia, CBC, and testing for HIV, hepatitis B, and syphilis).

Gynecologic Problems: Bartholin's Duct Cyst/Abscess

MAJ Timothy Pellini, MC, USA

Introduction: The mucus-secreting Bartholin's glands drain by way of a 2cm duct into a groove between the hymen and labia minora at the 4:00 and 8:00 position. The most common large cyst of the vulva is a cystic dilation of an obstructed Bartholin's duct. Obstruction of the duct leads to an asymptomatic or painful vulvar mass. Obstruction of the duct, even those resulting in Bartholin's abscess formation, is less likely the result of a sexually transmitted disease. Cultures from Bartholin's abscesses are often polymicrobial and contain a range of bacteria similar to the natural vaginal flora.

Subjective: **Symptoms**

Most will be asymptomatic, may have pain with walking, sitting, tight clothing, or intercourse; mass presents right or left outside of the vagina.

Focused History: *How did you discover the mass?* (caused pain or incidentally found) *Have you had any accompanying symptoms of vaginal discharge, fevers, bowel/bladder difficulty?* (febrile episodes suggest infection) *Has this happened before and how was it treated?* (not uncommon for these to recur)

Objective: **Signs**

Using Basic Tools: Inspection: Cystic mass, red overlying skin in the area of the Bartholin's duct and gland. Palpation: Warm, may be tender, induration if an abscess. A chronic duct obstruction will often be asymptomatic and an incidental finding on pelvic exam. If incidental finding, no treatment required.

Using Advanced Tools: Labs: Gram's stain. If available, aerobic/anaerobic cultures from mass cavity (after incised).

Assessment: **Differential Diagnosis:**

Mesonephric cyst: Most commonly single but can be multiple, 1-5cm, usually seen in upper half of vagina, benign, most asymptomatic

Epithelial inclusion cyst: Usually multiple, <1cm diameter, mostly asymptomatic, no treatment needed

Fibroma: Most common benign solid vulvar tumor, all age groups, mostly in labia majora

Lipoma: Benign and slow growing, usually softer and larger than fibromas, but like fibroma mostly asymptomatic

Trauma: Hematoma formation after blunt trauma (straddle injury, MVA, assault), manage conservatively (ice pack) if <10cm and not rapidly expanding

Tumor: Benign examples (fibroma, lipoma) mentioned previously, vulvar cancer usually ulcerative lesion

Scar: Usually resulting from birth trauma or gynecologic surgery; often inclusion cysts will form in these areas.

Plan:

Treatment: Only if symptomatic

Primary:

1. Incision & drainage (*see Part 3: General Symptoms: Gynecologic Problems: Incision and Drainage of Bartholin's Gland Mass*)
2. Pain control with **ibuprofen** 800mg po tid (or other NSAID). Patient will likely need a narcotic, such as **acetaminophen/codeine #3** or **acetaminophen/oxycodone**, 1-2 tabs po every q4-6h prn for the first 24-48 hours.
3. Antibiotics If abscess present: Give **ceftriaxone** 250mg IM x one dose and **clindamycin** 300mg po tid x 7days. Add **doxycycline** 100mg po bid x 7days if chlamydia clinically suspected (unless pregnancy suspected).

Alternative: Sitz baths, warm compress, pain control, +/- antibiotics.

Primitive: Supportive treatment listed under alternative section; without therapy most abscesses tend to spontaneously rupture/drain by the 3rd-4th day.

Patient Education

General: Wear loose clothing.

Activity: Avoid sexual activity, douching or tampons until wound healed. Limit physical activity for 48-72 hours.

Medications: Avoid doxycycline in pregnancy, breastfeeding and children. Avoid sun exposure with doxycycline.

No Improvement/Deterioration: Return ASAP for purulent or foul-smelling drainage, increased pain over baseline discomfort, redness and persistent heat in the area.

Follow-up Actions:

Wound Care: Sitz baths or warm compresses tid. Keep area clean and dry.

Return Evaluation: 48 hours and two weeks post-op.

Evacuation/Consultation Criteria: Evacuate immediately for worsening pain or signs of expanding infection. Evacuate if no improvement in 48 hours or if abscess recurs.

Notes: Asymptomatic cysts in women under 40 may be observed. A gynecologic exam should be performed yearly. Women over age 40 with new-onset Bartholin's cyst have a slightly increased risk of Bartholin's gland cancer. Biopsy is necessary. If lab evaluation positive for gonorrhea or chlamydia, treat as outlined in *Part 3: General Symptoms: Gynecologic Problems: Pelvic Inflammatory Disease*.

Gynecologic Problems: Incision and Drainage of Bartholin's Gland Mass

When: When a Bartholin's mass is symptomatic (cyst or abscess)

What You Need: Sterile prep and drape; local anesthetic agent such as 1% **lidocaine** (with or without **epinephrine**); 5cc syringe; 18 gauge needle to draw up the lidocaine; 22-26 gauge needle for injection; scalpel with 15 or 11 blade; Kelly clamp or other instrument to insert into abscess and break up any loculations or adhesions; Word catheter or silver nitrate cauterization sticks or iodoform gauze (if available); suture with needle (if available)

What To Do:

1. Discuss and describe procedure with the patient. Keep her informed as you move along.
2. Give dose of antibiotics; *see Treatment section in Part 3: General Symptoms: Gynecologic Problems: Bartholin's Duct Cyst/Abscess*.
3. Gather materials and set up surgical site.
4. Fill 5cc syringe with lidocaine using 18 gauge needle; replace 18 gauge with smaller gauge needle for injection
5. Protect yourself since the abscess may spray when opened and decompressed. Wear mask, gloves, and gown if available.
6. Place patient in low lithotomy position (patient lies on her back with her buttocks at the end of the table and her feet supported in stirrups). If table with stirrups not available, then patient may lie on table or bed with feet drawn up to buttocks and ankles together in midline. It may help to place a pillow underneath the buttocks.
7. Apply sterile prep and drape
8. Inject anesthesia (3-5cc of **lidocaine** should be sufficient) in triangular pattern around abscess. Wait 5 minutes.
9. Test for numbness by pinching skin lightly with Adson forceps or other sharp object. Inject 2-3cc more anesthetic if necessary
10. Identify incision site in the vaginal mucosa, ideally inside the hymenal ring.
11. Make a stab incision in the vaginal mucosa. It must enter the mass cavity. If something (fluid, pus, etc) is not draining out, then you are not there yet. Gradually deepen the incision until reaching the abscess.
12. Insert Kelly clamp into the cavity to a depth of 2-3cm if possible, and break up any loculations or adhesions. Allow the cavity to drain. Irrigate, irrigate, irrigate!
13. Evacuate patient to a gynecologist for definitive care. If evacuation not possible, proceed with the following steps:
    A. Insert Word catheter (leave in place for 2-4 weeks) or use silver nitrate sticks to cauterize the cavity base (sclerotherapy) or cut a 15cm length of iodoform gauze and loosely pack the cavity (for 24-48 hrs). The listed steps will help promote a fistulous tract to allow continuous drainage. Simple I&D will often result in reapproximation of the incision edges and prevent recurrence. Have the patient return in 24 hours for reassessment.
    B. If the mass and symptoms recur, you can repeat the previous steps or marsupialize the gland. Open the cyst as before, and then suture the everted edges of the cavity to the vaginal mucosa. Use absorbable, interrupted suture of 3-0 or 4-0 Monocryl. This allows for continuous drainage and a permanent open path.

What Not To Do

1. Do not open a Bartholin's mass through normal skin. Enter via the vaginal mucosa.
2. Do not make too large or deep an incision.
3. Do not attempt marsupialization of the gland unless evacuation is not available to a gynecologist.

Figure 3-12. Marsupialization of Bartholin's (Greater Vestibular) Gland

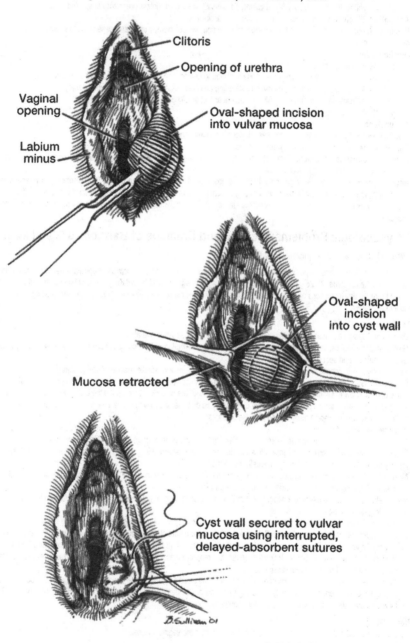

Headache

CAPT David Llewellyn, MC, USN & Maryann Hoftiezer, MSN, FNP-C

Introduction: Most headaches are non life-threatening/low risk, have no identifiable cause and are termed primary headaches (eg, migraine, cluster headache, tension headaches). Secondary headaches can be caused by virtually hundreds of conditions including referred pain from the ears, nose, throat, jaw, teeth, sinuses, neck, or tongue and generalized illness with fever can also cause a headache. Most of these secondary headaches are also non life-threatening. There are a few specific life-threatening/high-risk conditions that can present as a secondary headache. Bleeding in the central nervous system (CNS) from any cause (eg, subarachnoid bleeding, ruptured aneurism) or CNS infection (meningitis) is life-threatening. A careful history, including asking about deployed environments, and a physical examination with focus on the HEENT, neck, and the nervous system is crucial to identify these life-threatening conditions. The primary goal is to identify the small number of patients who present with a headache from a life-threatening condition from the overwhelming majority of patients who present with either a primary headache (migraine, cluster, tension) or secondary headache from a non-life threatening condition.

Subjective: Symptoms

Life-Threatening (high risk): Sudden onset (CNS bleed), no history of similar headache, coincident infection (meningitis), altered mental status, age >50 (increased risk for CNS bleeding), underlying problem with immune system (eg, AIDS increases risk of meningitis).

Non Life-Threatening (low risk): Patients usually have a history of similar headaches in the past. No changes in mental status, no stiff neck, no underlying illness or serious medical condition. **Migraine:** Pounding/throbbing pain, usually but not always unilateral, moderate to severe in intensity, often with nausea/vomiting, often with light or noise sensitivity; routine activities make it worse, patient wants to lie down in a quiet, dark room; builds up over minutes to hours and lasts hours to days; some patients have an "aura", such as flashing lights; women affected more than men. **Tension-type:** Global, squeezing headache; less severe than migraine; can last hours to weeks; no nausea or aversion to light and sound.

Cluster: Less common, but affects young men predominantly; severe, short-lived unilateral headaches, usually around the eye, lasting at most a few hours; can occur many times in a day and even wake the patient at night; may want to pace the halls (compare to migraine).

Sinus: Sinus headaches are relatively uncommon. Migraine can give sinus symptoms. Sinus headaches should have fever and purulent discharge, etc. Sudden barometric pressures changes from flying or diving can cause sinus pains.

Focused History: *Have you been at high altitude, or flying or diving?* (Exposure to extreme changes in atmospheric pressure seen at high altitude or diving may also indicate serious problems [eg, acute mountain sickness, decompression illness, breathing contaminated gases, etc.]) *Have you had a similar headache before?* (This makes a benign headache more likely.) *Have you taken headache medications? What have you tried in the past?* (use same treatment if effective) *Do you have other symptoms such as nausea, vomiting, sensitivity to light or sound?* (typical migraine) *Have you been hit in the head, or been in an accident? Do you have a fever, stiff neck or rash?* (Affirmative answer suggests meningitis, stroke, other CNS damage.) *Do you have any neurologic symptoms such as: trouble thinking/talking, loss of consciousness, visual blurring, double vision, vertigo, numbness, weakness, trouble walking or staying balanced?* (Positive answers suggest an intracranial problem.) *Does bending over make it better, worse, or have no effect?* (Pains increased by bending over or coughing could be from increased intracranial pressure, but are most likely migraine. The typical tension headache is not affected by position change. Pains worsened by standing up could be from low intracranial pressure, as can occur sometimes after a lumbar puncture or spontaneously.)

Objective: Signs

Using Basic Tools:

Life-Threatening: Inspection: Tachycardia, bradycardia, hypertension, fever (subarachnoid bleed, meningitis or increased intracranial pressure from any cause); fever (meningitis, CNS trauma, increased intracranial pressure); neck stiffness (meningitis or CNS bleed); abnormal neurological examination (including mental status examination [MMSE is adequate]; (*see Appendices: Table A-6. Mini-Mental Status Exam*) suggests a life-threatening abnormality; neurological exam may change over time, indicating a worsening condition.

Non Life-Threatening: Look for secondary causes of headache from the head, ears, eyes, nose, sinuses, temporal-mandibular joint (TMJ), throat, neck. Palpation: Trigger point tenderness to palpation (tension-type headache) or point tenderness over the TMJ area; swollen submandibular, periauricular and/or cervical lymph nodes (suggests infection or inflammation in oral pharynx, ear, or other HEENT).

Using Advanced Tools: Labs: WBC for infection. Papilledema suggests intracranial swelling, which is life-threatening. Neuro imaging and/or lumbar puncture will most likely be required if history and physical exam suggest a life-threatening condition.

Assessment: Differential Diagnosis:

Life-Threatening: Bleeding in the CNS from any cause (eg, subarachnoid bleed, ruptured aneurism); infection in the CNS (eg, meningitis).

Non Life-Threatening: Most headaches are benign and are probably migraine or tension-type headaches. Cluster headaches are more unusual but can be very painful. Secondary headaches can be referred pain from HEENT, etc. Most brain tumors do not initially cause headaches.

Post-concussive Syndrome and Mild Traumatic Brain Injury (mTBI): Head injuries are common in those exposed to IED (Improvised Explosive Devices) blasts. A very high index of suspicion should be maintained for a post-concussive syndrome in those with mild to moderate TBI. Typical symptoms include persistent headaches; cognitive complaints such as poor memory, decreased concentration, increased distractibility; dizziness; and behavioral complaints such as increased impulsiveness, irritability, fatigue, and sleep disturbances, etc. All patients suspected of suffering a head injury should be referred for further evaluation. *See Part 7: Trauma: Chapter 26: Mild Traumatic Brain Injury/Concussion*

Headaches after being at high altitude or diving: *See Part 6: Operational Environment: Chapter 20; Chapter 21 & Chapter 22*

Plan:

Treatment

1. Meningitis should be treated as soon as suspected. *See Part 4: Organ Systems Chapter 5: Meningitis*
2. First or worst headache needs emergent evacuation (CT, MRI and/or spinal tap may be needed).
3. Treat source of secondary headache, such as sinusitis, if recognized. *See Part 3: General Symptoms: ENT Problems: Sinusitis*
4. Treat primary headache symptomatically (early intervention is more effective). Patients with recurrent symptoms will require more than abortive/acute therapy and a condition of rebound migraine may develop in a patient with recurring history of headaches treated with only pain medication (eg, **acetaminophen**) for the acute event.
   a. Behavioral/nonpharmacologic: Ensure patients sleep regularly, get aerobic exercise, manage stress constructively and eat a healthy diet. Avoid caffeine or analgesic withdrawal. Local application of an ice pack or frozen bag of peas/corn may help, as may local massage or physical therapy.
   b. Prophylactic medications (oral): For all prophylactic medications, the general principle is to start at a low dose and gradually titrate to effect. "Start low and go slow." Ask women about pregnancy before prescribing these. Do not give valproic acid to a pregnant woman for headache. Most tension-type headaches are easily treated with simple over the counter medications. Once you have ruled out serious/secondary causes of headache, the condition most likely to cause problems for the most people is migraine. Migraine is a common, familial disorder related to neurotransmitter dysfunction, central sensitization to pain, and over-activity of the trigeminovascular system. If headaches are frequent, prophylactic medications could be considered. Common medications used in out-patient clinical practice are listed but, many of these medications may affect cognitive function and not appropriate in specific operational situations. Clinical judgment is needed. **Propranolol** 40 –160mg po per day, in 3 or 4 divided doses, or **verapamil** 120-360mg po per day are the only prophylactic medications that are currently on SOF Drug list. It may not be advisable to use these medications in some operational environments. Other medications (as available): **nortriptyline** 25-75mg po q hs, or **gabapentin** 300mg po tid or **valproic acid** extended release 500-1000mg po q hs, or **topiramate** 25-100mg po q day.
   c. Abortive or acute therapy: **Aspirin** 650-1000mg po, **acetaminophen** 1000mg po, **ibuprofen** 800mg po or **naproxen** 500mg po with food. Caffeine in coffee or cola sometimes helps. Some helpful combination drugs are **Midrin (acetaminophen/ dichloralphenazone/isometheptene)** 2 tabs initially, then 1 q1h to max of 5 in 12h or **Fiorinal (aspirin, butalbital, caffeine)** or **Fioricet (acetaminophen, butalbital, caffeine)** 1-2 tabs po q6h prn. Combinations of medication are more effective in some patients: **promethazine** 25mg po (which has anti-nausea and analgesic effects) + **diphenhydramine** 50mg po + **ibuprofen** 800mg po and/or **acetaminophen** 1000mg po. For management of nausea and vomiting with migraines: **Metoclopramide** 10mg po q8h prn or **prochlorperazine** 5-10mg IM q3-4h, max 40mg/day. Co-administration of **diphenhydramine** can reduce potential akathisia and dystonia, and may increase successful reduction in headache symptoms. **Ketorolac** 60mg IM is an option for those with nausea and vomiting unable to tolerate po meds. The following triptan medications specifically target migraine pathophysiology and when available are excellent for acute therapy of migraine headache: **Sumatriptan** 50-100mg po, 20mg in a nasal spray, (or 6mg in a sq auto-injector; max dose is 2 injections/incident at least 1 hr apart) or **zolmitriptan** 2.5-5.0mg po, or **rizatriptan** 5-10mg po are the most effective migraine medications, but nothing works for everyone. Limit triptan use to no more than 2 x week. **Naratriptan** 2.5mg po q day during the days of flow may be more effective for women with menstrual related headaches. The addition of **naproxen** 500mg po to triptan therapy may provide additional beneficial. Narcotics are rarely needed. Beware that overuse of analgesic medications (eg, acetaminophen) can produce rebound headaches. Supplemental magnesium and riboflavin helps some patients.

Patient Education

General: Migraine is not curable and will recur. Medications and behavioral interventions can decrease frequency, severity or duration. Most prophylactic medications take weeks to months to work, therefore patience is necessary. Smoking can worsen migraine. For women, menses often worsen migraines.

Activity: Regular aerobic exercise is helpful. Regular, adequate sleep is advised.

Diet: Avoid red wine, cheeses, aspartame, preservatives (in bologna, salami, hot dogs, sausage), and chocolate.

Medications: NSAIDs can cause GI problems. The triptans can cause a chest tightening sensation and should not be used in those with a risk of vascular disease. Ergots should also not be used in those with vascular disease or risk factors. Ergot products and triptans should not be given within 24 hrs of each other. Prophylactic medications like nortriptyline or gabapentin can cause sedation, usually manageable if titrated up slowly. Propranolol can cause fatigue, bradycardia, and is contraindicated in asthma. Valproic acid can cause weight gain. Most migraine medications are FDA categories C (toxic in animals) and D (risk of human toxicity) for pregnancy, and ergots (Cafergot and others) are X (contraindicated in pregnancy).

No Improvement/Deterioration: Reconsider your diagnosis. Unfortunately, some patients have no response to treatment or find the side effects intolerable. Refer those who do not respond for imaging and neurology evaluation.

Follow-up Actions

Return Evaluation: Reevaluate to assess effectiveness of treatment. Some patients may be depressed, and pain may be a manifestation of their depression. Treating the depression is the best treatment of the headache. Be careful not to cause a bigger problem by getting the patient hooked on narcotics.

Evaluation/Consultation Criteria: Evacuate if first or worst headache. Evacuate patient with headache and other specific neurological abnormality on history or physical exam. Evacuate if patient has history consistent with Post-Concussive Syndrome and Mild Traumatic Brain Injury (mTBI). Evacuate in other situations if service member unable to perform mission due to pain. Refer if patient fails adequate trials of standard prophylactic medications.

Jaundice
COL Peter McNally, MC, USA (Ret)

Introduction: Jaundice is the condition characterized by yellow discoloration of the skin, sclera of the eyes and mucous membranes. It results from systemic accumulation of bilirubin due to significant dysfunction of the liver and/or biliary tract. Under normal conditions, the heme protein from old red blood cells (RBCs) is broken down in the reticuloendothelial system (macrophages and other phagocytic cells) into unconjugated bilirubin, which is transported by the blood to the liver. There the liver cells (hepatocytes) conjugate the bilirubin and excrete it into the bile, where it is eventually eliminated from the body in the stool. Bilirubin is an end-product of heme degradation.

Figure 3-13. Normal Bilirubin Metabolism

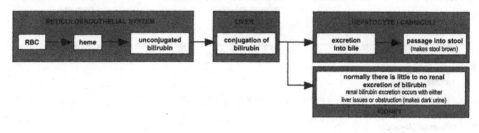

Figure 3-14. Situations of Altered Bilirubin Metabolism

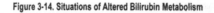

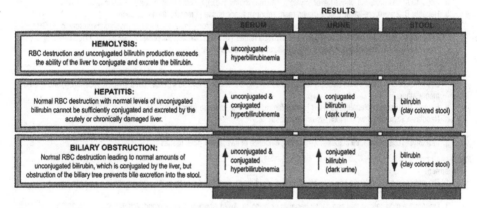

	RESULTS		
	SERUM	URINE	STOOL
HEMOLYSIS: RBC destruction and unconjugated bilirubin production exceeds the ability of the liver to conjugate and excrete the bilirubin.	↑ unconjugated hyperbilirubinemia		
HEPATITIS: Normal RBC destruction with normal levels of unconjugated bilirubin cannot be sufficiently conjugated and excreted by the acutely or chronically damaged liver.	↑ unconjugated & conjugated hyperbilirubinemia	↑ conjugated bilirubin (dark urine)	↓ bilirubin (clay colored stool)
BILIARY OBSTRUCTION: Normal RBC destruction leading to normal amounts of unconjugated bilirubin, which is conjugated by the liver, but obstruction of the biliary tree prevents bile excretion into the stool.	↑ unconjugated & conjugated hyperbilirubinemia	↑ conjugated bilirubin (dark urine)	↓ bilirubin (clay colored stool)

Subjective: Symptoms
Itching, confusion, abdominal pain, fever, weight loss, fatigue

Focused History: *When did you first notice this?* (Acute onset of symptoms with pain suggests stones. Painless jaundice with gradual onset over months suggests malignancy.) *Have you had any recent weight loss or gain?* (Rapid loss of >10% of body weight suggests malignancy and malnutrition.) *Have you recently been sick?* (Gastroenteritis symptoms of nausea, GI upset and diarrhea may suggest acute viral hepatitis. Progressive anorexia, significant weight loss [>10%], anorexia suggest malignancy. Pain, jaundice and fever [>101°F] suggests cholecystitis or cholangitis.)

Objective: Signs
Using Basic Tools:
Inspection: Frank jaundice of skin and scleral icterus (icterus of one eye only may indicate other eye is glass); fatigue, confusion and suppressed sensorium in fulminant hepatitis; spider angiomata over the blush area of the upper thorax and gynecomastia in chronic liver disease. Auscultation: Usually normal. Palpation: Enlarged and tender liver due to inflammation; spleen may also be enlarged. Ascites is uncommon in acute hepatitis, but may occur if fulminant hepatic failure occurs. A small, hard and nodular liver is typical of chronic hepatitis, cirrhosis and submassive necrosis. Percussion: Shifting abdominal dullness and fluid wave is suggestive of ascites.

Table 3-9. Comparison of Common Causes of Jaundice

Symptom/Sign	Acute Hepatitis	Chronic Hepatitis	Obstruction - stones	Obstruction - cancer
Viral prodrome	Yes	No	No	No
Pain	Tender liver	No	Yes	No
Fever	Low grade	No	Yes	No
Hepatomegaly	Yes, often tender	Often shrunken, may be enlarged and nodular	Normal	Enlargement suggests metastasis
Weight loss	Mild, anorexia	Variable	No	Yes if >10%
Stigmata of cirrhosis: • spider angiomata • gynecomastia • ascites	Usually not	Invariable, yes	No	Usually not

Using Advanced Tools: Labs: CBC for anemia, infection; urinalysis for urobilinogen

Assessment:
Differential Diagnosis
Hemolysis or hemoglobinopathy (sickle cell, G6PD, thalassemia)
Hepatic Causes (*see Part 5: Specialty Areas: Chapter 12: Viral Infections: Hepatitis A & Hepatitis B [and Hepatitis D]*): Acute or sub-acute
  hepatitis usually shows no signs of cirrhosis
  a. Hepatitis A: Influenza-like illness (fever, myalgia, nausea, vomiting, etc); tender hepatomegaly; splenomegaly in 10%.
  b. Hepatitis B: 2 week pre-icteric phase (fever, rash, arthritis); icteric phase (1 month); then resolution.
  c. Liver cell toxicity: Drugs (isoniazid, methyldopa, acetaminophen and chlorpromazine); Amanita mushroom poisoning; ETOH.
     Chronic hepatocellular disease: Show signs of cirrhosis (small, hard liver; ascites; esophageal varices; etc.) Hepatitis B or C
     (never hepatitis A): Ethanol, autoimmune hepatitis, other rare diseases
Obstructive:
  a. Stones in the gall bladder (cholecystitis), or stone in the bile duct: abdominal pain and/or fever. Charcot's triad of fever, jaundice,
     and right upper quadrant pain clinically identifies ascending cholangitis. Reynold's pentad adds shock (hypotension) and altered
     mental status.
  b. Primary sclerosing cholangitis: 80% will have inflammatory bowel disease (diarrhea)
  c. Neoplasm: Associated weight loss; usually painless
  d. Inflammation: Primary biliary cirrhosis usually seen in females 40-60 yrs, drugs (chlorpromazine, erythromycin)
  e. Infiltrative: Tuberculosis, sarcoidosis, lymphoma; evidence of invasion of other tissues

Plan:
Treatment
  1. Prevent spread of infectious hepatitis by using body fluid precautions, and managing all acute cases in an isolation area.
  2. Encourage po fluid and nutrition intake.
  3. Discontinue medications that can cause hepatitis or jaundice. Avoid all acetaminophen and alcohol.
  4. For suicide attempt with acetaminophen overdose, give **N-acetylcysteine** 140mg/kg po then 70mg/kg q4h for 17 doses
     and evacuate immediately.
  5. If clinical picture is consistent with obstructive jaundice with cholangitis (fever, RUQ abdominal pain), start IV antibiotics: **ticarcillin**
     or **piperacillin** 4g IV q6h and **metronidazole** 1g IV q12h.
Patient Education
  General: Follow body fluid precautions (*see Part 5: Specialty Areas: Chapter 12: Viral Infections: Hepatitis A & Hepatitis B [and
  Hepatitis D]*). Obtain vaccination for hepatitis A and B.
  Diet: High carbohydrate diet as tolerated. May need to limit protein to 1mg/kg per day if hepatic encephalopathy is present.
  Medications: Vitamin K 5-10mg po qd x 3 days for signs of hepatic decompensation (bleeding). Lactulose for hepatic encephalopathy
  15-30mL bid/tid (titrate to 3 loose bowel movements per day). Avoid acetaminophen.
  Prevention and Hygiene: Pre and post exposure vaccination for hepatitis A and B (*see Part 5: Specialty Areas: Chapter 13:
  Immunization Chart*). Household contacts, preschool children, barracks mates should be vaccinated for Hepatitis A. Good hand
  washing and sanitation are mandatory. Avoid promiscuous sexual contact.
  Wound Care: Blood and secretions are potentially infectious.
Follow-up Actions
  Return Evaluation: Acute viral hepatitis usually requires 2-3 months of convalescence to recover. Monitor symptoms.
  Evacuation/Consultation Criteria: Evacuate urgently if signs of hepatic decompensation such as encephalopathy, bleeding, easy
  bruisability, ascites, peripheral edema, or fever with RUQ abdominal pain. Evacuate more stable jaundiced patients when possible.
  Consult with GI specialist early and as needed.

Joint Problems: Joint Pain

LTC Michael Rossman, MC, USA

Introduction: Arthritis (joint inflammation) is not only painful, but also causes fear of disability and deformity. The pain may be mono (1 joint), oligo (2-4), or poly (≥5) articular. It may be related to trauma, overuse, degenerative processes, systemic inflammatory disease, or infection. The pain may come from the joint itself, nearby soft tissue structures, or referred from neurovascular structures. Most musculoskeletal or joint pain can be characterized as either mechanical or inflammatory. Mechanical processes can usually be treated conservatively with rest, ice, heat, or other physical therapy modalities and rehabilitative exercise. Inflammatory conditions tend to be more chronic, limiting, and require referral for specialty management. History, physical exam and evolution of the process over time are generally sufficient to distinguish mechanical from inflammatory disease. Psychosocial stresses may aggravate musculoskeletal pain. See individual sections in *Part 3: General Symptoms: Joint Problems.*

Subjective: Symptoms

Localized to joint: Pain, stiffness, swelling, warmth.

Systemic: Fever, fatigue, weight loss, loss of appetite, myalgias, and rash

Focused History: *Where does it hurt?* (Pain around a joint, with tenderness in soft tissue is likely muscle, tendon, ligament, or the bursa.) *How many joints hurt?* (The more joints, more likely it is systemic disease.) *How suddenly did the pain occur?* (In seconds or minutes, consider fracture and/or internal derangement. In hours or 1-2 days, consider infection, crystal deposition disease, or inflammatory arthritis syndromes. In days to weeks, consider indolent infections, osteoarthritis, or inflammatory arthritis syndromes.) *How long does it take to limber up in the morning to reach your best for the day?* (Stiffness resolving in <1 hr. more likely mechanical, eg, osteoarthritis; >1 hr. suspect inflammatory disease) *Any recent infections?* (consider infectious etiology.) *Have you had prior acute attacks of joint pain and swelling that resolved spontaneously in any joint?* (consider crystal deposition diseases and other inflammatory arthritis syndromes.)

1. Red, hot, swollen joint is a septic joint until proven otherwise. Gout and other crystal arthritides can mimic infection.
2. Symptoms of knee giving way or locking is usually mechanical (cartilage or ligament tear or loose body).
3. Complaints of numbness and tingling related to a sore joint are not typical arthritis complaints. Consider alternate diagnoses (eg, neurologic or neurovascular etiology).
4. There are only a few conditions that are so painful that the patient cannot put weight on the extremity: fracture, septic joint, or gout.

Objective: Signs

Using Basic Tools:

Fever: Often present with infection, but not always. Fever can also be seen with other inflammatory and crystal induced arthritis as well.

Rash: A new rash associated with arthritis usually indicates systemic disease, either infectious or inflammatory. Lesions include: papules that progress to vesico-pustules to larger hemorrhagic or bullous lesions (gonorrhea); scaly, red, hypertrophic lesions (psoriasis; discoid lupus–on face, scalp or elsewhere; reactive arthritis–on palms and soles; circinate balanitis—on penis); diffuse maculopapular rash (allergic reaction, drug reaction, serum sickness or virus); maculopapular rash on palms and soles (syphilis, Rocky Mountain spotted fever); large, red, tender subcutaneous nodules on shins that may coalesce into a more diffuse, red, swollen lower extremity, resembling cellulitis, or ankle periarthritis (erythema nodosum), hives (hepatitis B, C, or other viruses).

Eye: Conjunctivitis and iritis (Reiter's syndrome, vertebral arthritis); dry eyes and dry mouth (Sjögren's syndrome, and other connective tissue diseases).

Oral Cavity: Painless ulcers (Reiter's syndrome, lupus, syphilis)

Joint: Inspection: Examine the joint for swelling, effusion, deformity, erythema, and active range of motion. Inability to bear weight on the effected extremity suggests a fracture, septic joint, or gout. Palpation: Palpate for tenderness (joint versus surrounding tissue) and warmth (suggestive of inflammation and maybe infection). Perform passive ROM (Reduced active ROM with preserved passive ROM suggests soft tissue disorders such as bursitis, tendonitis, or muscle injury. If both active and passive ROM decreased, then soft tissue contracture, synovitis, or structural abnormality should be considered.) Joint stability: laxity with valgus or varus stress on a joint (usually elbow or knee) or a drawer sign (usually knee or ankle) or repeated joint dislocations is generally a sign of ligament or tendon injury.

Using Advanced Tools: Joint aspiration and Gram's stain of effusion: In the absence of a history of trauma, infusion or other signs of inflammation are infection until proven otherwise. Septic joints are almost always monoarticular; a significant joint effusion in a single accessible joint should be aspirated. For patients unable to be evacuated who have pain secondary to accumulation of infected fluid, joint aspiration may be both diagnostic and therapeutic. Diagnostic indication for joint aspiration is to differentiate bacterial (septic) from other inflammatory conditions. Operational realities and clinical condition may require a presumptive diagnosis of septic arthritis, initiation of antibiotic therapy and medical evacuation with re-evaluation of requirement for joint aspiration at next levels of care.

Labs:

1. Synovial fluid cell count with hemacytometer:
   a. WBC <2000 with <25% PMNs = noninflammatory fluid - osteoarthritis, trauma, avascular necrosis.
   b. WBC >2000, but <50,000 (5000 - 15,000 common) with 20-70% PMNs = inflammatory fluid - gout, pseudogout, viral, Lyme disease, rheumatoid arthritis, other arthritis
   c. WBC>50,000 = septic joint until proven otherwise
   d. RBC: TNTC = hemarthrosis - major trauma including fracture, internal derangement (ACL, meniscal tear), bleeding disorder
2. Gram's stain: Positive if infected with staph or strep; in gonococcal arthritis Gram's stain positive <25% of time
3. WBC: Elevated WBC with a left shift favors infection but does not rule out gout or inflammatory process.
4. Urinalysis: Proteinuria, hematuria, and RBC casts are seen in glomerulonephritis, which is associated with many types of polyarthritis including lupus, and some infections like endocarditis, hepatitis B&C, osteomyelitis, or HIV.

5. Monospot in the appropriate clinical setting can confirm the diagnosis of mononucleosis.
6. RPR in the appropriate clinical setting can confirm the diagnosis of syphilis.

Assessment: Differential Diagnosis

Monoarthritis: Septic joint: red, hot swollen joint is septic joint until proven otherwise and requires immediate treatment. History of crystalline disease (gout and pseudogout) helps, but does not rule out infection. Fracture and internal derangement are usually associated with significant trauma to affected joint. Tendonitis, bursitis and other soft tissue inflammation usually involves one joint region and can be distinguished from true arthritis by physical exam. Chronic mono- or oligoarticular pain (>6 weeks) is unusual. Degenerative disease (osteoarthritis) presents without inflammation or effusion. Chronically inflamed joints are likely septic with fungus or TB as the most likely organisms.

Oligoarthritis: The spondyloarthropathies, or vertebral arthritides, share common features of asymmetric oligoarthritis, inflammatory back pain, oral lesions, and inflammation of attachment tendons and ligaments. The group includes ankylosing spondylitis, reactive arthritis, psoriatic arthritis, and the arthritis associated with inflammatory bowel disease. Ankylosing spondylitis presents as insidious onset of inflammatory low back pain in young men (onset <age 40 yr.) and is often mistaken for mechanical lumbar sprain or strain for years before the diagnosis of inflammatory arthritis disease is entertained. Also can involve uveitis of the eyes. Reactive arthritis (previously referred to as Reiter's syndrome) begins after an infection, often a nonspecific urethritis, a post-gonococcal urethritis or a bacterial bowel infection with bloody diarrhea. In the weeks following the infection, the patient develops conjunctivitis and/or shallow, painless oral ulcers. These symptoms may be mild and overlooked or not reported. Shortly after, the patient develops an asymmetric oligoarticular inflammatory arthritis, usually involving large joints of the lower extremity, eg, knee or ankle. Psoriatic arthritis precedes psoriasis or occurs simultaneously 33% of the time. 67% of the time psoriasis precedes the arthritis. Approximately 95% of patients with psoriatic arthritis have peripheral disease. The other 5% have only axial involvement. Arthritis associated with inflammatory bowel disease usually is seen in people previously diagnosed with ulcerative colitis or Crohn's disease. Arthritis flares coincide with bowel flares 60-70%. Inflammatory low back pain awakens patient at night, causes profound morning stiffness lasting >1 hr., localizes to sacroiliac joint with tenderness, improves with exercise, radiates into the buttocks, posterior thigh and knee (not below the knee) and may alternate buttocks.

Polyarthritis: Involves both small and large joints in a symmetric fashion. Acute polyarthritis is often self-limited and resolves within 6 weeks without clear-cut diagnosis (viral, post-viral or post-vaccination arthritis). If the process last >6 weeks, it is most commonly rheumatoid arthritis.

Plan:

Treatment

General (mechanical, as well as some inflammatory causes of arthritis):

1. Rest, compress and elevate inflamed joints.
2. Apply ice and/or heat (alternating for 20 min each). Heat may feel better on a sore joint, but do not use within 48 hours of an acute injury.
3. Immobilize and protect joint with splint, brace, or cast and use crutches or cane, as appropriate.
4. Perform (active or passive) gentle range of motion exercises bid/tid early in treatment to retain mobility.
5. Later, perform strengthening and isometric exercises for supporting muscles followed by isotonic and weight bearing exercises as soon as tolerated.
6. Provide analgesia:
   A. **Acetaminophen:** Up to 1g po qid prn
   B. Severe joint pain may require narcotics (**codeine** or **oxycodone**) until patient can be transported for further evaluation.
   C. Nonsteroidal Anti-inflammatory drugs (NSAIDs) will also decrease inflammation at full strength and regular dosing.
      1. **Ibuprofen** 800mg po tid
      2. **Naproxen** 500mg po bid (often provides better compliance with less frequent dosing)
      3. **Piroxicam** 20mg po q day (better compliance but slower onset)
      4. **Indomethacin** 50mg po tid (preferred for intense inflammation as in gout or spondyloarthropathy)
      5. **Tolmetin** 400mg po tid (good alternative if indomethacin not tolerated due to CNS side effects)
7. Consider muscle relaxants, which may reduce muscle spasm and back pain associated with sacroiliitis, and may improve sleep disturbances and early morning pain and stiffness. **Cyclobenzaprine** 10mg po tid, or q hs for sleep effects.
8. Aspirate knees for comfort and to assist ambulation.

For septic joint:

1. Immobilize joint and allow no weight bearing or exercise until infection treated. Consider early medical evacuation based on clinical evaluation and response to therapy.
2. **Antibiotics:**
   a. If Gram's stain of synovial fluid is not available, treat empirically. *Neisseria gonorrhoeae* is the most common cause of acute non-traumatic septic arthritis in young adults. If you suspect based on history or Gram's stain of urethral discharge, treat as disseminated gonococcal infection. Give **ceftriaxone** 1g IV/IM q day or **cefotaxime** 1g IV q8h and continue through medical evacuation. If medical evacuation is not possible, continue IV antibiotic therapy until the patient is free of clinical disease for at least 24 hours and follow with **ciprofloxacin** 500mg po bid x 7 days. Treat patients with presumed gonorrhea for presumptive concomitant *Chlamydia trachomatis* with **doxycycline** 100mg po bid x 7 days or **azithromycin** 1g po x 1. If there is no history, signs or symptoms of STD, treat as presumed bacterial (non-gonococcal) arthritis, which is the most potentially dangerous and destructive form of acute septic monoarthritis. Give **nafcillin** or **oxacillin** 2g IV q4h and continue antibiotic through medical evacuation. If methicillin-resistant *Staphylococcus aureus* (MRSA) is suspected or prevalent in your location, start **vancomycin** 1g IV q12h. If medical evacuation is not possible, the duration of IV antibiotic therapy for non-gonococcal septic arthritis is typically 14-28 days followed by **ciprofloxacin**

500mg po bid or **doxycycline** 100mg po bid x 14 days. Total **vancomycin** dose should not exceed 2g/day >14 days unless serum levels are monitored. In patients in which IV access is absolutely not possible, **dicloxacillin** 500mg po ac qid or **ciprofloxacin** 750mg po + **rifampin** 300mg po bid may be useful. Continue antibiotic therapy for at least 2 weeks following resolution of clinical disease.

b. If Gram's stain of synovial fluid is available, treat as follows:

1. For gram-positive cocci (*Staphylococcus aureus* is the most common bacterium infecting adult joints, followed by *Streptococcus pneumoniae*.) Treat as presumed bacterial non-gonococcal arthritis (ie, as previously mentioned, **nafcillin** or **oxacillin** or **vancomycin** if MRSA is suspected).

2. For gram-negative organisms: (typical gram-negative intracellular diplococci of *N. gonorrhoeae*), treat as above for presumed disseminated gonococcal infection. Other gram-negative cells (ie, not gram-negative intracellular diplococci), give **ceftazidime** 1 to 2g IV q8h or **ceftriaxone** 2g IV q12h. If medical evacuation is not possible, continue IV therapy x 2 weeks followed by **ciprofloxacin** 500mg po bid x 2 weeks.

3. Gram-negative (no organisms seen) and no other clinical indications to suggest gonorrhea (*see Part 4: Organ Systems: Chapter 6: Bacterial Infections: Disseminated Gonococcal Infection*): Treat as presumed bacterial non-gonococcal arthritis (ie, as previously mentioned, **nafcillin** or **oxacillin** or **vancomycin** if MRSA is suspected).

Gout:

1. Current preferred treatment for an acute attack is **indomethacin** 50mg po tid, or other NSAID as above.
2. Alternatively, use **colchicine** 1mg po q2h prn until pain is relieved, or until diarrhea or vomiting presents. No more than 6mg should be given in 24 hours for a given attack.
3. Do NOT start chronic suppressive therapy during an acute attack. It could worsen attack. Obtain consultation before initiating chronic therapy with **probenecid** or **allopurinol** to prevent attacks (suppress serum uric acid levels).

Other Inflammatory Arthritis (non-infectious):

1. **Prednisone** 40mg po given once in the morning tapered (decrease 5mg/day) over a week to 15mg daily. The **methylprednisolone** dose-pack does this over a 5-day period.
2. If evacuation is delayed, prednisone can be further tapered by 2.5–5mg per week as tolerated.
3. Rheumatoid and lupus patients often respond well to 5-15mg daily.
4. Once the patient has been on prednisone for more than a week, it should be tapered slowly and not stopped suddenly.
5. Do not give steroids in trauma or for ankylosing spondylitis.
6. Steroids may benefit some patients with peripheral joint inflammation by improving their ability to function and ambulate until they can be transported for definitive care.
7. Alternate taper: **Prednisone** 40mg x 5 days, then 30mg x 5 days, then 20mg for 5 days, etc.
8. Patients with potentially life-threatening illnesses like systemic lupus erythematosus, allergic reactions with anaphylaxis, and drug hypersensitivity reactions (serum sickness like responses) need high dose steroids (**prednisone** 1mg/kg po in split dose, example: 20mg tid or qid) and immediate transport.

Patient Education

General: Discuss appropriate illness with patient:

1. Natural history of gout: attacks of 7-10 days average duration with multiple recurrences.
2. Acute polyarthritis: May be the reaction to an infection or an exposure; frequently resolves within weeks with unknown cause. If it is symmetric, involves small joints of the hands and wrists and persists >6 weeks, it may be rheumatoid arthritis.
3. Ankylosing spondylitis may lead to significant limitation of spinal motion. The initial inflammatory phase may cause severe pain and stiffness over many years. While symptoms wax and wane, the disease seldom goes into spontaneous remission with return to unrestricted function.
4. Reactive arthritis flares often lasts 6-24 months. 25% of the time it is a chronic disease never completely remitting. Avoiding chlamydial STDs may reduce the risk of recurrences.

Activity: Rest the inflamed joints but include range of motion, strengthening, and aerobic exercise as tolerated.

Diet: Emphasize caloric restriction, especially in overweight patients; limit red meat and fish and replace with low fat dairy products. Limit alcohol.

Medications: NSAIDs: Gastritis, ulcer, GI bleed if not taken with food; indomethacin may cause CNS side effects (headache, drowsiness, confusion)

Cyclobenzaprine: Daytime drowsiness if used tid; side effects tend to lessen after 2 weeks on the drug. Prednisone: The goal of steroid treatment is to use the lowest dose that is necessary for as short a time possible. Steroid side effects are multiple and potentially severe: weight gain, increased appetite, peripheral edema from salt and water retention, hypertension, hyperglycemia, osteoporosis, avascular necrosis of bone, nervousness, emotional lability, psychosis, yeast infections.

Prevention and Hygiene: Practice safe sex and use a condom use to decrease the risk of chlamydial STD and/or reactive arthritis.

No Improvement/Deterioration: Return for prompt reevaluation.

Follow-up Actions: Follow any acutely inflamed joint until resolution or referral.

Evacuation/Consultation Criteria: Promptly evacuate patients with septic joints, pain undiagnosed after 6 weeks or not adequately controlled with conservative therapy, steroid treatment required, acute tendon/muscle rupture, or severe internal derangement.

Joint Problems: Joint Dislocations

COL Winston Warme, MC, USA (Ret) & Alexander Bertelsen, PA-C

Introduction: Joint dislocations occur when joints are stressed beyond the normal range of motion. Although dislocations occasionally occur spontaneously (eg, patella), they are usually associated with some degree of trauma. A dislocation is a complete joint disruption such that the articular surfaces are no longer in contact. Dislocations may be associated with marked swelling/edema and may cause injury to adjacent blood vessels and nerves. For this reason, most dislocations should be reduced as soon as possible. This minimizes the morbidity to the patient, but caution is required because there may be associated fractures. Gentle examination of the distal limb for crepitus or abnormal motion due to fracture is prudent prior to attempting a reduction maneuver. Attempts at reducing a fracture dislocation can cause more harm than good and you probably need x-rays and an orthopedic consultation. Table 3-10 presents an overview of common dislocations and their management.

Table 3-10. Common Dislocations

Body Part	History and Usual Mechanism of Injury	Objective Findings	Treatment (Details below)
Shoulder: Anterior	Common; may be recurrent; frequently associated with athletics, hyperabduction/hyperextension most common or from direct impact on posterior shoulder	Pain and splinting of the extremity. Arm slightly abducted; unable to move arm across chest; inability to rotate arm; anterior medial, inferior displacement of humeral head to subcoracoid position	Reduce ASAP (see technique), providing no crepitus is noted with gentle IR/ER of the arm
Shoulder: Posterior	Rare; direct blow to front of shoulder, translational injury from falling on outstretched arm, ballistic movements with internal rotation during convulsion/seizure activity or electric shock	Pain and splinting of the extremity. Arm held at side; near total loss of ability to rotate externally; posterior "fullness" when compared with contralateral side	As above
Elbow: Posterior	Fall or forceful impact on outstretched hand with arm in full extension; generally posterior and lateral displacement of radius and ulna	Foreshortening of the forearm with posterior deformity at the elbow; marked pain; rapid swelling. Ulnar N. injury possible from valgus stretch.	Longitudinal traction followed by anterior translation of the forearm relative to the humerus (see technique); posterior splint
Elbow: Anterior	Direct impact on the posterior forearm with the elbow in flexion. Anterior displacement of radius and ulna	Fullness/deformity of antecubital fossa; inability to flex/extend forearm; may have associated brachial artery injury and/or ulnar, median and radial neuropraxias	Longitudinal traction followed by anterior translation of the humerus relative to the forearm. Apply posterior splint
Radial head subluxation (RHS) in children	AKA "nursemaid's elbow"; commonly caused by a sudden jerk or yank on a child's wrist or hand during discipline.	Pain, refusal to use arm; able to flex and extend elbow but unable to fully supinate; may have minimal swelling and no visible deformity. Be alert signs/symptoms of abuse!	Reduce (see technique); place in sling, advise parents that the problem may recur until age five
Hand: PIPJ or DIPJ	Direct trauma in athletics	Obvious, usually dorsal deformity	Longitudinal traction to reduce. Splint in Alumafoam or buddy tape. X-ray for associated fractures when able.
Hip: Usually posterior	Massive impact to knee while hip is flexed and adducted; common dashboard injury to front seat passengers during auto accidents.	Hip flexed, adducted, internally rotated, and shortened, may have associated fracture of femur, sciatic nerve injury is common as nerve lies posterior to joint.	Reduce (see technique) if unable to MEDEVAC STAT.
Patella: Spontaneous	May occur spontaneously following predictable specific leg movements in people with loose connective tissues and/or abnormal anatomy.	Knee flexed; patella palpable lateral to femoral condyle.	Reduce; reduction may occur spontaneously; immobilize with long leg splint or knee immobilizer. Refer to ortho if possible.
Patella: Traumatic	Associated with trauma: "cutting" laterally while sprinting, etc.	Moderate swelling, tenderness especially medial to the patella; patella palpable lateral to the femur.	Reduce gently as above. Refer for x-rays, possible. Arthroscopy and surgical repair of soft tissue injury or fractures.

Table 3-10. Common Dislocations, continued

Body Part	History and Usual Mechanism of Injury	Objective Findings	Treatment (Details below)
Knee (rare)	Direct, massive blow to upper leg or forced hyper-extension of knee. Exam of a knee that is reduced post injury but really swollen and "floppy" probably represents a dislocation that has spontaneously reduced and should be treated as such.	Dislocation cannot occur without ligamentous and capsular disruptions; inability to straighten leg; injury to peroneal nerve and popliteal artery are common.	Immediate distal neuro/vascular assessment and gentle reduction with longitudinal traction. Stabilize with long leg splint and frequent vascular (q15min) re-checks. MEDEVAC ASAP! LIMB THREATENING INJURY!
Subtalar Joint: Medial	Most common type. AKA "basketball foot" due to frequency of injury when one player lands on another's foot and inverts it. Dislocation can be associated with osseous or osteochondral fractures.	Swelling, tenderness, and medial displacement of the foot in plantar flexion.	Flex the knee and have an assistant hold the thigh. Apply longitudinal traction and gently evert, abduct and dorsiflex foot. Splint once reduced, may require open reduction.
Subtalar Joint: Lateral	Rare	Similar to above but with lateral displacement of the abducted and plantar flexed foot	Flex the knee and have an assistant hold the thigh. Apply longitudinal traction and gently abduct and dorsiflex foot. Splint once reduced; may require open reduction.

Techniques

Anterior and Posterior Shoulder Dislocations:

Assessment: Examine the affected joint and determine the sensation of over the deltoid muscle to rule out injury to the axillary nerve. Also confirm the sensation, circulation, and motor function of the forearm and wrist. Repeat these evaluations post-reduction.

Differential Diagnosis: Fractures as previously mentioned, combined fracture/dislocation; muscular contusion; brachial plexopathy; acromioclavicular separation

Plan:

Diagnostic Tests: X-ray, if available to confirm dislocation and rule out fractures of the humerus, clavicle, and scapula. (True AP scapula; scapular lateral; and an axillary view.)

Procedure:

A. Many dislocations can be reduced without anesthesia, especially if the reduction is performed immediately after the dislocation occurs. However, if anesthesia is required, develop a sterile injection site, and with a 1-1/2 in 20 gauge needle, inject 1% **lidocaine** 20mL inferior and lateral to the acromion process in the depression left by the displaced humeral head. Allow the local 10 min. to set up and the patient to begin to relax.

B. Reduction maneuvers: Reassure the patient that you will not make sudden, unexpected moves, and that you will stop momentarily if pain occurs. Halt all efforts at reduction if there is marked pain, or crepitus noted that would suggest a concomitant fracture.

   1) Self-reduction: Instruct the patient to sit on the ground with his back to a tree, wall, etc. and flex the knee to the body on the same side as the injured shoulder. Have the patient grasp the knee with both hands (fingers interlaced) and then slowly extend the leg. The slow extension of the leg may provide all the traction required to reinsert the humeral head back into the glenoid. This technique works especially well if instituted early with acute injuries, or on recurrent dislocators and requires minimal assistance. However, for the first time dislocator, assistance may be required as detailed.

   2) Stimson: Place patient on table in prone position with affected arm hanging off the table. Hang about 10-15 lbs from the wrist (holding weights diminishes capacity to relax shoulder) to provide traction and slowly (in about 10-15 minutes) return the shoulder to its normal configuration.

   3) "Dirty Sock" or "Water Ski" Technique: Instruct the patient to lie flat on the ground. Sit down beside the patient on the affected side with your hip touching the patient's hip. Place your sock covered foot in the patient's axilla, grasp the patient's wrist with both hands, and slowly lean back as if rowing or water skiing. Maintain slow, steady traction along an axis directly parallel to the patient's leg. (Do not pull laterally. Remember that the anterior shoulder dislocation is anterior and inferior.) The firm, steady traction with your foot in the axilla providing counter traction will gradually overcome the shoulder muscle spasm and the arm will often "clunk" into the socket after several minutes.

   4) Successful reductions will be recognized by marked pain relief, an audible "clunk", restoration of normal anatomic appearance of the shoulder, and return of more normal range of motion. Verify reduction by having the patient touch the opposite shoulder with his hand.

C. Post Treatment: Post reduction x-rays

Patient Education

General: Avoid the motion that contributed to the injury. Consider use of sling +/- swath to restrict abduction and external rotation. Refer to ortho if possible.

Prevention: The recurrence rates for anterior shoulder dislocations vary markedly with age: <20 y/o = >80% recurrence rate; >40 y/o = <25 % rate; higher if very active. If young (<35) and active in sports, etc. consider orthopedic consultation ASAP for acute arthroscopic stabilization to alter the natural history. Instruct in self-reduction technique described previously.

Activity: Restore motion and strength/endurance with physical therapy

Diet: No limitations

Medications: Control pain and inflammation with NSAIDs on regular basis (ibuprofen 800mg po tid x 7 days or diclofenac sodium 150mg po am and hs x 7 days).

Follow-up Actions

Consultation Criteria: Failure to reduce the shoulder is a requirement for reduction under anesthesia and possible surgical stabilization.

Elbow Dislocation:

Assessment: Examine the affected and confirm the distal sensory, motor, and circulatory status. Repeat these evaluations post reduction.

Differential Diagnosis: Elbow fractures; combined fracture/dislocation; muscular contusion; ulnar nerve injury.

Diagnostic Tests: AP and lateral x-rays if available to confirm dislocation and rule out fracture.

Plan:

Procedure:

A. Reduction of a dislocated elbow is straightforward. A local injection of 1% **lidocaine** w/o epi 10cc in the posterior prominence from the lateral side can be helpful if the reduction has been delayed. Premedication with an opiate or benzodiazepine may be desirable.

B. Apply longitudinal traction with the patient in the prone position.

C. Position the patient so that an assistant can grasp the upper arm or torso and apply countertraction. Grasp the forearm at the wrist and apply anterior traction along the axis of the forearm with the elbow slightly flexed and the forearm at the original degree of pronation or supination and attempt to move the forearm anteriorly, relative to the humerus, to its proper position. In the case of an anterior dislocation, move the humerus anterior relative to the forearm.

D. If the reduction is not complete after three vigorous attempts, or if there is evidence of nerve or vascular injury, splint the arm for comfort and evacuate ASAP.

E. Successful reductions may be recognized by marked pain relief, an audible "clunk", restoration of normal anatomic appearance and some mobility in the joint.

F. Post treatment:

1. Insure integrity of sensory, motor, and circulatory structures. Damage to the median, ulnar, and radial nerves has been reported, and entrapment of the median nerve following the reduction of a dislocated elbow has also been reported. Most injuries occur to the ulnar nerve, which sustains a valgus stretch during dislocation.

2. Apply a posterior splint with the elbow in 90° of flexion and the forearm in the neutral position.

3. Obtain post reduction x-rays when possible.

Patient Education

General: Avoid the motion that contributed to the injury.

Medications: Control pain and inflammation with NSAIDs on regular basis (ibuprofen 800mg po tid x 7 days or diclofenac sodium 150mg po am and hs x 7 days)

Follow-up Actions

Consultation Criteria: Failure of all the previous maneuvers suggests the requirement for reduction under anesthesia or surgical stabilization. Acute indications for surgery include open or irreducible dislocations, those associated with vascular injuries, and fractures, or entrapment of bony/ligamentous fragments in the joint space.

Radial head subluxation (RHS):

Assessment: Usually there is no history of significant trauma. Be mindful to pick up clues of non-accidental trauma in all injured children! Parents may admit that the toddler has received a sudden tug or pull on the arm, usually by an adult. The injury appeared to cause instant pain, and the child holds the arm motionless. Although comfortable at rest, the arm is splinted limply at the side with mild flexion in the elbow and pronation of the forearm. Examination reveals no deformity, discoloration, crepitation, or swelling. There is little palpable tenderness present. However, the child is likely to begin crying and splinting the arm with any forced movement, especially supination. Further exam of the arm should be entirely normal.

Differential Diagnosis: Elbow fractures; combined fracture/dislocation; muscular contusion.

Plan:

Diagnostic Tests: X-ray the elbow

Procedure:

A. Advise the parents that you believe the child's elbow is slightly "out of joint" and that this is a common and not serious problem but may hurt the child for a few moments until it snaps back into place.

B. To elicit parental assistance, ask the mother or father to hold the child comfortably in their lap.

C. Place your thumb directly over the head of the radius on the "tender spot" and press down gently while you smoothly supinate the forearm and extend the elbow. Then, fully flex the elbow as you continue to press against the radial head in the supinated forearm.

D. You will recognize a "click" or "thunk" under the pressing thumb which will indicate that the radial head has slipped back into normal position. The child is also likely to begin using the limb normally.
E. Advise the parents that you think the problem is resolved
F. Return when the child is calm and reevaluate the elbow.
G. Post treatment: Avoid repeating the mechanism that caused it. There is no reason to immobilize the arm.

Patient Education

General: Advise the parents that the dislocation is a common problem and admonish them to handle the child gently. If problem is recurrent, consider the potential of abuse.

Medications: Acetaminophen, dose according to age, if child is "fussy"

Prevention: Do not lift child by outstretched arms.

Recurrence or no improvement: return ASAP for recurrence

Follow-up Actions

Consultation Criteria: Consider potential of abuse if multiple recurrences. Examine for other evidence to support suspicion.

Hip Dislocations (Anterior and Posterior)

Assessment: Posterior dislocations of the hip result from direct blows to the front of the knee or upper tibia, typically in an unrestrained passenger in a motor vehicle. If the leg is adducted at the time of impact, the pure dislocation is more common. If the leg is abducted, then posterior wall acetabular fractures are more likely. Typical appearance of patient with a posterior hip dislocation is with the hip flexed, adducted, internally rotated, and resistant to movement in marked pain. If a fracture is present, this posture is less likely. Anterior dislocations result from forced abduction and external rotation. They are quite rare (only 5% of all hip fractures) and tend to present showing the abduction and external rotation.

Differential Diagnosis: Combined fracture/dislocation; muscular contusion; concomitant sciatic nerve injury; pelvic fractures.

Plan: **Diagnostic Tests:** AP pelvis film and cross table lateral x-rays needed.

Procedure:

A. Follow ATLS protocols. If able to MEDEVAC, do so STAT. If not, and injury is uncomplicated by ipsilateral fractures distal or pelvic fractures, proceed as follows.
B. Evaluate for crepitus with gentle IR/ER/log rolling of limb. Sedate with **morphine** 2-10mg IV if available. Place patient on the ground/floor and have an assistant stabilize the pelvis by pushing down on the iliac wings. Flex the hip and knee 90° each. Position yourself between the patient's legs and grasp the affected leg in both arms and pull the hip and leg on a 90° axis to the floor. This will take lots of force and may take 5-10 minutes of work, so use your legs and gently IR/ER the leg as you distract. Reduction should be manifested by a satisfying clunk. If you are unable to reduce the joint, it may be more complicated than you expect, so splint the patient in situ with pillows and evacuate.
C. Reduction may require general anesthesia. Rapid reduction in less than 8 hours is necessary to minimize the risk for neurologic dysfunction and avascular necrosis of the femoral head.
D. Post treatment: Even if you get the hip to reduce, keep the patient non-weight bearing until a CT exam is acquired to rule out incarcerated bony fragments.

Patellar Dislocation:

Assessment: History may reveal that there was direct blow to the medial aspect of the patella, or the ailment began suddenly, following a "cutting movement" away from the fixed foot, which causes contraction of the quadriceps and external rotation of the tibia on the femur. Patient will usually present in considerable pain with the knee slightly flexed, and the patella obviously located adjacent to the lateral femoral condyle. Some patients may report that this is a periodically repeated occurrence.

Differential Diagnosis: Fractures; soft tissue contusion

Plan:

Diagnostic Tests: X-ray with patellar views if available, to rule out concomitant fractures (28-50%)

Procedures:

A. If traumatic, perform ATLS protocols.
B. Provide immediate reduction.
   1. Address patient's concerns that you will not execute any sudden painful movements.
   2. Anesthesia/analgesia is generally not required, but you can aseptically put 1% **lidocaine** 15-20cc in the knee to make them more comfortable. Inject right under the laterally displaced patella after a good prep.
   3. Gently grasp the patella while stabilizing it with mild lateral traction and maintaining its position to prevent sudden movement.
   4. Support the limb and flex the patient's hip to relax the quads. Request the patient to slowly extend the knee.
   5. When knee is fully extended, release traction on the patella, which will usually slip comfortably back into its normal anatomic location.
C. Post treatment:
   1. Provide patient with a knee immobilizer or a long leg splint and crutches to maintain straight leg position. Weight bearing as tolerated is authorized.
   2. Provide NSAIDs

Patient Education

General: Avoid the motion that contributed to the injury.

Medications: Control pain and inflammation with NSAIDs on regular basis (ibuprofen 800mg tid x 7 days or diclofenac sodium 150mg am and hs x 7 days)

Recurrence or no improvement: Return NLT 24 hours, or ASAP after recurrence

Follow-up Actions
Return Evaluation: ASAP if recurrence
Consultation Criteria: Schedule orthopedic evaluation within 72 hours if available and particularly if related to trauma
Note: Although it is possible to reduce a patellar dislocation by simply "pushing" the patella back into the original position, resist the temptation, as it may cause cartilage damage and it is unnecessarily painful for patients.

Joint Problems: Shoulder Pain

CAPT Scott Flinn, MC, USN

Introduction: The shoulder is an inherently unstable, complex and intricate joint that is easily injured by trauma or overuse. A good history and physical examination are the basis for proper initial management. Shoulder pain is usually related to the following structures: muscles, bones, acromioclavicular (AC) joint, and the glenohumeral joint. Referred pain from neck (eg, nerve impingement), heart (eg, myocardial ischemia, pericarditis) or lungs (eg, pneumothorax or tumor) can also present as shoulder pain. Patients with multidirectional instability (MDI) have more motion than normal in the glenohumeral joint and often present with shoulder dislocations, subluxations, and impingement syndrome. A young, otherwise healthy active person with a traumatic anterior dislocation has roughly an 80% chance of recurrence.

Subjective: Symptoms
Acute shoulder pain (immediate onset) is usually due to trauma. Chronic or recurrent intermittent pain is usually due to overuse (or other repeated trauma). Constitutional: Pain at night: Rotator cuff injury can present as shoulder pain that is most noticeable at night. (Note: If there is diaphoresis, shortness of breath, and pain in the left shoulder, consider an acute myocardial infarction, neoplasm, or lung injury.) Fever and redness of the shoulder: Septic shoulder joint (rare) Numbness or tingling: Referred pain from nerve impingement in the cervical spine or brachial plexus. Location: AC joint injury presents with pain over the AC joint. A rotator cuff impingement or tear produces deep pain in the anterior shoulder. Fractures may produce pain that is not localized initially and severely aggravated with movement. Shoulder dislocations usually present with obvious deformity and severe pain especially with attempted abduction. A subluxation of the shoulder occurs when the humerus partially comes out of normal joint alignment and then relocates spontaneously. Dislocations and subluxations of the shoulder may cause a tear in the labrum (cartilaginous ring around the glenoid fossa) causing a deep, aching pain that may be associated with a painful click on movement of the shoulder.
Focused History: *Was there an acute injury?* (Trauma may cause dislocation, subluxation, muscle tear or fracture.) *Is the pain worse with overhead motion and at night?* (This suggests impingement syndrome.) *Is there numbness, tingling, or weakness?* (This is consistent with a nerve impingement.) *Can the arm be moved?* (If not, the possibility of fracture or dislocation is very high.) *Is there a painful, reproducible click?* (Clicks that are associated with pain suggest a labrum tear.)

Objective: Signs
Using Basic Tools: Inspection: Look for obvious deformity, suggesting a fracture or dislocation. In anterior dislocation, the head of the humerus slips inferiorly and anteriorly out of the glenohumeral joint and is seen as a prominence in the AC area. A prominent clavicle may be the result of an AC separation or clavicle fracture. Have the patient attempt to touch their opposite shoulder with the affected arm. If they are unable to do so, think anterior shoulder dislocation or fracture. Auscultation: A painful click may represent a labrum tear or a loose body in the joint. Listen to the lungs for abnormal lung sounds (tumor, infection) or absent lung sounds (pneumothorax). Palpation: Palpate for edema from contusions or fractures. Feel along the clavicle from midline to the AC joint for obvious deformity or crepitus from a clavicle fracture. Feel the AC joint for point tenderness or deformity. If injury is acute, tenderness may represent an AC joint separation; if chronic it could be due to AC joint capsulitis. Check sensation on the lateral deltoid (axillary nerve root, C5 nerve root impingement). Check shoulder strength for internal and external rotation, abduction, and in the "empty can" position (thumb at 2 and10 o'clock) to check the rotator cuff muscles. This sign is positive in rotator cuff tendonitis (impingement syndrome) or tear.

Assessment: Differential Diagnosis: Acute pain is usually due to trauma.
Fractures: History of forceful, direct blow.
Anterior shoulder dislocations: Most frequently caused by forceful abduction and external rotation of the arm.
AC joint separation: History of being tackled and driven into the ground onto the shoulder.
Acute biceps tear: Acute pain and deformity following a sudden lift or catching activity.
Rotator cuff tear: Following acute trauma in a young otherwise healthy patient or an overuse injury in an older patients.
Overuse injuries: Rotator cuff tear or impingement (tendonitis), AC joint capsulitis, degenerative joint disease (eg, osteoarthritis), and subacromial bursitis.

Plan:
Diagnostic Tests
1. X-rays are not necessary prior to reducing an anterior shoulder dislocation and the shoulder should be empirically reduced (see Part 3: General Symptoms: Joint Problems: Joint Dislocations). AP and lateral x-rays are useful to rule out fractures. In high-speed trauma, cervical spine x-rays may be required.
2. Gram's stain of joint aspirate: In cases of suspected septic arthritis, Gram's stain of aspirated joint fluid may be useful to confirm diagnosis and select antibiotic therapy.

Procedures
Injection of a local anesthetic into the subacromial region or AC joint (injecting the AC joint can be very difficult) may confirm impingement syndrome or AC joint capsulitis. Injection of anesthetic and steroid may provide longer-term relief, but should not replace PRICEMM (Protection, Relative Rest, Ice, Compression, Elevation, Medication, Modalities).

Treatment

1. Overuse injuries without significant damage such as rotator cuff tendonitis (impingement syndrome), AC joint capsulitis, sprains and strains can be treated with PRICEMM; protect from harm, appropriate activity modification, icing for 20 minutes tid, and administration of NSAIDs, if not allergic.

2. Shoulder dislocations can be reduced prior to obtaining x-rays. There are many techniques to do this (*see Part 3: General Symptoms: Joint Problems: Joint Dislocations; Techniques*). Following reduction, the arm is usually put in a sling for a minimum of 2 weeks and then gradual rehabilitation is performed over the next 6-8 weeks.

3. Fractures: Initial treatment includes splint, sling and swathe, and administration of pain medicines. Grossly deformed fractures or those causing neurovascular compromise may require reduction by in-line traction. Clavicle fractures and AC joint separations should also be placed in a sling and swathe. Pinning or somehow affixing the arm sleeve to the shirt just above the navel can accomplish this if no sling or other material is available. Open fractures: Clean gross debris and cover with a dressing. Do not reduce open fractures; when possible splint in place until definitive surgical care is available. For prevention of infection in combat related trauma for skin, soft tissue, open fractures, exposed bone or open joints, give **cephazolin** 1g IV q8h or **clindamycin** 900mg IV q8h x 72 hours or until definitive care reached.

Septic Joint: *See Part 3: General Symptoms: Joint Problems: Joint Pain; Septic Arthritis*

Patient Education

General: The severity of the injury will dictate the length of time necessary for full recovery

Activity: The activity level should be modified to prevent further injury, often pain can be the guide ("doc, it hurts to do this" - "so don't do that")

Diet: NSAIDs should be taken with food.

Medications: Narcotics cause sedation and NSAIDs may cause severe bleeding, kidney, or liver damage. All medications can produce allergic reactions.

Prevention and Hygiene: Avoid offending activities for overuse injuries; include rehabilitation program (strengthening).

Wound Care: Grossly contaminated wounds should be cleaned (flushed with cleanest water available) and dressed until definitive care is available.

Follow-up Actions

Return Evaluation: Overuse injuries, follow-up in 2-3 weeks. Anterior shoulder dislocations will require immobilization for 2-3 weeks for patients under 30 years old. In patients over 30 years old, rate of redislocation is lower and early mobilization (after 1 week) will limit joint stiffness. Gentle pendular motion exercises performed during the immobilization period will reduce the risk of frozen shoulder. Period of immobilization is followed by gradual increased range of motion and strengthening exercises.

Consultation Criteria: Fractures, rotator cuff tears, and suspected septic joints should be referred ASAP for surgical evaluation and treatment.

Notes: Rehabilitation exercise guide to minimize recurrence of overuse injuries: Use light weights and safety "spot."

Table 3-11. Rehabilitation Exercise Guide

STOP IMMEDIATELY IF PAIN IS FELT WITH ANY EXERCISE

Dumbbell Shoulder Flies	1. Hold the dumbbells down at the waist with thumbs pointing down.
	2. Raise the dumbbells up at 10 o'clock and 2 o'clock to shoulder height.
	3. Perform three sets of 10 every other day.
	4. As strength improves, increase the weight, and keep repetition number the same.
Dumbbell Shoulder Lateral Flies	1. Hold a dumbbell in the hands at waist level, thumb pointing forward.
	2. Slowly raise the dumbbell to shoulder height.
	3. Perform 3 sets of 10 every other day.
	4. As strength improves, increase the weight, not the number of repetitions.
Bench Press	1. Lie on the back with weights in a rack.
	2. Lift the barbell off the rack with hands shoulder width.
	3. Slowly lower the weight to the mid chest and then push it up again slowly during exhalation.
	4. Perform 3 sets of 10, every other day.
	5. As strength improves, increase the weight.

After the initial injury has healed, a strengthening program is essential to prevent additional injury.

Joint Problems: Hip Pain

CAPT Scott Flinn, MC, USN

Introduction: Hip and pelvic injuries may occur as a result of overuse or trauma. Knowing the mechanism of injury and evaluating the degree of functional impairment provides the basis for appropriate treatment. Sudden onset of pain with an inability to bear weight is an obviously worrisome presentation. Acute pain may result from trauma, change in degenerative disease or infection. Chronic pain may be due to osteoarthritis, bursitis, referred pain, or aseptic necrosis of the femoral head. The need for more advanced diagnostic tests requiring removal from the operational environment is based on the history and exam. **Risk Factors:** Recent increases in activity/training, biomechanical, or anatomic variations, and females with the "female athlete triad" (amenorrhea, eating disorder, and osteoporosis) are predisposing factors that contribute to overuse injuries including stress fractures.

Subjective: **Symptoms**

Constitutional: Fever (joint infection); non-ambulatory. Local: Ecchymosis. Traumatic nerve damage causes loss of sensation, cold leg.

Focused History: *Can you walk?* (determine if serious problem requiring crutches and/or evacuation) *How quickly did the pain come on?* (Sudden onset of severe pain and inability to walk suggest fracture/completed stress fracture or joint infection.) *Did you fall or get hit on your hip or back?* (suggests mechanism of injury) *Do you have back pain, or numbness or tingling in your leg?* (suggests pinched nerve from herniated disc or nerve damage from other etiology)

Objective: **Signs**

Using Basic Tools: Inspection: deformity indicates obvious severe injury. Palpation: tenderness over the greater trochanter, anterior superior or anterior inferior iliac spines (hip flexors), or deep in the joint area (tendonitis, bursitis, fracture); pain with gentle logrolling (suspect hip fractures); absent or diminished distal pulses (fracture or dislocation); diminished muscle strength relative to normal side (suggests muscle strain, tendonitis, or nerve injury). Range of motion (ROM): limitations in active or passive full ROM suggest possible serious injury. Always try active range of motion first, and then passive range of motion should be done gently and stopped if patient is experiencing pain.

Using Advanced Tools: X-rays: imperative for a definitive diagnosis if fracture suspected; Labs: Gram's stain of joint fluid if infection is suspected.

Assessment: **Differential Diagnosis**

Traumatic fractures: Deformity, pain, inability to ambulate

Femoral neck stress fracture: Pain at the extremes of internal and external hip rotation

Greater trochanteric bursitis: Pain located immediately over greater trochanter

Hip joint infection (extremely rare): In the absence of trauma, unable to conduct any active or passive ROM without severe pain.

Osteoarthritis: History of chronic overuse (eg, excessive weight bearing) or trauma. If has x-ray, may see degeneration late in process of disease.

Strains and tendonitis, such as hip flexor strain: Superficial tenderness and diminished strength of muscle.

Pyriformis syndrome: Chronic posterior hip and thigh pain, numbness or tingling; pain with passive internal rotation; no back pain

Herniated disc with nerve impingement: May have back pain but not always; numbness and tingling in distribution of a nerve, including sciatic nerve (sciatica) and others

Referred pain: Lower leg ailments (injuries, malalignments, etc.) may place abnormal stresses on the hip.

Aseptic necrosis: Chronic pain and/or limp typically in pediatric patients; also seen in sickle cell disease. Other injuries and degenerative changes of the hip, which can be diagnosed only with x-rays or specialty referral.

Plan:

Treatment

1. If the patient is unable to ambulate, use either crutches or a litter for transport.
2. Give pain medication, including **morphine**, as required. *See Part 8: Procedures: Chapter 30: Pain Assessment and Control*
3. Treatment for specific conditions:
   A. Trochanteric bursitis: After sterile preparation, inject a mixture of 1cc **lidocaine**, 1cc **bupivacaine**, and 1cc **triamcinolone** with a 25 gauge 1½ needle using a lateral approach. Insert the needle directly over the palpable greater trochanteric bursa on the lateral proximal thigh, push in until the greater trochanter is reached, and then slightly withdraw off the bone. Aspirate slightly to ensure the tip of the needle is not in a vessel, then inject the mixture, which should flow in very easily. If not, it is in muscle or tendon tissue and should NOT be forced. If resistance is met, reposition the needle by going back down to bone, backing off only slightly, and repeating the attempt to inject. Injection may produce excellent pain relief for a prolonged period of time.
   B. Strains, tendonitis, arthritis and other bursitis: Use PRICEMM, (*see Part 3: General Symptoms: Joint Problems: Joint Pain*). Always check for allergies prior to giving medications.
   C. Fractures: Apply traction splint (eg, Hare traction splint), give IV fluids if needed (*see Part 7: Trauma: Chapter 27: Resuscitation Fluids*) and evacuate urgently.
   D. Herniated disc: Use relative rest (bed rest has been shown to be more harm than good), ice, NSAIDs (*see Part 3: General Symptoms: Joint Problems: Joint Pain*). Later, use stretching, strengthening, and ROM exercises.
   E. Aseptic necrosis: Apply splint, allow no weight bearing, give NSAIDs (*see Part 3: General Symptoms: Joint Problems: Joint Pain*) and ROM exercises, evacuate.
   F. Septic arthritis of hip: Do not aspirate hip joint. Start antibiotics as seen in *Part 3: General Symptoms: Joint Problems: Joint Pain; Septic Arthritis.*

Patient Education

General: If a fracture is suspected, inform patient of probable need for surgical treatment.

Activity: If a femoral neck stress fracture is suspected, allow no further weight bearing to prevent completing the stress fracture that may necessitate surgical correction. Recommend crutches and total non-weight bearing on that hip until x-rays and/or bone scan or MRI can be obtained.

Diet: Additional calcium if suspect stress fracture

Medications: All medications may produce allergic reactions. Long-term use of anti-inflammatory medications may produce GI bleeds or kidney problems.

Prevention and Hygiene: Proper training may prevent development of stress fractures.

Follow-up Actions

Return Evaluation: If pain persists, reconsider diagnosis and consult specialist or evacuate patient.

Evacuation/Consultation Criteria: Evacuate cases of joint infection, fracture or suspected fracture, and aseptic necrosis. Also, evacuate any unstable patient or any team member unable to complete the mission due to inability to ambulate. Consult orthopedics for any patient to be evacuated and for others as needed.

Joint Problems: Knee Pain
CAPT Scott Flinn, MC, USN

Introduction: Knee pain is a very common complaint with numerous underlying causes. The correct diagnosis can be made by considering the timing and mechanism of injury (acute/trauma vs. chronic/overuse), symptoms and physical signs. Acute knee pain, that occurs within minutes to hours, is usually due to trauma or infection. Chronic knee pain may not have an obvious specific initiating event, but may be preceded by a long history of minor complaints. Anterior knee pain is usually due to an overuse condition (eg, patellofemoral syndrome [PFS] or patellar tendonitis). Pain from injuries to the collateral ligaments or menisci is referred to the side of injury. Other less common causes of (posterior) knee pain include Baker's cyst or extension of a deep vein thrombosis in a patient with trauma to the lower extremity. In addition to local causes, knee pain may be due to referred pain from the hip or thigh (eg, femoral shaft stress fracture). Malformations or variations in anatomic structures may predispose to overuse injuries. Examination by an experienced clinician may be as helpful as an MRI. Learn, practice and be able to perform an excellent history and physical examination of the extremities.

Subjective: Symptoms
Patient may present with specific localized pain or complaint of "limping", swelling, grinding or popping noises, buckling or "knee giving out." General symptoms of not "feeling well", fever and/or chills suggest infection. In a young patient with an acute single joint, septic arthritis is due to gonorrhea until proven otherwise.

Focused History: *What was the position of your leg/knee when the injury occurred?* (Direct trauma suggests structural injury; overuse syndromes suggest tendonitis or PFS.) *Did it swell immediately?* (eg, cruciate ligament tear, patellar dislocation, or fracture) *Did it swell within 12-24 hours?* (eg, meniscal tear, osteochondral defect, or capsule) *Did you feel or hear a "pop"?* (eg, anterior cruciate ligament (ACL) tear) *Does your knee give way or buckle due to pain or is it unstable?* (ACL tear or more rarely meniscal tear.) *Does your knee lock or catch?* (eg, meniscal tear, loose body, or ACL tear with stump "catching" in joint) *Did you hit your knee on something or have you been crawling on your knees?* (eg, prepatellar bursitis) Can you walk and/or bear weight? (eg, fracture or knee dislocation)

Objective: Signs
Using Basic Tools: Inspection: Swelling, erythema, bruising, ability to walk and range of active motion. Palpation: Compare knees for temperature differences. Increased warmth suggests infection or prepatellar bursitis. Note any swelling in the joint (trauma [blood] or inflammation [gout, arthritis, infection or reactive effusion from PFS]). Perform passive range of motion with hand on knee feeling for abnormal limitations in motion, clicking or popping (cartilage, ligament or meniscal injury). **Note:** Popping without pain is a normal thing in knee. Perform Lachman (drawer) test for ACL and posterior sag test for posterior cruciate ligament (PCL) to indicate tears of the respective ligaments. Assess meniscal integrity (tears cause joint line tenderness, effusion, and positive McMurray sign, which is pain with passive extension of knee while externally rotated). Palpate the collateral ligaments. If tender, bend the knee medially and laterally at 0 and 30° of flexion (increased opening suggests more severe tear). Palpate patella. Try to gently slide patella laterally; if apprehension, suggests patellar dislocation or subluxation. Evaluate mobility of patella (PFS) by pushing it medially and laterally while quadriceps is flexed. Feel the patellar tendon for intactness and tenderness (rupture or tendonitis). If patellar tendon ruptured, patient will not be able to extend leg. Assess distal pulses and sensation.

Using Advanced Tools: Labs: CBC and Gram's stain of aspirated joint fluid to rule out infection. Urinalysis: Urate crystals in sediment under polarized light microscopy in gout. X-ray: For fractures, dislocations, alterations of joint space.

Assessment: Differential Diagnosis
Acute traumatic knee pain: Evaluate for damage to ligaments (ACL, PCL, MCL, LCL), bone (eg, fracture or osteochondral defect), muscle (eg, quadriceps tear), cartilage (eg, meniscal tear) or capsule (eg, patellar subluxation or dislocation). One-third of all traumatic knee dislocations (39% of anterior dislocations) include popliteal artery damage. A rapidly expanding popliteal hematoma and/or a diminished pedal pulse suggest popliteal artery damage. **Note:** Infection and other inflammatory conditions (eg, gout) may also present acutely.

Chronic knee pain: Consider an old untreated injury, PFS, iliotibial band syndrome (ITBS), arthritis, tendonitis, bursitis or stress fractures.

Plan:
Treatment
1. If patient unable to walk, use crutches, cane and/or splint.
2. Reduce/inhibit swelling in the injured joint: RICE: Rest, Ice, Compression (wrap, brace or splint), Elevation
3. NSAIDs as necessary for pain and inflammation. For severe pain, *see Part 8: Procedures: Chapter 30: Pain Assessment and Control.*
4. Gonococcal arthritis is the most likely cause of infection in an otherwise intact knee without a history of trauma. If septic arthritis is suspected, give IV antibiotic. (*see Part 3: General Symptoms: Joint Problems: Joint Pain; Antibiotics for Septic Arthritis*) Because of high probability of simultaneous infection with *Chlamydia trachomatis* as an STD, treat with **azithromycin** 1g po in a single dose, or **doxycycline** 100mg po bid x 7 days. Gram's stain of cervical or urethral discharge may suggest GC but Gram's stain of fluid obtained by joint aspiration is preferred, when possible, to confirm the diagnosis. *See Part 8: Procedures: Chapter 30: Joint Aspiration.*
5. Aspirate pus/fluid and consider injecting anesthetic to enable member to walk out in combat conditions (*see Part 8: Procedures: Chapter 30: Joint Aspiration*). Injecting steroids is contraindicated as steroids may allow infection to rapidly worsen.

Patient Education
General: Most common knee injuries will resolve with conservative treatment and rehabilitation. Laparoscopic surgery may be required for specific injuries.
Activity: Depending on severity of injury, gradually advance range of motion, then add strength program with weight bearing as tolerated.
Medications: Use of NSAIDs may cause bleeding ulcers, kidney and liver damage. Do not provide unlimited quantities of NSAIDS and insist on follow up.

Prevention and Hygiene: Risk of overuse injuries can be minimized by "smart training," (eg, program that includes diet, proper stretching, strength and aerobic conditioning). If STD (eg, GC) is considered, review sexual history and provide appropriate treatment for sexual contacts.

No Improvement/Deterioration: Return to clinic if symptoms do not improve or persist despite conservative management.

Follow-up Actions

Return Evaluation: Update history and repeat physical examination. If diagnosis remains in question or symptoms fail to resolve with conservative management refer for orthopedic evaluation.

Evacuation/Consultation Criteria: Evacuate individuals whose physical limitations increase risk of mission failure. Aspiration of the knee joint may be indicated in instances of delayed evacuation. Traumatic knee dislocations cause tears of ACL, PCL and one or both of the collateral ligaments. Greater than 30% of traumatic knee dislocations involve popliteal artery injury that may result in vascular compromise and whenever possible these injuries require emergent referral for evaluation and treatment. Consult Orthopedics for case of severe knee pain or recurrent, persistent or undiagnosed injuries.

Joint Problems: Ankle Pain
CAPT Scott Flinn, MC, USN

Introduction: The most common cause of ankle pain is acute trauma (eg, sprain, fracture, fracture dislocation). Chronic ankle pain may indicate repeated injury, overuse injury, injury to a nerve, an inflammatory process (eg, gout or pseudo gout, rheumatoid), infection (eg, GC) or other type of chronic arthritis (eg, degenerative joint disease). Risk factors include previous injury (eg, fast roping, hard parachute landings) especially a history of previous high ankle (syndesmotic) sprain or walking long distances over rough terrain.

Subjective: Symptoms

Acute pain (immediate onset to a few hours) is most often due to trauma, infection (rarely) or acute flare of an underlying inflammatory condition. Sub-acute pain suggests re-injury or a chronic inflammatory condition. Chronic pain is usually due to old recurrent trauma with possible associated degenerative arthritis of the ankle. Constitutional symptoms: Fever, chills, malaise, suggests infection. If more than one joint is involved (polyarthritis), an underlying infectious or other inflammatory process should be considered. Location: Ankle trauma will cause sprains, fractures and fracture-dislocations, which include midfoot (Lisfranc's joint), metatarsals (especially the fifth metatarsal), the navicular tarsal bone, and the fibular head.

Focused History: *How did you hurt your ankle?* (If twisting injury, think sprain versus fracture; no trauma, suspect infection or inflammation) *Did you hear a "pop" or feel a tearing sensation? Can you walk?* (provides some description of extent of injury) *Have you had this before?* (eg, gouty arthritis in a patient known to have gout)

Objective: Signs

Using Basic Tools: Inspection: Confirm adequate distal blood flow, document abrasions, swelling, deformity, erythema, ecchymosis, and range of motion. Palpation: Locate distal pulse, normal temperature (increased local skin temperature suggests infection or inflammation, decreased skin temperature may suggest vascular compromise), note extent of edema. Palpate the posterior aspect of the medial and lateral malleolus and the base of the fifth metatarsal and the navicular bone for point tenderness as sign of fracture.

Using Advanced Tools: X-rays, Labs: Gram's stain of aspirated joint fluid if infection is suspected or to identify crystals (eg, gout, pseud- gout). Ottawa Ankle Rules: Obtain x-rays ASAP to rule out fracture when any of the following are present:

1. Pain/tenderness on posterior aspect or tip of medial malleolus
2. Pain/tenderness on posterior aspect or tip of lateral malleolus
3. Unable to walk 5 steps immediately after injury (by history) and during physical examination

Assessment: Differential Diagnosis
The history and physical will almost always lead to an accurate diagnosis.

Acute pain: Fracture, fracture dislocation essentially always includes history of trauma; may have localized point tenderness, possible deformity, moderate to severe swelling and limited ability to support weight. High ankle (syndesmotic) sprain (tibiofibular, posterior tibiofibular, transverse tibiofibular ligaments, and interosseous membrane) suspected based on history of severe dorsiflexion and/or eversion of the ankle with mod to severe swelling and pain. This injury can contribute to chronic ankle instability with increased risk of recurrent ankle sprain and calcified scarring. Joint infections are very rare without pre-existing trauma (including penetrating injury) and patient with infection in the joint space will avoid all movement of the ankle. Patient with acute flare of underlying inflammatory process will almost always have past medical history (PMH) that suggests correct diagnosis.

Chronic pain: Evaluate for PMH of recurring injury (eg, high ankle sprain), inflammatory joint disease (gout, pseudo-gout, rheumatoid) or degenerative joint disease (DJD). *See Part 3: General Symptoms: Joint Problems: Joint Pain*

Plan:

Treatment

1. If ambulatory, encourage ambulation. Leaving patient's boot on may help control swelling, pain management and provide additional support. Splint or cast if necessary.
2. If unable to walk or bear weight (under operational conditions), ambulation with improvised crutches or cane can avoid or delay immediate MEDEVAC.
3. If infection is suspected, start antibiotics (*see Part 3: General Symptoms: Joint Problems: Joint Pain; Septic Arthritis*) and consider early medical evacuation.
4. Manage pain with RICE: Rest, Ice, Compression (Ace wrap), Elevation; splint if required and give appropriate medication (NSAIDs for sprains, narcotics for fracture).

Patient Education

General: Explain underlying cause of pain (eg, suspected fracture/sprain vs. non-traumatic cause). Encourage patient to report additional symptoms (eg, numbness, increased pain, cool extremity) and follow up for rehabilitation and re-evaluation.

Activity: Rest, ice, compression and elevation if possible.

Diet: NSAIDs should be taken with food.

Medications: NSAIDs may cause bleeding ulcers, narcotics may cause respiratory depression and all drugs may cause allergic reactions.

Prevention and Hygiene: If compound fracture, try to keep as clean as possible to prevent infection.

No Improvement/Deterioration: If infected joint or compound fracture, concern for systemic infection/sepsis. Monitor blood pressure and mental status.

Wound Care: Keep wounds clean, dry and report signs of infection (increased pain, swelling, redness).

Follow-up Actions

Return Evaluation: Rehabilitation program should be started ASAP and return to full duty permitted when patient is able to run a figure 8 at full speed pain-free. The theory is to use the ankle as rapidly as possible while protecting from re-injury. Under normal conditions (eg, min–mod initial swelling, without PMH of high ankle sprain or other severe ankle injury); recovery from ankle sprain will require 3-6 weeks. A "slip on" figure 8 brace with laces can fit inside a boot and may help speed return to activity.

Evacuation/Consultation Criteria: Fracture with dislocation, penetrating injury to joint space, compound fracture, infected joints will require medical evacuation and orthopedic consultation as soon as operationally reasonable for optimal medical care and to minimize risk of long term loss of function.

Joint Problems: Finger Problems

COL Michael M. Fuenfer, MC, USAR

Introduction: The field environment presents many opportunities for injuries to the fingers. Care should be taken to keep the hands clean, utilizing gloves to prevent injury to the skin and soft tissue whenever feasible. Troops should avoid wearing rings into the field, on convoys and during deployments to avoid de-gloving injuries caused by rings becoming caught on nuts, bolts and other objects. Rings can be worn on dog-tag chains or carried when safety is an issue. Early recognition and treatment of infections involving the fingers will prevent progression to deep spaces of the hand which may rapidly result in extension of the infectious process and debilitating sequelae. The goal in treating infections of the fingers is to drain loculated collections of pus, débride the wound of devitalized tissue, remove any foreign bodies and contamination, and administer antibiotics if indicated.

Subjective: Symptoms

Pain with movement of the digit, tenderness, swelling, redness, and loss of function are all indicative of infections involving the fingers

Objective: Signs

In addition to subjective findings, expression of purulent material is an obvious indication of infection. Unrelieved pus under pressure may be extremely painful.

Assessment and Plan: Differential Diagnosis and Treatment

1. Felon
   - A. Definition: Closed space infection of the finger tip pulp. May or may not result in an expanding abscess involving the pulp of the finger, usually caused by penetrating trauma and most frequently due to *Staphylococcus*. Untreated or incorrectly treated, this condition may result in osteomyelitis.
   - B. Assessment: Early infection; mild erythema with a "tight or prickling" pain. Late infection; (extreme throbbing pain), induration of the pulp due to localized infection under pressure (abscess) within the fibrous septae anchoring the distal phalanx that will require incision and drainage.
   - C. Treatment:
     1. For mild/early infection (without abscess or severe swelling): May respond to warm soaks and oral antibiotics. Give **cephalexin** 500mg po bid or tid x 7-10 days or **dicloxacillin** 250mg po tid x 7-10 days. If suspicion of MRSA infection present, give **trimethoprim/sulfamethoxazole DS** po bid x 10-14 days or **tetracycline** 500mg po bid x 10-14 days or **doxycycline** 100mg po bid x 10-14 days. **Clindamycin** 300mg po tid x 10-14 days may be appropriate (although resistance to this class is seen in some locales).
     2. For late/severe infection (abscess): Make longitudinal incision on the midline of the volar pulp distal to the flexion crease plus IV antibiotic therapy. Give **nafcillin** or **oxacillin** 2g IV q4h or alternate: **cephazolin** 2g IV q8h or **clindamycin** 600-900 mg IV q8h (not to exceed 4.8g/day) and continue antibiotic through medical evacuation. If MRSA is suspected, substitute with **vancomycin** 1g IV q12h or as alternate, **clindamycin** 600-900mg IV q8h (not to exceed 1.8g/day). Urgent medical evacuation. Without adequate treatment this condition may result in significant skin necrosis and osteomyelitis. If medical evacuation is not possible in cases of severe infection; continue IV therapy until obvious signs of clinical improvement (usually 3-4 days) followed by oral antibiotic (eg, **dicloxacillin** 500mg po q6h or **erythromycin** 500mg po q6h) for an additional 7-10 days. If **vancomycin** is required for presumed MRSA, IV vancomycin therapy is followed by **clindamycin** 300-450mg po qid (not to exceed 1.8g/day) for an additional 7-10 days.

2. Herpetic Whitlow
   - A. Definition: An infection of the soft tissues of the distal phalanx by the herpes simplex virus. In children the primary source of infection is the orofacial area, and it is commonly due to HSV-1 transferred by the chewing or sucking of fingers or thumbs. In adults, it is more common for the primary source to be the genital region, with a corresponding preponderance of HSV-2.
   - B. Assessment: Intense pain and cutaneous vesicles or blisters containing clear fluid which may become cloudy after 40-72 hours
   - C. Treatment: Usually resolve within 3-4 weeks without treatment. A topical antibiotic (eg, **bacitracin**) may prevent secondary infection. If secondary bacterial infection without abscess, may treat as for paronychia. If abscess develops, incision and drainage will be required

3. Paronychia
   - A. Definition: An infection of the lateral and posterior fingernail folds often associated with hangnails, nail biting, and prolonged immersion in water. May or may not include abscess. Usually caused by *Staphylococcus*.
   - B. Assessment: Pain, erythema, induration adjacent to the nail bed

C. Treatment:
  1. If without abscess, may respond to local care that includes compresses or soaks to affected digit for 20 minutes tid plus antibiotic therapy (eg, **dicloxacillin** 250mg po tid x 7-10 days, or **cephalexin** 500mg po tid x 7-10 days, or **azithromycin** 500mg po day one then 250mg q day x 4 days)
  2. If abscess is superficial, a large gauge needle can be "run bevel down" along the nail into the abscess.
  3. For more well-formed abscess, use a scalpel to incise and drain by opening the involved lateral sulcus and treat with antibiotics as previously mentioned. Frequent warm soaks can be used to maintain patency of the incision and support wound drainage.

4. Tenosynovitis
  A. Definition: A closed-space infection of the tendon sheath usually due to direct trauma. Often caused by *Staph aureus* or Streptococcal species, but may be gram-negative or polymicrobial depending upon the source of inoculation.
  B. Assessment: Kanavel's cardinal signs of tenosynovitis are confirmed by aspiration of the tendon sheath. The 4 signs are:
    1. Fusiform swelling of the digit
    2. Semiflexed position of the finger
    3. Severe pain with passive extension
    4. Tenderness along the entire flexor sheath
  C. Treatment:
    1. Antibiotic therapy and urgent medical evacuation. Give **nafcillin** or **oxacillin** 2gm IV q4h or alternate: **cephazolin** 2g IV q8h or **clindamycin** 600-900mg IV q8h (not to exceed 4.8g/day) and continue antibiotic through medical evacuation. If MRSA is suspected, substitute with **vancomycin** 1g IV q12h or as alternate, **clindamycin** 600-900mg IV q8h (not to exceed 1.8g/day). Urgent medical evacuation.
    2. In cases of severe infection where <u>medical evacuation is not possible</u>, continue IV therapy until obvious signs of clinical improvement (usually 3-4 days) followed by oral antibiotic (eg, **dicloxacillin** 500mg po q6h or **erythromycin** 500mg po q6h) for an additional 10-14 days.
    3. If **vancomycin** is required for presumed MRSA, IV vancomycin therapy is followed by **clindamycin** 300-450mg po qid (not to exceed 1.8g/day) for an additional 10-14 days.
    4. If no resolution with antibiotics after 24 hours, surgical drainage will be required.

Anesthetizing the Finger:
  1. NEVER inject local anesthetic agents containing epinephrine into digits
  2. Perform a digital block by injecting anesthetic into the medial and lateral aspects of the base of the finger. *See Part 5: Specialty Areas: Chapter 19: Local/Regional Anesthesia: Digital Block of Finger or Toe*.
  3. Apply a 1 inch latex tourniquet proximal to the level of injury to minimize bleeding during procedure.

Male Genital Problems: Genital Inflammation
LTC Steve Waxman, MC, USA & LTC (P) Douglas Soderdahl, MC, USA

Introduction: Genital ulcers and urethral discharge are covered in the STD chapter. Most inflammation of the penis is related to the presence of foreskin and may be an early sign of diabetes mellitus. Skin infections in the genital area are similar to cellulitis in other parts of the body, in that they present with pain and redness and are usually caused by staphylococcal, streptococcal or fungal organisms. Skin inflammation/infection in this region can lead to scrotal, perineal or peri-rectal abscess. This later infection can involve multiple organisms, including gram-negative rods, that can lead to life-threatening necrotizing fasciitis (Fournier's gangrene), particularly in the severely injured or diabetic patient. With severe inflammation of the penis, patients may have difficulty voiding or may experience symptoms of septicemia: fever, fatigue and shock.

Subjective: **Symptoms**
Phimosis/paraphimosis: Phimosis refers to an abnormally tight foreskin. These patients may not be able to retract their foreskin, and in severe cases, the glans penis and urethral meatus cannot be seen. In paraphimosis, the foreskin is trapped behind the glans penis resulting in a doughnut-shaped swelling of the skin on the distal shaft and glans penis. Phimosis is usually due to prior scarring of the distal foreskin most often secondary to balanitis. Paraphimosis is usually iatrogenic following the placement of a Foley catheter in an uncircumcised male where the foreskin is pulled back behind the glans penis for placement and then not pulled back over the end of the penis when completed.
Balanitis: Inflammation of the foreskin in the uncircumcised male is called balanitis. Inflammation of the glans penis and foreskin occurs primarily in the uncircumcised male and is rare in the circumcised male. The glans will look wet, red and may have multiple small red bumps and a whitish material on the surface consistent with yeast. This condition should raise suspicion for diabetes mellitus. If the foreskin cannot be retracted easily, leave it extended. There are a number of non-infectious causes of a wet, red patch of skin on the glans penis. Differentiation often requires a biopsy to rule out cancerous or pre-cancerous lesions. When in doubt, treat for infection and refer for biopsy if the condition does not resolve. Common organisms: yeast and *Gardnerella*.
Thrombosed penile vein and sclerosing lymphangitis: The shaft of the penis just under the skin and on the surface of the erectile bodies contains numerous large veins that can develop clots. They will appear as dark, hard, raised bumps that follow the course of the vein. Lymph channels can also become hard cords, but will be clearer or lack color. These conditions probably result from overly vigorous intercourse.
Fournier's gangrene: This condition is life-threatening and is most likely to occur in the severely infected patient with poor circulation or diabetes. It presents as a rapidly spreading skin and subcutaneous inflammation with development of necrotic/purplish tissue. Crepitance (air in the subcutaneous tissues) in the face of infection is another hallmark sign of Fournier's gangrene.
Candida **infection:** Most cases will present as balanitis. Occasionally, the patient will present with a red scrotum with satellite red lesions. The rash will be itchy, painful and tender.

Cellulitis: Patients will have diffusely red and painful scrotal or penile skin. The skin may be weeping, thickened and have pustules. When the skin lacks pustules, it is important to determine if the skin changes are a reaction to underlying inflammation such as epididymo-orchitis or torsion of the testis. In the latter cases, the testis and epididymis are markedly tender. The patient can usually differentiate testis pain from skin pain. If the inflammation shows dark areas suggestive of necrosis, the patient is developing Fournier's gangrene.

Contact dermatitis: Contact with chemicals and even some ointments may cause a profound inflammation of the scrotal skin. The skin may have the appearance and tenderness of cellulitis. History of exposure is extremely important.

Focused History: *Any prior history of skin lesions on the penis or scrotum?* (may give a hint at the diagnosis if the patient has had similar lesions before) *Describe the location and duration of the symptoms. Any history of any sexually transmitted disease. Last sexual intercourse?* (may raise the possibility of STD as the etiology)

Objective: Signs

Using Basic Tools: Swelling, tenderness and redness; purulent discharge in the case of severe phimosis; swollen lymph nodes.

Using Advanced Tools: Labs: Urinalysis for presence of glucose, leukocytes, blood or nitrite; KOH prep of the weepy material on the skin may show the presence of yeast elements such as budding yeast or strands called hyphae. A good clean catch urine may be difficult to obtain due to the phimosis.

Assessment: Differential Diagnosis

Sexually transmitted disease lesions are usually much more focal than these inflammatory conditions. Acute onset of genital herpes can result in severe genital inflammation but is usually heralded by multiple clear vesicles.

Plan:

Treatment

Phimosis: Keep the penis clean with soap and water several times per day. Broad-spectrum antibiotics such as **ciprofloxacin** 500mg po bid or **cephalexin** 500mg po qid x 1 week may be used if purulent discharge is noted from the meatus.

Paraphimosis: Try to reduce the foreskin by pushing the glans in and pulling the edematous skin forward. You may be able to decrease some of the swelling with direct compression of the glans penis prior to reducing the foreskin. If the constricting band around the penis is very tight, it may be necessary to put some local anesthetic and incise the band with a dorsal slit (*see Dorsal Slit Procedure*). Refer for circumcision.

Balanitis: Wash the penis several times a day and apply antifungal cream such as **nystatin, nystatin/triamcinolone acetonide** or **clotrimazole** bid until resolved. If a wet prep shows no yeast elements, can give **metronidazole** 500mg po bid x 1 week.

Thrombosis of penile vein and sclerosing lymphangitis: Refrain from any sexual activity. Use NSAIDs such as **ibuprofen** 400mg po q6h prn and if available, apply warm moist compresses bid.

Fournier's gangrene: Perform emergent aggressive surgical incision and debridement. Broad-spectrum IV antibiotics such as **ampicillin** 2g q8h and **gentamicin** 5mg/kg q day and **metronidazole** 500mg q6h are usually warranted.

Candida **fungal infection:** Keep skin dry and antifungal medications such as **nystatin, nystatin/triamcinolone acetonide** or **clotrimazole** cream or ointment bid for 1 week or single dose **fluconazole** 150mg po. *See Part 5: Specialty Areas: Chapter 12: Fungal Infections: Candidiasis (Thrush)*

Cellulitis: For mild cases, give **dicloxacillin** 500mg po q6h x 1 week or **cephalexin** 500mg po q6h x 1 week. For severe cases, treat with **oxacillin** 2g IV q4h x1 week or **vancomycin** 1g IV q12h x 1 week

Contact dermatitis: For mild, treat with topical 1% **hydrocortisone** bid x 1 week and **diphenhydramine** 25mg po bid up to 1 week. In severe cases, add **prednisone** 50mg po q day and wean by 10mg/day over 5 days. If there is a question of infection, avoid steroids and treat with antibacterial or antifungal medications.

Alternative: Yeast infections can be treated with alkaline washes to the glans penis, if no oral agent is available. Dissolving a few sodium bicarbonate tablets in a small container of water can make an alkaline solution, which can be directly applied to the skin bid for a week as needed.

Patient Education

General: If the patient has recurrent balanitis, or symptomatic phimosis, consideration of elective circumcision should be entertained. Activity: Until the inflammation has subsided, activity that would cause the genital region to be wet should be avoided. Refrain from any sexual activity until healed. Prevention and Hygiene: Circumcision and general cleanliness will largely prevent much of the inflammatory problems. IT IS VERY IMPORTANT TO KEEP THE GENITAL REGION DRY.

No Improvement/Deterioration: If the genital swelling and erythema spreads rapidly, return for immediate re-evaluation.

Wound Care: Keep area clean and dry.

Follow-up Actions:

Return Evaluation: Reevaluate in 1 week: Phimosis/paraphimosis, balanitis, genital fungal infections. Re-evaluate as needed: Thrombosis of penile vein (takes several weeks to months to resolve). Rapidly spreading inflammation may be Fournier's gangrene, requiring immediate evacuation.

Evacuation/Consultation Criteria: Evacuate as for Fournier's gangrene, phimosis/paraphimosis. When lesions on the skin persist, refer for biopsy. Consult urology or dermatology, as needed.

Dorsal Slit Procedure:

Essential: If a Foley catheter is needed in a patient with severe phimosis, which obscures the meatus, cannulation is sometimes possible with manipulation of the catheter tip inside the foreskin. If catheterization is not possible, a dorsal slit procedure or supra-pubic catheter placement may be necessary. If the patient has para-phimosis which cannot be reduced, a dorsal slit procedure may be necessary to prevent compromise to blood flow to the glans penis.

1. Attempt non-surgical reduction with anti-inflammatory medications, ice water and lubricants. Evacuate patient to a trained provider for this procedure if possible. If there are signs of systemic infection (fever, nausea, fatigue, etc.), and prompt evacuation is not available, perform a dorsal slit.
2. Assemble equipment: 1% **lidocaine** (w/o epi), needle and syringe, clamp, forceps, scalpel or surgical scissors, needle driver, 4-0 suture, prep solution, alcohol.
3. Prep the penis as with any surgical procedure (sterile scrub, povidone-iodine, drape), and attempt to clean between the head and the foreskin, especially on the dorsal side.
4. Use 1% **lidocaine** 5-10cc and a small needle (25-26 gauge) to infiltrate the skin about mid-shaft and extend the wheal at least halfway around the shaft of the penis.
5. Confirm the top of the penile shaft (dorsal side) is numb with forceps or needle.
6. Use a straight clamp to crush the skin from the phimotic area back to the glans (head). Make sure the jaw stays between the glans and the foreskin. Do NOT pass the jaw into the meatus. The glans will still have sensation and the patient should be able to tell you if the meatus is being cannulated.
7. Leave the clamp on for 5 minutes to compromise blood flow in the area to be incised.
8. Remove the clamp and use scissors to cut the crushed skin where the clamp had been. Do not incise the glans.
9. This should expose the glans. Control bleeding with simple or figure of 8 stitches using 3-0 or 4-0 chromic sutures.
10. Clean the penis with sterile prep solution between the head and foreskin, and then wipe prep solution away with alcohol. Allow to air dry and apply a sterile dressing leaving the meatus clear.
11. Monitor the patient, as this maneuver is only temporary and the slit can contract. He should have an elective circumcision later.

Male Genital Problems: Testis/Scrotal Mass

LTC Steve Waxman, MC, USA & LTC (P) Douglas Soderdahl, MC, USA

Introduction: Testicular cancer occurs most commonly in young men ages 20-39 and can grow rapidly. Early detection and referral is necessary to avoid treatment delays. A solid, non-transilluminating mass located below the testicular surface and inseparable from the testis is cancer until proven otherwise.

Subjective: Symptoms
Painless testicular mass that gets larger over a short period of time (weeks to months). Scrotal masses (may be painful or not painful) outside the testis are usually cystic and benign.
Focused History: *When did you first notice the abnormality in your scrotum? Is the lesion changing in size?* (Tumors tend to increase in size over time.) *Is it painful or painless?* (Pain may be associated with an inflammatory etiology but does not rule out a tumor.) *Have you suffered any injury to the area or did the lesion present after heavy activity?* (may be due to a hematoma from trauma or a mass from an inguinal hernia.)

Objective: Signs
Using Basic Tools: Palpable mass in testis may appear smooth or irregular, be located on the surface or deep in the testis. Mass is usually hard and does not transilluminate. A solid testicular mass is testicular cancer until proven otherwise and requires immediate urologic evaluation and treatment.
Using Advanced Tools: Labs: Urinalysis: Typically normal. Ultrasound can confirm or rule out a solid intratesticular mass.

Assessment: Differential Diagnosis
Hydrocele (around the testis), spermatocele or epididymal cyst (above the testis): Smooth spherical masses that transilluminate and are benign
Cysts or fibromas of the tunica albuginea (capsule of the testis): Small 1-4mm size nodules on the surface of the testis that are usually benign. Ultrasound of the testis may or may not see these lesions so it is imperative to follow these patients closely (in a few weeks to months) to make sure the lesions are not enlarging.
Varicoceles: "Wormy" mass above the testes-usually on the left side but sometimes on the right or bilateral.They typically decompress when the patient shifts from the standing to the supine position. Varicoceles that do not compress or are present on the right side should also have renal imaging (most often ultrasound) to rule out a mass.
Other masses in the scrotum: On the cord, in the scrotal skin or in the midline area near the penis are almost always benign.
Epididymitis: Painful area behind the testis. *See Part 3: General Symptoms: Male Genital Problems: Epididymitis*
Torsion of the testicle: If the pain in the scrotum is severe. *See Part 3: General Symptoms: Male Genital Problems: Torsion of the Testicle*

Plan:
Treatment
Primary: If an intratesticular mass is suspected, immediate urologic evaluation is required to rule out malignancy. If the mass is extratesticular on physical examination, ultrasound is useful to further characterize the lesion. If the patient is suspected to have epididymitis: treat appropriately. *See Part 3: General Symptoms: Male Genital Problems: Epididymitis*
Patient Education
General: Instruct patient to perform monthly testicular self-exams and return if change in size. Activity: If the patient has epididymitis, treat appropriately and avoid activities that increase testicular pain until resolved. Avoid lifting more than 10-15 lbs., prolonged standing (>30 min.) or walking >¼ mile. Use an athletic supporter.
Follow-up Actions
Return Evaluation: Check patient in 2-4 weeks for change in masses that are felt to be benign.
Evacuation/Consultation Criteria: Urgently evacuate patients with a solid testicular mass (ie, suspected cancer). Any mass that

prevents examination of the entire testis that is increasing in size, or appears to be inseparable from the testis should be referred for further evaluation immediately. Patients with suspected testicular cancer should have tumor markers and chest x-ray performed prior to undergoing emergent inguinal orchiectomy (removal of the testis and spermatic cord).

Male Genital Problems: Prostatitis

LTC Steve Waxman, MC, USA & LTC (P) Douglas Soderdahl, MC, USA

Introduction: Prostatitis is often used liberally to describe voiding problems and pain associated with the prostate. Prostatitis may be secondary to an infection, so an empiric trial of antibiotics is useful. Urinalysis is suggestive but not conclusive.

Subjective: Symptoms

Prostatitis may present acutely with high fevers, chills, dysuria, pelvic or perineal pain or more subtly with obstructive symptoms that include problems initiating the urinary stream, low flow and dribbling; irritative symptoms include frequency (>q2 hours) and/or urgency; pain in the head of the penis or under the scrotum; low back pain; fever. The symptoms may come on acutely or be of a chronic nature.

Focused History: *When did the symptoms begin? Any prior history of prostatitis?* (This condition tends to be recurrent.) *Pelvic or peri rectal pain or discomfort?* (May represent an abscess which may require more aggressive therapy) *Difficulty urinating?* (may need a Foley catheter to drain urine) *Fever? Chills?* (These may indicate a systemic infection involving the bloodstream.)

Objective: Signs

Using Basic Tools: Physical exam. Digital rectal exam: Tender prostate with/without tender pelvic floor or coccyx (palpate 360° on rectal exam); Boggy or spongy feeling prostate and tender to palpation. Do not do a vigorous prostate exam or prostate massage on a patient with acute inflammation of the prostate as this could result in bacteremia and sepsis. Patients may go into urinary retention from prostatic obstruction due to inflammation. Men may also have pain and tenderness in the epididymides with a concurrent bout of prostatitis.

Using Advanced Tools: Labs: Urinalysis: heme and leukoesterase positive urine suggest infection. Urine can be completely normal in the face of prostate infection, inflammation or pain (prostatodynia). If available, bladder scan or sonogram of bladder to rule out urinary retention.

Assessment: Differential Diagnosis

Irritative voiding symptoms with or without fever: Urinary tract infection until proven otherwise, distal ureteral stone, urethral stricture, bladder neck dysfunction, bladder or prostate cancer, foreign body in bladder, overflow incontinence

Obstructive voiding: Enlarged prostate, urethral stricture, and neurologic disease of the spine or peripheral nerves

Painful prostate: Urinary tract infection, bladder neck dysfunction/prostatodynia/pelvic floor dysfunction, musculoskeletal pain, coccydynia, seminal vesiculitis

Plan

Treatment: Acute Prostatitis

Primary:

1. Patients who appear acutely ill (eg, high fevers, chills, dysuria, pelvic or perineal pain): begin high dose **ampicillin** 1-2g IV q6-8h and **gentamicin** 5mg/ kg IV q day. If penicillin allergic, use IV fluoroquinolones (**levofloxacin** 250mg IV q day or **ciprofloxacin** 400mg IV bid) or **vancomycin** 1g IV bid and **gentamicin** 5mg/kg IV q day. Hydrate aggressively. If the pt. is able to take oral fluids well, then push fluids. If pt. is appears septic, then hydrate with IV fluid at 150cc/hour and monitor urine output closely. If patient is having difficulty voiding or is unable to void, then place a Foley to gravity drainage. When the patient is afebrile, switch to oral fluoroquinolone (*see Part 4: Organ Systems: Chapter 8: Urinary Tract Infection*) for a total of 30 days.
2. Patient with fewer clinical signs of acute illness: (eg, low-grade fever or no fever), treat with fluoroquinolones po. *See Part 4: Organ Systems: Chapter 8: Urinary Tract Infection*
3. Treat any male suspected of having an infection for 30 days regardless of the location of symptoms (kidney, prostate or scrotum). Infected urine can easily reflux into prostatic ducts, therefore assume the prostate is infected.
4. If symptoms persist and urinalysis continues to be abnormal without improvement after 3-5 days, suspect bacterial resistance and change antibiotics.
5. If a bladder is palpated, attempt to pass a Foley catheter (*see Part 8: Procedures: Chapter 30: Urinary Bladder Catheterization*). Inability to pass catheter suggests a stricture or other obstruction. If unable to pass catheter and urologist is available within a short time period, then transfer immediately. If the patient's bladder is full and urethral catheter placement is not possible and urologist is not near, consider supra-pubic aspiration or catheter placement. *See Part 8: Procedures: Chapter 30: Suprapubic Bladder Aspiration (Tap) or Catheter Placement*
6. Add alpha-blocker if patient is having difficulty voiding.

Alternative:

Antibiotics: Sulfamethoxazole-trimethoprim DS po tid until fever resolves, followed by **sulfamethoxazole trimethoprim DS** po bid x 30 days, or **amoxicillin/clavulanate** 500mg po bid x 30 days, or **cephalexin** 500mg po qid x 30 days. **Doxycycline** is not as effective since it is bacterio-static, and should only be used (100mg po bid) if there is no other alternative. Nitrofurantoin has minimal tissue penetration and should not be used in prostatitis.

Treatment: Chronic Prostatitis

Primary:

1. Antibiotics, with or without alpha-blockers. **Levofloxacin** 500mg po q day has broad coverage for both C. *trachomatis* and urinary pathogens. Treat for 30 days. Alpha blockers include the following: **Alfuzosin** 10mg po daily or **tamsulosin** 0.4mg po q day and can increase to 0.8mg po daily, if necessary.

2. Patients who complain of frequency should be given bladder antispasmodics with caution since they can cause urinary retention. **Tolterodine LA** 4mg po q day or **oxybutynin** 5mg po tid prn. Treatment should continue based on clinical response and patient scheduled for urology referral.

Adjunctive measures: Sitz baths (sitting in a tub of warm water) can relax the pelvic floor musculature and decrease pain.
Empiric: If the patient has had multiple sexual contacts and initial symptoms of urethritis (urethral discharge) after finishing levofloxacin, a trial of **erythromycin** 500mg po qid x 30 days can be given. If symptoms persist, include **metronidazole** 250mg po tid x 30 days. The empiric usage of levofloxacin, erythromycin and metronidazole covers most STDs that would affect the lower urinary tract. Without urethral discharge or abnormalities on urinalysis or physical exam (no genital ulcers, lymphadenopathy, etc.), STDs are very unlikely.

Patient Education
Activity: Bedrest and IV antibiotics for septic patients with close monitoring of vital signs.
Medications: Alpha-blockers may make sinus conditions worse. Likewise, sinus medications may make voiding more difficult.
Prevention and Hygiene: Void on a regular basis and avoid lifting or straining with a full bladder. Refer to urology for recurrent symptoms or relapses.
No Improvement/Deterioration: If fever persists beyond 48-72 hours, return promptly. Some prostatitis symptoms or syndromes are slow to resolve. Do not draw PSA during acute episode of prostatitis as it will be elevated and not helpful to the screening for prostate cancer. PSA should be drawn at least 4 weeks after prostatitis has been treated and the patient asymptomatic. Prostatitis does not make a patient more susceptible to prostate cancer later in life. A prostate nodule on rectal exam should prompt a urologic referral.

Follow-up Actions
Return Evaluation: Fever can be expected to last 1-3 days.
Evacuation/Consultation Criteria: Aggressively rehydrate unstable patients in shock (*see Part 7: Trauma: Chapter 27*) and evacuate immediately. If urinary frequency and urgency persist after initial 30 days, continue treatment for another 30 days. Stable patients should eventually follow-up with an urologist electively to assess the need for further evaluation.

Male Genital Problems: Torsion of the Testicle
LTC Steve Waxman, MC, USA. & LTC (P) Douglas Soderdahl, MC, USA

Introduction: Rapid identification and treatment of testicular torsion is necessary to preserve testicle function. All patients require immediate scrotal exploration with detorsion of the affected side and tacking or fixation of the opposite testicle to the scrotal skin since it is also at risk of future torsion. Loss of both testicles not only results in sterility but loss of testosterone, which requires lifelong supplementation for normal body function. Salvage of the affected testicle can usually be achieved if blood flow is restored within 4 hours. Although testicular salvage is possible after 12 hours of torsion, the chances of success markedly decrease after 6 hours without arterial blood flow.

Subjective: Symptoms
Acute (<2 hr): Severe scrotal pain, onset can be at night while asleep, may have prior history of scrotal pain lasting less than 1 day, may have nausea/vomiting/anorexia, testicle is extremely painful, and spermatic cord may be tender.
Sub-acute (2-48 hr): Scrotal pain increases over several hours. After 24 hours, some of the pain may start to subside.
Chronic (>48 hr): History of acute onset of pain. Testicular pain is improved but not gone.
Focused History: *When did the pain begin? Sharp or dull? Does the pain vary in intensity? Does the pain change with sitting or standing? Is the pain getting better, worse or staying the same? Prior history of similar pain?* (Torsion of the testicle usually presents with sudden onset with no inciting influence, however, the classic presentation is not always the case and torsion should always be in the differential of testicular pain.)

Objective: Signs
Using Basic Tools: Extreme, diffuse tenderness of the entire testicle (typically "high riding" testicle) with no improvement with elevation of the testicle. Loss of cremasteric reflex on the affected side.
Using Advanced Tools: Labs: Urinalysis: usually normal. Strongly heme or leukoesterase positive sample suggests kidney stone or infection. Testicular ultrasound with color flow Doppler. Usually accurate and shows no blood flow to the affected testis. In longstanding torsion greater than several days, there may be blood flow to the capsule of the testicle. There may still be blood flow seen to the acutely torsed testicle if early on so the test is not 100%. Always refer for immediate surgical exploration if you suspect torsion.

Assessment: Differential Diagnosis
Orchitis: Fatigue, muscle aches, sore throat or other flu-like symptoms with gradual onset and normal spermatic cord. Mumps orchitis is extremely rare with modern vaccinations.
Severe epididymo-orchitis: Voiding symptoms with leukoesterase and nitrite positive urine. However, urinalysis can be normal with no voiding symptoms.
Tumor in the testicle: Consider when there is a mass typically without pain.
Torsion of the appendix testis/epididymis: Point tenderness on the superior portion of the testicle/epididymis with the remaining testicle being non-tender.
Ruptured testis: History of trauma
Kidney stone: Especially if lodged in the distal ureter, can have referred pain to the ipsilateral testicle, but a normal scrotal exam.
Incarcerated hernia: Most of the discomfort will be above the testicle. A hydrocele may be present, making it difficult to examine the testicle. If omentum is in the hernia, there may not be any bowel symptoms.

Plan:

Treatment

Primary: If urological or general surgical support is not immediately available, manual detorsion, with or without injection of the spermatic cord with local anesthesia. Torsion may be 180-720° (2 full twists).

1. Attempt to detorse the testicle first by rotating the testicle outward (like opening a book). If the pain worsens or does not improve, rotate the other direction. The torsion may be 2 full twists. If the testicle hangs lower but pain persists, continue untwisting the cord.
2. If **lidocaine** is available, inject into the cord using a long needle or spinal needle in the spermatic cord. This can be accomplished by straddling the cord on the affected side between 2 fingers just as the cord crosses over the pubic bone lateral and superior to the penis. Make multiple passes through the cord and down to the pubic bone injecting a total of 10cc of 1% **lidocaine**. This should numb the testis. This may relieve the pain, causing the cremasteric muscles to relax and may result in spontaneous de-torsion. If the pain is gone, check the testicle for descent to the normal position and if the testicle has become less tense. Also try to palpate the vas deferens posteriorly. This tube is about the consistency and size of uncooked spaghetti and is located behind and is easily separable from the bulk of the spermatic cord. If the tube is in its normal location, spermatic cord torsion is unlikely. You can use the vas deferens as a guide to untwist the cord. The vas deferens should lie posteriorly to the cord. Palpate the vas high in the scrotum and try to follow it down.

Patient Education

If the patient has spontaneous detorsion or the testicle is manually detorsed and the pain completely resolved, urologic consultation should be sought in as timely a fashion as possible.

General: Wear a scrotal support and await definitive surgery to prevent recurrence

Activity: Light activity with supporter until problem surgically corrected

Diet: NPO if surgery is imminent

Prevention and Hygiene: Preventive surgery is required to avoid similar torsion on the opposite side. Examine testicle regularly.

No Improvement/Deterioration: Prompt evacuation and surgical correction.

Follow-up Actions

Wound Care: Light activity for 3-4 weeks after surgery.

Return Evaluation: If the testicle was salvaged, the risk for shrinkage or atrophy increases with the length of time the testicle was torsed.

Evacuation/Consultation Criteria: All cases of suspected torsion should be referred. The patient is at risk for torsion on the opposite side as well. He should be evacuated as soon as possible to prevent this calamity, particularly if one testicle was not salvaged. The testicles both need to be surgically explored and fixed to the scrotal wall to prevent rotation. Loss of both testicles results in significant hormonal changes and infertility and should be avoided.

Male Genital Problems: Epididymitis

LTC Steve Waxman, MC, USA & LTC (P) Douglas Soderdahl, MC, USA

Introduction: The epididymis, usually located behind each testicle, is the site of final maturation and conduit of sperm. It can become painful from either mechanical or infectious irritation. Treatment involves both medication and scrotal support which may require strict bed rest in severe cases. Prior vasectomy is a potential risk factor.

Subjective: **Symptoms**

Pain in the scrotum behind the testis with tenderness of the epididymis, with or without pain in the testis. The pain may be similar to that of testicular torsion so this must also be in the differential diagnosis. Most commonly presents sub acutely with history of recurrent episodes but can present acutely (uncommon and primarily seen in older patients) with swelling, pain, fever, chills and other signs of a serious infection.

Focused History: *Any prior episodes of scrotal pain or epididymitis?* (Patients with a prior history of epididymitis are at increased risk of having another episode.) *Any recent heavy lifting, trauma or increased activity?* (These may promote epididymal inflammation.) *Did the pain come on gradually?* (may help differentiate from torsion)

Objective: **Signs**

Using Basic Tools: Swelling of the hemi-scrotum, urethral discharge, frequent and urgent urination, fever. Use penlight or otoscope to transilluminate the scrotum to differentiate swelling due to a solid mass (testis and epididymis) vs. fluid (bright, diffuse glow; seen with spermatocele or hydrocele).

Using Advanced Tools: Labs: Urinalysis: nitrite and leukoesterase positive urine (infection). Perform a urine culture if available and dipstick is positive. Perform a urethral swab for culture and Gram's stain to rule out gonorrhea and chlamydia.

Assessment:

Pain and tenderness in other areas of the scrotum suggests other causes (eg, hernia, varicocele, musculoskeletal pain or entrapped nerve). Intermittent testicular pain could be referred from a hernia, ureteral stone or even intermittent torsion.

Differential Diagnosis

Trauma: History or signs of trauma.

Torsion of testicle: Usually acute onset of severe pain, without fever. In early stages, may be able to localize pain to testicle with non-tender epididymis. *See Part 3: General Symptoms: Male Genital Problems: Torsion of the Testicle*

Hernia: May hear bowel sounds over mass in scrotum

Testicular tumor: Painless mass in testicle. *See Part 3: General Symptoms: Male Genital Problems: Testis/Scrotal Mass*

Plan:
Treatment
1. Scrotal support/elevation, bed rest.
2. NSAIDs such as **ibuprofen** 800mg po tid with food.
3. Antibiotics for 10-30 days.
   a. **Levofloxacin** 500mg po daily or **ciprofloxacin** 500mg po bid or **trimethoprim-sulfamethoxazole DS** po bid or **doxycycline** 100 mg po bid. In severe cases, give **ampicillin** 1g IV q6h plus **gentamicin** (loading dose of 1.5mg/kg followed by 1mg/kg IV q8h) or **ceftriaxone** 5mg/kg IV q day (**ceftriaxone** 500mg to 1g IV bid). Should be given until fever resolves, then convert to oral antibiotics.
   b. If there is a urethral discharge, give **ceftriaxone** 250mg IM (or **ciprofloxacin** 500mg po) single dose to treat gonorrhea, and follow with 7-10 days of **doxycycline** 100mg po bid (or **levofloxacin** 500mg po q day).
   c. If neither fever nor discharge is present, treat empirically with **doxycycline** 100mg po bid or **levofloxacin** 500mg po q day or **ciprofloxacin** 500mg po bid or **trimethoprim-sulfamethoxazole DS** po bid for 2-4 weeks.

Patient Education
General: Use condoms
Activity: Light duty until swelling has resolved. Scrotal support with briefs or jockstrap
Diet: Regular
Medications: Be alert for allergic reactions to some antibiotics. Use sunscreen with doxycycline, Septra, Cipro and Levaquin.
Prevention and Hygiene: The epididymis is susceptible to repeated inflammation, so recommend a comfortable athletic supporter for all high-impact activities. If symptoms occur on the other side, be suspicious that the first episode was torsion.

Follow-up Actions
Return Evaluation: Follow up in 1 month for re-evaluation of the scrotum. Refer to urology if symptoms persist or progress despite adequate course of treatment.
Evacuation/Consultation Criteria: Evacuation is not usually necessary. If there is a persistent mass in the scrotum, refer patient for ultrasound and urologic consultation.

Memory Loss
CDR Christopher Jankosky, MC, USN

Introduction: Memory dysfunction is a frequent cognitive problem brought to the clinician and is common in deployed active duty forces. 34% of Persian Gulf veterans indicated in a survey that they had symptoms of memory problems. Determining the etiology of the symptoms and whether they represent a life-threatening condition can be difficult. Memory loss may occur in isolation, or may be associated with difficulties in attention, concentration, naming, or language. Sorting out these symptoms is very complex. Head injury is the most common cause of amnesia.

Subjective: **Symptoms**
Decreased ability to recall events. Associated symptoms may include headache, neck pain, weakness, fatigue, delusions, hallucinations, changes in sleep pattern, and physical/emotional stresses. Medical personnel in the field must focus on the patient's general level of attention, as there are a number of acute events (trauma, toxins, hypoxia, infection) that may cause a diminished level of consciousness. Diminished attention may be the earliest indication of a patient progressing to unconsciousness. Medical personnel may query the patient or his comrades about his current level of attention compared to baseline. Be aware that patients with delirium may also manifest difficulties in memory, but instead of reduced alertness they may manifest increased vigilance, psychomotor and autonomic overactivity, agitation, tremulousness, hallucinations, fantasies, or delusions.
Focused History: *What is your name?* (It is rare for a patient to forget his own name, and if this occurs it is unlikely to represent an organic etiology.) *Have you had this problem before? Have you had any physical or psychological illnesses in the past?* (can suggest diagnosis, or related illnesses; also tests memory) *Have you had any recent head injuries, infections, fevers, medication change, alcohol use, or toxic exposure?* (can explain etiology of symptoms)

Objective: **Signs**
Using Basic Tools: Perform vital signs assessment, HEENT exam, and a complete neurological exam, including a Mini-Mental Status Examination (*see Appendices: Table A-6. Mini-Mental Status Exam*). Assess memory function in detail. May have obvious head injury, odor of alcohol, fever. Difficulty with immediate recall is generally seen in patients with confusion or delirium. Test this aspect of memory with the simple test of digit span. A normal individual should have a digit span of 5 or more. Slowly recite to the patient a string of 5 digits, and then immediately ask them to repeat them to you. Document the longest string that he can correctly repeat. Additional tests can include counting backwards from 20, or reciting months in reverse order. Normal patients should be able to perform these tests correctly. A patient with amnesia may have difficulty with the learning ability function of memory. Ask the patient to retain 3 unrelated words for 5-10 minutes, during which you perform other testing. Although an anxious patient may need prompting to recall one of the 3 words, most patients should be able to recall all 3. Testing of retrieval ability is more difficult because the examiner may not know the patient's fund of knowledge. Testing can include standard information questions such as national leaders and dramatic news events. Knowledge specific to his individual military unit can also be asked. If the patient is able to successfully pass these memory tests, then his primary problem is unlikely to be with memory function. Further assessment of other cognitive functions will need to be performed as indicated by the clinical situation and his response to the MMSE. If there is an indication of diminished alertness during administration of the MMSE, ensure that more detailed questioning is performed to ascertain level of consciousness. Documentation of specific deficits will assist later examiners in determining if clinical situation is improving or deteriorating.
Using Advanced Tools: Labs: WBC for infection. Blood glucose if considering hypoglycemia. Pulse oximetry for hypoxia. Papilledema (an indication of increased intracranial pressure) should cause immediate concern for intracranial hemorrhage, swelling, or mass. Chemistry panel for electrolyte abnormalities (if I-stat is available)

Assessment: **Differential Diagnosis**

Traumatic brain injury: Memory problems following head trauma are common, so patient may not remember the injury. Intracranial bleeding may lead to severe symptoms within minutes, but may also progress slowly over hours to days, requiring close follow-up. *See Part 7: Trauma: Chapter 26: Mild Traumatic Brain Injury/Concussion*

Infection: Herpes simplex encephalitis is the most common infection causing predominantly memory problems. There are usually associated behavioral deviations, disorientation, seizures, or weakness. Most patients will be febrile.

Stroke (ischemic from blocked vessel, or hemorrhagic from bleed): Uncommon in young individuals without other neurologic signs or symptoms. Ask about stroke risk factors: hypertension, smoking, diabetes, positive family history, hyperlipidemia, oral contraceptives, binge alcohol drinking, atrial fibrillation, and coronary heart disease.

Seizure disorder: Rarely manifested as isolated memory and cognitive problems. *See Part 4: Organ Systems: Chapter 5: Seizure Disorders and Epilepsy*

Hypoxia: Can result in permanent damage to the memory systems of the brain. History may reveal a recent hypoxic event.

Inflammatory: Consider multiple sclerosis or CNS sarcoidosis, although these rarely cause isolated memory problems.

Transient global amnesia: Uncommon in young adults; no associated symptoms, and the condition resolves within 24 hours.

Migraine: Memory problems are transient (hours), and usually associated with a headache; prior history of migraines.

Psychiatric: Causes can include sleep deprivation, stress, anxiety, PTSD, delirium, and depression. Psychiatric etiologies usually present as a retrograde amnesia. Other psychiatric symptoms are usually present. This category should be strongly considered if the patient does not know his own name.

Decompression sickness: History of recent diving and/or flying; may have other associated neurological findings, including subtle (soft) signs. *See Part 6: Operational Environment: Chapters 20 & 21*

Other: Metabolic (such as thiamine deficiency), hypoglycemia, toxic, degenerative, or neoplastic causes may also be considered.

Plan:

Treatment

1. Secure all weapons.
2. Confirm stability of physical and neurological status, especially changes in level of consciousness. Frequent communication with detailed questions will assist in early detection of diminished alertness leading to loss of consciousness.
3. Provide supportive treatment: rest, fluids (by po or IV), reassurance, and observation will improve or stabilize many conditions.
4. Closely supervise military personnel who return to duty. If given significant independent responsibilities, they can be a danger to themselves or others if memory problems remain.
5. Herpes simplex encephalitis has a high mortality and demands early and aggressive treatment with IV antiviral medication, such as **acyclovir** (if available) 30 mg/kg/day IV in 3 divided doses for at least 10 days, and evacuate immediately.
6. Intracranial bleeding, swelling, or mass requires neurosurgical intervention.

Patient Education

General: Significant memory problems may be due to an organic or psychiatric etiology.

No Improvement/Deterioration: Return for evaluation daily initially, as symptoms may worsen rapidly in some illnesses.

Follow-up Actions

Return Evaluation: If traumatic head injury occurred and symptoms worsen over days, suspect a slow intracranial bleed. Medically evacuate ASAP. Repeat funduscopic exams to look for papilledema on follow up exams.

Evacuation/Consultation Criteria: Evacuate if patient unable to function, if unstable or if deteriorates. Consult psychiatry or neurology if needed.

Note: Definitive diagnosis may require lumbar puncture, neuroimaging, EEG or use of specialty consultation.

Obstetric Problems: Pregnancy

LTC Marvin Williams, MC, USA & CPT Jesse P. Reynolds, SP, USA

Subjective: **Symptoms**

In women with regular menstrual cycles, a history of one or more missed cycles (periods) is suggestive of pregnancy. Associated symptoms include fatigue, nausea with or without vomiting, breast tenderness, backache, heartburn, constipation, frequent urination, urgency, urinary incontinence (caused by the enlarged uterus compressing the bladder), and "quickening" (first movements of a fetus felt in utero usually between 16-20 weeks).

Focused History: *What was the first day of your last menstrual period?* (Add 7 days to the first day of the last normal menses and subtract 3 months to calculate the estimated date of delivery.)

Objective: **Signs**

Spider angiomata (branched capillaries on the skin, shaped like a spider) and blotchy or patchy palmar erythema (more than 50-60% of patients), regress after delivery. Striae gravidarum (stretch marks) develop in 50% of pregnant woman. Hyperpigmentation of nipples, areolae, umbilicus, axillae, perineum and midline of lower abdomen (linea nigra), breast enlargement due to increased hormone levels which later causes release of colostrum (thin, yellowish fluid seeping from the nipple) and lactation, hemorrhoids, ankle swelling, varicose veins.

Using Basic Tools: Fetal heart tones can be auscultated (using the bell side of stethoscope) at or beyond 18-20 weeks of gestation.

Using Advanced Tools: Pregnancy tests can be used in the field. Most are nearly as accurate (97-99%) as a laboratory test on serum.

Assessment:

Palpation of fetal parts and the appreciation of fetal movement and heart tones are diagnostic.

Plan:

Treatment: *See Part 3: General Symptoms: Obstetric Problems for appropriate treatment sections*

Obstetric Problems: Induction of Labor

LTC Marvin Williams, MC, USA

What: It will be very rare for you to attend a normal childbirth. Your presence will more than likely be requested for the "worse case scenario" birthing experience (ie, fetal demise or eclampsia). That said, it is imperative that you have a basic understanding of induction of labor. Given your limited choices of induction agents, we will focus on misoprostol, which is a synthetic prostaglandin (PG1) available as 100 or 200 microgram tablets. The current FDA recommended use for misoprostol is the treatment of peptic ulcer disease secondary to NSAID therapy. The formulation gained popularity as an "off label" induction agent because of its inexpensive cost and stability at room temperature. Misoprostol is also present endogenously within the uterine muscle and fetal membranes during pregnancy. When utilized as an induction agent, misoprostol is typically administered intravaginally or under the cervix because of fewer side effects (fever, chills, vomiting, and diarrhea).

What You Need: **Misoprostol** 25 micrograms (you will have to cut the tablets into quarters [for 100mg tablets]—use a sharp instrument as the tablets are small). Dose the tablets q4h not to exceed 12 doses (48 hours).

When: Some of the more common indications for induction that you may have to deal with in theater are preeclampsia/eclampsia, intraamniotic infection, fetal demise, or fetal distress. Perform induction when the benefits of delivery outweigh the risks of continuing the pregnancy, and when there are no contraindications to a vaginal delivery.

What To Do:
1. Determine gestational age of fetus. *See Part 3: General Symptoms: Obstetric Problems: Vaginal Delivery*
2. Check abdomen for scars of previous Cesarian delivery. If present, do not induce labor.
3. Examine genitals for signs of active genital herpes outbreak. If present, do not induce labor.
4. Evaluate cervix by visualizing and palpating. The condition of the cervix will determine the success of the induction. The more dilated and thin the cervix, the greater the chance of a successful induction.
5. Palpate the mother's abdomen to determine how the fetus is positioned. Induce only if the baby is in a cephalic (head first) lie.
6. If the uterus is unscarred and the baby is term, insert **misoprostol** 25 micrograms intravaginally (next to cervix) q4h (up to 12 doses). (Misoprostol is not scored and the tablets must be divided to provide the dose needed for induction.) Onset of labor and subsequent delivery is variable but most patients will deliver within 36 hours.
7. Upon initiating an induction of labor, refer to the section "vaginal delivery" for direction on fetal monitoring and the delivery procedure.

What Not To Do:
1. Do not attempt to induce labor if there is a history of a classical cesarean delivery; an active outbreak of genital herpes; known placental abnormalities such as the placenta covering part or most of the cervix or has implanted too deeply into the uterine wall, or if the fetus is in a tranverse or oblique lie.
2. Do not attempt induction if you think the pregnancy is less than 37 (term) weeks along.

Obstetric Problems: Vaginal Delivery

LTC Marvin Williams, MC, USA & CPT Jesse Reynolds, SP, USA

When: Labor is defined as progressive dilation of the uterine cervix in association with repetitive uterine contractions resulting in complete dilation (10 cm) and effacement (thinning) of the cervix. Normal labor is a continuous process.
    First stage: Onset of labor through full dilation and effacement of cervix
    Second stage: Full cervical dilation and delivery of the infant
    Third stage: Interval between the delivery of the infant and delivery of the placenta
    Fourth stage: Recovery of the uterus after delivery of the placenta

What You Need: 1% **lidocaine without epinephrine** (approx. 20-30cc), **misoprostol**, sterile gloves (several pairs), gauze bandages and prep solution, 2-0, 3-0, and 4-0 absorbable suture (vicryl or chromic) for the repair, scissors or a scalpel to make the episiotomy incision, sterile (or clean) towels, suction device (bulb syringe), suture forceps, and needle holders

What To Do:
During the First Stage of Labor:
1. Assess baby's gestational age by asking the mother the date of the 1st day of her last normal menstrual period, subtracting 3 months and adding 7 days (40 weeks +/- 2 weeks). Palpate and measure the height of the uterine fundus (top) from the pubic bone. Up to about 36 weeks, this distance in centimeters approximates gestational age (ie, 32cm from pubic bone to top of fundus equals approximately 32 weeks gestational age). If not >36 weeks by dates or measurement, *see Part 3: General Symptoms: Obstetric Problems: Preterm Labor.*
2. Listen for fetal heart rate (FHR). Normal rate is approximately 120-160 bpm. Periodically reassess during labor. A good rule of thumb is during the first stage of labor, FHR should be evaluated q15 minutes recorded during and immediately after a contraction. The rate normally decreases during contractions but should recover.
3. Encourage the mother to walk as gravity and motion will encourage cervical dilation.
4. Read this section and others related to birth (*see Part 3: General Symptoms: Obstetric Problems: Episiotomy and Repair & Breech Birth*).
5. Periodically assess progression of labor by timing contractions. Eventual delivery is likely when contractions are <3 minute apart.
6. Check the birth canal with a sterile gloved hand once before birth to ensure the cervix is fully dilated and effaced (fully thinned out).

Figure 3-15. Key Anatomical Landmarks for a Normal Delivery

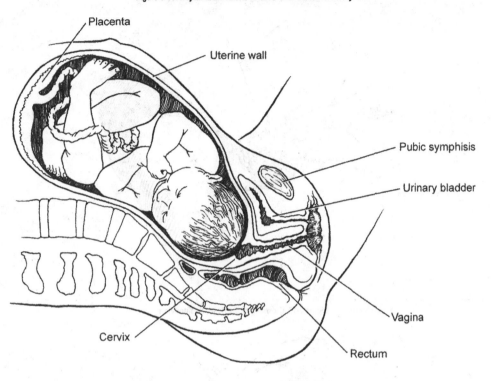

Placenta

Uterine wall

Pubic symphisis

Urinary bladder

Vagina

Cervix

Rectum

During the Second Stage of Labor: (*see Figures 3-16 & 3-17*)

1. As the cervix progresses to complete dilation, place the patient in the dorsal lithotomy position (patient is on her back with her thighs flexed on the abdomen). Women from some cultures may prefer to squat.
2. With each contraction, the patient should be urged to push and the care provider should perform perineal massage. During the second stage, check FHR at least q5 minutes, during and immediately after each uterine contraction. The rate normally decreases during contractions but should recover.
3. As the fetal head crowns (ie, distends the vaginal opening), consider an episiotomy if massage has failed to stretch the tissue adequately. Although not routinely required, an episiotomy may facilitate the delivery of a large infant, or one with shoulder dystocia. In selected cases, an episiotomy will decrease the risk of a tear of the perineal tissue into the rectum. *See Part 3: General Symptoms: Obstetric Problems: Episiotomy and Repair*
4. As crowning continues, it is very important to support the fetal head via a modified Ritgen maneuver. This is accomplished by placing your hand over the fetal head while your other hand exerts pressure through the perineum onto the fetal chin. Use a sterile towel to avoid contamination of this hand by the anus.
5. After the head is delivered, suction the mouth and nose with the bulb syringe.
6. Check the neck for the presence of an umbilical cord around it, which should be reduced if possible. If the cord is too tight, it should be doubly clamped and cut.
7. Place your hands on the chin and head, applying gentle downward pressure, delivering the anterior shoulder. Avoid injury to the brachial plexus; avoid excessive pressure on the neck.
8. Deliver the posterior shoulder by upward traction on the fetal head.
9. Delivery of the body should occur easily (*see Figure 3-18*).
10. Cradle the infant in your arms, suction once again and the umbilical cord is clamped and cut. If no clamps are available, suture may be used. *See Part 5: Specialty Areas: Chapter 15: Newborn Resuscitation*
11. To avoid significant heat loss, dry the newborn completely and wrap in towels or blankets.
12. If the mother (or another person) can hold the baby safely, put the baby to the mother's breast. This will help the uterus contract.

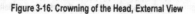

Figure 3-16. Crowning of the Head, External View

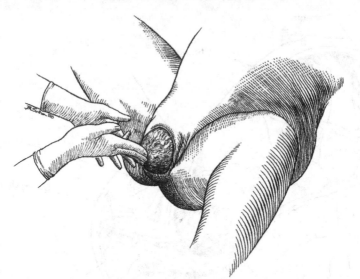

Figure 3-17. Crowning of the Head, Sagittal View

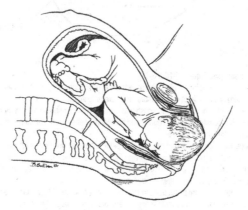

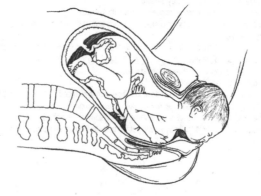

Figure 3-18. Delivery of the Body

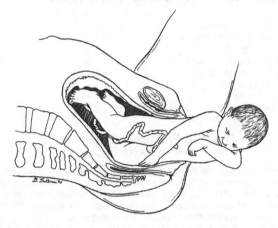

During the Third Stage of Labor:

1. Soon after delivery of the infant, the placenta will follow. Placental delivery is imminent when the uterus rises in the abdomen, the umbilical cord lengthens, and a "gush" of blood is noted. AVOID excessive traction on the umbilical cord to avoid uterine inversion (pulling the uterus "inside-out"), which will cause profound blood loss and shock. Instead, wait up to 30 min. for spontaneous delivery of the placenta. *See Figure 3-19*

2. If spontaneous placental separation does not occur, remove the placenta manually. Pass a gloved hand into the uterine cavity and gently apply traction to the umbilical cord, using the side of the hand to develop a cleavage plane between the placenta and the uterine cavity.

3. Inspect the placenta to ensure it is complete. Inspect the cord for the presence of the expected two umbilical arteries and one umbilical vein.

4. After the delivery of the placenta, palpate the uterus to ensure that it has reduced in size and become firmly contracted. If the uterus does not seem firm after the initial uterine massage, administer **misoprostol**, which is a synthetic prostaglandin (PGE1). This drug is given as an initial dose of 800-1000 micrograms rectally or orally. The dose may be repeated in one hour and maintenance therapy should then be instituted at 200 micrograms q4h for 24 hrs. There are no known contraindications to the medication and it can be administered to hypertensive as well as asthmatic patients. Side effects include fever and tachycardia.

5. Inspect the birth canal in a systematic fashion. Evaluate lacerations of the vagina and/or perineum and extensions of the episiotomy, and repair if necessary. *See Part 3: General Symptoms: Obstetric Problems: Episiotomy and Repair*

Figure 3-19. Delivery of the Placenta

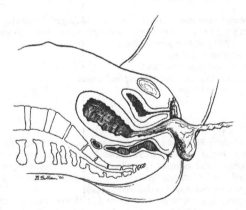

During the Fourth Stage of Labor:

1. The likelihood of serious postpartum complications is greatest in the first hour or so after delivery. Palpate the uterus to ensure that it is firm. Repeat uterine palpation through the abdominal wall frequently during the immediate postpartum period to ascertain uterine tone.

2. Monitor pulse, blood pressure and the amount of vaginal bleeding q15 minutes for the first hour, then q30 min. for 3 hours after delivery to identify excessive blood loss.

3. Manage pain with **ibuprofen** 800mg po tid with food or **Tylenol #3** (**acetaminophen + codeine**) 1-2 tablets po q4-6h
4. Apply ice to the perineum for 20-30 minutes q4-6h to decrease swelling after the delivery.

What Not To Do:

1. Do not contaminate the birth canal prior to birth.
2. Do not allow the episiotomy to tear into the rectum.
3. Do not forget to reduce umbilical cord.
4. Do not forget to suction the baby's mouth and nose.
5. Do not forget to clamp and cut the umbilical cord.
6. Do not forget to clean and dry the baby.
7. Do not forget to deliver the placenta.
8. Do not forget to repair an episiotomy and any tears.
9. Do not forget to monitor the mother's vital signs.

Obstetric Problems: Preterm Labor

LTC Marvin Williams, MC, USA & CPT Jesse Reynolds, SP, USA

Introduction: Preterm birth (PTB) as a result of preterm labor (PTL) is the most common cause of infant morbidity and mortality. Complications include respiratory distress syndrome (RDS), intraventricular hemorrhage (IVH), necrotizing enterocolitis (NEC), sepsis, and seizures. Long term morbidity associated with PTL and delivery includes chronic lung problems (bronchopulmonary dysplasia or BPD) and developmental abnormalities. PTL is defined as regular uterine contractions occurring with a frequency of 10 minutes or less between 20 and 36 weeks gestation, with each contraction lasting at least 30 seconds. When contractions are accompanied by cervical effacement (thinning), dilation (opening), and/or descent of the fetus into the pelvis, it becomes increasingly difficult to stop labor. The cause of PTL is unknown but many factors have been associated with it and some include: dehydration, rupture of membranes, infections, uterine enlargement (twins), uterine distortion (fibroids), and placental abnormalities (previa and abruption), smoking and substance abuse. Approximately 5% of women will rupture the amniotic membrane around the fetus prior to the onset of labor. This is called premature rupture of membranes (PROM). Preterm PROM (pPROM) refers to this occurrence in pregnancies prior to 37 weeks of gestation and accounts for 15-25% of cases of PROM. Preterm PROM is responsible for about one third of all preterm births. In women with pPROM who have a viable fetus (>24 weeks gestation), every effort should be made to evacuate the patient to a hospital with neonatal intensive care support. If this is not possible, delivery may need to be completed within 24 hours of pPROM to avoid infection in fetus and mother. One of the most important causes of early onset neonatal infection is group B streptococcus (GBS).

Subjective: Symptoms

Menstrual-like cramps, low back pain, abdominal or pelvic pressure, painless uterine contractions, and increase or change in vaginal discharge (mucus, watery, light bloody discharge).

Objective: Signs

Using Basic Tools: Palpable uterine contractions; palpable cervical dilation and effacement; visualization of amniotic fluid "pooling" in the vagina (PROM)
Using Advanced Tools: Labs: Urinalysis and a saline wet preparation to evaluate for bacterial vaginosis. Fern test (amniotic fluid dries on a slide to resemble the leaves of a fern plant) to assess for PROM.

Assessment: Assess for PTL risk factors, and treat those found.

Differential Diagnosis

Low back pain/spasm: Palpate for back spasm; evaluate for associated neurological symptoms (leg tingling, radiation, etc)
Infection: Evaluate for urinary tract infection (urinalysis, fever), GI infection (diarrhea, fever) and vaginosis (saline wet prep).
Ureter/kidney stone: Evaluate flank pain, fever; perform urinalysis
True labor: Verify dates of last menstrual period
PROM: History of vaginal gush or leak, positive Fern test
Constipation: History of infrequent bowel movements; retained fecal material
Diarrhea: Infection, food poisoning, and others

Plan:

Treatment

1. Arrest labor: (Tocolytic Therapy)
   Primary: Administer **nifedipine** 30mg po as a loading dose, followed by an additional 20mg po in 90 minutes. An alternative regimen is to administer 10mg po q20 minutes for up to 4 doses. After the initial treatment, the maintenance dose is 20mg po q4-8h. Watch for symptoms such as nausea, flushing, headache, dizziness, palpitations, and tachycardia. Do not use in women with cardiac disease (left ventricular dysfunction or congestive heart disease). Do not use this medication in conjunction with magnesium sulfate (may cause respiratory paralysis).
   Alternative (32-34 weeks): For 2nd line therapy of pregnancies at 32–34 weeks of gestation, administer **terbutaline** as a 0.25mg subcutaneous injection, q20-30 minutes for up to 4 doses or until tocolysis is achieved. Withhold if the maternal heart rate exceeds 120 bpm. Once labor is inhibited, 0.25mg can be administered q3-4h until the uterus is quiescent (no contractions) for 24 hours. Watch for maternal tachycardia, palpitations, and a lowered BP. Target maternal pulse rate >100 and <120 bpm. Do not use this drug in women with maternal cardiac disease, poorly controlled hyperthyroidism or diabetes mellitus.

Alternative (<32 weeks): For 2nd line treatment of PTL in pregnancies <32 weeks of gestation, administer **indomethacin** 50-100mg po loading dose, followed by 25mg po q4-6h. Watch for GI side effects (nausea, esophageal reflux, gastritis, and emesis). Do not give to women with bleeding disorders, liver disease, GI ulcerative disease, renal dysfunction, and asthma (in women with hypersensitivity to aspirin). Do not administer this medication greater than 48 hours as prolonged use increases the risk to the fetus. **Note:** Contraindications to Tocolytic Therapy: Maternal: Significant hypertension (*see Part 3: General Symptoms: Obstetric Problems:* Preeclampsia Eclampsia), antepartum hemorrhage, cardiac disease. Fetal: Gestational age >37 weeks, fetal death, chorioamnionitis (intrauterine infection)

2. Prevent infection (PROM; PTL >12 hours; history of UTI, vaginal infections in last 2 weeks):
    Primary: Penicillin G 5 million units IV initially, then 2.5 million units q4h until delivered
    Alternates: Ampicillin 2g IV q4-6h or **ceftriaxone** 1g IV q12h.
    For those patients who are penicillin allergic, **clindamycin** 600mg po q6h or 900mg q8h or **erythromycin** 1-2g po q6h or **vancomycin** 500mg po q6h or 1000mg po q12h.

3. Help fetus mature: After postponing delivery, many fetuses less than 34 weeks gestation will benefit from administering steroids to the mother. The effect of the steroids on the fetus is to accelerate fetal lung maturity, lessening the risk of respiratory distress syndrome at birth. Give **dexamethasone** 6mg IM q12h x 4 doses.

4. Evacuate the mother: Keep her rolled over on her left or right side, with a pillow between her knees, with an IV securely in place. If IV access is lost during a bumpy truck or helicopter ride, it will be nearly impossible to restart it without stopping or landing. Consider tocolytic therapy in all mothers being transported unless contraindications exist or greater than 37 weeks gestation.

Patient Education
Activity: Decreased activity and bedrest may be required to avoid further PTL.
Prevention and Hygiene: Avoid emotional stress.
No Improvement/Deterioration: Report recurrent symptoms immediately. Early intervention is more effective in stopping PTL.
Follow-up Actions
Return Evaluation: Follow weekly to assess for recurrent symptoms and risk factors for PTL.
Evacuation/Consultation Criteria: Evacuate after initial PTL symptoms if possible. Avoid emergent evacuation if possible. Consult expert if available.

Obstetric Problems: Relief of Shoulder Dystocia
LTC Marvin Williams, MC, USA & CPT Jesse P. Reynolds, SP, USA

What: Shoulder dystocia is a labor complication caused by difficulty delivering the fetal shoulders. Although this is more common among women with gestational diabetes and those with very large fetuses, it can occur with babies of any size. Unfortunately, it cannot be predicted or prevented. Improperly relieving the dystocia can result in unilateral or bilateral clavicular fractures. As it will be very rare for you to be present for a normal childbirth, you will probably only be involved with this problem very late in its course. Fetal demise may have occurred. The obstruction must be relieved or eventually the mother will die of uterine rupture or sepsis.

When: After delivery of the head, the fetus seems to try to withdraw back into the birth canal (the "turtle sign"). Further expulsion of the infant is prevented by impaction of the fetal shoulders within the maternal pelvis. Digital exam reveals that the anterior shoulder is stuck behind the pubic symphysis. In more severe cases, the posterior shoulder may be stuck at the level of the sacrum.

What To Do: If you are not present for the delivery, check for fetal life. If you are present for the delivery, take the following steps:
1. Check for the umbilical cord wrapped around the baby's neck and reduce it.
2. Suction the infant's mouth and nose to clear the airway of amniotic fluid and other debris.
3. Do not apply excessive downward traction on the head to get the baby out. This action can injure the nerves in the neck and shoulder (brachial plexus palsy) and must be avoided. While most of these nerve injuries heal spontaneously and completely, some do not. Do not apply pressure to the mother's uterus. This only pushes the shoulder more tightly against the pubic bone.
4. Although routine episiotomy is discouraged, controversy exists as to whether episiotomy is necessary during a shoulder dystocia since shoulder dystocia is not typically caused by soft tissue obstruction. It may assist with particular maneuvers, such as delivering the posterior arm during a shoulder dystocia. *See Part 3: General Symptoms: Obstetric Problems: Episiotomy and Repair*
5. Have mother stop pushing and apply gentle downward traction on the infant's chest and back in an effort to free the shoulder. If this unsuccessful, try some alternative maneuvers to free the shoulder.
6. Place the mother in the McRoberts' position, and apply gentle downward traction on the baby again. This position involves flexing the mother's thighs tightly against her abdomen. This can be accomplished by the woman herself or by assistants. By performing this maneuver, the axis of the birth canal is straightened, allowing a little more room for the shoulders to slip through.
7. If the McRoberts' maneuver fails, have an assistant apply downward, suprapubic (above the bony pubic arch) pressure to drive the anterior fetal shoulder downward, to clear the pubic bone. This should be strong pressure and may lead to a clavicular fracture which is usually of no consequence. Again, apply coordinated, gentle downward traction on the baby.
8. If pressure straight down is ineffective, have the assistant apply it in a more lateral direction. This tends to nudge the shoulder into a more oblique orientation, which usually provides more room for the shoulder to deliver. Again, apply coordinated, gentle downward traction on the baby.
9. Often, the baby's posterior arm has entered the hollow of the sacrum. Reach in posteriorly, identify the posterior shoulder, follow the humerus down to the elbow and identify the forearm. Grasping the fetal wrist, draw the arm gently across the chest and then sweep the arm up and out of the birth canal, freeing additional space and allowing the anterior shoulder to clear the pubic bone. Once again, apply coordinated, gentle downward traction on the baby.

10. An electric light bulb cannot be removed by simply pulling it out - it must be unscrewed. This concept can be applied to shoulder dystocia problems. Rotate the posterior shoulder, allowing it to come up outside of the subpubic arch. At the same time, bring the stuck anterior shoulder into the hollow of the sacrum. Continue rotating the baby a full 360° to rotate (unscrew) both shoulders out of the birth canal. Two variations on the unscrewing maneuver include:
    a. Rotating/shoving the shoulder towards the fetal chest ("shoving scapulas saves shoulders"), which compresses the shoulder-to-shoulder diameter, and
    b. Rotating the anterior shoulder first rather than the posterior shoulder. The anterior shoulder may be easier to reach and simply moving it to an oblique position rather than the straight up and down position may relieve the obstruction.
11. Consider a symphysiotomy. *See Part 3: General Symptoms: Obstetric Problems: Symphysiotomy*
12. If the mother is sedated, to perform any of these procedures fundal pressure can be applied to the uterus in place of her expulsive efforts.

What Not To Do: Do not pull the baby straight out.

Obstetric Problems: Breech Birth
LTC Marvin Williams, MC, USA

What: Breech presentation is an abnormality in which the buttocks or legs of the fetus, rather than the head, appear first in the birth canal. There are several breech variations, including buttocks first, one leg first or both legs first. "Frank breech" means the buttocks are presenting and the legs are up along the fetal chest—the safest position for breech delivery. In any breech birth, there are increased risks of umbilical cord prolapse and delivery of the feet through an incompletely dilated cervix, leading to arm or head entrapment. These risks are greatest when a foot is presenting ("footling breech").

When: Because of the risks of breech delivery, many breech babies are born by Cesarean delivery in developed countries. In operational settings, Cesarean section may not be available or may be more dangerous than performing a vaginal breech delivery. It is up to the care team to decide which option will be the safest mode of delivery for both mother and infant.

Figure 3-20. Key Anatomical Landmarks for Breech Delivery

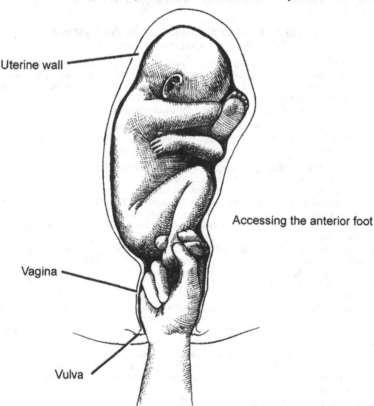

Uterine wall

Accessing the anterior foot

Vagina

Vulva

Figure 3-21. Key Anatomical Landmarks for Breech Delivery: Pubic Symphysis

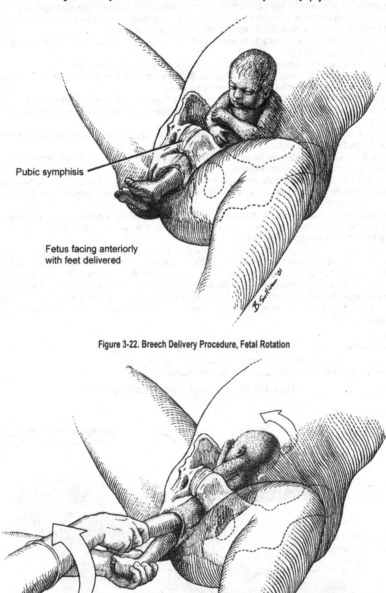

Pubic symphisis

Fetus facing anteriorly
with feet delivered

Figure 3-22. Breech Delivery Procedure, Fetal Rotation

Gentle rotation of
fetus to face posteriorly

What To Do: See Figures 3-20 – 3-24

1. The simplest breech delivery is a spontaneous breech. The mother pushes the baby out with normal bearing down efforts and the baby is simply supported until it is completely free of the birth canal. These babies essentially deliver themselves. This works best with smaller babies, mothers who have delivered in the past or frank breech presentation.
2. If a breech baby gets stuck halfway out or if you need to speed the delivery, perform an "assisted breech" delivery. It is very helpful to have a second person assist you.
3. A generous episiotomy will give you more room to work, but may be unnecessary if the vulva is very stretchy and pliant.
4. Grasp the baby so that your thumbs are over the baby's hips. Rotate the torso so the baby is face down in the birth canal. A towel can be wrapped around the lower body to provide a more stable grip.
5. Have your assistant apply suprapubic pressure to keep the fetal head flexed, expedite delivery and reduce the risk of spinal injury.
6. Exert gentle outward traction on the baby while rotating the baby clockwise and then counterclockwise a few degrees to free up the arms.
7. If the baby's arms are trapped in the birth canal, you may need to reach up along the side of the baby and sweep them one at a time, across the chest and out of the vagina.
8. It is important to keep your hands low on the baby's hips. Grasping the baby above the hips could easily cause soft tissue injury to the baby's abdominal organs including the kidneys.
9. During the delivery, always keep the baby at or below the horizontal plane or axis of the birth canal. If you bring the baby's body above the horizontal axis, you risk injuring the baby's spine. Only when the baby's nose and mouth are visible at the introitus is it wise to bring the body up.
10. At this stage, the baby is still unable to breathe and the umbilical cord is likely occluded. Without rushing, move steadily toward a prompt delivery. Place a finger in the baby's mouth to control the delivery of the head. Try not to let the head "pop" out of the birth canal. A slower, controlled delivery is less traumatic.
11. It will be very rare for you to be present for the initial attempt at delivery. Therefore, you must be prepared to see the most catastrophic complication of a failed breech delivery, an entrapped head with fetal demise. The head must be delivered or the mother will eventually die of uterine rupture or sepsis. If evacuation is available, this problem meets the criteria to be life-saving. If evacuation is not available in the near future, the head must be delivered. Palpate the vagina to see if a fetal arm is trapped behind the head (nuchal arm). If so, pushing the arm back over the fetal head may allow room for delivery. If the fetus died some time ago, firm traction on the body may cause the head to distort and deliver. If all else fails, consider a symphysiotomy as a life-saving measure for the mother.

What Not To Do:

1. Do not assist too early. Only intervene if a breech baby gets stuck part way out of the pelvis.
2. Do not place your hands too high on the abdomen. Keep hands low on the baby's hips.
3. Do not raise baby above the horizontal plane until the nose and mouth are delivered.

Figure 3-23. Breech Delivery Procedure, Fetal Extraction

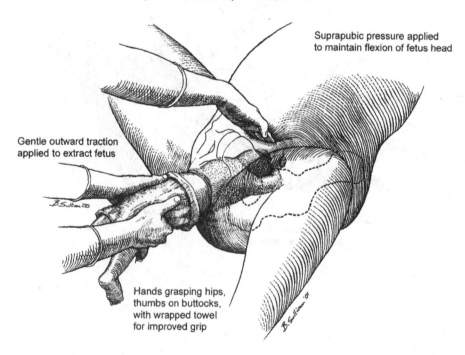

Suprapubic pressure applied to maintain flexion of fetus head

Gentle outward traction applied to extract fetus

Hands grasping hips, thumbs on buttocks, with wrapped towel for improved grip

Figure 3-24. Breech Delivery Procedure, Fetal Extraction

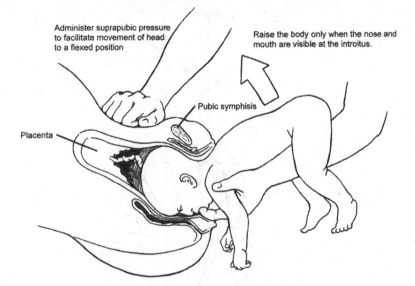

Administer suprapubic pressure to facilitate movement of head to a flexed position

Raise the body only when the nose and mouth are visible at the introitus.

Pubic symphisis

Placenta

Obstetric Problems: Symphysiotomy
LTC Marvin Williams, MC, USA

What: Symphysiotomy is a procedure that is performed to increase the size of the pelvic outlet to facilitate a vaginal delivery of a baby. Although effective in opening the maternal pelvis and relieving obstruction, the procedure is associated with high maternal morbidity.

When: Performed during the second stage (full dilation of the cervix) of labor to enlarge the pelvis when dystocia (difficult delivery) is encountered (ie, shoulder dystocia, head entrapment of a breech delivery, fetal heart rate <90 bpm for more than 5 minutes) or any medical condition that worsens during labor in which a delayed delivery would harm the mother (eg, eclampsia).

What You Need: IV access, Foley catheter, scalpel, 10cc of 1-2% **lidocaine with epinephrine**, 2.0-3.0 absorbable suture, needle driver, tissue forceps, scissors

What To Do:
  Surgical Procedure:
1. Place the patient in an exaggerated lithotomy position with proper support of the legs.
2. Insert a Foley catheter.
3. Inject approximately 10cc of **lidocaine** with epinephrine over the area of the pubic symphysis.
4. Place your index and middle finger into the vagina along the urethra and displace it laterally (palpate the Foley). *See Figure 3-25*
   Make a 2-3cm vertical incision over the cephalad portion of the symphysis with a scalpel blade. *See Figure 3-26*
5. After the delivery is performed, close the skin with simple interrupted stitches utilizing the 2.0 suture.

What to Expect:
1. The patient will experience difficulty walking after the procedure for approximately 2 weeks, and may require assistance when ambulating for the first few days after the procedure.
2. The pelvis will be permanently enlarged after the procedure. The procedure IS NOT a contraindication for future vaginal deliveries.
3. The patient will experience a significant amount of pain. *See Part 8: Procedures: Chapter 30: Pain Assessment and Control*
   Administer:
   a. **Meperidine** 25-50mg IM q3-4h for pain plus
   b. **Ibuprofen** 800mg po q8h with food or
   c. **Hydromorphine** (or equivalent) 2-3mg po q4-6h for pain.

What Not To Do:
1. Do not cut the baby when making your incision.
2. Do not attempt to reapproximate the pubic symphysis when repairing the incision. Close only the skin.

Figure 3-25. Symphysiotomy Procedure, Palpation of the Foley Catheter

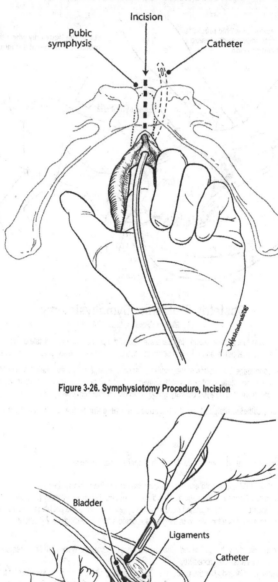

Figure 3-26. Symphysiotomy Procedure, Incision

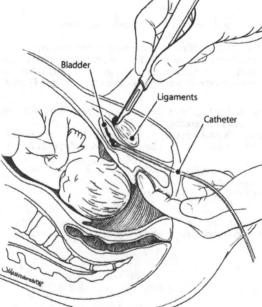

Obstetric Problems: Cesarean Delivery
LTC Marvin Williams, MC, USA

What: The delivery of a fetus by abdominal surgery (laparotomy) requiring an incision through the uterine wall (hysterotomy).

When: Perform this procedure only when it is absolutely necessary, and is the only life saving measure for mother! PERFORM THE SYMPHYSIOTOMY FIRST. The decision to perform a Cesarean delivery (CD) must be based on the health and stability of the mother and fetus. Recognize that performing the procedure in the field as an untrained provider is extremely dangerous and will likely result in significant morbidity or mortality for both mother and infant. In this setting, the SOF medic should always consider the health and welfare of the mother prior to that of the fetus. If a CD is anticipated, prepare equipment and read this material, since the procedure must often be performed emergently when vital signs become unstable.

The following are relative indications for CD under field conditions:

1. **Fetal Complications:**
   a. Non-vertex (not head first) such as a transverse lie or breech presentation. Attempt vaginal delivery first. *See Part 3: General Symptoms: Obstetric Problems: Breech Birth*
   b. Multiple gestation: triplets or greater, twins in which the first twin is not head first (vertex). Attempt vaginal delivery of at least one fetus. *See Part 3: General Symptoms: Obstetric Problems: Breech Birth*
   c. Large fetus: Attempt vaginal delivery first.
   d. Fetal distress: Fetal heart rate (<90 bpm) for more than 5 minutes

2. **Placental Complications:**
   a. Placenta previa (placenta lies over cervical os)
   b. Placental abruption (premature placental separation).
   c. Although these conditions cannot be diagnosed in the field, any large vaginal hemorrhage during labor, or hemorrhage accompanied by fetal distress should be reason to suspect them and consider CD.

3. **Uterine Complications:**
   a. Previous CD with midline incision (classical).
   b. Other surgery (eg, for fibroids) where the uterine cavity was entered. There is an increased risk for uterine rupture in this situation. Cesarean deliveries with low transverse incisions are much less risky. Attempt vaginal delivery first.

4. **Vaginal Complications:**
   a. Obstructive conditions (eg, genital warts, cervical cancer). If noted, these conditions may hinder dilation of the cervix and descent of the fetus through the birth canal. Attempt vaginal delivery first.
   b. Vaginal infections (eg, Group B *Streptococcus*, genital herpes). Delivering the infant through the birth canal will greatly increase the baby's risk of contracting these infections, which will likely be fatal.

5. **Maternal Complications:** Any medical condition that worsens during labor in which a delayed delivery would harm the mother (eg, eclampsia).

6. **Abnormal Labor (failure to progress):** Labor that does not progress (continued cervical changes and fetal descent) over several hours endangers the fetus by increasing the risk of cord compression and neurological damage.

What You Need: Surgical assistants (two if possible); prep solution; sterile gloves; 0 (Vicryl and chromic), 2-0 non-absorbable, and 3-0 or 4-0 Vicryl absorbable suture; scalpel to make the incision; IV access; anesthesia: (*see Part 5: Specialty Areas: Chapter 19: Total Intravenous Anesthesia*), or use 1-2% **lidocaine** with **epinephrine** ONLY if TIVA is not available. Do not exceed 300cc or 5mg/kg (usually requires 30-50cc; be aware of lidocaine toxicity. Two grams of **cefazolin** or 1g of **ceftriaxone** or any equivalent IV antibiotic 30-45 minutes prior to surgery if possible; administer **oxytocin** 10 units IM after delivery of the placenta; sterile (at least clean) bandages; sterile surgical instruments: needle driver, forceps, retractors, clamps, scissors and a Foley catheter if available.

What To Do: Surgical Procedure
1. Place the patient in supine position with a roll under her left side (leftward tilt for uterine displacement).
2. Prep her with some sort of cleaning solution (povidone-iodine or equivalent), and catheterize her with a Foley catheter, if available.
3. Provide anesthesia. If TIVA sedation is not available, use **lidocaine** to infiltrate just below the skin and into the subcutaneous tissue following a vertical pattern from 2-3cm above the pubic bone to 1-2cm below the umbilicus.
4. Take the scalpel blade and make a vertical incision beginning 1-2cm below the umbilicus to approximately 2-3cm above the pubic bone. The incision should initially cut through the skin and some of the subcutaneous tissue (fat). Carefully cut through the remaining fat with shallow strokes. Be careful not to cut directly through the uterus!
5. Once you reach the rectus fascia (shiny white tissue), make a shallow midline vertical incision through it, being careful not to injure the rectus muscles. Have your assistant (if you have one) elevate the fascia with a retractor or hands while you cut. Separate the abdominal muscles in the midline.
6. The next layer you encounter is the peritoneum, a clear, thin layer of tissue. If you look closely, you may be able to see bowel (intestines) through it. Pick up the peritoneum with forceps or a clamp; with scissors, make a small incision into the peritoneum being careful not to injure the bowel. Extend the incision vertically (both superiorly and inferiorly) exposing the abdominal contents. Make sure you can visualize everything before cutting to avoid potential injury to bowel or bladder.
7. Visualize the uterus and notice the shiny peritoneal surface located on the lower aspect of it (uterovesical peritoneum). Grasp and elevate this area in the midline with forceps or clamp. Make a small incision laterally. With your fingers, bluntly dissect the peritoneum off of the uterus, creating a bladder flap, which decreases the chance of injury to the bladder. After the bladder flap has been developed, use a retractor to retract the bladder anteriorly and inferiorly to facilitate exposure of the intended incision site.
8. Make an incision at the inferior margin of the lower segment of the uterus and insert your first 2 fingers toward the fundus (top

of the uterus). QUICKLY extend the incision toward the fundus by cutting between the spread fingers (vertical incision) with scissors (or a scalpel). Have an assistant frequently suction or wipe the area with each cut to help you visualize the incision. Be careful not to cut the infant! Perform the remainder of steps prior to giving oxytocin quickly to avoid massive blood loss.

9. Remove all retractors and insert a hand into the uterine cavity to elevate and flex the fetal head through the incision. Should the head be deeply wedged into the pelvis, an assistant can apply upward pressure through the vagina to dislodge the head.
10. Once the head is present through the incision, suction the infant's nose and mouth.
11. When suctioning is complete, deliver the baby by applying moderate fundal pressure on the uterus from the abdomen.
12. Doubly clamp or tie the cord with suture or use hemostats then cut between the clamped areas and hand the infant off to your assistant. See Part 5: Specialty Areas: Chapter 15: Newborn Resuscitation
13. Following delivery of the newborn, 10 units of **oxytocin** IM or 20 units can be mixed with a 1L bag of lactated Ringer's and run via IV. (Do not exceed more than 500-600cc/hr with the first bag. Decrease the rate to 100-125 cc/hr for the second bag.)
14. Remove the placenta manually by applying gentle traction on the cord until the placenta is expelled from the uterus. Exteriorize (lift it out of the abdominal incision) the uterus and place it on the abdomen. Cover the top of the uterus (fundus) with a sterile, moist sponge (bandage). Use a sterile, dry sponge to wipe the uterine cavity clean of all clots and placental debris. Do not expose the uterus or other intraperitoneal structures to any non-sterile objects, if at all possible.
15. Inspect the uterine incision and control any bleeding points temporarily with clamps (ring/sponge forceps or Allis clamps) or have your assistant hold direct pressure until you are ready for the repair of the uterus. Next, take a number 0 suture and begin just inferior to the lower margin of the incision, tie your suture and with subsequent stitches, run them toward the fundus in a continuous locking manner. Place stitches 1cm from the edge of the incision, 1cm apart and attempt to keep them out of the uterus. Use a second inverting layer only if hemostasis (control of bleeding) is not obtained with the first layer. The bladder peritoneum need not be closed.
16. Inspect for any bleeding from the incision, and control it with interrupted figure-of-eight stitches. The uterus can then be returned to the abdomen. Irrigate the pelvis and lower abdomen with at least 1L of sterile fluid. Make sure that all sponges (bandages) and needle counts are correct or have been accounted for prior to closing the abdomen.
17. There is no need to reapproximate the peritoneum. Using 0 Vicryl (not chromic due to its inability to maintain tensile strength) begin closing the fascia. The initial suture should be placed inferior to the lower margin of the vertical incision and in a running fashion, close the fascia. Irrigate and inspect the subcutaneous tissue for bleeding. If there is significant fat tissue, reapproximate the subcutaneous tissue with several interrupted stitches with 3-0 or 4-0 vicryl. Close the skin using staples (if applicable) or 2-0 non absorbable sutures in an interrupted fashion. Apply a sterile dressing and leave it in place for approximately 24 hrs.
18. If the bladder is inadvertently lacerated, use a 2-layer technique to close it (running layers like the fascia) as well as leaving the Foley in for 7-10 days. Put the patient on a prophylactic antibiotic: **nitrofurantoin** 100mg po bid x 7 days or **azithromycin** 500mg po daily x 7 days while the Foley catheter is in place.
19. Counsel the patient that she will not be a future candidate for a trial of labor. SHE WILL ALWAYS HAVE TO HAVE A CESAREAN DELIVERY FOR EACH SUBSEQUENT PREGNANCY, or risk uterine rupture and death for both mother and fetus.

Post-Operative Orders:
1. Diet: NPO except sips of water. May begin clear liquids 24 hrs after surgery if bowel sounds present, then advance diet as tolerated.
2. List allergies to medications.
3. Initial vital signs (BP, P, RR) q15 minutes for the 1st hour, then VS q 2h X 2, then q4h X 72 hours.
4. Bedrest for 8 hrs, then out of bed with assistance.
5. Turn, cough and deep breathe q2h while awake.
6. Ice pack to the incision q4-6 hrs for 30-45 minutes
7. Strict monitoring and recording of intake and output (fluids).
8. Leave the Foley catheter in place for 24 hours to monitor urine output. A patient should make at least 30cc/hr.
9. **Meperidine** 25-50mg IM q3-4h for pain
10. **Promethazine** 25mg IM q8h for nausea and vomiting
11. Once patient tolerating clear liquid diet well, remove IV, change IM pain management to oral, and remove Foley catheter.
12. **Ibuprofen** 800mg po q8h with food
13. **Hydromorphine** (or equivalent) 2-3mg po q4-6h for pain.
14. CBC 6-8 hrs post op and again at 24 hrs post-op to check for bleeding (low HCT), infection (increased WBC, bands).
15. Remove stitches at 7 days

What Not To Do:
1. Do not get too excited. It will impede decision-making.
2. Do not cut into the intestines, bladder or baby.
3. Do not forget to retract the bladder once you have developed your flap so as not to injure it.
4. Do not expose the uterus or other intraperitoneal structures to any non-sterile objects if at all possible.
5. Do not operate too slowly. Once the uterus is entered, the baby must be delivered and the uterus closed quickly to achieve control of bleeding before significant hemorrhage endangers the mother's survival.

Obstetric Problems: Episiotomy and Repair
LTC Marvin Williams, MC, USA & CPT Jesse Reynolds, SP, USA

What: Incision of the perineum to enlarge the vaginal opening, and subsequent repair of the incision. Episiotomies can be performed in the midline or starting in the midline and extending laterally. The mediolateral episiotomy is more painful, but is less likely to extend into the rectum and when required, the mediolateral episiotomy is the preferred procedure in the emergent, field setting.

When: Routine episiotomy is discouraged. Median (midline) episiotomy is associated with a higher risk of lacerations to the anal sphincter or rectal mucosa than mediolateral episiotomy or spontaneous obstetrical lacerations. Controversy exists as to whether episiotomy is necessary during a shoulder dystocia since shoulder dystocia is not typically caused by soft tissue obstruction. It may assist with particular maneuvers, such as delivering the posterior arm during a shoulder dystocia. If determined to be required at the time of delivery, perform an episiotomy when 3-4cm of fetal scalp is visible at the vaginal opening. The most common practice is to repair the episiotomy after the delivery of the placenta.

What You Need: 1-2% lidocaine with **epinephrine** (approx. 20-30cc), sterile gloves, gauze bandages, prep solution, 2-0, 3-0, and 4-0 absorbable suture (Vicryl or chromic) for the repair, scissors or a scalpel to make the episiotomy incision, suture forceps and needle holders.

Figure 3-27. Episiotomy, Midline

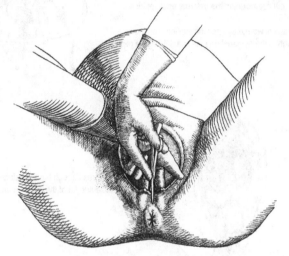

What to Do:

Episiotomy: Indicated to prevent severe perineal lacerations, increase the diameter of the soft tissue outlet to relieve dystocia, and facilitate delivery of fetuses with nonreassuring status. It is better to cut an episiotomy than to have the baby tear the perineal tissue into the rectum.

1. If no anesthesia has been given, administer 5-10cc of **lidocaine** along the midline of the perineum and posterior vagina. Remember not to administer more than 50cc of **lidocaine** total, and to aspirate prior to injecting. If the perineum is very thin and well stretched, anesthesia may not be necessary.
2. Place the first two fingers into the posterior vagina between the fetal head and the vaginal wall.
3. Cut between the fingers, through the vaginal wall extending to the right at a 45° angle (approximately 4:30 on a clock face). **Note:** Figure 3-27 demonstrates a midline, not a medial lateral episiotomy
4. If pressure from the fetal head does not control bleeding, press a 4x4 bandage against the incised tissue to stop hemorrhage.
5. An alternate site for the episiotomy is the in the midline, but this risks extension into the rectum.

Repair of the mediolateral episiotomy

1. Place the first stitch (2-0 or 3-0 absorbable) proximal to the vaginal apex of the incision.
2. Using a running locking stitch, close the vaginal portion of the episiotomy down to the vaginal introitus taking care to close the full depth of the incision. Tie this suture.
3. Using interrupted stitches, close the deep perineal and gluteal portions of the episiotomy giving an anatomical closure. Place the first suture at the top bringing the vaginal opening together to prevent lopsided closure.
4. Close the perineal skin with a subcutaneous stitch technique starting at the apex most distant from the introitus.

Classifications of perineal episiotomies and lacerations

First degree: Extends only through the vaginal and perineal skin
Second degree: Extends deeply into the soft tissues of the perineum down to, but not including, the external anal sphincter
Third degree: Extends through the perineum and anal sphincter
Fourth degree: Extends through the perineum, anal sphincter, and rectal mucosa to expose the lumen of the rectum

First Degree Episiotomy or Laceration Repair

1. Test the area to be sutured for residual sensation. If necessary, administer **lidocaine** into the tissue as with typical wound repair.
2. If the edges of lacerated tissue are less than 1cm apart and not bleeding, repair is not necessary.
3. Place the first stitch (2-0 or 3-0) 1cm deep (proximal) to the end of the vaginal portion of the episiotomy (or laceration) and tie it.
4. Continue with locking, continuous sutures 1cm from each wound edge, 1cm apart and 0.5cm deep through to the introitus or hymenal ring (or distal end of the laceration). Ensure the edges of the hymenal ring lay approximated. Do not cut the suture in episiotomy repair.

5. With another suture, sew a running subcuticular suture from the anal end of the skin wound back up toward the vagina to close the perineum.
6. Take the end of the suture back under the hymenal ring and tie it in the vagina.

Figure 3-28. Repair of 2nd Degree Episiotomy

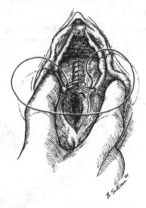

Laceration extends deeply into soft tissuesof the perineum down to, but not including,the external anal sphincter.

Repair vaginal wound by applying locking, continous suture through to the hymenal ring, as in a 1st degree repair.

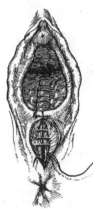

3-4 interrupted sutures through the subcutaneous fascia, muscle and fat of the peritoneum

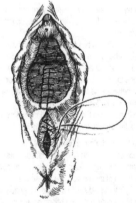

Approximate the edges of the perineal fascia with continuous, non-locking suture sewing towards the anus

Second Degree Episiotomy Repair: (see Figure 3-28)
1. Repair vaginal wound as in First Degree Repair down to the hymenal ring. Do not cut the suture.
2. With another suture, sew 3-4 deep, interrupted stitches in the subcutaneous fascia, muscle and fat of the perineum.
3. Take the suture from the vagina under the hymenal ring and approximate the edges of the perineal fascia with continuous non-locking suture sewing toward the anus.
4. Sew a running subcuticular suture back up toward the vagina to close the perineum.
5. Take the end of the suture back under the hymenal ring and tie it in the vagina.
6. Do not suture any tear near the ureter without inserting a Foley catheter to avoid inadvertent urethral closure.

Third and Fourth Degree Repair: (see Figure 3-29)
1. Reapproximate the rectal mucosa with interrupted, fine 4-0 sutures (usually two layers), taking care not to puncture the mucosa and to leave the ends of the suture in the tissue, not the rectal lumen.
2. Repair the torn ends of the doughnut-shaped anal sphincter with four well-spaced interrupted sutures that traverse through the capsule of the muscle.
3. Then repair the wound as in a second-degree laceration or an episiotomy.

Figure 3-29. Repair of 3rd and 4th Degree Episiotomy

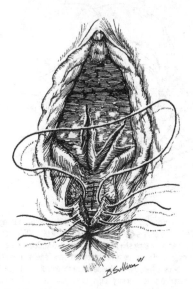

Reapproximate rectal mucosa with
interrupted, fine 4-0 sutures (usually two layers),
taking care not puncture the mucosa
and to leave the ends of the suture
in the tissue, not the rectal lumen.

Repair the torn ends of the donut-shaped
anal sphincter with four well-spaced
interrupted sutures that traverse
through the capsule of the muscle.

Management after Episiotomy
1. Apply ice to the affected area tid to control swelling.
2. Relieve pain with **Tylenol#3 (acetaminophen + codeine)** 1-2 tabs po q3-4h.
3. Pain may be an indication of a large hematoma or perineal cellulitis. Examine these areas carefully if pain is severe or persistent.
4. Give stool softeners for approximately 7-14 days and direct increased intake of fiber and water.
5. Do not give enemas.

What Not To Do:
1. Do not fail to restore anatomical features.
2. Do not use too many sutures.
3. Do not fail to achieve hemostasis.

Obstetric Problems: Postpartum Hemorrhage
LTC Marvin Williams, MC, USA & CPT Jesse Reynolds, SP, USA

When: PPH is defined clinically and described as any excessive bleeding that causes the patient to become symptomatic. These signs and symptoms are related to the degree of blood loss during the delivery and can be present with as little as 15% (1000mL) loss of blood volume. Some of the most common presenting symptoms are palpitations, lightheadedness, and vertigo which may lead to oliguria, vascular collapse, and death. In order to control bleeding after a vaginal delivery, two events occur. The uterine muscle contracts causing a marked decrease in blood flow to the area locally and clotting factors are released within the circulation to prevent excess hemorrhage. These are some of the causes of PPH:
1. Uterine atony occurs when the uterus fails to contract after delivery of the fetus and is the most common cause of PPH. Risk factors for uterine atony are: uterine overdistention (large baby, multiples, excessive amniotic fluid); rapid or prolonged labor; over 5 pregnancies; infection; leiomyomas (uterine fibroids).
2. Trauma from lacerations (perineal, vaginal, cervical, and uterine), episiotomies, or uterine rupture
3. Retained membranes or placenta
4. Uterine inversion, which can occur as a result of excessive traction on the umbilical cord

What You Need: Ringer's lactate (RL), 2 16 gauge or larger IV catheters, **misoprostol**, scalpel, #0 absorbable suture, gauze, Kerlix (to pack the vagina)

What To Do: The key to success is early recognition of a symptomatic patient and the institution of treatment measures. Begin by stabilizing the patient's vital signs and stopping the bleeding.
1. Obtain IV access with 2 large-bore (16 gauge or greater) if possible. Begin to correct the patient's volume deficit initially with a crystalloid (RL) solution given at a 3:1 ratio for each milliliter of estimated blood loss (EBL). For example, if EBL is 1200mL, then the patient would receive 3600mL of RL.
2. Evaluate uterine tone by palpating the uterus for firmness. If it seems soft or boggy, begin fundal massage or bimanual manipulation (*see Figure 3-30*) as this stimulates the uterus to contract.

Figure 3-30. Fundal Massage   **Figure 3-31. Removal of Retained Placenta**

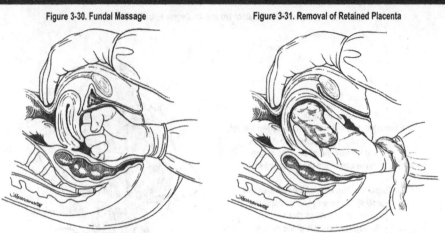

3. If the uterus does not seem firm after the initial uterine massage, administer **misoprostol**, which is a synthetic prostaglandin (PGE1). This drug is given as an initial dose of 800-1000 micrograms rectally or orally. The dose may be repeated in one hour and maintenance therapy should then be instituted at 200 micrograms q4h for 24 hours. There are no known contraindications to the medication and it can be administered to hypertensive as well as asthmatic patients. Side effects include fever and tachycardia.

4. If the uterus is firm, then look elsewhere for bleeding source. Quickly evaluate the entire birth canal (perineum, vagina, cervix, and lower uterine cavity) for lacerations or hematomas. Lacerations from the vagina or cervix that are bleeding heavily should be repaired with an absorbable #0 suture in a running fashion beginning above the level of the laceration. It is very important to obtain adequate exposure, retraction, and lighting in order to repair this type of injury. Upon completion of the repair, repeat another examination to make certain that all areas of hemorrhage are controlled.

   a. Avoid draining vaginal or vulvar hematomas unless they continue to expand, become infected, or unresponsive to pain medication. A good rule of thumb to practice for drainage of vulvar hematomas is make a wide a linear incision within the skin and evacuate the clot. Close the "dead space" in layers using #0 absorbable suture and apply a sterile pressure dressing. Evacuation of vaginal hematomas is performed in a similar manner with the exception of closing the incision. Vaginal hematomas require packing the incision to tamponade the edges.

   b. The packs should be left in place for 24 hours. Give a broad spectrum penicillin such as **ampicillin-sulbactam** 3g IV (reconstitute the antibiotic in 5mL of normal saline or sterile water and inject it into a one liter bag of LR) q6h until the patient is afebrile for 24 hours If allergic to penicillin or sulfa, may substitute **ciprofloxacin** 200-400mg IV q8h.

5. If no lacerations are observed and bleeding above the cervix continues, perform a careful bimanual examination and uterine exploration. By wrapping the hand with a moist gauze, the removal of any retained placenta or membranes can be facilitated (*see Figure 3-31*). In cases of uterine rupture, the patient may experience intermittent episodes of uterine atony with uncontrolled bleeding. In this setting, an exploratory laparotomy is required for repair. Vaginal and uterine packing with evacuation to a surgical facility is in order.

6. A uterine inversion occurs when the top of uterus (fundus) collapses into the uterine cavity. With this, you will feel a mass at the cervix or within the vagina. Fortunately, a uterine inversion is a rare event and should be expected with the onset of brisk vaginal bleeding and the inability to palpate the uterine fundus abdominally. Once diagnosed, administer **terbutaline** 0.25mg slow IV push (over one minute). Once relaxed, use uterine pressure to return the prolapsed portion of the uterus to its proper position (*see Figure 3-32*).

Figure 3-32. Returning Prolapsed Portion of the Uterus to Proper Position

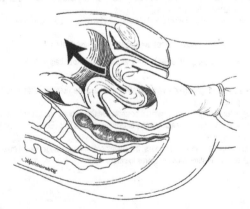

What Not To Do:
1. Do not delay in providing resuscitative measures.
2. Do not forget to evaluate the entire birth canal.
3. If packing is utilized, remember the total number of Kerlix, sponges, etc., and perform a count upon completion to ensure that all packing has been recovered.

Obstetric Problems: Intraamniotic Infection and Endometritis
LTC Marvin Williams, MC, USA & CPT Jesse Reynolds, SP, USA

Introduction: Intraamniotic infection (IAI) is an infection of the amniotic fluid, membranes, placenta or uterus. IAI is usually caused by an ascending infection of normal vaginal flora (*E. coli* and group *B streptococci*). The most common risk factors for IAI are: preterm delivery, nulliparity, young age, prolonged rupture of fetal membranes (>12-18 hours), sexually transmitted infections, and multiple cervical examinations.

Subjective: Symptoms
Malaise, headache, fever, abdominal discomfort.
Focused History: *Are you pregnant?* (IAI is a condition associated with pregnancy.) *Has your water broken?* (IAI is found most often after rupture of the membranes.) *Do you have a UTI?* (Women often have a history and recognize the symptoms.) *Do you have your appendix?* (if no, appendicitis less likely) *Do you or have you recently had the "flu"?* (Pneumonia usually presents following symptoms of "a cold" or "the flu".)

Objective: Signs
Using Basic Tools: Vital signs: The diagnosis of IAI is made clinically based upon maternal temperature (>100.4°F) and 2 of the following findings; maternal tachycardia (>100 bpm), fetal tachycardia (>160 bpm) uterine tenderness, foul odor of the amniotic fluid. Inspection: Most patients will appear to be "normal."
Using Advanced Tools: Labs: CBC (a WBC >15,000 cells/cubic millimeter is an independent criteria). Maternal temperature >100.4°F, a WBC >15,000 and one other of the criteria noted above is consistent with a diagnosis of IAI.

Assessment: Differential Diagnosis
Pneumonia: *See Part 4: Organ Systems: Chapter 3: Respiratory: Pneumonia*
Upper urinary tract infections (pyelonephritis): *See Part 4: Organ Systems: Chapter 8: Urinary Tract Infection, Pyelonephritis*
Viral syndrome: *See Part 5: Specialty Areas: Chapter 12: Viral Infections*
Appendicitis: *See Part 4: Organ Systems: Chapter 7: Appendicitis*

Plan:
Treatment:
Primary: Give **ampicillin-sulbactam** 3g IV (reconstitute the antibiotic in 5mL of normal saline or sterile water and inject it into a liter bag of LR) q6h until the patient has delivered. The treatment can then be discontinued after the first postpartum dose.
Alternative: Clindamycin 900mg IV q8h.
Patient Education
General: Most patients do very well and recover quickly after delivery. The patient should be monitored for continued infection.
Activity: As tolerated and no lifting greater than 10 pounds for 6 weeks if possible as well as vaginal rest for 6 weeks.
Diet: As tolerated
No Improvement/Deterioration: Instruct patient to return if persistent temperature (>100.4°F) in spite of antibiotic therapy; uterine tenderness and foul-smelling lochia.
Follow-up Actions
Return Evaluation: Return in 6 weeks for postpartum visit with routine provider.
Evacuation/Consultation Criteria: Patients not demonstrating definite improvement of symptoms should be referred for specialty care.
Puerperal Endometritis is an infection of the decidua (ie, pregnancy endometrium) caused by bacteria that are part of the normal vaginal flora. Endometritis has risk factors, symptoms and signs similar to IAI. The diagnosis is established when the patient displays a fever of 100.4°F within 36-48 hrs of delivery. Other symptoms include uterine tenderness, tachycardia, foul-smelling lochia (vaginal bleeding), and malaise. The differential for endometritis is essentially the same as IAI with the addition of atelectasis. Treat with **ampicillin-sulbactam** 3g IV q6h until the patient improves clinically and is afebrile for at least 24 hrs. For those patients who fail to respond to initial therapy, consider adding **clindamycin** 900mg IV q8h until symptoms improve or afebrile for 24 hrs. Another alternative is **metronidazole** 500mg IV q12h. Definite improvement should be apparent within 48-72 hrs.

Obstetric Problems: Preeclampsia/Eclampsia
LTC Marvin Williams, MC, USA & CPT Jesse Reynolds, SP, USA

Introduction: Preeclampsia is maternal hypertension accompanied by proteinuria, seen from the 20th week of gestation through delivery in a previously normotensive woman. Preeclampsia is classified as mild or severe. If these symptoms are complicated by seizures or coma, the mother has eclampsia. Other forms of hypertensive disorders include:
Chronic hypertension (or preexisting hypertension) is defined as systolic pressure 140mmHg, diastolic pressure 90mmHg, or both, that predates pregnancy, is present before the 20th week of pregnancy, or persists greater than 12 weeks postpartum.
Preeclampsia superimposed upon chronic hypertension is diagnosed when a woman with preexisting hypertension develops new onset proteinuria after 20 weeks of gestation. Women with both preexisting hypertension and proteinuria are considered preeclamptic if there is an increase of blood pressure to the severe range (SBP 160mmHg or DBP 110mmHg) in the last half of pregnancy, especially if accompanied by symptoms or new onset abnormalities in laboratory values.
Gestational hypertension refers to hypertension (usually mild) without proteinuria (or other signs of preeclampsia) developing in the

latter part of pregnancy which usually resolves by 12 weeks postpartum. If the hypertension persists beyond 12 weeks postpartum, then the diagnosis is chronic hypertension.

Hypertensive disorders are the most common medical complications of pregnancy, effecting approximately 5-14% of pregnancies, and are more common in first-time mothers. The etiology of preeclampsia is unknown and it can be defined as mild or severe. Approximately 1% of patients with preeclampsia develop eclampsia.

Subjective: Symptoms

Visual disturbances (usually irregular luminous patches in the visual fields after physical or mental labor), headaches, nausea, vomiting, epigastric pain and, seizures or coma

Objective: Signs

Mild Preeclampsia:

1. Blood pressure changes (measure on two occasions at least 6 hours apart):
   a. Systolic blood pressure (SBP) of 140mmHg or greater or
   b. Diastolic blood pressure (DBP) of 90mmHg or greater (<110) or
   c. Mean arterial BP (MAP) (calculated as 1/3 the difference between SBP and DBP, plus the DBP) of 105mmHg and/or an increase of 20mmHg over baseline
2. Proteinuria 2+ or > on a urine dipstick
3. Pathologic edema: generalized or involving the hands or face (**Note:** Moderate edema is a feature of approx. 70-80% of normal pregnancies and is no longer used as clinical criteria to diagnose preeclampsia.) Weight gain greater than 4 pounds week in the 3rd trimester may be one of the first signs of preeclampsia.

Severe Preeclampsia:

1. Blood pressure changes (measure on two occasions at least 6 hours apart)
   a. SBP of 160mmHg or greater or
   b. DBP of 110mmHg or greater
2. Proteinuria 3+ OR 4+ on dipstick
3. Severe edema, including pulmonary edema
4. Evidence of end organ compromise (cerebral or visual disturbances)
5. Persistent abdominal pain with nausea and vomiting. May also see:
   a. Oliguria (<400mL in 24 hr).
   b. Decreased platelet count (thrombocytopenia <100,000) or elevated liver function tests
   c. Hyperreflexia

Eclampsia:

1. Convulsions (seizures) during pregnancy with history of preeclampsia, or without other explanation.
2. Hypertension. May also see weight gain, edema, proteinuria, visual disturbances, and right upper quadrant/epigastric pain.

Using Advanced Tools: Labs: Urinalysis for urine protein (dipstick); platelet count

Assessment:

Differential Diagnosis

Appendicitis, diabetes, gallbladder disease, gastroenteritis, glomerulonephritis, hyperemesis gravidarum (excessive vomiting in pregnancy), kidney stones, peptic ulcer, pyelonephritis, lupus, viral hepatitis.

Plan:

Stabilize and evacuate. Definitive therapy in the form of delivery is the only cure for preeclampsia. The difficulty in therapy is deciding when to deliver the infant. The decision to deliver will depend on the severity of the disease, the status of the mother and the fetus, and the gestational age at the time of the evaluation. Take the severity of the condition and the fetal gestational age into consideration, and either deliver the pregnancy or place the patient on bed rest. Perform close surveillance until the pregnancy reaches term or the preeclampsia worsens, dictating the need to deliver. There is no advantage to cesarean delivery over vaginal delivery for preeclampsia. Therefore, delivery route should be based on obstetric indications (worsening condition). In the field setting, the patient will usually present either after having a seizure or with difficulty breathing due to pulmonary edema. At this point, evacuation for delivery is the best option. If this is not possible, consider induction of labor. Inform the family of the expected poor outcome.

Treatment:

Mild Preeclampsia:

1. Observe for worsening signs of the disease.
2. If patient's condition does not progress, discharge and follow on a twice weekly basis.
3. In a field or remote setting, (between 24–34 weeks of gestation) give **dexamethasone** 6mg IM q12h for a total of 4 doses to accelerate fetal lung maturity.
4. **Magnesium sulfate** is the standard medication given to prevent seizures. If it is available, the safest method of administration is 5g deep IM into each buttock (10g total) followed by 5g deep IM q4h. Concurrent use of magnesium sulfate with calcium channel blockers may result in hypotension or respiratory paralysis. Evaluate the patient every hour for the presence of patellar reflexes (loss of reflexes being the first manifestation of magnesium toxicity), respiratory depression (<12 per minute), and the urine output (should exceed 100mL per 4 hours). Magnesium sulfate is usually continued for 24 hours postpartum. Toxic levels cause muscle weakness, respiratory paralysis, and cardiac arrest. Administer **calcium gluconate** 1g slow IV push over 2-3 minutes to counteract magnesium toxicity.
5. Deliver at term (≥ to 38 weeks gestation) or sooner if maternal or fetal condition worsens.

Severe Preeclampsia:

1. With SBP >180mmHg or the DBP >110mmHg, the possibility of intracerebral damage increases warranting antihypertensive medication. Give **hydralazine** 5-10mg IV q20 min. as indicated, or **labetalol** 20mg IV q10 min. with a max dose of 300mg, to reduce BP. Monitor BP q5 min. for at least 30 min. after giving the drug. Please note that some of the side effects with labetalol are maternal tachycardia, headache and flushing.
2. Give **magnesium sulfate** as described previously.
3. Evacuate if possible.
4. If evacuation is not possible deliver the fetus (*see Part 3: General Symptoms: Obstetric Problems: Induction of Labor*).
5. Treat the pulmonary edema by fluid restriction and gentle use of diuretics (ie, **furosemide** 10mg IV push q6h not to exceed 20mg).

Eclampsia:

1. Give magnesium sulfate as above (as an alternative if magnesium sulfate is not available, **phenytoin** 10-15mg/kg IV at a rate of less than 50mg/min, then 100mg IV/po q6-8h x 24 hours).
2. Provide oxygen and airway support as needed.
3. Evacuate.
4. If evacuation not feasible, deliver the fetus after seizure activity has abated (remember ACLS).
5. If anticonvulsants are not available, consider cesarean delivery as life saving procedure (*see Part 3: General Symptoms: Obstetric Problems: Cesarean Delivery*).

Patient Education:

Activity: Remain at bedrest on left side to minimize symptoms.

Prevention: Increase water intake, but maintain normal salt intake.

Follow-up Actions

Evacuation/Consultant Criteria: Evacuate early to avoid complications of eclampsia. Consult experts for management in remote settings (to include cesarean delivery if necessary).

Palpitations

BG Joseph Caravalho, Jr., MC, USA

Introduction: Palpitation is the uncomfortable awareness of one's heartbeat. This generally occurs when the heart rhythm becomes irregular (eg, "skipped beats" or fast beats, whether short or sustained runs). Palpitations represent a fairly common complaint, and can be related to numerous systems and conditions. Cardiac (eg, arrhythmias, valve disease, cardiomyopathies), psychiatric (eg, panic, anxiety, depression), metabolic (eg, thyrotoxicosis, hypoglycemia, scombroid food poisoning), high output states (anemia, fever, pregnancy), medications (sympathomimetic agents, anticholinergics, vasodilators), habits (cocaine, nicotine, caffeine) or catecholamine excess (stress from any cause or exercise). The overwhelming majority of patients that present with the isolated complaint of palpitations will not have a serious underlying disease process. The presence of additional significant symptoms or signs (eg, dizziness, syncope, decreased BP) should prompt further evaluation of the specific underlying cause (eg, VT, WPW, prolonged QT interval). The primary goals are to rule out a potentially life-threatening condition (rare), decrease any inciting causes of the palpitations (eg, caffeine, nicotine, stress) and reassure patient of the generally benign nature of most palpitations. SOF medics should in most cases be able to rule out life-threatening conditions based on history and physical exam without the need for more invasive tests.

Subjective: **Symptoms**

Focused History: Ask questions in a logical order, use the "PQRS&T" mnemonic (*see Part 3: General Symptoms: Chest Pain*) to ensure you can fully characterize the symptoms. *What makes the palpitations start/worsen? What makes them decrease/stop?* (Caffeine, alcohol, nicotine, over-the-counter cold remedies and lack of sleep are the most common aggravating factors. Some members utilize anabolic steroids, weight reduction supplements or other health food supplements that contain ephedrine or similar drugs. Asthma medications are largely derivatives of adrenaline and can cause palpitations. Non-sedating antihistamines and hypermotility agents can cause ventricular premature beats [VPBs] and ventricular tachycardia [VT]. Discontinuation of these factors will usually make the symptoms go away. Fear and anxiety worsen the symptoms but not necessarily the rhythm disturbance.)

Is either related to exercise, stress, lack of sleep, body position, alcohol, Valsalva maneuvers (ie, "popping ears", "bearing down"), body position, carotid massage, cold water? (Sitting down, lying down, or taking a nap will often stop the symptoms. Bearing down will abruptly terminate a paroxysmal supraventricular tachycardia [PSVT]. Splashing cold water on one's face, which invokes the diving reflex, may also abruptly stop PSVTs. Occasionally, patients will nap in the setting of prolonged episodes, and it is not uncommon for a PSVT to resolve during the nap.)

Does it start/stop abruptly and without apparent reason? What do the palpitations feel like? (Do not simply accept the fact that the palpitations "hurt" or that they are uncomfortable. With tachydysrhythmias, the patient may describe a "fluttering," "pounding," or "like worms under the chest" sensation or he may acknowledge tachycardia, whether regular or irregular in rhythm. With sporadic events, such as with VPBs and premature atrial contractions [APBs], the patient may describe the heart "turning over," "flopping," or "stopping.")

Where else does the sensation travel? (With chest discomfort that may concern you for underlying coronary artery disease, see if the pain travels to the arm, shoulder, back or jaw.)

How strong/devastating are the symptoms? (Use a 1-10 scale to characterize severity. I find the semi-quantitative severity scale more useful than descriptive words, as most patients cannot easily describe minor changes in discomfort. The self-reported severity scale also allows the patient to be his/her own barometer over time. Do not let the patient give you a number greater than 10.)

What appears whenever the palpitations occur? (Nausea, thirst, frequent urination, and complaints of pain in the chest are non specific and of little value in determining the cause. Additionally, the patient may be extremely anxious during these events. With poor cerebral perfusion associated with very fast tachydysrhythmias, the patient may describe lightheadedness or syncope. If the heart rate goes over 180, the member usually must sit or lie down. With underlying coronary artery disease, the patient may report nausea, vomiting or diaphoresis [cold, clammy sweat]).

How do the episodes start and stop? How long do the episodes last? How frequently do they recur? (VPBs and APBs may occur as frequently as multiple times per minute. Atrial fibrillation and flutter may be extremely short-lived, or can last for hours or days. The patient may not sense isolated VPBs or APBs, and symptoms may relate only to frequent or sustained events. Certain tachydysrhythmias typically start and stop abruptly and without warning. Most runs of PSVT are self-limited and the member finds that lying down or bearing down stops them. If the rapid heart beating lasts for hours, they usually are gone after a nap.)

Objective: Signs
Using Basic Tools: Pulse, VPBs and APBs. Atrial fibrillation is irregularly irregular. Hypotension with dizziness indicates the rhythm is compromising cardiac output. A fever can cause sinus tachycardia, as can hypovolemia (look for orthostatic hypotension on the tilt test), hypoxia. Respirations >30 may result from anxiety and hyperventilation, which can cause dysrhythmias. Both pneumonia and pneumothorax are important causes of tachycardia. Auscultation will provide a more accurate reflection of the patient's heart rate. Tachycardic rhythms may produce low amplitude, non-palpable pulses. An enlarged, tender thyroid, associated with hand tremor, strongly suggests hyperthyroidism as the cause of the tachydysrhythmia.
Using Advanced Tools: Obtain an ECG to identify the underlying rhythm, even if symptoms have resolved. Pulse Ox: <93% consistent with a serious condition.

Assessment:
Determine whether palpitations are life-threatening or non life-threatening:
  Life-Threatening: All patients with palpitations associated with significant symptoms or signs (chest pain, SOB, dizziness, syncope, decreased blood pressure) and or any heart rhythm or rate with symptoms or signs of hemodynamic compromise
  Non Life-Threatening: No other significant signs or symptoms of hemodynamic compromise:
   Tachycardia: HR >100 bpm (without associated decrease in blood pressure) can be a physiologic response to anemia, fever, exercise, anxiety, hypovolemia, hypoxia.
   Bradycardia: HR <60 bpm (without associated decrease in blood pressure) is often seen in well trained athletes with HRs as low as 40 bpm with skips due to premature beats or second degree AV block.
   Isolated VPBs: Wide (>3 little boxes) QRS complexes that occur out of synchronization with the other complexes.
   Isolated APBs: Narrow QRS complexes look similar to, but out of synchronization with, the baseline complexes.
   Heart Block: Dropped or missing QRS where one would have been expected
   Atrial Fibrillation: Irregularly irregular QRS rhythm; no P waves
   Atrial Flutter: Characteristically presents with a saw tooth baseline and regular QRS rhythm. May appear as an irregular rhythm if variable atrioventricular (AV) nodal conduction.
   Stable Narrow Complex Tachycardias (narrow QRS pattern at a rate 100 >150): eg, Paroxysmal Supraventricular Tachycardia (PSVT), in a hemodynamically stable patient. Some maneuvers to slow rate for better diagnosis (also may convert some PSVT to normal a sinus rhythm) are:
     a. Valsalva maneuver: Bearing down like having a bowel movement will terminate or transiently slow all supraventricular tachycardias.
     b. Carotid sinus pressure: While standing to the right of the supine patient, place your left arm under his neck and grasp his left shoulder. When the patient looks to the left, his hyperextended neck exposes his right carotid sinus. Locate the carotid artery pulsation just under the angle of the right jaw. After listening for carotid bruits, rest the stethoscope's diaphragm on the patient's precordium. Then, while listening to the heart beat, press on the carotid sinus vigorously (it should be uncomfortable for the patient) with your right index and middle fingers for 3-5 seconds, allowing 5-10 seconds between repetitions.
     c. Diving reflex: Place the member's face in a basin of cold or ice water

Plan:
Treatment
Life-Threatening (unstable):
   Immediately stabilize as per ACLS procedures and evacuate. The diagnosis and management of Wide QRS Complex dysrhythmias is beyond the scope of this handbook and these patients should be stabilized and evacuated as operational situation permits. *See Part 4: Organ Systems: Chapter 1: Cardiac: Resuscitation*
Non Life-Threatening:
   1. Reassure patient that their symptoms (palpitations) are not a life-threatening condition.
   2. Remove likely causes (caffeine, sleep deprivation, over-the-counter medications).
   3. If other symptoms of another condition (eg, hyperthyroid, hyperglycemia, anemia, pregnancy), identify underlying cause and manage appropriately (see relevant section).
   4. **Propranolol** 20-40mg po qid can be used for ventricular rate control (as required to improve symptoms, eg, palpitations, fatigue) of otherwise stable and documented narrow-complex tachydysrhythmias, or stable atrial fibrillation or flutter to meet operational requirements. **Note:** Beta blockers (or calcium channel blockers) may cause or worsen hypotension in patients with atrial fibrillation and patients should be monitored closely if beta blocker is used to control ventricular rate.

Patient Education

General: Palpitations are ALMOST always non life-threatening. The patient is not having a myocardial infarction.

Activity: If no syncope or near syncope symptoms, then no restriction is indicated. When the symptoms of rapid heart beating come on, the member should sit down and bear down.

Diet: Avoid caffeine and other stimulants

Medications: Propranolol may cause fatigue.

Prevention: Avoid those medications and foods that cause symptoms. Get plenty of rest.

No improvement/Deterioration: If symptoms persist, worsen, or are associated with syncope or pre-syncope return to the clinic.

Follow-up Actions

Return Evaluation: Confirm absence of other symptoms, reassure patient. If symptoms continue, remove the member from the field.

Evacuation/Consultation Criteria: Evacuate if unable to perform duties, if symptoms are not controlled or underlying heart disease is suspected. The presence of stable VPBs, APBs, PSVT, or AF should not be the sole cause to remove the member from the field while performing critical mission executions. Consult cardiology or internal medicine as needed.

Note: Onset of new atrial fibrillation, flutter or other abnormal rhythm requires specialty evaluation for optimal diagnosis and management which may include electrical or chemical cardioversion with or without anticoagulation as soon as operational considerations permit. See service specific Aviation and Diving Medicine guidelines for operators performing special duty.

Rash with a Fever

LTC (P) Daniel Schissel, MC, USA

The sudden appearance of a cutaneous eruption and a fever is frightening and an often intimidating clinical challenge. Rarely does one have to rely solely on their morphologic assessment as when confronted by an acutely ill patient with a fever and a rash. If a diagnosis is not established quickly in certain patients (eg, septicemia) life-saving treatments may be delayed unnecessarily. Furthermore, rapid diagnosis and isolation of patients with contagious disease prevents spread to other persons and preserves the fighting force. Contagious cutaneous diseases presenting with fever and a rash include viral infections (eg, adenovirus, echovirus, herpes simplex, measles, rubella, varicella/ chicken pox) and bacterial infections (eg, meningococcal, staphylococcal, streptococcal, and secondary syphilis). As mentioned in the Dermatology Introduction (*see Part 4: Organ Systems: Chapter 6*), the morphologic diagnosis of cutaneous eruptions is a discipline based on detailed observation, with precise identification of the primary and secondary skin lesions being paramount. The differential diagnosis of an acutely ill febrile patient with a rash may be broken down into three main categories according to the primary lesion(s) observed. *See Part 4: Organ Systems: Chapter 6 or Part 5: Specialty Areas: Chapter 12* for more diagnostic and treatment information.

Table 3-12. Differential Diagnosis of Acutely Ill Patient with Rash

Disease	Macules or Papules	Vesicles, Bullae, or Pustules	Purpuric Macules, Papules, or Vesicles
BACTERIAL:			
Cat-Scratch	X	X	
Gonococcemia			X
Meningococcemia	X	X	X
Pseudomonas aeruginosa		X	X
Staphylococcal			
Erysipelas	X	X	X
Scalded Skin Syndrome	X	X	
Toxic Shock Syndrome	X	X	
Streptococcal (scarlet fever)	X		X
Tularemia	X	X	
RICKETTSIAL:			
Boutonneuse Fever	X		
Rickettsialpox	X	X	
Rocky Mountain Spotted Fever	X	X	X
Trench Fever	X		
Typhoid Fever	X		
Typhus, Louse-borne/epidemic	X		
Typhus, Murine/endemic	X		
Typhus, Scrub	X	X	
VIRAL:			
Adenoviral infections	X		
AIDS/HIV	X		X
Coxsackievirus (hand-foot-and-mouth disease)	X		
Enterovirus Infections; Echo, Coxsackie	X	X	X
Erythema Infectiosum	X		

Table 3-12. Differential Diagnosis of Acutely Ill Patient with Rash, continued

Disease	Macules or Papules	Vesicles, Bullae, or Pustules	Purpuric Macules, Papules, or Vesicles
VIRAL: (continued)			
Erythema Multiform (HSV)	X	X	
Gianotti-Crosti (papular acrodermatitis)	X		
Herpes Simplex/Disseminated		X	
Herpes Zoster/Generalized		X	
Measles (rubeola)	X		
Roseola Infantum	X		
Rubella (German measles)	X		
Varicella (chickenpox)	X	X	
OTHER:			
Drug Hypersensitivity	X	X	X
Kawasaki Disease (mucocutaneous lymph node syndrome)	X		
Lyme Disease	X		
Psoriasis	X		
Secondary Syphilis	X		
Serum Sickness	X		
Stevens-Johnsons Syndrome	X	X	
Systemic Lupus Erythematosus	X	X	X
Toxic Epidermal Necrosis	X	X	

Pruritus (Itching)
LTC (P) Daniel Schissel, MC, USA

Introduction: Rash and pruritus sometimes present together and may be related (*see Part 3: General Symptoms: Rash with a Fever*). The intensity of itching can vary from mild to severe, and can interfere with sleep at night and the ability to focus during the day. Suicide due to intractable pruritus has been reported. In some cases, the cause may be obvious, such as exposure to an irritant or allergen known to the patient. Other cases, especially the more chronic and generalized ones may be more difficult to understand and/or treat. A thorough history and physical is needed to unravel such cases. Begin by determining whether the pruritus is due to a local skin condition or a systemic problem.

Subjective: **Symptoms (in addition to itching)**
   Variable: Pain, insomnia, rash (virtually any type of skin lesion), fever, erythema
   Focused History: *Have you been in contact with plants, chemicals, shoes or other sources of leather or rubber?* (suspect contact dermatitis) *Do you have any personal history or family history of allergy, asthma, hay fever or childhood eczema?* (suggests atopic allergic diagnosis) *Have you changed medications or dosages lately? Have you had significant, recent exposure to sunlight, biting insects or sick people?* (may suggest diagnosis) *Have you had a viral illness in the last 2-6 weeks?* (Pityriasis rosea is characterized by herald patch and pruritus.) *Have you noticed any hair loss, dry skin or pigment changes?* (consider thyroid disease) *Have you had any jaundice, or clay-colored stools?* (consider liver disease) *Where have you noticed the rash?* (Specific sites are more likely in some conditions, eg, finger web spaces, axillae, nipples, umbilicus and genitals for scabies; sun-exposed areas for sunburn, some drug reactions.)

Objective: **Signs**
   Using Basic Tools: Agitation, excoriation, thickened and/or hyperpigmented skin, fatigue, possible rash (varied presentations but if there are no lesions where the patient cannot reach [eg, mid-back], the condition is likely systemic), erythema, fever, lymphadenopathy, jaundice, hives; others also possible.
   Using Advanced Tools: Labs: CBC with differential for infection (eosinophils in parasitic infestations), anemia; Urinalysis for urobilinogen, protein, casts, sugar; Stool specimens for occult blood and/or O&P; KOH to identify tinea infections; Gram's stain and/or culture for cellulitis; CXR: To rule out complications.

Assessment:
   Differential Diagnosis:
      Pruritus with rash: See separate sections on scabies, lice, psoriasis, contact dermatitis, fungal/tinea infections and many of the infectious cutaneous diseases.
      Xerosis (dry skin is itchy skin!): Dry, flaky, macular lesions over large area.
      Atopic dermatitis: Affects the popliteal and antecubital fossae; dry, hyperkeratotic, confluent papules.

Psoriasis: Found in scalp, external auditory canals, genitals and superior aspect of the intergluteal cleft; plaques of dry, hyperkeratotic skin

Drug eruptions: Erythematous, generalized, fine rash; history of drug/medication use

Urticaria: Edema, erythema, wheal reaction to allergen/irritant; may be generalized

Seborrheic dermatitis: Oily, flaking skin; often in the hair

Sunburn: Sun exposed areas; erythema and edema, with pain

Contact dermatitis (allergic or irritant): Edema, erythema, pain on areas exposed at work (hands, face, etc.)

Pityriasis rosea: History of viral illness; oval, macules and papules on trunk and extremities

Insect bites: Single or multiple erythematous, edematous macules

Scabies: Linear burrows with excoriations in finger web spaces, axillae, nipples, umbilicus and genitals

Pediculosis (head, body or pubic lice): Excoriations in appropriate areas; visible lice or nits

Fungal infections: Erythematous, hyperkeratotic plaques in moist body areas; KOH positive scrapings

Folliculitis: Cellulitis around hair shaft

Lichen simplex chronicus: Single or confluent papules with mosaic pattern

Pruritus ani or vulva: Often due to unknown causes, or from infections (peri-anal strep), infestations (pinworms), trauma, contactants, cancer, lichen planus or lichen sclerosis, or psychological factors

Contagious diseases: Fever and rash (usually macular/papular); include viral infections (eg, adenovirus, measles, rubella, varicella/chickenpox); bacterial infections (eg, meningococcal, staphylococcal, streptococcal, and secondary syphilis)

Pruritus without rash: See separate sections on jaundice, hypothyroidism, diabetes, anemia

Thyroid disease: Thinning of the lateral eyebrows, loss of skin pigment

Uremia/kidney failure: Proteinuria, casts on urinalysis (UA)

Obstructive biliary disease: Urobilinogen on UA, jaundice, abdominal pain

Diabetes mellitus: Glucose on UA; polyphagia, polyuria, polydipsia.

Microcytic anemia

Drug side effects: History of medication use.

Neurologic disorders: Such as paroxysmal pruritus in multiple sclerosis

Several cancers: Lymphadenopathy in many types, low blood cell lines

Pregnancy: *See Part 3: General Symptoms: Obstetric Problems: Pregnancy*

Plan:

Treatment

1. Treat infectious agents (tinea, parasitic, viral and bacterial) as discussed in their respective sections.
2. Treat other rashes (psoriasis, etc.) and systemic diseases (diabetes, etc.) as discussed in their respective sections.
3. Treat dry skin with a gentle regimen of less bathing (every other day instead of daily) with warm, not hot water, for short duration (<5 minutes), and either gentle soap like Dove for Sensitive Skin or a soap substitute (Cetaphil lotion). Cleanse only the areas needing it, like the face, axillae and anogenital region. Pat dry gently with a towel, taking care not to rub. Immediately apply an emollient like Moisturel or Eucerin or Vaseline or Crisco. Aveeno Colloidal Oatmeal bath can help but be sure to rinse off the residual matter.
4. Relieve itching:
   A. Sarna lotion (camphor and menthol) and cool compresses can relieve itch for short periods of an hour or so.
   B. Avoid extensive applications of topical steroids when the etiology of pruritus is unclear.
   C. Antihistamines (eg, **hydroxyzine** 25-50mg po) or the antidepressant **doxepin** 25mg po can be helpful at bedtime, but tend to cause drowsiness, so use with caution.
   D. Ultraviolet sunlight (UVB or PUVA) can help. Avoid midday sun with burning infrared rays.
   E. Anxiety and stress, as well as depression can elicit or worsen pruritus. Psychiatric consultation may be helpful, but work hard to get the patient's confidence before even suggesting this.

Patient Education

General: Do not use water to moisten skin. It causes further drying. Take medication as indicated. Do not scratch.

Prevention: Keep skin moist during winter by avoiding hot water, excessive washing, harsh soap.

Follow-up Action

Evacuation/Consultant Criteria: Evacuation is not normally necessary. Consult dermatology as needed.

Note: Skin biopsy by dermatologist is sometimes necessary for accurate diagnosis.

Shortness of Breath (Dyspnea)

LCDR Tim Quast, MC, USN & MAJ Christopher J. Lettieri, MC, USA

Introduction: Dyspnea is a sensation of difficult or labored breathing and may be related to a primary airway (eg, presence of foreign body, trauma, paralyzed vocal cords) or other causes such as: pulmonary (eg, asthma, COPD, pneumonia, pulmonary embolus); cardiac (eg, ischemia, tamponade, CHF), metabolic (eg, lactic acidosis seen in diabetic ketoacidosis, drug overdose), exposure to occupational/CBR agents (eg, decompression sickness, chemicals), neurologic (eg, effect on CNS respiratory centers, Guillain-Barré), or psychogenic (eg, anxiety attack). Do not confuse dyspnea with stridor, which is a high-pitched noise emanating generally from the upper airway. Although stridor may be present in the case of airway obstruction, it is not necessarily present in the setting of dyspnea. The clinician should focus on time of onset of dyspnea: did dyspnea come on over a period of time and is long-standing (eg, emphysema) or did it come on rapidly (eg, pulmonary embolus, acute exacerbation of asthma)? Determine the underlying cause responsible for the dyspnea (ie, airway, pulmonary, cardiac, metabolic, neurologic, occupational/CBR exposure, or psychogenic) and treat appropriately.

Subjective: **Symptoms**

Usually anxious, complaining of shortness of breath (SOB) possibly even demonstrating obvious difficulty maintaining a conversation during questioning.

Focused History: *How long have you had your SOB? Is your SOB getting progressively worse?* (distinguish between acute or chronic process) *Is anyone else experiencing similar symptoms?* (possible occupational other CBR exposure) *Is there chest pain associated with your SOB and if so, where in particular? Are you having pain right now?* (Myocardial infarction or pulmonary emboli may cause chest pain and dyspnea.) *Have you had a recent respiratory illness?* (Pneumonia may follow a URI.) *Have you had fevers or chills? Have you coughed up any mucus or blood recently?* (COPD, pneumonia or pneumothorax) *Have you noticed yourself wheezing or do you notice it is difficult for you to get the air out of your lungs as opposed to into your lungs?* (eg, asthma or chemical irritant) *Do you smoke?* (increased risk for COPD, spontaneous pneumothorax, or cardiac ischemia) *Has there been a period of prolonged sedentary activity such as flying?* (increased risk of pulmonary embolus) *Is it difficult for you to sleep on your back or do you awaken at night with SOB? Have you had any lower leg or ankle swelling?* (congestive heart failure) *Has it been difficult or painful for you to swallow?* (retropharyngeal mass or abscess, epiglottitis with obstruction) *Have you had any recent weight loss?* (TB or lymphoma) *Is fatigue a primary, or the primary, co-symptom?* (anemia or hypothyroidism) *Have you noticed lower extremity or upper extremity weakness?* (neuromuscular disorders, myositis) *Have you had trauma to the neck or chest?* (pneumothorax or pulmonary contusion) *Did the symptoms start while you were eating or holding something in your mouth?* (aspiration) *Do you have a history of heart problems, diabetes, vascular disease, asthma, COPD? What medications or drugs are you taking?* (may point to underlying disease, side effects or non-compliance taking medications) *Have you ever had any mental health problems, including suicide attempts?* (anxiety, drug abuse) *Do you have numbness around your mouth?* (occasionally seen in psychogenic hyperventilation)

Objective: **Signs**

Using Basic Tools: Vital signs: Temperature: Elevation suggests infectious processes (pneumonia, epiglottitis). **Note:** Low grade fever may be seen with pulmonary embolus, MI and in those patients "working" to breathe (asthma, COPD, psychogenic). Hypotension: (eg, cardiac cause, pulmonary embolus). Hypertension: (eg, chronic vascular disease-related dyspnea or in psychogenic dyspnea). Inspection: Anxious patient, sitting upright, (unless there is a decrease in mental status, eg, drugs, head trauma, stroke, diabetic coma). There may be evidence of trauma with open wounds, distorted anatomy, bruising, and swelling. Rapid, labored breathing, use of accessory muscles of respiration with anxiety or sensation of doom suggests imminent requirement for immediate action with focus on airway and ventilation and additional specific action as required (eg, ACLS, ATLS). Psychogenic dyspneic patients (as well as those which are drug-related) may also appear tachypneic, tachycardic and diaphoretic (sweating). Tachycardia and tachypnea (except in CNS/drug related hypoventilation). Level of mental status is variable depending on degree and underlying mechanism causing of hypoxia and may range from anxious (asthma, psychogenic dyspnea to comatose. (drugs, stroke, head trauma, diabetic coma). Auscultation: Rales or rhonchi (eg, pneumonia, CHF); wheezing (obstructive airway disease), decreased breath sounds (severe asthma, emphysema). Pulse oximetry: Decreased oxyhemoglobin saturation (eg, SaO_2 <92%) may correlate to level of dyspnea in some circumstances, although dyspnea may be present when oxyhemoglobin saturations are within normal limits. SaO_2 levels less than 92% may be seen in numerous disorders such as PE, pneumonia, and CHF, but low SaO_2 is not necessary to make these diagnoses. **Using Advanced Tools:** CXR: Pulmonary edema (increased vascular markings) in CHF, infiltrate (increased local density) in pneumonia, effusion (fluid in pleural space) with pulmonary embolus or pneumonia; neck x-ray (if available) for epiglottal swelling or foreign body in airway; ECG (*see Part 8: Procedures: Chapter 30: ECG: Three-Electrode Rhythm Tracings*) to assist with evaluation of AMI, arrhythmia.

Assessment:

Differential Diagnosis

Airway: A primary problem of inspiration involving the upper airway level (eg, foreign body, trauma, edema of the glottis, paralysis of vocal cords)

Pulmonary: Airflow restriction or obstruction within the pulmonary airways or parenchyma (eg, asthma, COPD, pneumonia, atelectasis, pneumothorax, pleural effusion, hemothorax, pulmonary embolism) causes an increase in the work or effort required to breathe, producing dyspnea.

Cardiac: Problems that slow or impede the delivery of oxygenated blood cause dyspnea. Etiologies include valvular malfunction, ischemia/infarction (eg, acute coronary syndrome, tamponade, and congestive heart failure).

Metabolic changes: Diseases or ingestion of specific substances can cause a change in blood pH, and subsequent increase or decrease in rate and depth of respiration (eg, blow off CO_2), that may be perceived as dyspnea (eg, diabetic ketoacidosis, ingestion of antifreeze). Identify history of disease or exposure to specific substances.

Nervous system: Diseases or processes that depress the brain's respiratory control center can result in dyspnea. Some causes include narcotics stroke or head trauma. Also, neuromuscular disorders must be considered such as myositis, myasthenia gravis, or Guillain-Barré syndrome.

Psychogenic: Anxiety is a well-known cause of tachypnea. Patients may interpret tachypnea as dyspnea, which further increases their level of anxiety. They may develop muscle (myoclonic) spasms.

Occupational/CBR exposure: History or increased risk of exposure (eg, diving, flight, exposure to chemical or CBR); determine if others are having symptoms of exposure.

Plan:

Treatment

Airway: Provide and secure an adequate airway, provide supplemental oxygen and verify adequate oxygenation using pulse oximetry. *See Part 8: Procedures: Chapter 30: Initial Airway Management and Ventilatory Support; Intubation & Pulse Oximetry Monitoring*

Foreign object: Remove object if possible (Heimlich maneuver or sweep/grasp object); do NOT intubate with object in airway!

Neck trauma: After checking for foreign bodies (eg, teeth), intubation or cricothyroidotomy as required.

Epiglottitis: Carefully evaluate status of airway. Cricothyroidotomy may be preferred in severe cases. *See Part 4: Organ Systems: Chapter 3: Epiglottitis*

Tumor: May require intubation or emergency airway, ie, cricothyroidotomy. Tumor location may influence choice of airway.

Retropharyngeal abscess/hematoma: Intubate or perform cricothyroidotomy if necessary. Do NOT drain abscess or hematoma; give antibiotics (**cefuroxime** 1g IV q8h, or **cefotaxime** 2g IV q4-8h through medical evacuation). This is a surgical emergency and a surgeon should be notified immediately.

Pulmonary: Asthma, COPD, pneumonia: See appropriate respiratory section.

Pneumothorax/tension pneumothorax/hemothorax: O_2; needle thoracotomy; address underlying condition; place chest tube. *See Part 8: Procedures: Chapter 30: Thoracotomy, Needle and Chest Tube*

Pleural effusion: O_2; needle thoracentesis to drain pleural effusion; address underlying illness. *See Part 4: Organ Systems: Chapter 3: Pleural Effusion*

Cardiac: Acute Coronary Syndrome (ACS), CHF, Tamponade: Evaluate and provide advanced cardiac life support (ACLS) as required. *See Part 4: Organ Systems: Chapter 1: Acute Coronary Syndrome (Acute Myocardial Infraction and Unstable Angina); Congestive Heart Failure (Pulmonary Edema) & Pericarditis*

Metabolic: Identify underlying disease or substance causing metabolic abnormality (eg, diabetes, methanol, ethylene glycol, aspirin toxicity). *See Part 4: Organ Systems: Chapter 4: Diabetes Mellitus*

Nervous system (eg, narcotic/substance abuse, stroke, head trauma, Guillain-Barré): May require intubation and ventilatory support.

Psychogenic: Have patient breathe into a bag (will reverse myoclonic spasms in 10-15 minutes). Rule out underlying medical condition. Treat anxiety with an anxiolytic. *See Part 3: General Symptoms: Anxiety*

Occupational/CBR exposure (eg, decompression sickness, high altitude pulmonary edema, exposure to chemical irritant/CBR): Provide supplemental oxygen. *See Part 6: Operational Environment: Chapter 20: Decompression Injuries; Chapter 22 & Chapter 25*

Patient Education

General: Return for reevaluation if symptoms recur, worsen or new symptoms. Reassure the patient whenever possible (anxiety worsens the symptoms).

Follow-up Actions

Evacuation/Consultant Criteria: Unless the cause is known and patient responds to therapy evacuation for definitive diagnosis and therapy will be required. Evacuate when patient has been stabilized.

Syncope (Fainting)
CDR Christopher Jankosky, MC, USN

Introduction: Syncope (fainting) is the sudden transient loss of consciousness and motor tone followed by spontaneous return to patient's baseline condition. The underlying basic mechanism is most commonly hypoperfusion of the brain. A decrease in intravascular volume (eg, blood loss, dehydration, adrenal insufficiency); a cardiac arrhythmia (eg, V-Fib, V-Tach, asystole, profound tachycardia [>180 bpm] or bradycardia [<40 bpm], WPW, prolonged QT); metabolic disturbance (eg, hypoglycemia, hypercapnia from hyperventilation) or severe pain (eg, ectopic pregnancy, migraine headache, or chest pain) may present as syncope. The most common (25-65%) cause of true recurrent syncope is vasovagal or vasodepressor (neurocardiogenic syncope). Although the long term prognosis for patients with recurrent vasovagal syncope is excellent (no increase in mortality or morbidity), the short term potential adverse effects on individual operational readiness can be significant. Specialty referral is required for definitive diagnosis and management of recurrent neurocardiogenic syncope. Although there are many possible causes of syncope; the SOF medic's primary responsibility is to determine whether a life-threatening cause of syncope is present, provide appropriate management, and minimize the risk to the team's mission.

Subjective: **Symptoms**

Sudden, unexplained loss of consciousness possibly preceded by light-headedness, nausea, sweating, sudden fatigue, hunger or "seeing stars." Loss of consciousness is of brief duration and usually resolves with spontaneous return to baseline condition soon after the patient is placed in a supine, horizontal position.

Focused History: *Do you have any symptoms now?* (headache, focal neurological deficit, consistent with intracranial process; confusion consistent with post-ictal state following seizure) *What were you doing when you passed out?* (Syncope during or following exercise could suggest dehydration/hypovolemia, arrhythmia or cardiac structural defect; standing at attention in formation for prolonged period suggests vasovagal syncope.) *Has this ever happened before?* (If repeatedly associated with exercise, could suggest arrhythmia or cardiac structural abnormality; history of recurrent episodes with prolonged standing or other stimulus [eg, shots] most consistent with vasovagal syncope.) *Did anyone see you pass out?* (Observer may confirm loss of consciousness, seizure activity, timing of any apparent injuries.) *Did you soil your clothing?* (consistent with loss of consciousness related to seizure) *Are you taking any medications?* (Insulin or other diabetic medication increases risk of hypoglycemia, diuretics, sleep medication, muscle relaxants, medications [eg, Wellbutrin for depression or smoking cessation] that lower threshold for seizure activity.) *Have you been drinking alcohol?* (dehydration/hypovolemia) *Have you been having vomiting and diarrhea?* (dehydration/hypovolemia) *Have you ever been pregnant? Are you pregnant?* (History of unusual abdominal pain or vaginal bleeding could suggest blood loss hypovolemia.)

Objective: **Signs**

Using Basic Tools: Vital signs (record blood pressure, pulse, and temperature). General exam may reveal fatigued patient with cool, clammy skin. Consciousness should return once patient is in a horizontal position and cerebral blood flow restored. Auscultation: May reveal structural cardiac abnormalities. Assess for any area of localized pain. A specific neurological deficit following a syncopal event may indicate a stroke whereas a transient confusional state could indicate a post-ictal condition following a convulsion.

Using Advanced Tools: Labs: blood glucose, hematocrit for anemia; ECG for arrhythmia; pregnancy test for female, if possible ectopic pregnancy.

Assessment:
Differential Diagnosis
Cardiac: Rhythm, conduction or specific evidence of cardiac ischemia (eg, V-Fib, V-Tach, prolonged QT, profound tachycardia >180 or profound bradycardia <40 or ST elevation suggesting acute MI on ECG). Structural abnormality: Significant cardiac murmur (eg, aortic stenosis, mitral regurgitation)

Hemorrhage: Trauma, GI bleed, ruptured aortic aneurysm, ruptured spleen, ruptured ovarian cyst, ruptured ectopic pregnancy

Hypoglycemia: Low blood glucose on finger-stick Glucometer. Chemstrip urinalysis positive for ketones in starvation, diabetic ketoacidosis (DKA), others.

Hypovolemia: Tilt test positive with BP dropping >20mm and HR rising >10 bpm

Heat injury: Heat exhaustion may be triggered by excessive sweating and inadequate fluid replacement.

Seizure disorder: May have evidence of tongue biting, urinary and bowel incontinence, post-ictal confusion

Pulmonary embolism: Hemodynamically significant pulmonary embolism is uncommon but a well documented cause of syncope.

Subarachnoid hemorrhage: Syncope in patients following a new or most severe headache ("the worst headache of my life")

Vasovagal/Vasodepressive (neurocardiogenic syncope): Most common cause of syncope, excellent long term prognosis, may be an operational concern for reliable function in the short term.

Many medications and recreational drugs: Can cause syncope and alterations in consciousness, especially if taken in combination with alcohol.

Plan:
Treatment:
Primary:
a. Protect patient from injury and place with feet elevated.
b. Obtain ECG to evaluate for conduction disturbances and abnormal intervals (eg, WPW, prolonged QT, short PR). Follow standard treatment protocols for any identified cardiac condition.
c. If dehydrated, start IV and deliver D5NS bolus infusion of 500cc. Continue 200cc/hr until systolic BP >90.
d. If hypoglycemia is suggested by the Chemstrip or the history, give one ampule of D50 IV.
e. Identify possible occult source of loss of blood (trauma, GI bleed, ruptured spleen, ruptured ovarian cyst, ruptured ectopic pregnancy)
f. If concern for pulmonary embolism or subarachnoid bleed, stabilize vital signs and consider medical evacuation. *See Part 3: General Symptoms: Chest Pain & Headache*
g. If concern that patient has had a seizure, *see Part 4: Organ Systems: Chapter 5: Seizure Disorders and Epilepsy.*

Empiric: Start IV with Normal Saline and reevaluate clinical effects of first 1000mL NS.

Primitive: Elevate the feet and cover with warm blanket.

Patient Education
General: Transient loss of consciousness with spontaneous return to baseline condition in a young person is most likely vasovagal and not serious. If recurrent (more than one per month), or results in bodily injury, then consult higher authority. When an aura occurs, lie down or sit down and place your head between your knees.

Activity: Wherever possible avoid conditions that precipitate the event (eg, prolonged periods of standing "at attention") Patient should not stand duty alone for 48 hours after a syncopal event. They should not drive, jump, or dive after a second event until evaluated at a higher echelon of care.

Diet: Drink plenty of fluids, restrict refined sugars; avoid alcohol.

Prevention and Hygiene: Maintain hydration. Advise unit to prevent other heat or drug related injuries.

No Improvement/Deterioration: Return for reevaluation promptly.

Follow-up Actions
Return Evaluation: Repeat evaluation, including ECG, Chemstrip, blood pressure, and hematocrit.

Consultation Criteria: Any patient with life-threatening rhythm disturbance, seizures or severe headache followed by syncope should be referred to higher level of care immediately. More than two syncopal episodes or dysrhythmias should be evaluated further once out of the field.

Chapter 1: Cardiac/Circulatory: Acute Coronary Syndrome (Acute Myocardial Infarction and Unstable Angina)

BG Joseph Caravalho, Jr., MC, USA

Introduction: Acute coronary syndrome (ACS) is caused by decreased blood flow to the heart (myocardial ischemia) and is the most common of 6 life-threatening conditions that can present as chest pain (*See Part 3: General Symptoms: Chest Pain*). Acute myocardial infarction (AMI) is myocardial ischemia with injury to myocardial tissue. Unstable angina (UA) is reversible myocardial ischemia without myocardial tissue injury. In the field, it may be impossible to determine whether or not the myocardial ischemia is myocardial infarction or unstable angina. Initial management of both conditions is the same and whenever possible patients should be evacuated to advanced medical care. ACS is the leading cause of death in the US and in most of the developed world. Although usually thought of as a disease of older people, almost half of the cases of ACS in the US occur in people under the age of 65. ACS can and does occur in people in their 20s and 30s. Early aggressive management can significantly improve mortality and morbidity but approximately 25% of AMI patients will die from the inciting event. A significant number will die within 1 hour of symptom onset, usually due to a malignant cardiac dysrhythmia, whereas another large subgroup will die within several days, most likely related to heart failure. While some of the diagnostic and therapeutic procedures noted in the chapter are currently not possible in the SOF environment, advances in miniaturization of ECG machines, blood chemistry machines and pharmacology allow remarkably advanced diagnosis and treatment in austere environments. **Cardiac Risk Factors:** Prior ACS or history of coronary artery disease, smoking/tobacco use, hypertension, ACS before age 55 in parents or siblings, diabetes, high total cholesterol, low HDL cholesterol, obesity and history of peripheral vascular disease.

Subjective: Symptoms *See Part 3: General Symptoms: Chest Pain*

Chest pain associated with ACS is often defined as dull, diffuse, and may be described as a pressure sensation or discomfort rather than pain. Pain of ACS may occur at rest or with exercise, may be prolonged, recurrent and with increasing frequency where as the chest pain of a patient with routine angina (non life-threatening) is usually brought on by exercise, lasts less than 5 minutes and is relieved with rest. ACS pain may be accompanied by diaphoresis, SOB, nausea and feelings of dread. Atypical presentations of ACS are not uncommon and it is a mistake to base diagnosis (or rule out ACS) on the basis of history alone.

Focused History: *Have you ever had this type of pain before? When?* (eg, "Yes, the first time was yesterday when I ran to the 3rd floor of HQ" is ACS until proven otherwise). *Has anyone in your family had a heart attack?* (eg, Family history of AMI in young 1st degree relatives indicates increased risk of underlying cardiac disease in patient.) *What do you think this is?* (Patient's level of concern may indicate ischemic or other life-threatening condition.)

Objective: Signs

Using Basic Tools: Tachycardia or bradycardia, hypertension or hypotension; diaphoresis in association with chest pain; inspiratory rales and S-3 gallop (left-sided cardiac failure); hepatojugular reflux, jugular venous distension and peripheral edema (right-sided cardiac failure).

Using Advanced Tools: ECG: ST segment elevation is the hallmark of myocardial infarction, while ST depression and T-wave inversion are signs of myocardial ischemia. Pattern of ST segment elevation may be used to identify the location of the infarction. Elevation in leads I, AVL, and V-1 through V-3 indicate an anterior MI. Elevation in leads II, III and AVF usually indicate an inferior MI. ST elevation in V-2 through V-6 indicates an anterolateral MI. A normal ECG does not rule out AMI. With a high index of suspicion, repeat the ECG several times (q5 minutes), and then monitor continuously for dysrhythmias. *See Figure 4-1*

Assessment: Differential Diagnosis

Determine if ACS or stable angina or non-ischemic chest pain. *See Part 3: General Symptoms: Chest Pain* for discussion of 5 other life-threatening causes of chest pain and 6 categories of non life-threatening causes of chest pain.

ACS: A diagnosis of ACS should be made if onset or PQRST questions (*see Part 3: General Symptoms: Chest Pain*) suggest ischemic pain. Symptoms consistent with AMI, a 1mm of ST segment elevation in contiguous leads or new-onset left bundle branch block (LBBB) are considered presumptive evidence of an AMI. ST segments can be falsely elevated in several conditions, including myocarditis, left ventricular hypertrophy, ventricular aneurysms, early repolarization, hypothyroidism, and hyperkalemia.

Stable angina: Although presumably rare in deployed SOF US forces, this may be seen in indigenous population

Non-ischemic chest pain: Includes other potentially life-threatening causes of chest pain such as aortic dissection, pulmonary embolism and esophageal rupture.

Plan: Treatment (Acute Coronary Syndrome)

1. Assess airway, breathing and circulation. *See Part 4: Organ Systems: Chapter 1: Cardiac: Resuscitation*
2. Provide supplemental oxygen to bring the oxygen saturation above 95%.
3. Attach cardiac monitor if available and treat any malignant dysrhythmias. *See Part 4: Organ Systems: Chapter 1: Cardiac: Resuscitation*
4. **Nitroglycerin** 0.4mg sublingual q5 minutes x 3 doses, or until pain relief. Use caution in patients with suspected inferior wall AMI and involvement of the right ventricle as nitrates may cause severe hypotension in these patients.
   a. Check BP between doses; do not give if systolic BP below 90
   b. If BP drops below 90, give 500cc normal saline boluses until BP returns to >100 systolic.
5. IV of normal saline at 100cc/hr to maintain urine output.
6. **ASA** 325mg po chewed immediately, and then 325mg po q24h, if not contraindicated.
7. For severe pain, **morphine** 2mg IV q5 minutes up to 5 doses, pain relief, hypotension, or sedation. Monitor respiratory status closely.
8. **Low molecular weight heparin** 1mg/kg SC q12h (if no underlying kidney disease)

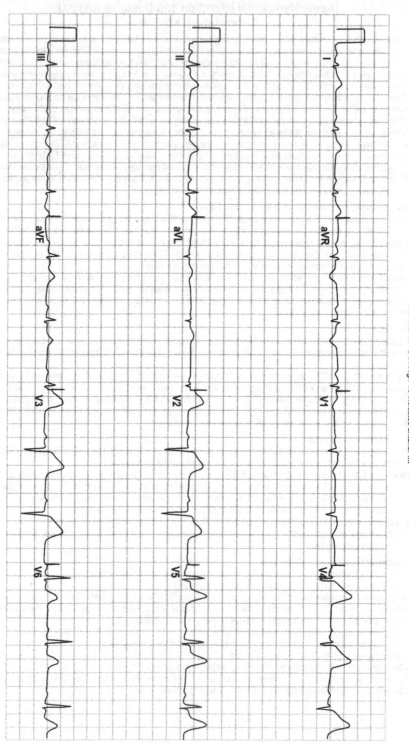

Figure 4-1. ECG Showing ST Segment Elevation in Leads V2 through V5
Elevation in V2 through V5 indicated anterior MI

9. If available, **clopidogrel** 150mg po immediately, and then 75mg po q day.
10. Beta blocker therapy should be given to patients without contraindications (eg, history of asthma, evidence of congestive heart failure). Give **metoprolol** 50mg po bid or **propranolol** 40-80mg po qid (to keep HR <80). Do not give if systolic BP is below 90. If history of asthma precludes use of beta blocker and BP is adequate, **verapamil** 80mg po qid may provide benefit.
11. **Lisinopril** 5mg po q day, starting on day 1, and then advanced up to 20mg po q day, as tolerated by BP.
12. If compromise in pulmonary function (eg, rales), give **furosemide** 40mg po. *See Part 4: Organ Systems: Chapter 1: Congestive Heart Failure*
13. If patient is symptomatic with HR <40bpm, give **atropine** 1mg IV, which may be repeated x 1 in 5 minutes.

Patient Education

Activity: Maintain bedrest to minimize cardiac oxygen demand.
Diet: Sips of water only for first 6-12 hours, then small, light meals, preferably clear liquids only.
Prevention: Make lifestyle changes to minimize cardiac risk factors.

Follow-up Actions

Evacuation/Consultant Criteria: Evacuate patients suspected of ACS immediately after stabilization treatment. Keep patient under close observation at all times. Establish phone or radio contact with medical control as early as possible and continue contact until the patient reaches definitive care. A patient with an AMI may benefit from primary percutaneous intervention or thrombolysis if less than 12 hours has elapsed from the time of onset of symptoms. In the event medical evacuation is not possible, attention should be paid to complete relief of chest pain using methods described previously. Beta blocker therapy and ASA should be continued indefinitely as tolerated and any symptoms suggesting CHF should be managed. *See Part 4: Organ Systems: Chapter 1: Congestive Heart Failure* A majority of patients who remain asymptomatic after an uncomplicated acute MI can return to prior level of "nonphysical" work, safely within two weeks. In these patients daily walking and other physical activity should be encouraged and gradually increased as tolerated by the patient.
Note: Several enzyme markers are routinely used for diagnosis of AMI but they are not available in the field. Thrombolytic therapy is considered only in cases of confirmed AMI, and their use is beyond the scope of the SOF medic in an austere environment.

Table 4-1. Killip Classification

The Killip classification is a useful tool for assessing prognosis in association with AMI:

Killip Class I:	No clinical signs of heart failure. Prognosis good, <5% mortality.
Killip Class II:	Bibasilar rales bilaterally in up to 50% of lung fields, isolated S-3. Prognosis good.
Killip Class III:	Rales in all lung fields; consider acute mitral regurgitation. Prognosis fair to poor.
Killip Class IV:	Cardiogenic shock. Decreased LOC, SBP less than 90mmHg, decreased urine output, pulmonary edema, cold, clammy skin. Prognosis poor, mortality near 80%.

Chapter 1: Cardiac/Circulatory: Congestive Heart Failure (Pulmonary Edema)

BG Joseph Caravalho, Jr., MC, USA

Introduction: Congestive heart failure (CHF) is the heart's inability to pump enough blood to meet the body's demands. CHF may be seen following any of these conditions: pulmonary embolism, sepsis, anemia, thyrotoxicosis in pregnancy, dysrhythmias, myocarditis, endocarditis, hypertension and myocardial infarction (MI). Other associated causes include fluid overload due to acute renal failure, shock lung due to toxic fumes/smoke/heat inhalation of a fire or blast that causes destruction of the alveolar surfactant, and high altitude pulmonary edema. It is easier to treat CHF after recognizing and treating any of these precipitating causes.

Subjective: Symptoms

Shortness of breath (SOB); dyspnea on exertion (DOE), dyspnea when supine (orthopnea), or suddenly awakening from sleep with a sense of breathlessness (paroxysmal nocturnal dyspnea, or PND); swelling of the ankles and legs (pedal edema); fatigue and nausea.
Focused History: *Have you been recently injured or seriously ill?* (ie, infection associated endocarditis, myocarditis, pericarditis, pneumonia, ARDS or injury increasing risk for pulmonary embolism or ARDS) *Are you taking any medications?* (eg, birth control pills may increase risk of pulmonary embolism or illegal drugs [numerous cocaine associated cardiac and pulmonary problems] or alcohol [arrhythmias or myocardiopathy]) *Have you ever been told you have a heart condition?* (History of coronary artery disease, CHF, murmur or valve disease suggests recurrence or worsening of that specific condition.) *Have you been exposed to major changes in atmospheric pressure recently?* (History of rapid ascent or descent might suggest symptoms of acute mountain or decompression sickness.)

Objective: Signs

Using Basic Tools: Vital signs: Fever >101°F; tachycardia >120bpm, tachypnea >30rpm, hypotension or pulsus paradoxus, (eg, valvular infection). Pulsus paradoxus is an abnormally large inspiratory decline in systemic arterial pressure (ie, >10mmHg drop in SBP during inspiration). Head/Neck: Jugular venous distension (JVD); lip cyanosis. Lungs: Rales (fine crackling breath sounds); productive cough with pink, frothy fluid; pleural effusion. Heart: Sounds of a galloping horse (all four hoofs striking the ground S4,S1,S2,S3); holosystolic murmur (eg, mitral regurgitation); diastolic murmur (eg, aortic regurgitation). Extremities: Cyanosis, pitting edema of the ankles and legs.
Using Advanced Tools: ECG: Look for ST elevation or new bundle branch block. Labs: Elevated WBC suggests infection; casts on urinalysis suggest renal failure.

Assessment: **Differential Diagnosis**
Acute myocardial infarction: >1mm ST elevation in 2 or more ECG leads. *See Part 4: Organ Systems: Chapter 1: Acute Coronary Syndrome (Acute Myocardial Infarction and Unstable Angina)*
Myocarditis: ST elevation in all ECG leads; PR depression; ST/TW changes
Acute infective endocarditis: Loud murmur of mitral regurgitation or aortic insufficiency with a fever and WBC >14K
Hypertensive emergency: Diastolic BP >110. *See Part 4: Organ Systems: Chapter 1: Hypertensive Emergencies*
Acute blast injury and/or smoke inhalation: Sputum contains carbon particles. *See Part 4: Organ Systems: Chapter 3: Inhalation Injury due to Smoke and Toxic Chemicals*
Multilobar pneumonia: Fever, WBC>15K, thick yellow/green sputum with WBCs. *See Part 4: Organ Systems: Chapter 3: Pneumonia*
Mountain sickness: History of recent arrival at >5000 feet AGL. *See Part 6: Operational Environment: Chapter 22: Acute Mountain Sickness*

Plan:
Treatment
Primary:
1. Oxygen at 3-5 L/min to raise oxygen saturation to 93-95%
2. **Furosemide** 20mg IV and doubling q30 minutes until diuresis ensues, up to 200mg total. There is no additional benefit in giving more than 200mg if diuresis has not ensued.
3. **Nitroglycerin** 0.4mg sublingual, repeating q5 minutes for a total of 3 doses.
4. Sit patient up with legs dangling to ease dyspnea.
5. Monitor urine output and body weight (2.2 pounds, or 1 kilogram, equals a liter of fluid loss).
Alternative: Intubation with positive pressure breathing (bag-valve-tube forced inhalation) and 100% oxygen flows, if oxygen saturation remains <85%.
Empiric: Antibiotics if infective endocarditis is suspected from fever, heart murmur, and red spots on the fingers. Give **cephalothin** 2gm IV qid and **gentamicin** 1.5mg/kg IV q8h through medical evacuation. If medical evacuation is not possible, continue IV antibiotic therapy for 4 weeks.
Primitive: Last resort for the management of severe pulmonary edema:
1. Rotating BP cuffs: Inflate BP cuffs to a pressure between the patient's systolic and diastolic pressures on three of the four limbs, and then rotate the cuffs every 5min in order to sequester venous blood and reduce venous return to the heart. Ensure that no limb is compressed continuously for more than 15-20 minutes at a time. And/or (based on clinical conditions):
2. Venesection: Removing 300-500mL of blood into an empty infusion bag will reduce the circulating blood volume and pulmonary vascular pressure. However, it also creates the problem of decreasing the patient's oxygen carrying capacity, which worsens his tissue oxygenation. This technique must not be used when other care is available.
Patient Education
General: Salt restriction is necessary and weight should not increase over 2 pounds in a day.
Activity: Rest, sitting upright until diuresis ensues
Diet: Clear liquids until oxygen sat >93-95% and breathing easier, then allow low sodium foods
No Improvement/Deterioration: Evaluate immediately for evacuation
Follow-up Actions
Evacuation/Consultation Criteria: Evacuate immediately if unable to achieve diuresis or oxygen sat >90%, for persistent cyanosis, or if HR remains over 150bpm (dysrhythmia) or suspicion of endocarditis. Sedation, intubation with 100% oxygen by bag-valve-tube ventilation and ECG monitoring (if available) is required for transport. The key is to maximize oxygen transport to the tissues. Continue to work aggressively on treatment options listed. Request medical evacuation at lowest altitude levels possible. Even a healthy 28 year old cannot remain in CHF over 2-4 hours without risk of developing life-threatening heart rhythms.

Chapter 1: Cardiac/Circulatory: Hypertensive Emergencies
CDR John Hammes, MC, USN

Introduction: Chronic hypertension may have long term effects but usually does not warrant intervention in the field. Patients should have further evaluation and treatment upon completion of the mission. A hypertensive emergency is defined as acute hypertension with damage to organs such as the brain, eye, heart, or kidney. The diastolic blood pressure (BP) is usually at least 110-120mmHg. Marked hypertension accompanying head trauma is a compensatory response.

Subjective: **Symptoms**
Headache; blurred vision; neurologic deficits; decreased urination; shortness of breath while walking or sitting that worsens when lying down; fatigue; nausea; lack of energy; confusion and chest pain.
Focused History: Most patients with hypertension are asymptomatic. In a patient whose blood pressure is elevated (BP usually >110-120mmHg) the following symptoms are consistent end organ damage and a hypertensive emergency: *Are you having chest pain?* (myocardial ischemia) *Difficulty breathing?* (suggests pulmonary edema) *Back pain?* (aortic dissection) *Weakness/numbness/altered thinking?* (encephalopathy or stroke)

Objective: **Signs**
Using Basic Tools: BP >220/120; bounding pulses; swelling of the legs; cyanosis; tachypnea, tachycardia or bradycardia; lungs may be clear or have rales of CHF or pulmonary edema; forceful heartbeat on chest wall; loud bruit in peri-umbilical area in renal artery stenosis; decreased urinary output from renal dysfunction (as either a cause or an effect); neurologic defects (encephalopathy). Organ damage of note includes effects on heart, brain, eyes and kidneys.

Using Advanced Tools: Labs: Protein and casts on urinalysis (renal failure); ECG may reveal atrial and/or ventricular enlargement and/or ischemic/strain changes of ST segments or T-wave inversions. Funduscopic exam: Blurring of the optic disc or red splotches of hemorrhage on the retina.

Assessment: Differential Diagnosis
Acute renal failure: Casts seen in the urine sediment
Stroke: Focal neurologic deficit or altered level of consciousness
Aortic dissection: >10mm difference in systolic BP between the arms
Closed head trauma with elevated intracranial pressure: History of trauma, wound on the head, pupils different in size

Plan:
Treatment
Treat acute hypertension if there is evidence of organ damage, or if BP reaches 220/120mmHg. There is no evidence that treating patients with a BP below 200/110 in the absence of symptoms of end organ damage is beneficial. While attempts at lowering BP to a safer level (eg, 160s/90s) may be appropriate in absence of end-organ damage, the questionable benefit must be balanced against the potential for harming the patient by lowering the BP too rapidly and thus causing inadequate perfusion of vital organs.
Primary: Labetalol 300mg po qid or **lisinopril** 10mg po or **enalapril** 5mg po qid or **clonidine** 0.1mg po q1 up to 6 doses may be tried to lower the diastolic BP to 100-110, (do not lower diastolic BP to <90mmHg, in the first 24 hours):
Note: that if BP is not controlled with 1 medication, it is OK to add an additional medication from a second class, with the caveat that time (approximately 1 hour) should be given to observe the effect of adding a medication so as not to lower the BP too rapidly.
Alternative: Diuresis: **furosemide** 20mg IV (or po) and double q30 minutes until diuresis occurs. Give **nitroglycerin** 300-400mcg sublingual q5 min x 3 doses if patient has anginal symptoms. Sedate with **diazepam** 5-10mg po q6h if agitated or evidence of alcohol withdrawal.
Primitive: Sitting or elevating the head is essential if head trauma is suspected. Phlebotomy of 500cc (withdraw one unit by gravity into an empty IV fluid bag) if pulmonary edema is present and diuresis not possible.
Patient Education
General: Hypertension is a common, chronic disease that can be controlled with diet, exercise and medications to minimize the risk of stroke, kidney failure or heart failure. There is no need to acutely treat hypertension unless organ damage is evident.
Activity: Rest will lower the BP. Strenuous physical exertion will raise the pressure and should be minimized until BP stable.
Diet: Avoid salt and salty foods.
Medications: Antihypertensive medications are often sedating and can cause orthostatic hypotension.
Prevention and Hygiene: Exercise, weight control, and salt avoidance.
No Improvement/Deterioration: Return for reevaluation.
Follow-up Actions
Wound Care: Clean and dress any wounds appropriately.
Return Evaluation: Daily BP checks after initial lowering until resolution of end organ findings. If evidence of end organ damage is present or worsening, additional medications not available in the field will be needed to treat the member.
Evacuation/Consultation Criteria: Progression of neurologic deficits, CHF or anuria should prompt urgent consultation and evacuation if possible. Hypertensive Emergency: Funduscopic findings of flame hemorrhages, or ECG findings of lateral ischemia.
Note: Significant elevations in BP may be an appropriate response to the increase in intracranial pressure that may occur in pressure. A primary concern in the management of head trauma is to avoid hypotension. Maintaining a mean arterial pressure (MAP)* of 90-100mmHG is a primary goal in the management of patients with closed head injury. *See Part 7: Trauma: Chapter 22: Mild Traumatic Brain Injury/Concussion: Assessment and Management*

*MAP = [(2 x DBP) + (SBP)]/3

Chapter 1: Cardiac/Circulatory: Pericarditis
BG Joseph Caravalho, Jr., MC, USA

Introduction: Acute pericarditis is inflammation of the pericardial sac surrounding the heart that results in chest pain. The majority of cases are idiopathic or post-viral. Other causes are acute myocardial infarction, uremia, bacterial infection, tuberculosis, collagen-vascular disease, neoplasm (lung, breast, melanoma, lymphoma, leukemia) or trauma.

Subjective: Symptoms
Precordial chest pain (typically sharp) with a pleuritic component (worse with respirations); fever; shortness of breath on exertion or rest; fatigue; and malaise
Focused History: Describe your chest pain. *When and how did it begin? What makes it better or worse?* (The chest pain of acute pericarditis is typically relatively acute in onset, occurs over the anterior chest and is often pleuritic, that is, exacerbated by inspiration and frequently described as "sharp or stabbing." Pain is decreased when sitting up or leaning forward.)

Objective: Signs
Using Basic Tools: Vital signs: May have low fever. Severe restriction of heart motion because of cardiac tamponade or constrictive pericarditis can sometimes be picked up by noticing that the pulse is felt during expiration but not during inspiration (or is much weaker during inspiration). This observation (pulsus paradoxus) may be measured while taking the BP, using very careful auscultation. During deflation of the BP cuff, the first Korotkoff sounds are audible only during expiration. With further deflation, the Korotkoff sounds are heard throughout the respiratory cycle. The difference between the systolic pressure at which the first Korotkoff sounds are heard during expiration and the pressure at which they are heard throughout the respiratory cycle is a measurement of pulsus paradoxus. A difference of >10mmHg

is considered abnormal. Repeated careful measurements of the blood pressure using this method can be used to identify an increased level of constriction in either cardiac tamponade or constrictive pericarditis (**Note:** It may be present also in a severe asthma attack.) Inspection: Diaphoresis, pallor, increased prominence of neck vein distension. Auscultation: Pericardial friction rub (squeaky leather sound) is loudest leaning forward on held expiration, with the diaphragm of the stethoscope over the left lower sternal edge; possible pleural rub ("Velcro" sound).
Using Advanced Tools: ECG: Diagnostic ST elevation in most leads and PR depression in II, III, aVF. Labs: WBC >15K suggests infectious cause; urinalysis showing protein and casts suggests uremic cause.

Assessment: Differential Diagnosis
Pleurisy: Pleural rub without pericardial rub or ECG abnormality. *See Part 4: Organ Systems: Chapter 3: Pleurisy*
Aortic dissection: Different pulse pressures between the arms
Pulmonary embolism: Typically unilateral calf tenderness and swelling consistent with phlebitis. *See Part 4: Organ Systems: Chapter 3: Deep Vein Thrombosis and Pulmonary Embolism*
Pneumothorax: Absence of breath sounds on one side is typical. *See Part 4: Organ Systems: Chapter 3:* Pneumothorax
Acute myocardial infarction: ECG shows typical ST elevation in 2 or more contiguous leads only. *See Part 4: Organ Systems: Chapter 1: Acute Coronary Syndrome (Acute Myocardial Infarction and Unstable Angina)*
Pericardial tamponade: Falling BP with rising neck veins and signs of hypovolemic shock

Plan:
Treatment
Primary: Rest. **Ibuprofen** 800mg po tid. Perform pericardiocentesis for tamponade. *See Part 8: Procedures: Chapter 30: Pericardiocentesis*
Alternative: Consider giving **prednisone** 60mg po q day x 5 days for protracted cases.
Primitive: Morphine: Titrate dosage beginning at 2mg IV. Repeat q5 minutes until pain is relieved, without over-sedation.
Empiric: If bacterial infection is suspected, the most common cause is *Staphylococcus*. Give **nafcillin** or **oxacillin** 2g IV q4h or **cephazolin** 2gm IV q8h or **clindamycin** 600-900mg IV q8h (not to exceed 4.8 gm/day) and continue antibiotic through medical evacuation.

Patient Education
General: Inflammation of the pericardial sac is often idiopathic or viral and self-limiting over 5-7 days. Pericarditis is not life-threatening unless fluid starts to accumulate in the sac. Exertion, even though it hurts, will not worsen the condition.
Activity: Rest and limit heavy exertion when possible
Diet: Low-sodium
Medications: Take NSAIDs and prednisone with food.
No Improvement/Deterioration: Return for re-evaluation if pain persists >7 days on ibuprofen. Pericardiocentesis may need to be repeated for recurrent tamponade.

Follow-up Actions
Return Evaluation: Consider tamponade if increasing SOB and fatigue. Perform pericardiocentesis if falling BP and rising neck veins associated with a pericardial rub.
Evacuation/Consultation Criteria: Following stabilization (ie, pericardiocentesis), evacuate patients with history of cardiac tamponade.

Chapter 1: Cardiac/Circulatory: Cardiac Resuscitation
BG Joseph Caravalho, Jr., MC, USA

What: Resuscitation of sudden cardiac death or patient with hemodynamically unstable cardiac condition, which, if left untreated, would likely result in sudden cardiac death (SCD). SCD is a common presentation of coronary artery disease, and may be its first sign. Approximately 75% of SCD is due to cardiovascular disease. Sudden syncope may or may not be preceded by chest pain, fluttering sensation in chest, diaphoresis or dizziness. Frequently, arrest is due to malignant cardiac dysrhythmias, most commonly ventricular fibrillation (VF) and pulseless ventricular tachycardia (VT). Early defibrillation of VF or cardioversion of pulseless VT is closely correlated with neurologically intact survival. The most important goal in SCD treatment is to diagnosis and defibrillate/cardiovert VF/VT as soon as possible after onset.

When: A patient is unresponsive and in cardiac arrest. All patients with palpitations associated with significant symptoms or signs (chest pain, sob, dizziness, syncope, decreased blood pressure) and/or any heart rhythm or rate with symptoms or signs of hemodynamic compromise.

What You Need: Defibrillator/Monitor or Automatic External Defibrillator (AED), oxygen, airway adjuncts as needed and ACLS drugs as needed.

What To Do: Basic and advanced cardiopulmonary resuscitation should be performed according to 2005 American Heart Association (AHA) Guidelines for Cardiopulmonary Resuscitation and Emergency Cardiovascular Care. Circulation 2005; 112:IV1. The following principles are meant to highlight specific points and not to replace the 2005 AHA Guidelines.
1. Do a rapid scene survey/tactical assessment to determine any threats in the immediate area.
2. Establish that the patient is unresponsive.
3. Send for help; send for AED or defibrillator/monitor.
4. Open the patient's airway, check for breathing.
5. If the patient is not breathing, give rescue breaths that cause the chest to rise.
6. Check carotid pulses.
7. If no pulse, begin CPR (rate of 100 continuous chest compressions/min; 2 breaths after every 30 compressions), complete at least 2 full cycles, even if monitor/defibrillator or AED arrives before then. Ventilations: Only enough tidal volume to confirm initial chest rise. Care must be taken to avoid excessive ventilation.
8. Intubate and give oxygen, if possible.

9. With AED, attach leads to patient and turn on AED as per instructions.
10. Stop CPR while AED analyzes rhythm.
11. Institute therapy based on 2005 American Heart Association Guidelines for Cardiopulmonary Resuscitation and Emergency Cardiovascular Care
12. Transport victim to highest-level of medical care available as soon as possible.
13. Establish IV access en route if not already done.

Defibrillation: In adults use the highest available energy (200-360 J with a biphasic defibrillator and 360 J with a monophasic defibrillator). Remember the goal in cardiac resuscitation is preventing ischemic brain injury while restoring the normal circulatory action of the heart. When evaluating a possible cardiac patient, have your resuscitation medications and equipment set up and ready to go. If the patient goes into arrest, the appropriate action can be taken with a minimum of confusion.

What Not To Do:

1. Do not initiate CPR on an obviously dead patient.
2. Do not initiate CPR under direct enemy fire. A patient in cardiopulmonary arrest during a firefight is dead.
3. Do not touch the patient while AED is analyzing the cardiac rhythm.
4. Do not use the "Analyze" function on an AED while in a moving ground vehicle or during moderate/heavy turbulence if in an aircraft
5. Do not leave your patient alone. Patients with acute myocardial infarctions can develop a malignant dysrhythmia (frequently VT or VF) without warning.
6. Do not assume that a "normal" ECG rules out heart disease as a cause of chest pain. It is reasonable to repeat the ECG within 5-10 minutes.
7. Do not assume that all "heartburn" pain is due to indigestion. In particular, do not assume that pain relieved with a "GI Cocktail" is non-cardiac in origin.
8. Do not withhold aspirin if there is a chance of cardiac chest pain. Most people can tolerate a single dose of aspirin without difficulty. Exceptions are cases of true aspirin allergy, asthma with aspirin sensitivity, and active ulcer, GI bleeding or hemorrhagic stroke.

Resuscitation Algorithms:
Cardiac resuscitation algorithms have been developed by the American Heart Association. *See* http://heart.org for more information.

Chapter 2: Blood: Introduction
COL Richard Tenglin, MC, USA (Ret)

Blood is made up of solid (cellular) and liquid (plasma) components. Cellular elements originate from bone marrow, and may be broken down as follows: white blood cells (WBCs) that fight infection, red blood cells (RBCs) that transport oxygen and platelets that stop bleeding. Symptoms result due to low numbers of cells or deficient cell function (which paradoxically may occur with increased numbers of abnormal cells, such as with leukemia), or when cell numbers build up to such a point that they obstruct blood flow. Low cell numbers are caused immunoglobulins, electrolytes, protein and water. Evaluation of blood disorders often requires performing a spun hematocrit and a Wright (Camco Quik Stain) stained peripheral smear.

Chapter 2: Blood: Anemia
Col Richard Tenglin, MC, USA (Ret)

Introduction: Anemia refers to an abnormally low amount of the oxygen-carrying protein hemoglobin (may also have low number or volume of red cells) in peripheral blood. "Hematocrit" is the percent volume of whole blood occupied by the red cells, and is determined by spinning a sample of blood and measuring the volume of the "packed" red cells divided by the total volume of the sample. It is a rough measure of the amount of oxygen-carrying protein (hemoglobin) in the sample, but is subject to many problems with technique that can lead to numbers that do not reflect the true hemoglobin content of blood. Modern Coulter Counters used in clinical labs actually measure the amount of hemoglobin, and calculate, but do not actually measure, the hematocrit. The SOF medic will actually measure the hematocrit, but must be aware that bad technique (not spinning the sample sufficiently), or some diseases will give results that do not reflect the actual hemoglobin content of the patient's blood. Anemia may be acute (traumatic blood loss) or chronic (due to chronic disease), and results from either increased loss/destruction of red cells or failure of the bone marrow to produce sufficient quantities of hemoglobin/red cells to make up for normal red cell loss. Anemia can be determined by a spun hematocrit. The procedure for obtaining a hematocrit and "normal" values are specific to the machine used. Normal hemoglobin levels differ among ethnic populations and between men and women, with males and whites averaging higher values. Worldwide, the most common cause of acquired anemia is iron deficiency due to chronic blood loss from hookworm and menstruation. Other important causes are lack of important nutrients (protein, Vitamin B12, folic acid) and suppression of the bone marrow from chronic infection or inflammation. The presence of sickle cell disease or sickle cell trait is an increased risk factor for potentially life-threatening complications during strenuous exercise or exposure to hypoxic environments (altitude). The causes of anemia are extensive and beyond the ability of the medic to accurately diagnose in the field environment.

Subjective: **Symptoms**
Acute: Lightheadedness, pallor, shock, syncope, altered mental status.
Chronic: Lethargy, fatigue and decreased energy, rapid heartbeat and shortness of breath/dyspnea with exertion.
Focused History: *Have you had headaches, feeling tired, told you looked pale? When did you first notice the symptoms?* (Is this an acute or chronic problem?) *Have you had vomiting or diarrhea?* (blood in vomit, or black, tarry stools with GI bleeding) *Have you had recent trauma?* (abdominal trauma risk of rupture of the spleen) *Where have you traveled recently?* (increased risk of infection, eg, malaria, hookworm) *Have you made any changes to your diet? What is your diet?* (possible nutritional deficiencies) *Have you had a recent pregnancy or change in menstrual blood loss?* (iron deficiency anemia, especially in developing countries)

Objective: Signs

Using Basic Tools: Acute: shock, hypotension, weak pulse, syncope, altered mental status. Chronic (compensated for intravascular volume loss): pale skin, mucous membranes (eyelids, under the tongue), nail beds and palm creases (compare color of normal palmar crease to patient's).

Using Advanced Tools: Labs: Spun hematocrit or hemoglobin; stool for occult blood; peripheral smear (see Laboratory Procedures Chapter on the electronic version)

Assessment: Differential Diagnosis

Bacterial infection: Peripheral smear of patient with fever and chills with elevated total white blood cell (WBC) count with great preponderance of polymorphonuclear leukocytes (PMNs).

Viral infection: Fever, plus or minus chills, malaise with peripheral blood smear showing significantly low lymphocytes (to include HIV and others).

Parasitic infection: Increased eosinophils with history of risk to exposure to parasites, (eg, visceral larval migrans or chlamydia). Hypersensitivity or allergic reactions: History of exposure to allergen. Peripheral blood smear shows increased number of eosinophils.

Increased basophils: Uncommon (suggest a problem with the stain or staining procedure)

Folic acid or vitamin B12 deficiency: Macrocytosis, history to suggest absorption problem or dietary deficiency

Iron deficiency: Microcytosis, history of blood loss (pregnancy, chronic blood in stools, abnormal menstrual flow)

Thalassemia: Microcytosis, anisocytosis, poikilocytosis and target cells

"Sickle cell conditions: Banana or "sickle" shaped cells. May have family history or history to suggest previous "sickle cell crisis". People with sickle cell disease or sickle cell trait are at increased risk of life-threatening symptoms during strenuous exercise and or exposure to hypoxic (altitude) environments.

Note: Confirmatory testing for these anemias is beyond the scope of the SOF medic. Unusual hemoglobins or hemoglobin levels may be common within certain ethnic groups. Attempting to correct these presumed anemias is inappropriate.

Plan:

Treatment

1. Iron supplementation is appropriate only for menstruating females and patients whose stool is positive for occult blood (requires additional studies to identify underlying cause). Iron supplementation is not otherwise appropriate without laboratory determination of iron deficiency.
2. Correct obvious nutritional deficiencies and treat infections or inflammation.
3. Blood replacement in the face of rapid loss is addressed in Part 8: Procedures: Chapter 30: Field Blood Transfusion.
4. Treat acute sickle crisis with:
   A. Fluids: orally if possible and IV if needed – 3-4L/day in adults
   B. Liberal use of medications for pain. Selection of medications is determined by the severity of the pain. NSAIDs like **ibuprofen**, **acetaminophen** with **codeine**, or IV **morphine** are appropriate for mild, moderate and severe pain, respectively, and should be continued until pain levels decrease. See Part 8: Procedures: Chapter 30: Pain Assessment and Control
   C. Treatment of predisposing conditions, such as infections
   D. Steroids and antibiotics are not routinely indicated.

Note: No non-US sources of blood can be trusted for accuracy of blood types, freedom from infection, or deterioration from improper storage. US Embassies can often provide information on where the safest blood products may be obtained within a specific country or region, but use of these products always entails a significant risk of both immediate and delayed life-threatening consequences.

Patient Education

General: The medic should inform the patient whether of not a clear cause of the anemia has been found, and what specific next steps are required for diagnosis and management.

Activity: Activities that cause symptoms (eg, lightheaded, fatigue) should be limited.

Diet: A healthy diet needs to be maintained so that deficiencies in diet do not arise during treatment for the anemia. Other dietary modifications may be required based on definitive diagnosis of type of anemia present.

Medications: Dark stools and constipation are typical of iron repletion.

No Improvement/Deterioration: Worsening of symptoms or failure of symptoms to improve require evaluation.

Follow-up Actions

Evacuation/Consultation Criteria: Evacuate patients with acute anemia and acute sickle crisis after initial stabilization. There is usually no need to evacuate patients with other anemias. Consult hematologist as needed.

Chapter 3: Respiratory: Common Cold (Viral Upper Respiratory Tract Infections

COL Duane Hospenthal, MC, USA

Introduction: Hundreds of viruses and bacteria can infect the mucous membranes, leading to symptoms which included nasal congestion, sore throat, and cough (see Part 3: General Symptoms: Cough; ENT Problems: Pharyngitis, Adult; Part 5: Specialty Areas: Chapter 12: Adenovirus & Infectious Mononucleosis). This section focuses on the relatively mild, acute viral upper respiratory tract infections (URI) called colds. URIs are most commonly acute localized infections secondary to rhinovirus which involve the nose and throat. The frequency of these infections generally decreases with age, 5-7 episodes a year in preschoolers, 2-3 per year in adults.

Subjective: Symptoms

General: Rhinitis (clear secretions) and nasal congestion are common. May also suffer malaise, sneezing, scratchy or sore throat, cough, hoarseness, and headache. Fever is less common.

Focused History: Have you had a fever? (URIs are typically associated with normal or low-grade temperature increases.) Do you have a headache? (Mild headache that worsens upon standing is typical; severe headache signals other potential illness.) Where is the *headache?* (If located over sinuses and worsens when head is lowered, may have sinusitis with or without cold.) *Do you have a productive cough?* (Cough associated with colds are generally non-productive or produce only clear mucus.) *Is the cough worse at night or when you lie flat?* (typical for post-nasal drip from cold, sinusitis, allergic or irritant rhinitis) *Do you have itchy or watery eyes?* (Itchy, watery eyes is more typical of allergies.) *How long have you had the symptoms?* (Colds usually do not last longer than a few days, and not over 2 weeks.) *How often do you get colds?* (Frequent colds may suggest allergies, increased susceptibility to infection due to immunocompromise, anatomical defect, etc.) *What makes the symptoms better or worse?* (Medications including decongestants and acetaminophen may improve symptoms.)

Objective: Signs
Using Basic Tools: Inspection: Secretions in nose; inflamed nasal mucosa; pharyngeal erythema, with or without exudate; normal to low-grade fever (temperature increase) Palpation: Non-tender sinuses (tender sinuses are seen in sinusitis) Auscultation: Clear chest
Using Advanced Tools: Otoscope: Eardrums appear normal with no fluid behind them; Labs: Monospot negative; WBC with differential is normal or may demonstrate an increase in atypical lymphocytes.

Assessment: Differential Diagnosis
Influenza: Is characterized by fever and systemic symptoms such as myalgias. Cold symptoms are much more mild and are limited to the nasopharynx.
Allergic rhinitis: Recurrent and/or seasonal symptoms of itchy eyes and/or nose; increased tearing and/or watery nasal discharge, sneezing, due to postnasal drip, nasal membranes pale or violaceous and swollen
Irritant rhinitis: Non-seasonal history of exposure to irritant, rhinorrhea without ocular symptoms or sore throat
Sinusitis: Tender sinuses; red, swollen nasal membranes; green or yellow discharge from nose and throat; can follow a cold
Diphtheria: Seen typically in children but can attack non-immune adults; gray membrane may be seen on pharynx.
Adenovirus: Fever, pharyngitis, and/or conjunctivitis; usually in epidemics in non-immune recruits or displaced persons
Streptococcal pharyngitis: Erythematous pharynx with exudate about tonsils, cervical lymphadenopathy, often with fever
Gonococcal pharyngitis: Often asymptomatic, but may have sore red throat, painful swallowing and history of exposure

Plan:
Treatment
1. Treatment is based on symptom control or relief.
2. Use decongestants to relieve nasal congestion. **Oxymetazoline** nasal spray 0.05% solution. Use for no more 3 days, or just at night, to avoid rebound congestion. Adults and children ages 6 and up: 1-3 sprays/nostril q12h. **Pseudoephedrine:** Adults, 60mg po q6h; Children 2-6 years, 15mg q6h; 6-12 years, 30mg po q6h.
3. **Ibuprofen** 200-600mg po q8h or **acetaminophen** 350-700mg po q4-6h are commonly used for symptomatic relief of pain and fever.
4. **Nasal ipratropium bromide** (nasal **Atrovent** 0.06% in adults, 0.03% in children) 2 sprays/nostril tid or qhs has been shown to reduce local symptoms and shorten duration of rhinorrhea symptoms by one day.
5. Antibiotics are not indicated unless secondary bacterial infection occurs.

Patient Education
General: Infections can spread via airborne droplets (cough, sneeze) and contact (contaminated hands and objects). The usual course of a cold is 3-7 days; incubation period is 1-3 days.
Activity: Rest is important to speed recovery. Strenuous activity can delay recovery.
Medication: Use based on symptoms.
Prevention: Hand washing can reduce transmission.
No Improvement/Deterioration: Return if symptoms worsen or do not resolved in 2 weeks, or if fever develops.

Follow-up Actions
Return Evaluation: Evaluate for alternative diagnoses and complications, including secondary bacterial infection, if still symptomatic after 72 hours or if fever develops.
Evacuation/Consultation Criteria: Evacuation not usually necessary. Consult primary care physicians as needed.

Chapter 3: Respiratory: Influenza
COL Duane Hospenthal, MC, USA

Introduction: Influenza virus infection of the upper and lower respiratory tract (ie, nose, throat, lungs), the "flu", typically presents with sudden-onset fever, chills, headache, and fatigue. While people are able to continue most activities with a cold virus, influenza almost always impacts ability to perform typical tasks (mission capability). Elderly patients, infants, expectant mothers (3rd trimester), the immunosuppressed, and patients with chronic heart and lung diseases more frequently suffer life-threatening complications, such as secondary bacterial pneumonia. 30,000-50,000 people die annually in the US due to influenza.

Subjective: Symptoms
Fever, chills, malaise, headache, fatigue, and sore throat. Muscle aches (myalgias) of the back, arms, and legs are especially prominent symptoms.
Focused History: *Have you been exposed to anyone with similar symptoms?* (Incubation period is 1-4 days, average 2, from exposure to symptoms.) *Did your illness begin suddenly?* (Acute onset of fever and illness is typical of influenza, but not of viral upper respiratory tract infections [URI/common cold]). *Were you vaccinated for the flu this season?* (Influenza is much less common in vaccinated persons.)

Objective: Signs
Using Basic Tools: Vital signs: Fever often runs higher than 101°F but typically subsides within 3 days. Inspection: No rash. Palpation: Muscle tenderness is common. Auscultation: Clear chest (Wheezes occur in patients with known asthma or in 10% of cases of viral influenza.)

Using Advanced Tools: Otoscope: Eardrums appear normal with no fluid behind them. Labs: Monospot negative; WBC without leukocytosis.

Assessment: Differential Diagnosis

Common cold: The common cold is not characterized by fever or systemic symptoms such as myalgias. Symptoms limited to the nasopharynx.

Leptospirosis and rickettsial diseases: Also present with sudden-onset fever and myalgias; look for exposure history

Atypical pneumonia (see Part 4: Organ Systems: Chapter 3: Pneumonia): Fatigue, mild respiratory symptoms.

Infectious mononucleosis: Positive Monospot; less acute onset, malaise, sore throat, swollen cervical lymph nodes.

Sinusitis: Tender sinuses; red, swollen nasal membranes; green or yellow discharge from nose and throat; tooth pain; can follow a cold or complicate allergic rhinitis.

Adenovirus: Fever, pharyngitis, and/or conjunctivitis; usually in epidemics in non-immune military recruits or displaced persons.

Plan:

Treatment

1. **Oseltamivir** 75mg po bid or **zanamivir** 2 oral inhalations (10mg) daily x 5 days started within 2 days of the onset of symptoms. Avoid zanamivir use in persons with asthma. Oseltamivir is approved for children 1 year of age or older, zanamivir for $\geq$7 years. Oseltamivir is dosed based on weight in children (<40kg). **Amantadine** or **rimantadine** are both dosed 100mg bid po for 3-5 days, started within 2 days of the onset of symptoms. Because of resistance to this class of antivirals, neither is recommended currently in the US. Antivirals can be used for prophylaxis during outbreaks, especially in high-risk populations (ie, nursing homes, daycare, the immunocompromised). Length of therapy is usually at least 2 weeks or 1 week after end of outbreak. Oseltamivir is given at 75mg po once daily for prophylaxis; zanamivir is given at its regular treatment dose.
2. **Ibuprofen, naproxen,** and other NSAIDS, as well as **acetaminophen** may be used symptomatic relief of fever and arthralgia.

Patient Education

General: Infections can spread via airborne droplets (cough, sneeze) and contact (contaminated hands and objects). The usual course of influenza is 3-7 days in adults. Persons are infectious from 1 day before symptoms until about 5 days into the illness.

Activity: Rest is important to speed recovery. Strenuous activity can delay recovery.

Medication: Avoid aspirin therapy in children because of risk of Reye syndrome.

Prevention: Hand washing can reduce transmission. Vaccination will prevent specific strains of influenza, but not all influenza. The vaccine cannot cause influenza, but some side effects (myalgia, headache) may mimic mild influenza or cold symptoms. Two types of vaccine are currently available. These include the classic trivalent inactivated (killed), IM administered vaccine (TIV) and a newer live attenuated, nasally administered vaccine (LAIV). Both of these are modified annually to contain the most likely disease-causing seasonal strains (2 influenza A and 1 influenza B strains). The TIV is approved for persons 6 months of age and older. The LAIV is approved for ages 2-49.

No Improvement/Deterioration: Return if symptoms worsen, recur, or do not resolve in two weeks. Recurrence of fever often indicates secondary bacterial infection (ie, pneumonia).

Follow-up Actions

Return Evaluation: Evaluate for alternative diagnoses and complications, including secondary bacterial infection, if still symptomatic after 72 hours of treatment (particularly if in high-risk group).

Evacuation/Consultation Criteria: Evacuation not usually necessary, except for moderate to severe influenza. Consult primary care physicians as needed.

Note: Avian influenza/pandemic influenza: The introduction of new strains of influenza into the population can result in pandemic disease. There is little cross-protection afforded by seasonal immunization to novel strains. Most new strains arise from avian influenza viruses. Key to these becoming potential pandemic strains is adaptation (mutation) to be easily transmitted between people. Currently, two similar H5N1 avian strains with high human mortality (>50%), but poor human-to-human transmission have spread from Asia into Europe and Africa. Human cases of avian influenza are chiefly associated with handling of infected birds. Influenza symptoms in persons with exposure to poultry in Asian and other risk locations (check World Health Organization website for most up-to-date information: www.who.int) should raise concern for infection with these potentially pandemic strains.

Chapter 3: Respiratory: Pneumonia

CPT Samuel Burkett, MC, USA

Introduction: Pneumonia, an infection of the lung, is the 6th leading cause of death in the United States, 4th leading cause of death worldwide, and is the most common infectious cause of death. Promptly assessing severity and avoiding delays in initiating treatment decreases the risk of mortality. Treatment should include antibiotics that cover typical and atypical organisms.

Subjective: Symptoms

Common symptoms include fever, rigors (shaking chills), night sweats, malaise, cough (may be either productive and non-productive), shortness of breath, and occasional myalgias. Less common symptoms include nausea, vomiting, abdominal pain, mental status changes, and pleuritic chest pain.

Focused History: *Do you have a cough? Are you coughing up any blood or sputum? What color is it?* (Green, brown, or bloody sputum can indicate a bacterial pathogen, although the absence of color does not exclude bacterial pneumonia.) *Does coughing or deep breathing make your chest hurt?* (Chest pain of pneumonia characteristically worsens with cough and deep breathing.) *Do you have fever or shaking chills?* (Atypical pneumonia can present with low-grade fever, but typical pneumonia classically presents with high fever that follow rigors.) *Do you have trouble breathing?* (may be mild and only with exertion or more severe and occurs at rest [typically seen with pneumonia]) *What other symptoms do have?* (Viral pneumonia is typically associated with other head and neck symptoms, such as runny nose and sore throat. Atypical pneumonia may be associated with nausea, vomiting or abdominal pain.)

Objective: **Signs**

Using Basic Tools: Vital signs: Fever>101°F or <96°F, Resting pulse>90 beats/min, Respiratory rate>18. Inspection: Conversational dyspnea (difficulty speaking in full sentences); central cyanosis with severe hypoxia (bluish discoloration of lips, extremities); splinted respirations; altered mental status; use of accessory respiratory muscles. Bullous myringitis on ear exam or erythema multiforme on skin exam may be suggestive of *Mycoplasma pneumoniae*. Auscultation and Percussion: Localized changes, such as decreased intensity of breath sounds, dullness to percussion, or rales/rhonchi may indicate lobar consolidation, collapsed lung, or a pleural effusion. Pulse oximetry <90%.

Using Advanced Tools: Labs: WBCs >12,000 cell/mm³ (typical pneumonia in immunocompetent patients); WBCs <4,000 cell/mm³ (atypical pneumonia in immunocompromised patients). Creatinine >1.2mg/dL or BUN >20mg/dL (indicating volume depletion) Sputum: Gram's stain (>25 WBC/LPF, <10 Epithelial cells/LPF indicates infection) CXR: Typically unilateral lobar alveolar infiltrate. Other findings include diffuse infiltrates (atypical pneumonia), multiple lobar involvement, interstitial infiltrates (viral pneumonia), cavitary lesions, rapid change from a prior radiograph, or the presence of a pleural effusion.

Note: The typical findings for pneumonia include fever, productive cough with purulent sputum, elevated white blood cell count, and unilateral infiltrate on chest x-ray. Absence of these findings does not rule out pneumonia.

Assessment:

Severity: Patients should be considered for hospitalization based on Pneumonia Severity Index (PSI) risk factors:
1. Patient's age >65, nursing home resident
2. Co-morbid conditions
   a. Neoplastic disease, congestive heart failure, central nervous system, renal or liver disease
3. Abnormal physical exam
   a. Altered mental status
   b. Pulse >125, RR >30, Sys BP <90
   c. Temp <95°F, or >104°F
   d. Pulse oximetry <90%
4. Intensive Care Unit admission criteria include mechanical ventilation, multilobar pneumonia, hypotension, or high oxygen requirement.

Differential Diagnosis

Pleurisy: Pneumonia is one of a number of conditions that can present with pleuritic chest pain. *See Part 4: Organ Systems: Chapter 3: Pleurisy*

Pulmonary Embolism: Acute onset with dyspnea and pleuritic chest pain; may include a low grade fever. *See Part 4: Organ Systems: Chapter 3: Deep Vein Thrombosis and Pulmonary Embolism*

Bronchitis: Auscultation of all lobes of the lung should still be possible despite transmitted upper airway sounds.

Plan:

Treatment

Always check for medication allergies
1. Outpatients (no PSI risk factors). May use <u>one</u> medication. Choose from:
   A. Macrolides: Safe in children and pregnant women
      1. **Azithromycin** 500mg po x1, then 250mg po once daily x 4 days
      2. **Erythromycin** 500mg po qid x 7 days
   B. Fluoroquinolones: Not for children <12 or pregnant women
      1. **Levofloxacin** 500mg po once daily x 7 days
      2. Do not use ciprofloxacin alone for pneumonia
   C. Tetracyclines: Not for children <12 or pregnant women
      1. **Doxycycline** 100mg po bid x 7-10 days

2. Outpatients (age >65 or one co-morbid condition) treat with 2 oral medications: One beta-lactam AND either a macrolide or doxycycline.
   A. Beta-lactam (2nd, 3rd, or 4th generation cephalosporin or extended spectrum penicillin) (one of the following)
      1. **Amoxicillin/Clavulanate** 875/125mg po bid x 10 days
      2. **Cefaclor** 500mg po tid x 10 days
      3. **Cefuroxime** 250mg po bid x 10 days
   PLUS
   B. Macrolide or Doxycycline (one of the following)
      1. **Azithromycin** 250mg po once daily x 10 days
      2. **Erythromycin** 500mg po qid x 10 days
      3. **Doxycycline** 100mg po bid x 10 days

3. Hospitalized patients (age >65 and co-morbid condition OR abnormal physical exam) Use combination IV beta-lactam AND macrolide. May use IV **levofloxacin** as a single agent. Start treatment as soon as possible. Change to a po antibiotic combination 24-48 hours after the patient clinically improves. Treat for a total of 10 days.

A. IV Beta-lactam (2nd, 3rd, or 4th generation cephalosporin or extended-spectrum penicillin) (one of the following):
1. **Ceftriaxone** 1g IV once daily
2. **Cefotaxime** 2g IV q6h
3. **Cefuroxime** 750mg IV q8h
4. **Ceftazidime** 2g q8h
5. **Piperacillin** 4g q6h

PLUS

B. IV Macrolide (one of the following)
1. **Erythromycin** 500mg IV q 6h
2. **Azithromycin** 500mg IV once daily

OR

C. IV Fluoroquinolone as single agent
1. **Levofloxacin** 750mg IV once daily

4. Other treatments
A. IV fluid: Give 1-2L of normal saline or lactated Ringers to everyone upon presentation. Give more IVF to maintain SBP >90
B. Supplemental oxygen to maintain pulse oximetry >90%
C. Antipyretics for fever above 101˚F or myalgias: **Acetaminophen** 650mg po q4h or **ibuprofen** 400mg po q4h
D. Bronchodilators for shortness of breath or wheezing in patients with asthma or chronic obstructive pulmonary disease
1. **Albuterol** metered dose inhaler 2 puffs q4h
2. **Albuterol** 2.5mL (via nebulizer) q4h

Patient Education
General: Stop smoking
Medication: Complete a full course of antibiotics as prescribed
Activity: Bedrest while on IV antibiotics. Limited activity for 1-2 weeks (temporary profile, T-2).
Prevention: Vaccinate all personnel and all recruits for influenza (yearly) and adenovirus. Vaccinate asplenic individuals with Pneumococcal vaccine (Pneumovax) and *Haemophilus influenzae* vaccine (Hib). Everyone over 65 years old should receive a Pneumovax vaccine once every 5 years.

Follow-up Actions
No Improvement/Deterioration: Return if symptoms do not improve in 48 hours.
Return Evaluation: Reevaluate or refer patients with delayed recovery. If poor response or late deterioration (5-10% of patients), suspect inadequate antibiotic dosing or a complication such as empyema or pleural effusion. All patients should have a follow-up chest x-ray in 6-8 weeks to ensure complete resolution of infiltrate.
Evacuation/Consultation Criteria: Evacuate if unstable, respiratory rate >30/min, falling blood pressure (SBP<90 or DBP<60) or increasing tachycardia after 2L of IVF, altered mental status, cyanosis or decreasing oxygen saturation. Evacuate patients with no underlying lung disease who require supplemental oxygen to higher level of care (a supplemental oxygen requirement in young healthy individual indicates severe pneumonia.) An increased amount of supplemental oxygen may be required while flying. Consult a pulmonologist, internal medicine, or infectious disease specialist for pleural effusion, empyema, and hemoptysis.

Chapter 3: Respiratory: Pleurisy
LTC Ethan E. Emmons, MC, USA

Introduction: "Pleurisy" (also called pleuritis) is acute inflammation of the parietal pleura, or the outer lining of the lung, that is manifest by a distinct type of chest pain called pleuritic pain. It is distinctive in its typical pattern of onset, location, and relationship to respiratory movements. Pleurisy may result from a number of injuries and/or conditions and treatment should focus on pain relief and treatment of the underlying condition. **Geographic Associations:** There is no geographic association with pleurisy per se. However, tuberculosis (TB) is a common cause of pleurisy and should be considered when operating in areas where TB is endemic. Parasitic diseases (amebiasis, paragonimiasis) are a less common cause but should also be considered where appropriate. **Seasonal Variation:** There is no seasonal variation with pleurisy per se. However, viral infections are a common cause of pleurisy and tend to occur commonly in the winter and spring seasons. **Risk Factors:** A prior history of pleuritis, especially if it was associated with a pneumothorax or pulmonary embolism. Travel to areas endemic for TB and parasitic diseases or a history of immunosuppression (HIV) should also be considered a risk factor.

Subjective: Symptoms
1. Localized distribution that is nearly always specific to one side or the other and follows intercostal nerve distributions
2. Clear relationship to respiratory movements with worsening during inspiration
3. Pain that may be described as "sharp" or "burning" when breathing quietly, but will worsen with deep breathing and can be excruciating when sneezing or coughing
4. Posturing of the patient to limit motion of the affected area. Additionally, pain from "diaphragmatic pleurisy" is often referred to the same side shoulder and neck. Patients with pleurisy or pleuritic pain will also present with symptoms specific to the underlying cause, such as fever, dyspnea, purulent sputum, h/o trauma, acute versus sub-acute onset, etc.
Focused History: *Where is the pain located and does it worsen when you take a deep breath?* (Localized pain that worsens with inspiration confirms the presence of pleurisy or pleuritic pain and would reduce the likelihood of pain secondary to a myocardial infarction or heart attack.) *Did the pain come on acutely or slowly over time?* (Acute onset of pleuritic pain suggests spontaneous or traumatic pneumothorax, traumatic hemothorax, pulmonary embolism, or pneumococcal/bacterial pneumonia. Gradual onset over several days is more suggestive of viral infections, TB, pleural effusions, or other infectious and/or inflammatory processes. Onset over weeks would suggest malignancy or connective tissue disease.) *Are you having significant dyspnea or shortness of breath?* (Dyspnea associated with pleuritic pain should raise suspicion for pulmonary embolism, pneumothorax, or bacterial pneumonia.) *Do you have*

symptoms of an upper respiratory infection either now or previously? (A recent respiratory illness or unknown febrile illness is suggestive of viral pleurisy, one of the most common causes of pleurisy.) Are you coughing up purulent sputum? (The presence of purulent sputum would suggest bacterial pneumonia.) Does the pain increase while supine and decrease when upright? (Pleuritic pain from pericarditis is often positional in this way.) Where have you traveled in the last 2 years? (TB, parasitic diseases and other rare bacterial diseases that cause pleuritic pain are often only endemic to specific regions.)

Objective Signs

Using Basic Tools: Vital Signs: Although almost any cause of pleuritic pain can cause at least a low grade fever, a temperature of >101° should suggest an infectious etiology such as bacterial pneumonia. Hypotension may be seen with pulmonary embolism, tension pneumothorax, severe trauma and patients severely ill from pneumonia. Myocardial infarction may reveal hypo- or hypertension. Most other patients will be mildly hypertensive secondary to pain. Inspection: Unless the pleuritic pain is secondary to a traumatic pneumothorax, in most cases there are no overt findings on simple inspection. One may occasional observe the patient maintaining one body position in an effort to minimize movement of the affected area. Palpation: The affected area may be tender to palpation. Percussion: The affected area will likely be painful for the patient. Findings with percussion may be secondary to known causes of pleurisy, such as hyper-resonance of the affected side in pneumothorax and dullness to percussion of the affected side in bacterial pneumonia or pleural effusion. Auscultation: Is the most important basic tool available in the evaluation of pleurisy. Unilateral decreased breath sounds should suggest pneumothorax. A localized decrease in breath sounds would be more consistent with a pneumonia or pleural effusion. The presence of a pleural rub (rough scratching sound heard with inspiration and expiration) or pericardial rub (rough scratching sound heard with the cardiac cycle) would suggest viral pleurisy or pericarditis, respectively. A myocardial infarction may reveal a new S3 heart sound on exam.

Using Advanced Tools: Pulse ox: A reduced oxygen saturation of <92% would be suggestive of pulmonary embolism or pneumonia. Pneumothorax may also occasionally show reduced oxygen saturation. ECG may be used to assess for evidence of myocardial infarction or pericarditis. Labs: WBC: If elevated and/or with neutrophilic shift, then consider infectious etiology (bacterial or parasitic). Feces for ova & parasites: If appropriate parasites identified, this may suggest the etiology of pleuritic pain. Microhematocrit determination: A reduced hematocrit in the setting of trauma without another obvious source of blood loss may suggest hemothorax.

Assessment: Differential Diagnosis See Part 3: General Symptoms: Chest Pain

Myocardial infarction (MI): Accurate history is most important since MI pain is often described as a sub-sternal squeezing or pressure with radiation to the neck or arm that is most often WITHOUT variation to respiration and most often cannot be reproduced by palpation. An ECG is the most beneficial test in assessing for an MI.

Pneumonia: Often includes pleuritic type chest pain, but there will be evidence of pulmonary infiltrate (decreased breath sounds) or infiltrate on CXR.

Pneumothorax: Acute onset of pleuritic chest pain, dyspnea and decreased breath sounds on auscultation.

Pulmonary embolism: Typically includes acute onset of pleuritic chest pain with significant dyspnea and possible history (prolonged immobilization) or signs (swollen lower leg)

Diving/Aerospace injuries: History of exposure to changes in atmospheric pressure. See Part 6: Operational Environment: Chapters 20 & 21

Rib fracture: Accurate history suggesting trauma and most often point tenderness to exam. Need to rule out pneumothorax by exam (equal and symmetric breath sounds present, equal resonance to percussion and no evidence of tracheal deviation).

Costo-chondral pain: May be secondary to muscle/chest wall injury or herpes zoster. Former can be determined by accurate history suggesting trauma or over exertion and by ruling out pneumothorax. Latter would present with pain in typically only one dermatomal or intercostal distribution and would be followed by the associated skin lesions a few days later.

Plan

Diagnostic Tests: Diagnostic testing should focus on identifying the underlying cause of the patient's pleuritic pain.

Procedures: Any treatment procedures must be based on underlying etiology and are described elsewhere. A tension pneumothorax must be treated by emergent needle decompression or chest tube placement. Non-tension pneumothorax may be treated by needle aspiration or chest tube placement. Suspected pleural effusions or hemothorax should be assessed radiographically and drained if indicated.

Treatment

Primary:

Primary treatment should be directed at control of the pleuritic chest pain, and treatment of the underlying cause. Pain control for viral pleurisy, pericarditis, and mild to moderate pain may be accomplished with NSAIDs such as **indomethacin** 100mg po tid or **naproxen** 500mg po bid. More severe pain may require the use of narcotics such as **oxycodone/aspirin** (1 tab po q6h prn) or **morphine** 1-2mg IV q4-6h prn (see Part 8: Procedures: Chapter 30: Pain Assessment and Control). Antibiotics/anti-parasitics should be given empirically based on suspected organisms (see Part 4: Organ Systems: Chapter 3: Pneumonia). Procedures should be performed as discussed previously (See appropriate section for further discussion of specific procedure).

Alternative:

Corticosteroids (**prednisone** 50mg po q day x 5-7 days and then tapered over 4-6 weeks) may be given to those with viral pleurisy or pericarditis and who are intolerant or experience no improvement with NSAIDs. Corticosteroids generally should not be used in cases of suspected bacterial or parasitic infection.

Empiric: If the etiology of the pleurisy is unknown, empiric treatment (initially with NSAIDs) of pain control is indicated

Primitive: Attempt to control pain by whatever modalities are available.

Patient Education

General: Education should be geared toward underlying cause. Viral pleurisy is expected to resolve on its own over 1-2 weeks.

Activity: Activity as appropriate for the underlying cause or as tolerated.

Diet: No special diet indicated.

Medications: NSAIDs may cause stomach upset and should be taken with food. Long-term NSAID use increases the risk of bleeding ulcers and kidney disease. Prednisone may promote weight gain, fluid retention, euphoria, difficulty sleeping, easy bruisability, increased risk of bleeding ulcers and increased susceptibility to infections. Antibiotics may cause allergic reactions and other drug specific reactions.

Prevention and Hygiene: Underlying disease specific. Suspected tuberculosis or other infectious causes should be addressed appropriately (ie, isolation, droplet precautions, precautions handling feces, etc.).

No Improvement/Deterioration: Persistent pain and/or symptoms despite "appropriate" therapy may suggest misdiagnosis and a need for reassessment. Similarly, in a patient with pneumonia a persistent fever with increasing lethargy and malaise despite antibiotics is suggestive of deterioration or misdiagnosis.

Follow-up Actions

Return Evaluation: If indicated by the underlying etiology or if the pleuritic pain does not improve.

Evacuation/Consultation Criteria: Evacuation/consultation should be considered for any pneumothorax or suspected pleural effusion or pulmonary embolism. Patients with pneumonia should also be considered for consultation if they do not show rapid improvement on appropriate antibiotics. Any pleuritic pain that does not improve despite appropriate treatment should also be referred for evaluation.

Note: Pleurisy or pleuritic pain should be considered a symptom of some underlying process and not considered a primary diagnosis.

Chapter 3: Respiratory: Pneumomediastinum
COL Kenneth R. Kemp, MC, USA

Introduction: Pneumomediastinum is a condition that occurs when air tracks along bronchovascular sheaths of the lung into the mediastinum. It most often occurs as a result of barotrauma, defined as abnormally high pressure within the airways of the lungs. Barotrauma may occur with a vigorous Valsalva maneuver, such as could occur during childbirth or with inhalation of illicit drugs. It can occur with overly vigorous bagging during bag-valve-mask resuscitation, as a result of over expansion of the alveoli during mechanical ventilation, or during decompression after diving. Pneumomediastinum may also occur after trauma resulting in tracheobronchial disruption or fracture of the bones around the upper airways. Esophageal rupture associated with recurrent vomiting may also cause pneumomediastinum. Occasionally, extrathoracic air can enter the chest and travel along tissue planes into the mediastinum such as could occur after chest tube placement. Rarely, it occurs after teeth extraction or dental drilling. Pneumomediastinum must be considered as a possibility whenever a patient has suffered trauma to the chest, there has been particular difficulty in securing an emergent airway, it is difficult to bag a patient during bag-valve-mask ventilation, or high airway pressures are detected during mechanical ventilation. Patients most often have chest pain when pneumomediastinum occurs. However, patients who are sedated on mechanical ventilation may not have any symptoms so a high index of suspicion is required when risk factors for this condition are present. While pneumomediastinum itself may not warrant emergent therapy, its presence should alert the provider that barotrauma has occurred or that tracheal disruption might be present in cases of trauma. A diligent search for the underlying cause and very close monitoring is necessary when pneumomediastinum is detected.

Subjective: Symptoms

Within minutes to hours after the inciting event, the patient may have increased shortness of breath (SOB), chest pain, or rapid swelling of the face and neck. The chest pain may be described as substernal and pleuritic with radiation into the back, neck, shoulder, or arms. The patient may have dysphagia (difficulty swallowing) or dysphonia (difficulty speaking) due to air tracking in the neck.

Focused History: *Have you been diving?* (Pneumomediastinum may occur within minutes after diving.) *Are you having SOB? Do you have chest pain?* (In the proper setting, the patient may develop rapid symptoms as described previously. Often, patients may be unable to give a good history due to acute distress or sedation. Not uncommonly, patients may be asymptomatic.) *How long have you had these symptoms?* (A rapid deterioration after bagging, intubation, trauma, Valsalva maneuver, or chest tube placement or a sudden increase in airway pressures during mechanical ventilation should alert the provider to the possibility of pneumomediastinum.)

Objective: Signs

Using Basic Tools: Acute illness: Vital signs: Low grade fever, tachypnea, tachycardia, hypertension or hypotension. Inspection: Subcutaneous emphysema may be present in the upper torso and neck, detected by the finding of crepitus (a crackling sound or sensation when palpating the skin). Marked and rapid swelling of the face, neck, or upper torso may also be present. Auscultation: Most often will be normal with pneumomediastinum alone, but Hamman's crunch may be present, which is a crunching or clicking sound heard over the precordium during the heartbeat. If pneumomediastinum occurs with a pneumothorax, breath sounds will be decreased on the side of the injury. Pneumomediastinum does not present as a chronic illness. If it does not resolve, it may lead to acute pneumothorax or pneumopericardium, both of which can lead to cardiovascular collapse.

Using Advanced Tools: CXR: A thin line of radiolucency along the left heart border is the most common finding. Air outlining the borders of the trachea, esophagus, aorta and great vessels, and/or the pericardium would be indicative of pneumomediastinum. A continuous line of radiolucency from one hemidiaphragm to the other underneath the heart, the continuous diaphragm sign, is also indicative of pneumomediastinum. Patients who are on mechanical ventilation may have high airway pressures when on a volume cycled mode.

Assessment:

Definitive diagnosis is made by the proper clinical context along with the CXR abnormalities as described above.

Differential Diagnosis

Pneumothorax: Symptoms may be similar but the CXR will differentiate a pneumothorax, which is lung collapse due to air escaping between the chest wall and the lung.

Pneumopericardium: Sudden cardiovascular collapse with distended neck veins and quiet heart sounds would indicate possible pneumopericardium. Also, a CXR will demonstrate air around the cardiac silhouette in pneumopericardium.

Pulmonary interstitial emphysema: This is a condition that occurs typically in newborns on mechanical ventilation within hours of birth. Air collects in the perivascular spaces and may precede pneumothorax or pneumomediastinum. It would not typically be found in the combat environment.

Esophageal rupture: In esophageal rupture, there is usually a history of recurrent vomiting or heaving and a CXR will show a pleural effusion with an air-fluid level: a hydropneumothorax.

Radiographic artifact: The CXR will suggest a pneumomediastinum but the clinical history and physical findings will not support the diagnosis. This may occur due to the effect of overlying skin folds or due to clothing or other items that are outside of the thorax.

Plan:

Treatment

Primary:

1. Initial therapy: Administer 100% oxygen if available, which may accelerate resorption of mediastinal air.
2. Reduce any elevation in airway pressure. This may require less vigorous bagging or a reduction in tidal volume if the patient is on mechanical ventilation.
3. Close observation in a monitored setting. Most cases will resolve spontaneously. Obtain serial CXRs q4-6h until stable, then at least once daily until resolved. If tracheobronchial disruption is suspected, evacuate immediately to Echelon III for bronchoscopy and/or surgical repair.
4. If symptoms progress to pneumothorax, perform emergent decompressive needle thoracostomy and/or insert chest tube(s).
5. For cases related to exposures to extreme changes in barometric pressure; *see Part 6: Operational Environments: Chapter 20 & 21*

Patient Education

General: Avoid potential inciting events and trauma as much as possible.

Activity: Bed rest in a closely monitored setting until pneumomediastinum is resolved.

Prevention: Avoid overly vigorous bagging. Use good technique during intubation, chest tube insertion, and tracheostomy.

No Improvement/Deterioration: Evaluate for pneumothorax or pneumopericardium. Evacuate to echelon III as soon as possible.

Follow-up Actions

Return Evaluation: Symptoms that do not improve should be referred for specialty care and additional special studies.

Evacuation/Consultation Criteria: Evacuate patients who cannot complete the mission, or whose symptoms do not resolve. Consult internist or pulmonologist prn.

Chapter 3: Respiratory: Pneumothorax
COL Jackie A. Hayes, MC, USA

Introduction: A pneumothorax is a collection of air that occurs in the pleural space and causes collapse of the lung. The pleural space is the potential space between the 2 layers of pleura, the parietal (covering the chest wall) and visceral (covering the lung) pleura. Under normal conditions, the pressure within the pleural space is less than that within the lungs. When air enters the pleural space, the pressure increases to greater than the pressure of the lung and the lung collapses. This collapse can be partial or complete depending on the amount of air within the pleural space and the pleural pressure. A pneumothorax can occur spontaneously with no identifiable reason or they may be caused by specific injury or trauma to the lung or chest wall. Frequently they are caused by a defect in the periphery of the lung known as bullae. This area may be more vulnerable to rupture when there are pressure changes within the thorax. A spontaneous pneumothorax can occur with extreme changes in pressure of the lungs that may occur with activities such as scuba diving or sky diving. When there is no known underlying lung disease and a spontaneous pneumothorax occurs, it is known as a primary spontaneous pneumothorax. If there is underlying lung disease such as emphysema, cystic fibrosis, cavitary pneumonia or tuberculosis, it is known as a secondary spontaneous pneumothorax. The most common types of trauma to cause a pneumothorax are penetrating injuries such as stab wounds or gunshot wounds but a pneumothorax can occur with blunt force trauma especially if there is an associated rib fracture. When a pneumothorax causes increased thoracic pressure, it can lead to a shift in the structures within the mediastinum. This leads to compromise of cardiopulmonary function and is life threatening if not immediately treated. **Risk Factors:** The most common risk factors for pneumothorax are penetrating and blunt trauma to the chest. Secondary spontaneous pneumothorax most commonly occurs in individuals with underlying bullous or cystic lung disease such as emphysema or cystic fibrosis. Individuals with primary spontaneous pneumothorax are usually younger males most commonly in their 20s and rarely over 40 years old. A history of smoking has also been associated with an increased risk of primary spontaneous pneumothorax. Medical and surgical procedures that require penetration of the thorax are risk factors for pneumothorax as well. Mechanical ventilation can cause pneumothorax due to increased intrathoracic pressures.

Subjective: Symptoms

Most commonly present with chest pain (90%) and dyspnea (80%). Symptoms are usually sudden in onset and chest pain is most commonly pleuritic with a sharp or stabbing character. Patients may also have increased anxiety and cough. Some individuals may have more nonspecific symptoms such as fatigue and malaise.

Focused History: *Are you having shortness of breath?* (Most patients with a pneumothorax present with shortness of breath [SOB]. The SOB usually acute in onset but may also be gradual in onset. In many cases, the SOB continues to worsen overtime and may become severe.) *Do you have chest pain?* (Most patients with pneumothorax will also have chest pain. It may develop rapidly. Some patients may also describe neck or back pain. Many patients may have difficulty providing a good history due to severity of symptoms and acute distress.) *How long have you had these symptoms?* (Many patients will have a rapid onset of symptoms and distress after an inciting event such as trauma, medical or surgical procedures or while on mechanical ventilation. The presence of rapid onset of symptoms and a history of a potential inciting event should cause concern for the presence of a pneumothorax. Even if there is no history of a potential risk factor, a spontaneous pneumothorax should be considered.)

Objective: Signs

Using Basic Tools: Acute illness: Vital signs: Tachypnea, tachycardia, hypertension or hypotension. A pulsus paradoxus (*see Part 4: Organ Systems: Chapter 1: Pericarditis*) may be present. Palpation: Subcutaneous emphysema may be present in the upper torso and neck, detected by the finding of crepitus (a crackling sound or sensation when palpating the skin). Percussion: There may be hyperresonance (a hollow sound) over the involved side. Inspection: There may be asymmetric expansion of the chest wall. Marked and rapid swelling of the face, neck, or upper torso may also be present. Patients may also be diaphoretic, have cyanosis or display splinting of the chest wall (to relieve pain). With a tension pneumothorax, there may be jugular vein distention (JVD) and shift of the trachea to the opposite side of the pneumothorax. Auscultation: Breath sounds may be decreased or absent on the affected side.

Using Advanced Tools: CXR will show a pleural line that is moved away from the chest wall. Between the pleural line and the chest wall, there will be an area that will be without lung markings. This indicates the presence of a pneumothorax and associated collapsed lung. In supine patients, an area of radiolucency along the costophrenic angle may be seen. This is known as a deep sulcus sign.

Assessment:

Diagnosis of pneumothorax should be suspected in someone presenting with symptoms of chest pain and SOB with associated findings on exam. The diagnosis is confirmed with CXR or in some cases, chest computed tomography. Tension pneumothorax is a clinical diagnosis and the diagnosis should be made if the appropriate symptoms and exam findings (hyperresonance, decreased breath sounds, tracheal shift and JVD) are present.

Differential Diagnosis:

Pleurisy: Is suggested by the symptoms and clinical scenario. Physical exam may reveal dullness to percussion or a friction rub on auscultation. Signs of a pneumothorax would be absent such as hyperresonance to percussion and crepitus. CXR would not show evidence of a pneumothorax but it may show evidence of pneumonia which can cause pleurisy.

Pulmonary embolism (PE): Cannot be effectively ruled out using basic tools. If an alternative diagnosis such as pneumonia or pneumothorax can be made using basic tools, the possibility of pulmonary embolism is decreased. CXR may reveal an alternative diagnosis such as pneumothorax or pneumonia but it is not diagnostic of PE. Computed tomography of the chest, ventilation-perfusion scanning or pulmonary angiogram is required for definitive diagnosis.

Myocardial infarction (MI): Obtaining a reliable history is essential in ruling out acute MI. The pain will be often described as a substernal squeezing or pressure with radiation to the neck or arm that is usually without respiratory variation and not reproduced by palpation. An ECG is the most beneficial test in assessing for an MI. *See Part 4: Organ Systems: Chapter 1: Acute Coronary Syndrome (Acute Myocardial Infarction and Unstable Angina)*

Pneumomediastinum: Signs and symptoms associated with a pneumomediastinum are similar to those of a pneumothorax. On physical examination, crepitus may be present but there will not be the presence of hyperresonance on percussion or decreased breath sounds. CXR will not show evidence of a pneumothorax.

Esophageal spasm or rupture: Although patients may present with acute onset of chest pain, SOB is not a common symptom with esophageal spasm or rupture. The physical signs of pneumothorax are also absent. Some patients with esophageal rupture may also have a pneumomediastinum and the signs and symptoms or this diagnosis may be present. The CXR may show evidence of a pneumomediastinum but it will not be consistent with a pneumothorax.

Pericarditis: Chest pain may be present but there will be no signs of a pneumothorax on physical examination. ECG can be helpful in making a diagnosis of pericarditis and may show diffuse ST segment elevation. CXR will be negative for evidence of a pneumothorax.

Radiographic artifact: In some situations, radiographic artifact may suggest the presence of a pneumothorax. In many cases, the patient with radiographic artifact will not have any other signs or symptoms of a pneumomediastinum. The most common cause of radiographic artifact mimicking pneumothorax is skin folds. One clue is that the skin fold will extend beyond the thorax or does not extend to the ribs. Also, pulmonary vessels can be seen extending beyond the skin fold which suggests that a pneumothorax is not present. If the patient is stable and treatment can be deferred, the patient should be repositioned and the radiograph should be repeated.

Plan:

Treatment

Primary:

1. Initial therapy: <u>Administer oxygen if available</u> and in the highest concentration available. This can accelerate resorption of the pneumothorax by 4-fold over room air and treat respiratory distress and hypoxia if present.
2. Treat the pneumothorax by placement of a chest tube (tube thoracostomy). Once the chest tube is placed, it should be attached to a pleural drainage system with suction or water seal. A one-way valve known as a Heimlich valve can also be used to drain the pneumothorax. If it is a spontaneous or iatrogenic pneumothorax that is small and stable (less than 15% of the hemithorax), it may be treated with observation only or in some cases, simple needle aspiration of the pneumothorax. Tension pneumothorax is a medical emergency that requires immediate evacuation of the pneumothorax. Initially this can be done by needle decompression pending placement of a chest tube. *See Part 8: Procedures: Chapter 30: Thoracostomy, Needle and Chest Tube*
3. <u>Reduce any elevation in airway pressure for patients receiving mechanical ventilation</u>. This may require a reduction in tidal volume if the patient is on mechanical ventilation or less vigorous bagging if they are being manually ventilated.
4. Close observation in a monitored setting. A small pneumothorax may resolve slowly with only supportive treatment. Serial CXRs should be obtained if possible to document stability and/or resolution
5. Patients with recurrent or non-resolving pneumothorax may need surgical treatment to close a defect in the pleura.

Primitive: A tension pneumothorax is life-threatening and a medical emergency. In this situation, a needle thoracostomy should be performed as soon as possible. In this procedure, a large bore needle or catheter is passed into the 2nd intercostal space at the midclavicular line. This will allow for partial decompression until a chest tube can be placed.

Patient Education

General: Patients with pneumothorax should avoid air travel unless a chest tube is in place as the air will expand at altitude and cause enlargement of the pneumothorax.

Activity: Bed rest initially in a closely monitored setting until pneumothorax is improved or resolving.

Prevention: For patients receiving mechanical ventilation, avoid high airway pressures and large tidal volumes. Avoid overly vigorous bagging during manual ventilation. Use proper technique during medical procedures in an attempt to avoid complications to include pneumothorax.

No Improvement/Deterioration: Evaluate for tension pneumothorax or associated hemothorax. If a chest tube has been placed make sure that the tubing has not become disconnected or dislodged allowing the pneumothorax to enlarge and develop into a tension pneumothorax.

Evacuate to higher levels of care as soon as possible.

Wound Care: Provide routine care of any traumatic wounds present. If a chest tube is placed, secure it with suture and cover with a sterile dressing to keep it clean and dry. Once the chest tube is removed, close the site with a suture.

Follow Up Actions
Return Evaluation: Patients should be followed closely until resolution of the pneumothorax. If a chest tube is in place, if the pneumothorax is resolved, stable and there is no longer an air leak, it should be placed to water seal. If the lung remains inflated on water seal for 24 hours or longer, the chest tube can be removed. If pneumothorax is recurrent, patients should be referred for specialty care for consideration of surgical treatment.

Evacuation/Consultation Criteria: In almost all cases, patients with a pneumothorax should be evacuated for more definitive management. If evacuation is by air, a chest tube should be in place to prevent enlargement or recurrence of the pneumothorax. Otherwise, evacuation should be by ground. Consult a surgeon, cardiothoracic surgeon or pulmonologist as needed.

Note: A tension pneumothorax is a medical emergency and is life-threatening. Diagnosis should be made by clinical criteria and a CXR should not be needed to confirm before treatment is initiated with needle thoracostomy/decompression and chest tube thoracostomy.

Chapter 3: Respiratory: Pleural Effusion
CPT Michael Perkins MC, USA & MAJ Christopher Lettieri, MC, USA

Introduction: A pleural effusion is fluid in the space between parietal pleura on the chest wall and visceral pleura around the lungs. If the fluid accumulation is large (>1/3 of the hemithorax or over 1-2L), it can interfere with the mechanical ability to breathe. The 2 major types are transudative effusions, which are passive fluid accumulations, and exudative effusions due to irritation and inflammation. Transudative effusions are usually bilateral, slightly greater on the right side and are usually caused by heart failure, low albumen in circulation, excessive volume replacement (IV fluids) and rapid loss of albumen in the urine (nephrotic syndrome). Exudative effusions are caused by inflammatory involvement (including infections, trauma and malignancies) of the overlying visceral pleura, which often results in acute pleurisy (chest pain with inspiration) and the leakage of serous fluid into the pleural space. The type of cells in the fluid may indicate the cause of the effusion. Exudative effusions are typically associated with an increased amount of protein or leukocytes resulting from the inflammatory condition.

Subjective: Symptoms
Stabbing or sharp chest pain with breathing or cough (pleuritic pain), chest pressure or tightness that changes with position, or shortness of breath (SOB) on exertion.

Focused History: *Have you had a recent respiratory illness?* (typical for an effusion) *Do you have chest pain during every deep breath?* (Chest pain worsens with inspiration.) *Do you have SOB? Have you had fever?* (indicates a complicated or infected effusion or empyema) *What makes the symptoms better?* (Pain may be minimized by shallow breathing, minimal talking or exercise, or by holding/lying on the affected side.)

Objective: Signs
Using Basic Tools: Inspection: May lean towards or lie on affected side, and use arms to support and minimize chest movement (splinted respirations). Palpation: Warm skin over affected area. Abnormally large or small liver with possible ascites. Peripheral edema in heart failure. Percussion: Dullness means a pleural effusion or empyema. Auscultation: Chest: Absent breath sounds over pleural effusion, although occasionally a pleural friction rub may be heard. If rales and rhonchi are heard, a pneumonic process such as pneumonia is possible. Heart: Extra sounds (murmurs, rubs and gallops) may indicate signs of cardiac failure.

Using Advanced Tools: Determining whether the effusion is transudative or exudative can help determine the underlying cause and required treatment. This requires special laboratory tests. If not available, grossly purulent fluid typically indicates an infection and should be drained by tube thoracostomy (*see following section*). Labs: Elevated WBC or increased neutrophils on differential supports infection; sputum for Gram's stain and culture; effusion fluid for Gram's stain and WBC differential. A large number of neutrophils containing bacteria indicate an empyema (*see Part 4: Organ Systems: Chapter 3: Empyema*) while large cells of abnormal shape may indicate cancer. Atypical lymphocytes can occur with viral infections. CXR: Effusion shadow overlying lungs, and possible enlarged heart.

Assessment: Differential Diagnosis
Transudative effusion: Congestive heart failure, liver failure (any cause), nephrotic syndrome (any cause)
Exudative effusion: Infection: bacterial (empyema), fungal, tuberculosis; cancer (lung or metastatic); collagen vascular disease: rheumatoid arthritis, lupus; vascular: pulmonary embolus; unknown: granulomatous

Plan:
Treatment
1. Treat the primary disorder if possible
   a. Give antibiotics for pneumonia. *See Part 4: Organ Systems: Chapter 3: Pneumonia*
   b. If a transudative effusion is suspected, give a trial of **furosemide** 20-60mg po q day or bid (if required)
2. Perform thoracentesis (*see following section*) to improve breathing, if **furosemide** ineffective or in the face of pneumonia that does not improve.

      a. Withdraw 30cc of fluid for diagnostic laboratory evaluation <u>or</u>

      b. Draw off the effusion if fluid accumulation compromises respiratory status. Try not to remove more than 1000cc of fluid in the first 24 hours (can repeat procedures). Removing too much fluid can cause rapid fluid shifts in the lung tissue, which worsens hypoxemia (newly expanded lung is poorly perfused) and causes hypotension.

      c. A chest tube thoracostomy MUST be performed if the fluid is infected, but is typically not indicated for other causes. *See Part 8: Procedures: Chapter 30: Thoracostomy, Needle and Chest Tube*

3. Administer supplemental oxygen since these patients are commonly hypoxic.

Patient Education
Activity: Bedrest with indwelling chest tube initially.
Diet: High protein diet unless liver failure is present, then diet must be modified to avoid hepatic encephalopathy

Follow-up Actions
Return Evaluation: Refer patients that do not improve for specialty care and additional special studies.
Evacuation/Consultation Criteria: Evacuate unstable patients, or those who require on-going thoracenteses. Consult internist or pulmonologist.

Chapter 3: Respiratory: Procedure: Thoracentesis
CPT Michael Perkins MC, USA & MAJ Christopher Lettieri, MC, USA

What: Thoracentesis is the removal of pleural fluid percutaneously by needle aspiration to determine the cause of fluid accumulation or to relieve the symptoms associated with the fluid accumulation.

When: Perform a diagnostic thoracentesis when the presence of fluid in the pleural space is confirmed by physical examination (and preferably by CXR), and the likelihood of bacterial infection in the fluid is high (worsening condition despite broad spectrum antibiotics, lying with affected side down, progressive fever and lethargy).

Risks: Thoracentesis is a relatively safe procedure; however, some relative contraindications include history of coagulopathy (increase risk of bleeding), pleural effusion of insufficient volume (less than one centimeter of fluid layering on lateral decubitus chest film), active skin infection where the needle will be inserted, and underlying severe respiratory disease.

Complications of thoracentesis include pneumothorax, bleeding, infection, puncture of abdominal organs, and pulmonary edema of the re-inflated lung. Re-expansion pulmonary edema can occur if too much fluid is removed too quickly. Typically, no more than 1000mL of fluid should be removed. The most common major complication is pneumothorax.

Thoracentesis can cause a pneumothorax in two ways: by introducing air through the back of the syringe or needle hub into the pleural space (it does not progress to complete pneumothorax and does not require treatment), or by an accidental puncture of the lung.

If the patient is symptomatic, keep him under observation and follow the patient's progress with a serial CXR. Normally the puncture in the lung seals and air is absorbed spontaneously. More severe leaks are caused by coughing or needle movement, which causes a larger tear in the lining of the lung. These injuries may require a chest tube to re-inflate the lung.

What You Need: Essential: 1½ inch needle 18–21 gauge (21 may be too small if pus is in the pleural space), 10-30cc syringe to aspirate fluid, topical antiseptic (iodine-based cleanser followed by alcohol wipe). Recommended: 1-2% lidocaine for SC anesthesia in a 10cc syringe with 23 gauge needle, sterile drape, sterile gloves, clamp, sterile laboratory tubes.

What To Do:
1. Determine the point of entry. The posterior approach is most common because the interspaces between ribs are wider in the back. The ideal location is the 7th or 8th interspace posteriorly, midway between the posterior axillary line and midline. This site avoids possible accidental puncture of the liver, spleen or diaphragm. Tap with finger and listen with or without a stethoscope to identify where the percussion becomes dull (height of pleural fluid accumulation). Mark this location by pressing the tip of an ink pen (point retracted) into the skin below where dullness begins and superior to any underlying rib (avoid the neurovascular bundle immediately below the inferior rib margin). Gently apply pressure for 30 seconds to leave a small red circle that will last during the procedure. Loculated or small effusions may not always be accessible with this approach and should be evacuated if possible for advanced care.
2. Have the patient straddle a chair backwards; resting their arms on the back of the chair.
3. Disinfect the skin around the insertion site and drape the area.
4. Anesthetize the tissues. Begin by anesthetizing the skin at the mark. Aspirate to ensure no blood return before injecting **lidocaine**, then advance slightly and repeat. Aim the needle towards the upper margin of the rib and anesthetize the top of the rib, then the parietal pleura. Advance the needle gently and carefully while keeping suction, then stop and inject lidocaine, and advance again. anesthesia needle is generally a 23–25 gauge, and you can use it to withdraw several cc's of fluid if you enter the pleural space, The confirming your landmarks for introduction of the larger needle and syringe.
5. Insert the thoracentesis needle with syringe. Aim for the top of the rib below your mark and inch your way past, continuing at a 30° angle downwards toward the pleural. A slight "give" will indicate that you have pierced the parietal pleura. Aspirate 50cc's of fluid or more (*see Part 4: Organ Systems: Chapter 3: Pleural Effusion*). The clamp may be used to stabilize the needle at the skin to prevent accidental additional penetration of the needle down to the lung.
6. Withdraw the needle and syringe.
7. Write a procedure note. Be sure to describe the site and approach used, the appearance of the fluid and how much fluid was removed.
8. Complications appear with in the first 24 hours. Have the patient remain in bed for at least 2 hours after the procedure, avoid coughing or lifting objects for 24 hours, and inform you immediately if they cough up blood, experience shortness of breath, dizziness, a tight feeling in the chest, or any other problems.
9. Send sample of fluid for the most important tests first, which are Gram's stain and differential count of inflammatory cells in a field setting.
10. Repeat as needed.

What Not To Do:
1. Do not move the plunger end of the syringe laterally during the procedure. This swings the needle around inside the patient, tearing the pleura and causing a large pneumothorax.
2. Do not take off the syringe and leave the needle hub in the patient. This can also result in pneumothorax, allowing air to enter the pleural space. If it is necessary to change syringes while leaving the needle in, have the patient "hum" to produce positive pleural pressure.

Chapter 3: Respiratory: Empyema
MAJ Thomas Zanders, MC, USA

Introduction: An empyema is a pleural effusion of pus caused by progression of infection into the pleural cavity. In approximately 60% of cases, the empyema is the life-threatening complication of pneumonia. Direct inoculation of the pleural cavity by penetrating chest trauma, esophageal trauma, thoracentesis or chest tube placement causes the remainder of cases. An empyema typically starts as sterile fluid associated with pneumonia (para pneumonic effusion) in which there is bacterial translocation into the fluid. This pleural infection produces significant inflammation. Aggressive treatment of an empyema must be rapidly initiated in order to reduce associated significant morbidity and mortality.

Subjective: Symptoms
Fever, chills, rigors, cough, chest pain especially with inspiration, shortness of breath, malaise, nausea, vomiting, poor appetite
Focused History: *Have you had pneumonia or a respiratory illness?* (Empyema is a complication of untreated or ineffectively treated pneumonia.) *How high is your fever?* (Anaerobic empyemas may have low-grade fever, but high fever is more common.) *What makes the symptoms better or worse?* (Shallow breathing and holding or lying on the affected side minimizes chest pain.)

Objective: Signs
Using Basic Tools: Vital signs: Fever >101.5°F, tachycardia, tachypnea, hypotension. Inspection: Generally ill-toxic appearance. Patient may be somnolent or gravely ill. Mental status changes are common in impending sepsis. Patient may have shallow respirations or splinting the affected side. Palpation: Warmth over local area of chest, tenderness to chest wall palpation or while patient takes deep breath suggests an empyema or other effusion. Enlarged axillary lymph nodes may be present. Evaluate for evidence of recent trauma or instrumentation. Percussion: Dullness to percussion suggests a pleural effusion which can represent an empyema. Auscultation: Rales and rhonchi may be heard from surrounding areas of pneumonia. Pleural friction rub may be heard. Dull respirations with shifting margins of dullness (change in position) indicate fluid effusion; unchanging pattern of dullness is consistent with empyema and/or consolidative pneumonia; decreased tactile fremitus may be present with both pleural effusion and empyema but will be increased with lobar consolidation.
Using Advanced Tools: Serum lab tests are similar to those patients with significant infection; leukocytosis with left shift sputum. Gram's stain may show bacterial and WBCs, hemoglobin and hematocrit may be elevated due to hemoconcentration. Key to diagnosis is made with a diagnostic thoracentesis. Pus (cloudy purulent smelling fluid) within the pleural cavity is diagnostic with the exception of thoracic duct damage causing a chylothorax (chylothorax will not have purulent smelling fluid). The pleural fluid will have large amount of WBCs and bacteria (gram-positive, gram-negative or both) seen on Gram's stain. A low pH <7.20 and glucose less than 60mg/dL is also frequently seen.

Assessment: Differential Diagnosis
Other causes of pleural effusions: congestive heart failure (usually bilaterally), cirrhosis (evidence of longstanding liver disease), parapneumonic effusion, hemothorax (usually evidence of trauma and blood return on thoracentesis), malignancy, and chylothorax.

Plan:
Diagnostic Tests: The diagnostic tests are focused on obtaining pleural fluid via thoracentesis. If radiographs are available, a posterior-anterior, lateral and lateral decubitus films should be performed prior to thoracentesis to evaluate for flowing pleural fluid.

Procedures: If there is concern for an empyema and the physical exam is consistent with a pleural effusion, the patient should undergo a diagnostic thoracentesis. *See Part 8: Procedures: Chapter 30: Thoracostomy, Needle and Chest Tube*

Treatment: Overall treatment is focused at complete drainage of the infected pleural fluid AND the administration of antibiotics. Acute onset of symptoms and preceding pneumonia or upper respiratory infection usually indicates aerobic bacterial infection. Slowly progressive symptoms especially in those patients with history of aspiration, alcoholism, and poor dentition are more likely to have anaerobic bacterial infection.
  Primary:
  1. Chest tube drainage (*see Part 8: Procedures: Chapter 30: Thoracostomy, Needle and Chest Tube*) is the <u>most important treatment</u>. Ideally use 26-36 French chest tube size. Give IV antibiotics if possible before inserting chest tube. Where medical evacuation is delayed or not an option, reaccumulation of fluid will require repeated drainage.
  2. Antibiotics: (Aerobic coverage): **Cefotaxime** 1gm IV or IM (if necessary) q12 h or **ceftriaxone** 2g IV q day (or 1g IM q12h) plus, for anaerobic coverage, give **clindamycin** 600mg IV q8h or **ampicillin-sulbactam** 3g IV or IM (if necessary) q6h. Continue IV antibiotic therapy through medical evacuation to higher level care. Where medical evacuation is not an option, continue antibiotic therapy for a minimum of 14 days. Reaccumulation of fluid and persistence of infection are significant risks and requires close clinical observation with repeated aspiration of empyema and antibiotic therapy continued if required.
  3. Supportive: supplemental oxygen, aggressive crystalloid IV fluids to maintain good urine output and reverse hemodynamic instability, change patient positioning and mild chest physiotherapy with close attention to not accidentally remove chest tube.
  Secondary: If antibiotics are not available, any antibiotic will likely partially treat causative organism. If chest tube placement is not available, remove as much infected pleural fluid as possible with a thoracentesis. This procedure can be repeated daily if the fluid reaccumulates and may be performed in conjunction with pleural cavity saline lavage (through thoracentesis needle).

Primitive: Give any antibiotic available, humidified environment, prevent patient from lying on one side, and attempt to maintain hydration.

Patient Education

Activity: Restrict activity to bed rest and attempt to prevent accidental chest tube removal

Diet: High calorie with adequate protein to replace body stores.

Follow-up Actions

Return Evaluation: All patients with an empyema should be evacuated to higher level of care.

Evacuation/Consultation Criteria: Evacuate unstable patients. Consult internist or pulmonologist.

Notes: Pleurectomy/decortication (pleural stripping) in cases of "trapped lung" is a definitive procedure only done by surgeons when a large scar forms and impairs normal lung function.

Chapter 3: Respiratory: Epiglottitis
COL Michael J. Morris, MC, USA

Introduction: Epiglottitis (or supraglottitis) is a rapidly progressive infection of the epiglottis and adjacent tissues usually caused by bacteria. The local inflammation and edema from this infection lead to airway obstruction that can result in death without emergent intervention. Most cases were in children due to *Haemophilus influenzae* type b (Hib) but have been reduced dramatically since 1991 with the introduction of infant Hib vaccination. It is becoming increasingly recognized in the adult population due to other bacterial organisms and other non-infectious etiologies. **Geographic Associations:** It is more frequently found in countries or regions where there is no pediatric Hib vaccination program. There is no specific association with any geographic region for adults. **Seasonal Variation:** There is no established seasonal predilection for epiglottitis and it may occur any time of the year. **Risk Factors:** In adults, epiglottitis has been associated with hypertension and diabetes mellitus.

Subjective: **Symptoms**

Epiglottitis is characterized by an abrupt onset and rapid progression. Many patients may have minor antecedent upper respiratory tract symptoms; the usual duration of illness prior to hospitalization is less than 24 hours and frequently less than 12 hours. Sudden onset of the constellation of fever, severe sore throat, dysphagia, and drooling is common. Airway obstruction is rapidly progressive. The affected patient experiences a choking sensation, is distressed on inspiration, and is anxious, restless, and irritable. Speech can be muffled and is often described as a "hot potato" voice, which sounds as if the patient is speaking with a hot potato in the mouth. However, hoarseness and stridor are not prominent features. The patient usually assumes a sitting position with arms back, trunk leaning forward, neck hyperextended, and chin thrust forward in an effort to maximize the diameter of the obstructed airway.

Focused History: The clinical diagnosis of epiglottitis is highly suggested when a patient presents in the characteristic sitting position with anxiety, drooling, sore throat, dysphagia, and inspiratory distress without significant stridor. The provider should have a low threshold for considering the diagnosis if any is present since epiglottitis progresses rapidly. *When was your onset of symptoms?* (usually less than 12-24 hours after mild upper respiratory infection) *Does your throat hurt?* (increased pain in the throat with cough and swallowing) *Do you have fever or shaking chills?* (Epiglottitis is associated with fevers greater than 102°F.) *Do you have trouble speaking?* (complaints of muffled voice and difficulty talking with characteristic "hot potato" voice) *Do you have trouble breathing?* (Patients will complain of being SOB or not able to take deep breath, will note increased symptoms when lying down.) *Do you have trouble swallowing?* (Patients may complain of difficulty swallowing or painful swallowing, may note inability to swallow secretions or drooling).

Objective: **Signs**

Using Basic Tools: Vital signs: Elevated temperature above 102°F, increased RR above 20, HR generally elevated, normal BP, normal pulse oximetry. Inspection: Anxiety, irritability. Patients will prefer to be in a sitting position with the trunk leaning forward and neck hyperextended. Drooling due to pain with swallowing; muffled, hoarse voice; mild respiratory distress with marked retractions; mouth open with tongue protruding. The epiglottis may be readily seen by simple depression of the tongue with a tongue blade. The diagnosis is confirmed by visualization of an edematous, erythematous epiglottis upon careful examination of the oropharynx. An endotracheal tube should only be used in extreme circumstances if the patient is nearing respiratory failure. Cyanosis is a late findings (indicates severe airway compromise). Palpation: Normal findings on neck and chest examination. Percussion: Normal findings on examination. Auscultation: Upper airway stridor; decreased breath sounds.

Using Advanced Tools: Direct or indirect laryngoscopy also can be performed and may be needed to confirm the diagnosis in adults. Concerns have been raised about the safety of visualizing the epiglottis in patients with suspected epiglottitis, since respiratory arrests have occurred during such efforts. The optimal method to visualize the epiglottis is by direct laryngoscopy under anesthesia and controlled conditions in the operating room by an experienced otolaryngologist or anesthesiologist. Labs: Leukocytosis is the rule; the white blood cell count is often $\geq$20,000 cells/mm^3 with an increased percentage of neutrophils and band forms.

Assessment

Diagnostic efforts should be individualized according to the severity of illness of the patient. In those with mild symptoms in whom the diagnosis is suspected, but for whom other diagnoses are also strong possibilities, the patient may be gently approached in the upright position and examined with careful application of a tongue blade or indirect laryngoscopy. Fever between 102 and 104°F is nearly universal, and patients with epiglottitis usually appear "toxic."

Differential Diagnosis: Other infectious etiologies in the upper airway may also cause similar symptoms and can be:

Laryngotracheobronchitis: May be either viral or bacterial in nature. It is a common complaint after an antecedent upper respiratory infection. It is generally a diagnosis of exclusion in a patient who does not the physical signs or symptoms of pneumonia. Patients may complain of a mild to moderate cough with sputum production over several days. They do not appear ill and generally have a normal lung examination except for a few coarse upper airway rhonchi.

Uvulitis: Can be diagnosed on upper airway examination based on the appearance of a large, swollen uvula.

Foreign body lodged in the larynx or vallecula: Should be suspected in a patient with a reported aspiration event with symptoms of upper airway obstruction. Requires examination of the larynx (either direct or indirect) to identify foreign body and establish diagnosis.

Peritonsillar or retropharyngeal abscesses: On physical examination it may be possible to appreciate midline or unilateral swelling of the posterior pharyngeal wall. The evaluation is complicated by inadequate visualization due to the patient's inability to open the mouth widely. Examination of the oral cavity may reveal a fluctuant mass. *See Part 3: General Symptoms: ENT Problems: Peritonsillar Abscess Needle Aspiration*

Angioedema: Affects the skin and mucosal tissues of the face, lips, mouth, and throat, larynx, extremities, and genitalia, often in an asymmetric pattern. It may occur in isolation, accompanied by urticaria, or as a component of anaphylaxis. Associated facial, lip or tongue swelling on examination in association with airway distress favors angioedema as the diagnosis. *See Part 7: Trauma: Chapter 27: Anaphylactic Shock*

Plan:
Treatment
1. Provide and maintain an adequate airway: Attempts at intubation should not be made by inexperienced personnel due to further airway compromise. Establish an artificial airway as soon as possible in all patients in whom the diagnosis of acute epiglottitis is made. Endotracheal intubation is the procedure of first choice using a tube 0.5-1.0mm smaller than otherwise indicated. This is generally done in the operating room under general anesthesia. Alternative methods to gain immediate control of the airway, such as needle cricothyrotomy, are considered temporary until a more permanent procedure (tracheostomy) can be performed.
2. Give antibiotics. Preferred initial IV antibiotic regimens now include a combination of **oxacillin** 2g IV q4h or **nafcillin** g IV q4h or **cefazolin** 2g IV q8h or **clindamycin** 600mg IV q8h or **vancomycin** 1g IV q12h PLUS **ceftriaxone** 2g IV q day or **cefotaxime** 2g IV q4-8 h or **cefuroxime** 1.5g IV q8h or **ampicillin-sulbactam** 2-3g IV q6h. All recommended antibiotic regimens should initially be given IV (patients will be unable to take oral meds initially). The decision to switch to oral medications is generally made after the first 48-72 hours of IV antibiotics and based on patient response with decreased upper airway inflammation. All doses provided are for adults. The optimal duration of antibiotics for the treatment of epiglottitis is unknown. Recommended treatment is 7-10 days.

Patient Education
General: Once the patient has been intubated and hospitalized, most patients will require sedation and mechanical ventilation for 48-72 hours. The general length of antibiotic treatment and hospitalization is 7-10 days.

Activity: No activity until recovery from acute illness (after 72 hours)

Diet: No special diet is indicated

Medications: Some patients may develop allergic reactions to antibiotics in the future but are generally well tolerated with few side effects.

Prevention and Hygiene: No specific hygiene measures are indicated.

No Improvement/Deterioration: Any patient with suspected epiglottitis should be hospitalized and observed for possible airway compromise.

Wound Care: No wound care indicated

Follow-up Actions
Return Evaluation: Patients who are managed appropriately from their acute illness generally have no long-term sequelae.

Evacuation/Consultation Criteria: Epiglottitis, if suspected, is a true airway emergency. The mortality can be 10% in patients who do not undergo endotracheal intubation or managed in an intensive care unit. If epiglottitis is suspected, the patient needs to be immediately transported to a medical facility that has the capability to manage a compromised upper airway.

Note: Do not attempt to treat or manage epiglottitis unless in a facility (with the right equipment) where a compromised airway can be properly treated. Attempts at airway evaluation or intubation by non-experienced personnel can lead to further airway compromise and respiratory arrest.

Chapter 3: Respiratory: Inhalational Injury Due to Smoke or Toxic Chemicals
MAJ Thomas B. Zanders, MC, USA

Introduction: Inhalational Injury represents tissue injury of the upper and lower respiratory tracts due to thermal injury, toxic byproducts of combustion, and irritant gas inhalation. Broadly, the type of inhalational injury is defined by the anatomic location; supraglottic, subglottic and systemic intoxication. Supraglottic structures (nares, pharynx, and epiglottis) sustain primarily thermal injury. Subglottic structures (trachea, bronchi, and alveoli) sustain mucosal injury due to smoke particulate matter and irritant chemicals (exception is steam injury which can produce thermal injury to entire respiratory system). Finally, toxic gasses such as carbon monoxide, cyanide, and methane lead to cellular hypoxia and cell death. The diagnosis of early inhalational injury can be difficult but is essential to improve the high mortality rate due to rapid airway obstruction. **Risk Factors:** Inhalational injury can occur with and without cutaneous burn injury. The likelihood of sustaining inhalational injury rises as degree of cutaneous burns increases. Those burned within closed space, found unconscious or loss of consciousness during injury, the young, and the elderly are all at increased risk of sustaining inhalational injury.

Subjective: Symptoms
Symptoms can be highly varied but are all related to upper and lower respiratory tracts. Severe coughing, dyspnea, hoarseness, excessive lacrimation or rhinorrhea all may indicate inhalational injury.

Focused History: *Where was the fire?* (Injury in a closed space, house or vehicle, significantly increases the risk of inhalational injury.) *What was burning?* (Rubber, plastic, and petroleum products can produce sulfur dioxide, ammonia and chlorine which can cause severe subglottic injury.) *Did you lose consciousness for any period of time?* (Loss of consciousness increases risk of inhalational injury.) *Do you feel short of breath or are you coughing up soot?* (Dyspnea and production of carbonaceous sputum are indicators of inhalational injury.)

Objective: Signs

No one test or sign is highly sensitive or specific to the diagnosis of inhalational injury. The diagnosis relies heavily on clinical history and basic physical exam findings.

Using Basic Tools: Vital signs: Tachypnea, tachycardia, hypoxia (may not have significant hypoxia especially with carbon monoxide exposure). General Evaluation: Potential altered level of consciousness or coma, anxiety-agitation, significant coughing. Inspection: Facial burns, singed nasal vibrissae, singed facial hair, significant rhinorrhea and/or lacrimation, carbonaceous sputum production, bronchorrhea (copious watery sputum production), labored breathing with accessory muscle use, tripod positioning (leaning forward with labored breathing), mucosal erythema of nares or pharynx, significant cutaneous burns. Percussion: The exam may be normal shortly after injury. Auscultation: Stridor, wheezing, and hoarseness, are highly concerning for inhalational injury. A patient may also have diffuse rales and rhonchi if severe subglottic injury is present.

Using Advanced Tools: There is no utility in basic tests to make diagnosis of inhalational injury. Soon after injury, the majority of patients will have normal lab studies as well as normal chest radiographs.

Assessment:

The patient should have history consistent with fire or chemical exposure. Always evaluate for co-existent trauma. Typically airway and mucosal edema peaks at 24-48 hours following injury.

Differential Diagnosis:

Pulmonary contusion, pneumothorax, abdominal trauma, aspiration, and upper airway trauma.

Plan:

Treatment

Primary:

1. Endotracheal intubation should be performed (nasotracheal or orotracheal route) if the patient is not spontaneously breathing or breathing is severely labored. Prophylactic early intubation should be performed in those patients with significant symptoms, severe facial burns, burns with loss of consciousness, and those with >40% TBSA burns.
2. Primary treatment is focused on supportive care and typical ABCs of resuscitation.
3. For spontaneously breathing patients, elevate head of bed and provide humidified 100% oxygen (improves clearance of carbon monoxide and decreases mucosal thermal injury). If respiratory therapy equipment is available, give bronchodilators: Nebulized albuterol 2.5mg diluted to 3cc with normal saline nebulized over 10 minutes and repeated q20 minutes x 3 doses then 2-4 hours as needed depending upon symptoms or inhaled **racemic epinephrine** (7.5mL of 1.125% nebulized over 10 minutes. May be given q1-2hrs.
4. The patient should also undergo standardized therapy for cutaneous burns. *See Part 7: Trauma: Chapter 29: Burns (Thermal, Scald or Chemical)*

Empiric: Aggressive pulmonary toilet, humidification of supplemental oxygen, close monitoring for progressive pulmonary and upper airway edema (especially during resuscitation of cutaneous burns)

Primitive: Limit further smoke injury, elevation of head, chest percussion to promote secretion clearance, perform cricothyroidotomy if unable to perform endotracheal intubation.

Patient Education

General: Any hoarseness, mucosal swelling or dyspnea needs to be evaluated immediately.

Activity: Restrict activity to minimal duties for mild injury and bed rest for moderate or severe injury.

Diet: Moderate and severe injury should remain NPO

No Improvement/Deterioration: Same symptoms as initial evaluation.

Follow-up Actions

Return Evaluation: Those with mild resolving symptoms should be re-evaluated in 24-48 hrs for complete resolution of symptoms and evaluation for return to duty.

Evacuation/Consultation Criteria: Evacuate unstable patients as well as those with moderate to severe facial burns and/or progressive symptoms. Consult burn center and pulmonologist.

Notes: Those sustaining burn injuries in combat are more likely to have head and neck burns, inhalational injury and other non-burn traumatic injuries. Circumferential full thickness burns of the chest should be treated with thoracic escharotomies to relieve thoracic restriction. Steroids should not be given in inhalational injury since this significantly increases risk of infection.

Chapter 3: Respiratory: Hypersensitivity Pneumonitis

Capt Dara Regn, USAF, MC

Introduction: Hypersensitivity pneumonitis is an immunologic induced inflammatory lung disease resulting from sensitization and subsequent re-exposure to any of a wide variety of inhaled organic dusts or inorganic chemicals. The disease results in a diffuse inflammation of the lung parenchyma, particularly the terminal bronchioles, interstitium, and alveoli, with little or no involvement of the larger airways. Eventually the inflammation can result in granuloma formation and may progress to fibrosis with permanent restrictive disease. In cases where the allergen is inhaled repeatedly, recurrent pneumonia can be sudden and life threatening. Thermophilic actinomycetes is a mold that causes several types of hypersensitivity pneumonitis: farmer's lung, air conditioner lung (exposure to moldy air filter) and bagassosis or cotton worker's lung (inhalation of fibers or moldy cotton). Other common types include bird breeder's lung (inhalation of avian protein, blood or dander), isocyanate lung (exposure to toluene diisocyanate [TDI] or methylene diisocyanate [MDI] used in polyurethane, plastics and some spray paints) and washing powder lung (*Bacillus subtilis* enzymes).

Subjective: **Symptoms**

Acute illness (within 4-8 hours of exposure): May be mistaken for "24 hour flu" with cough, dyspnea, fever, chills, headache, malaise, and body aches. Symptoms last for 12-24 hours. Between attacks, the patient is usually asymptomatic. Chronic/sub-acute illness:

Resembles progressive chronic bronchitis with cough, dyspnea, exercise limitation, anorexia, weight loss, and fatigue

Focused History: *Do you get sick after a specific activity or exposure* (eg, hay, textile mill, other organic dusts)? *What is your occupation? Do symptoms go away when on vacation or visiting relatives in a distant city or state?* (Diagnosis based on history of symptoms only occurring at work or in a certain environment that would expose Soldier to organic dusts. Sometimes a patient will need to keep a diary to log all their activities and exposures.) *How long do your symptoms last?* (Generally, pneumonitis will start to improve over 24 hours, unless there is additional exposure.)

Objective: Signs

Using Basic Tools: Acute illness: Vital signs: Fever up to 104°F, tachypnea, tachycardia. Inspection: Acute sputum production (clear, white or colored), cyanosis. Auscultation: Fine, mid- to end-inspiratory crackles in chest. Signs may improve without treatment if removed from the offending agent. Chronic illness: Vital Signs: Afebrile or low-grade fever. Inspection: Progressive cyanosis and clubbing of fingers. Auscultation: Fine, mid- to end-inspiratory crackles in chest; right heart failure with extremity swelling. Signs will not acutely improve when removed from the offending agent due to lung scarring from chronic exposure.

Using Advanced Tools: CXR: Normal to reticulonodular pattern that is widespread or predominantly in the lower lungs. May also present at patchy interstitial infiltrates. Pulmonary function studies (if available) may show restriction and reduction in diffusing capacity of the lung. Lab studies are neither sensitive nor specific for this disease process.

Assessment:

Definitive diagnosis can only be made based on high clinical suspicion through a combination of characteristic symptoms, exposure history, signs, CXR findings, pulmonary function testing, and immunologic test results.

Differential Diagnosis:

Acute illness resembles typical and many atypical pneumonias which all require CXR for further evaluation.

Viral pneumonia: Symptoms of fever, chills, cough

Influenza pneumonia: Symptoms of fever, chills, cough, sore throat

Mycoplasma pneumonia: Symptoms of intractable cough that is not productive, sore throat, runny nose

Non-pulmonary signs include anemia, joint pains, skin rash.

Chronic illnesses:

Non-resolving or recurrent pneumonia

Tuberculosis (TB): Symptoms of fever, chills, cough, coughing up blood, unintentional weight loss, night sweats. If this is suspected, soldier MUST immediately be placed in respiratory isolation. *See Part 5: Specialty Areas: Chapter 12: Mycobacterial Infections: Tuberculosis*

Sarcoidosis: Symptoms include cough, shortness of breath

Fungal infections: Symptoms vary depending on type of fungal infection from being asymptomatic to coughing up blood.

Pneumocystis carinii pneumonia with HIV: Symptoms of shortness of breath, fever, chills, weight loss, fatigue

Plan:

Treatment

Primary:

1. Initial therapy: Prevention through avoidance of re-exposure. Improvement in ventilation, air filtering systems, or masks may help in some circumstances.
2. Corticosteroids: **Prednisone** 0.5-1mg/kg/day po for 1-4 weeks.
3. Antipyretics: **Acetaminophen** 500mg po q4h. DO NOT exceed total of 4000mg in a 24 hour period.
4. Supplemental oxygen via nasal cannula to maintain oxygen saturation >90%

Primitive: Avoid offending agent. Breathe humidified air from steam kettle or shower.

Patient Education

General: Avoid offending agent. There is risk of irreversible lung damage with continued exposure. Note that chronic exposure may lead to a loss of acute symptoms previously experienced on exposure, ie, patient may lose awareness of exposure-symptom relationship.

Activity: Restrict if symptoms worsen after exposure to antigen

Prevention: Use appropriate masks and filters when exposed to offending agent. Keep ventilation systems clean and well maintained.

No Improvement/Deterioration: Return for worsening symptoms or those that do not resolve after 3-4 days of treatment.

Follow-up Actions

Return Evaluation: Symptoms that do not improve should be referred for specialty care and additional special studies.

Evacuation/Consultation Criteria: Evacuate patients who are not able to complete the mission, or whose symptoms do not resolve. Consult internist or pulmonologist as needed.

Chapter 3: Respiratory: Asthma

CPT James Woodrow, MC, USA & MAJ Christopher Lettieri, MC, USA

Introduction: Asthma is a condition characterized by a reversible obstruction to air flow caused by increased resistance in the medium sized bronchi. This reaction is a response to some external trigger or stimuli that induces bronchial smooth muscle spasm, mucosal edema, heavy secretions, and inflammation. Some common triggers include cold air, exercise, smoke, animal dander, or respiratory tract infections. Asthma differs from other diseases of the airways (eg, bronchitis, emphysema) in that it is at least partially reversible when the triggers are removed or when treatment is initiated. If asthma is poorly controlled, then over time, these airway changes can become permanent. Asthma is most commonly diagnosed during childhood but can present at any age. Asthma typically presents as discrete episodes interspersed with asymptomatic periods. Frequency is highly variable ranging from daily symptoms to symptoms that occur less than once per year. Disease can also vary greatly; symptoms can range from a mild discomfort to a life-threatening condition.

Subjective: Symptoms

Cardinal features of asthma include dyspnea, wheeze, cough, and chest tightness. Symptoms are episodic and most patients are asymptomatic between episodes.

Focused History: *When do you have the most trouble breathing? Have you identified any triggers that will lead to trouble breathing?* (There are typically one or more clear precipitating events or triggers that are easily identified by the patient. Unprovoked symptoms typically occur at night or in the early morning.) *Do you have any other symptoms such as pains in your chest or trouble breathing when you lie flat?* (Asthma should be distinguished from other causes of shortness of breath. Asthma is not typically worse when lying flat and does not present with chest pain.) *Have you had a fever?* (Asthma does not typically cause fever of chills.) *How long have you been having these symptoms?* (Chronic, stable disease should be distinguished from an acute attack.) *How many nights are you awakened by wheezing or cough?* (Once a potentially life-threatening exacerbation is ruled out, chronic disease severity should be assessed. A well controlled asthmatic should not wake up with symptoms more than twice per month.) *How often do you use your rescue inhaler?* (If asthma is well controlled, rescue inhaler should only be required 2 x wk, not counting use prior to exercise.) *How many days of work or school have you missed in the last month because of asthma?* (It is also important to note how symptoms are affecting the patient's life. Any interference with normal activity suggests poor control.) *Do you have heartburn or frequent sinusitis?* (Exacerbating conditions such as gastroesophageal reflux, post nasal drip, sinusitis, and vocal cord dysfunction should be sought out and treated.) *Do you have a history of allergies or a recurrent itchy rash?* (Asthma is commonly associated with other atopic conditions such as eczema and allergic rhinitis. Presence of these conditions would support the diagnosis of asthma.) *Do you smoke? Do you live with someone who does?* (Smoking history, including exposure to second-hand smoke is important because it can make asthma more difficult to control. A long smoking history can also suggest alternative diagnoses including COPD.) *Do you own a cat or a dog? Do you have cockroaches in your quarters?* (Exposure to common removable antigens should be sought out.) *Does anyone in your family have asthma?* (A family history of asthma or atopic disease should be noted as support for the diagnosis.)

Objective: Signs

Using Basic Tools: Vital signs: Signs of respiratory distress include increase respiratory rate and/or tachycardia. A physical exam typically has normal findings between asthma attacks. During an attack however, a physical exam will help gauge severity and rule out alternative explanations for dyspnea. Inspection: During normal respiration, the scalene and sternocleidomastoid muscles are not used. Use of these muscle groups is a sign of respiratory distress. When the diaphragm begins to tire, paradoxical abdominal movements occur. The abdomen should move out with respiration. When the diaphragm stops contracting forcefully it is pulled up by accessory muscles, which causes the abdomen to move inward during inspiration. Auscultation: Lung sounds may be normal between attacks. Also, during an acute attack, lung sounds may become clear as the obstruction worsens, which is often a sign of impending respiratory arrest. Presence of expiratory wheezing suggests either poorly controlled asthma or an acute attack. No other lung sounds, other than wheezing, should be heard. The presence of localized rhonchi, for example, will suggest a diagnosis of pneumonia. Congestive heart failure can mimic asthma and even present with wheezing. On exam, you would hear basilar crackles and an extra heart sound (S3). The length of the expiratory phase should be noted and, if prolonged, taken as a sign of active asthma. Palpation: Pulsus paradoxus is defined as a 10mmHg or greater drop in systolic BP during inspiration and is a sign of severe inspiratory airflow resistance. Percussion: Dullness to percussion is not typical of asthma and should suggest an alternative diagnosis, such as a pleural effusion.

Using Advanced Tools: Low oxygen saturation should be interpreted as a sign of a severe asthma attack. CXR is useful to help rule out alternative etiologies but will commonly be normal during an acute asthma exacerbation. Spirometry if available: A drop in peak expiratory flow (PEF) may precede onset of symptoms of an asthma exacerbation. Although normal values differ with gender, height, and age, a <u>PEF rate below 200L/min indicates severe obstruction for all but unusually small adults</u>. Baseline spirometry, performed before and after bronchodilation, can help establish a diagnosis, classify disease severity, and gauge response to treatment.

Assessment: Differential Diagnosis

Foreign body aspiration: Always consider in children!

COPD: Presents with constant instead of episodic symptoms. Consider in older patient with history of smoking CXR: Hyperinflation. Spirometry: Little response to bronchodilation. *See Part 4: Organ Systems: Chapter 3: Chronic Obstructive Pulmonary Disease*

Infections such as pneumonia or bronchitis (croup or bronchiolitis in children): Fevers, chills, cough, and sputum production. CXR: Focal infiltrate. *See Part 4: Organ Systems: Chapter 3: Pneumonia; Chronic Obstructive Pulmonary Disease & Part 5: Specialty Areas: Chapter 15: Most Common Pediatric Diseases: Throat Problems: Croup*

Epiglottitis: Fevers, chills. Toxic appearance. Drooling. Inspiratory stridor. *See Part 4: Organ Systems: Chapter 3: Epiglottitis*

Vocal cord dysfunction (paradoxical adduction of vocal cords during inspiration): Lack of response to asthma treatment. Spirometry: Truncation of inspiratory flow volume loop.

Congestive heart failure: Difficulty breathing while lying flat. Physical exam: Basilar rales. Extra heart sound (S3). Jugular venous distension. CXR: Diffuse pulmonary edema. *See Part 4: Organ Systems: Chapter 1: Congestive Heart Failure (Pulmonary Edema)*

Pulmonary embolus: Sudden onset following surgery, trauma, or long periods of immobilization. Physical Exam: Typically normal. CXR: Typically normal. *See Part 4: Organ Systems: Chapter 3: Deep Vein Thrombosis and Pulmonary Embolism*

Plan:

Treatment

Acute attack: Measure initial PEF to provide a baseline for repeated measures. Doubling of the initial peak flow value, measured hourly, is a reliable indicator of improvement.

Initial therapy

1. Give **albuterol** as a metered dose inhaler (MDI). Give 4-8 puffs (90mcg/puff) q20 minutes for up to 4 hours, then q1-4h prn. **Albuterol** can also be given as a nebulized inhaler. Dilute 2.5-5mg (1mL of 5% **albuterol** contains 5mg of albuterol) with saline to a total of 3mL and give over 5-15 minutes, tid-qid. Children under 2, use nebulizer or MDI with valved spacer and mask.

Children 2-4 years use MDI and valved spacer. Children over 5 years use MDI or powder inhaler.

2. Short course of oral corticosteroids, 2mg/kg po q am x 5-7 days. (eg, **prednisone** 40-80mg po q day for adults)

Long term management based on NAEPP (National Asthma Education and Prevention Program) asthma severity categories.

1. Mild intermittent asthma: Symptoms no more than twice per week with nocturnal symptoms no more than twice per month. Adult dosing: Give **albuterol** (short-acting beta-agonist). The preferred route of administration is by metered dose inhaler (MDI). If the patient cannot use the device, albuterol can be inhaled via a nebulizer. Dosing: Inhaler: 2-4 puffs (90ug/puff) q4-6h prn. Nebulizer: Dilute ½ mL (1mL of 5% albuterol contains 5mg of albuterol) to 3mL total volume, with sterile normal saline. Deliver nebulized solution over 5-15 minutes q4-6h prn. No regular treatment required for children <5 years old.

2. Mild persistent asthma: Symptoms >2 x per week, but <1 time per day or nocturnal symptoms greater than twice/month but not more than once per week. Preferred medication is a low dose inhaled corticosteroid in addition to an as needed short acting beta agonist. **Fluticasone** is dosed in 44mcg, 110mcg, or 220µg/puff MDI. Low dose (adult) 88–264µg; (child) 88–176µg given bid. Alternative options include: **montelukast** (leukotriene modifier) 10mg po q day for adults, 5mg for children 6-14 yrs old, and 4mg for children <6 yrs old or **cromolyn** MDI 2-4 puffs tid-qid (adults); 1-2 puffs tid-qid (children <12).

3. Moderate persistent asthma: Daily symptoms or nocturnal symptoms more than once per week. Preferred regimen is a medium dose inhaled corticosteroid with a long acting beta agonist in addition to an as needed short acting beta agonist. **Fluticasone** (inhaled corticosteroid) plus salmeterol is available in a combination dry powder inhaler (DPI). Medium dose (adult and child) 250mcg/50mcg bid. Alternative regimens: Medium dose inhaled corticosteroid plus **montelukast** (leukotriene modifier)10mg po q day for adults, 5mg for children 6-14 years old, and 4mg for children <6 years old.

4. Severe persistent asthma: Continuous symptoms with frequent nocturnal symptoms. Preferred regimen is the same for moderate persistent asthma except the inhaled corticosteroid should be increased to a high dose. **Fluticasone/salmeterol** should be increased to 500µg/50µg dosed bid. Consider adding oral steroids (**prednisone**) at 2mg/kg/day to existing regimen.

Manage conditions that may make asthma worse.

1. Seasonal allergies: Consider referral to an allergist in order to test for potentially avoidable allergens such as animal dander or dust mites.

2. Rhinosinusitis. Chronic sinusitis and allergic rhinitis can make asthma worse through a variety of mechanisms including post-nasal drip. Consider treatment with upper airway decongestants such as pseudoephedrine and/or antihistamine. *See Part 3: General Symptoms: ENT Problems: Rhinitis/Rhinorrhea*

3. Gastroesophageal reflux. Microaspiration of gastric contents can exacerbate asthma. Consider treatment with H$_2$ receptor antagonists or proton pump inhibitors. *See Part 4: Organ Systems: Chapter 7: Acute Peptic Ulcer Disease*

4. Vocal cord dysfunction: Consider referral to pulmonologist to rule out paradoxical closing of vocal cords during inspiration.

Patient Education

General: Patient must understand their disease: symptoms, medications, inhalers, nebulizers and peak flow meters and be able to monitor symptoms and PEF rates. Have a pre-arranged action plan for exacerbations or emergencies. Give a written action plan and school plan to caretakers of asthmatic children.

Prevention: Investigate and control triggering factors (pollutants, exercise, house-dust mite, molds, and animal dander). Get annual influenza immunization. Avoid aspirin and aspirin containing medications. Avoid sulfites and tartrazine (food additives).

No Improvement/Deterioration: Return immediately if symptoms worsen.

Follow-up Actions

Return Evaluation: Evaluate for on-going control of symptoms, and alter medications as outlined previously.

Evacuation/Consultation Criteria: Evacuate severe asthmatics and those with a history of emergent attacks, once they are stable. Evacuate moderate asthmatics that are not able to complete the mission, since they may worsen and require intensive therapy during the mission. Consult primary care physician, internist or pulmonologist as needed.

Chapter 3: Respiratory Chronic Obstructive: Pulmonary Disease

CPT James Woodrow MC, USA & MAJ Christopher Lettieri, MC, USA

Introduction: Chronic obstructive pulmonary disease (COPD) includes emphysema, chronic bronchitis, and a mixture of these two, as well as long-standing, poorly controlled asthma. All of the causes of COPD reduce the patient's ability to ventilate by increasing obstruction to expiratory airflow. In emphysema, airways collapse during exhalation, causing air trapping. Only about 25% of cigarette smokers develop emphysema, but those that show early disease will continue to lose function for as long as they smoke and for some time after they quit. In chronic bronchitis and in some long-standing asthma, airways are narrowed by reactive smooth muscle constriction, mucus and secretions. By definition, chronic bronchitis is the presence of a productive cough for 3 months in each of 2 consecutive years with all other causes of chronic cough excluded. Spirometry is also required to confirm expiratory airflow obstruction (reduced FEV1/FVC ratio). Most patients will demonstrate features of both chronic bronchitis and emphysema.

Subjective: **Symptoms**

Chronic, productive cough; shortness of breath (SOB)

Focused History: *Do you have trouble breathing? Is your trouble breathing intermittent or persistent?* (COPD is distinguished from asthma by persistent instead of intermittent symptoms.) *How much can you exert yourself without trouble breathing? Do you cough up any mucus?* (emphysema - dry, non-productive cough; chronic bronchitis - almost always productive) *What color is your sputum?* (A sudden change in amount of sputum or sputum color indicates a bacterial infection.) *How long have you been coughing up mucus or sputum?* (Productive cough daily for 3 months in each of 2 consecutive years is evidence of chronic bronchitis.) *What seems to improve your symptoms?* (Bronchodilators will help partially; avoiding smoking is the best alleviator.) *How long have you smoked tobacco? How* *many cigarettes or packs per day did you smoke? When did you quit?* (Most will have a long smoking history.) *Have you had the influenza and pneumonia vaccinations?* (important preventive measures for all COPD patients)

Objective: Signs

Using Basic Tools: Vital signs: RR >18. Pulmonary: Inspection. Labored breathing or use of accessory muscles suggests an active exacerbation. A "barrel" shaped chest or increased anteroposterior diameter due to air trapping indicates presence of emphysema. Patients may lean forward and breathe through pursed lips. Auscultation: Breath sounds may be distant. Expiratory phase may be prolonged and wheezes may be heard especially with forced expiration.

Using Advanced Tools: Labs: CBC for polycythemia (HCT over 52% suggests chronic hypoxia or nocturnal hypoxia). Sputum for Gram's stain and culture is not generally helpful unless an infection with a resistant pathogen is suspected. CXR: May be normal in mild to moderate COPD. Typical x-ray abnormalities include hyperexpanded lungs and flattened diaphragms. Also look for conditions predisposed by COPD such as pneumonia and lung cancer. Pulse oximetry: <90% saturation during rest or ambulation (6 minute walk). Pulmonary function tests (if available) will show an obstructive defect prior to symptom onset and can help grade severity of obstruction.

Assessment: Differential Diagnosis

Persistent asthma: Distinguished by inability to reverse obstruction with treatment.

Gastroesophageal reflux disease (GERD): Those with recurrent aspiration present with symptoms resembling chronic bronchitis.

Bronchiectasis: Chronic scarring and dilation of the airways causing frequent bouts of bacterial pulmonary infection.

Bronchogenic carcinoma: May mimic chronic bronchitis.

Plan:

Treatment

Primary:

1. **All patients:** Counseling on smoking cessation is the most important intervention. All patients should also be up to date with Pneumovax and influenza vaccines. If patient desaturates to below 88% while breathing room air, supplemental oxygen should be administered. Give as needed bronchodilators as first line therapy: albuterol 1-2 puffs from the metered dose inhaler q4-6h, which may be increased to q3h in more severe cases. (Use of spacer device [AeroChamber, InspirEase] may be beneficial.) The toxicity of theophylline precludes its use in the field. **Ipratropium** 2-4 puffs qid and prn can be used as an alternative or in combination with **albuterol.**

2. **Moderate disease:** Defined as FEV1 between 50 and 80%. Consider adding a long-acting bronchodilator, such as **salmeterol** 2 puffs bid. Indications for adding inhaled corticosteroids, such as **fluticasone** include a reversible component on spirometry after administration of bronchodilator; recurrent exacerbations requiring hospitalization; and FEV1<60% predicted or <1L (absolute volume).

3. **Severe disease:** Defined as FEV1 below 50% predicted. Consider adding combination long acting beta agonist and inhaled corticosteroid combination such as **fluticasone/salmeterol** which should be used at a high dose (250mcg/50mcg or 500mcg/50mcg bid). Long term treatment of COPD with oral steroids is not recommended and may actually make respiratory status worse.

4. **Exacerbations:** Most exacerbations are due to infection but a change in air quality is another common trigger. Treatment should include short acting inhaled bronchodilators such as **albuterol** with or without **ipratropium** along with steroids such as **prednisone** 30-40mg po q day x 7 days. Consider antibiotics (**doxycycline** 100mg po bid or **trimethoprim-sulphamethoxazole** DS 1 po bid x 5-10 days) for signs of airway infection such as increased sputum or sputum purulence Severe exacerbations may require hospitalization, IV administration of medications, and possible positive pressure ventilation (either BiPAP or IPPV via endotracheal tube)

Empiric: Oxygen (low flow 1-2L/min) if pulse oximetry shows <88% saturation. Antibiotics (*see Part 4: Organ Systems: Chapter 3: Pneumonia*)

Primitive: Caffeine has some bronchodilation effects and can be effective in some patients. Belladonna plant (deadly nightshade) was administered in the past by smoking the dried plant for the anticholinergic effects of the atropine found in the plant. (Not recommended as atropine can have severe nervous system side effects.)

Patient Education

General: Avoid inhaled pollutants. Stop smoking tobacco. This treats emphysema better than medications.

Prevention: Immunize with pneumococcal vaccine and influenza vaccine.

Follow-up Actions

Return Evaluation: Symptoms that do not improve should be referred for specialty care and additional special studies.

Evacuation/Consultation Criteria: Evacuate unstable patients. Consult primary care physician, internist or pulmonologist as needed.

Chapter 3: Respiratory: Deep Vein Thrombosis and Pulmonary Embolism

CPT Michael Perkins MC, USA & MAJ Christopher Lettieri, MC, USA

Introduction: A deep vein thrombosis (DVT) is a blood clot that forms in one of the large veins within the upper or lower extremities. A pulmonary embolism (PE) occurs when a DVT dislodges and travels to the lung, causing a loss of oxygenation of the blood flowing in that area of the lung. A PE is a life-threatening complication of DVT. PE presents as 3 different syndromes: embolism without infarction (most common and causing acute unexplained dyspnea until clot is lysed/dissolved); pulmonary infarction (complete obstruction of a distal branch of the pulmonary arterial circulation causing necrosis of part of the lung); or acute cor pulmonale (a massive clot obstructing a majority of both the pulmonary arteries and right ventricle of the heart, causing right heart failure). Patients will usually have signs and symptoms of either a

DVT or a PE, but can have signs and symptoms of both at the same time. Often, symptoms may be subtle and overlooked and confirming this diagnosis is frequently difficult. **Risk Factors:** Trauma, prior injury to an extremity, central venous catheters, prolonged bed rest, prolonged travel (especially on airplanes), oral birth control pills, and underlying hypercoagulable states that make people more prone to clot formation (such as malignancy or genetic predisposition), dehydration.

Subjective: Symptoms

DVT: Pain and swelling in an extremity, usually in one leg. However, it can occur in the arms or in both legs simultaneously.

PE: Three different clinical presentations are possible, depending on which PE syndrome is present.

1. Embolism: Acute unexplained shortness of breath (SOB) without other significant symptoms.
2. Infarction: Chest pain associated with labored breathing, anxiety, occasional low-grade fever and cough (possibly with bloody sputum) for which no other cause (chest trauma, pneumonia, angina, etc.) can be determined.
3. Massive PE: Catastrophic cardio-pulmonary failure in patients who have risk factors for venous thromboembolism

Focused History: *Did the SOB start suddenly?* (PE is an acute condition. Symptoms may progress over several days, but it starts suddenly.) *Do you feel anxious?* (A sense of foreboding or anxiety without clear reason is common.) *Have you had any recent lower extremity or pelvic injury?* (DVT and PE are usually associated with stasis or an injury to a great vein.) *Did you strain with a bowel movement before the symptoms began?* (Straining can dislodge lower abdominal clot.) *Have you or anyone in your family had blood clots before?* (may be prone to form clots—hypercoagulable) *Have you recently become active after a time of bedrest or a long plane trip where you were sitting for several hours?* (PE typical after 2-3 days bedrest or long periods of immobility.)

Objective: Signs

Using Basic Tools: Vital signs: Low-grade fever if any (<101°F), respiratory rate >18, resting pulse over 90 bpm.

Inspection: Cyanosis, hypotension and distended neck veins may indicate massive PE; anxiety, dyspnea and splinted breathing (due to pleuritic chest pain) are typical. Peripheral edema, pain, and warmth in one leg suggest the presence of a DVT. Edema in both legs may indicate right heart failure. Auscultation: Area of rales or absent breath sounds may indicate location of an infarct or large PE. S3 gallop may indicate PE or CHF. Distant heart sounds with tamponade. A cardiac rub suggests pericarditis.

Using Advanced Tools: An ECG should be obtained in all patients: It can be used to rule out other diagnoses including pericarditis or MI that can mimic the presenting symptoms. Pulse oximetry will show the low oxygen saturation that usually occurs with PE. CXR may reveal a wedge-shaped infiltrate suggestive of infarction or an infiltrate(s) in the lower lungs that may be seen with PE. Massive PEs cause "pruning" or absence of the lung blood vessels which may be seen on CXR.

Assessment: Differential Diagnosis

A history of risk factors (ie, trauma, long periods of immobilization, dehydration) may suggest DVT & or PE. *See Part 3: General Symptoms: Chest Pain*

DVT may mimic:

Cellulitis: Skin infection with warmth and swelling and skin erythema.

Baker's cyst: A benign cyst in back of knee; nontender, non-acute

Pulmonary embolism may appear to be:

Myocardial infarction: Typical history and ECG changes. *See Part 4: Organ Systems: Chapter 1: Acute Coronary Syndrome (Acute Myocardial Infarction and Unstable Angina)*

Pneumothorax: May include history of trauma. *See Part 4: Organ Systems: Chapter 3: Pneumothorax*

Severe acute bronchospasm: Acute onset of dyspnea with wheeze and coughing. Occurs in asthma attack, severe systemic allergic reaction (anaphylaxis), or after inhaling a high concentration of toxic gas or smoke. With asthma, may have a family history of asthma or recurrent rashes. If anaphylaxis is present, additional symptoms may include pruritus, flushing, urticaria/angioedema, and sense of choking, and there is a history of allergy with recent exposure to inciting agent (eg, drug, insect sting, food). With inhalation injury, there is a history of recent inhalation of a noxious agent. *See Part 4: Organ Systems: Chapter 3: Asthma; Inhalation Injury Due to Smoke and Toxic Chemicals & Part 7: Trauma: Chapter 27: Anaphylactic Shock*

Pneumonia: Toxic clinical appearance, history of URI with auscultatory and CXR findings of pneumonia. *See Part 4: Organ Systems: Chapter 3: Pneumonia*

Pericarditis with tamponade: Distant heart sounds, elevated neck veins, hypotension. *See Part 4: Organ Systems: Chapter 1: Pericarditis*

Thoracic aortic dissection: Pain is a "tearing" quality and radiates to the mid or upper back. CXR often shows widening of the mediastinum.

Severe gastroesophageal reflux: Pain is a "burning character", may have acid taste in mouth and/or food regurgitation, worse in supine position or after spicy or large meals. *See Part 4: Organ Systems: Chapter 7: Acute Gastritis*

Plan:

Treatment

Primary:

1. Prevent DVT and PE in high-risk post-op patients by:
   1) frequent and early ambulation
   2) use **heparin** 5000U subcutaneously q8-12h or low-molecular weight heparin (**enoxaparin**) 30mg subcutaneously q12h
   3) external pneumatic compression, and gradient elastic stockings
2. Evacuate patients with PE or DVT and those with risk factors and suspicion of PE
3. For PE or DVT, if the risk of bleeding is low, give **enoxaparin** 1mg/kg subcutaneously q12h. Alternate (if lab available for PTT measurement): **Heparin**, initial bolus of 80units/kg, followed by a drip of 18units/kg/hour as IV drip. PTT should be measured q6h and the drip titrated to maintain a PTT between 70-90. Both treatments can cause bleeding and patients should be monitored for this complication.

4. Administer supplemental oxygen 2L to maintain the SpO$_2$ above 92%.
5. Administer IV fluids (see Part 7: Trauma: Chapter 27: Resuscitation Fluids) to help maintain cardiac function in massive PE.

Patient Education
General: Avoid thrombus in high-risk patients.
Activity: Early ambulation to avoid DVT and PE. No activity during PE or DVT until patient receives anticoagulation therapy at referral facility.
Medications: Avoid aspirin or NSAIDs while on heparin to minimize bleeding risks or enoxaparin.
Prevention: Avoid lower extremity activity or intra-abdominal strain that could dislodge additional thrombus if already have PE. Maintain blood flow during prolonged travel or bedrest by walking and stretching to avoid DVT and PE.

Follow-up Actions
Evacuation/Consultation Criteria: Emergently evacuate patients with PE, and those with risk factors (eg, DVT) or suspicion of PE. Consult pulmonologist or internist.

Chapter 3: Respiratory: Acute Respiratory Distress Syndrome
MAJ Christopher Lettieri, MC, USA

Introduction: Acute Lung Injury is a sudden, diffuse inflammatory process of the pulmonary parenchyma. It results from numerous causes. Non-cardiogenic pulmonary edema (fluid not resulting from heart failure) and the inflammatory process impair the lungs ability to exchange gases and severe hypoxia frequently ensues. Acute Respiratory Distress Syndrome (ARDS) is the extreme form of acute lung injury. ARDS is defined by 4 criteria:

1. Sudden, diffuse, bilateral pulmonary (alveolar) infiltrates
2. Non-cardiogenic pulmonary edema (no evidence of left ventricular dysfunction/congestive heart failure)
3. Hypoxia with a P/F ratio <200 (divide the PaO$_2$ obtained from ABG by the FiO$_2$ [% of delivered air that is oxygen])
4. Precipitating etiology known to cause ARDS

ARDS may result from a number of underlying conditions, including pneumonia, inhalation of toxic substances, aspiration or near-drowning, pancreatitis, massive transfusions, burns and septic shock. ARDS is a common manifestation of the systemic inflammatory cascade causing multi-organ dysfunction syndrome which may occur with septic shock and trauma. Mortality from ARDS is high. Untreated individuals frequently experience rapid deterioration and death (nearly 100% mortality). Even with ICU and ventilatory support, mortality is typically 40-60% depending on the underlying etiology.

Subjective: **Symptoms**
Difficulty breathing and severe shortness of breath, rapidly progressive hypoxemic respiratory failure, agitation, mental status depression.
Focused History: Patient may be too ill to provide comprehensive information. However, precipitating factors as listed should be explored. How long ago did you start feeling sick? (ARDS usually begins 24-48 hours after the initial insult [ie, septic shock].) Alleviating or Aggravating Factors: As previously stated, precipitating factors should be addressed as they may guide therapy.

Objective: **Signs**
Using Basic Tools: Vital signs: Fever may be present and does not necessarily indicate infection. Tachypnea and tachycardia are nearly universally present. Hypoxia helps define the condition and may be profound. In cases of shock (septic or hemorrhagic), hypotension and tachycardia are common. Inspection: The patient will be ill-appearing and typically unstable. Cyanosis (blue/gray/purple skin discoloration) may be present. Use of accessory respiratory muscles may imply impending respiratory failure. Auscultation of chest: Rales or crackles may be heard.
Using Advanced Tools: Pulse Ox: O$_2$ saturation <90% and not responsive to O$_2$ therapy; CXR: Diffuse, fluffy infiltrates & pulmonary edema.

Assessment: **Differential Diagnosis**
Any cause of pulmonary edema or acute lung injury may present similarly to ARDS. As such, ARDS should be considered as a severe consequence at the end of the spectrum of these other causes of acute lung injury (ie, pneumonia, drowning, drug overdose, sepsis, pancreatitis, massive transfusions, etc.). Supportive care with supplemental O$_2$ or mechanical ventilation is the same. The major determining factor is to distinguish non-cardiac causes of pulmonary edema from acute cardiac dysfunction as this requires different treatment. Cardiogenic pulmonary edema (from congestive heart failure, acute ventricular dysfunction or pericardial disease) is suggested by peripheral edema, orthopnea, respiratory crackles and other findings. See Part 4: Organ Systems: Chapter 1: Congestive Heart Failure (Pulmonary Edema)

Plan:
Treatment
Primary:
1. Treat the underlying etiology when possible (ie, initiate antimicrobial therapy for pneumonia and sepsis).
2. Deliver supplemental O$_2$ to maintain normal oxygenation. This will frequently require mechanical ventilator support. Non-invasive methods are not preferred but may be used en route to more definitive care.
3. Unless mandated to treat the underlying cause, administer fluid and blood products sparingly to minimize further pulmonary edema.
4. Evacuate for ICU care and ventilator support as soon as possible. Without evacuation to intensive care support patients with the multiorgan dysfunction seen in ARDS will not do well and should be made as comfortable as possible within the context of operational considerations.

Patient Education
Activity: Bed rest.
Prevention: Suspect this complication with severe injuries and evacuate early.

Follow-up Actions
   Evacuation/Consultation Criteria: Urgently evacuate patients with severe injuries, particularly those who are elderly, very young, have underlying chronic diseases or who are immunocompromised. Consult an intensivist, pulmonologist or internist.

Chapter 3: Respiratory: Chronic Obstructive Sleep Apnea
MAJ Christopher J Lettieri, MC, USA

Introduction: Apnea is a state of no airflow, either with or without respiratory effort, and is defined as a cessation of airflow for ≥10 seconds. Hypopneas are diminished or inadequate airflow and may cause similar physiologic manifestations as apneas. Apnea and hypopneas may result in insufficient respiration with impairments in both ventilation and oxygenation. There are 2 forms of apnea. Central apneas occur when there is no effort to breathe. This is due to a loss of central drive and may occur with head injuries or as a side effect of hypnotics or analgesics, most commonly narcotics and benzodiazepines. Obstructive apneic events occur when there is no airflow despite an intact drive to breath with respiratory muscle activity attempting to breathe. As per the name, this results from an obstruction occurring along the upper respiratory tract. While foreign bodies and blood may obstruct the airways, the most common cause of obstruction is the tongue. The tongue may obstruct the upper airways with mental status depression. This may occur with profound illnesses, trauma or as a consequence of sedating medications or alcohol. Relaxation of pharyngeal and palatal muscles from alcohol, sedatives, muscle relaxants or other CNS depressants can diminish the caliber of the upper airways resulting in apnea or hypopnea. Perhaps the most common reason occurs during sleep in a large number of individuals. This is known as obstructive sleep apnea (OSA). It is known to occur in 2-4% of the adult population but speculations place the prevalence as high as 20-25%. While obesity, age, male gender and habitual snoring are common associated findings, OSA occurs in young, physically fit individuals as well. OSA is a chronic condition with numerous consequences to both health and quality of life. It may cause excessive daytime sleepiness, inattentiveness, depression, GERD, sexual dysfunction, weight gain headaches and sinus congestion. It is also an independent risk factor for heart attack, stroke, heart failure, hypertension and diabetes. Early cardiovascular events and death are significantly more common among individuals with OSA. In susceptible individuals, nasal/sinus congestion and sedation from drugs and alcohol may precipitate or worsen OSA.

Subjective: **Symptoms**
   Early: Disrupted sleep with frequent arousals or repetitive awakenings with transient sensation of shortness of breath (SOB), frequent nocturia (awakening to urinate), morning headache poor memory or concentration, erectile dysfunction or decreased libido, recent weight gain, irritability and habitual loud snoring. Excessive daytime sleepiness is the hallmark of this syndrome.
   Late: Depression, hypertension, heart disease, heart failure, stroke
   Focused History: *Are you sleepy during the day? Have people told you that you snore?* (Excessively sleepiness in a habitual snorer strongly suggests OSA.) *What seems to worsen your symptoms?* (Alcohol or sedatives, and additional weight gain will worsen sleep apnea. These precipitating factors should be avoided until further evaluation or treatment occurs as they may worsen the underlying condition.)

Objective: **Signs**
   Using Basic Tools: Vital signs: For all causes of apnea, the absence of airflow (or breathing) with resulting hypoxia define the condition. Hypertension commonly develops in chronic obstructive sleep apnea. Inspection: Narrowed airway, large tonsils, low-hanging soft palate or uvula may predispose to airway blockage at night. An inability to see the uvula with the mouth open has been shown to increase the risk of OSA. Neck: a neck circumference of greater than 17 inches in men and 15 inches in women increase the risk of OSA. Auscultation: Turbulent airflow during sleep may produce stridor or snoring. Extra heart sounds or crackles at the lung bases may suggest heart failure.
   Using Advanced Tools: Labs: An elevated hematocrit (polycythemia) on CBC may be a consequence of chronic hypoxemia. When resources are limited, OSA can be empirically diagnosed by observing episodic and recurrent episodes of hypoxia (oxygen desaturations) during sleep. A definitive diagnosis requires polysomnography (sleep study) and referral to a sleep medicine or pulmonary specialist.

Assessment: **Differential Diagnosis**
   Narcolepsy: Usually associated with sudden loss of muscle tone during emotional moments, and/or hallucinations on awakening, inadequate sleep (review history), depression/anxiety disorder (*see Part 3: General Symptoms: Depression and Mania & Anxiety*).
   Asthma, COPD, CHF, GERD, prostatic enlargement: Are all causes of nocturnal awakening. See respective sections in this book. If nocturnal awakening occurs suddenly, see panic attacks in *Part 3: General Symptoms: Anxiety*.
   Hypothyroidism: Causes sleep disturbances and sluggishness. *See Part 4: Organ Systems: Thyroid Disorders*
   Medications: Many meds produce daytime sleepiness or sleep disruptions, most commonly sedatives, analgesics, beta-blockers, bronchodilators, steroids, anti-depressants, antihistamines and anti-seizure agents.

Plan:
   Treatment
      Primary:
      1. For acute airway obstruction, removal of the foreign body or repositioning of the tongue (by jaw thrust or adjuvant airway devices) must be done immediately as this is an acute life-threatening condition. When in doubt, securing a definitive airway with endotracheal intubation should be done without hesitation. Minimize sedatives if possible. *See Part 8: Procedures: Chapter 30: Initial Airway Management and Ventilatory Support*
      2. For OSA, treatment options include oral appliances, surgery and Continuous Positive Airway Pressure (CPAP). These are done following referral for specialty care. Short-term therapy can be effective while evacuation or further evaluation is pending. Positional therapy (sleeping on the side) and empiric use of non-invasive ventilation should be attempted. Weight loss should be encouraged and sedating agents should be avoided. Patients should not drive, operate heavy machinery or engage in unsafe activities if excessively sleepy.

Alternative: CNS stimulants provide some short-term effect. For excessive sleepiness, **modafinil** 200mg po q morning has been shown to promote wakefulness and alertness and does not have the same unwanted side effects as amphetamine-based stimulants. **Protriptyline** 10-30mg po or **fluoxetine** 20-60mg po daily may reduce the severity of mild to moderate sleep apnea.

Patient Education

General: Treat obesity with behavior modification. Regaining lost weight will generally cause a return of symptoms.

Activity: Encourage exercise after ensuring cardiorespiratory system is healthy enough to tolerate the stress.

Prevention: Avoid sedatives and alcohol, which act as central nervous system depressants and worsen sleep apnea. Avoid driving while excessively sleepy.

Follow-up Actions

Return Evaluation: Long-term compliance is not high for CPAP unless the patient has severe sleep apnea syndrome. Consider alternate therapies listed previously in these patients.

Evacuation/Consultation Criteria: Evacuation is not typically necessary. Consult primary care physician, internist or pulmonologist as needed. Enlarged tonsils and anatomic abnormalities usually require surgical correction by an ENT surgeon.

Note: A diagnostic sleep study is recommended to make definitive diagnosis.

Chapter 4: Endocrine: Adrenal Insufficiency

MAJ Abel Alfonso, MC, USA & COL Robert Vigersky, MC, USA

Introduction: Primary adrenal insufficiency (AI) is a deficient production of cortisol, and aldosterone that can occur acutely due to hemorrhage, infarction involving the adrenal circulation, gram-negative bacterial sepsis, and blunt or penetrating abdominal trauma. Acute adrenal insufficiency is a medical emergency associated with severe orthostatic hypotension, shock, hyponatremia and often hyperkalemia. Sub-acute or chronic primary adrenal insufficiency is usually the result of an autoimmune process (Addison's disease, or other autoimmune disease), metastatic cancer (in developed countries), or replacement of normal adrenal tissue by tuberculous (TB) infection (in TB endemic areas). Secondary adrenal insufficiency, characterized by deficient production of cortisol but normal production of aldosterone, is most commonly due to adrenal gland suppression from chronic glucocorticoid therapy (eg, prednisone for treatment of chronic obstructive pulmonary disease [COPD]) but can also be caused by disease (eg, malignancies) or injury to or near the hypothalamus or pituitary gland.

Transection or infarction of the hypothalamus or pituitary gland caused by closed or penetrating head trauma can cause and acute form of "secondary" adrenal insufficiency.

Subjective: **Symptoms**

Acute: Severe orthostatic hypotension or shock; severe, poorly localized abdominal pain; nausea; vomiting; weakness; mood change; confusion or psychosis. Sub-acute and chronic: Fatigue, malaise, weight loss, poor appetite, nausea, postural faintness or lightheadedness, loss of libido, depression, anxiety, confusion or acute psychosis.

Focused History: *Do you feel faint or pass out when you stand up?* (orthostatic hypotension) *Do you have nausea and vomiting?* (poor general condition) *Have you lost interest in sex?* (Loss of libido is common.) *Are you having trouble thinking clearly?* (Decreased concentration/mental slowness may be present.) *Do you feel sad or depressed?* (common finding) *Do you have any abdominal pain? Where?* (usually diffuse and poorly localized) *How long have you felt ill?* (If less than four weeks, it may reflect an emergency.) *Do you feel better if you eat salty foods? Do you crave salty food and drink?* (Since sodium loss through the urine is responsible for volume depletion, salt craving is an adaptive response.)

Objective: **Signs**

Using Basic Tools:

Acute Presentation (< 2-4 weeks onset): Orthostatic hypotension*, tachycardia, flank ecchymoses (bruises), fever >100.4°F, confusion/disorientation, ileus/abdominal tenderness (mimicking "acute abdomen").

Sub-acute/Chronic Presentation (>4 weeks): Orthostatic hypotension* (mild), hyperpigmentation (especially palmar creases and scars; primary AI only), loss of muscle mass/loose skin folds; vitiligo (skin depigmentation) goiter (enlargement of the thyroid)

*Systolic BP <20mmHg standing than supine, change in HR >10bpm standing compared to supine

Using Advanced Tools: Labs: **Acute:** Elevated WBC, platelets, eosinophils on CBC with differential, hypoglycemia. **Chronic:** Elevated platelets on CBC, hypoglycemia

Assessment:

Definitive diagnosis will be beyond the capabilities of field laboratories (low sodium, high potassium, low serum AM cortisol, others).

Differential Diagnosis

Acute: Other hypotensive states, including blood loss hypovolemia, volume depletion from gastroenteritis-related vomiting and diarrhea, pancreatitis, and diabetic ketoacidosis.

Sub-acute/chronic: Chronic infections (such as TB, cytomegalovirus [CMV], and fungal infections), metastatic cancer, diabetes mellitus, hyperthyroidism, depression or psychotic states such as bipolar disorder or schizophrenia

Plan:

Treatment

Primary: Acute: Rapidly infuse **normal saline solution** (2L rapidly, then 250-500cc/hour, adjust rate of infusion based on pulse, blood pressure, and overall state of well-being); administer **dexamethasone** 4mg IV as a single dose. Replacement therapy with **hydrocortisone** 20mg po each morning and 10mg po each evening should be administered after resolution of acute symptoms until a definitive medical evaluation by a physician.

Alternative: Prednisone 5-7.5mg po once daily in the morning may be substituted as replacement therapy in lieu of hydrocortisone.

Primitive: If no glucocorticoid medication is available, attempt hemodynamic stabilization by aggressive intravenous hydration using normal saline solution at 250-500cc per hour or more.

Empiric: In any case of shock or severe hypotension without obvious blood loss, render empiric treatment to cover the possibility of adrenal insufficiency. Accompany wide-open intravenous infusion of isotonic saline [0.9% NaCl (NS)] solution with the administration of **dexamethasone** 4mg IV bolus q24 hours (alternatively, **hydrocortisone** 100mg may be given IV q8h).

Patient Education

General: Taking medication daily is essential to preserving health. If an additional acute illness develops, double the daily dose of steroid medication for the duration.

Activity: No restrictions.

Diet: No restrictions. If steroid medication is unavailable, a high-salt diet can help minimize symptoms, preserve blood pressure and overall functional status.

Medications: Chronic corticosteroid use can result in weight gain and other side effects.

Prevention and Hygiene: In developing countries, test the patient and their close contacts for TB, the most common cause of this syndrome worldwide.

No Improvement/Deterioration: Seek medical care promptly for any acute illness resulting in vomiting or if an illness persists for more than a day on double-dose steroid therapy.

Follow-up Actions

Return Evaluation: Expect rapid improvement in symptoms after initiating steroid therapy. After starting maintenance therapy, reassess symptoms and vital signs, including weight and blood pressure within one week. If improved, re-evaluate every 1-3 months.

Evacuation/Consultation Criteria: Referral to a medical center for appropriate confirmatory testing, and treatment.

Chapter 4: Endocrine: Diabetes Mellitus

MAJ Abel Alfonso, MC, USA & COL Robert Vigersky, MC, USA

Introduction: Diabetes mellitus (DM) is a chronic disease that causes abnormally high blood glucose levels and is the leading cause of blindness, amputations, and end-stage renal disease in the United States. Coronary heart disease is the main cause of death in persons with diabetes. Diabetes mellitus results from either absolute deficiency of insulin (type 1 diabetes), or from subnormal target cell response to insulin (insulin resistance) combined with failure to compensate for this insulin resistance because of the inability to produce higher concentrations of insulin (relative insulin deficiency) (type 2 diabetes). Type 2 diabetes accounts for up to 90% of all cases of diabetes. In the Americas and Western Europe, most cases of type 2 diabetes are associated with obesity, a sedentary lifestyle and/or a genetic predisposition. Most patients with type 2 DM have had insulin resistance and asymptomatic hyperglycemia for years before being diagnosed. Type 1 diabetes develops acutely and is most often caused by autoimmune destruction of the insulin-producing beta cells within the pancreatic islets. Patients with type 1 diabetes may exhibit other autoimmune diseases, such as hypothyroidism, rheumatoid arthritis or hyperthyroidism due to Graves' disease. DM due to another endocrine disease (such as Cushing's syndrome or acromegaly) is called secondary diabetes mellitus. Gestational DM is DM that begins during pregnancy, and usually reverses at the time of delivery. Affected women are often overweight and have increased risk of developing type 2 DM later in life. Patients with new or uncontrolled diabetes may occasionally present as an acute medical emergency due to severe dehydration related to a prolonged hyperglycemic condition or severe ketoacidosis related to an inadequate production of insulin.

Subjective: **Symptoms**

Classically: Excessive thirst (polydipsia), excessive urination, especially at night (polyuria/nocturia), weight loss despite increased appetite and food intake (polyphagia), blurred vision. To have these symptoms, blood sugars are typically 300mg/dl and above. Patients with newly diagnosed type 2 DM frequently have no acute symptoms since their blood sugars are not that high but long-standing mild hyperglycemia may cause complications of diabetes, such as foot ulcers, peripheral neuropathy or erectile dysfunction (ED) in men if present for long periods of time (5 or more years).

Focused History: Quantity: *How many times do you wake up to urinate each night?* (>1 is suspicious) *How much weight have you lost?* (Weight loss despite increased food intake is suspicious.) *Is your appetite increased? Are you unusually thirsty?* (polyphagia/polydipsia) *Do you notice any blurring of your vision? Have you had sores on your feet or other wounds that are slow to heal?* (typical in type 2 DM) *Do your feet feel numb or as if you were walking on pins and needles?* (Loss of sensation and pain suggest neuropathy, a possible complication of diabetes.) *Is it difficult or impossible for you to have an erection (males)?* (ED is common.) **Duration:** *When did your symptoms begin?* (Type 1 diabetics may present acutely ill with diabetic ketoacidosis [DKA].) **Other:** *Age?* (Type 1 DM is most common in young [<30 years], slim individuals; type 2 DM is most common in older, overweight individuals.) *Does anyone in your family have diabetes?* (There is a strong family predisposition, particularly with type 2 DM.)

Objective: **Signs**

Physical examination is usually unreliable for diagnosis of DM.

Using Basic Tools: Vital signs: BP drop >20mmHg systolic comparing supine vs. standing position (orthostatic hypotension), tachycardia (autonomic neuropathy)

Inspection: Central obesity ("beer belly" or "apple on a stick" configuration); dry mucous membranes (reflecting volume loss/dehydration); fruity/acetone breath smell (seen in type 1 diabetics with DKA); ulcers on the soles of the feet (secondary to peripheral neuropathy and poor wound healing); vitiligo (de-pigmented regions of skin) or goiter (enlargement of the thyroid gland) can be associated with type 1 diabetes and other autoimmune endocrine diseases. Palpation: "Tenting" of the skin (suggests volume depletion in young individuals); reduced or absent light touch sensation in distal legs and feet (reflects peripheral neuropathy, associated with diabetes).

Percussion: Absent ankle jerk or knee reflexes (may reflect peripheral neuropathy, associated with diabetes).

Using Advanced Tools: Labs: Test for glucose and ketones on urine dipstick (DM diagnosis); blood glucose by fingerstick; hemoglobin A1c which reflects the average blood glucose over the past 2-3 months (not available in the field).

Assessment: **Differential Diagnosis**

Malabsorption states, protein/calorie malnutrition, hyperthyroidism: Can also cause weight loss/increased appetite

Diabetes insipidus (polyuria due to hormonal or renal causes), urinary tract infection, and prostatic hypertrophy: Can also cause polyuria

Diabetes insipidus: Can cause polydipsia

Plan:

Treatment

Primary: Patients with severe hyperglycemia with blood glucose >250mg/dL (hyperosmolar shock) and/or large ketonuria (ketoacidosis) can present as an acute emergency. For severely ill patients, volume replacement and **NPH insulin** at an empiric starting dose of 0.3 units/kg body weight, IV may be required. Evacuate profoundly symptomatic patients; look for orthostatic hypotension, nausea and vomiting, "large" ketones and glucose on urine dipstick as major indications to evacuate. Give high volume **isotonic saline** (0.9 NaCl/ Normal Saline) fluid therapy and intravenous **regular insulin** (10 units preferably given IV although IM or SQ can be used initially, followed by 5 units per hour) while en route. Monitor finger-stick blood glucose (FSBG) prior to administering insulin, every hour during IV insulin therapy, and for major change in clinical condition. Do not give additional insulin if FSBG <200mg/dL due to possibility of insulin-induced hypoglycemia, but continue to monitor blood glucose every hour. Resume insulin therapy if follow up FSBG >250mg/dL. Although serum potassium levels might seem normal or elevated upon presentation, total body potassium stores are deplete and levels will likely fall rapidly following insulin administration and correction of acidosis. For this reason, serum electrolytes should be followed very closely and replenished whenever possible. When stable, insulin SC divided in two daily doses (every 12 hours) may be required to manage hyperglycemia. Management of diabetes may require an oral hypoglycemic agent for fasting blood sugar in the 200-250mg/dl range: **glipizide** 5-10mg/day or **glyburide** 5mg/day are effective and widely available. Give stable newly diagnosed diabetics appropriate dietary and exercise regimens (*see Patient Education section*).

Primitive: Severely symptomatic patients who are volume depleted can be treated with aggressive isotonic saline (0.9 NaCl/Normal Saline) infusion IV (1-2L over one hour, followed by 150-250cc/hour), pending transport to a definitive care facility. Urine output is the best indicator of hydration status

Empiric: Empiric drug or insulin therapy is potentially dangerous and should be avoided in the absence of blood glucose testing. Patients with positive urine ketones and a rapid respiratory rate probably have profound metabolic acidosis (ketoacidosis) and need to be transported to a skilled medical facility as soon as possible.

Patient Education

General: DM is usually a permanent condition, but careful self-management offers long-term benefit in minimizing occurrence and severity of micro- and macrovascular (small and large blood vessel) complications.

Activity: Stable patients benefit from 45-60 minutes of moderate aerobic exercise. Walking 2-3 miles daily is usually well tolerated in the absence of foot lesions.

Diet: Acutely ill patients such as those with DKA should be kept NPO while en route to a definitive care facility. In stable patients, limit intake of simple sugars in favor of a balanced diet comprised of 45-60% of total energy intake in the form of complex carbohydrates (fruits, vegetables, whole grains and low-fat dairy products). Severe restriction of dietary carbohydrates in diabetes is not indicated. Even modest weight loss (5%-10% of total body weight) can have beneficial effects in overweight and obese diabetics. A reduction from usual intake of approximately 500kcal/day is recommended with a goal of losing approximately 2 lbs/week.

Prevention and Hygiene: Patients should return for a urinary dipstick test bid until urinary glucose and ketones are negative or trace. No Improvement/Deterioration: Patients should be referred for definitive medical care.

Follow-up Actions

Return Evaluation: Daily to twice weekly initially, as dictated by severity of hyperglycemia and ketonuria.

Evacuation Consultation Criteria: Immediately evacuate all severely hyperglycemic, severely ketonuric or pregnant patients. All other patients with diabetes mellitus should be evacuated at the earliest availability.

Chapter 4: Endocrine: Hypoglycemia

MAJ Abel Alfonso, MC, USA & COL Robert Vigersky, MC, USA

Introduction: Hypoglycemia is an abnormally low blood glucose level. The level that individual patients experience signs and symptoms of low blood sugar varies. It usually occurs below 60mg/dL; blood glucose ≥70mg/dL is not considered hypoglycemia. Normal body function depends on glucose, the primary energy source for most cells. Metabolism of glucose is mediated by glucagon and epinephrine (which stimulate the liver to change stored glycogen into glucose for use as an energy source) and by cortisol and growth hormone.

Collectively, glucagon, epinephrine, cortisol and growth hormone are called counter-regulatory hormones because they oppose the action of insulin on glucose metabolism. Insulin promotes uptake of glucose by muscle and other tissues and removal of excess circulating blood glucose for storage in the liver as glycogen. A blood sugar at any given point in time is a function of 3 factors: the amount of food eaten, the amount of insulin, and amount of counter-regulatory hormones. Therefore, hypoglycemia is caused by an imbalance among these 3 factors.

Subjective: **Symptoms**

Signs of severe hypoglycemia (needing assistance of others to correct hypoglycemic episode) include abrupt change in mental status, a decline in the level of consciousness, seizures and coma. Other symptoms include amnesia, bizarre behavior, hemiparesis (muscular weakness or partial paralysis affecting one side of the body), poor coordination, double or blurred vision, and headaches. Early signs of low blood glucose include anxiety, hunger, generalized sweating, palpitations and tremor. Some individuals have been mistaken for being drunk.

Focused History: *Do you feel shaky or nervous?* (suggests adrenergic nervous system response to hypoglycemia) *Do you have a craving for sugar or foods?* (appetite stimulated by falling blood glucose level) *Are you having difficulty thinking clearly?* (Cental nervous system [CNS] dysfunction results from significant hypoglycemia.) *When did your symptoms begin? Has it ever happened before?* (True hypoglycemia begins abruptly, and can recur in similar circumstances over time.) *Do you have symptoms in the mornings before* *eating breakfast? Do you have symptoms before or after meals?* (Timing the onset of symptoms may point to the underlying cause of hypoglycemia.) *When was your last meal? Were you more active today than usual?* (Decreased food intake or unaccustomed exercise are common precipitants of hypoglycemic attacks.) *Do you have diabetes? Are you taking insulin or pills to control your diabetes?* (Most patients with hypoglycemia are receiving drug treatment for diabetes mellitus.) *How long after eating did your symptoms improve?* (Hypoglycemia reverses rapidly with ingestion of carbohydrate.)

Objective: Signs

Using Basic Tools: Notoriously non-specific symptoms that resolve WITHIN MINUTES after giving IV or oral glucose. Vital signs: Tachycardia, hypertension, tachypnea. Inspection: Diaphoresis, dilated pupils, confusional or psychotic state, drowsy or comatose, ataxic gait, coma, generalized seizure. Auscultation: Aortic or pulmonic flow murmurs. Palpation: Left- or right-sided facial/upper extremity/lower extremity weakness or paralysis; decreased visual acuity or visual fields. Percussion: Brisk deep tendon reflexes

Using Advanced Tools: Labs: Glucose and ketones on urine dipstick. The glucose should be negative and the ketones might be positive. (Lack of food intake for more than 8-10 hours can cause starvation ketosis.)

Assessment:

Always consider hypoglycemia as an easily treatable form of mental status impairment. ALWAYS check for it in patients presenting with coma, seizure, confusion or focal neurologic signs.

Differential Diagnosis: Drug overdose with sedative or narcotic agents, alcohol intoxication, idiopathic seizure disorder, closed head trauma, CNS infection (meningitis, encephalitis), and a variety of metabolic insults (uremia, metabolic alkalosis, respiratory acidosis or severe hyponatremia) can all produce severe confusion or coma and cannot be visually distinguished from hypoglycemia. At times hypoglycemia can provoke focal neurologic signs such as hemiparesis, which reverse with treatment of hypoglycemia.

Plan:

Treatment

Primary: 1 amp of 50% **dextrose in water (D50W)** should be injected IV push, rapidly.

Alternative: Mild symptoms and cooperative: 8 oz of sweetened fruit juice, non-diet colas or sports drink (ie, Gatorade)

Empiric: 1 amp of **D50W** rapid IV push for any form of mental status impairment when blood glucose testing is unavailable

Emergent: Glucagon 1mg may be reconstituted (comes as two vials, a powder and a diluent, which must be combined) and injected IM if IV access is difficult or impossible.

Patient Education

General: Wear a medical alert bracelet or necklace if prone to hypoglycemia.

Activity: Except as noted, normal unrestricted activity is permitted.

Diet: Normal diet unless frequent hypoglycemia, then add mid-morning, mid-afternoon, and bedtime snacks and eliminate "free sugars" (ie, regular sodas, candy, cakes, pies, juices, etc.).

Medications: Patients with history of severe hypoglycemia need glucagon self-injection kit for IM administration; family members and roommates should be instructed on proper use as well.

Prevention and Hygiene: Do not miss meals or exercise strenuously after 4 or more hours of fasting. Check finger-stick blood glucose prior to exercise or driving.

No Improvement/Deterioration: Give patients with severe symptomatic presentations (coma, seizures, focal neurologic signs) IV 5% dextrose (in normal or half-normal saline) after recovery. Observe 12-24 hours.

Follow-up Actions

Return Evaluation: Routine diabetes-oriented care and education should suffice for most patients with diabetes mellitus an episodes of hypoglycemia. Recurrent hypoglycemia following treatment mandates additional **D50W** and evacuation. Consider pituitary or adrenal insufficiency, renal or hepatic failure.

Evaluation/Consultation Criteria: Severe (coma, seizure, focal neurologic presentation) or frequent (>1 severe episode per month) hypoglycemia should be evacuated.

Chapter 4: Endocrine: Thyroid Disorders

MAJ Abel Alfonso, MC, USA & COL Robert Vigersky, MC, USA

Introduction: Goiter is an enlargement of the thyroid gland, which can usually be appreciated visually or by palpation. The presence of a goiter does not indicate whether there is too much, too little, or the correct amount of thyroid hormone being produced. For example, goiter may be an adaptive process, reflecting increased size and number of thyroid follicles in an attempt to overcome deficient production of thyroid hormones by individual cells with a net normal thyroid hormone level. It can also be a result of autonomous excessive or diminished thyroid hormone production. Worldwide, a common cause of simple goiter is iodine deficiency. This usually results in an insufficient amount of thyroid hormone being produced. This condition is not expected in island or coastal regions where seafood or kelp (iodine-rich foods) is consumed regularly, but may occur inland in large continents. Areas of the world where iodine deficiency is known to be a significant problem include mountainous regions, parts of sub-Saharan Africa and central China. **Hyperthyroidism** (an overactive thyroid which is sometimes referred to as thyrotoxicosis) is most commonly due to Graves' disease, an autoimmune disease caused by one or more antibodies stimulating the thyroid stimulating hormone (TSH) receptor. TSH itself comes from the pituitary gland and is responsible for stimulating the thyroid to make thyroid hormones such as l-thyroxine. Another cause of hyperthyroidism, toxic multinodular goiter, results when thyroid hormone is produced independently. It can also be caused by too much exogenous administration of l-thyroxine. Finally, hyperthyroidism can result from leakage of thyroid hormones from a gland damaged in trauma or from viral infection in a self-limited process called thyroiditis or from exogenous administration. TSH-induced hyperthyroidism is extremely rare. **Hypothyroidism** (an underactive thyroid) most commonly results from autoantibodies directed against thyroid enzymes, resulting in decreased production of thyroid hormones. Other causes include iatrogenic (occurring as the result of treatment by a physician or surgeon) due to radioactive iodine therapy or thyroidectomy, transient hypothyroidism after a period of thyroiditis, and certain drugs. TSH deficiency is uncommon and rarely occurs without other evidence of pituitary disease.

Subjective: **Symptoms**

Simple goiter: Mass in the anterior neck; dysphagia; dysphonia (hoarseness); stridor, cough or wheezing as a result of compression of the esophagus, recurrent laryngeal nerves or trachea by the goiter.

Hyperthyroidism: Excessive sweating, heat intolerance, fatigue, muscle weakness, reduced exercise tolerance, nervousness, irritability, tremor, weight loss, increased frequency of bowel movements (hyper-defecation rather than diarrhea), oligomenorrhea (infrequent menstruation), palpitations, insomnia, and eye irritation/discomfort. See notes for comments on pregnancy and thyroid storm.

Hypothyroidism: Fatigue, depressed mood, poor memory, somnolence, cold intolerance, weight gain, hair loss, constipation, menorrhagia (menstruation with excessive flow), and muscle cramps.

Focused History: Goiter: *Are you aware of a lump in your neck?* (Many patients with goiter are unaware.)

Hyperthyroidism: *Do you have more bowel movements per day than you did before?* (Increased frequency suggests hyper-defecation.) *Does your heart race at night or does a rapid heartbeat wake you from sleep?* (Persistent rapid heart rate is typical.) *Have you become thinner or lost weight?* (typical) **Hypothyroidism:** *Have you recently gained weight?* (common) *How many hours are you sleeping each day? How long have you required this much sleep? Do you fall asleep or feel tired during the day?* (Increased sleep requirement is typical.) *Are you having fewer bowel movements each week than you did before?* (Constipation is typical.)

Mass Effect of Goiter: *Do you have any difficulty when you breathe in?* (stridor) *Do you cough or feel as if you are choking when you lie down?* (compressing trachea) *Do you have difficulty swallowing solid food like meat?* (esophageal compression) *Do you have persistent hoarseness or change in your voice?* (compression of vocal cord nerves) **Hyperthyroidism:** *Do you feel "hotter" than other members of your family and do you feel sick when it is hot?* (heat intolerance) *Do you feel nervous or irritable most of the time? Do your hands tremble most of the time?* (typical symptoms) **Hypothyroidism:** *Do you notice any change in your hair? Is it falling out by handfuls? When did you become aware of hair loss? Do you seem "colder" than other members of your family?* (typical symptoms) *Do you have trouble concentrating or being alert while you are working?* (decreased state of alertness and mental slowing) *Do you have cramps in your legs when you walk or run?* (neuromuscular dysfunction)

Goiter: *How long have you been aware of a mass in your neck?* (Benign goiter may be present for many years; sudden appearance suggests possibility of cancer.) *Do other members of your family have a lump like this?* (Goiter may manifest heritable thyroid dysfunction.) *Any history of ionizing radiation exposure?* (increased likelihood of developing thyroid cancer) *When did you first begin to feel different from normal?* (Sudden onset suggests thyroiditis or a dietary exposure, such as iodine.)

Alleviating and Aggravating Factors: *Do you feel/function better or worse when it is warm (or cold)?* (hypothyroidism: poor tolerance for cold; hyperthyroidism: poor tolerance for heat)

Objective: **Signs**

Simple Goiter: Using Basic Tools: Vital signs should be normal. Inspection: Look for an obvious lump or mass in the anterior neck, below the thyroid cartilage ("Adam's apple"). Palpation: Enlarged, smooth or nodular, fleshy or firm to hard mass in the anterior neck, between the thyroid and cricoid cartilages.

Hyperthyroidism: Using Basic Tools: Vital signs: Tachycardia (HR >100 bpm or significantly higher than baseline); Diastolic BP might be elevated (>90mmHg). Inspection: Fine tremor of hands at rest, stare, proptosis (projecting globe of the eye, creating a "bug-eyed" appearance), eyelid lag. Palpation: Diffuse or nodular goiter (thyroid enlargement), diaphoresis (warm, moist palms and generalized increased sweating) Auscultation: Bruit over thyroid gland or supraclavicular space, systolic ejection murmur (reflect increased cardiac output), sinus tachycardia or atrial fibrillation (irregular heart rhythm/pulse). Percussion: Brisk deep tendon reflexes (reflects increased neuromuscular irritability).

Hypothyroidism: Using Basic Tools: Vital signs: Temperature <97°F; bradycardia <60/min. Inspection: Pale, thin, dry skin; "droopy" eyelids; loss of lateral eyebrow, periorbital and facial edema; coarse voice; slow response to questions; depressed affect. Palpation: Diffuse, firm goiter (thyroid enlargement) in anterior neck; cool, dry skin. Percussion: Delayed deep tendon reflex return phase, especially at ankles (return is like a "ratchet").

Assessment:

Patients with goiters require serum TSH and thyroid hormone (thyroxine or free thyroxine) measurement, which are not available in the field, for accurate differentiation between hyper- and hypothyroidism.

Differential Diagnosis

Goiter: Other anterior neck masses are frequently either solid tumors (may be benign or malignant) or cysts (usually benign). Goiter will usually be distinguished by moving up and down with swallowing, whereas other neck masses may remain fixed.

Hyperthyroidism: Anxiety states, factitious disorder, starvation/malnutrition, pheochromocytoma (tumor of the adrenal medulla or sympathetic paraganglia), stimulant drug abuse (cocaine, amphetamines), and congestive heart failure may produce similar symptoms. The finding of a goiter and the absence of prior psychiatric history and drug abuse history strongly favors hyperthyroidism.

Hypothyroidism: Depression, chronic fatigue syndrome, bereavement, hypothermia, sedative drug abuse (barbiturates, benzodiazepines, etc.) may cause similar symptoms. Most patients with hypothyroidism are not acutely ill, and can begin empiric treatment on a cautious basis. This is especially true in the elderly with possible underlying coronary heart disease. Very sick individuals require urgent evacuation, including patients in coma and those with profound hypothermia (temp <96°F).

Plan:

Treatment

Simple Goiter

Primary: Definitive treatment is dependent on the results of blood tests not available in the field.

Primitive/Empiric: Iodine supplementation (low dose if in goiter-endemic area)

Hyperthyroidism

Primary: Propranolol 10-40mg po qid to render pulse <80bpm and decrease tremors. An alternative beta-blocker would be **atenolol** 50-100mg po bid. **Verapamil** 40-80mg po tid may be used in patients with contraindications to beta-blockers.

Hypothyroidism
   Primary: Definitive treatment is dependent on the results of blood tests not available in the field.
   Primitive: Provide warmest possible environmental temperature and encourage physical activity.
Patient Education
   General: Definitive blood testing is an important aspect of care and follow-up is essential to well-being.
   Activity: Normal activities are permitted without restriction for patients with simple goiter. Patients with suspected or confirmed hyperthyroidism should not perform strenuous exercise or employment-related activity until the condition is improved. Acceptable activities include light duty in a cool (preferably indoor) environment, and clerical duties.
   Diet: Avoid dietary goitrogens (see note) in patients with simple goiter or hypothyroidism.

Follow-up Actions
   Return Evaluation: Most patients with minor symptoms can be followed at two to four-week intervals. For patients with hyperthyroidism, emphasis should be on heart rate control (goal is <80 bpm) and tremor control. Definitive therapy includes oral medications (usually methimazole or propylthiouracil), radioactive iodine therapy, or surgical intervention (thyroidectomy).
   Evacuation/Consultation Criteria: Severe symptoms, including high fever, confusion or delirium, congestive heart failure, hypothermia, coma, severe bradycardia, or local compressive symptoms in the neck (especially choking or stridor) require urgent evacuation to a referral center attended by an endocrinologist (a specialist in gland and hormone disorders).
   Notes: Dietary goitrogens: Cassava meal, cabbage, rutabaga, and turnips impair the action of the enzyme thyroid peroxidase, and may worsen simple goiter and induce hypothyroidism. Pregnancy: Normal pregnancy results in mild symptoms that can be confused with hyperthyroidism. Severe symptoms suggest the presence of hyperthyroidism in pregnancy and expedient consultation is required if at all possible. Slight enlargement of the thyroid gland is expected in normal pregnancy. Thyroid Storm: Most cases of hyperthyroidism are not emergencies, but the medic should be alert to the possibility of the syndrome of thyroid storm. Thyroid storm is a symptom constellation including fever, delirium (or confusion, also known as encephalopathy), very marked tachycardia, and a generally "toxic" appearance. Individuals with these features require emergent evacuation to a skilled medical facility. Interim treatment in the field should include beta-blocker medication (**propranolol**), antipyretic therapy with **acetaminophen** (theoretically, aspirin may worsen the condition by releasing thyroid hormone from binding sites on plasma proteins) and/or ice packs, and sedation using benzodiazepines or **haloperidol.**

Chapter 5: Neurologic: Seizure Disorders and Epilepsy
CDR Robert Wall, MC, USN

Introduction: A seizure is an uncommon event that can be caused by many different ailments and processes. Not all convulsions become an epileptic condition, and most are brief and self-limited. Once a "diagnosis" of epilepsy is documented, it will follow the patient for the rest of their life and greatly impact their employability, insurability, driving status and many other areas.

Subjective: Symptoms
   Abrupt onset of abnormal muscle activity, or prodrome of confusion, déjà vu, peculiar behavior, automatisms, or other psychic phenomena preceding onset.
   Focused History: *Did injury or illness precede the seizure ?* (trauma, infection) *Was there an aura prior to the seizure?* (prodrome, complex partial seizure) *How long did the seizure last? Did you bite your tongue or were you incontinent?* (frequently seen in seizure) *How did you feel after the seizure?* (post ictal phase) *Have you had seizures before including childhood?* (recurrence suggestive of epilepsy) *What medications are you taking?* (Some may decrease seizure threshold.) *What is your alcohol history?* (association with seizures)

Objective: Signs
   Using Basic Tools: Sudden onset of loss of consciousness, followed by abnormal motor activity such as tonic rigidity, clonic rhythmic movements of the limbs, urinary incontinence, frothing at the mouth, and biting the tongue and mouth; may last seconds to minutes, and is usually followed by a period of weakness, somnolence and confusion (post-ictal state); seizure will spontaneously stop without any intervention after a few minutes.
   Using Advanced Tools: Labs: WBC for infection; urinalysis for glucose level; ECG for arrhythmia etiology for syncope.

Assessment: Differential Diagnosis
   The differential diagnosis of a convulsive event is extensive: idiopathic epilepsy, alcohol or drug associated seizures, post concussive syndrome, convulsive syncope, heat stroke, infectious (meningitis), brain mass lesions, nerve gas exposure and metabolic abnormalities, eclampsia in pregnancy. Wellbutrin, INH and other medications may lower seizure threshold. *See index and appropriate sections of this book for discussions of most of these conditions.*

Plan:
   Treatment
   Many of these medications and procedures may not be available in the field.
   Primary: Symptomatic treatment initially.
   1. Remove the patient from an area where he could injure himself or others. Keep sharp and breakable objects away from the patient. Pad objects to avoid injury.
   2. Do not put anything in the patient's mouth. Never put your fingers in the patient's mouth.
   3. MEDICATIONS ARE RARELY INDICATED FOR A FIRST TIME SEIZURE.
   4. After the seizure, evacuate the patient to an appropriate treatment facility for a neurological examination and further evaluation. The exam will usually be normal, other than confusion and somnolence in the immediate post-ictal period, which may last for hours. After focal motor seizures, there may be a period of Todd's paralysis, which is focal weakness of the affected limb.

Alternate: For recurrent seizures:

1. If the seizure lasts more than 10 minutes, immediate medical intervention is indicated.
2. Begin an IV access line.
3. EEG monitoring if available.
4. Administer benzodiazepine: **Lorazepam** 4-8mg IV.
5. If lorazepam unavailable, consider **diazepam** 5-20mg IV. (Lorazepam has slightly longer onset [~3 min], but longer half-life [12-24 hours]. Diazepam acts slightly more rapidly [~2 min] but shorter half-life [15-30 min]).
6. If this does not stop the seizure, consider **phenytoin** 1000mg IV as an infusion over 30 minutes, not to exceed 50mg/min. When giving phenytoin as an infusion, do not mix it with D5W because it will precipitate. Clear the IV tubing with normal saline first.
7. If this does not stop the seizure, consider **phenobarbital** 10mg/kg IV over 10 minutes. May be repeated one time. Must have a secure airway. Closely monitor breathing.
8. If this does not stop the seizure, general anesthesia or barbiturate coma may be required. Advanced care will be required.
9. Transport to the nearest MTF for further evaluation and disposition. Use **phenytoin** 300mg po or IV q day for MEDEVAC transport. Always monitor the airway as these drugs may cause respiratory suppression. If IV unavailable, **phenobarbital** may be given IM. Do not give phenytoin or diazepam IM.

Note: If seizure lasts more than ten minutes, there is the possibility of status epilepticus. These seizures must be stopped ASAP. This is a life-threatening event and may produce significant brain injury if the patient survives. Emergency medical assistance and intervention must be rapidly sought.

Patient Education

General: NO DRIVING, WEAPONS HANDLING, OR OTHER DANGEROUS ACTIVITIES UNTIL MEDICALLY CLEARED. DMV reporting per state requirements.

Activity: Normal as tolerated. Avoid sports/activities such as scuba diving, skiing, horseback riding, or activities where there could be injury to self or others should a seizure occur. Weight lifting with a spotter only.

Diet: Avoid alcohol.

Prevention and Hygiene: Low stress, good diet, exercise, and good sleep hygiene (8 hours per night, regularly).

Follow-up Actions

Return Evaluation: In 2-4 weeks as necessary.

Evacuation/Consultation Criteria: Urgent evacuation is not normally required for a patient with a single seizure that spontaneously resolved. Patients should ultimately be referred for a non-emergent, ROUTINE Neurological Consultation.

Note: Though epilepsy afflicts up to 1% of the population, non-epileptic convulsive events are considerably more common.

Chapter 5: Neurologic: Meningitis

CDR Robert Wall, MC, USN

Introduction: Meningitis is an acute, life-threatening infection of the lining of the brain and spinal cord. It can be caused by a virus, bacteria, fungus, parasite, or more complex organism. Travel to exotic places, especially those with questionable sewage and pest control, increases the risk of acquiring and disseminating this disease. Bacterial meningitis is rapidly progressive and should be considered an emergency. Aseptic meningitis (normally caused by viruses) has a less acute course. Meningitis is a treatable and potentially curable disease if diagnosed and treated early. However, delays in diagnosis and treatment can lead to permanent neurological disability and possibly death. *Also see Part 5: Specialty Areas: Chapter 15: Serious Pediatric Diseases: Meningitis*

Subjective: **Symptoms**

Fever, stiff neck, headache, photophobia, malaise; later: delirium, coma, seizures, nausea, vomiting, dizziness

Focused History: *How fast did your symptoms progress?* (period of hours for bacterial meningitis, but longer for viral) *Have you been exposed to others who have been ill or had meningitis?* (Ear infections, sinus disease, pneumonia, UTIs, bronchitis, sepsis, infected wounds may harbor meningitis organisms.) *Have you taken any antibiotics recently?* (Presentation may be masked.) *Have you had meningitis in the past?* (increased susceptibility) *Do you have any immune deficiency?* (increases susceptibility) *Does it hurt to bend your neck or touch your chin to your chest?* (typically positive in infection) *Have you noticed any new rash?* (petechiae in early meningococcal meningitis)

Note: US Military Personnel are generally immunized against meningococcal meningitis.

Objective: **Signs**

Using Basic Tools: Fever; cervical meningismus (stiff neck, painful to move); prostration; toxic appearance; positive Kernig's sign (inability to completely extend the knees straight – stretches spinal cord); positive Brudzinski sign (forward flexion of the head produces flexion at hip and knee – stretches spinal cord); rash (may indicate activation of the clotting cascade—hemorrhagic fevers; or petechial with meningococcus). Chronic infection: deafness.

Note: Do complete neurological examination, including Glasgow Coma Scale (*see Appendices: Table A-5. Glasgow Coma Scale*), looking for alterations of mental status or ambulation, and focal neurological deficits. Perform a thorough examination for possible sources of infection, such as middle ear, sinus, lungs, urinary tract, and wounds.

Using Advanced Tools: Labs: WBC count or blood smear (may show leukocytosis in bacterial meningitis), urinalysis; RPR, blood cultures; CXR

Assessment:

Differential Diagnosis: Other than by using the presence of systemic signs of infection and meningeal signs, these diagnoses will be very difficult to distinguish in the field. If in doubt, treat for bacterial meningitis. Meningitis comes in many forms that are infectious, the most common including bacterial and viral. Fungal, cryptococcal and coccidioidal forms also may occur in immunocompromised patients, but may also occur in the immunocompetent as well. Other more rare forms include tuberculous, parasitic, and spirochetal.

Rickettsial infection: Usually no leukocytosis; no meningeal signs; "tache noire" lesion (an ulcer covered with black, adherent crust)
Leptospirosis: Look for conjunctival discharge; history of exposure to water which might be contaminated with animal urine
Cerebral malaria: No meningeal signs; positive blood smear; thrombocytopenia
Malignancy: Variable symptoms based on lesion location.
Severe viral or bacterial sepsis: With headache, high fever, but without meningeal seeding
Brain abscess: Focal neurologic findings; low-grade temperatures; no neck stiffness or tenderness
Subdural/epidural hematoma: History of trauma with rapid or progressive development of symptoms
Subarachnoid hemorrhage: Often low-grade temperature; acute onset preceded by severe headaches; focal neurologic findings
Stroke: Variable symptoms based on lesion location

Plan:
Treatment
Important Note: Certain procedures and medications may be limited or unavailable in the field setting.

1. Begin antibiotics as soon as possible if bacterial meningitis is suspected (time to antibiotic administration is correlated with outcome).
   Empiric Choices: Adult dosages:
   Ceftriaxone (first line if available) 2g IV q12h. May require as much as 14 days or longer as indicated.
   Cefotaxime 2g IV q4-6h. May require as much as 14 days or longer as indicated.
   Penicillin 24 million units/day IV in 6 divided doses. May require as much as 14 days or longer as indicated.
   Ampicillin (Not recommended as monotherapy due to pneumococcal resistance. Consider adding in the very young, elderly, or immunocompromised to cover listeriosis) 12g/day IV in 6 divided doses. May require as much as 14 days or longer as indicated.
   Vancomycin (Consider adding in infants and small children, as well as to cover PRSP. Not recommended as monotherapy; no meningococcus coverage.) 2g/day IV in 2 divided doses. May require as much as 14 days or longer as indicated.
2. Evacuate immediately.
3. Airway support and oxygen. Intubate as needed.
4. Fluid hydration with IV NS or LR.
5. Control fever with **acetaminophen** 650mg po q4-6h prn.
6. If HSV encephalitis is suspected, give **acyclovir** 12.5mg/kg/day IV divided tid x 10 days.
7. Consider steroids (**dexamethasone** 0.15mg/kg/day IV q6h x 4 days), with first dose prior to starting antibiotics, if bacterial meningitis is likely present (based on an acute presentation).
8. Additional pain medication and sedation may be necessary. Be aware that such medications may affect the mental status examination and should not be confused with an encephalitis presentation.

Patient Education
Activity: Bedrest
Diet: As tolerated.
Prevention and Hygiene: Meningococcal vaccine: Required for personnel deploying to countries within the EUCOMAOR where the risk of meningococcal disease is significantly elevated above the US baseline, including: ALL OF AFRICA EXCEPT: South Africa, Botswana, Swaziland, Lesotho, and Zimbabwe. Meningococcal vaccine is not required for personnel deploying only to other countries in the EUCOM AOR. Meningitis may be contagious and good personal hygiene is mandatory. Respiratory isolation for first 24 hours of therapy (possible droplet spread of organism). Consider meningococcal vaccine pre-deployment. Give intimate/household contacts of suspected meningococcal or *Haemophilus influenzae* type b (Hib) meningitis patients prophylaxis with **ciprofloxacin** 500mg po x 1 dose in adults (CONTRAINDICATED IN PREGNANT PATIENTS). Alternate prophylaxis regimens: **ceftriaxone** 250mg IM x 1 dose, or **rifampin** 600mg po q12h x 4 doses, or **azithromycin** 500mg po x 1 dose, or **ofloxacin** 400mg po x 1 dose. No Improvement/Deterioration: Return to the medic for persistent fever or mental status changes.

Follow-up Actions
Return Evaluation: Return to medic 3-5 days after discharge for reevaluation, including repeat neuro exam.
Evacuation/Consultation Criteria: Evacuate immediately after starting antibiotics, if meningitis is suspected. Refer to Infectious Disease or Internal Medicine for definitive treatment. Consult Neurologist in difficult cases. A lumbar puncture with evaluation of spinal fluid, which is not available in a field environment, is the definitive test to diagnose meningitis.
Note: Penicillin allergic patients may also have allergic reactions to ceftriaxone.

Chapter 5: Neurologic: Trigeminal Neuralgia
CDR Christopher Jankosky, MC, USN

Introduction: Trigeminal neuralgia represents one of the most painful conditions in the orofacial area. It affects approximately 5 people per hundred thousand per year. There is a slight female predominance. Incidence peaks in middle age. The etiology is related to injury to the trigeminal (fifth cranial) nerve or brainstem trigeminal pathways. Microvascular compression of the trigeminal nerve root in the posterior fossa is thought to be the most common etiology. The diagnosis is made clinically, based on signs and symptoms, as well as excluding other possible causes of facial pain.

Subjective: **Symptoms**
Characterized by the abrupt onset of paroxysmal episodes of unilateral lancinating pain in the distribution of one or more divisions of the 5th cranial nerve. The 2nd or 3rd division of the trigeminal nerve (mid and lower face) are most commonly affected. Pain confined to only

the 1st division (upper face, including the eye region) is rare. More than one division may be affected. These brief lightning-like spasms of pain last for seconds (usually less than 2 minutes), but may occur in rapid succession for a period of several hours. Episodes can recur throughout the day or night. Between attacks there are no symptoms. Episodes are commonly initiated by nonpainful physical stimulation of specific facial "trigger points." Chewing food, talking, brushing the teeth, or washing the face may also aggravate trigger points.

Focused History: History should focus on onset, duration, character, and intensity of pain. *Does the patient have a trigger point?* (Inquire about past dental, facial, or cranial injuries or surgical procedures.) *Are there any underlying symptoms such as chronic headache, facial pain, fevers, chills, or fatigue?* (In the young active duty population, focus on possible underlying multiple sclerosis [previous transient neurologic symptoms lasting greater than 24 hours] or a brain stem tumor [headaches, vertigo, visual changes, or other neurologic symptoms].)

Objective: Signs
Using Basic Tools: Perform a complete neurologic exam, with attention to the cranial nerves. Although the patient may describe a subjective area of altered sensation on the face, there should be no objective sensory or motor deficits on the examination. Carefully examine the teeth, gums, sinuses, and oropharynx to rule out an infectious or inflammatory disease processes.

Using Advanced Tools: Laboratory exams are normal in trigeminal neuralgia, with labs determined by the need to rule out other potential diagnoses (for example, an ESR to evaluate for temporal arteritis).

Assessment:
Differential Diagnosis: There are many conditions that on initial evaluation may be mistaken for trigeminal neuralgia. Many of these conditions have continuous pain. Alternate conditions may have associated sensory loss, diminished corneal reflex, involvement of adjacent brainstem structures, fever, fatigue, or additional findings on examination.

Multiple sclerosis: Signs of neurological deficit, localized to different CNS locations, separated over time.

Brainstem region tumors or vascular lesions: Specific neurological symptoms or signs will suggest location

Infections: Should include other signs of infection

Herpes zoster or post herpetic neuralgia: Evaluate for facial skin lesions over painful area.

Hemicranial migraine, cluster headache: *See Part 3: General Symptoms: Headache*

Dental caries: Identified by thorough dental exam

Temporal arteritis: Generally a disease seen in patients >60 years old, associated with visual disturbance.

Sinus infection: Would likely include history and physical exam consistent with sinus problem

Glaucoma: Decreased vision, halos around lights.

Plan:
Diagnostic Test: At a tertiary center, a brain MRI may help identify other potential etiologies.

Treatment
Primary: Carbamazepine 100mg po on day one, then 100mg po bid on day two. Add 100mg/day q2 days, to a maximum of 1200mg/24hrs. 200mg bid, tid, or qid is effective for most patients. Carbamazepine in rare cases has resulted in agranulocytosis (5-8 x more than in general public). When prescribing carbamazepine, obtain baseline and periodic CBC and liver function tests to monitor for possible hematologic suppression or hepatic dysfunction.

Alternatives: In selected cases, the skeletal muscle relaxant **baclofen** has been used alone or in combination with **carbamazepine**. The starting dose for **baclofen** is 5-10mg po tid, with gradual increase to a maintenance dose of 50-60mg per day. Sedation, dizziness, and dyspepsia can occur with treatment, and the drug should be discontinued slowly since seizures and hallucinations have been reported upon withdrawal. If field formulary is limited, a trial of benzodiazepines is reasonable and should be individualized to minimize side effects. Initiate **diazepam** at low dose of 2mg po tid. Anti-seizure medications **phenytoin** and **gabapentin** have also been used to relieve symptoms but these medications are usually not readily available in the field and patients will require observation to determine optimal therapeutic dose.

Patient Education
General: Patient should be aware of potential side effects of medication and communicate frequently with his medic so as to ensure that medication side effects do not impair his occupational functioning,

Medications: Carbamazepine will result in side effects, most prominently sedation, nausea, and dizziness.

No Improvement/Deterioration: Significant improvement may take days. Always consider re-examination for new signs/symptoms that may suggest an alternative diagnosis.

Follow-up Actions
Return Evaluation: Monitor for medication efficacy and side effects. Chronic pain and antiseizure medications are both associated with an increased risk of depression and suicide and patients will require closer monitoring than is routinely available in the deployed operational setting. The paroxysms of pain, combined with the initial medication side effects, will likely impede the service member's occupational functioning. Duty limitations need to be determined on a case by case basis.

Evacuation/Consultation Criteria: If the medic is unclear as to the diagnosis or symptoms not well controlled, further consultation should be sought. Consider medical evacuation early on for:
1. Impairment of the patient's occupational capabilities
2. Need for laboratory monitoring while on treatment medications
3. Specialist consultation for confirmation of diagnosis and consideration of surgical therapy if medication treatment does not successfully alleviate the excruciating paroxysms of unilateral facial pain

Neurologic: Chapter 5: Bell's Palsy (Idiopathic Facial Nerve Palsy)
CDR Christopher Jankosky, MC, USN

Introduction: Bell's palsy is a common peripheral mononeuropathy involving the 7th cranial nerve. It usually follows a benign course, has no obvious underlying cause and is a condition from which 85% of patients recover fully. **Risk Factors:** Consider Lyme disease if in an endemic area.

Subjective: Symptoms
Onset of weakness in muscles of facial expression, slurred speech and drooling when drinking; diminished or altered taste, increased sensitivity to sound or pain behind the ear on the involved side; evolves over 1-2 days; bilateral involvement and numbness are rare. **Focused History:** *When did you first notice the symptoms? Any other neurologic symptoms? Recent head trauma?*

Objective: Signs
Using Basic Tools: Unilateral weakness (paresis) of the entire half of the face including the forehead, slurred speech and drooling. Remainder of full neurologic exam should be normal.

Assessment: Abrupt onset of unilateral facial muscle weakness in a young adult without other explanation is likely to be Bell's palsy.
Differential Diagnosis: Bilateral involvement can occur, but is rare and suggests more serious disease such as sarcoidosis, Lyme disease or Guillain-Barré syndrome.
Sarcoidosis: There will be paralysis of additional parts of the nervous system.
Lyme disease: A history of tick bite and characteristic rash (erythema migrans)
Guillain-Barré syndrome: An absence of reflexes is typical of Guillain-Barré.
Herpes zoster: Simultaneous characteristic vesicular eruptions in the ear canal or on the face
Myasthenia gravis: Weakness of additional muscles (especially the eye muscles, causing double vision)
Central nervous system lesion: Weakness of unilateral facial muscles from a central lesion in the cerebrum or brainstem is often associated with additional neurological signs and symptoms outside of the 7th cranial nerve distribution

Plan
Treatment
Primary:
1. Protect the eye from exposure keratitis (dryness, erythema, poor vision) and foreign bodies by wearing eyeglasses when outdoors and taping or patching the eye during sleep. Instill artificial tears several times throughout the day and viscous artificial tears (if available) at bedtime to help keep the eye surface lubricated and free of debris.
2. Most young adults will make a full recovery with no pharmaceutical treatments, but there is evidence that early administration of steroids will improve outcome. Recommend **prednisone** administration in a 9-day course that includes a taper. Administer 60mg/day po x 5 days, followed by doses of 40, 30, 20, and 10 on days 6-9.
3. If herpes zoster is suspected etiology, give **acyclovir** 800mg po five times a day x 5 days.

Patient Education: Expect full recovery in several weeks. Protect the eye until able to close it fully.
Follow-up Actions:
No Improvement/Deterioration: Weakness may worsen during the first couple of days but then stabilize, with recovery over 1-3 months.
Return Evaluation: Evaluate patient once a week or until recovery is imminent.
Evacuation/Consultation Criteria: Refer to ophthalmology if signs of exposure keratitis develop. Refer to neurology for gradual worsening (over several days to weeks), failure to improve by three months and/or involvement of other parts of the nervous system

Chapter 6: Skin: Introduction to Dermatology
LTC (P) Daniel Schissel, MC, USA
Classical Elements of the Clinical Approach to Dermatologic Disease Diagnosis and Disposition

Subjective: Gather information just as in the approach to other organ systems, including skin symptoms like pain, pruritus and paresthesia, and constitutional symptoms like fever.

Objective: Diagnose skin eruptions visually based on primary and secondary type, shape, arrangement, and distribution of skin lesions. Always include a thorough evaluation of all the mucous membranes, hair and nails.
I. Type of Skin Lesion
   a. Primary Lesions
   (1) **Macule:** A circumscribed area of change in normal skin color that is flat and less than 0.5cm in diameter. Example: freckles
   (2) **Patch:** A circumscribed area of change in normal skin color that is flat and >0.5cm in diameter. Examples: café-au-lait spots, port-wine stains
   (3) **Papule:** A solid lesion, usually dome-shaped, <0.5cm in diameter and elevated above the skin. Examples: verrucae, molluscum contagiosum
   (4) **Nodule:** A solid lesion, usually dome-shaped, >0.5cm in diameter and elevated above the skin. Examples: neurofibromas, xanthomas, and various benign and malignant growths
   (5) **Plaque:** An elevation above the skin surface occupying a relatively large surface area in comparison with its height. Frequently formed by a confluence of papules. Examples: lichen simplex chronicus and psoriasis
   (6) **Vesicle:** A circumscribed, thin walled, elevated lesion <0.5cm in diameter and containing fluid. Examples: herpes, dyshidrotic eczema, varicella, and contact dermatitis

(7) **Bulla:** A circumscribed, thin walled, elevated lesion >0.5cm in diameter and containing fluid. Examples: burns, frostbite, pemphigus

(8) **Comedo:** Retained secretions of horny material within the pilosebaceous follicle. Examples: open (blackheads) and closed (whiteheads), the precursors of the papules, pustules, cysts and nodules of acne

(9) **Pustule:** A circumscribed elevation containing pus. Examples: sterile lesions as in pustular psoriasis or bacterial as in acne and impetigo

(10) **Cyst:** A circumscribed, thick walled, slightly elevated lesion extending into the deep dermis and subcutaneous fat. Examples: epidermal inclusion and pilar cysts

(11) **Wheal/Hive:** A distinctive white to pink or pale, red, edematous, solid elevation formed by local, superficial, transient edema. They characteristically disappear yet may reappear within a period of hours. Examples: dermographism, insect bites, and urticaria

(12) **Telangiectasia:** Blanchable (fades with fingertip pressure), small, superficial dilated capillaries. Examples: rosacea, lupus erythematosus and basal cell skin cancer

(13) **Purpura:** Non-blanchable, purple area of the skin that may be flat/nonpalpable or raised/palpable. Examples: hemorrhagic lesions of some fevers

b. **Secondary lesions** represent evolution (natural) of the primary lesions or patient manipulation of primary lesions. Although helpful in differentiating lesions, they do not offer the same diagnostic descriptive power as the primary lesion.

(1) **Atrophy:** Thinning and wrinkling of the skin resembling cigarette paper

(2) **Crust (Scab):** Dried serum, blood, or pus

(3) **Erosion:** Loss of part or all of the epidermis that will heal without scarring

(4) **Ulcer:** Loss of epidermis and at least part of dermis that results in scarring

(5) **Excoriation:** Linear or hollowed-out crusted area caused by scratching, rubbing, or picking

(6) **Lichenification:** Thickening of the skin with accentuation of the skin lines

(7) **Scale:** Accumulation of retained or hyperproliferative layers of the stratum corneum

(8) **Scar:** Permanent fibrotic changes seen with healing after destruction of the dermis

II. **Shape of Lesion**

a. **Annular:** Ring shaped, round or circular

b. **Nummular:** Coin shaped

c. **Oval:** Oblong

d. **Polycyclic:** Rings within rings

e. **Polygonal:** Geometric shaped

f. **Round:**

g. **Serpiginous:** Snake-like

III. **Arrangement of the lesions** in relationship to each other

a. **Grouped Arrangement**

(1) **Annular:** Circular, round or like a ring

(2) **Arciform:** Shaped in curves

(3) **Herpetiform:** Like or in the shape of a herpetic lesion

(4) **Linear:** Geometrically forming a straight line

(5) **Reticulated:** Net-like

(6) **Serpiginous:** Shape or spread of lesion in the fashion of a snake

b. **Disseminated Arrangement:** Diffuse involvement without clearly defined margins or scattered discrete lesions

IV. **Distribution of Lesions**

a. **Isolated single lesions**

b. **Localized to specific body region**

c. **Universal over the entire body surface**

d. **Patterned**

e. **Sun-exposed areas**

f. **Symmetrical**

g. **Follicular based**

h. **Flexure or extensor surfaces**

Assessment:

Synthesize, integrate, and form a hypothesis by combining the history and the primary and secondary characteristics of the lesion(s) together with their shape, arrangement and distribution. *See Appendices: Color Plates: Figure A-24.D*

Plan:

Find treatments that allow troops to complete their mission, treat the process, and prevent recurrence. Explain the disease process and treatment thoroughly in words the patient can understand.

Chapter 6: Skin: Bacterial Infections: Staphylococcal Infections

MAJ Charles M. Moon, MC, USA

Introduction: Staphylococcus infections (SI) of the skin, most commonly caused by *Staphylococcus aureus* (SA), are often seen in the deployed setting and in military recruits where poor hygiene and close quarters living may promote disease transmission. Rates of SA infections, especially methicillin-resistant *Staphylococcus aureus* (MRSA), are on the rise in most areas of the US and across all branches of the military. SA may infect the superficial portion of the hair follicle causing a folliculitis or infect deeper causing a furuncle, commonly referred to as a boil. Multiple furuncles coalescing with interconnecting sinus tracts are called carbuncles, and are often found on the posterior neck. Furuncles and carbuncles are commonly caused by MRSA, which are typically deeper seated than ordinary SA infections and best treated with surgical incision and drainage (I&D). When lesions are deep seated and inflamed, they may develop surrounding cellulitis, which can require urgent medical care to prevent sepsis and tissue destruction. This section will not focus on superficial staphylococcal infections such as impetigo (*See Part 4: Organ Systems: Chapter 6: Bacterial Infections: Impetigo Contagiosa*) or streptococcal skin and soft tissue infections (*See Part 5: Specialty Areas: Chapter 20: Bacterial Infections: Streptococcal Infections, Life Threatening*). **Geographic Associations:** Worldwide distribution. SA infections are common during all seasons but anecdotal reports of increased infection rates during times of higher temperatures exist. **Risk Factors:** Immunocompromise, poor hygiene, crowded living conditions (barracks, prison), high prevalence of MRSA/ SA in the community, recurrent skin diseases (like eczema), recent incarceration, participation in contact sports, recent/frequent antibiotic use, IV drug use, men having sex with other men, shaving of body hair, previous history of SA infections.

Subjective: Symptoms

Superficial follicular infections may cause itchy or asymptomatic pimples/pustules. With deeper seated infections (furuncles/carbuncles/ ecthyma), expect enlarging tender erythematous lump that may be hot to the touch. May complain of being bit by a spider. Ulceration with thick, black crust can be seen with ecthyma. In advanced cases, expanding redness around the nodule and/or fever, chills, and general malaise may develop.

Focused History: *Have you or anyone near you had something similar before?* (may be a carrier of SA or have close contact with someone that is carrier) *Does the lesion hurt?* (MRSA infections are typically deeper seated, associated with more edema/ inflammation, and hence are painful.) *Has redness been spreading away from the initial lesion; have you been having fever or malaise?* (impending cellulitis, sepsis, or toxic shock syndrome)

Objective: Signs

Using Basic Tools: The most common signs are detected with visual inspection and palpation.

Folliculitis: Often asymptomatic pustule that may be centered on a hair follicle; can be confused with acne. Minimal edema or tenderness

Ecthyma: Ulceration with punched out appearance and necrotic base, often overlying black crust/ eschar. May be multiple

Furuncle/Carbuncle: Enlarging painful, erythematous nodule. May eventually develop overlying pustule, vesico-bullae, or spontaneously rupture purulent material. Coalescing furuncles are termed carbuncles and are often recurrent/ chronic. Pressing on one portion of a carbuncle may eject purulent discharge from other interconnected areas.

Cellulitis: Expanding area of erythema, pain, edema, and warmth often on the feet, legs, cheeks, or around furuncle sites; possible fever, malaise

Using Advanced Tools: Gram's stain of purulent discharge may demonstrate gram-positive cocci in pairs (staphylococcus) or chains (streptococcus). Wound culture will probably not be available in the deployed/field setting, but would be most helpful to aid in antibiotic selection.

Assessment: Differential Diagnosis

Folliculitis: Acne, hot tub folliculitis caused by *Pseudomonas* species (itchy red papules in bathing suit distribution/on torso), dermatophyte/fungal infections of the hair follicle (often seen in patients mistakenly treating fungal infections with a topical steroid), pityrosporum yeast (acne like eruption with follicular based pustule, erythema; itching), pseudofolliculitis barbae (shaving bumps), acne keloidalis nuchae (folliculocentric scaring flesh colored papules on occiput or posterior neck; keloids), miliaria (heat rash), keratosis pilaris (papules; sandpaper texture on the thighs, upper out arms, and buttocks), bug bites

Furuncle/carbuncles/ecthyma: Deeper/soft tissue infections.

Hidradenitis suppurativa: This typically found in the axilla, buttock, and groin; chronic/recurrent; may need wound culture to differentiate

Dissecting cellulitis of the scalp: Only found on the occiput of the scalp

Deep fungal infections: Often on leg/foot; chronic; seen in central and south America or Caribbean.

Brown recluse spider bite: Not common; dusky erythema progressing to a necrotic expanding ulceration with severe pain. *See Part 4: Organ Systems: Chapter 6: Bug Bites and Stings: Spider (Black Widow, Brown Recluse) Bites*

Plan:

Treatment

Primary:

I&D, daily packing with iodoform strips until healed. (*See Part 8: Procedures: Chapter 30: Skin Mass Removal*). IV placement if IV antibiotics are required. For uncomplicated, non-invasive infections eg, impetigo/superficial folliculitis, give **cephalexin** 500mg po bid or tid x 7-10 days or **dicloxacillin** 250mg po tid x 7-10 days. The treatment of choice for skin abscess causes by SA (including MRSA) is I&D. For deeper/soft tissue infection not amendable to I&D or suspicion of MRSA infection present, give **trimethoprim/ sulfamethoxazole DS** po bid x 10-14 days or **tetracycline** 500mg po bid x 10-14 days or **doxycycline** 100mg po bid x 10-14 days. **Clindamycin** 300mg po tid x 10-14 days may be appropriate (although resistance to this class is seen in some locales). Avoid using fluoroquinolones due to rapid emergence of resistance with this antibiotic class. Often deeper seated/soft tissue infections will become fluctuant and can then be easily incised and drained. I&D remains the treatment of choice for MRSA soft tissue infections. Failure to I&D early can have catastrophic consequences. Clinical indications for systemic antibiotic use in addition to I&D include extremes of age, surrounding cellulitis (especially if expanding), immunocompromise, central facial lesions, and failure to respond to drainage alone. Many providers (author included) will initiate antibiotics in the absence of the afore-mentioned indications despite lack of clear evidence of effectiveness of this approach; as mentioned previously, I&D is usually adequate to treat deeper/soft tissue infections.

Patient Education

General: Advise of the infectious nature of condition; ability to transmit to close contacts through direct contact or via inanimate objects used by others (chair, computer, bed, razor, nail clippers)

Diet: Maintain adequate hydration, especially if febrile.

Prevention and Hygiene: Antibacterial soap (chlorhexidine gluconate solution 4%) when showering. Apply mupirocin ointment to nostrils and fingernails which are common sites of SA carriage: antibiotic suppression may be required long term (30-90 days) if recurrences; despite aggressive prevention strategies many patients (up to 50%) who are SA/MRSA carriers will become re-infected. Avoid sharing clothing, bedding, and inanimate objects with others, sanitize/dispose of these items.

Wound Care: If I&D performed that requires packing of wound, have patient follow up daily for dressing changes and observe closely for expanding erythema, fever, worsening pain. At each dressing change, remove and discard packing material, cleanse the surrounding skin with isopropyl alcohol or hydrogen peroxide, irrigate wound cavity with sterile NaCl, re-pack, and cover wound with bandage. Continue until the wound cavity has healed and no longer requires packing material. If ulceration/open wound not requiring packing is present, advise patient to cleanse the wound and surrounding skin daily with soapy water, cover with petrolatum jelly and apply occlusive bandage; repeat 1-2 x/day until healed.

Follow-up Actions

Evacuation/Consultant Criteria: Evacuation to higher level of care for patients not responding (persistent fever; expanding edema/erythema) to I&D and oral antibiotics that would cover for MRSA, toxic appearance, sepsis, extremes of age, immunocompromised patients, other co-morbid illnesses (ie, diabetes).

Chapter 6: Skin: Bacterial Infections: Disseminated Gonococcal Infection
LTC (P) Daniel Schissel, MC, USA

Introduction: Gonococcemia is a systemic infection with *Neisseria gonorrhoeae* following the blood-borne spread (dissemination) of the gram-negative diplococci from infected sites (0.5 to 3% of untreated cases). The majority of patients will have arthritis or arthralgia and although most are <40 years old, DGI can occur in the elderly or newborns. DGI is 3 times more common in females.

Subjective: **Symptoms**
Usually includes a prodrome of fever and chills, anorexia, malaise during the 7-30 day incubation period. Patients typically present with tenosynovitis, dermatitis, and polyarthralgia (without purulent arthritis), or purulent arthritis without associated skin lesions.
Focused History: *Do you have a history of STD or unsafe sexual practices?* (history of exposure to GC) *Are you pregnant?* (Pregnancy, immediate post-partum status and recent menstruation are risk factors.)

Objective: **Signs**
Using Basic Tools: Lesions: 1-5mm erythematous macules (2-20 lesions) that evolve to slightly tender, deep-seated, hemorrhagic pustules within 24-48 hrs; center may become necrotic; located on arms and hands more often than legs or feet, in regions near the joint spaces. *See Appendices: Color Plates: Figure A-21.D.* Tenosynovitis of the extensors/flexors of the hands and feet is common. Septic arthritis occurs with asymmetrical, erythematous, hot, tender knee, elbow, ankle or metacarpophalangeal joints. Other organ systems may also be infected: hepatitis, carditis, meningitis, and others. Evaluate for other STDs.
Using Advanced Tools: Labs: Gram's stain of mucosal surfaces may yield gram-negative diplococci; culture mucosal sites (80-90% yield).

Assessment: **Differential Diagnosis:**
Hepatitis B: Rash if present is likely urticarial and joint involvement is symmetrical.
Other bacterial arthritis: May be difficult to differentiate clinically
Acute rheumatic fever (ARF): Rash is generally transient and never pustular or vesiculo-pustular. *See Part 5: Specialty Areas: Bacterial Infections: Acute Rheumatic Fever*
Infective endocarditis: Many will have symptoms of significant cardiac abnormalities.
Connective tissue diseases: Systemic lupus erythematosus (multiple joints, multiple organ effects); rheumatoid arthritis, psoriasis generally insidious onset (**Note:** Reiter's syndrome presents acutely.)
Meningococcemia: Severe presentation and CNS/meningeal symptoms may predominate.
Secondary syphilis: Involvement of palms and soles, generalized pustular lesions, generalized lymphadenopathy

Plan:
Treatment
See Part 3: General Symptoms: Joint Problems: Joint Pain
Patient Education
Prevention: Re-educate patient on safe sexual habits
Follow-up Actions
Evacuation/Consultant Criteria: Evacuate patients if possible. Consult as needed.

Chapter 6: Skin: Bacterial Infections: Meningococcemia
LTC (P) Daniel Schissel, MC, USA

Introduction: *Neisseria meningitides* is a gram-negative coccus found in the nasopharynx of approximately 5–15% of the general population. The bacteria invade the blood stream presenting as meningitis with meningococcemia (70%) or meningococcemia without meningitis (27%). Transmission is through person-to-person inhalation of droplets of infectious nasopharyngeal secretions. The highest incidence is observed midwinter in children age 6-12 months, while the lowest is in adults over 20 years during the midsummer. Infants, asplenics, immunodeficient or complement (blood proteins important in immune response) deficient individuals are considered at increased risk. A rash that may progress from non-specific to petechial to hemorrhagic over several hours in an acutely ill patient with severe arthralgia/myalgia should raise the index of suspicion for infection by Neisseria meningitides. *See Part 4: Organ Systems: Chapter 5: Meningitis*

Subjective: **Symptoms**
Prodrome of spiking fever, chills, myalgia, arthralgia; rash, photophobia, headache
Focused History: *When did you first begin to feel ill?* (Early treatment is critical, untreated meningococcemia can progress to death within hours of onset of symptoms) *Do you have leg pain, cold hands/feet, noticed abnormal skin color?* ("Early" signs of sepsis that occur at a median of 8 hours after onset of illness.)

Objective: **Signs**
Using Basic Tools: Vital signs: High fever, tachypnea, tachycardia, mild hypotension. Inspection: Rash: small, palpable, petechial lesions with irregular borders and pale gray, vesicular centers most commonly observed on the trunk and extremities (but may be seen anywhere, including the palms, soles and mucous membranes); posterior neck rigidity and tenderness with stretching; photophobia; altered consciousness; severely ill patients may display ecchymosis and coalescence of the purpuric lesions into bizarre shaped gray-to-black necrotic areas associated with disseminated intervascular coagulation.
Using Advanced Tools: *See Part 4: Organ Systems: Chapter 5: Meningitis*

Assessment: **Differential Diagnosis**
See Part 4: Organ Systems: Chapter 5: Meningitis

Plan:
Treatment
See Part 4: Organ Systems: Chapter 5: Meningitis
Patient Education
General: Recovery rate is >90% if adequately treated, and 50% or lower if not treated.
Prevention and Hygiene: Exercise protective measures for patient and provider by using a surgical mask (or other respiratory protection) on both the patient and support staff exposed. Close contacts of patient and others exposed should receive prophylaxis.
See Part 4: Organ Systems: Chapter 5: Meningitis
Follow-up Actions
Evacuation/Consultation Criteria: Evacuate cases after instituting immediate IV antibiotic therapy.

Chapter 6: Skin: Bacterial Infections: Erysipelas and Cellulitis
LTC (P) Daniel Schissel, MC, USA

Introduction: Erysipelas and cellulitis are skin infections that present with redness, warmth and tenderness without the associated suppurative (pus) foci seen in an abscess (eg, carbuncle, folliculitis). Both may include lymphangitis and involvement of regional lymph nodes and both are frequently the result of Group A beta-hemolytic *Streptococcus pyogenes* or *Staphylococcus* aureus. Erysipelas is an acute infection of the upper dermis and superficial lymphatics characterized by an erythematous, warm, raised, tender area of the skin often presenting acutely with associated fever and chills. Cellulitis involves the deeper dermis and subcutaneous fat that generally presents more gradually over several days. Inoculation of bacteria for both erysipelas and cellulitis is through a break in the skin barrier (puncture, laceration, abrasion, surgical site), or underlying dermatosis (pitted keratolysis, tinea, or stasis dermatitis/ulcer). Predisposing factors include penetrating wounds or other trauma to the skin, previous skin conditions, prior surgery resulting in lymphedema, diabetes mellitus, hematologic malignancies and other immunocompromised states. For additional discussion of specific areas, *see Part 4: Organ Systems: Chapter 6: Bacterial Infections; Part 3: General Symptoms: Eye Problems: Orbital/Periorbital Inflammation & Male Genital Problems: Genital Inflammation*

Subjective: **Symptoms**
Erysipelas: Prodrome of malaise, anorexia, fever and chills is occasionally observed. More common is the rapid development of high fever and chills coincident with the acute development of local signs of infection.
Cellulitis: Typically symptoms of redness, warmth and tenderness develop at the initial site of infection and progress in severity over a several day period.
Focused History: *When did you first notice symptoms?* (Erysipelas typically presents over a period of hours vs the typically more indolent presentation of a cellulitis.) *Did you injure the area?* (Infection may follow a minor cut or insect bite). *Have you had similar symptoms in the past?* (may indicate an underlying predisposing condition.)

Objective: **Signs**
Using Basic Tools: The primary lesion of erysipelas is a bright erythematous, edematous, raised, warm, tender plaque with sharp, palpable leading margins. *See Appendices: Color Plates: Figure A-21.E.* The distribution of lesion varies from the face (eg, "butterfly sign" on the face; sharply demarcated area of the ear "Milian's ear sign") to the lower extremities. Usually there is associated regional lymphadenopathy. Cellulitis generally is not as sharply demarcated but includes essentially all of the other local manifestations of infection (redness, warmth, tenderness) with our without associated lymphangitis and regional lymph node swelling.
Using Advanced Tools: Labs: WBC count consistent with infection.

Assessment:
Differential Diagnosis: Diagnose based on clinical findings.
Early allergic or irritant contact dermatitis: Will be pruritic but not painful
Fixed drug eruption: Non-painful
Deep venous thrombosis: *See Part 4: Organ Systems: Chapter 3: Deep Vein Thrombosis and Pulmonary Embolism*
Thrombophlebitis: Patient may have a history of venous puncture with redness, warmth, tenderness spreading along a specific vein. There may be a palpable cord (ie, vein) that persists even when the limb is raised.
Rapidly progressive necrotizing fasciitis: May present as a well-demarcated dusky purpuric lesion that is caused by thrombosis of

the vessels. *See Part 5: Specialty Areas: Chapter 12: Streptococcal Infections, Life Threatening*

Gout: Patient has a history of similar symptoms in the same location (eg, big toe). *See General Symptoms: Joint Problems: Joint Pain*

Herpes zoster: History of pain in a dermal distribution prior to onset of skin lesion is typical. *See Part 4: Organ Systems: Chapter 6: Viral Infections: Herpes Zoster (Shingles)*

Plan:
Treatment
Primary:
Early mild cases of erysipelas or cellulitis: Give **dicloxacillin** 500mg po q6h or **cephalexin** 500mg po q6h x 7-10 days. If MRSA is suspected by history of previous infection or prevalence in area, give **clindamycin** 150-300mg po q6h or **penicillin** 500mg po q6h PLUS either **TMP-SMX DS** 1 po q8-12h or **doxycycline** 100mg po q12h x 10-14 days. Classic erysipelas (eg, systemic symptoms of fever and chills) or severe cellulitis (eg, systemic symptoms or rapidly progressing skin lesion): Give **nafcillin** or **oxacillin** 2 gm IV q4h or alternate: **cephazolin** 2g IV q8h or **clindamycin** 600-900mg IV q8h (not to exceed 4.8g/day) and continue antibiotic through medical evacuation. If MRSA is suspected, substitute with **vancomycin** 1g IV q12h or as alternate **clindamycin** 600-900mg IV q8h (not to exceed 1.8g/day). Urgent medical evacuation. If medical evacuation is not possible in cases of severe infection, continue IV therapy until obvious signs of clinical improvement (usually 3-4 days) followed by oral antibiotic (eg, **dicloxacillin** 500mg po q6h or **erythromycin** 500mg po q6h) for an additional 10-14 days. If vancomycin is required for presumed MRSA, follow IV vancomycin therapy with **clindamycin** 300-450mg po qid (not to exceed 1.8g/day) for an additional 10-14 days. Supportive: Elevation of infected extremity will promote lymph drainage, decrease swelling and facilitate resolution of infection.
Patient Education: Good hygiene, immediate attention (eg, washing and bandaging) skin lesions decreases risk of serious infection. Prevention: Keep wounds clean, dry and protected.
Follow-up Actions
Evacuation/Consultation Criteria: Evacuate urgently cases that present with systemic signs of infection (fever and chills) or those cases that do not show good response to initial therapy. Consult dermatology or infectious disease if possible.

Chapter 6: Skin: Bacterial Infections: Staphylococcal Scalded Skin Syndrome
LTC (P) Daniel Schissel, MC, USA

Introduction: Staphylococcal scalded skin syndrome (SSSS) is a fairly distinctive pediatric dermatosis caused by an epidermolytic (epidermis-destroying) toxin. The reason for the association with children appears to be related to the fact that most adults and children over the age of 10 can localize, metabolize, and excrete the toxin more efficiently. They may develop bolus impetigo instead but will limit the hematogenous dissemination of the toxin. This condition is most common in children 5 years of age and younger.

Subjective: **Symptoms**
Prodrome: Fever, malaise, extreme irritability, and anorexia; irritable child with low-grade fever.
Focused History: *When did the lesions first occur?* (SSSS typically appears after 3-7 days of birth and essentially never at birth, lesions of congenital syphilis may be present at birth.) *Is there a family history of similar lesions in other children in infancy?* (Certain congenital conditions may present with lesions that can mimic SSS.) *Are there similar lesions in other family members at this time?* (Scabies and other infestations may affect infants as well.)

Objective: **Signs**
Using Basic Tools: Generalized macular erythema, with fine, stippled, "sandpaper" appearance, rapidly progressing to a tender scarlatiniform phase over 24-48 hrs; spreads from the intertriginous and perioral facial areas to the rest of the body. The exfoliative phase is heralded by a characteristic perioral crusting that often cracks in a radial fashion. Within 48-72 hours, the upper epidermis may become wrinkled or slough off with light stroking of the skin (Nikolsky's sign). Shortly thereafter, flaccid bullae and desquamation of the upper layers of the epidermis are noted. Unless subsequent infective processes are present, the entire skin will re-epithelialize with scarring within 2 weeks. *See Appendices: Color Plates: Figure A-22.F*
Using Advanced Tools: Labs: *Staph aureus* cultured only from colonized site of infection; umbilical stump, external ear canal, conjunctiva, or nasal mucosa.

Assessment:
Diagnosis based on clinical criteria and verified by culture from a primary infection site.
Differential Diagnosis
Erythema multiforme: Classic target lesions that tend to affect distal extremities including palms and soles.
Drug-induced toxic epidermal necrosis: History of drug ingestion prior to symptoms (eg, sulfonamides).
Pemphigus vulgaris: An autoimmune disease seen primarily in middle age or older individuals. Lesions typically begin in the oropharynx.

Plan: **Treatment:**
Primary:
Supportive: Reliable home care, including cool baths or compresses and oral fluid replacement.
Antibiotics: **Dicloxacillin** 30-50mg/kg/day po in divided doses. In newborns and infants where extensive sloughing has occurred: **oxacillin** IV 200mg/kg/day q4h until clear clinical evidence of healing is apparent. Apply **mupirocin** ointment or **silver sulfadiazine** to affected areas bid until healing is observed for more irritated and inflamed areas.
Follow-up Actions
Reevaluation: Change antibiotics or evacuate if not improving. Ensure normal healing is taking place at follow-up exams.
Evacuation/Consultant Criteria: Evacuate if unstable or not responding. Consult dermatology as needed.

Chapter 6: Skin: Bacterial Infections: Impetigo Contagiosa

LTC (P) Daniel Schissel, MC, USA

Introduction: Impetigo is an acute, contagious, superficial infection caused by *Staphylococcus aureus* (bolus/ulcerative), or group A beta-hemolytic streptococci (vesiculopustular), or both. Although seen in all age groups, impetigo is most common in infants and children, occurring most frequently on the exposed parts of the body, especially the face, hands, neck and extremities. Predisposing factors include crowded living conditions, neglected minor wounds, and poor hygiene.

Subjective: Symptoms
Itching, honey yellow crusting and weeping lesions

Focused History: *Does anyone else have similar symptoms?* (often spread between close contacts). *Did you have trauma to the area prior to symptoms?* (may be a complication of minor trauma)

Objective: Signs
Using Basic Tools: Lesions: 1-2mm erythematous macules, which quickly develop into vesicles or bullae surrounded by a narrow halo of erythema. The vesicles rupture easily and release a thin, yellow, cloudy fluid which subsequently dries to a characteristic "honey crust" (*see Appendices: Color Plates: Figure A-22.B*). Scattered, discrete lesions located most frequently on the exposed parts of the body, especially the face, hands, neck and extremities. Groups of lesions may have satellite auto-inoculated lesions at the periphery. There may be associated regional lymphadenopathy.

Using Advanced Tools: Labs: Gram's stain of early vesicular lesions reveals gram-positive intracellular cocci in clusters or chains.

Assessment: Differential Diagnosis
Varicella: *See Part 5: Specialty Areas: Chapter 15: Most Common Pediatric Diseases: Skin Problems: Viral Exanthems*

Herpes simplex: *See Part 5: Specialty Areas: Chapter 10: Oral and Dental Problems: Herpetic Lesions (Cold Sores, Fever Blisters)*

Bullous tinea: *See Part 4: Organ Systems: Chapter 6: Superficial Fungal Infections: Dermatophyte (Tinea) Infections*

Allergic contact dermatitis: History of recent exposure to irritant (eg, solvent, other chemical exposure). *See Part 4: Organ Systems: Chapter 6: Contact Dermatitis*

Plan:
Treatment

Primary: Dicloxacillin 250-500mg po tid-qid x 10 days

Alternative: Cephalexin 500mg po tid-qid x 10 days or **erythromycin** 250mg po qid x 10 days

Empiric: A high bacterial load may stimulate a super antigen reaction and aggravate the disease process. To decrease the bacterial load, wash the area with **chlorhexidine gluconate** soap once daily until cutaneous lesions clear. Appy **mupirocin** to the nose each night for suspected Staph A carrier states.

Patient Education

Wound Care: Keep lesions covered and moist with antibiotic ointment or petrolatum to aid in rapid healing,

Prevention and Hygiene: Very contagious process. Hand washing and wound care are paramount.

No Improvement/Deterioration: Lack or response to appropriate coverage may indicate MRSA carrier state or infection.

Follow-up Actions

Evacuation/Consultation Criteria: Evacuation not usually indicated. Consult dermatology or infectious disease as needed.

Chapter 6: Skin: Mycobacterial Infections: Buruli Ulcer

LTC (P) Kurt Maggio, MC, USA

Introduction: Buruli ulcer begins as a single, hard, painless subcutaneous nodule that ulcerates to form a lesion with a characteristic necrotic whitish or yellowish base (cotton wool appearance) with an undermined border. Most commonly seen on the arms and legs, the lesion is caused by *Mycobacterium ulcerans* which produces a toxin that contributes to the ulcer's extensive necrosis. Infection is believed to be caused by inoculation of bacteria contaminated soil or water. **Geographic Associations:** The disease has been reported to occur in Africa, especially the Buruli district of Uganda, Nigeria, Ghana, and Benin, as well as Australia, Mexico, and Malaysia. **Seasonal Variation:** None. **Risk Factors:** Exposure to contaminated soil and fresh water in an endemic area

Subjective: Symptoms: None or mild tenderness
Focused History: *Was the onset slow and progressive over several years?* (suggests slow growing bacterial process) *Is your ulcer painful?* (painful would suggest other processes such as cancer or other infections) *Where have your been deployed or traveling?* (geographically restricted distribution of disease)

Objective: Signs
Using Basic Tools: Inspection: Extensive area of ulceration with undermined borders and necrosis centrally with erythema peripherally

Using Advanced Tools: Direct smear examination of swabs from ulcers using Ziehl-Neilson stain. Aerobic, anaerobic, and mycobacterial cultures.

Assessment:
Diagnose based on the appearance of the lesion, history of exposure in an endemic area.

Differential Diagnosis: Other sources of ulceration including **skin cancer, leishmaniasis, syphilis, tuberculosis, tropical ulcer**; **cellulitis with ulceration** (fever, hot wound, advancing erythema)

Plan:
Diagnostic Tests: Visual inspection of the lesion

Treatment
Treat ulcer that is <5cm in width with antibiotics alone. For ulcer >5cm, give antibiotics plus wide excision (may require skin graft). Antibiotic therapy: **Rifampin** 10mg/kg of body weight (up to 600mg/day) po daily x 8 weeks and **streptomycin** 15mg/kg body weight (0.75–1g/day) IM daily x 8 weeks.

Patient Education
General: Local wound care and covering the ulcer will prevent secondary infection by bacteria, botflies, etc.
Activity: No restrictions
Diet: No restrictions
Medications: Side effects rare but may include: Ototoxicity (tinnitus, high frequency hearing loss) with streptomycin 1%. With rifampin, pseudomembranous colitis, nephric toxicity, hemolytic anemia, and flu-like symptoms if taken irregularly; may discolor urine, sweat, tears to orange-brownish.
Prevention and Hygiene: Avoid exposure to soil and water in endemic areas.
No Improvement/Deterioration: Fever (may indicate secondary infection) or bleeding (may indicate ulceration to depth of underlying vital structures)

Follow-up Actions
Return Evaluation: Follow-up if able to evacuate and treat.
Evacuation/Consultation Criteria: Whenever possible for diagnosis and treatment (eg, extended antibiotic therapy with or without excision).

Zoonotic Disease Considerations
Agent: *Mycobacterium ulcerans*
Principal Animal Hosts: None known
Clinical Disease in Animals: Buruli ulcer can be seen in koala bears
Probable Mode of Transmission: Inoculation into open wound
Known Distribution: Restricted to Africa (especially the Buruli district of Uganda, Nigeria, Ghana, Benin), Australia, Mexico, and Malaysia.

Chapter 6: Skin: Mycobacterial Infections Cutaneous Tuberculosis
MAJ Charles Moon, MC, USA

Introduction: Cutaneous tuberculosis (TB) is caused by infection with *Mycobacterium tuberculosis*, an acid fast, aerobic, gram-positive organism. This is a relatively rare condition and only approximately 1% of all TB patients demonstrate skin lesions. Skin lesions can develop after primary skin inoculation but more commonly they represent hematogenous or lymphatic dissemination from a pulmonary focus. TB infects almost 2 billion people in the world (about 1 out of 3 living humans). 1 in 10 people infected with TB will develop active TB in their lifetime and the disease is responsible for approximately 1.6 million deaths per year worldwide. Most cutaneous TB indicates systemic TB infection, especially in patients with HIV infection or immunocompromise. The incidence of all forms of TB has increased due to the HIV epidemic and a rise in resistant strains of TB.

Subjective: **Symptoms**
Most skin lesions are asymptomatic; some have a painless nodule progressing to an ulcer; itching is uncommon.
Focused History: *Have you been exposed to someone with tuberculosis?* (This might indicate a potential source of infection.)

Objective: **Signs**
Using Basic Tools: Inspection: **Primary skin inoculation lesion:** Ulceroglandular complex is a non-tender, reddish brown papulonodule, which slowly enlarges and erodes to form a well-circumscribed ulcer. Patient may develop non-tender lymphadenopathy (3-8 weeks later). Warty TB is a warty papule that can become fluctuant and purulent. This is a common dermatologic presentation following primary skin inoculation in individuals with previous immunity to TB. **Miliary TB skin lesion:** Caused by the spread of TB from a primary internal focus (often lung, lymphatic or bone). Variable presentations: boggy, indurated, erythematous skin and purulent ulcerations overlying infected subcutaneous tissue and enlarged lymph nodes (scrofuloderma); brown-red papules, soft and apple-jelly like, most common on the face, ears, buttocks and breasts (lupus vulgaris); discrete, blue-red to brown, tiny papules, some capped with minute vesicles, which rupture to leave a crust and may affect all body parts, but the trunk, thighs, buttocks and genitalia are most common. Using Advanced Tools: Place a PPD. A positive test does not indicate active TB, only previous exposure. A negative PPD does not completely rule out TB of the skin since the patient could be immunocompromised and not mount an appropriate immune response.

Assessment: **Differential Diagnosis**
Primary skin inoculation (rare): Primary syphilis, tularemia, cat scratch disease, sporotrichosis/deep fungal infections, atypical mycobacterial infections, leishmaniasis, and many others.
Cutaneous manifestations of pulmonary TB: Extensive list including tertiary syphilis, deep fungal infections, chronic granulomatous disease, leishmaniasis, sarcoidosis, squamous cell carcinoma, and many others

Plan: **Treatment**
Primary: There are multiple agents to choose from. Many organisms are multi-drug resistant. *See Part 5: Specialty Areas: Chapter 12: Mycobacterial Infections: Tuberculosis*
Primitive: None effective.
Empiric: Basic health measures, including clean and nutritious food and water, immunizations, and sanitation to help fight the infection. Conservative wound care and bandage if skin breakdown or ulceration
Patient Education:
General: Cutaneous TB, in general, is not an emergency. The risk of developing TB in healthy individuals is very low after exposure, but evaluation within 1-2 months or upon redeployment from endemic/epidemic regions should be performed. Meat handlers,

veterinarian workers, and persons involved in autopsies (or undertaker duties) are at increased risk for cutaneous TB.

Medications: Some medications can be toxic, so periodic blood tests are necessary during treatment.

Prevention and Hygiene: If exposed to an infected individual (several days of living or working in close quarters), test with PPD. Those who test positive will require a CXR to evaluate for active infection. These individuals should also receive prophylaxis therapy for TB.

See Part 5: Specialty Areas: Chapter 12: Mycobacterial Infections: Tuberculosis

Follow-up Actions

Evacuation/Consultation Criteria: Immediate medical evacuation is usually not required for patients with cutaneous TB but patients should be evaluated for active TB and started on TB prophylaxis. (*see Part 5: Specialty Areas: Chapter 12: Mycobacterial Infections: Tuberculosis*). Within 1-2 months, refer to an appropriate specialist for complete evaluation and choice of multiple drug therapy. Confirmation of cutaneous TB will more than likely require a biopsy with special stains, interpretation by a dermato-pathologist, and culture of a tissue sample. Due to the broad differential and varied appearance of skin lesions, this diagnosis may be difficult to establish without advanced clinical testing.

Chapter 6: Skin: Mycobacterial Infections: Leprosy (Hansen's Disease)

LTC Joseph Wilde, MC, USA

Introduction: A chronic infectious disease caused by the acid fast bacillus, *Mycobacterium leprae*. It commonly affects the skin, cutaneous nerves or eyes but may also involve internal organs. Leprosy is endemic in India, sub-Saharan Africa, South and Central America, the Pacific Islands and the Philippines. India accounts for 70% of all the cases in the world. It is also found in the Southeastern US and Hawaii.

Subjective: Symptoms

Hypopigmented, brown, or reddish skin lesions with decreased or no sensation. Ulcerations of the hands/feet. Paresthesias or loss of sensation in peripheral nerves. Muscle weakness or wasting.

Focused History: *Do you have any hypopigmented (white) skin lesions that have not healed?* (may be a subtle finding in intermediate or tuberculoid type leprosy) *Have you ever traveled to area known to have high risk of leprosy?* (Brazil, India, Madagascar, Mozambique, Myanmar, and Nepal are 6 of the top 11 countries with highest incidence of leprosy.) *Have you been in direct or close contact with patient known to have leprosy?* (increased risk factor) *Do you have a history of frequent infections or illnesses?* (could suggest decreased immune response eg, HIV, and increased risk of infection)

Objective: Signs

Using Basic Tools: Inspection: Examine skin for patches and plaques with variable color including erythema, hyperpigmentation, or hypopigmentation; tissue swelling with nodules or ulcerations; lesions are common on the face, ears, and extremities. Palpation: Assess for areas of hypoesthesia (light touch, pinprick, temperature and anhidrosis), especially peripheral nerve trunks and cutaneous nerves. The most common nerve affected is the posterior tibial nerve. Others commonly damaged are the ulnar, median, lateral popliteal, and facial nerves. Besides sensory loss, there may be associated tenderness and motor loss.

Using Advanced Tools: Slit-skin smears: A very superficial, and preferably bloodless, 3-4mm incision is made in the skin using a blade to obtain fluid from lesional or normal skin overlying the earlobes, elbows, or knees. Place the fluid is placed on a glass slide. Stain using the Ziehl-Neelsen acid-fast method or the Fite method to look for organisms.

Assessment: Differential Diagnosis

Tinea corporis: KOH positive

Mycosis fungoides: Requires skin biopsy

Cutaneous TB: May also have cough/night sweats

Other causes of erythema nodosum (GI infections, drug reactions, sarcoidosis, others)

Plan:

Treatment

Primary: For paucibacillary disease (negative skin smears with 5 or fewer characteristic skin lesions), give **dapsone** 100mg po q day PLUS **rifampin** 600mg po q day x 12 months. For multibacillary disease (positive skin smears with any characteristic skin, nerve, or eye findings), give **dapsone** 100mg po q day PLUS **rifampin** 600mg po q day PLUS **clofazimine** 50mg po q day x 24 months.

Empiric: Dapsone 100mg po q day PLUS **rifampin** 600mg po q day x 12 months

Primitive: Keep skin lesions clean with soap and water. Cover with bandages to minimize potential disease spread and aid in wound healing. Splints or crutches may be needed for patients having bony deformities, foot ulcers, or loss of digits. Provide patients with proper footwear to protect feet.

Patient Education

General: Most persons are immune to leprosy. Subclinical disease is common in endemic areas, and the infection progresses to clinical disease in only a select few.

Activity: Based on level of neurologic deficit, skin lesions, ocular, or bony/joint involvement. Patients may need crutches or splints to minimize weight bearing.

Diet: Normal

Medications: Dapsone: hemolysis, decreased WBC count. Rifampin: red/orange discoloration of urine. Clofazimine: blue/brown pigmentation of the skin

Prevention and Hygiene: Isolate known patients until therapy is instituted. Keep skin lesions clean with soap and water. Cover with bandages to minimize potential disease spread and aid in wound healing.

No Improvement/Deterioration: Medical treatment of the disease may result in significant inflammatory sequelae termed "reactional states" in up to 30% of patients. These usually occur within three months of instituting drug therapy. Patients at the highest risk are those with multibacillary leprosy and/or preexisting nerve impairment. Reactional state symptoms include: erythema/edema/tenderness of peripheral nerves, fever, malaise, arthralgia, and painful subcutaneous nodules. The reactional states may require treatment with systemic corticosteroids, NSAIDS, or other medications to minimize further damage to the peripheral nervous system. Consult specialty care for guidance.

Wound Care: Keep skin lesions clean with soap and water. Cover with bandages to minimize potential disease spread and aid in wound healing.

Follow-up Actions

Return Evaluation: If possible, follow patients every month for the first 3 months of therapy to monitor for reactional states or drug toxicity. The visits can be less frequent after that based on specific patient needs.

Evacuation/Consultation Criteria: Diffuse skin involvement, severe ocular involvement, or debilitating reactional states following institution of therapy.

Chapter 6: Skin: Viral Infections: Ecthyma Contagiosum
LTC (P) Daniel Schissel, MC, USA

Introduction: Ecthyma contagiosum (EC) infections (milkers' nodules, human orf) are caused by a genus of Parapoxviruses, which normally infect animals world wide. Humans contract these infections from handling infected livestock or working in infested areas where the virus may be harbored on fences, feeding basins, and other surfaces in the livestock areas. Human-to-human infection does not occur.

Subjective: Symptoms

Pruritus in an abraded area. This lesion enlarges and becomes painful. Occasional complaints of fever and chills.

Focused History: *Have you been around sheep, goats, yaks, or cattle?* (usually reports a history of contact with ungulates) *If so, when?* (EC has 5-7 day incubation period.)

Objective: Signs

Using Basic Tools: Inspection: In milkers' nodule, the primary lesion is a deep erythematous papule or small group of papules that enlarges gradually into a firm, smooth, hemispherical nodule varying in size up to 2cm in diameter. As with other viral processes, the lesions usually become umbilicated. In human orf (HO) infections, there are 6 classic clinical stages of the usually solitary lesion that last approximately 1 week; erythematous papular stage, targetoid plaque with central crusting, tender nodular, acute weeping nodular stage, regenerative stage, and regressive stage that heals without scarring. An ascending regional lymphangitis may be observed. The most common location is the dorsum of the index finger on the dominant hand due to handling the livestock or items with the livestock area. Other exposed skin sites of the arm, face, and leg are also at risk of infection.

Assessment: Diagnosis based on clinical morphologic criteria and history of exposure to infected bovine or ungulate livestock or livestock areas.

Differential Diagnosis

Erysipelas: See Part 4: Organ Systems: Chapter6: Bacterial Infections: Erysipelas and Cellulitis

Erysipeloid: May include history of minor trauma to fingers or hands and history of exposure from handling seafood

Atypical mycobacterium: Mycobacterium marinum following minor trauma and exposure to fresh or salt water

Bacillary angiomatosis: History may include vascular skin lesion in a person suspected of an immunodeficiency condition (eg, HIV)

Cat-scratch disease: See Part 5: Specialty Areas: Chapter 12: Bacterial Infections: Bartonella Infections (Cat Scratch Disease, Oroya Fever, Trench Fever)

Leishmaniasis: See Part 5: Specialty Areas: Chapter 12: Parasitic Infections: Leishmaniasis

Pyogenic granuloma: May include a history of a friable (freely bleeding) lesion on the gingiva during 1st half of pregnancy

Plan:

Treatment

Primary: Symptomatic treatment for pain and pruritus.

Alternative: Antibiotic for secondary wound infections.

Patient Education

General: There are no effective vaccines for milkers' nodules or human orf available for livestock. The highest risk of HO is in workers slaughtering sheep, infecting approximately 5% of workers. Spontaneous, non-scarring, healing occurs generally in 4-6 weeks.

Prevention and Hygiene: Keep wounds clean and covered to aid in healing and decrease secondary infection.

No Improvement/Deterioration: Referral for biopsy and histological confirmation of process.

Follow-up Actions

Reevaluation: Refer for biopsy and histological confirmation of diagnosis.

Evacuation/Consultation Criteria: Evacuation not necessary. Consult dermatology as needed.

Zoonotic Disease Considerations

Contagious Ecthyma (Orf)

Agent: Orf virus (Parapox)

Principal Animal Hosts: Sheep, goats

Clinical Disease in Animals: Lesions on skin of lips and oral mucosa of lambs; udders of nursing ewes

Probable Mode of Transmission: Occupational exposure

Known Distribution: Worldwide; common

Chapter 6: Skin: Viral Infections: Herpes Zoster (Shingles)
LTC (P) Daniel Schissel, MC, USA

Introduction: Herpes zoster (HZ) is an acute, localized, reactivation of a latent infection with varicella-zoster virus (VZV) that remains in the sensory ganglia after the initial infection (chickenpox). HZ is characterized by clustered vesicles on an erythematous patch in a dermatome distribution of one or more sensory nerves. The most frequently involved dermatomes are the 2nd cervical to lumbar nerves (C2-L2) and the 5th and 7th cranial nerves. HZ is most commonly seen in elderly patients over the age of 50. Immunocompromised patients with HZ may have more extensive involvement with multiple dermatomes being affected and a higher risk of viremia and visceral dissemination.

Subjective: Symptoms

A prodrome of pain, tenderness, itching, burning, and/or tingling in a dermatomal distribution (band or "belt-like" pattern) precedes the eruption by 2-7 days. Intense pain in the dermatome usually persists throughout the eruption and resolves slowly (post-herpetic neuralgia). Constitutional symptoms of headache, fever and chills occur in approximately 5% of patients.

Focused History: *Did you have pain in the area prior to the development of skin lesions?* (Most patients who develop HZ lesions will describe a deep burning, throbbing or stabbing pain in area of a single dermatome within several days to weeks prior to onset of lesions.) *How is your health in general?* (eg, weight loss, resistance to infection) (Incidence of HZ is higher in immunocompromised patients, eg, HIV, malignancy.) *Have you noticed pain or skin lesions on the nose or upper face?* (Patients with lesions in this part of the face are at high risk of developing ophthalmic involvement.)

Objective: Signs

Using Basic Tools: Erythematous papules or plaques, that evolve to umbilicated vesicles and bullae that commonly progress to pustules (over 48-72 hours) and crust over by 7-10 days; new lesions may continue to appear for up to 1 week; lesions typically cluster in the distribution of a single unilateral dermatome. *See Appendices: Color Plates: Figure A-22.C*

Using Advanced Tools: Labs: Tzanck smear of vesicle (undersurface of the vesicle or bullae has the highest yield) with multinucleated giant epidermal cells.

Assessment:

Differential Diagnosis: Pain can be intense and may resemble that of:

Cardiac disease: *See Part 3: General Symptoms: Chest Pain*
Acute abdomen: *See Part 3: General Symptoms: Acute Abdominal Pain*
Vertebral disk herniation: *See Part 3: General Symptoms: Back Pain, Low*

The eruption of zoster can resemble:

Allergic contact dermatitis/irritant contact dermatitis: *See Part 4: Organ Systems: Skin Disorders: Contact Dermatitis*
Localized bacterial infection: *See Part 4: Organ Systems: Chapter 6: Bacterial Infections*

Plan:

Shorten course of illness and subsequent development of notalgia paresthetica (back pain numbness and tingling) - a painful prolonged sequelae

Treatment

Primary: Acyclovir 800mg po 5 x day x 7-10 days decreases vesicle formation, time to crusting and days of pain when instituted within 72 hours of exanthem eruption. Antihistamines may be useful for pruritus (eg, **loratadine** 10mg po daily) and in some cases opioid analgesics (eg, **oxycodone/acetaminophen** or similar) may be required for pain. *See Part 8: Procedures: Chapter 30: Pain Assessment and Control*

Prevention: Prompt treatment during prodrome can lessen severity and shorten course of illness. Although contact precautions are not routinely recommended in the general population, in a deployed operational setting covering of lesions with clothing or dressings and avoiding direct contact may reduce risk of spread of the varicella virus to others. Individuals who have not been exposed to varicella (chickenpox) exposed to patients with HZ are more likely to develop primary varicella (chickenpox) than HZ. A specific vaccine for HZ has been approved by FDA and is currently recommended for patients >60 years old.

Follow-up Actions

Evacuation/Consultation Criteria: Evacuate troops whose condition interferes with mission performance.

Ophthalmic zoster: Look for vesicles on the eyelids and tip of the nose (Hutchinson's sign) - occur in 30% of patients with involvement of the nasociliary branch. Start antiviral therapy and initiate URGENT MEDEVAC/Refer. Blindness may develop if not treated appropriately and quickly.

Ramsay Hunt syndrome: Initiate antiviral therapy and URGENT MEDEVAC individuals who have suspected HZ involvement of the facial nerve and auditory nerves resulting in same-side facial paralysis and vertigo with vesicular lesions on the tongue, buccal mucosa, floor of the mouth, lips, ear, and external auditory canal.

Chapter 6: Skin: Viral Infections: Molluscum Contagiosum

LTC (P) Daniel Schissel, MC, USA

Introduction: Molluscum contagiosum (MC) virus is endemic in school age children through casual contact and spread of the poxvirus. Lesions are discrete, characteristically umbilicated, pearly, red papules. Involvement of the diaper area, trunk, face, and axilla is common. In the adult population, MC is usually transmitted sexually, and may resolve spontaneously after several months or may reappear. Shaving in the pubic area or other involved areas can cause spreading of the lesions through microabrasion in the skin. In addition, patients with underlying atopic dermatitis/eczema, the lesions may be more extensive, wide spread and autoinoculation more prominent given the extensive pruritus associated with this condition. HIV infected patients may have hundreds of small (2-3mm) papules or develop giant 1-2cm lesions.

Subjective: Symptoms

Asymptomatic, slow growing papules; commonly irritated by trauma or scratching, which can cause local spreading and/or secondary infection.

Focused History: *Do you have a history of atopic dermatitis or eczema?* (molluscum contagiosum more common) *Do you have a history of STD or history of increased risk of STD?* (may be associated with underlying immunodeficiency, eg, HIV)

Objective: Signs

Using Basic Tools: Sharply circumscribed single or more commonly multiple, superficial, pearly to translucent, dome-shaped papules with a characteristic umbilication that may be seen easily with a hand-held lens. They initially present as pinpoint papules, increase slowly to 2-3mm in size, and are often found in the genital region. *See Appendices: Color Plates: Figure A-22.E*

Using Advanced Tools: Hematoxylin and eosin staining shows keratinocytes with eosinophilic cytoplasmic inclusion bodies.

Assessment: Diagnosis is most frequently made by characteristic appearance of lesion.

Differential Diagnosis

Flat warts (verruca plana) or condylomata acuminata (venereal warts): Application of a dilute solution of acetic acid (3-5%) will induce a characteristic acetowhite appearance thought to be the result of coagulation of epithelial cytokeratins. *See Part 4: Organ Systems: Chapter 6: Viral Infections: Warts (including Venereal Warts/Condyloma)*

Squamous cell or basal cell skin cancers: Past history of skin cancer or extensive sun exposure increases risk of skin cancer. *See Part 4: Organ Systems: Chapter 6: Skin Disorders: Skin Cancer (Basal, Squamous Cell and Malignant Melanoma)*

Sebaceous gland hyperplasia: Primarily seen in elderly

Epidermal inclusion cyst: Discrete fully movable cyst or nodule, often with a central punctum. *See Part 8: Procedures: Chapter 30: Skin Mass Removal*

Plan:

Treatment

Primary:

Treatment depends on location on body. Facial lesions should be treated less aggressively to decrease the risk of scarring.

Retinoid gel 0.01%-0.25% applied to affected area each night will cause a minor irritation to the lesion and works well for the face, as does **potassium hydroxide** topically. Apply to lesion daily until cleared.

Alternative: Curettage, followed by **imiquimod** 5% cream applied to the lesion each day until cleared.

Patient Education

General: Patient will likely continue to develop new lesions (in or around the area of old ones) that are not clinically visible at the initial visit. Return for additional treatment as needed

Medication: Avoid sun exposure or use sunblock when using retinoid gel.

Prevention: Keep all skin surfaces well hydrated/emolliated to avoid spread of the lesions. *See Part 5: Specialty Areas: Chapter 11: Introductions to STDs*

Follow-up Actions

Return Evaluation: Consider alternate treatment or diagnosis, or refer for biopsy to rule out cancer if not responding to treatment

Evacuation/Consultation Criteria: Evacuation not usually necessary. If not responding to appropriate therapy, refer to dermatologist or primary care physician for biopsy to rule out cancer.

Chapter 6: Skin: Viral Infections: Warts (including Venereal Warts/Condyloma)

LTC (P) Daniel Schissel, MC, USA

Introduction: The common wart is a benign growth in the epidermis seen in 7-10 % of the population. It is caused by the human papilloma virus (HPV) and commonly presents as papules and/or plaques in school age children. Some HPV strains have been associated with malignant transformation (ie, cancer of the cervix, penis and esophagus).

Subjective: Symptoms

Usually slow growing; commonly irritated with minor trauma or excoriations.

Focused History: *When did you notice the first notice lesions? Do close contacts have similar lesion?* (If venereal warts are diagnosis, discussion of close contacts, history of STDs and discussion of safe sexual practice is appropriate.)

Objective: Signs

Using Basic Tools:

Verruca vulgaris: Appear predominately on the dorsal aspect of the hands and periungual region of the nail but may occur anywhere on the skin. They vary from solitary isolated lesions to vast numbers in any given individual. The normal progression of the primary lesion is from a small, round, discrete, flesh colored papule to a larger yellowish tan to black lesion that measures from several millimeters to a couple of centimeters. The surface of the lesion commonly takes on a rough finely papillomatous (verruciform) surface with many characteristic "reddish-black seeds" (thrombosed capillary loops).

Verruca plana: Appear predominately as smooth, flesh-colored to slightly tan, elevated papules, 2-5 mm in diameter, with a round or polygonal base on the face, neck, arms, and legs. In the bearded area of men and on the legs and axilla of women, irritation from shaving tends to cause the warts to spread in linear arrays (Koebner effect).

Verruca plantaris: Appear initially as small, shiny, skin colored, sharply marginated papules that evolve to plaques with a rough hyperkeratotic surface. They commonly present over the weight bearing points of the foot and therefore are commonly tender to palpation. They may be distinguished from calluses by noting the loss of the normal dermography (skin lines) that calluses usually retain. *See Part 5: Specialty Areas: Chapter 9: Plantar Warts*

Venereal wart/condyloma acuminatum: Appear initially as tiny, pinpoint, flesh-toned, papules that may grow rapidly to cauliflower-like masses in any region of the anogenital area and the oral mucosa.

Using Advanced Tools: Skin biopsy may be required in some cases to confirm diagnosis (eg, Bowen's disease, squamous cell or other carcinoma)

Assessment: **Differential Diagnosis:** See appropriate sections in this book for most of the conditions listed under differential diagnosis of various types of warts.

Verruca vulgaris: Seborrheic keratosis, lichen planus, simple callus, molluscum contagiosum, carcinoma with verrucous (wart-like appearance

Verruca plana: Simple callus, foreign body, lichen planus, carcinoma with verrucous (wart-like) appearance

Venereal warts: Condyloma lata (syphilis), intraepithelial neoplasm (Bowen's disease), invasive squamous cell skin cancer, molluscum contagiosum, lichen planus, skin tag

Plan:
Treatment
Primary:
Verruca vulgaris: Trim warts; apply liquid **nitrogen** to the lesion (for 5 seconds, slowly thaw, repeat x 1) if available; or apply 40% **salicylic acid** to area once daily after trimming lesions; apply duct tape if unable to keep acid plaster on lesion; may need to treat for 8-10 weeks until dermography (skin lines) returns.

Verruca plana: Trim warts; apply liquid **nitrogen** to the lesion for 5 seconds, slowly thaw, repeat x 1; or apply 40% **salicylic acid, retinoic acid,** to the lesions as described previously.

Venereal warts: Apply **podophyllin** (10-25%) to the lesions every 2-3days; after applying, leave on for 6 hours and then wash off. Large areas should not be treated in a single application and podophyllin should not be applied to cervix, vaginal epithelium or other mucosa and is contraindicated in pregnancy or patient at risk of pregnancy.

Alternative: Apply liquid nitrogen. Liquid nitrogen can be combined with topical treatments to speed clearance.
Verruca plantaris: Trim warts; recommend against apply liquid **nitrogen** to the lesion for secondary pain with ambulation apply 40% **salicylic acid** to area once daily after trimming lesions; apply duct tape if unable to keep acid plaster on lesion; may need to treat for 8-10 weeks until dermography (skin lines) returns.

Patient Education
General: Venereal warts are one of the most common forms of STDs and the benefits of safe sexual practices should be emphasized. Prevention and Hygiene: Safe sexual practices. A vaccine for prevention of HPV has been developed and where available, is expected to significantly reduce risk of some cervical cancers in populations at risk.

Follow-up Actions
Return Evaluation: Consider alternate treatment or diagnosis, or refer for biopsy to rule out cancer if not responding to treatment.

Evacuation/Consultation Criteria: Evacuation not indicated, unless venereal warts cannot be treated and are large enough to interfere with mission. If condyloma involves the meatus of the penis, refer to urologist.

Chapter 6: Skin: Superficial Fungal Infections: Dermatophyte (Tinea) Infections
LTC (P) Daniel Schissel, MC, USA

Ringworm - Tinea corporis	Jock itch - Tinea cruris
Athlete's foot - Tinea pedis	Some Dandruff - Tinea capitis
Finger/toenails - Tinea unguium	Dandruff of beard - Tinea barbae/faciale
Palms and soles - Tinea manuum	

Introduction: Dermatophyte infections are superficial, caused by fungi that invade only dead outer layers of the skin or its appendages (stratum corneum, nails, hair). *Microsporum, Trichophyton* and *Epidermophyton* are the genera most commonly involved. Some dermatophytes produce only mild or no inflammation. In such cases, the organism may persist indefinitely, causing intermittent remissions and exacerbations of a gradually extending lesion with a scaling, slightly raised leading border. In other cases, an acute infection may occur, typically causing a sudden, vesicular and bullous reaction of the feet or an inflamed, boggy lesion of the scalp (kerion) due to a strong immunologic reaction to the fungus. Transmission of dermatophyte infections may be grouped into 3 main categories: from animals, from the environment, and from one another. Infections are seen worldwide.

Subjective: Symptoms
Rash, itching and flaking; severe cases: Painful, pruritic blisters.

Focused History: *Have you ever had this before? What was used to treat it? Was that effective?* (may indicate source of infection and indicate appropriate management)

Objective: Signs
Using Basic Tools:
Tinea corporis: Scaling, sharply demarcated plaque with or without vesicles or pustules that develops a central clearing and peripheral enlargement producing an annular configuration, commonly on forearm and neck. *See Appendices: Color Plates: Figure A-21.B*

Tinea pedis: Various patterns: Slightly erythematous plaque on the plantar surface of the foot; dry, superficial, white scale is observed in an arciform pattern; moist patch of erythema, small fissures and erosions usually localized to the fourth and fifth interdigital spaces and the lateral sole.

Tinea unguium (onychomycosis): Whitish/yellow/brown, thick, dry, subungual (under nail) accumulation of friable keratin debris; the great toe is commonly affected first. *See Appendices: Color Plates: Figure A-21.A*

Tinea capitis: 3 main groups: Focal patch of alopecia with minimal scale and erythema; "Black dot" appearance of broken off hair shafts also seen with minimal scale and erythema; kerion: a boggy, purulent, inflamed group of pustules that is often tender to touch and heals with severe scarring.

Tinea cruris: Similar to Tinea corporis but restricted to the intertriginous area of the groin.

Tinea barbae: Similar to Tinea corporis but restricted to the facial area.

Tinea manuum: Similar to Tinea corporis but restricted to the hands and feet.

Using Advanced Tools: Labs: KOH preparation for characteristic fungal hyphae is recommended in all suspected cases. *See Appendices: Color Plates: Figure A-21.C*

Assessment: See appropriate sections and index in this book. Diagnosis requires a KOH preparation. Woods Lamp exam for groin and foot lesions is strongly recommended to rule out secondary bacterial infections. Coral red fluorescence is commonly observed with secondary Corynebacterial infections.

Differential Diagnosis

Pityriasis rosea: May start with a "herald" patch. *See Part 4: Organ Systems: Chapter 6: Superficial Fungal Infections: Tinea (Pityriasis) Versicolor*

Discoid eczema: Patient will often have personal or family history to suggest allergic conditions (eg, asthma, allergic rhinitis, atopic dermatitis).

Psoriasis: Distribution of lesions frequently includes elbows, knees, palms, soles of feet and appearance of red scaling lesions in these areas can suggest the diagnosis.

Secondary syphilis: History of STDs, lesions often involves soles of feet or palms of hands and do not demonstrate hyphae on KOH prep

Plan:

Treatment

Primary: Lac-Hydrin and clotrimazole topically bid for 2-4 weeks for tinea pedis and onychomycosis. **Lac-Hydrin** decreases the dryness and increases the barrier properties of the skin preventing re-infection. **Griseofulvin** 500mg po bid with fatty meals (aids absorption) for 2 weeks for tinea corporis to 2-3 months for tinea capitis. Not effective against candidiasis or tinea versicolor.

Clotrimazole topical preparations (cream and solution) are effective against most fungal infections when applied bid/tid to affected areas and washed off before reapplication.

Alternate: Itraconazole and terbinafine are not recommended in the field due to the inability to properly evaluate side effects and rapid recurrence. A more effective treatment of onychomycosis is prevention and daily topical **ciclopirox** nail lacquer (**Penlac**) as it also promotes good daily foot care habits.

Note: Nystatin treats only candidal infections, not dermatophytes.

Patient Education

Prevention and Hygiene: Good foot maintenance: change socks frequently, dry out boots, use antifungal soaps, use shower shoes. For patients with hyperhidrosis, topical aluminum chloride at night on air dried surfaces is recommended.

Follow-up Actions

Reevaluation: Repeat KOH and Woods Lamp evaluation and clinical assessment.

Evacuation/Consultation Criteria: Evacuation should not be necessary.

Zoonotic Disease Considerations

Dermatophytosis (Ringworm)

Principal Animal Hosts: Dogs, cats, cattle

Clinical Disease in Animals: Dogs: focal alopecia, scaly patches with broken hairs; cats - focal alopecia, scaling, crusting; cattle: scaling patches of alopecia with gray-white crust; calves: periocular lesions

Probable Mode of Transmission: Direct contact with fomites and infected animals

Chapter 6: Skin: Superficial Fungal Infections: Tinea (Pityriasis) Versicolor

LTC (P) Daniel Schissel, MC, USA

Introduction: Tinea versicolor (pityriasis versicolor) is a chronic, asymptomatic fungal infection caused by *Pityrosporum orbicularis*. The fungus, found worldwide, is seen most commonly in young adults in temperate zones, and accounts for up to 5% of all reported fungal skin infections. The fine scales of this lesion are teeming with hyphae and spores that transmit the disease. The lesions are best appreciated during the summer months when sun exposure leads to increasing discrepancies in skin pigmentation between affected and unaffected areas. Predisposing factors for infection include warm humid climate, genetic predisposition, high plasma cortisol levels (ie, patients taking corticosteroids), serious underlying disease or immunocompromise, and pregnancy.

Subjective: Symptoms

Asymptomatic to slightly pruritic depigmentation of skin is the common chief complaint.

Focused History: *When did you first notice symptoms?* (Lesions are typically more evident in the summer.) *Are you, or have you been on medications?* (history of corticosteroids) *Have you had similar symptoms in the past? Have you been treated for these symptoms in the past?* (may suggest diagnosis and management) *Do you have any history of STD?* (possible secondary syphilis)

Objective: Signs

Using Basic Tools: White, tan, brown, or pink coalescing macules, patches and thin plaques with a peripheral fine scale; found most commonly on the upper torso and neck (or face in children). Lower extremities and genitals are rare sites of involvement.

Using Advanced Tools: Labs: KOH prep of scales reveals numerous short, straight or ring-shaped hyphae.

Assessment:

History and clinical features are often sufficient to differentiate these various conditions.

Differential Diagnosis

Allergic contact or irritant dermatitis: History of exposure or allergic reaction. *See Part 4: Organ Systems: Chapter 6: Skin Disorders: Contact Dermatitis*

Tinea (various): *See Part 4: Organ Systems: Chapter 6: Superficial Fungal Infections: Dermatophyte (Tinea) Infections*

Pityriasis rosea: Headache, malaise, and pharyngitis may occur (small number of cases) but except for itching, condition is usually asymptomatic. May start with a "herald" patch (2-5cm, single round or oval, rather sharply defined pink or salmon-colored lesion on the chest, neck, or back). The lesion soon becomes scaly and clears centrally, leaving a cigarette paper-like scale directed inwards toward the center. May be indistinguishable from tinea and will often require KOH preparation to rule out tinea.

Post inflammatory changes: History of previous inflammation (trauma, infection) in area of lesion (hyper- or hypo-pigmentation)

Vitiligo: Familial, autoimmune hypopigmentation, with only cosmetic effects

Secondary syphilis: History of STDs, lesions often involves soles of feet or palms of hands and do not demonstrate hyphae on KOH prep.

Plan:

Treatment

Primary: Ketoconazole 400mg po with orange juice to aid in absorption, wait one hour, exercise, leave sweat on body till the morning, then wash with **selenium sulfide** suspension. Repeat in one week

Alternative: Fluconazole 200mg po as described previously.

Primitive: Apply **propylene glycol** 50% in water bid for 2 weeks.

Patient Education

General: Relapse may require weekly washing with selenium sulfide suspension for it helps prevent re-infection. Repigmentation of the affected areas takes up to 90 days.

Diet: No alcohol use with oral medications due to increase liver damage

Prevention and Hygiene: Use antifungal soaps. Wash weekly with selenium sulfide.

Follow-up Actions

Evacuation/Consultation Criteria: Evacuation is not necessary. If lesions do not respond to appropriate therapy, refer patient to dermatologist or to endocrinologist to rule out endocrine disorders.

Chapter 6: Skin: Parasitic Infections: Loiasis
LTC Joseph Wilde, MC, USA

Introduction: A parasitic infection caused by the *Loa loa* worm and transferred to humans by the bite of an infected blood-sucking tabanid flies (deer fly, horse fly, or mangrove fly); found in damp, forested areas of West and Central Africa.

Subjective: Symptoms

Migrating sensations in the skin described as itching, tingling, pricking or creeping; recurrent temporary edema of hands and upper extremities (Calabar swellings); painful irritation of the conjuctiva and eyelids.

Focused History: *Have you noticed any itchy, warm, painful swellings on the hands or upper extremities that may have come and gone over the past weeks, months, years?* (Worms can survive for more than 10 years with symptoms recurring several times a year.)

Objective: Signs

Using Basic Tools: Localized subcutaneous edema/erythema of the extremities; injected/ edematous bulbar conjunctivae with direct visualization of adult worms.

Using Advanced Tools: Labs: CBC for eosinophilia; peripheral thick blood smear for microfilaria (*see Appendices: Color Plates: Figure A-26.J.*). Ophthalmoscopic exam: Microfilaria of the anterior chamber.

Assessment: Differential Diagnosis

Gnathostomiasis: May also cause recurrent hand swelling; due to the ingestion of certain types of raw fish. *See Part 5: Specialty Areas: Chapter 12: Parasitic Infections: Gnathostomiasis*

Toxocariasis (ocular and visceral larva migrans): Hepatomegaly, chronic abdominal pain, pneumonitis

Onchocerciasis: Subcutaneous nodules on head and shoulders; pigment changes; atrophy; edema of skin. *See Part 4: Organ Systems: Chapter 6: Superficial Fungal Infections: Onchocerciasis (River Blindness)*

Plan:

Treatment

Primary: Diethylcarbamazine 9mg/kg po tid after meals x 21 days; not available in US

Alternative: Albendazole 200mg po bid x 21 days

Patient Education

Prevention: Personal protective measures against insect bites (permethrin, DEET, insect netting, etc.).

Follow-up Actions

Evacuation/Consultant Criteria: Evacuation not usually indicated. Consult dermatology or infectious disease as needed.

Chapter 6: Skin: Parasitic Infections: Myiasis
LTC Joseph Wilde, MC, USA

Introduction: A parasitic infestation of the skin by the larvae of flies. Infestation can occur in any open wound or uninjured exposed intact skin. The human bot fly (*Dermatobia hominis*) is the fly species that most often infests humans with its larvae, although it also parasitizes a wide range of wild and domestic animals, including cattle, sheep, goats, pigs, dogs, cats, rabbits, monkeys, buffalo, and even some birds. *D. hominis* sometimes goes by other names, including the torsalo and American warble fly. It measures approximately ½-inch in length. *D. hominis* is only found in the Americas. It is distributed from southern Mexico down throughout Central America and parts of South America to northern Chile and Argentina. *D. hominis* is especially common in Mexico and Belize.

Subjective: **Symptoms**
Painful or pruritic skin boils with sensation of movement under the skin
Focused History: *Do you have any "insect bites" that aren't healing?* (a typical presenting complaint) *Have you had any trauma or open wounds or diseases (eg, diabetes or other peripheral vascular disease) especially to lower extremities?* (common risk factor and site of infestation)

Objective: **Signs**
Using Basic Tools: A single or localized group of furuncular (boil-like) lesions typically seen on the face, arms, legs, or scalp, with a central punctum draining serosanguineous fluid. Close observation of the central punctum reveals the posterior portion of a fly larva.

Assessment: Diagnose by clinical presentation or recent travel to an endemic area
Differential Diagnosis
Bacterial furunculosis: No larvae in lesion
Deep fungal infection: KOH positive
Atypical mycobacterial infection: No larvae in lesion

Plan:
Treatment
Primary: Place occlusive material such as petrolatum, mineral oil, butter, or raw pork to cause the larvae to exit the skin (also diagnostic).
Alternative: Surgical excision of the larvae may be required in some cases. Antibiotics may also be necessary in cases of concurrent secondary skin infection.
Patient Education
Activity: Limitation of activity may be required depending on location and extent of the infestation
Diet: Normal
Prevention and Hygiene: Proper use of insect repellents and mosquito netting will decrease transmission.
No Improvement/Deterioration: Monitor closely for any new skin lesions or signs of secondary infection
Wound Care: Wash bid with soap and water and apply antibacterial or sterile white petrolatum ointment
Follow-up Actions
Return Evaluation: Re-examine in 24 hours and 7 days after treatment.
Evacuation/Consultation Criteria: Evacuation normally not necessary for localized infestations. Consult dermatology or infectious disease if skin lesions do not heal or spread beyond the original area of involvement.

Chapter 6: Skin: Parasitic Infections: Onchocerciasis (River Blindness)
LTC Joseph Wilde, MC, USA

Introduction: Onchocerciasis is a filarial parasitic disease of humans caused by *Onchocerca volvulus*. Black flies, the vectors of the disease, require fast-flowing streams or rivers for reproduction. Most cases are found in sub-Saharan Africa along the fifteenth parallel from Senegal to Ethiopia. The geographic distribution of onchocerciasis in Latin America is sporadic, with foci in Ecuador, Guatemala, Venezuela, Colombia, southern Mexico, and the state of Amazonas in northern Brazil.

Subjective: **Symptoms**
Severe pruritus starting in one location (usually an extremity) which generalizes to the body and worsens with itching; deep painful skin nodules; ocular symptoms (photophobia, excessive tears, pain, blurred vision)
Focused History: *Have you recently visited or lived in an endemic area? Did the itching begin in one area and then spread?* (indicates spread of the parasite) *Do you have any problems with blurred vision, eye pain, or photophobia?* (may indicate infection of eyes)

Objective: **Signs**
Using Basic Tools: Acute cases may present only with pruritus, which is often worse on the buttocks, abdomen, and lower extremities. The resulting dermatitis may have a variable appearance. It tends to be a papular eruption with overlying superficial erosions due to constant scratching. Chronic skin changes, such as lichenification and scarring, are seen in long-standing cases. Deep subcutaneous nodules measuring pea-sized or larger develop later. These are filled with microfilariae and may occur anywhere on the body.
Using Advanced Tools: Labs: CBC for eosinophilia, microscopic examination superficial skin snip showing filariae (lift the skin with an inserted needle, clip off a small superficial portion of the skin with a sharp knife or scissors, place specimen on microscope slide with a drop of normal saline, cover with a coverslip, and examine under microscope). Filariae can be visualized moving at the edges of the skin slice.

Assessment: Diagnose with clinical findings and history of travel to endemic areas.
Differential Diagnosis
Scabies: Common in groin area and fingers
Insect bites: Pruritus eases with scratching
Miliaria rubra: Small papules and vesicles at opening of sweat glands

Plan:
Treatment
Primary: Ivermectin 100-200mcg/kg po single dose. A single dose is not curative, but decreases the parasite load significantly. It may need to be repeated every 6 months to suppress dermal and ocular microfilaria counts. Patients with known eye involvement should be pre-treated with **prednisone** 1mg/kg/day po daily x 3-5 days prior to ivermectin treatment.
Note: Treatment of onchocerciasis with **ivermectin** therapy can facilitate entry of *Loa loa* microfilariae ("eye worm") to the central

nervous system with encephalopathy and other severe neurologic complications. In areas where co-infection is likely to exist, noontime blood should be obtained to evaluate for evidence of *L. loa* microfilariae (sheathed microfilariae with prominent nuclei that extend all the way to tip of the tail) prior to initiation of ivermectin therapy for onchocerciasis. *See Part 4: Organ Systems: Chapter 6: Superficial Fugal Infections: Loiasis*

Alternative: Doxycycline 100mg po daily administered x 6-8 weeks has demonstrated efficacy in reducing micro filarial loads, sterilizing adult worms, and decreasing adult worm viability. It targets bacteria of the *Wolbachia* species, known endosymbionts in *O. volvulus.*

Empiric: Ivermectin 100-200mcg/kg po x one dose.

Primitive: Excise nodules and examine for adult worms

Patient Education

Activity: As tolerated. Painful subcutaneous onchocercomas may limit some motor activity.

Diet: Normal

Medications: Patients on ivermectin may experience allergic and inflammatory reactions to dead microfilariae. These reactions may include facial and peripheral edema, headache, myalgia, arthralgia/synovitis, lymph node enlargement, orthostatic hypotension, and tachycardia. Ocular toxicity includes eyelid edema, conjunctivitis, or inflammation of any structure within the globe.

Prevention and Hygiene: Avoid river areas, especially riverbanks, in endemic areas. Maximize personal protective measures (insect repellents and mosquito netting, etc.). Institute vector control methods if available.

No Improvement/Deterioration: Signs of worsening disease include: spread of dermatitis to new areas of body, increased numbers of painful subcutaneous nodules, or increased ocular symptoms as mentioned previously.

Wound Care: Surgical wounds following nodule excision should be kept clean with soap and water followed by application of sterile wound dressings daily.

Follow-up Actions

Return Evaluation: Follow-up in 6-12 months for re-treatment with ivermectin if patient lives in an endemic area

Evacuation/Consultation Criteria: No need to evacuate. Consult dermatology if unsure of diagnosis or if patient does not respond to treatment.

Chapter 6: Skin: Parasitic Infections: Swimming Dermatitis (Sea Bather's Eruption [salt water], Swimmer's Itch [fresh and salt water])

LTC (P) Daniel Schissel, MC, USA

Introduction: Swimming dermatitis occurs globally and takes 2 forms. Sea bather's eruption or "sea lice" is caused by a hypersensitivity reaction to the stinging nematocysts of a cnidarian larva from marine jellyfish, Portuguese man-o-war, sea anemone, or fire coral. It typically presents in areas covered by clothing or swim wear, unlike swimmer's itch, which usually occurs in exposed areas. Cercarial dermatitis is more commonly known as swimmer's itch in the fresh waters of the north central US, and clam digger's itch along the coastal salt waters. It is caused by the penetration by immature forms (cercariae) of a schistosome that normally infest birds, into the skin of an unsuspecting swimmer or bather causing an inflammatory dermatosis. The cercariae die later in the skin, self-limiting the infection.

Subjective: Symptoms

Complaints of a prickly eruption within a few minutes to hours where the larvae sting or the cercaria penetrate; repeated exposure (allergic response) cause larger, longer lasting, and more pruritic lesions in cercarial swimmer's itch dermatitis. Other symptoms in sea bather's eruption may include fatigue, headache, fever, chills, and nausea. With sea bather's eruption, many patients recall seeing small 2-3cm jellyfish in the water or small "black dots" on the water's surface.

Focused History: *Have you recently been bathing, swimming, or walking in water?* (exposure risk)

Objective: Signs

Using Basic Tools: Fine, papular rash in covered areas (sea bather's eruption) or exposed areas (swimmer's itch); lasts hours (swimmer's itch) to days; scratches often become secondarily infected; repeated cercaria exposures cause larger, longer lasting papules, that may advance to pustules and vesicles over 3-4 days.

Assessment:

Diagnosis based on clinical presentation and history of exposure in infested waters.

Differential Diagnosis

Allergic or irritant contact dermatitis: *See Part 4: Chapter 6: Skin Disorders: Contact Dermatitis*

Plan:

Treatment

Primary: These are self-limited diseases. Treatment consists of cleaning area involved (and any clothes worn during presumed exposure), symptomatic relief of pruritus with antihistamines (eg, **loratadine** 10mg po q day) and prevention of secondary infection in areas of excoriation. Topical steroids: **Triamcinolone** q day to bid until resolved or 10 days of treatment can alleviate more advanced allergic reactions to repeated exposures to cercaria.

Patient Education

General: Prevent cercarial dermatitis by avoiding prolonged immersion in infested waters and treating infested fresh water streams and lakes with a mixture of copper sulfate and carbonate, or sodium pentachlorophenate. Dry briskly after potential exposure to remove cercaria before they have sufficient time to penetrate. Apply 20% copper sulfate solution to the skin and allow to dry prior to potential exposure.

Follow-up Actions

Evacuation/Consultant Criteria: Do not evacuate patients. Generally no need to consult specialists.

Chapter 6: Skin: Bug Bites and Stings: Bed Bugs

LTC (P) Daniel Schissel, MC, USA

Introduction: The bed bug (*Cimex lectularius*) is a 3-5mm, wingless, 6 legged, reddish brown, flattened, oval bodied, blood-sucking nocturnal insect. It hides in crevices, bedding, or furniture, and normally emerges to feed at night in the dark. It is capable of traveling very long distances in search of its blood meal, often from one house to another. Under normal conditions, it feeds about once a week but has been known to survive 6-12 months without feeding. It characteristically leaves 3 bite marks in succession on its victim: "breakfast, lunch and dinner." It has been cited as a possible vector for trypanosomiasis, hepatitis B, and other infectious agents.

Subjective: **Symptoms**

Bite is not felt while sleeping; small asymptomatic macule at bite site; if sensitized (having developed an allergic reaction to the salivary secretions) have intensely pruritic papules that may evolve into a nodule that persists for weeks.

Focused History: *Have other individuals reported similar symptoms?* (Infestation of areas near general sleeping quarters is common.) *Do you have bites on unexposed skin?* (Bed bugs typically feed on unexposed skin, whereas scabies and other arthropods generally feed on both exposed and unexposed skin.) *Have you noticed specks of blood on linens?* (Bed bugs are usually not found in the bed, but specks of blood may be found on linens.) *Have you noticed an odor in sleeping quarters?* (Bed bugs produce a pungent odor that may be recognized.)

Objective: **Signs**

Using Basic Tools: Lesion is variable from a small, erythematous macule in non-sensitized individuals to an intensely pruritic papule or wheal, often with a central hemorrhagic dimple, in sensitized individuals. Characteristically 2-3 lesions grouped in a linear fashion on the exposed areas of the face, neck, arms, or hands. Bullae are more common in younger patients that have been sensitized. Secondary infection of the excoriated lesions often clouds the clinical presentation.

Assessment:

Diagnosis based on clinical morphologic criteria and history of exposure.

Differential Diagnosis

Scabies: Usually on both exposed and unexposed skin, lesions often demonstrate burrows.

Mites: Bites may appear in clusters in both exposed and unexposed skin or along sock or belt lines as opposed to linear bites in exposed skin seen with bed bugs.

Nummular dermatitis: As lesions get older, they may clear in the center and get scaly to resemble ringworm or psoriasis.

Irritant or allergic dermatitis: History of ectopy or exposure to irritant. *See Part 4: Organ Systems: Chapter 6: Skin Disorders: Contact Dermatitis*

Plan:

Treatment

Relieve pruritus with antihistamines (eg, **loratadine** 10mg po q day). Topical steroid cream (1% **hydrocortisone** or **triamcinolone** bid - tid) may be useful where inflammation is not related to secondary infection. Topical antibiotic lotion, (eg, **bacitracin** bid – tid x 5-7 days) should be used for bites with secondary infection.

Patient Education

General: Bedbugs commonly inhabit cracks and crevices of mud houses and thatched roofs. Infestation is common with up to 80-90% of the residents of the refugee camps having wheals from bedbug bites.

Prevention: Eliminate the bug and intermediate hosts (eg, birds, bats) from the environment with insecticides (consult preventive medicine). Clothes and bed netting may be treated with permethrin.

Follow-up Actions

Evacuation/Consultation Criteria: Evacuation is not necessary. Consult as required for diagnosis and assistance with management of infestation.

Chapter 6: Skin: Bug Bites and Stings: Centipede Bites

LTC (P) Kurt L. Maggio, MC, USA

Introduction: Centipedes are elongated, cylindrical arthropods having a single pair of legs ending in claws on each body segment (millipedes have 2 leg pairs per segment). Centipedes have been reported up to 26cm long, and are frequently more colorful (red, yellow, black, and blue) than millipedes and thus more likely to be sought as trophies. Most have very poor or non-existent vision. Unlike millipedes, centipedes are carnivorous. The legs on the first body segment are modified into fangs that bite and channel venom into prey. In addition to the venom, some species discharge defensive substances from glands along the body segments that may cause skin blistering similar to that seen with millipede exposure. A single fatality has been reported in a child bitten on the head by a large centipede. Most small species are harmless. They are widely distributed, especially in warm, temperate and tropical regions, live in moist environments (most commonly in forests among leaf litter or rotting timber), in caves, along the beach (under damp seaweed and other debris). **Risk Factors:** Exposure of uncovered skin to moist vegetation/forested areas during conditions of limited visibility.

Subjective: **Symptoms**

Within minutes to hours, severe local pain, swelling and redness; swollen, painful lymph nodes; headache; palpitations; nausea/vomiting; anxiety.

Focused History: *Abrupt onset of pain at site?* (suggests arthropod bite) *One region (especially an extremity) affected?* (Most centipede bites occur on the extremities.) *Any arthropod seen resembling a centipede?* (Visual clue suggesting centipede.)

Objective: **Signs**

Using Basic Tools: Inspection: Paired hemorrhagic puncture wounds with edema, erythema, tenderness and local necrosis at site of bite; lymphangitis/lymphadenopathy may be present. General: Significant anxiety, possible systemic toxic reaction (unlikely)

Assessment:
Diagnosis is based on the bite history or identification of the centipede.
Differential Diagnosis
    Anaphylaxis: *See Part 7: Trauma: Chapter 27: Anaphylactic Shock*
    Other bug bites and stings including hymenoptera and spiders: *See Part 4: Organ Systems: Chapter 6: Bug Bites and Stings*
    Cellulitis: Fever, hot wound, advancing erythema

Plan:
    Treatment
        Primary: Supportive. Apply ice/cold for pain, 1% **hydrocortisone** cream tid x 7 days, and **acetaminophen** 650mg po qid x 7 days or NSAIDs (*see Part 3: General Symptoms: Joint Problems: Joint Pain*) for inflammation. There is no known antivenin.
    Patient Education
        General: Further exposure should be limited. Insect repellents should be applied.
        Activity: No restrictions
        Diet: No restrictions
        Medications: No significant side effects
        Prevention and Hygiene: Avoid exposure to and never handle centipedes. Use caution when turning soil and when moving or climbing over rocks. Use work gloves in endemic areas.
        No Improvement/Deterioration: Return for fever, or reddening or blackening of the skin.
    Follow-up Actions
        Return Evaluation: Monitor for secondary infection (pain, crust, fever) or skin blackening (necrosis is uncommon). Follow-up if lesion persists more than 3 weeks or develops secondary infection.
        Evacuation/Consultation Criteria: Evacuation not necessary unless bite complicated by necrosis or cellulitis, or generalized reaction to bite (uncommon). Consult primary care or preventive medicine physician, or entomologist as needed.

Chapter 6: Skin: Bug Bites and Stings: Millipede Exposure
LTC (P) Kurt L. Maggio, MC, USA

Introduction: Millipedes are elongated, worm-like arthropods having 2 pairs of legs on each body segment (centipedes have one pair of legs per segment). They range in size from almost microscopic to 30cm in length, with 100-300 pairs of legs. They are generally brown/black/gray in color, slow moving, nocturnal herbivores that live in humid environments. Millipedes sense primarily with their antennae, having only rudimentary eyesight. When threatened, they coil up into a ball to protect their more vulnerable underbelly. Millipedes do not have biting mouth parts or fangs, but they secrete an irritating, repellent liquid from pores along the sides of their bodies when they feel threatened. In large doses, these secretions can be corrosive and cause blistering of skin. No deaths have been reported from millipede exposures, and it is unlikely that any such exposure, even to a small child, would prove fatal. **Geographic Associations:** They are widely distributed, especially in warm, temperate and tropical regions. Millipedes can be found in soil, leaf litter, under stones or decaying wood. **Seasonal Variation:** Millipedes are more prevalent and active in warm, wet conditions. **Risk Factors:** Unprotected skin exposure to moist vegetation/forested areas; conditions of limited visibility

Subjective: **Symptoms:**
    Within minutes to hours, painful, irritated skin, eye irritation and pain (ocular exposures).
    Focused History: *Did you have abrupt onset of pain at site?* (suggests arthropod bite) *Where is the bite located?* (Most millipede bites occur on the extremities.) *Did you see what bit you?* (Visual clue suggesting millipede.)

Objective: **Signs:**
    Using Basic Tools: Inspection: Brown staining of the skin at the site of contact, along with erythema, mild edema and vesicle formation; may have characteristic curved shape corresponding to millipede's shape. Skin may later crack, slough and heal; conjunctivitis may progress to ulceration of the conjunctiva and cornea (ocular exposures).

Assessment:
Diagnose based on the history of millipede handling or identification of the specimen.
Differential Diagnosis: Bites from other arthropods
    Cimex (bed bugs): Series of bites in a row ("breakfast, lunch and dinner"). *See Part 4: Organ Systems: Chapter 6: Bug Bites and Stings: Bed Bugs*
    Hymenoptera (fire ants): Multiple painful hive-like swellings develop into sterile pustules. *See Part 4: Organ Systems: Chapter 6: Bug Bites and Stings: Hymenoptera (Bee, Fire Ant, Hornet, Yellow Jacket, Ant) Stings*
    Centipedes: Paired hemorrhagic puncture wounds. *See Part 4: Organ Systems: Chapter 6: Bug Bites and Stings: Centipede Bites*
    Caterpillar (Lepidoptera) "sting": Hive-like swelling at site of bite with intense pain, pattern of caterpillar's spines seen on skin resembling railroad tracks

Plan:
    Treatment
    1. Irrigate exposed eye promptly with copious amounts of water or saline to dilute toxin. If conjunctival ulcer, *see Part 3: General Symptoms: Eye Problems: Eye Injury*
    2. Wash exposed skin thoroughly with soap and water to remove any remaining toxin.
    3. Apply 1% **hydrocortisone cream** to skin tid a day x 7 days. Do not use steroids in the eye.
    4. Supportive therapy with ice/cold; **acetaminophen** or NSAIDs may be comforting. *See Part 3: General Symptoms: Joint Problems: Joint Pain*

Patient Education:
General: Further exposure should be limited. Insect repellants should be applied.
Activity: No restrictions
Diet: No restrictions
Medications: No significant side effects
Prevention and Hygiene: Avoid exposure to and never handle millipedes. Use caution when turning soil and when moving or climbing over rocks. Use work gloves in endemic areas.
No Improvement/Deterioration: Return promptly for continuing eye pain or deteriorating vision.
Follow-Up Actions
Return Evaluation: Examine involved eye(s) daily until healed. No further exams needed for skin lesions.
Evacuation/Consultation Criteria: Evacuation not necessary unless conjunctival ulcer is large or does not heal in 24-48 hours. Consult ophthalmologist or primary care physician, or entomologist as needed.

Chapter 6: Skin: Bug Bites and Stings: Hymenoptera (bee, fire ant, hornets, yellow jackets, ant) Stings

LTC (P) Kurt L. Maggio, MC, USA

Introduction: The stinging insects of the order Hymenoptera include bees, wasps, hornets, yellow jackets and ants. Hymenoptera stings are a nuisance for most victims who usually recover without sequelae. 17-56% of patients will have a local reaction and 1-2% will have a generalized reaction. Hymenoptera are so ubiquitous and live in such close proximity to humans that they are responsible for more human deaths each year than all other venomous animals combined. 50% of fatalities occur within the 1st hour, and 75% occur within 4 hours after the sting. The venom load from 30 wasp stings or 200 honeybee stings may be sufficient to cause death. Alternately, a single sting may provoke a generalized anaphylactic reaction (the proteinaceous venom is a potent activator of the immune system) and death in a sensitized individual, particularly if there was an earlier, milder generalized reaction. The shorter the time interval is since the previous challenge, the more likely a severe subsequent reaction will occur. Additionally, cross-reactions to the venoms of various members of the Hymenoptera family have been reported. (ie, individual who suffers an anaphylactic reaction to a wasp bite may also simultaneously develop anaphylaxis to ant bites). Hymenoptera are social insects that live in colonies or hives located in caves, hollow trees or in the ground; most often found among flowers and fruit where they feed and are probably attracted by bright colors, perfumes and colognes. They are widely distributed, especially in warm, temperate and tropical regions. Fire ants have a more limited distribution. All are more prevalent and active in warm conditions. Bees have a stinger with a specialized tip that not only penetrates the skin and delivers venom, but possesses a barb that anchors the stinger in the skin. The bee is able to sting only 1 time, because the barbed stinging apparatus remains in the victim when the bee flies away causing evisceration and death of the insect. The so-called "killer bees" are hybrids of species (eg, European bees and African bees) that evolved under different environmental conditions. While the individual venom and sting are no different from other species, "killer bees" tend to be overtly aggressive, are prone to "gang up" on victims, and may chase intruders up to 150 meters. Wasps, hornets, and yellow jackets are generally more aggressive than bees, and have a barbless stinger that allows them to inflict multiple stings. Yellow jackets are carnivores that congregate around dead meat or foodstuffs. Fire ants typically bite and hold onto the victim with their mandibles and then swivel their abdomen in an arc around the fixed mouthparts, inflicting multiple stings. The venom of most ants is less potent than that found in flying Hymenoptera, causes much less tissue destruction and is much less likely to elicit a generalized allergic reaction (about 80 anaphylactic deaths reported). The venom of fire ants is almost 95% alkaloid and exerts a direct toxic effect on human and animal systems. A number of human deaths from the toxins contained in multiple fire ant bites have been reported, especially in old and debilitated persons. However, other individuals have been known to survive as many as 5,000 fire ant stings.

Subjective: **Symptoms**
Instantaneous stinging pain, warmth (vasodilation) and pruritus at site of sting(s), nausea and vomiting, visceral pain following ingestion of insect and stings to the GI tract. urticaria, shortness of breath, wheezing airway (tongue, soft palate, etc.) weakness, syncope, anxiety/confusion, chest pain
Focused History: *Did you have instantaneous onset of pain at site?* (suggests Hymenoptera sting) *Did you receive multiple near-simultaneous stings in portion of body exposed?* (Most Hymenoptera stings occur on exposed skin but can occur through clothing.) *Did you see any insects resembling Hymenoptera species?* (visual clue suggesting cause)

Objective: **Signs**
Using Basic Tools: Inspection; stinging apparatus from bees and bleeding may be seen in the wound, confluent red rash, rapidly spreading edema (as large as 10-15cm), hypotension, tachypnea, tachycardia, shock and cardiorespiratory arrest, distal sensory loss if stung over peripheral nerve, delirium.
Using Advanced Tools: Corneal ulceration following corneal injury

Assessment: Diagnose based on history of exposure and/or captured specimens.
Differential Diagnosis
Angina: *See Part 3: General Symptoms: Chest Pain*
Rheumatoid arthritis: *See Part 3: General Symptoms: Joint Problems: Joint Pain*
Corneal abrasion/laceration: *See Part 3: General Symptoms: Eye Problems: Eye Injury*
Snake bite: *See Part 5: Specialty Areas: Chapter 17: Toxicology: Venomous Snake Bites*
Cat scratch disease: *See Part 5: Specialty Areas: Chapter 12: Bacterial Infections: Bartonella Infections (Cat Scratch Disease, Oroya Fever, Trench Fever)*
Cellulitis: *See Part 4: Organ Systems: Chapter 6: Bacterial Infections: Erysipelas and Cellulitis*
Honey exposure in susceptible individual: If known to be allergic by history of prior exposure

Plan:
Treatment
Primary: Anaphylactic or Generalized Toxic (Anaphylactoid) Reaction: *See Part 7: Trauma: Chapter 27: Anaphylactic Shock*

Single Sting from Flying Hymenoptera (bees, wasps, hornets, and yellow jackets):
1. Remove stinger and venom sac intact as quickly as possible (stinging apparatus may actively inject venom into the wound for one minute), regardless of method.
2. Apply ice or cold water for anesthesia and to control swelling.
3. Apply topical **benzocaine** 20%/**menthol** 0.5% spray as a local analgesic and topical 1% **hydrocortisone** cream tid for up to 7 days as desired (*see Part 3: General Symptoms: Rash with a Fever*). Other remedies to include ammonia, sodium bicarbonate, and papain (meat tenderizer) have minimal proven effectiveness.
4. Elevate extremity to limit spread of edema.

Fire Ant Stings:
1. Do not unroof vesicles.
2. Apply topical **bacitracin** ointment and/or **benzocaine** 20%/**menthol** 0.5% spray for secondary infections tid a day for up to 7 days. *See Part 3: General Symptoms: Rash with a Fever.* Use prophylactic **cephalexin** suspension (250mg/5mL) one teaspoon po qid x10 days for children with >30 fire ant stings.
3. **Ibuprofen** 400-800mg po tid for up to 7 days may reduce the degree of inflammation; **diphenhydramine** 25mg po tid for up to 7 days may diminish itching but promote tiredness.

Massive Multiple Stings:
1. Be prepared to treat for anaphylaxis or anaphylactoid reaction from venom load. *See Part 7: Trauma: Chapter 27: Anaphylactic Shock*
2. Do NOT use massive doses of parenteral steroids or antibiotics in individuals not having anaphylactic or toxic reaction.
3. Give **ibuprofen** 400-800mg po tid for up to 7 days to reduce inflammation (*see Part 3: General Symptoms: Joint Problems: Joint Pain*) and **diphenhydramine** 25mg po tid for up to 7 days to reduce pruritus (*see Part 3: General Symptoms: Pruritus/Itching*).
4. Use topical 1% **hydrocortisone** cream tid for 7 days and topical anesthetics (eg, **benzocaine** 20%/ **menthol** 0.5%) prn.

Patient Education
General: If attacked or stung by flying bees or wasps, do not flail arms, etc. Crushing one insect may incite others to attack even more vigorously. Although the insects may defend an area up to 150 meters from their nests, they can only fly about 4 mph. Therefore, healthy individuals can easily outrun the swarm and escape.

Activity: Restrict movement of affected area/extremity.

Diet: No restrictions.

Medications: Any individual with a generalized reaction should be referred for allergy testing and desensitization, and should thereafter wear a medic-alert tag and carry an emergency medical kit containing at least an antihistamine and aqueous epinephrine in a pre-filled syringe for immediate self treatment. Continue immuno therapy indefinitely as long as risk of exposure is substantial.

Prevention and Hygiene: Avoid nests, hives, bee trees, locations around flowers, fruit, etc. Avoid bright colored clothing, perfume/cologne, etc. Wear shoes (ground nests are common). Do not use noisy equipment (mowers, etc.) in vicinity of "killer-bee" colonies.

No Improvement/Deterioration: Return promptly for emergence of anaphylactic signs (*see Signs: Generalized*)

Follow-Up Actions
Return Evaluation: Be alert for rebound anaphylaxis as medication levels diminish. Observe stings for secondary infection. Be alert for serum sickness up to 14 days post-sting.

Evacuation/Consultation Criteria: Immediately evacuate cases with anaphylactic or generalized reactions. Other cases do not require evacuation, even with multiple stings. Consult primary care physician and allergist as needed. Consult entomologist for insect identification if available.

Chapter 6: Skin: Bug Bites and Stings: Mites
LTC (P) Daniel Schissel, MC, USA

Introduction: Mites are tiny parasitic arachnids that burrow under or attach themselves to the skin where they inflict small bites that cause much larger rashes. The best known mite, *Sarcoptes scabiei* or scabies, is covered in another section of this chapter. Other common mites are dust mites, which cause respiratory allergic symptoms, and harvest mites, also called chiggers or redbugs. The chigger is distinct from other mites in that only the larval stage is parasitic to humans and animals. When chiggers meet an obstacle in the clothing, like a belt or boot top, they inject an irritating secretion that causes the itching sensation and then drop off or are scratched off. The pruritus peaks on the 2nd day and gradually subsides in a week.

Subjective: **Symptoms**
Local pruritic, burning or stinging sensation accompanying erythematous lesions.
Focused History: *Have you been walking in the woods, grass or undergrowth?* (Chiggers live in grain stems, in grasses or undergrowth waiting to attach to a passing victim.)

Objective: **Signs**
Using Basic Tools: Discrete, 1-2mm, erythematous papules often with a hemorrhagic center commonly seen along the belt line or boot top. The primary lesion of other mites follows a spectrum from erythematous papules, pustules, vesicles, to general urticaria. Secondary linear excoriations are common with all mite infestations. In children, these eruptions are often widespread, with urticaria, and even bullae formation. The pruritus may persist for weeks and may progress to impetigo in children.

Assessment: Diagnosis based on clinical morphologic criteria and history of exposure.
Differential Diagnosis
Bed bugs: Usually limited to exposed areas of skin.

Nummular dermatitis: As lesions get older, they may clear in the center and get scaly to resemble ringworm or psoriasis.

Irritant or allergic dermatitis: History of ectopy or exposure to irritant. *See Part 4: Organ Systems: Chapter 6: Skin Disorders: Contact Dermatitis*

Plan:
Treatment
Primary: Relief of pruritus (loratadine 10mg po q day); cool baths or compresses, topical steroid cream (1% **hydrocortisone** or **triamcinolone** bid - tid) may be useful where inflammation is not related to secondary infection. Topical antipruritics (eg, **calamine** lotion, aloe or **Chig-a-rid**) may also be helpful.

Primitive: Household vinegar (5% acetic acid) has been a useful measure for post-exposure prophylaxis and treatment or pruritus.
Patient Education
General: Material employed for protection against mites function more as toxicants than true repellents. DEET provides the best protection when applied to the clothing. Benzyl benzoate is an excellent chigger toxicant and remains effective after rinsing, washing, or submersion in water.
Follow-up Actions
Evacuation/Consultant Criteria: Evacuation is not normally necessary. Dermatology consultation may be helpful for further treatment options.

Chapter 6: Skin: Bugs Bites and Stings: Spider (Black Widow, Brown Recluse) Bites
LTC (P) Daniel Schissel, MC, USA

Introduction: The Black Widow (BW) spider (*Latrodectus mactans*) may be found from southern Canada to Mexico and Cuba. The female is easily recognized by her coal black globular body and red-orange hourglass marking on the underbelly. It favors cool, dark, little-used places to set its web, including outdoor toilet seats. The **Brown Recluse** (BR) (*Loxosceles reclusa*) has a 1cm oval light tan to dark brown body, and a leg span over 2.5cm. A classic dark brown violin-shaped dorsal marking extending from the 3 sets of eyes (rather than 4 seen in other spiders) to the abdomen differentiates it from other brown spiders. It is found across the United States, like the BW, only bites in self-defense. It is commonly found in storage closets, old shoes or boots, rock bluffs and barns. BR venom is hemolytic and necrotizing and contains a spreading factor. Other species of *Latrodectus* and *Loxosceles* are found in other areas of the world. Several species of funnel-web spiders (*Atrax and Hadronyche*) and the red-black spider have been reported to induce fatal bites in Australia, and the *Phoneutria fera* (banana spider) from South America can cause neurotoxic and necrotic lesions. Most spider bites can be treated supportively as with the BW or with wound care and shock precautions as with BR.

Subjective: Symptoms
Spider bites fall into one or more of the follow categories: local reactions, systemic reactions or allergic reactions.

BW: Pinching bite followed by local swelling and burning at the puncture site; abdominal cramping and pain begins within 10-60 minutes, peaking at about 3 hours.

BR: Painful, stinging bite with gradual development of severe pain in 2-8 hours; slow progression over the following weeks of a necrotic ulcerating process spreading from the bite; 25% of patients will also have a systemic reaction also, with nausea, vomiting, fever, chills, muscle aches and pains.

Focused History: *Was the spider seen during the bite?* (Review of 600 cases of suspected spider bites found that in 80% of cases other causes were identified.) *When were you bitten and when did you notice the lesion?* (Initial lesion from brown recluse bite can be noticed within 10 minutes following bite.) *Did you have trauma to the area prior to symptoms?* (may indicate an infection from previous injury) *Have you ever had a similar reaction?* (may indicate history of severe allergic reaction to other agents)

Objective: Signs
Using Basic Tools:
BW: Bite with 2, red, punctate markings on an erythematous plaque most commonly found on the buttocks or groin area. Within 10-60 minutes, severe abdominal cramping and spasmodic muscular contractions may develop and peak up to 3 hours after the bite. Irritability, agitation, and sweating may develop in children. Hypertension in 20-30% of patients within the initial hours following the envenomation of adults may be observed.

BR: Tender, swollen bite that progresses to hemorrhagic vesicle or bullae (sinking blue macule) that may be seen within 10 minutes of the initial bite, and later (5-7 days) to a slowly enlarging gangrenous eschar with a border of erythema and edema; lymphangitis; wound granulates, leaving a large fibrous scar; systemic symptoms (loxoscelism) are observed in up to 25% of patients and include fever, chills, nausea, and joint pain, generalized erythema, purpuric macular eruption, thrombocytopenia, hemoglobinuria, hemolytic anemia, renal failure and shock. "Black urine" may be seen in severe hemolysis.

Using Advanced Tools: Spider may be sent to entomologist for identification.

Assessment:
Diagnose based on history of exposure to a spider bite, clinical symptoms and signs and identification of spider by expert entomologist.
Differential Diagnosis
BW
Acute abdomen: Patients with acute abdomen are more likely to appear tired, flaccid and hypotensive compared to those with history of BW bite (latrodectism) who tend to be hyperactive, hypertensive and have muscle spasms. *See Part 4: Organ Systems: Chapter 7: Acute Peritonitis*

Tick or other arthropod bite: History of exposure to tick or other arthropod.

BR
Phoneutria banana spider: Exposure in South America or related to fruit imported from South America
Atrax funnel-web spider: Exposure to a spider bite in Australia.
Necrotizing fasciitis (staphylococcus, streptococcus, other): Prior history of skin trauma or infection. *See Part 4: Organ Systems: Chapter 6: Bacterial Infections*
Pyoderma gangrenosum: History of inflammatory bowel disease.
Anaphylaxis: Acute onset of cough, wheezing, dyspnea, urticaria/angioedema, tachycardia, hypotension, sense of impending doom, and collapse. *See Part 7: Trauma: Chapter 27: Anaphylactic Shock*
Rabies: History of animal bite. *See Part 5: Specialty Areas: Chapter 12: Viral Infections: Rabies*
Tetanus: History of trauma. *See Part 5: Specialty Areas: Chapter 12: Viral Infections: Tetanus*

Plan:
Treatment
General: Clean with soap and water; apply ice; calm patient; observe for 24 hours to rule out signs of systemic involvement and provide tetanus prophylaxis.
Specific:
BW: Diazepam 2-10mg po q6-8h, or 5-10mg IM or IV may be used for relief of muscle spasm; in cases with latrodectism, **calcium gluconate** 10% solution, 10mL IV (given over 3-4 minutes) and repeated in 2-3 hours may be given for relief of muscular pain. Provide tetanus prophylaxis.
BR: Elevate bite site to decrease the localized reaction; pain control (eg, **acetaminophen** 500mg po q4-6h); good wound care to minimize scarring. Topical steroids may be useful for large localized lesions. In cases of viscerocutaneous loxoscelism with extensive hemolysis, IV hydration and careful monitoring of renal function will be required.
Patient Education
General: Most patients recover fully in 2-3 days from a BW bite, but it has been fatal in children. Return if new symptoms or symptoms persist.
Follow-up Actions: Observe for signs of systemic involvement for 24 hours. Identify and appropriately manage secondary infection.
Evacuation/Consultation Criteria: Urgently evacuate unstable patients including those with systemic reaction to BR bite. Advanced treatment of bites, including dapsone and or antivenin, requires evacuation to a medical treatment facility.

Chapter 6: Skin: Bug Bites and Stings: Scabies
LTC (P) Daniel Schissel, MC, USA

Introduction: Scabies is a transmissible parasitic skin infection caused by the mite *Sarcoptes scabiei* and is characterized by superficial burrows, intense pruritus and secondary infections. The female mite tunnels into the epidermis layer and deposits her eggs along the burrow. The adult female mite has a lifespan of approximately 15-30 days and lays 1-4 eggs per day, which hatch in 3-4 days. After hatching, the larva mature into adult mites in 10-14 days, and their whole life cycle is 30-60 days. The survival for an adult mite apart from the human host is estimated at several days. Scabies is most commonly transmitted by skin-to-skin contact or through fomites such as clothing and bedding from an infected person.

Subjective: **Symptoms**
Continuous low-grade pruritus of the genital areas to include the areola (nipple region) in females, with increased itching at night.
Focused History: *Is anyone else complaining of similar symptoms?* (commonly transmitted by skin-to-skin or clothing contact) *What is the itching like?* (typically widespread and severe, worse at night, seems to be out of proportion to extent of visible lesions on the skin, spares the head except in infants and young children)

Objective: **Signs**
Using Basic Tools: Presentation ranges from papules, vesicles, and linear burrows, intermingled with or obliterated by scratches, dried skin, and secondary infection. The burrow is the home of the female mite, the papules are the temporary invasion of the developing larvae, and the vesicular response is believed to be a sensitization to the invader. The primary locations of invasion include the web spaces of the fingers and toes, the axillae, the flexures of the arms and legs, and the genital regions to include the areola. The head and face are commonly spared in adults but not children. The papules of the genital region may persist for weeks to months after the mite has been cleared.

Assessment: Base diagnosis on clinical exam with history of severe pruritus, a papular or papulovesicular eruptions with burrows, and a characteristic distribution pattern. The definitive diagnosis can only be made with isolating evidence from the patient of an infestation "scabies prep."
Differential Diagnosis
Mites: Milder pruritus than scabies
Bed Bugs: Usually limited to exposed areas of skin and commonly seen as 3 bites ("breakfast, lunch and dinner")
Nummular dermatitis: As lesions get older, they may clear in the center and become scaly to resemble ringworm or psoriasis.
Irritant or allergic dermatitis: History of ectopy or exposure to irritant. *See Part 4: Organ Systems: Chapter 6: Skin Disorders: Contact Dermatitis*

Plan:
Treatment
Primary:
1. Apply **permethrin** 5% cream from the neck down and leave on the skin overnight (8-14 hours) followed by thorough rinsing. A 2nd treatment 1 week following is suggested despite the high cure rate after a single application. Not to be used on children under 2 months of age.

2. Clip the nails and scrub under the distal nail to dislodge any excoriated mites.
3. Change and wash all undergarments and bedding in hot water prior to showering off the permethrin cream. Dry-clean (or seal in an airtight bag for 2 weeks) clothing items that cannot be washed.
4. Treat all family members and personal contacts at the same setting.

Alternative: The antihelmintic **ivermectin** (as an off-label use) has been very effective. (Do not use in pregnant or lactating women.) Give **ivermectin** 200ug/kg po x 1 with a repeat dose in 2 weeks or give 10% **crotamiton** (massage into skin of entire body from chin down; repeat application in 24 hr with a cleaning bath taken 48 hrs after last application) A 2nd line alternative is **benzene hexachloride**. Apply to total body from neck down, leave on 8-12h (adults), 6-8h (children), 6h (infants) then remove by thorough washing.

Secondary: Relieve pruritus with oral antihistamines (eg, **loratadine** 10mg po q day), cool baths or compresses, and topical steroids. Topical antipruritics like **Sarna** lotion or **PrameGel** are alternatives.

Patient Education

General: Do not clean the hair or body excessively, as this can lead to excessively dry skin and a secondary focus of pruritus. Often the pruritus persists despite normal hygienic routines if the patient has a hypersensitivity to the mite or its products.

Follow-up Actions

Reevaluation: Repeat examination for those with continued nocturnal exacerbation of their pruritus. This is the feeding time of the scabies mite and will help differentiate between a hypersensitivity reaction and persistent infestation. Consult dermatology.

Evacuation/Consultation Criteria: No need to evacuate. Consult dermatology as needed.

Zoonotic Disease Considerations

Principal Animal Hosts: Cattle, dogs, and cats

Clinical Disease in Animals: Intense pruritus, lesions start on head, neck and shoulders and can spread to the rest of the body.

Probable Mode of Transmission: Contact with infected animals.

Chapter 6: Skin: Bug Bites and Stings: Flea Bites
LTC (P) Kurt L. Maggio, MC, USA

Introduction: Fleas are small wingless insects, tan brown in color, with long hind legs to allow for jumping from host to host. Virtually all animals, as well as, humans have associated fleas, but they are not strictly species-specific. The most common fleas afflicting humans include the human flea *Pulex irritans*, the dog flea *Ctenocephalides canis*, the cat flea *Ctenocephalides felis*, and the oriental rat flea *Xenopsylla cheopis*. They are able to bite and extract a blood meal from the host's superficial capillaries. Irritation is produced when the flea's saliva is injected into the skin. Fleas can remain dormant for months. Fleas can be vectors of several diseases, including bubonic plague, endemic typhus, brucellosis, melioidosis, and erysipeloid. Fleas are widely distributed throughout the world wherever there are animal hosts present; more active in warmer conditions. **Risk Factors:** Exposure to animals, refugee populations, crowded sleeping conditions especially in previously vacant buildings.

Subjective: Symptoms

Intense itching, swelling and redness at sites of bites, usually on the lower extremities and waist, within hours of exposure.

Focused History: *Onset abrupt?* (suggests external exposure such as from bites) *Eruption mostly on legs, wrists and hands?* (suggests areas where fleas are able to jump) *Pet, rodent, or other animal exposure?* (suggests appropriate means of exposure)

Objective: Signs

Using Basic Tools: Inspection; scattered grouped lesions or extensive areas with erythema, edema, urticarial papules.

Assessment:

Based on the distribution of the lesions, history of exposure, or visual identification of the flea.

Differential Diagnosis:

Other bug bites and stings including hymenoptera and spiders: *See Part 4: Organ Systems: Chapter 6: Bug Bites and Stings*

Cellulitis: Fever, hot wound, advancing erythema. *See Part 4: Organ Systems: Chapter 6: Erysipelas and Cellulitis*

Plan:

Diagnostic Tests: Visual identification of the flea

Treatment

Primary: Supportive. Apply ice/cold; 1% **hydrocortisone** tid for 7 days as needed to skin for comfort. Lesions take several weeks to resolve. Monitor for secondary infection (pain, crust, fever).

Alternative: Camphor and menthol or any available anti-itch cream would be helpful.

Patient Education:

General: Further exposure should be limited. Insect repellents containing N, N-diethyl-3-methylbenzamide (DEET) should be applied to exposed skin surfaces, and uniforms and clothing must be treated with permethrin. Pets or other animals can be administered commercially available products in spray or collar form to control fleas.

Activity: No restrictions

Diet: No restrictions

Medications: No significant side effects

Prevention and Hygiene: Avoid exposure to affected animals. Animal flea control measures can prevent recurrence.

No Improvement/Deterioration: Return promptly for fever (may indicate secondary infection or vector transmission of plague or typhus)

Follow-up Actions:

Return Evaluation: Follow-up if lesions persist more than 3 weeks or continued crops of new lesions (suggests ongoing exposure).

Evacuation/Consultation Criteria: If infection (cellulitis) occurs or eruption becomes generalized

Zoonotic Disease Considerations
Agent: Flea
Principal Animal Hosts: Humans, dogs, cats, rodents
Clinical Disease in Animals: Plague, typhus
Probable Mode of Transmission: Bite
Known Distribution: Worldwide where animal hosts are present

Chapter 6: Skin: Bug Bites and Stings: Pediculosis (crab lice, head lice, body lice)
LTC (P) Daniel Schissel, MC, USA

Introduction: Pediculosis is a parasitic infestation of the skin (scalp, trunk, or pubic areas) that usually occurs in overcrowded dwellings. Head and pubic lice are found on the head and in the pubic area. Body lice are seldom found on the body (only getting on the skin to feed), but can be found in the seams of clothing.

Subjective: **Symptoms**
Pediculus humanus capitis (head louse): pruritus of the sides and back of the scalp. *Pediculus humanus corporis* (body louse): localized or generalized pruritus on the torso. *Pthirus pubis* (crab louse): asymptomatic or mild to moderate pruritus in the pubic area for months.
Focused History: *Have you had itching or noticed lesions around the back of your neck or ears, or itching and linear marks on trunk, or itching in pubic area, axilla or periumbilical area?* (common symptom of head lice, body lice and crab lice) *Does anyone else in the family or other closes contacts have similar symptoms?* (Cross reinfection is common unless close contacts are treated.)

Objective: **Signs**
Using Basic Tools:
Head Lice: <10 organisms usually identified with naked eye or hand lens. The nit (1mm oval, gray, firm capsule) cemented to the hair is the egg remnant of a hatched louse. New, viable eggs have a creamy yellow color. The infestation can be dated from the location of the nit, since they are deposited at the base of the hair follicle and the hair grows 0.5mm daily. Also: excoriation, secondary infection and adenopathy.
Body Lice: Excoriated, small erythematous papules localized to the torso area. Nits and lice are found in the seams of clothes.
Crab Lice: 1-2mm brown to gray specks in the hair-bearing areas of the genital region. Nits appear as tiny white adhesions to the hair. Small erythematous papules at the sites of feeding, especially in the periumbilical area. Secondary excoriation and lichenification may be present. Maculae caerulea are non-blanchable blue to gray macules, 5-10mm in diameter, at the site of a bite that result from the breakdown of heme by the louse saliva. These lesions may be found from the groin to the eyelash. Adenopathy may be observed with secondary infections.

Assessment: Diagnose based on clinical findings and confirm with identification of lice or nits.
Differential Diagnosis: Irritant or allergic dermatitis, arthropod reaction, seborrheic dermatitis, scabies, eczematous dermatitis, folliculitis. Differentiate by finding lice or nit.

Plan:
Treatment
Primary:
1. Wash bedding in hot water. Clothing items that cannot be washed should be sealed in an airtight bag for 2 weeks or dry-cleaned.
2. Apply **permethrin** 1% rinse to the affected area (eg, scalp/pubic area/axilla as clinically indicated) and wash off after 10 minutes.
3. Examine and treat all family members and personal contacts at the same time. Remove nits with a very fine-toothed nit comb. **"Step-2"** or Clear Lice Egg remover Cleansing Concentrate applied to the hair will help aid in nit removal. (No pediculicide is 100% ovicidal.)

Alternative: Lindane shampoo 1.0% (may not be available in US), and **pyrethrin** shampoo 0.3% used in a similar fashion as previously mentioned.
Secondary: Relieve pruritus with oral antihistamines, cool baths or compresses, and topical steroids. Topical antipruritics like **Sarna** lotion or **PrameGel** are alternatives.
Patient Education
General: Do not clean the hair or body excessively, as this can lead to excessively dry skin and a secondary focus of pruritus. Reinfection from untreated family members or other close contacts is common and these individuals should be treated at the same time as the patient.
Follow-up Actions
Evacuation/Consultant Criteria: No need to evacuate. Consult dermatology as needed.

Chapter 6: Skin: Spirochetal Diseases: Yaws
LTC Joseph Wilde, MC, USA

Introduction: *Treponema pallidum* subspecies pertenue causes this chronic relapsing infectious disease. It is found primarily in children less than 15 years of age who live in warm rural areas along the Tropic of Cancer. Specifically: Africa (Ghana, Benin, and Ivory Coast), Southeast Asia (Papua New Guinea, Indonesia, South Pacific Islands), South central Asia (India, Sri Lanka), and Central America (low prevalence in Ecuador, Columbia, Brazil, Guyana, and Surinam). Yaws is transmitted by broken skin (ie, cut, abraded, or inflamed) coming in direct contact with active skin lesions.

Subjective: **Symptoms**
Single, exophytic skin lesion that tends to ulcerate and crust; may be followed by period of healing, then reappearance or multiple raspberry-like lesions. Finally, untreated patients may have bone involvement, resulting in joint pain, difficulty walking or fractures.

Focused History: *Have you been in contact with any person having open skin lesions in the past 3 months?* (Incubation stage may last 10-90 days.)

Objective: Signs

Using Basic Tools: Patients having early disease may present with a primary papular lesion, headache and malaise. The secondary stage follows with more diffuse skin lesions described in this section. Inspection: Yaws may have 3 clinical phases. The primary stage (3-6 months) shows a single erythematous, infiltrated plaque, which eventually heals with scarring. The secondary stage (2 weeks to 6 months after appearance of initial lesion) emerges rapidly, with multiple papules that ulcerate and form yellowish crust. The tertiary stage develops in approximately 10% of infected patients after 5-15 years and shows deep ulcerated nodules with underlying involvement of bone.

Assessment:

Diagnose based on clinical findings in an endemic region and confirm with darkfield microscopic exam of the exudates from skin lesions.
Differential Diagnosis: Specifically, any patient in an endemic area who has thick hyperkeratotic/fissuring skin of the hands and feet should be suspected of having yaws. This may also result in a crab-like gait. Genital lesions are not common and most likely represent incidental/nonsexual contact.

Syphilis: Genital lesion and symptoms or history of sexual contact with infected person. *See Part 5: Specialty Areas: Chapter 11: Genital Ulcers*

Leishmaniasis: History of black fly bite, travel to endemic area. *See Part 5: Specialty Areas: Chapter 12: Parasitic Infections: Leishmaniasis*

Plan:

Treatment

Primary: Benzathine penicillin 1.2-2.4mu IM x 1 dose (0.6-1.2mu for children under 10 years)
Alternative: Tetracycline or **erythromycin** 500mg po qid x 15 days (for children, **erythromycin** 8-10mg/kg po qid x 15 days).
Empiric: Benzathine penicillin 1.2mu IM x 1 dose
Primitive: Keep skin lesions clean with soap and water. Cover with bandages to minimize spread. Splints or crutches may be needed for patients having bone/joint pain.

Patient Education

General: Avoid contact with infected persons having active lesions.
Activity: Normal for patients without bony involvement. Patients with bony involvement may require crutches/splints to ambulate as tolerated.
Diet: Normal
Medications: Penicillin (hypersensitivity reaction; doxycycline (photosensitivity, GI upset); erythromycin (GI upset)
Prevention and Hygiene: Avoid close contact with infected persons.
No Improvement/Deterioration: Progression of skin lesions beyond the initial primary papule or symptoms of joint/bone swelling/pain which may indicate progression to tertiary disease
Wound Care: Clean open wounds daily with soap/water. Cover affected areas with clothing/bandages if possible.

Follow-up Actions

Return Evaluation: Follow up 2 weeks after initial treatment to ensure resolution of all skin lesions. Patients with bony involvement may require consultation with orthopedics or rheumatology for other therapy
Evacuation/Consultation Criteria: Progression of skin lesions beyond the initial primary papule or symptoms of joint/bone swelling/pain which may indicate progression to tertiary disease. Refer to dermatology, rheumatology, or orthopedics

Chapter 6: Skin: Spirochetal Diseases: Pinta
LTC Joseph Wilde, MC, USA

Introduction: Pinta is a chronic infectious disease affecting of the skin caused by *Treponema pallidum* subspecies *carateum*. It is found only in some areas of the Brazilian rainforest. Transmission occurs by repeated direct skin or mucous membrane contact with infected individuals. It is usually acquired during childhood.

Subjective: Symptoms

Nonspecific, diffuse, red scaling papules which may coalesce and become hypopigmented over several years.
Focused History: *Have you been in contact with any other person having similar skin lesions?*

Objective: Signs

Using Basic Tools: Acute: Multiple erythematous macules that may be slightly raised on exposed skin. Chronic: After a lapse of months or years, mottled hypopigmentation skin appears.
Using Advanced Tools: Definitively diagnose by darkfield microscopy.

Assessment: Differential Diagnosis

Vitiligo (autoimmune hypopigmentation): Common skin condition not limited to geographic area of known risk for exposure to pinta.
Tinea corporis: Fungal infection shown as confirmed by KOH positive skin prep.

Plan:

Treatment

Primary: Benzathine penicillin 1.2-2.4mu IM x 1 dose (0.6-1.2mu for children under 10 years)
Alternative: Tetracycline or **erythromycin** 500mg po qid x 15 days (for children, erythromycin 8-10mg/kg po qid x 15days).
Empiric: Benzathine penicillin 1.2mu IM x 1 dose
Primitive: Clean wounds with soap and water daily. Use clothing, bandages, or occlusive dressings to cover open wounds if possible

Patient Education
General: Avoid contact with infected persons.
Activity: Normal
Diet: Normal
Medications: Penicillin (hypersensitivity reaction; doxycycline (photosensitivity, GI upset); erythromycin (GI upset)
Prevention and Hygiene: Avoid close contact with infected persons. Clean open wounds daily with soap/water. Cover affected areas with clothing/bandages if possible.
No Improvement/Deterioration: Spread of skin lesions beyond original site of infection with onset of characteristic darkening or lightening of the skin.
Wound Care: Clean with soap and water. Place moist dressings to facilitate wound healing.
Follow-up Actions
Return Evaluation: Follow-up weekly after initial treatment to ensure that all open skin lesions have healed completely.
Evacuation/Consultation Criteria: No need to evacuate. Consult dermatology if skin lesions do not resolve within 2 weeks or continue to spread to new body locations.

Chapter 6: Skin: Skin Disorders: Psoriasis
LTC (P) Daniel Schissel, MC,USA

Introduction: Psoriasis is a multifactorial genetic disorder of the skin that affects approximately 2-3% of the adult population in western countries, with onset before age 20 in 1/3 of cases. There are many clinical manifestations, but the most common (vulgaris) is typically expressed as chronic scaling papules and plaques in a characteristic extensor surface distribution.

Subjective: **Symptoms**
Chronic history (months to years) chronic scaling papules and plaques in a characteristic extensor surface distribution. Acute exacerbations occur in guttate psoriasis and generalized pustular psoriasis; fever, chills, arthritis, and weakness will accompany acute onset of generalized pustular psoriasis. Subtle cases may be suspected in patients with only a slight gluteal crease "pinkening" and nail findings.
Focused History: *Have you noticed any changes in summer months?* (Psoriatic lesions tend to improve with increased exposure to ultraviolet light.) *Have you noticed lesions on elbows, knees?* (typical location for psoriatic lesions) *Do you smoke or drink alcohol?* (increased incidence of psoriasis) *Have you had a recent illness or other increased stress?* (Various triggers have been identified that may affect the course of the disease.)

Objective: **Signs**
Using Basic Tools: Skin: sharply demarcated, "salmon pink" erythematous, round to oval papules and plaques with characteristic "silvery-white" scale. The arrangement ranges from a few scattered discrete lesions to diffuse involvement without identifiable borders. Lesions generally are seen in a bilaterally symmetrical pattern with a distinct predilection for the extensor surfaces of the knees and elbows. The central portion of the plaques may resolve and involute leaving nummular, annular, gyrate, or arcuate patterns. Scalp, lumbosacral and anogenital lesions are also common. When one excoriates the "silvery-white" scale, there is pinpoint bleeding (Auspitz sign).
Fingernail: pitting, subungual hyperkeratosis (thickening of the nail material), onycholysis (loosening of the nail plate from the nail bed), and "oil spot" (yellowish-brown) spots under the nail.
Using Advanced Tools: Labs: KOH of scale from lesion to ensure the process is not fungal.

Assessment: Diagnose based on the characteristic clinical presentation.
Differential Diagnosis
Seborrheic dermatitis: Dry scalp, seborrheic lesions normally remain within the hairline
Lichen simplex chronicus: Small, very itchy, papule(s)
Candidiasis: KOH positive
Drug reaction: History of drug exposure

Plan:
Treatment: Only with topically administered agents. Ointments tend to penetrate the psoriatic plaques better and are preferred.
Primary:
1. NEVER GIVE ORAL STEROIDS as they may cause a systemic pustular eruption and kill the patient.
2. Use topical fluorinated corticosteroids (**betamethasone, fluocinolone, clobetasol**) in an ointment or cream base q day x 2 weeks. Apply after soaking off the scale in a salt-water bath bid x 2 weeks. Then move to non-fluorinated steroid ointments due to the risk of developing permanent striae and local atrophy. Apply the ointment to the skin when still wet, then pat dry.
3. Never apply fluorinated steroid to the face or in occluded areas like the groin or axilla for they are at higher risk for developing atrophy and striae
Alternative: Triamcinolone ointment, topical **calcipotriene**, tar preparations
Symptomatic: **Hydroxyzine** 25-75mg po q4-6h for pruritus.
Empiric: Ultraviolet exposure (20 min exposure to noonday sun) will accelerate the resolution of the lesions.
Patient Education
General: Lesions can be exacerbated by stress and illness. Minimize friction increases and folds by maintaining appropriate weight and avoid irritating underarm deodorants. Avoid irritating facial soaps and burning from sun exposure. Avoid irritation from tight garments in the genital area as well as exposure to accumulated feces and urine. Avoid vigorous brushing, combing, or scratching of the scalp.
Medications: NO oral steroids, beta-blockers, lithium, NSAIDs. All can exacerbate the lesions, as can antimalarials.
Prevention and Hygiene: Use antifungal soaps.

Follow-up Actions
  Re-evaluation: If lesions do not start to resolve in 2-3 weeks referral is needed.
  Evacuation/Consultation Criteria: Referral is not usually indicated, unless unstable.

Chapter 6: Skin: Skin Disorders: Pseudofolliculitis Barbae
LTC (P) Daniel Schissel, MC, USA

Introduction: Pseudofolliculitis barbae (PFB) is a common disorder of the pilosebaceous unit of the beard and commonly known as "razor bumps" or "shave bumps." It is caused by multiple factors and is more common in those with very curly beard hair. Affected persons may have a genetic predisposition due to abnormal formation of the hair follicle. When hair is lifted and shaved, it retracts into the pilosebaceous unit. Curly hair can then penetrate the side of the follicular unit and cause a mechanical irritation in the skin, or the curly hair may exit appropriately and then curl back into the surface of the face again, causing an irritation. PFB like lesions can develop in any area in men and women that is shaved or the hair is removed. At least 50% of black males and 3% of white males who regularly shave have tendency to develop these lesions.

Subjective: **Symptoms**
  Development of papules and pustules in the beard area after shaving.
  Focused History: *Have you ever noticed these lesions before?* (Typically pseudofolliculitis barbae is a chronic condition that may be associated with acute inflammatory flares.)

Objective: **Signs**
  Using Basic Tools: Follicular-based papules and pustules below the jaw line and on the anterior neck. Number of lesions may vary from a dozen to >100. A piece of hair may be seen protruding from the lesions. Long-standing lesions may become hyperpigmented, nodular (eg, keloid formation), cystic or granulomatous.

Assessment: Diagnose based on predisposition to condition, history and clinical findings.
  Differential Diagnosis
    Acute folliculitis: Pyoderma of hair follicles secondary to microbial infection (seen in patients with or without previous history of PFB) and possibly associated with predisposing factors (nasal carriage of *S. aureus*, exposure to whirlpools, swimming pools with inadequate chlorination contaminated with *Pseudomonas aeruginosa*, antibiotic or corticosteroid therapy that predispose to *Candida* folliculitis)
    Acne: Lesions seen in other areas.
    Irritant contact dermatitis: Lesions in other areas, possible history of exposure to irritant (eg, change in shaving lotion)

Plan:
  Treatment
    Primary: Manage mild cases with proper shaving techniques. Allow the hair to grow out onto the surface of the skin and then trim with a safety razor or clipper. Gently lift out remaining buried ingrown hair tips onto the surface and clip; do not pluck or pull.
    Alternative: A chemical depilatory with strict adherence to the time it is left on the skin to avoid secondary chemical irritation.
    Empiric: Minocycline 100mg po bid will help decrease the irritation and secondary infection.
  Patient Education
    General: Shave gently with "bump fighter" razor, without pulling the skin taut or repeating over the same area; shave "with the grain" of the hair. Close shaving promotes oblique penetration of the sharpened hairs into the skin and should be avoided whenever possible. Prevention and Hygiene: Apply moist heat after shaving, followed by a moisturizer (like razor bump fighter), and avoid strong astringents like alcohol that will only dry the face and cause more irritation. Use a soft brush (toothbrush will work) 2-3 x a day to lift the hair and prevent them from penetrating the skin
  Follow-up Actions
    Evacuation/Consultation Criteria: No need to evacuate.

Chapter 6: Skin: Skin Disorders: Skin Cancer (Basal & Squamous Cell, Malignant Melanoma)
MAJ Charles Moon, MC, USA

Basal Cell Carcinoma (BCC)

Introduction: BCC is by far the most common cancer in the world, with well over 1 million cases diagnosed each year in the US alone. BCCs are virtually 100% curable if found early and appropriately treated since metastasis are very rare. Early detection and treatment are paramount in order to avoid extensive tissue destruction, damage to adjacent structures, and complex surgical reconstruction. Sun exposure and fair complexion are the main risk factors for BCC skin cancer development. Unfortunately, much ultraviolet radiation (sun) exposure occurs before age 18 when most people believe they are not affected by skin cancer. Patients diagnosed with a BCC have a 45% risk of developing at least one more within the subsequent 2 years.

Subjective: **Symptoms**
  Very slow-growing, small, pearly or waxy papule, usually in a sun-exposed area. Patient may complain of a sore that will not heal. There may be a history of trauma preceding the lesion.
  Focused History: *Do you have any skin lesions that are not healing, enlarging, or bleed easily?* (BCCs are often slow growing, friable, and may ulcerate.) *Have you been diagnosed with skin cancer before?* (Previous skin cancer history is a marker for significant sun exposure, which places the patient at risk for additional skin cancer development.)

Objective: **Signs**

Using Basic Tools: Waxy or pearly papule with telangiectasias (small, dilated blood vessels) that can enlarge to several cm over time; superficial erosion or ulceration often with scabbing; some lesions appear like flat scars, usually without a history of trauma; some superficial lesions appear like a small patch of eczema (slight scale and erythema) often on the trunk; sun-exposed areas are the most common sites: ears, periauricular skin, eyelids and periocular skin, nose, cheeks, temples, forehead, upper chest, back, and arms forearms; can occur even in protected areas like the axilla, so skin exams should be thorough and complete.

Assessment: **Differential Diagnosis**

Actinic keratosis, squamous cell carcinoma, benign lichenoid keratosis, intradermal nevus, neurofibroma, irritated seborrheic keratosis, amelanotic (non-pigmented) melanoma, tricholemmoma. Differentiating these conditions in the field is nearly impossible, since they require expert microscopic evaluation of a biopsy.

Plan:

Treatment

Defer treatment until return from mission (tumors are very slow growing). Observation is preferable to any treatment. For local nationals, if evacuation or referral cannot be accomplished within 6 months, perform full thickness excision with 4-5mm margins all around the tumor. Store tumor in formaldehyde if possible for later study.

Patient Education

Prevention: Education about sun precautions is vital: avoid the sun during hours when the individual's shadow is shorter than their height (typically between 1,000-1,600); wear long sleeves, pants and broad-brimmed hats, apply sunscreen of SPF 30 or greater (with special attention to the nose, ears and lips).

Follow-up Actions

Evacuation/Consultant Criteria: Evacuate non-urgently (routine status) if on long deployment. Otherwise, delay treatment until return from mission. Consult dermatology as needed.

Squamous Cell Carcinoma (SCC)

Introduction: SCC is the 2nd most common skin cancer, affecting over 200,000 Americans each year. Metastasis may occur with invasive SCCs, especially on the lip or ear. Rates of metastasis range from about 1-5%. Non-invasive or in situ SCC (also termed Bowen's disease) can become invasive with time in about 5-26% of cases. SCC typically develops on sun-exposed skin and individuals with fair complexions are at higher risk for developing SCC. Other risk factors include a history of ionizing radiation exposure, immunocompromise such as in organ transplant recipients, or a history of arsenic ingestion. In sun-protected areas, chronic ulcers or scars predispose to SCC development and may carry a higher metastasis rate (around 30%). There is a variant of SCC called keratoacanthoma (KA), which grows very quickly and may spontaneously regress. Mid-facial KAs can be especially aggressive and destructive.

Subjective: **Symptoms**

KAs grow rapidly, while SCCs usually are slow growing and much more common; usually painless lesion; history of chronic sun exposure is common, fair complexion.

Focused History: *Do you have any skin lesions that are not healing, enlarging, crusted, or bleed easily?* (SCCs progressively enlarge, may be friable, are often hyperkeratotic, and may ulcerate.) *Have you been diagnosed with skin cancer before?* (This is a marker for significant risk factor exposure, which places the patient at risk for additional skin cancer development.)

Objective: **Signs**

Using Basic Tools: Red, scaly (hyperkeratotic) papules are most characteristic for SCC. Size varies from a few mm to several cm. SCCs, when more advanced, can present as tumor-like growths with central necrosis and scab. SCC in situ can occur on the glans penis or within the foreskin, and usually has a soft, red, velvety appearance, without hyperkeratosis (called erythroplasia of Queyrat). SCC in situ on the penis, perineum, and perianally may also present as red, brown, flat-topped verrucous papules/ plaques and can be confused with genital warts in sexually active adults (called Bowenoid papulosis). SCC on the penis or vulva may be associated with cancer-producing human papilloma virus strains (HPV type 16). In general, a biopsy may be warranted for any pigmented, erosive, bleeding, or therapy resistant genital lesion to exclude malignancy. SCC in situ or Bowen's disease on areas other than the genitals may appear like an erythematous (fiery appearing), scaly plaque on sun exposed sites. These lesions may be confused as areas of eczema, psoriasis, tinea, or a superficial BCC by untrained personnel. KAs arise rapidly (over weeks) and appear like a volcano with a central core of keratin surrounded by domed, rolled borders, usually ranging in size from 1-3cm. Metastatic SCC may present with palpable lymphadenopathy in the affected, draining lymphatic basin.

Assessment: **Differential Diagnosis**

BCC, actinic keratosis, ulcers, chronic ulcerative herpes, benign adnexal tumors, various dermatitides (in cases of Bowen's disease). Differentiating some of these conditions in the field is nearly impossible, requiring expert microscopic evaluation of a biopsy.

Plan:

Treatment

Evacuate and refer to dermatology. If evacuation is not possible in the foreseeable future (1-2 months: relatively slow growing tumor), perform full thickness excisions with 5mm margins all around the tumor. Store the tumor in formaldehyde, if possible, for later study. Prevention: Education about sun precautions is vital: avoid the sun during hours when the individual's shadow is shorter than their height (typically between 1,000-1,600); wear long sleeves, pants and broad-brimmed hats, apply sunscreen of SPF 30 or greater (with special attention to the nose, ears and lips).

Follow-up Actions
  Evacuation/Consultation Criteria: Evacuate non-urgently (routine status) if less than 2 months before return from deployment. Otherwise, delay treatment until return from mission. Consult dermatology as needed.

Malignant Melanoma

Introduction: The incidence of malignant melanoma, the most serious form of skin cancer resulting in 75% of skin cancer deaths, is rising faster than all other cancers in the US. In 1930, 1 in 5,000 Americans was likely to develop melanoma during their lifetime. In 2005, 1 in 62 Americans had a lifetime risk of developing invasive melanoma, a 2000% increase from 1930. In addition, with the inclusion of in situ melanoma (non-invasive), 1 in 34 Americans have a lifetime risk of developing melanoma. Today, melanoma is the 2nd most common fatal cancer in women aged 20 to 29. This type of skin cancer is characterized by the uncontrolled growth of pigment-producing cells (melanocytes). Melanomas may appear suddenly without warning but also can develop from or near a mole. They are found most frequently on the sun exposed head/neck, upper back, and legs (a location more commonly seen in women), but can occur anywhere on the body including non sun exposed sites like the soles, under nails, and on the buttocks. Although melanoma can metastasize and cause death, it is very curable with early detection and surgical excision. The depth of invasion into the skin is the best predictor of long term survival. For localized melanoma (melanomas that has not spread beyond the top layer of the skin), the average 5 year survival rate is 98%. Approximately 83% of melanomas are diagnosed at a localized stage. **Risk Factors:** Family history of melanoma in 1st degree relatives; childhood history of severe sunburns; personal history of many atypical nevi.

Subjective: Symptoms
  Often, the first sign of melanoma is a change in the size (enlargement), shape, color, borders, or feel of an existing mole. Most melanomas have a black or blue-black area. Melanoma also may appear as a "new mole." It may be black, abnormal, or "ugly looking." Melanomas in an early stage may be found when an existing mole changes slightly, for example, when a new black area forms or the pigmentation of changes. In more advanced melanoma, the texture of the mole may change; for example, it may become hard or lumpy. More advanced tumors may itch, ooze, or bleed, but melanomas usually do not cause pain or symptoms.
  Focused History: *Have you had melanoma in your family/childhood sunburns/unusual moles or freckles?* (typical risk factors)

Objective: Signs
  Using Basic Tools: Use the mnemonic ABCDE for lesion: "<u>A</u>"–asymmetry, "<u>B</u>"– border irregularity, "<u>C</u>"– color variegation or change, and "<u>D</u>"– diameter greater than 6mm, and "<u>E</u>"-elevation. The earliest of these is probably color variegation, which includes darkening of a lesion, or the appearance of red, white and/ or blue colors. Irregular areas which are very dark (brown-black), or which become very light in color are also bad signs. Amelanotic melanomas are difficult to diagnose because they have little pigment and can appear non-specifically as a flesh-colored papule/nodule. These are responsible for about 1/3 of melanomas found under the nail. Asymmetry and border irregularity come from uncontrolled growth of abnormal melanocytes at the edges of the lesion. Notched, grooved, or scalloped borders are suspicious and are usually apparent in a lesion of 6mm diameter or more. Early melanomas tend to be flat (macular) but can develop papular/nodular components indicating that the cancer is invading deeper into the skin and a hence has a higher risk to metastasize. Associated lymphadenopathy may suggest metastasis. Melanoma can also develop on acral locations (hands and feet) and is more commonly seen in darker skinned races such as Africans. Acral melanomas may present with dark brown-black discoloration in the nail beds and nail matrix (which is just proximal to the cuticle and between the skin and the bone of the distal phalanx) or non-specific nail changes such as lifting or splitting of the nail.

Assessment: Differential Diagnosis
  Seborrheic keratosis, pigmented basal cell carcinoma, atypical nevus, solar lentigo, subungual hematoma (in acral melanoma). Differentiating these conditions in the field is nearly impossible, since it requires expert microscopic evaluation of a biopsy.

Plan:
  Treatment
    Evacuate quickly (within 2 weeks) for evaluation and biopsy, preferably by a dermatologist. If emergent evacuation is not possible, perform initial excision with margins around the entire tumor. Store the tumor in formaldehyde for later review. Evacuate patient with biopsy specimen as soon as possible.
  Patient Education
    Prevention: Perform self-exam of the entire skin at least monthly. Avoid ultraviolet exposure as listed previously. If personal history of melanoma, a strong family history, or many atypical nevi, have routine full body checkup by a dermatologist with palpation of appropriate lymph node basins.
  Follow-up Actions
    Evacuation/Consultation Criteria: Evacuate immediately. Consult dermatology immediately.

Chapter 6: Skin: Skin Disorders: Seborrheic Keratosis
MAJ Charles Moon, MC, USA

Introduction: A seborrheic keratosis (SK) is a very common pigmented, benign tumor. These growths typically appear after the age of 30 and typically involve the face, neck and back. They may be seen in all races.

Subjective: Symptoms
  Strong hereditary predisposition; slightly more common in males; rarely pruritic or painful unless irritated or secondarily infected after trauma.
  Focused History: *Has the lesion enlarged or changed color?* (This may indicate melanoma, however SKs may enlarge and have varied dark colors.)

Objective: **Signs**

Using Basic Tools: Inspection: Lesion varies in size (2-20mm), round to oval, often elevated, "stuck-on" appearing, papule or plaque with variable pigmentary change. The surface of lesion commonly has "warty" (verrucoid) appearance as it matures and grows; face, trunk and extremities are common sites.

Stucco keratoses are a variant of SKs found symmetrically below the knees; often smaller in size (1-3mm), warty appearing, and grey to white in color.

Using Advanced Tools: Close inspection with a hand lens will often show epidermal cysts filled with keratin (horn cyst) or dark keratin plugs and the lesions should almost be able to be picked off with a no. 15 blade. Biopsy is necessary to confirm the diagnosis for atypical lesions.

Assessment: Diagnose based on clinical criteria

Differential Diagnosis: Early lesions: actinic keratosis, wart, malignant melanoma, squamous cell carcinoma, solar lentigo (if lesion is flat), nevus. Later lesions - malignant melanoma, pigmented basal cell carcinoma, squamous cell carcinoma, nevus, wart. Differentiating these conditions in the field can be very difficult without expert micro-scopic evaluation of a biopsy. Therefore, if concern exists for a cancerous lesion, shave biopsy should not be delayed.

Plan:

Treatment

None is required for this benign lesion. Cryotherapy if often employed to treat these lesions, however they often recur. Curettage with/without cryotherapy is also a common treatment modality. Most cases of melanoma, in which the diagnosis is missed or delayed, are often misdiagnosed initially as a SK, so ensure your diagnosis is accurate prior to destructive treatments.

Patient Education

This is a common proliferation of keratinocytes (skin cells). Follow up if change in color or growth of lesion to rule out a malignant melanoma. Melanomas can sometimes masquerade as benign appearing nevi or seborrheic keratoses.

Follow-up Actions

Evacuation/Consultation Criteria: No need to evacuate. Consult dermatology as needed.

Chapter 6: Skin: Skin Disorders: Contact Dermatitis

MAJ Charles Moon, MC, USA

Introduction: Contact dermatitis (CD) can be due to irritant or allergic reactions. Allergic contact dermatitis (ACD) develops when the skin becomes sensitized to a specific allergen and is then re-exposed to it. Tiny amounts of allergen can cause a reaction in these individuals, which is characterized by itching and rash in the distribution of contact. Conversely, an irritant contact dermatitis (ICD) occurs without previous sensitization, tends to be dose related, and may be characterized by burning/pain in addition to itching. ICD is more common and accounts for 80% of cutaneous contact reactions, while ACD is responsible for 20% of cases. Both can cause acute or chronic skin reactions; the history and pattern of eruption can provide clues to the nature of the contact.

Subjective: **Symptoms**

With CD, small vesicles or larger bullae may be present. These can weep a straw colored fluid, which will crust on the affected area giving the appearance of impetigo. Various skin reactions including wheals, erythema, hives, edema, papules, vesicles/bullae, and non-specific eczematous plaques can also occur with either ICD or ACD. Itching and burning of the skin are the most common symptoms with contact dermatitis. If the agent is also a systemic allergen (eg, latex), shortness of breath and wheezing may be seen, but this is rare.

Focused History: *Have you noticed any specific substances or environments that cause this rash?* (This may help uncover an offending irritant or allergen. Some patients with ACD or ICD know exactly what the offending agent is. Others may require keeping journals to correlate symptoms and exposures.) *Have you had this rash or similar ones in the past?* (CD is often recurrent and in cases of ACD, the dermatitis may worsen with subsequent exposures.) *Does your rash itch?* (ACD is often intensely pruritic; ICD may burn, while other dermatoses that can be confused with CD may be asymptomatic.)

Objective: **Signs**

Using Basic Tools: Inspection: The distribution of the eruption is often the most helpful clue in establishing the diagnosis of a contact dermatitis. With dermatitis on the hands or feet, CD should always be suspected. Not all sites exposed to an allergen will cause CD. For example, thinner more sensitive areas of the skin like the eyelids and neck may develop ACD from nail polish or fragrances, while thicker areas of the skin like the hands will not react when exposed to the identical irritant or allergic contactant. Cold dry environments may predispose individuals to ICD when the barrier function of the skin is cracked and less oily, while hot climates may allow sweat to solubilize allergens and enhance penetration of the skin, promoting ACD. Finally, patients may develop an allergy to substances they have been exposed to for years. These issues may cause confusion when trying to establish the diagnosis of CD. Common patterns of ACD and ICD are listed:

ACD: Plants such as poison oak can leave linear streaks of itchy, red papules and vesicles/bullae, corresponding to resin deposition from the plant on the skin. Nickel, commonly used as an alloy, is the most common cause of ACD, but other metals such as gold can cause ACD. ACD to metals often affects the earlobes from earrings, the neck from necklaces or dog-tags, and the abdomen from a belt buckle or button. Shoes and boots with leather have traces of tanning chemicals, rubber, chemicals involved in producing rubber, and adhesives. These can all cause ACD and may produce severe, incapacitating reactions on the bilateral, dorsal feet of Soldiers. Preservatives and fragrances in beauty and health care products are a common cause of ACD on the face, armpits, neck, and eyelids. Neomycin is a very common cause of ACD (sensitizing almost 10% of all people exposed to it) and can create a picture suggestive of an infection when patients apply first aid products containing neomycin (Neosporin) to wounds. Formaldehyde and formaldehyde releasing products are present in dry-cleaned clothes, permanent press/ wrinkle free fabric, and many skin/hair products. These chemicals are common allergens and can present as diffuse rashes that may mimic nummular eczema or other diffuse non-specific eruptions. If dermatitis develops around sites of the elastic band contact, like the beltline and proximal thighs, think of the "Bleached Rubber Syndrome." This results from contact of elastic with household bleach, creating a sensitizing chemical not present in new, unbleached underwear.

ICD: 90% of cases of hand dermatitis are due to ICD and are commonly seen in manufacturing, mining, food service, and healthcare industries due to occupational exposures. The most common causes of occupational ICD include soaps, frequent or vigorous hand washing, petroleum products, cutting oils, and coolants.

Assessment: Differential Diagnosis

Various conditions may be differentiated based on the symptoms, appearance, and distribution of the dermatitis.

Atopic dermatitis (eczema): Excoriated papules and plaques with thickened skin (lichenification); intermittent course; typical distribution of cheeks and extensor extremities in infants, antecubital and popliteal fossae in children, may have widespread skin or just dorsal hand involvement in adults; severe pruritus.

Seborrhea: Greasy, yellow scale and erythema on ears, scalp, brow, face, and chest; chronic and relapsing; mild pruritus

Xerotic eczema (winter itch): Fine scale, often on back and extremities; moderate pruritus; seen more often in drier climates and seasons (winter).

Stasis dermatitis: Erythematous scaling plaques; brown and copper colored discoloration of affected skin; pruritus; seen on lower extremities or elderly adults as result of chronic lower extremity swelling.

Nummular dermatitis: Circular scaling plaques that are often confused with tinea infections; lower legs commonly involved but can be widely distributed; pruritus; often chronic and intermittent.

Psoriasis: Erythematous plaques with thick white scale; scalp, ears, elbows, hands, feet, knees, umbilicus, and gluteal cleft; pruritus variable, but typically not severe; may be associated with chronic arthritis.

Pityriasis rosea: Salmon colored round to oval plaques with scale that trails the leading edge (tinea with scale on the advancing or leading edge); often on trunk in fir tree distribution; spontaneously resolves in week to months; significant pruritus; initial larger oval lesion may precede the more generalized eruption (herald patch).

Tinea: Annular scaling red plaques seen at most any location on body and scalp; often causes hair loss if affects scalp; pruritus

Scabies: Non-specific erythematous crusting papules on wrists, ankles, abdomen, thighs, and sometimes linear burrows in web spaces; in male patients will often see crusted papules on the penis and scrotum; severe pruritus; commonly seen in deployed or basic training population.

Impetigo: Erythematous papules and plaques with honey-yellow crusting; often asymptomatic; superficial skin infection with *Staphylococcus aureus*.

Cellulitis: Erythematous, often expanding plaque with deep seated edema; often on lower extremity, face, or hands; painful; may be accompanied by fever and malaise; commonly caused by *Staphylococcus aureus* or *Streptococcal* species.

Plan:
Treatment
Primary:
1. AVOIDANCE IS KEY! Protective clothing can help, but a change of occupation, hobby or exposure may be necessary.
2. Topical steroids (higher potency like **fluocinonide** ointment bid or medium potency like **triamcinolone** ointment bid) help suppress the inflammation while identifying the offending agent.
3. For exudative, weeping areas, a soothing astringent (drying) treatment such as Burow's solution compresses bid/tid can help. Minimize wet-dry cycles and avoid over-cleansing the skin. In generalized cases, bathe just every other day, with lukewarm water for less than 5 minutes. Use only a mild cleanser like Cetaphil lotion or Dove Sensitive Skin soap. Avoid scrubbing the affected areas.
4. Bland emollients like white petrolatum will help to moisturize and protect the skin.
5. Oral antihistamines like **hydroxyzine** 25-50mg tid/qid, or up to 50mg at bedtime can alleviate much of the itch. The antipruritic effects of hydroxyzine last 24 hours and the drowsiness usually only lasts 8-10 hours, which is a decided advantage over diphenhydramine. These medications may be best used at dinnertime, providing itching relief at bedtime and improving sleep. Due to the prolonged sedative effects, these medications should not be used in individuals on flying status and may be inappropriate for use in the deployed/field environment.
6. Oral steroids, like **prednisone**, may be needed in the most severe cases and are used in a tapering fashion for 3 weeks; starting at 60mg q day x 7 days, then 40mg q day x 7 days, then 20mg q day x 7 days. Reserve oral steroids for the most widespread, treatment resistant, or bothersome eruptions. Three weeks of treatment are often required to outlast the cutaneous hypersensitivity reaction. Avoid using short courses of oral corticosteroids or Medrol dose pack, since patients will often have rebound worsening of their dermatitis when the medication is discontinued.

Empiric: Empiric treatment should be focused on removal of a suspected allergen or irritant. Topical steroids may be used, as listed above, if one suspects CD.

Patient Education
General: Counsel patient that exposure to allergen, even if small/ minor, can trigger allergic contact dermatitis. Also patients need to know that they can develop CD to substances that they have used for a long duration, often making determination of the offending substance difficult.

Activity: In cases of severe CD on the feet, the patient may require a soft or open toe shoe profile. This may restrict the patient's ability to ambulate in a deployed setting. Generally cases of CD should not limit activity unless severe or if the hands or feet are significantly affected.

Medications: Patients should be counseled on the risk of skin thinning or striae (atrophy) with over-use of topical steroids; high potency topical steroids should not be used for longer than 4-6 weeks continuously on body sites without close monitoring for side effects.

Lower potency topical steroids should be used on the face, but also carry the risk of skin striae and atrophy with long term use. Use of topical steroids on the face can trigger acne like eruptions with long term use or quick discontinuation. Topical steroids are absorbed through the skin and may cause growth delay with widespread, long term application in pediatric patients with a high body surface to volume ratio. Oral corticosteroids can raise blood pressure and affect glucose metabolism; therefore use with caution in hypertensive or diabetic patients. Long term use of oral corticosteroids (greater than one month) is associated with a variety of metabolic side effects and should be managed by providers knowledgeable of the numerous side effects. Use caution in prescribing first generation antihistamines due to the sedating effects.

Prevention and Hygiene: Basic hygiene and avoidance of allergen/irritant. If exposed to a possible contact allergen, wash affected skin and affected clothes/equipment immediately with soapy warm water.

No Improvement/Deterioration: Evacuate for possible biopsy or allergic patch testing if the patient continues to worsen, fails to respond to treatment after one month, has frequent relapses of CD, or if the diagnosis is uncertain.

Wound Care: In cases of significant skin breakdown or ulceration, keep the area clean with warm, soapy water; covered with petrolatum ointment and an occlusive dressing until healed.

Follow-up Actions

Return Evaluation: Patient may f/u as needed if no response to allergen or irritant avoidance. Recheck in 4 weeks if dermatitis persists requiring frequent use of a high potency topical steroid.

Evacuation/Consultation Criteria: Evacuation is typically not necessary, except with systemic allergic symptoms. Consult as needed

Chapter 7: Gastrointestinal: Appendicitis

COL Peter McNally, MC, USA (Ret)

Introduction: Appendicitis is the most common abdominal surgical emergency. Between 5-10% of people develop this condition in life (lower percentage in developing world). Appendicitis can occur at ANY AGE, but is most common during ages 10-40. Consider the diagnosis of appendicitis in anyone with an appendix that develops acute abdominal pain.

Subjective: **Symptoms**

Classic sequence (occurs in only 50% of patients): (1) generalized abdominal pain; (2) anorexia, nausea or vomiting; (3) localized pain over the appendix; (4) fever (low-grade). About 95% of patients have anorexia, nausea or vomiting. Hunger or persistent eating is atypical in appendicitis. The sensation of constipation or "gas stoppage" is common, but defecation does not bring relief of symptoms and diarrhea is uncommon. With time the pain gradually increases, but may then subside for a period after the appendix perforates (usually after > 24 hours), and pain resumes with greater intensity and generalization. In the field environment, peritonitis and death are likely at that point.

Focused History: *When did the pain start?* Describe the pain. *Where does it hurt the most?* (Initially, the pain of appendicitis is usually colicky, vague and not severe. It reaches a peak at 4 hours only to gradually subside, and then reappear as a severe pain localized to the right lower quadrant [RLQ]. The shift in pain from generalized to the RLQ [McBurney's march] is a diagnostic clue.)

Objective: **Signs**

Using Basic Tools: Temperature: Fever (101-102°F) frequently develops over 24 hrs. Higher fever is atypical. Inspection: Guarding, abdominal pain with cough. Palpation: Abdominal tenderness: more common in RLQ, may be localized over the appendix at McBurney's point (2 inches from the anterior superior iliac spine along a line that intersects with the umbilicus); rebound tenderness; costovertebral angle tenderness (CVAT) in retrocecal appendicitis; positive psoas sign, which is pain extending the right hip while patient lies on his left side; positive obturator sign: with the patient supine and the right hip and knee flexed, pain when right leg passively crosses over left (internal rotation). Referred pain: Palpation of LLQ produces pain in RLQ. Perform pelvic and rectal exams: Lateral digital movement may assist to localize pain.

Using Advanced Tools: Labs: WBC with differential (>10,000/mL, in over 90% of appendicitis), pregnancy test, urinalysis.

Assessment:

Differential Diagnosis: Quite extensive. *See Part 3: General Symptoms: Acute Abdominal Pain*

Industrialized nations:

In females: Pelvic inflammatory disease, ovarian cysts, Mittelschmerz (pelvic bleeding from a ruptured ovarian follicle), ectopic pregnancy: *See Part 3: General Symptoms: Gynecologic Problems: Pelvic Pain, Acute*

Gastroenteritis, enterocolitis (eg, Yersinia), or mesenteric lymphadenitis: Nausea, vomiting precedes abdominal pain. Diarrhea more prominent than constipation.

Ureteral colic, acute pyelonephritis: Colicky pain, dysuria, abnormal urinalysis

Constipation: LLQ pain; positive rectal exam. *See Part 3: General Symptoms: Constipation*

Food poisoning: Vomiting and/or diarrhea. *See Part 4: Organ Systems: Chapter 7: Acute Bacterial Food Poisoning & Part 3: General Symptoms: Diarrhea, Acute*

Peritonitis: Multiple etiologies; usually higher fever or rigors, different pain profile. *See Part 3: General Symptoms: Acute Abdominal Pain & Part 4: Organ Systems: Chapter 7: Acute Peritonitis*

Bowel obstruction: Vomiting, different pain profile. *See Part 3: General Symptoms: Acute Abdominal Pain & Part 4: Organ Systems: Chapter 7: Acute Intestinal Obstruction*

Developing countries:

Intussusception (a section of the bowel telescoping into another): Much more common due to tubercular, parasitic and lymphoid adenopathy; diverticulitis less common because of high fiber diets. Colonic and even small bowel volvuli (twisting) are also common.

Typhoid fever: RLQ pain often with headache, fatigue, splenomegaly, normal WBC, and roseola-type rash. *See Part 5: Specialty Areas: Chapter 12: Bacterial Infections: Typhoid Fever*

Amebic hepatic abscess: May present as RUQ pain and following rupture, fluid may accumulate in the RLQ with associated RLQ symptoms.

Ascaris infestation: Found in Southern China, India and Central Africa; can lead to bowel obstruction or perforation, cholecystitis, and appendicitis. Similarly, filariasis (found in India) often mimics appendicitis but with higher (103-104°F) fevers, nausea, and RLQ pain. Peritoneal signs are rare. *See Part 5: Specialty Areas: Chapter 12: Parasitic Infections: Ascariasis (Roundworm) & Filariasis (Elephantiasis)*

Sickle cell disease (crisis): Usually includes neurologic symptoms, pain far out of proportion to physical findings

Acute porphyria: 20-40 year old females, southern Africa, precipitated by sulfa drugs, alcohol or barbiturates. Severe colicky pain with nausea, vomiting, and constipation, and neurologic symptoms. WBC often normal and abdominal exam more benign than the complaint of pain. The patients will have a low-grade fever and jaundice/dark urine.

Malaria: Fever, chills, vomiting, history of travel to a malaria-endemic area. *See Part 5: Specialty Areas: Chapter 12: Parasitic Infections: Malaria*

Lead poisoning/colic: Vague, persistent abdominal pain.

Plan:
  Treatment
  1. IV fluids to maintain adequate urine output (*see Part 7: Trauma: Chapter 27: Resuscitation Fluids*)
  2. Antibiotics:
      A. **Ceftriaxone** 2g IV q day or **cefotaxime** 2g IV q8h + **metronidazole** 500mg IV q6h or
      B. **Ciprofloxacin** 400mg IV q12h or **levofloxacin** 750mg IV q24h + **metronidazole** 500mg IV q6h or
      C. **Ertapenem** 1g IV q day or **moxifloxacin** 400mg po q day (where IV access not possible and patient is able to tolerate oral medications)
  3. Evacuation: Urgent medical evacuation to surgical care prior to perforation markedly decreases chances of morbidity and mortality. Elevate head and flex knees during evacuation.
  4. If evacuation is not possible, and patient's clinical condition continues to deteriorate despite 48-72 hrs of appropriate antibiotic therapy, consider appendectomy only as a last resort. *See Part 4: Organ Systems: Chapter 7: Emergency Field Appendectomy*
  5. Manage pain: *See Part 8: Procedures: Chapter 30: Pain Assessment and Control*

  Patient Education
  General: Appendectomy should cure the patient of symptoms if the diagnosis was correct.
  Diet: No dietary restrictions.

  Follow-up Actions
  Return Evaluation: Reevaluation for symptoms of pain, fever, diarrhea. Return for evaluation if appendectomy does not lead to prompt restoration of baseline good health.
  Evacuation/Consultation Criteria: Evacuate urgently for surgery. Incidence of perforation increases dramatically after 24 hrs of symptoms. Needs routine postoperative surgical follow up for evidence of wound complications, then primary care management.

Chapter 7: Gastrointestinal: Emergency Field Appendectomy
COL John Holcomb, MC, USA and SFC Dominique Greydanus, USA (Ret)

What: The removal or drainage of a suppurative or perforated appendix through an emergency laparotomy.

When: Only when the patient has failed 48-72 hours of appropriate antibiotic therapy, absolutely cannot be evacuated in time, is having high spiking fevers, has an elevated WBC count and peritonitis, and will die without the operation. Tell your commander this is a life or death maneuver, and the patient has only a small chance of living despite this operation.

Background: The ultimate goal should be to avoid operating in this environment. In a field setting without dedicated surgical support, acute appendicitis is treated with IV antibiotics until evacuation is possible. If evacuation is not possible, the majority of acute appendicitis patients can still be treated with IV antibiotics (only 30% will recur later). The patient with perforated appendicitis presents more difficulty, however they can still be treated with IV antibiotics in a non-operative fashion, and only 50% of these patients will require an emergency operation. The decision to perform an appendectomy without the support of personnel proficient in intra-abdominal surgery is extremely dangerous. This is essentially a triage decision, maximizing your limited resources, personnel and surgical experience by treating the majority of patients with antibiotics alone. Once the decision has been made to operate, it is important to adequately prepare the personnel assisting you. Discuss all steps of the procedure extensively and review all reference material available. No one on the surgical team should have more than one job. Practice on an animal immediately before doing the appendectomy. After all this preparation, it is still likely that unintentional complications (and perhaps death) will result from this type of field surgery. These guidelines apply to both US and local national patients.

What You Need: Personnel: A dedicated anesthesia technician experienced in performing IV anesthesia or general tracheal anesthesia is required. The patient must not move around and the abdominal wall must be relaxed during surgery. Two surgical assistants are required. Supplies: Surgical preparation solution (for the abdomen), sterile gloves (>3 sets), silk ties or ligatures, 0 (zero)-Vicryl (for the fascia) on a taper needle, sterile bandages (to pack the wound), sterile gauze bandages (for incisional bleeding), a large volume (6-10 liters) of sterile saline or water (to irrigate the peritoneal cavity), suction device, NG tube, Foley catheter. Instruments: Scalpel, 2 needle drivers, 2 tissue forceps, 2 retractors, 6 clamps and scissors. Additional things to do prior to surgery: Obtain a well-ventilated space with good lighting and a narrow tabletop that allows access to both sides of the patient. A headlight is extremely useful. Obtain good IV access and instill additional IV antibiotics, if not already given. Ensure that the NG tube and Foley catheter are in place prior to the first incision.

What To Do:

1. This procedure should not be performed without the radio consultation of a physician experienced in intra-abdominal surgery.
2. Stay calm.
3. Place the patient in the supine position on the table.
4. Have the anesthesia technician start the anesthetic.
5. Prep the patient's abdomen from pubic area to nipples and from side to side down to the level of the posterior axillary line.
6. Place NG tube and Foley if not already in place.
7. Place an incision between the umbilicus and the anterior superior iliac crest, transversely across the abdomen (*see Figure 4-2*). Make a larger, instead of smaller, incision to see better (at least 4-6 inches long). The incision should cut through the skin, and then down through subcutaneous fat. Apply clamps to bleeders as required. Ensure you are clamping a vascular structure before you do so. Using the silk ligatures, tie off bleeders whose clamps obstruct the incision. Carefully deepen the incision down to the fascia, which is the shiny white tissue (gristle). Make an incision through the anterior fascia (*see Figure 4-3*). Stay lateral to the rectus muscle seen beneath the fascia. At this point, take a hemostat and spread in the tissue lateral to the rectus muscle along the line of your incision. Using the spreading motion, progress deeper through the lateral abdominal wall, and into the peritoneal cavity. Once into the peritoneal cavity, fluid should come out. Place both index fingers into the peritoneal cavity and spread in the direction of your incision to widen the peritoneal opening (*see Figure 4-4*). Place the retractors at the medial and lateral portion of the incision, with the end of the retractor in the peritoneum. Have the assistants pull in opposite directions along the direction of the incision to enlarge access to the peritoneal cavity. Have your assistants keep the retractors in the wound.

Figure 4-2. Appendectomy: Incision Location

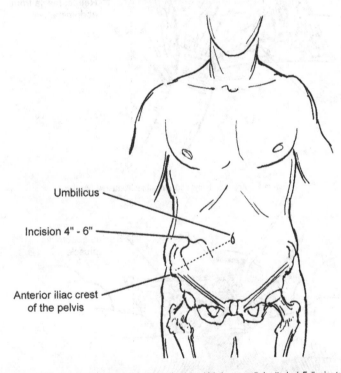

Umbilicus

Incision 4" - 6"

Anterior iliac crest
of the pelvis

8. The cecum is the part of the large bowel in the right lower quadrant, to which the appendix is attached. Following teniae (which are the longitudinal bands that are seen on the colon) on the colon down to the cecum, pull the cecum into the wound, and locate the appendix at the base of the cecum (*see Figure 4-5*). This maneuver is not as easy as it sounds and may take some time.
9. If the appendix is easily seen, and is acutely inflamed (red, swollen), it must be removed. Dissect the mesoappendix (where the artery to the appendix lies) from the appendix, doubly ligate the mesoappendix, and cut in between the two ligatures (*see Figure 4-6*). These ligatures must be tied down well to close the appendiceal artery running through the mesoappendix, and prevent significant bleeding. Now isolate the appendix by doubly ligating its base, adding a third ligature more distal to the proximal two and dividing between the ligatures (*see Figure 4-7*). Remove and dispose of the appendix. Inspect the base of the appendix left on the cecum to make sure both ligatures are tight, as a loose ligature will fall off and cause a cecal fistula, resulting in worsening intra-abdominal sepsis and death.

Figure 4-3. Appendectomy: Retraction of Fascia from Abdominal Wall

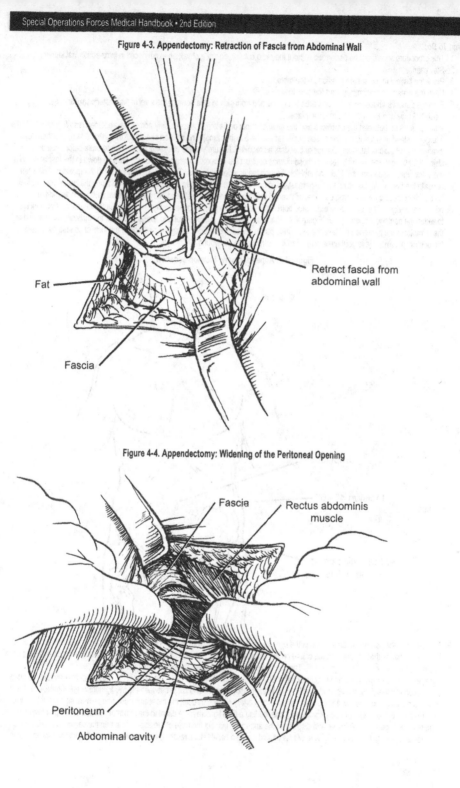

Retract fascia from
abdominal wall

Fat

Fascia

Figure 4-4. Appendectomy: Widening of the Peritoneal Opening

Fascia

Rectus abdominis
muscle

Peritoneum

Abdominal cavity

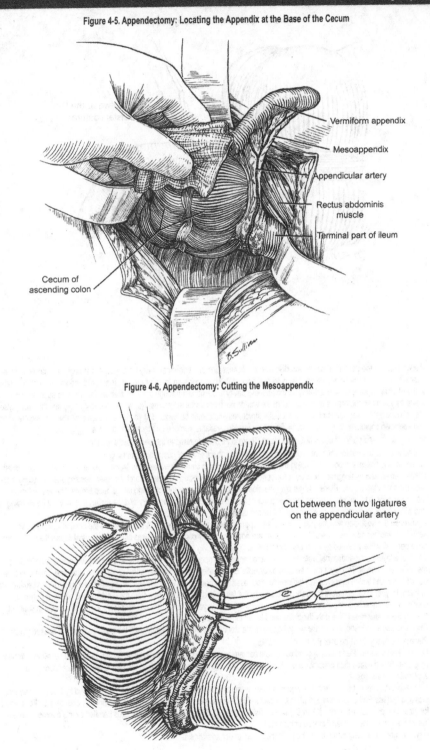

Figure 4-5. Appendectomy: Locating the Appendix at the Base of the Cecum

Vermiform appendix

Mesoappendix

Appendicular artery

Rectus abdominis muscle

Terminal part of ileum

Cecum of ascending colon

Figure 4-6. Appendectomy: Cutting the Mesoappendix

Cut between the two ligatures on the appendicular artery

Figure 4-7. Appendectomy: Cutting the Appendix

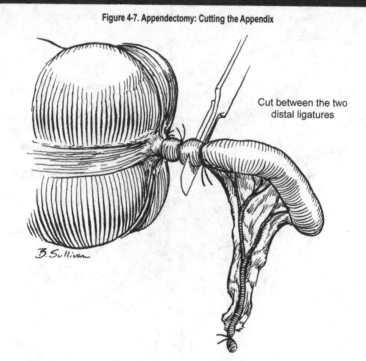

Cut between the two
distal ligatures

B.Sullivan

10. If upon entering the peritoneal cavity, you discover an abscess and an abdominal cavity full of pus, it is strongly recommended that this abscess cavity be drained out the right flank by placing a stab wound incision (carefully avoid organs and important structures) lateral to the original incision, placing a drain into the abscess cavity and exiting it through the flank stab wound. Palpate abdominal wall from inside as you make the drain site incision to insure you do not hit any vital structures. Remember the iliac artery and the ureter also reside in the right lower quadrant; both are tubular structures and should be avoided. If you have suction available, irrigate the abscess and abdomen copiously with 4-6L of sterile fluid. If no suction available, remove pus by repeatedly inserting gauze into the abscess cavity and pulling it out until it looks clean. There is no need to remove the perforated appendix.

11. If upon entering the peritoneal cavity you discover a localized abscess full of pus, drain it and irrigate.

12. Hemostasis is critically important. Closing the abdomen with ongoing bleeding will result in sepsis, hypotension and eventual death. Obtain hemostasis by tying the silk ligatures around any remaining clamped vessels. Search for other bleeding sites including those near the flank stab wound. Place a finger over the bleeding site, collect your thoughts and take a deep breath. This is a valuable maneuver prior to randomly clamping large, important structures (such as the iliac artery and the ureter) that may not be bleeding and will only cause further injury or damage if they are clamped.

13. If you enter the abdomen with the plan of doing an appendectomy and the appendix is normal, leave the appendix in place, and search for another obvious cause. However, there are not many easily correctable causes of intra-abdominal sepsis that would not have been effectively treated by 72 hours of antibiotics.

14. Close one layer of the abdominal wall, the fascia, to complete the operation. The difficulty here is closing without causing injury to the underlying bowel. This layer must be closed correctly, or the patient will eviscerate with coughing at a later time. Take your time, do not hurry, and watch every pass of the needle. Your assistants need to be as observant as you are. Take your O-Vicryl suture, start laterally, tie your knot, and work medially. Take bites of the fascia one centimeter back from the cut edge and advance only one centimeter at a time. It is imperative not to include loops of bowel in your sutures. It is not necessary to include muscle in your sutures; that weakens your repair. The only thing you need to put together is the fascia.

15. Once the fascia is closed, irrigate the wound again with a liter of sterile fluid and lightly pack the wound with saline soaked gauze. Place a sterile dry dressing over the top of the packs.

16. Do not close the skin. Perforated appendices create contaminated wounds that should not be closed, but should be allowed to heal by granulation. If evacuation becomes available in the next 48 hours, refrain from closing the skin to facilitate later abdominal exploration by a surgeon.

17. If the appendix was not perforated, the wound is clean without hemorrhage, and evacuation has not occurred by 5 days, close the skin and fat (see Part 3: General Symptoms: Obstetric Problems: Cesarean Delivery) as a delayed primary closure. Use **lidocaine** as for other skin procedures, such as Part 8: Procedures: Chapter 30: Skin Mass Removal. Wounds handled by this approach are less likely to become infected than if closed immediately.

18. Have the anesthesia technician bring the patient out from under anesthesia.

Post-Operative Orders:

1. Get the patient out of bed as soon as he can tolerate it to minimize pulmonary complications. Have patient inflate a surgical glove like a balloon several times an hour, for same reasons.
2. Keep the NG tube in place until the patient has return of bowel function. The patient is very ill, so do not anticipate that they will be eating for several days after surgery. Provide stress ulcer (*see Part 4: Organ Systems: Chapter 7: Acute Peptic Ulcer*) and DVT (*see Part 4: Organ Systems: Chapter 3: Deep Vein Thrombosis and Pulmonary Embolism*) prophylaxis if available. Once bowel function returns (bowel sounds and passing gas) pull the NG tube and begin a clear liquid diet. Advance the diet as tolerated.
3. Monitor vital signs frequently, as often as every 2-4 hours. This patient should require almost constant attention the first 24 hours.
4. Monitor the I & O to make sure the IV fluids are at a high enough rate. Leave the Foley catheter in place as a way to monitor their output (should be 0.5-1.0 cc/kg/hr). Remove the Foley when patient is tolerating liquid diet. Ensure he is able to urinate after Foley has been removed.
5. Provide pain control. *See Part 8: Procedures: Chapter 30: Pain Assessment and Control*
6. Keep the patient from vomiting by using anti-emetic as needed (eg, **prochlorperazine** 5-10mg IM q 3-4h, max 40 mg/d).
7. An elevated WBC count and spiking temperatures 3 days after operation may be concerning for evidence of continued sepsis. It is not unusual to have temperature spikes for 1-2 days after operation but these should decrease after 72 hours.
8. The drain output should decrease over 5 to 6 days, and the drain may be pulled at that time.
9. Continue antibiotics for 10-14 days after surgery.
10. Keep the wound clean and allow it to granulate closed over several weeks. Use dilute povidone-iodine or bleach for the first 48 hours, and then switch to new dressings soaked in sterile saline until a pinkish layer of granulation tissue covers the fascia.

What Not To Do

1. Take care not to cause unnecessary bleeding. There will be oozing from the surface of inflamed and cut tissue. Most of this will stop with pressure and time.
2. Do not cut into the intestines inadvertently. If you do, close it in a single layer with 000-silk or Vicryl suture.
3. Make sure your assistants retract and help you. You must see the layers of bowel as you close them.
4. Do not make your skin incision too small. If you have difficulty seeing, make the incision bigger.
5. Do not race through the operation. Take your time and operate safely. It is much better to be safe than to move too fast.
6. Do not operate without a dedicated anesthesia technician. The "surgeon" will have enough on his mind.
7. Do not operate without 2 assistants for retraction. They will also be accessory eyes and brains during this procedure.

Chapter 7: Gastrointestinal: Acute Cholecystitis

COL Peter McNally, MC, USA (Ret)

Introduction: Gallbladder stones are common in the United States, (10-15% of adults) and 2-3 times more common in women (4 Fs: fat, forty, female, and fertile). Cholecystitis (gall bladder inflammation) occurs more commonly in certain populations (eg, malaria, sickle cell, and ascaris infestations). Overall mortality from an acute case of cholecystitis is 3% but only 1% in young, otherwise healthy adults. Once a patient develops symptoms or complications (acute cholecystitis) from gall stones, surgery should be strongly considered. Otherwise healthy adults will generally receive cholecystectomy on the initial hospitalization 24-48 hrs after stabilization of symptoms with fluids, NSAIDs and antibiotics. Suspected acute cholangitis (fever + right upper quadrant pain+ jaundice) equals "pus in the biliary tree" and is a surgical emergency.

Subjective: Symptoms

Biliary colic pain: usually located in the upper abdomen, frequently in the right upper quadrant (RUQ), may radiate to the right scapula; may be precipitated by a meal, but more commonly there is no inciting event; gradually increases over 15-60 min., plateaus for 1 or 2 hrs before slowly going away; if persists longer than 4 hrs it is unlikely to spontaneously resolve. 75% of patients have a history of previous attacks of biliary colic before acute cholecystitis.

Focused History: *Does the pain get better with antacids?* (ulcer) *Does the pain radiate to the back and right scapula?* (gallstones) *Is the pain continuous and does not relent even in the "fetal" position?* (pancreatitis) *Have you experienced pressure or heavy weight on the chest that radiates to the left chin, shoulder or arm, especially with exertion?* (angina) *Have you lost more that 10 lbs in the last month?* (cancer)

Objective: Signs

Using Basic Tools: Inspection: Patients with acute cholecystitis appear uncomfortable and ill. Mild fever (<102°F) with mild jaundice may be seen in up to 20% of cases of cholecystitis. Auscultation: Bowel sounds should be present, unless gangrenous gallbladder or gallstone pancreatitis. Palpation: Murphy's sign: During palpation of the right subcostal region, pain and inspiratory arrest may occur when the patient takes a deep breath, bringing the examiner's hand in contact with the inflamed gallbladder. The obstructed and swollen gallbladder is palpable in 1/3 of acute cholecystitis.

Using Advanced Tools: Labs: WBC with differential will demonstrate infection.

Assessment: Differential Diagnosis

Ascending cholangitis: Fever, RUQ pain and jaundice (Charcot's Triad) is a surgical emergency.
Obstruction of the common bile duct (gall stone or tumor): Marked jaundice, dark urine, clay-colored stools
Pancreatitis: Diffuse abdominal pain with ileus and vomiting
Peptic ulcer disease: Vomiting, hematemesis or melena if bleeding
Cardiac pain: Angina, heart attack
Esophageal reflux, hiatal hernia: Acid taste, pain relieved with antacid
Pleurisy/pneumonia: Respiratory complaints, pain with deep inspiration
Liver mass (abscess, tumor, cirrhosis): Jaundice, RUQ pain, no fever, no relationship to meals

Plan:
Treatment
1. IV fluids: *See Part 7: Trauma: Chapter 27: Resuscitation Fluids*
2. Antibiotics: *See Part 4: Organ Systems: Chapter 7: Acute Peritonitis*
3. Pain management: **Ketorolac** 30-60mg IM initially, followed by 15-30mg IM q6h; alternatively 15-30mg IV initially, followed by 15-30mg IV prn; not to exceed 120mg/d and not to exceed 5 days of treatment (adjust for age and renal function if required). Narcotics may be required to control pain. *See Part 8: Procedures: Chapter 30: Pain Assessment and Control*
4. Suppress acid secretion. *See Part 4: Organ Systems: Chapter 7: Acute Gastritis*
5. Control fever with NSAIDs, (eg, **ibuprofen** 400-800mg po tid to qid, not to exceed 3.2g in one day)
6. For nausea, give **prochlorperazine** 5-10mg IM q3-4h, max 40mg/day or ondansetron 4mg IV q8h.
7. Medical Evacuation: High fever >102°F, jaundice, persistent pain, vomiting, worsening symptoms or failure to improve over 24 hours should prompt medical evacuation. Cholangitis is "pus in the biliary tree" and a surgical emergency.

Patient Education
General: Half of acute cholecystitis will resolve within 7-10 days without emergent surgery. Left untreated, 10% will be complicated by localized (retroduodenal) perforation and 1% by free (into the peritoneal cavity) perforation.
Diet: Dramatic weight reduction programs are associated with development of gallstones in 25-50%. Avoid greasy or fatty foods.
Prevention: Avoid foods that precipitate symptoms.

Follow-up Actions
Return Evaluation: Recurrent pain should be investigated promptly.
Evacuation/Consultation Criteria: See evacuation guidance. Suspected acute cholangitis (fever + RUQ pain + jaundice) is a surgical emergency.

Chapter 7: Gastrointestinal: Acute Bacterial Food Poisoning
COL Peter McNally, MC, USA (Ret)

Introduction: Bacterial food poisoning is any illness caused by the consumption of food contaminating bacteria or bacterial toxins. The major recognized causes of bacterial food poisoning are limited to 12 bacteria: *Clostridium perfringens, Staphylococcus aureus* (*see Appendices: Color Plates: Figure A-26.C*), *Vibrio cholera* (*see Appendices: Color Plates: Figure A-26.N*) & *parahaemolyticus, Bacillus cereus, Salmonella, Clostridium botulinum, Shigella, toxigenic E. coli* (*see Appendices: Color Plates: Figure 26.G*), certain species of *Campylobacter, Yersinia, Listeria*, and *Aeromonas* (*see Appendices: Color Plates: Figure A-26.A*). Most cases arise from ingesting contaminated food. The attack rates are high, with most persons ingesting the food becoming afflicted. Rapid onset of symptoms indicates the presence of pre-formed toxins liberated from contaminated food.

Table 4-2. Food Poisoning

Organism	Source	Average Incubation (hrs)	Clinical Features
Bacillus cereus	Fried rice, vanilla, sauce, meatballs, barbecued chicken, boiled beef	2	Vomiting, crampy abdominal pain, diarrhea Duration 1/2 - 1 day
Clostridium botulinum (toxin)	Canned foods, fermented fish	12-36	Visual disturbance, descending paralysis, non-specific GI symptoms dyspnea, potentially fatal
Clostridium perfringens	Beef, chicken, turkey	12	Diarrhea and crampy abdominal pain predominate symptoms. Duration 1 day
Vibrio cholera	Water	24-72	Watery diarrhea, in severe disease (epidemics) 50% mortality if massive fluid/electrolyte loss is not replaced (500–1000cc/hr may be required) Duration 4-6 days
Vibrio parahaemolyticus	Seafood	12	Nausea, vomiting, headache, fever, diarrhea and crampy abdominal pain. Duration 3 days
Staphylococcus aureus (toxin)	Ham, pork, canned beef	3	Vomiting, nausea, crampy abdominal pain > than diarrhea. Usually within 1-6 hrs after ingestion

Table 4-2. Food Poisoning, continued

Organism	Source	Average Incubation (hrs)	Clinical Features
Yersinia enterocolitica	Chocolate or raw milk, pork cole slaw, dairy, poultry beef	72	Fever, crampy abdominal pain, diarrhea and vomiting. Keys: pharyngitis, arthritis mesenteric adenitis and rash. Duration 7 days
Listeria monocytogenes	Milk, raw vegetables, cole slaw, dairy poultry, beef	3-70 days	Diarrhea, fever, crampy abdominal pain, nausea, vomiting. Duration depends on severity
Campylobacter jejuni	Milk, beef, chicken, pet animals	48	Diarrhea, fever, nausea, vomiting, headache, myalgia. Key: may see bloody diarrhea. Duration 7 days
Escherichia coli	Salad, beef (toxin)	24	Diarrhea, crampy abdominal pain, nausea, headache, fever, myalgias. Keys: may see hemolytic uremic syndrome and bloody diarrhea. Duration 3 days
Salmonella	Eggs, poultry, meat	24	Diarrhea, crampy abdominal pain, nausea, vomiting, fever, headache. Duration 3 days
Shigella	Milk, potato, tuna, turkey	24	Crampy abdominal pain, salads fever, diarrhea, bloody diarrhea, headache, nausea, vomiting. Duration 3 days

Subjective: Symptoms
Nausea, vomiting, crampy abdominal pain, fever, myalgias, headache, diarrhea (sometimes bloody).
Focused History: *What have you been eating? Is anyone else in your unit/village sick with these symptoms?*

Objective: Signs
Using Basic Tools: Inspection: Patients appear ill and dehydrated. Auscultation: Abdominal bowel sounds are often hyperactive. Palpation: Mild to moderate abdominal tenderness. Peritoneal signs (rebound, guarding, point tenderness) are atypical.
Using Advanced Tools: Labs: Elevated WBC with differential may indicate systemic infection; stool cultures, blood cultures.

Assessment: Differential Diagnosis: *See Part 3: General Symptoms: Acute Abdominal Pain*
When the predominant symptoms are crampy abdominal pain and diarrhea, consider non-food-poisoning etiologies like acute *Giardia lamblia* or antibiotic diarrhea. When a recurrent past history of symptoms is present, consider inflammatory bowel disease.

Plan:
Treatment
1. Rest
2. Rehydration (oral or intravenous) correction of electrolyte disturbances. *See Part 3: General Symptoms: Diarrhea, Acute & Part 7: Trauma: Chapter 27: Resuscitation Fluids*
3. Anti-emetics as necessary (eg, **prochlorperazine** 5-10mg IM q3-4h, max 40mg/day or **ondansetron** 4mg IV q8h)
4. Antibiotics are usually NOT necessary and may promote increased carrier rates for *Salmonella* and the incidence of hemolytic uremic syndrome (HUS) seen in patients with Shiga Toxin-producing E. Coli (STEC). **Note:** If operational conditions require antibiotic prophylaxis to mitigate risk of adverse acute symptoms of "traveler's diarrhea", **ciprofloxacin** 500mg po daily x 3 days can be used. Routine or chronic use of antibiotics for prophylaxis of traveller's diarrhea is not recommended.
5. If botulism poisoning is suspected, *see Part 6: Operational Environment: Chapter 26: Biological Warfare* for additional information re: diagnosis and management.
6. If non-food poisoning related diarrhea is suspected, see management in *Part 3: General Symptoms: Diarrhea, Acute*.
Patient Education
General: Be a cautious consumer. Food left at room temperature is a potential breeding source for bacteria. Proper hand washing is important in preparation of food, especially when handling raw meats, poultry and eggs. Wipe down counters before and after preparing

food. Avoid wooden cutting boards because they cannot be easily disinfected.

Diet: If the food smells bad or has not been refrigerated, avoid it.

Prevention; For large outbreaks, obtain stool cultures from patients. Obtain stool culture from food handlers when suspicious of *Yersinia enterocolitica, Salmonella* or *Shigella* to prevent further outbreaks.

Follow-up Actions

Return Evaluation: Only if symptoms persist, worsen or relapse. For protracted illness or signs of sepsis, blood cultures may be necessary.

Evacuation/Consultation Criteria: Evacuation is not usually necessary. Consult infectious disease or internal medicine for systemic toxicity, bloody diarrhea, high fever.

Chapter 7: Gastrointestinal: Acute Gastritis
COL Peter McNally, MC, USA (Ret)

Introduction: Inflammation of the stomach lining or acute gastritis is common. The causes of gastritis are numerous, but it is most commonly caused by consumption of alcohol, aspirin, non-steroidal anti-inflammatory drugs (NSAIDs) or by acute infections.

Subjective: Symptoms
Dyspepsia (epigastric discomfort or burning), nausea, vomiting, postprandial fullness/bloating and occasional GI bleeding; history of excess alcohol consumption or ingestion of aspirin, NSAIDs, corrosives or poorly prepared or preserved food.

Focused History: *Does the pain get better with antacids?* (ulcer) *Does the pain radiate to the back and right scapula?* (gall stones) *Is the pain continuous and does not relent even in the "fetal" position?* (pancreatitis) *Have you experienced pressure or heavy weight on the chest that radiates to the left chin, shoulder or arm, especially with exertion?* (angina) *Have you lost more than 10 lbs in the last month?* (cancer)

Objective: Signs
Using Basic Tools: Inspection: Vomiting and epigastric pain; appears pale and dehydrated; no fever. Palpation: Abdomen is usually soft but may have some mild to moderate tenderness in the epigastric region. Rectal examination: Look for black stools (melena) or blood.

Using Advanced Tools: Labs: CBC for evidence of infection or anemia; and urinalysis (elevated bilirubin).

Assessment: Differential Diagnosis
GI bleeding: Hematemesis or melena should suggest alternative diagnosis such as bleeding peptic ulcer, Mallory-Weiss tear (esophageal tear caused by retching), etc.

Peritonitis: Peritoneal signs (guarding, rebound, absent bowel sounds) suggest intra-abdominal infection. *See Part 4: Organ Systems: Chapter 7: Acute Peritonitis*

Hepatobiliary disease: RUQ pain. Murphy's sign (pain on deep inspiration), possible icterus (yellow sclera)

Possible malignancy: Significant weight loss

Plan:
Treatment

Primary: Discontinue gastric irritants such as alcohol and/or medications (aspirin/NSAIDs). Rehydrate with oral or IV fluids. Give short course (4 weeks) of H2-blocker (eg, **famotidine** 40mg po q hs) or proton pump inhibitor (eg, **omeprazole** 20mg po daily) to promote healing of gastritis.

Patient Education

Complications: If acute gastritis is associated with bleeding (hematemesis or melena), *see Part 4: Organ Systems: Chapter 7: Acute Peptic Ulcer.*

Diet: Take clear liquids initially, then progress to bland diet and then back to regular diet.

Medications: Antiemetics may be needed. Use short course of over-the-counter antacids or acid-blocking medications.

Prevention and Hygiene: Consume only properly prepared and preserved food, clean water.

No Improvement/Deterioration: Return for additional evaluation if fail to improve within 24 hours or signs of abdominal pain, fever, icterus.

Follow-up Actions

Return Evaluation: Repeat exams if worsening symptoms of pain, fever, signs of GI bleeding.

Evacuation/Consultation Criteria: Evacuation is not usually necessary unless GI bleeding develops. Consult for worsening symptoms of pain or fever, or for signs of GI bleeding.

Chapter 7: Gastrointestinal: Acute Pancreatitis
COL Peter McNally, MC, USA (Ret)

Introduction: Acute pancreatitis is an inflammatory process of the pancreas usually associated with severe pain in the upper abdomen. Gallstones and alcohol abuse cause about 80-90% of acute pancreatitis. Most mild to moderately ill patients with acute pancreatitis will get better, but the mortality rate is 50% for patients with severe (necrotizing) pancreatitis. Endoscopy and or surgery significantly decrease morbidity of patients with gallstone related pancreatitis.

Subjective: Symptoms
Pain: located in the epigastrium; may be localized to the right upper quadrant and radiate to the back; pain reaches a maximum intensity rapidly over 10-20 minutes described as unbearable, with little relief offered by position. Patients frequently assume a fetal position. Nausea and vomiting are common.

Focused History: *Do you drink alcohol/how much? Do you or your family have a history of gallstones?* (Alcohol and gallstones account for >90% cases of pancreatitis.) *Have you had any trauma to the abdomen?* (traumatic pancreatitis) *What medicines are you taking?* [list of medicines known to cause pancreatitis; use mnemonic "NO IDEA" N=NSAIDs; O=other, valproate; I = IBD drugs [sulfasalazine, 5-aminosalicylic acid [Immunosuppressants] azathioprine, 6-mercaptopurine]; D=diuretics [furosemide, thiazides]; E=Estrogen; S=Antibiotics [metronidazole, sulfonamides, tetracycline, nitrofurantoin and AIDS drugs [didanosine, pentamidine]]. *Do you have high triglycerides?* (4% of pancreatitis is caused by high triglycerides usually >500-1,000.) *Do you take aspirin or NSAIDs?* (These medicines, even when over the counter, can cause a penetrating ulcer and even pancreatitis.) *Have you passed any tarry, foul smelling, black stool or melena?* (Melena is a sign of gastrointestinal bleeding, from ulcer, gastritis, esophageal tear or esophageal varices.)

Objective: Signs

Using Basic Tools: Inspection: Appears acutely ill; mental status may be depressed, especially if associated with acute alcohol ingestion; fever, tachycardia and hypotension; ecchymosis along the flanks (Grey Turner's sign) or around the umbilicus (Cullen's sign) grave prognosis; jaundiced sclera (icterus); distended abdomen.

Auscultation: Decreased breath sounds from effusions or rales (ARDS)—grave prognosis; abdominal pain may cause splinting and shallow respirations; absent bowel sounds. Percussion: The abdomen is tympanic and diffusely tender.

Using Advanced Tools: Labs: CBC with differential (evidence of anemia and infection); Pulse oximetry (ARDS), Assess Ranson's criteria for severity. Do x-ray of chest and abdomen. Look free air (perforation of a hollow viscous organ), dilated loops of bowel, air-fluid levels (GI obstruction), calcified gallstones (cholecystitis) or calcification in the pancreas (chronic calcific pancreatitis).

Assessment: Differential Diagnosis

Gall stone vs. alcohol (or other) related pancreatitis: Patients without a history of alcohol abuse or other (see "NO IDEA" mnemonic above) cause may have gallstone related pancreatitis. **Note:** Early endoscopy and/or surgery significantly decrease morbidity of patients with gallstone related pancreatitis

Peritonitis: Rebound tenderness, rigid, board-like abdomen, septic appearance, no bowel sounds

Peptic ulcer disease: Vomiting blood, melena on rectal examination

Cholecystitis: Tenderness in the right upper quadrant, (+) Murphy's sign

Ischemic bowel: Absence of bowel sounds, disproportionate examination (abdomen softer that you expect from the degree of pain to palpation), poor peripheral pulses, signs of poor circulation

Aortic aneurysm: Abdominal bruit, pulsatile abdomen, shock, poor or absent distal pulses, mottled abdomen

Bowel obstruction: Signs of abdominal distention, hyperactive bowel sounds or absence of bowel sounds, tympany to abdominal percussion.

Bowel perforation: Signs of peritoneal irritation, rigid abdomen, fever, sepsis

Plan:

Treatment

Mild (edematous) pancreatitis will improve with NPO, IV fluid hydration and other supportive care over the course of a week. Severe necrotizing pancreatitis is a life-threatening condition.

Primary:

1. NPO until pain resolved.
2. Control pain: **Morphine** or **hydromorphone** may be required. *See Part 8: Procedures: Chapter 30: Pain Assessment and Control*
3. Give IV fluid resuscitation (D5-lactated Ringer's solution). A common error in managing pancreatitis is inadequate IV fluid resuscitation. During the initial 48 hrs, 250–500cc/hour may be required to maintain tissue perfusion and urine output (60cc/hr).

Note: Monitor I & O and closely follow clinical condition to minimize 3rd spacing and massive edema.

4. Insert NG tube for decompression to mitigate risk of vomiting/aspiration and distended abdomen.
5. Identify risk and manage possible delirium tremens (DTs) if underlying alcohol withdrawal is suspected. (*See note*)
6. Give antibiotic therapy for life-threatening complications. *See Part 4: Organ Systems: Chapter 7: Acute Peritonitis*
7. Suppress gastric acid secretion. *See Part 4: Organ Systems: Chapter 7: Acute Peritonitis*
8. Evacuate patients suspected of developing severe (necrotizing) pancreatitis.

Patient Education

General: If gallstones caused the pancreatitis, then definitive treatment (surgical removal) and cure may prevent future attacks. If the cause of pancreatitis is alcohol, abstinence is the key to prevent chronic relapsing pancreatitis. See CAGE questionnaire in Notes section.

Diet: NPO during acute pancreatitis, then as tolerated after resolution.

Medications Shown to Cause Acute Pancreatitis: Use the mnemonic "NO IDEA".

Prevention: Cessation of all alcohol. Stop medicines proven to cause pancreatitis indefinitely, see previous list.

Normalize high triglyceride or calcium levels to prevent additional attacks.

Follow-up Actions

Evacuation/Consultation Criteria: These patients need urgent evacuation. Any first attack of pancreatitis needs gastroenterology consultation. Mild isolated cases should undergo primary search for etiology. A gastroenterologist should see all second attacks of pancreatitis. If alcohol abuse is suspected etiology, initiate intervention and therapy.

Notes:

1. *Ranson's Criteria for severity of pancreatitis (1 point each)

   At Admission (5 criteria)

   Age >55 years; WBC >16,000/mm³; Glucose >200mg/dL, Lactate dehydrogenase > 350IU/L, and Aspartate transaminase >250U/L

During Initial 48 hours (6 criteria)
HCT decrease of 10mg/dL; PaO_2 <60mmHg; Blood urea nitrogen increase of >5mg/dL, Calcium <8mg/dL, Base Deficit >4mEq/L, Fluid sequestration >6L.

Table 4-3. Predicted Mortality Rates Based on Ranson's Criteria

Number of Ranson's Criteria	Predicted MORTALITY Rate
< 2	5%
3-5	10%
> 6	60%

2. Patients suspected of chronic alcohol dependence may require a benzodiazepine to control symptoms of alcohol withdrawal (eg, agitation, hallucinations) and mitigate risk of developing full blown delirium tremens (DTs) with hallucinations, disorientation, tachycardia, hypertension, low grade fever, agitation diaphoresis and seizures.
Lorazepam 1-2mg po with dosing adjusted as necessary. Monitor closely to avoid respiratory compromise. Assess level of sedation and withdrawal symptoms 1 hr after each oral dose and q4h. Full blown DTs occur in up to 5% of patients with alcohol withdrawal and have a mortality rate of 5%. Treatment of DTs will likely require an IV benzodiazepine (eg, **diazepam** 5-10mg IV) repeated prn to control symptoms. Patients require close monitoring for decreased level of consciousness and respiratory compromise. Hold the benzodiazepine dose when Ramsey Sedation score is >4. Patients should also receive **thiamine** 100mg IM x 1 dose. *See Part 5: Specialty Areas: Chapter 18: Substance Abuse*
Ramsey Sedation Score: 1 = Fully awake; 2 = Drowsy, but awakens spontaneously; 3 = Asleep but arouses and responds appropriately to verbal commands; 4 = Asleep, unresponsive to commands, but arouses to shoulder tap or loud verbal stimulus; 5 = Asleep and only responds to firm facial tap and loud verbal stimulus; and 6 = Asleep and unresponsive to both firm facial tap and loud verbal stimuli.
CAGE (Cut, Annoyed, Guilt, Eye Opener) Questions: Cut: *Ever felt you ought to cut down on your drinking?* Annoyed: *Have people annoyed you by criticizing your drinking?* Guilt: *Ever felt bad or guilty about your drinking?* Eye Opener: *Ever had an eye-opener to steady nerves in the AM?* Yes to 2 questions = Strong Indication. Yes to 3 questions = Confirms Alcoholism.

Chapter 7: Gastrointestinal: Acute Peritonitis

COL Peter McNally, MC, USA (Ret)

Introduction: Acute peritonitis is a potentially catastrophic illness caused by infectious organisms attacking the peritoneum. There are 2 types of acute peritonitis: primary and secondary. Primary acute peritonitis is associated with spontaneous bacterial infection of ascites seen in persons with cirrhosis. Secondary acute peritonitis most commonly occurs when some other medical condition causes bacteria to spill into the abdominal cavity and is associated with rapid medical deterioration. The 5 most common causes of acute secondary peritonitis are appendicitis, cholecystitis, diverticulitis, pancreatitis, and bowel perforation. Each has a characteristic pattern of symptoms to suggest the etiology. When abscess or perforation complicates any of these causes, generalized peritonitis ensues. Generalized peritonitis (other than that caused by penetrating injury) requiring surgical intervention is caused by perforated peptic ulcer (40%), appendicitis (20%), gangrene of bowel/gallbladder (15%), post-op complications (10%), or other causes (15%). Exact details of the onset of the pain, and associated symptoms (eg, change in bowel or menstrual habits) are helpful in drawing attention to the affected organ. Mortality is high in many groups, especially in the elderly and patients suffering organ failure before development of peritonitis. Peritonitis secondary to appendicitis or perforated duodenal ulcer is associated with >90% survival, whereas peritonitis from other causes, including postoperative peritonitis, has only approximately 50% survival.

Subjective: Symptoms

Pain and fever. **Appendicitis:** Generalized abdominal pain that becomes localized to the right lower quadrant (and eventually McBurney's Point); anorexia; sensation of "gas blockage" and need for BM, but no improvement after enema or defecation. *See Part 4: Organ Systems: Chapter 7: Appendicitis.* Cholecystitis: 90% of patients will be symptomatic, with epigastric or right upper quadrant pain that peaks over 30 minutes, then plateaus for 1-2 hours before gradual decreasing; some relate pain to fatty meals, or radiation to the right scapula. *See Part 4: Organ Systems: Chapter 7: Acute Cholecystitis.*
Diverticulitis: More common in the elderly; pain may occur after straining to have a BM, and is initially localized to the left lower quadrant (95%); associated with fever (60-100%) and elevated WBC count (70-80%). Pancreatitis: Chronic, excessive alcohol abuse and gallstones cause most pancreatitis, with acute onset of rapidly progressive, incapacitating, diffuse abdominal pain, radiating to the back; patients are typically in the fetal position for comfort. *See Part 4: Organ Systems: Chapter 7: Acute Pancreatitis.* Bowel Perforation. Immediate onset of severe abdominal pain; several causes, including perforation of gastric or duodenal ulcer, appendix, diverticula, or other hollow viscus (due to foreign body ingestion, abscess, etc.).

Focused History: *Have you been exposed to gunfire, explosion other source of trauma?* (possible injury extending to peritoneal cavity) *Do you have a history of peptic ulcer disease or abdominal pain?* (possible perforation of ulcer or diverticuli) *Have you had an appendectomy?* (may rule out appendicitis)

Objective: Signs

Using Basic Tools: Vital signs: Fever 100-101°F, tachycardia. Inspection: Evidence of penetrating trauma to any location should raise suspicion of peritoneal injury and risk of peritonitis. Patient in fetal position, because any movement worsens pain; visible peristalsis suggests bowel obstruction. Auscultation: Absence of bowel sounds in all 4 quadrants suggests peritonitis. Always auscultate before doing percussion or palpation. Percussion: Absence of dullness over the liver suggests free air and perforation. Palpation: Begin with very gentle palpation away from the area of maximal symptoms; board-like abdomen is unmistakable and indicates obvious peritonitis;

shake the pelvis to assess rebound tenderness; iliopsoas and obturator signs (see GI: Appendicitis) are suggestive for retroperitoneal inflammation. Rectal exam look for melena or bright red blood. Serial examinations: Diminishing bowel sounds with increasing tenderness and the development of rebound indicates peritonitis.

Using Advanced Tools: Labs: CBC (increased white count may suggest infarction). Abdominal x-ray: free air, dilated loops of bowel, air-fluid levels, (GI obstruction) calcified gallstones (cholecystitis), calcification seen in pancreas (seen in chronic pancreatitis)

Assessment: Differential Diagnosis

Most likely source will be identified by history and physical exam; *see specific comments in Subjective and Objective.*

Perforated peptic ulcer (40%)

Perforated appendix (20%)

Gangrene of the bowel or gall bladder (15%)

Post operative complications (10%)

Other causes (15%) rule out penetrating trauma. Gunshot, shrapnel or other penetrating wounds to the chest, back, abdomen, thigh can result in peritonitis if the effects of the penetration extend to the peritoneal cavity. A thorough history and physical examination is required on 100% of seriously ill or injured patients.

Plan:

Treatment

1. Intravenous antibiotics must cover both aerobic and anaerobic bacteria. Use one of the following options:
   A. **Ceftriaxone** 2g IV daily or **cefotaxime** 2g IV q8h plus **metronidazole** 500mg IV q6h.
   B. **Ciprofloxacin** 400mg IV q12 h or **levofloxacin** 750mg IV q24h plus **metronidazole** 500mg IV q6h
   C. **Ertapenem** 1g IV daily or **moxifloxacin** 400mg po daily (where IV access not possible and patient able to tolerate oral meds)
2. Give IV fluids to compensate for respiratory and third space losses. *See Part 7: Trauma: Chapter 27: Resuscitation Fluids*
3. Control pain. *See Part 8: Procedures: Chapter 30: Pain Assessment and Control*
4. Control nausea and vomiting. Give antiemetic (eg, **promethazine** 25mg IM/po q8h, or **ondansetron** 4mg IV q8h)
5. Suppress gastric acid secretion: Use one of the following methods (consistent with clinical and operational considerations): Oral: **Cimetidine** 400mg bid or **famotidine** 20mg bid or **ranitidine** 150mg bid for 8-12 wks. Alternative po antacids: **omeprazole** 20mg q day or **lansoprazole** 30mg q day.
   NG tube: (for patients on prolonged NPO with NG tube): **Famotidine** 20mg per NG tube q6h and follow with oral therapy when NG tube is removed (as required).
   IV: **Cimetidine** 300mg q6h or **famotidine** 20mg q12h or **ranitidine** 50mg q6-8 h or **pantoprazole** 40mg q24h and follow with oral therapy when IV is removed (as required).
6. Nasogastric tube decompression for significant abdominal distention or vomiting, and keep NPO.
7. Evacuate for definitive surgical treatment.

Patient Education

Activity: Bedrest.

Diet: Metabolic needs during acute peritonitis are great, equivalent to a 50% total body surface area burn. Caloric requirement is often in the 3000-4000 calorie range and must be given parenterally by IV (not available in field conditions).

Follow-up Actions

Return Evaluation: Postoperative follow up is contingent upon operative findings, treatment and hospital course.

Evacuation/Consultation Criteria: Evacuate ASAP. Consult general surgery.

Chapter 7: Gastrointestinal: Acute Peptic Ulcer

COL Peter McNally, MC, USA (Ret)

Introduction: Peptic ulcers are defects in either the gastric or duodenal mucosa. Almost all ulcers are caused by infection with *Helicobacter pylori*, consumption of aspirin or NSAIDs (ibuprofen, naproxen, sulindac, piroxicam, etc.) or severe physiologic stress (extensive trauma, burns or CNS injury). Some ulcers are related to ingestion of fish parasites. Most ulcers cause mid-epigastric pain, often associated with nausea or vomiting. Complications of ulcers include bleeding, perforation and obstruction. Generally, pain will herald the presence of an ulcer before complications occur. Ulcer pain is decreased by ingestion of alkali and patients often give a history of self-medication with bicarbonate of soda, antacids or over-the-counter acid blocking medicines.

Subjective: Symptoms

Gnawing epigastric pain between the umbilicus and the xiphoid, increased by food and relieved by alkali (gastric ulcer); awakening from sleep with pain that radiates to the mid-back (duodenal ulcer); anorexia, nausea and vomiting.

Focused History: *Does the pain get better with antacids?* (ulcer) *Does the pain radiate to the back and right scapula?* (gallstones) *Is the pain continuous and does not relent even in the "fetal" position?* (pancreatitis) *Have you experienced pressure or heavy weight on the chest that radiates to the left chin, shoulder or arm, especially with exertion?* (angina) *Have you lost more than 10 lbs in the last month?* (cancer)

Objective: Signs

Using Basic Tools: Vital signs: Pulse >100 bpm, systolic BP <90: probable hypovolemia. Orthostatic change in VS (systolic BP drop of 20mmHg or pulse rise 20 bpm): significant hypovolemia. Inspection: Pallor of anemia and diaphoresis suggests significant blood loss. Palpation: Tender epigastric area; vomiting bright red blood (hematemesis) or coffee grounds suggests active or recent bleeding from the upper GI tract; melena ("tarry" black, oily and odiferous stool that suggests upper GI tract bleeding); weight loss. Auscultate and palpate abdomen: Absent bowel sounds, rigid exam, peritoneal signs suggest perforated or penetrating ulcer. Rectal exam: Melena means recent UGI bleeding.

Using Advanced Tools: Labs: Hematocrit. Aspirate gastric contents: NG aspirate with bile, no blood or "coffee grounds" suggests no active bleeding. Coffee grounds may mean recent bleeding. If there is bright red blood, then has active bleeding.

Assessment: **Differential Diagnosis**
Dyspepsia: Usually, mild symptoms that respond to gut rest and oral antacids
Gallstones: Usually, associated with RUQ pain that radiates to the back, especially right shoulder
Pancreatitis: Usually, severe unrelenting abdominal pain radiates to back and patients will assume knee chest, "fetal position"
Angina: Usually, associated with chest pressure that radiates to left shoulder, arm, or chin; with diaphoresis & SOB
Malignancy: Usually associated with anorexia, significant weight loss (>10 lbs)

Plan:
Treatment
    1. Treat the uncomplicated ulcer:
        A. Stop aspirin or NSAIDs.
        B. Suppress acid secretion by one of the following methods (consistent with clinical and operational considerations):
            Oral therapy: **Cimetidine** 400mg bid or **famotidine** 20mg bid or **ranitidine** 150mg bid x 8-12 weeks.
            Alternatives include po proton pump inhibitors: **Omeprazole** 20mg q day or **lansoprazole** 30mg qd x 8-12 weeks.
            NG tube (for patients on prolonged NPO with NG tube): **Famotidine** 20mg per NG tube q 12h and follow with oral therapy when NG tube is removed (as required).
            IV therapy: **Cimetidine** 300mg q6h or **famotidine** 20mg q12h or **ranitidine** 50mg q6-8h or **pantoprazole** 40mg q24h and follow with oral therapy when IV is removed (as required).
    2. Management of actively bleeding ulcer (optimal management of bleeding and determination of risk for rebleed requires endoscopy and patients should be evacuated as soon as operational conditions permit)
        A. Obtain and secure IV access (18 gauge) and provide fluid resuscitation for tactical settings (Hextend 500mL IV bolus may be repeated x 1 after 30 minutes if required, continue resuscitation with packed red blood cells, lactated Ringers or normal saline) to maintain perfusion to CNS and urine output to 60cc/hr).
        B. Inhibit gastric acid secretion with IV proton pump inhibitor: **Pantoprazole** 80mg IV bolus followed by 8mg/hr infusion x 72 hr or 80mg bolus followed by 80mg q12h x 72 hr. Other proton pump inhibitors (at equivalent IV doses to inhibit gastric acid) may be used if available (eg, **lansoprazole, esomeprazole** or **omeprazole**)
        C. Evacuate with preparation to provide as aggressive fluid resuscitation as resources and conditions permit. *See Part 8: Procedures: Blood Transfusion*
    3. Eradicate *Helicobacter pylori* with "triple" therapy: For 14 days, give **omeprazole** 20mg bid or **lansoprazole** 3mg bid, plus **clarithromycin** 500mg bid or **amoxicillin** 500mg tid, plus **metronidazole** 500mg bid.

Patient Education
General: 90-95% of duodenal ulcers and ~80% of gastric ulcers are caused by infection with *Helicobacter pylori*. Most of the remaining ulcers are caused by ingestion of aspirin or NSAIDs. Emotional stress or food does not cause duodenal and gastric ulcers.
Diet: Consume a healthy diet and avoid foods that aggravate symptoms.
Medications: The ulcer should be treated with medicine to decrease stomach acid production. When H. pylori infection is suspected, as in recurrent ulcer disease, it should be treated with "triple therapy."
Prevention and Hygiene: Avoid aspirin and NSAIDs. Use acetaminophen instead for head, muscle or joint aches.
No Improvement/Deterioration: Return if symptoms worsen or persist after 2 weeks of treatment. Also, return immediately if vomiting blood or "coffee grounds", or passing blood or tarry stools from the rectum (hematemesis or melena).

Follow-up Actions
Return Evaluation: Patients with symptoms that increase or symptoms that persist after 2 weeks of treatment require upper endoscopy to excluded complicated ulcer disease or malignancy. Refer those with hematemesis or melena. Relapse of symptoms after successful treatment suggests failure to eradicate or reinfection with H. pylori or concurrent aspirin/NSAIDs use.
Evacuation/Consultation Criteria: Evacuate unstable and bleeding patients (melena, hematemesis). Consult gastroenterologist or internist for uncomplicated ulcer disease, and a general surgeon for patients with melena or hematemesis.
Note: Upper GI endoscopy or x-ray series may be required to confirm the diagnosis in garrison.

Chapter 7: Gastrointestinal: Acute Intestinal Obstruction
COL Peter McNally, MC, USA (Ret)

Introduction: Acute obstructions, which are partial or complete blockages in the bowels, are divided into small and large intestinal causes. Both cause an acute onset of severe abdominal pain, distention and nausea and vomiting. Prompt evaluation, decompression and surgical correction of the obstruction (before bowel infarction or perforation occurs) are the keys to management. The percentages listed in this section are for industrialized nations. Small intestinal obstruction is caused by: adhesions (56%), hernias (25%), neoplasm (10%), other (9%). Large intestinal obstructions are caused by: neoplasms (60%), volvulus (20%), diverticular stricture (10%), other (10%). Intussusception (20-30% of all obstructions in Africa and India where ascariasis is endemic) and volvulus are much more common than cancers and diverticulitis in the developing world.

Subjective: **Symptoms**
Acute onset of severe, crampy abdominal pain with associated vomiting (vomitus is usually foul smelling due to increased bacteria in the gut) and abdominal distention; pain is paroxysmal; proximal obstructions every 4-5 minutes; distal obstructions less frequently; strangulated bowel (both proximal and distal) cause consistent excruciating pain. Rectal bleeding is consistent with mucosal ulceration from intestinal ischemia, inflammatory bowel disease or malignancy.

Focused History: *Are you passing gas?* (partial obstruction) *Vomiting blood?* (ulceration or malignancy) *Vomiting fecal matter?* (distal bowel obstruction) *Have you had significant weight loss?* (malignancy or inflammatory bowel disease)

Objective: Signs

Using Basic Tools: Inspection: Febrile, toxic, dehydrated from vomiting, distended abdomen with possibly visible peristaltic waves (in small bowel obstruction). Presence of surgical scars suggests possible adhesions as cause of bowel obstruction. Auscultation: Frequent, high-pitched bowel sounds occur in waves early, but the bowel may be silent later due to peritonitis or bowel infarction. Borborygmi (loud bowel rumblings audible without stethoscope) correspond to paroxysms of pain. Percussion: Obstructed and dilated, gas-filled loops of bowel are often tympanic with percussion of the abdomen. Palpation: Pain. A mass suggests the location of obstruction. Check for hernias (inguinal, femoral, or umbilical), surgical scars (adhesions). Rectal exam: To evaluate for mass or bleeding.
Using Advanced Tools: Labs: CBC (increased WBC with left shift in strangulation of bowel associated with small bowel obstruction). X-ray of abdomen: dilated loops of bowel and/or air-fluid levels (obstruction of bowel), free air seen in abdomen (perforation of stomach or bowel), calcified gallstones (cholecystitis), chronic calcific pancreas (pancreatitis).

Assessment: Differential Diagnosis

Peritonitis (from any cause): Rebound tenderness, rigid, board like abdomen, septic appearance, no bowel sounds.
Peptic ulcer disease: Vomiting blood; melena on rectal examination
Cholecystitis: Tenderness in the right upper quadrant, (+) Murphy's sign
Ischemic bowel: Absence of bowel sounds, disproportionate examination (abdomen softer that you expect from the degree of pain to palpation), poor peripheral pulses, signs of poor circulation
Aortic aneurysm: Abdominal bruit, pulsatile abdomen, shock, poor or absent distal pulses, mottled abdomen.
Diverticulitis: Pain localized in left lower quadrant
Food poisoning: Diarrhea, vomiting following exposure to contaminated food, others with similar symptoms.
Neoplasms: Palpable mass

Plan:

Treatment
1. Place NG tube (if available). Keep NPO.
2. IV fluids to restore fluid and electrolyte losses caused by vomiting. *See Part 7: Trauma: Chapter 27: Hypovolemic Shock*
3. Give antiemetic (eg, **promethazine** 25mg IV/IM/po q8h, or **ondansetron** 4mg IV q8h), but no pain meds until sure of diagnosis and awaiting evacuation. *See Part 8: Procedure: Chapter 30 Pain Assessment and Control*
4. Suppress gastric acid to mitigate risk for stress gastritis. *See Part 4: Organ Systems: Chapter 7: Acute Gastritis*
5. Medical evacuation surgical evaluation and management of mechanical bowel obstruction, symptoms persist for >12 hours or if fever or peritoneal signs develop.
6. IV antibiotics should be administered if signs of peritonitis. *See Part 4: Organ Systems: Chapter 7: Acute Peritonitis*

Patient Education
General: If pain persists or reoccurs return for re-evaluation.
Diet: Low roughage if a history of recurrent partial small bowel obstructions.
No Improvement/Deterioration: Persistent pain or pain associated with vomiting, dehydration, bleeding, or fever should be evaluated promptly.

Follow-up Actions
Return Evaluation: Routine post-operative follow-up.
Evacuation/Consultation Criteria: Evacuate ASAP. Consult general surgery.

Chapter 7: Gastrointestinal: Anorectal Disorders: Anal Fissure
LTC Jeffery Nelson, MC, USA

Introduction: Anal fissure (acute or chronic) is a very common complaint that typically presents as a sharp pain and bleeding with bowel movements (BM). The initial fissure is usually caused by a hard BM. Most people have had anal fissures at some point in their lives and these lesions usually heal within one month. Why anal fissures become chronic (>1 month's duration) in some individuals and not in others is unknown. **Risk Factors:** Dehydration and hard stools can increase the risk of anal fissure.

Subjective: Symptoms

Sharp or cutting pain during BMs and bright red rectal bleeding are the classic symptoms associated with anal fissure. Patients report blood tinged toilet tissue or bright red blood in the toilet bowl following defecation or blood streaked stool. These symptoms can be acute (<30 days) or chronic.

Focused History: *When did your symptoms start?* (Patients may associate onset of initial symptoms with a hard BM.) *How long have you had pain and bleeding with BMs?* (If their symptoms have persisted for more than 30 days, the fissure is considered chronic and will require some intervention to achieve resolution.)

Objective: Signs

Using Basic Tools: Inspection: Do a rectal exam with the patient lying on their left side with their knees tucked up to their chest. Gently spread the buttocks and external anal tissues until the fissure is visible in the anterior or posterior midline position. Once the anal fissure is visualized, further exam (eg, digital rectal exam, anoscopy) is not required and will only inflict unnecessary pain.

Assessment:
Visual identification of an anal fissure in the anterior or posterior midline position. Anal lesions which raise concern (ie, that do not appear to be a simple anal fissure in the anterior or posterior midline position) or which are accompanied by additional symptoms (weight loss, bloody diarrhea, mass, lymphadenopathy) should be referred for further evaluation.

Differential Diagnosis
Infections: HIV, syphilis, gonorrhea, herpes simplex, etc. *See Part 5: Specialty Area: Chapter 11: Introduction to STDs*
Inflammatory conditions: Crohn's disease and ulcerative colitis usually are associated with additional symptoms (ie, abdominal pain, bloody diarrhea, peri rectal lesions, weight loss).
Malignancy: Lymphoma, leukemia, squamous cell carcinoma. Malignant lesions appear very different from a benign anal fissure. They typically cause large wounds with heaped up edges and may occur anywhere around the anal verge, not just in the midline. Digital rectal exam may reveal the lesion and/or mass to extend into the anal canal. These lesions also frequently produce a large amount of exudate and bleeding. Anal lesions which raise concern for one of these should prompt referral.

Plan:
Treatment
Primary: Topical anesthetic (**lidocaine**) jelly applied prior to BM can provide symptomatic relief. **Hydrocortisone** cream 2.5% applied bid to the fissure will relieve pain in the short term (<30 days). **Psyllium** seed fiber supplements one teaspoon mixed in water or juice bid will soften the stool and reduce tissue trauma. This treatment is appropriate for relief of symptoms in a patient who presents with a history of a chronic anal fissure, but these patients will require referral to achieve successful definitive management.
Primitive: Attention to hygiene, increased fluid intake and increased dietary fiber.

Patient Education
General: 90% of acute anal fissures will heal with conservative measures listed. Patient should return if new symptoms or symptoms persist.
Activity: No restrictions required
Diet: High fiber diet.
Medications: Anal steroid creams should not be used for more that 30 days to avoid skin breakdown.
Prevention and Hygiene: Normal use of soap and water is sufficient. Aggressive scrubbing only causes further skin breakdown and delays healing.
No Improvement/Deterioration: If the fissure is not healed within 30 days of conservative management, the patient should be referred.

Follow-up Actions
Return Evaluation: One or two follow-up visits within the 30 day healing period.
Evacuation/Consultation Criteria: If the patient has an atypical lesion that does not fit the description of an anal fissure, a referral evacuation is indicated.

Chapter 7: Gastrointestinal: Anorectal Disorders: Hemorrhoidal Disease
LTC Jeffery Nelson, MC, USA

Introduction: Hemorrhoidal disease is extremely common all over the world, varies in severity, occurs in any environment in all seasons, and is a frequent reason for troops to seek medical attention. Hemorrhoids are normal tissue (dilated veins) located in the submucosal layer of the lower rectum and thought to be involved in part of the anorectal continuance mechanism. Normal hemorrhoidal tissue is divided anatomically into internal and external components with the internal hemorrhoids above the anus in the lowest part of the rectum (above the dentate line). External hemorrhoidal tissue exists below the rectum underneath the anal skin itself. Internal hemorrhoids do not cause pain, because no nerves that carry pain signals to the brain exist over them. Hemorrhoidal disease may be caused by internal hemorrhoids, external hemorrhoids, or both and the provider must be able to tell the difference and know the different treatment options. **Risk Factors:** Patients often have a family history of hemorrhoidal disease. Repetitive activities which cause prolonged Valsalva maneuvers (eg, weight lifting, straining to defecate, and reading on the toilet). About 4% of any population (both sexes) will experience hemorrhoidal disease. In the general population, symptoms peak between 45-65 yrs and are less frequently seen in patients less than 20 yrs.

Subjective: **Symptoms**
It is important to realize that many patients with anorectal problems will complain of "hemorrhoids", when, in fact, their actual problem may be completely unrelated to their hemorrhoids. Internal hemorrhoidal problems present as bright red rectal bleeding, and/or prolapse of the hemorrhoidal tissue out of the anus (the patient will say that some kind of tissue falls out of their anus with a bowel movement). External hemorrhoidal problems manifest as thrombosis, which may or may not leave skin tags after the clot resolves. When external hemorrhoids thrombose they do cause pain, because the blood clot causes inflammation and irritates the overlying skin, which does have pain innervation. Patients will complain of a painful swollen lump close to the anal opening. Sometimes the patient will also complain of bleeding if the overlying skin necroses (dies) and the clot leaks out.
Focused History: *Are you in pain?* (The presence of pain points to a thrombosed external hemorrhoid [TEH] or some other non-hemorrhoidal problem, but not internal hemorrhoidal issues. The patient should also have a painful, swollen lump on the anus if they have a TEH.) *Do you have rectal bleeding? Is the bleeding bright red, or do you also have clots and dark blood? Is the blood just on the toilet paper, in the water, on the stool, mixed in the stool, or some combination of these?* (Red blood on the toilet paper and/or in the toilet water is typical of internal hemorrhoidal bleeding. Blood clots, dark blood, and blood mixed in the stool may be something more serious, like colorectal cancer, and should be aggressively investigated.) *Do you feel anything fall out of your anus when you strain to have a BM?* (This is hemorrhoidal prolapse. This means that their internal hemorrhoids are large enough to fall outside of the anal opening with a BM.) *Do you have to push this tissue back in with your fingers, or does it go back inside on its own?* (This will give you a sense of how large their internal hemorrhoids are, and may determine treatment.)

Objective: **Signs**

Using Basic Tools: Inspection: The easiest method of examining the anus and perineum in the field environment (or in the clinic, for that matter) is in the left lateral decubitus position. The patient lies on their left side with their knees up to their chest. An assistant may be required in some instances to help retract the buttocks to examine the anus. A TEH will appear as bluish, swollen bulge right at the anal opening. Prolapsed internal hemorrhoidal tissue may be visible at the anal opening and appears as a bright red bulge or bulges. Infrequently a patient's external hemorrhoids may thrombose circumferentially around the anus along with prolapse and incarceration (trapping) of the internal hemorrhoids outside the anus. This situation is known as a hemorrhoidal crisis. Massive swelling of the hemorrhoidal tissues will be visible. In most situations of internal hemorrhoidal bleeding, or even prolapse, the anus appears completely normal externally. Palpation: Do a digital rectal examination to feel for any masses in the anus and lower rectum. Hemorrhoidal tissue, unless very enlarged, is not easily palpable. One should also determine the patient's general sphincter tone (increased, normal or decreased) by having the patient squeeze down on the examining finger.

Using Advanced Tools: Hemoglobin and hematocrit in a patient who gives a chronic history that suggests significant blood loss.

Assessment:

Internal hemorrhoids are graded on a scale from I to IV:

Grade I: Internal hemorrhoids may bleed, but they do not prolapse

Grade II: Bleeding and prolapse that reduces spontaneously; the patient does not have to push their hemorrhoids back inside the anus.

Grade III: Bleeding and prolapse that does not reduce spontaneously; the patient must push their hemorrhoids back inside the anus.

Grade IV: The internal hemorrhoids are permanently prolapsed and cannot be reduced.

Hemorrhoidal crisis exists when all or most of the internal hemorrhoidal tissues are prolapsed through the anal sphincter and become incarcerated (trapped on the outside). This causes massive edema (swelling) of the hemorrhoids and thrombosis of the external hemorrhoids, as well. The patient typically is in significant pain (from the thrombosis) and discomfort.

External hemorrhoids are either thrombosed (clotted) or not. Many times patients will have skin tags around their anus from prior episodes of thrombosis (stretched out skin from the swelling), but these are not hemorrhoidal tissues. Irritation to persistent skin tags (from previously thrombosed external hemorrhoids) can result in irritation and pruritus.

Differential Diagnosis

Hemorrhoidal crisis (prolapsed, incarcerated internal hemorrhoid): As described previously.

Thrombosed external hemorrhoid: As described previously.

Anal fissure: Easily seen by spreading the anal tissues apart and looking in the posterior or anterior midline for a linear cut, or wound. Lesions not in the midline suggest other pathology. *See Part 4: Organ Systems: Chapter 7: Anorectal Disorders: Anal Fissures*

Perirectal abscess: Redness, tenderness and swelling over the abscess adjacent to the anus

Note: Abscess may be present with minimal external signs. *See Part 4: Organ Systems: Chapter 7: Anorectal Disorders: Peri-rectal Abscesses*

Anal pruritus: Difficulty maintaining optimal hygiene in the field, loose BMs increase fecal soilage and may result in anal pruritus that usually immediately responds to improved cleaning and conservative measures (see below).

Other causes of anal pruritus include: anorectal disease (eg, abscess, fistula, external hemorrhoids), dermatologic conditions (eg, contact dermatitis, atopic dermatitis), infections (eg, herpes, syphilis, gonorrhea, candida) and should be pursued if symptoms do not respond to conservative management or are associated with other symptoms.

Levator ani syndrome: Muscle spasm around the rectum. It is a diagnosis of exclusion that requires confirmation by specialist referral.

Plan:

Treatment

Hemorrhoidal crisis (prolapsed and incarcerated internal hemorrhoidal tissue): Inject a perianal block with 20cc of 1% **lidocaine** directly around the anal sphincter. This will release the spasm and allow manual reduction of the internal hemorrhoids. After placing the block with the smallest gauge needle possible, press on the hemorrhoidal mass with the examining hand for 5 minutes. This will relieve the patient's discomfort and allow for a less emergent evacuation or transfer to a higher level medical facility.

TEH: The first 72 hours of the thrombosis is the most painful period and is typically the time in which the patient optimally is referred for total hemorrhoid excision. After the first 72 hours, the painful symptoms begin to resolve, making excision unnecessary. All TEH will resolve if given enough time to do so. If referral is not possible, comfort measures are the most appropriate action and include NSAIDs (ie, **ibuprofen** 400-600mg po q6h prn pain) hot ("sitz") baths, or warm shower will provide temporary relief and improve hygiene. Anticipate that complete relief of symptoms typically takes about 2 weeks, but it does vary significantly from patient to patient.

Note: Simple incision and drainage (I & D) of the clot is inadequate for 2 reasons. First, it does not remove the whole thrombosed hemorrhoid, which may allow the thrombosis to recur later on. Second, it only removes one of the clots which make up the hemorrhoid. A TEH is actually a collection of many clotted veins, not just one. I & D of the clot frequently leads to no resolution of the patient's discomfort at all and will cause a bleeding wound in addition to the painful TEH. The only reason to excise a TEH is to relieve the patient's pain.

Alternative: None. There is virtually no role for any hemorrhoid creams or suppositories. They have no effect on pain, bleeding, or prolapse.

Anal pruritus: Treatment is based at underlying cause but conservative management and reassurance are successful in 90% of patients. Instruct patients re: anodermal care that includes keeping area clean and dry (but without excessive wiping or use of astringent cleaners), bathing or wiping with water following defecation. A short course (<1week) of 1% **hydrocortisone** cream applied bid plus a protective ointment (**zinc oxide**) will often help. In patients whose symptoms are worse at night, an antihistamine (eg, **diphenhydramine** 25mg po hs) is helpful until local measures take effect.

Patient Education

General: Most hemorrhoidal problems, such as internal hemorrhoidal prolapse and bleeding or a TEH will resolve. However, the normal course of hemorrhoidal disease is multiple recurrences and worsening over time of the same issues. The patient will require referral to a general or colo-rectal surgeon for definitive management (immediately for hemorrhoidal crisis).

Activity: As tolerated. Usually 1-2 days of rest is required.

Diet: No specific dietary or fluid restrictions are necessary, but a high fiber diet with adequate fluids is recommended to keep bowel movements soft.

Medications: Some sort of fiber supplementation is indicated, such as psyllium seed (2 teaspoons/day in water or juice), which will soften the stool and improve the regularity of bowel movements.

Prevention and Hygiene: Warm baths or showers bid-tid, and after every BM. No specific prevention measures are effective. The patient should avoid activities associated with worsening of their symptoms, such as reading on the toilet or weight lifting.

No Improvement/Deterioration: Anticipate recurrence of symptoms (eg, bleeding, prolapse, and/or pain) until patient is referred for definitive surgical management.

Wound Care: No wound issues exist here unless the provider creates a wound. Wounds around the anus should be left open and treated with frequent baths or showers.

Follow-up Actions

Return Evaluation: If the patient is not transferred immediately, then they should be seen again within one week for reevaluation.

Evacuation/Consultation Criteria: Hemorrhoidal crisis requires evacuation. A TEH may require evacuation if excision is desired and/or the pain is extreme and the Soldier is rendered ineffective.

Chapter 7: Gastrointestinal: Anorectal Disorders: Peri-rectal Abscesses
LTC Jeffery Nelson, MC, USA

Introduction: Peri-rectal abscesses result from the infection of anal glands (which are normal structures). These glands secrete a mucus substance that is responsible for lubricating the anal canal during defecation. Once an abscess forms in one of these glands, it may spread to the surrounding soft tissue of the anus and rectum. A peri-rectal abscess then typically presents as a painful, red swelling around the anus and sometimes even out on to the buttocks. As is the case for all abscesses, cure requires drainage. Because of the anatomical features of this area, infections can range from relatively benign to life threatening with requirement for significant surgical intervention. **Risk Factors:** No specific risk factors known although it has been observed that peri-rectal abscesses tend to occur more frequently in some individuals.

Subjective: **Symptoms**

Pain is the most common symptom, occurs early in the course of the disease and may be present before redness (erythema) or swelling around the anus is noted. The patient complains of fevers and chills.

Focused History: *When did you first notice pain? Have you ever had peri-rectal abscesses in the past? Have you ever had surgery of the anus or rectum? Do you have Crohn's disease, or is there any history of Crohn's disease in your immediate family?* (This disease frequently causes abscesses of the anus and can be very complicated to manage.) *Where around the anus does it hurt?* (This will complete the examination.)

Objective: **Signs**

Using Basic Tools: Inspection: Visualize peri-rectal area to identify redness and swelling. Describe location of the abscess as left, right, anterior, and posterior to the anus. Bilateral involvement (a "horseshoe" pattern) suggests a deep space infection that will require early advanced surgical management. Palpation: Peri-rectal abscesses are extremely tender and feel warm to the touch. A digital rectal exam may reveal induration (hardness) on the side of the anus where the abscess is located. Pus may also drain from the anus in some cases.

Assessment: Simple inspection and palpation with digital rectal exam are all that is required in the acute situation. There are no grading systems for peri-rectal abscesses.

Differential Diagnosis

Crohn's disease: An inflammatory bowel disease that can present as a perirectal abscess or perirectal fistula that typically also includes a history of abdominal pain, blood stools and weight loss.

Insect bites: Generally more superficial lesions with secondary infection

Carbuncles or furuncles:

Hidradenitis suppurativa: Infected sweat glands that may occur around the anus. If the patient has a history of many skin infections and has a scarred/pitted perineum, then hidradenitis is more likely than a peri-rectal abscess.

Pilonidal sinus disease: Infected hair follicles that occur over the sacral area in the gluteal cleft, not around the anus. *See Part 4: General Symptoms: Chapter 7: Anorectal Disorders: Pilonidal Sinus Disorders*

Bartholin's cyst: Inflammation of the Bartholin's gland duct. *See Part 3: General Symptoms: Gynecologic Problems: Bartholin's Cyst/Abscess*

Plan:

Treatment

Primary:

1. Incision and drainage: This is not a sterile procedure. Position the patient lying on their left side with their knees bent up to their chest (or as high as they can get them). This provides a stable and comfortable position for the patient, as well as excellent exposure to the anorectum. One other person is necessary to help hold the buttocks apart. Inject 1% **lidocaine** 2-5cc or 0.25% - 0.5% **bupivacaine** 2-5cc using the smallest gauge needle possible into the skin directly over the abscess. Any scalpel blade

       may then be used to cut into the abscess through the numb skin, but an 11 blade is ideal for this purpose. Make sure the incision is at least 1.5-2cm long to provide adequate drainage. No packing of the abscess cavity is necessary and will only cause undue pain to the patient. Simply place gauzes or a pad over the wound and let it drain.

2. Post procedure: The patient should sit in a tub of warm water or take a warm shower bid until it heals. Only 50% of drained abscesses will completely heal; the other half will become what is know as an anal fistula.

3. Pain control: Drainage of the abscess will relieve most, if not all, pain. **Ibuprofen** 400-600mg po tid-qid or **acetaminophen** (300mg)/**codeine** (30mg) po tid-qid prn may be useful as needed.

4. Antibiotics: Not routinely required for an uncomplicated and localized peri-rectal abscess without evidence of significant accompanying cellulitis. If cellulitis is present; **ciprofloxacin** 750mg po bid plus **metronidazole** 500mg po tid x 7-10 days may be useful.

Alternative: If incision and drainage is impossible, antibiotics may mitigate risk of systemic infection until drainage of the abscess can be achieved. **Note:** Antibiotics are not the cure and should be given only as a temporizing measure until definitive surgical management has been accomplished.

Primitive: Drainage may be achieved with any means available (eg, spontaneous).

Patient Education

General: After drainage of the abscess the patient should know that he/she has about a 50% chance of developing an anal fistula, which is a connection between the rectum and anal skin where the abscess was drained. If this occurs, the patient will require referral to a general or colon and rectal surgeon for a more definitive procedure.

Activity: As tolerated.

Diet: No special diet.

Prevention and Hygiene: As previously discussed – showers or baths bid-tid.

No Improvement/Deterioration: If the abscess cannot be drained, or is drained inadequately, the abscess may continue to grow resulting in rapid spread of infection. In severe cases, patients may become septic (systemic infection) with widespread necrosis of their perineal tissues around the anus, rectum, penis and scrotum (colloquially referred to as Fournier's gangrene). This is a life-threatening situation and requires immediate evacuation. *See Part 3: General Symptoms: Male Genital Problems: Genital Inflammation*

Wound Care: As previously discussed – simply keep it covered and clean. Do not pack the wound.

Follow-up Actions

Return Evaluation: This condition will likely eventually require definitive surgical treatment as directed by clinical and operational conditions. Initially (under field conditions) if the abscess drains and patient's symptoms resolve, follow-up once a week is adequate.

Evacuation/Consultation: Untreated or inadequately treated perirectal infection is a potentially life-threatening condition. Symptoms or signs that suggest a deep, expanding or systemic infection are indications for immediate medical evacuation.

Chapter 7: Gastrointestinal: Anorectal Disorders: Pilonidal Sinus Disease

LTC Jeffery Nelson, MC, USA

Introduction: Pilonidal sinus disease is a relatively common disorder that is characterized by acute and chronic abscess formation caused by hair burrowing into hair follicles in the gluteal cleft. Patients are typically young men who work outside and sit for prolonged periods of time. However, this disease can be seen in both men and women and can occur at any age. **Seasonal Variation:** May occur at any time of year, but is more common in hot environments. **Risk Factors:** Male sex; deep gluteal cleft; thick hair distribution over the buttocks; prolonged sitting and poor hygiene.

Subjective: **Symptoms**

Pain and swelling over the sacrum in the gluteal cleft (crease down the middle of the buttocks above the anus). Patients may also present with a chronic form of the disease where they have had abscesses in this region that have drained but failed to completely heal. In this case, they will have a draining wound, which represents the opening to the sinus cavity. Patients usually have some degree of discomfort with pain and drainage. Most also complain of difficulty sitting and doing some exercises, such as sit-ups.

Focused History: *When did you first notice the problem? Do you have pain, drainage, or both? Have you ever had a pilonidal abscess drained before? Have you ever had surgery for their pilonidal disease before? If so, do you know the nature of the surgery? Are you currently taking any antibiotics?* (These questions will help determine if the situation is acute or chronic. An acute abscess requires drainage in the short term, usually within 12 hours. A chronic abscess or draining sinus only requires good wound care in the short term, along with referral to a higher level of care for definitive management.)

Objective: **Signs**

Using Basic Tools: Inspection: On the sacral area of the buttocks, patients with pilonidal sinus disease should have some number of midline pits. These pits look like holes in the skin and occur in the exact middle of the gluteal cleft. They actually are stretched out hair follicles that are the source of the problem. These pits are the entry point of hair, debris and bacteria into the subcutaneous tissue that causes the infection. Hair may protrude from them. The abscesses or sinuses can either be in the middle, as well, or off the midline to one side or the other (as is most often the case). An acute abscess will appear much like any other abscess. It will be red, swollen, and tender to touch. It may also be draining if the overlying skin has necrosed. Palpation: An acute abscess will be very tender to the touch and also hot. A chronic abscess should not be as tender, or tender at all, since it already has been drained (but just has not healed). Subcutaneous induration (inflammation that feels hard) may also be present.

Assessment

There are no tools or scales used to grade this disease, but it is helpful to assess whether the disease is mild, moderate, or severe. This is a judgment call and highly subjective but will help the provider who receives the patient as a referral.

Differential Diagnosis

Perirectal abscess: These abscesses occur around the anus and are not associated with the midline gluteal cleft pits. They arise from infected anal glands. *See Part 4: Organ Systems: Chapter 7: Anorectal Disorders: Peri-rectal Abscess*

Crohn's disease: This is an inflammatory disease that can affect the entire GI tract including the anus, and as such, should not involve tissue over the sacrum. However, in severe cases with extensive tissue involvement, it may be difficult to discern.

Hidradenitis suppurativa: Inflammatory condition that affects apocrine sweat glands and only occurs where these sweat glands are located, such as the axilla, groin, and perineum (anus and genitalia). Many believe that this disease exists within the same spectrum as pilonidal disease, but with a different manifestation. It is most common in African-American individuals, but is known to occur in all races. There are no midline pits in this disease process, and usually simple drainage of the skin abscesses is all that is required in the short term. In the chronic form of the disease, extensive scarring will be present in the region where the acute abscess is located (eg, if the abscess is in the perineum, it would be common to see scarring from prior infections around the anus).

Plan:

Treatment

Chronic disease: A chronic abscess, or sinus, that is already an open, draining wound does not require further drainage. Only definitive surgery by a specialist can resolve this situation. Basic wound care and shaving is all that is indicated in the field environment. Shaving helps with basic hygiene, and may help heal uncomplicated cases and avoid a need for subsequent surgery. Any razor may be used to shave off all the hair around the pilonidal sinus and midline pits for 2 inches in all directions. This should be repeated at least every 2 weeks. Any hair sticking out of the pits should also be picked out with a forceps or small clamp at the same time.

Acute disease: Incision and drainage (I&D): Any acute abscess should be drained. Using a small needle (25 gauge or smaller) and a 10cc syringe, inject local anesthetic (1% **lidocaine**) just under the skin over the top of the abscess where the incision will be made. Any sterile scalpel blade may be used but a #15 blade is ideal. Make sure the incision is large enough to ensure adequate drainage. One of the most common mistakes is making too small an incision. Ensure that all material (eg, retained hair) is removed from the abscess cavity. Apply gauze wound dressing.

Wound care: The area around the wound (2 inches in all directions) should be shaved every 2 weeks until healing has occurred. Warm showers bid in between dressing changes is required (avoid use of soap over the immediate wound).

Note: Adjuncts (eg, peroxide or povidone-iodine) are not necessary and actually kill tissue and delay healing.

Antibiotics: If cellulitis extends from the area of the abscess, a course of antibiotics (eg, **cephalexin** 250mg po q6h x 7-10 days) may be required.

Patient Education

General: Patients must be dedicated to hygiene (to include shaving) and in many cases pilonidal wounds take months to heal. Although usually a self-limited process that burns itself out over time, in some cases the conditions becomes chronic requiring a definitive surgical procedure.

Activity: Some restrictions (especially related to carrying backpacks or other field equipment) can be anticipated in the initial stages of treatment.

Diet: No dietary restrictions

Prevention and Hygiene: Shaving the area every 2 weeks may be tried to limit incidence of recurrence

No Improvement/Deterioration: Refer patients if the lesion fails to improve within 2 weeks or sooner if clinical condition worsens.

Follow-up Actions

Return Evaluation: Every 1-2 weeks.

Evacuation/Consultation Criteria: Failure of progress towards wound healing within 2 weeks, extensive disease, or active infection that fails to resolve following abscess drainage and antibiotics should prompt referral.

Chapter 8: Genitourinary: Urinary Tract Problems

LTC Steve Waxman, MC, USA & LTC (P) Douglas Soderdahl, MC, USA

Introduction: This section will provide tips for the assessment and disposition of major symptoms associated with the urinary tract, excluding trauma.

Examination Tips

1. Assessing a patient with flank pain: Lightly tap or push with fingers on right or left upper back. If there is significant kidney irritation, this will elicit increased pain.

2. Abdominal exam:
   A. Percuss the region superior to the pubic bone. Distention with a dull tap suggests a distended bladder holding a large volume of urine. In the female, the pubis is much lower and a smaller volume of urine can be appreciated on percussion or bimanual exam.
   B. Look for peritoneal signs: increased pain with light tapping on the abdomen, pain with shaking of the abdomen and hips, pain when suddenly releasing pressure on the abdomen (rebound).

3. Scrotal exam:
   A. If possible, always exam the patient in both the standing and supine positions.
   B. Testis position and varicoceles are best appreciated in the standing position.
   C. If a bright light such as a penlight or an otoscope is available, transilluminate all scrotal masses to determine cystic (bright, diffuse glow) or solid nature of the mass.
   D. Try to determine if a mass is inside the testicle (possible tumor) or outside the testicle and whether the mass is painless or painful. Ask if the mass is new or old and whether it has changed in size. Try to determine if the mass can be reduced (hernia versus a hydrocele).

E. Severe testicular pain of sudden onset should be worked up immediately to rule out testicular torsion.

4. Rectal Exam

A. Prostates are generally the size of a walnut and about one or two fingerbreadths wide in a man under the age of 30.

B. With the patient standing and bending over an examination table, the top of the prostate should be easy to reach.

C. The prostate is usually soft, non-tender and without any nodules.

D. A tender and "boggy" prostate suggests prostatitis.

Urinalysis

1. Dilute urine with a specific gravity of 1.005 or less, or concentrated urine (dehydration, first morning void, etc.) of 1.015 or higher suggests normal renal function.

2. When there is visible blood in the urine, the protein from the blood can raise the urine dipstick protein value to 2+.

3. Nitrite positive urine can be from skin bacteria if the person (male or female) voided a small amount without doing a clean catch. Avoid this problem by starting to void, then sliding the cup into the stream.

4. Infections can be nitrite negative.

5. Trace heme on a urine dipstick can be due to strenuous activity or running but still requires further workup by an urologist if persistent.

6. Trace leukocyte urine can look significantly positive when viewed under the microscope.

7. Cloudy urine in specimens with an alkaline pH (6 or higher) can be amorphous phosphate and be normal in young individuals.

8. The presence of crystals in the urine does not automatically mean that the person has kidney stones.

Normal voiding

1. Normal first urge to urinate occurs with about 5oz (150cc) in the bladder.

2. Normal bladder capacity in an adult is 10-15oz (300-450cc).

3. Normal time between voiding averages greater than every 2 hours.

4. Average total 24-hour urine volume for adults is about 1 quart. Ideal would be 2 quarts/day. This translates to 40-80mL of urine per hour.

Blood in the urine (hematuria)

1. Trauma with visible blood in the urine suggests possibility of major injury. Stabilize and transfer for evaluation. If patient is able to void, severe injury to bladder and urethra is less likely (but not ruled out).

2. Hematuria with irritative voiding symptoms should be treated initially as an infection. Exposure to bodies of fresh water in Africa or the Middle East may lead to schistosomiasis as a cause of blood in the urine.

3. Hematuria with flank pain and:

A. No fever, no drug exposure and no trauma suggest a kidney stone.

B. Fever, but no trauma should be treated for a possible kidney infection.

C. Renal imaging with ultrasound or CAT scan is desirable to rule out obstruction or abscess in these patients.

D. High proteinuria, but no fever or drug or chemical exposure suggests nephritis.

4. Hematuria with painful scrotum should be treated initially as an infection.

5. Gross hematuria (visible blood) without any other symptoms can be a sign of cancer at any age.

Blood in the semen (hematospermia)

If there are no difficulties voiding, the physical exam (including rectal exam) is normal and the urinalysis several days after the event is negative, then this is likely an inflammation of the seminal vesicles. Treatment should be a 2 week course of sulfa or quinolone. Hematospermia usually takes 3-6 weeks to resolve. If the blood in the ejaculate persists, further urologic workup is warranted to rule out prostate cancer in patients older than 35. A PSA drawn at the time of urinary tract infection, prostatitis, urinary retention or catheterization is likely to be falsely elevated. First treat the acute event and then draw a PSA 1 month later to get an accurate reading. PSAs are not typically helpful in patients under the age of 35.

Cannot control urine (leaking, incontinence): See Part 4: Organ Systems: Chapter 8: Urinary Incontinence

Cannot urinate (anuria)

Catheterization (see Part 8: Procedures: Chapter 30: Urinary Bladder Catheterization) is one method of determining if there is urinary retention. Ultrasound is another method which is faster, easier and more comfortable for the patient if readily available. In a patient with large amounts of retained urine (greater than one liter), gross hematuria can result following decompression, which may require catheter irrigation to keep the bladder draining well. The urine should clear over several days following decompression. Monitor patient's electrolytes closely in cases of post obstructive diuresis (large urine outputs following relief of urinary obstruction). For a more detailed discussion, see the information on catheterization in the Prostatitis and Incontinence sections.

Discharge from the penis: Refer to STDs: Urethral Discharge

Lumps in the genital region or swollen scrotum: See Part 3: General Symptoms: Male Genital Problems: Testis/Scrotal Mass & Part 5: Specialty Areas: Chapter 11

Pain in the side (flank): See Part 4: Organ Systems: Chapter 8: Urolithiasis (Kidney or Ureteral Infections)

Pain in the scrotum

1. Tenderness located primarily in the testis: consider torsion, epididymitis.

2. Point tenderness on upper pole of testis: consider torsed appendix testis or cyst.

3. Tenderness primarily in cord above and or behind the testis: consider epididymitis or hernia.

4. Mass in testis: consider tumor.
5. Mass above testis or around testis that glows when a strong light is placed against it: hydrocele or spermatocele.
6. Large mass with history of direct blow to testis: fractured testis vs. hematoma.

Pain with urination

In most cases, it is safer to initially assume a urinary tract infection (UTI) and treat with antibiotics (*see Part 4: Organ Systems: Chapter 8: Urinary Tract Infections*). Treat vaginitis if found (*see Part 3: General Symptoms: Gynecologic Problems: Candia Vaginitis/Vulvitis*).

Persistent erections (priapism)

1. A tender, painful erection lasting more than four hours is the definition of priapism. This is an emergent condition best treated by an emergency room physician or urologist. Although this condition may resolve spontaneously, cold water immersion and manual compression of the penis may be successful. **Pseudoephedrine** 30mg po x 1 dose or **oxymetazoline** 0.05% nasal spray 2-3 sprays x 1 may be helpful while trying to get the patient to a higher echelon of care.
2. A painless partial or full erection especially with history of spinal cord injury can be observed. Similar treatment can be used.

Skin lesions in the genital region

Ulcers (*see Part 5: Specialty Areas: Chapter 11: Genital Ulcers*):
1. Ulcers that form immediately after intercourse are from trauma.
2. If always associated with the ingestion of one particular medication, the ulcer represents a fixed drug reaction.
3. Painful - chancroid, herpes
4. Painless - syphilis (hard or firm induration, chancre), granuloma inguinale, or LGV

Blisters and nodules

1. If there is any question of the diagnosis, assume it may be sexually transmitted (herpes) and avoid further sexual contact.
2. Persistent lesions should be evaluated electively to r/o cancer.
3. Most causes are benign and/or self-limited.

Generalized edema

1. Generalized swelling of the penile shaft skin with itching is usually either a contact allergic reaction or idiopathic. If an offending agent can be identified (or suspected), treat with **diphenhydramine** 25-50mg po q4-6h or other antihistamine. Avoid the chemical irritant.
2. Inflammation of the foreskin in an uncircumcised male suggests balanitis. Treat with anti-fungal medication such as **clotrimazole** cream tid. If the patient has phimosis and recurrent episodes of balanitis, he may need a circumcision on an elective basis.
3. Suspect a skin infection if there is significant erythema and pain, which may also involve the scrotum. Abscesses of the penis or scrotum need immediate incision and drainage. In some individuals this infection can be life-threatening and can also include skin necrosis and crepitance, called Fournier's gangrene. *See Part 3: General Symptoms: Male Genital Problems: Genital Inflammation*

Cannot Move Foreskin (Phimosis/Paraphimosis)

Inability to retract the foreskin (phimosis) or to pull it forward to its normal position (paraphimosis) can be problematic in the field. Often the foreskin is edematous from irritation or infection. Monitor this condition for excessive circumferential swelling which could compromise blood flow in the penis. Anti-inflammatory medications, ice water and lubricants may be helpful. If there are signs of systemic infection (fever, nausea, fatigue, etc.), and prompt evacuation is not available, a dorsal slit should be performed in the field. Most patients require circumcision later.

Dorsal Slit: Prepare the penis as with any surgical procedure (sterile scrub, povidone-iodine, drape), and attempt to clean between the head and the foreskin especially on the dorsal side. Anesthetize the dorsum of the foreskin with **lidocaine** (NO EPINEPHRINE!) 5-10cc using the smallest gauge needle (25-26) available. Use forceps or needle to ensure dorsal foreskin is numb. Clamp the dorsal foreskin tightly beginning at the tip and working back to where the foreskin meets the shaft. Leave the clamp in place for several minutes, as this will compromise blood flow in the area to be incised. Remove the clamp, and using sterile scissors or scalpel, carefully incise the dorsum of the foreskin through its entire thickness, through the line of devascularized tissue formed by the clamp. Do not incise the head of the penis. Fold the two sides of the incised foreskin back and away from the penis. Place chromic sutures on the cut edges to control bleeding.

Chapter 8: Genitourinary: Urinary Incontinence

LTC Steve Waxman, MC, USA & LTC (P) Douglas Soderdahl, MC, USA

Introduction: Incontinence, the inability to voluntarily control the flow of urine, is only a social nuisance in most cases. Incontinence can be categorized as stress incontinence, urge incontinence or mixed incontinence. Stress incontinence denotes leakage of urine during physical activity (ie, exercise, laugh, cough, sneeze). Urge incontinence denotes involuntary leakage of urine preceded by a strong urge to void. Mixed incontinence is a combination of both stress and urge components. A rarer form of incontinence is overflow incontinence which is when a patient is unable to empty his bladder and urine leaks out because the bladder is full. If the incontinence is not due to infection, and a physical exam including gross motor and sensory (numbness or muscle weakness) exam is normal, serious complications are unlikely. Incontinence is fairly common in women. Daytime incontinence in men is highly abnormal and suggests significant underlying disease.

Subjective: Symptoms

Uncontrollable loss of urine

Focused History: *Do you leak urine when you cough, lift heavy objects or jump up and down? Do you go to the bathroom often to prevent urine leaking out?* (Affirmative answers suggest stress incontinence.) *When you have to go to the bathroom, is the urge strong? Do you have a hard time holding your urine when you get the urge? When you leak, is it a lot?* (Affirmative answers suggest urge incontinence.) *Do you have a hard time emptying your bladder even though you feel like you have to? After you go to the bathroom, do you feel like you still have to go again? After you go to the bathroom, do you leak?* (Affirmative answers suggest urinary retention, which may be accompanied by overflow incontinence.) *Do you feel constantly wet? Do you feel that the wetness or dripping may be coming from your vagina?* (Affirmative answers suggest fistula or hole between the bladder or urethra and the vagina. Patients may have components of both diagnoses, such as mixed urge and stress incontinence.)

Objective: Signs

Using Basic Tools: Wet clothing; trauma or irritation to the vagina; neurologic deficits: difficulty walking, numbness in the perineum or increased deep tendon reflexes.

Using Advanced Tools: Labs: Urinalysis: moderately to strongly positive leukoesterase should be considered an infection. Moderate to strongly positive heme should be considered an infection initially, but may be cancer, urinary tract stone or other condition. Urinary catheterization (*see Part 8: Procedures: Chapter 30: Urinary Bladder Catheterization*) for suspected retention.

Voiding Diary: Time and amount of urinations over a 3-7 day period. Number of pads per day that the patient uses for their leakage. Gravida (Pregnancy)/ Para (Delivery) status.

Assessment: Differential Diagnosis

Stress incontinence, urge incontinence, mixed incontinence, and retention as described previously.

Stress incontinence: In females can be due to loss of support in the region of the bladder neck and proximal urethra or intrinsic sphincter deficiency or both.

Urge incontinence: Is often idiopathic (without known cause), and is usually more common with increasing age and multiple childbirth. It is important to rule out other causes of urge incontinence, specifically neurological disease or malignancy.

Overactive bladder: Frequent urination may also be accompanied by urgency and urge incontinence.

Continuous leakage in the setting of trauma or recent pelvic surgery (ie, hysterectomy): Suggests injury to the bladder

Co-morbidities: Advanced diabetes with neuropathy and overflow incontinence

Compression of the spinal cord: From disk disease, spinal tumors and brain disease (eg, stroke)

Multiple sclerosis or other neural tissue disease

Plan:

Treatment

Primary: Treat any urinary tract infection (*see Part 4: Organ Systems: Chapter 8: Urinary Tract Infection*). Any persistent microhematuria requires imaging of the upper tracts (preferably a CT IVP) and a cystoscopy by urology to rule out tumor or stone.

Treat specific type of incontinence:

Stress incontinence: Empty bladder frequently. Wear pad or panty liner. Practice Kegel exercises (tighten the muscles around the vagina 40-160 times per day).

Urge incontinence: Mild: **Hyoscyamine** 0.375mg po bid or **methenamine/methylene blue/phenyl salicylate/benzoic acid/atropine sulfate/hyoscyamine (Urised)** 1 po qid or **flavoxate** 100-200mg po bid. Moderate/Severe: **oxybutynin chloride** 5mg po tid-qid or **tolterodine tartrate LA** 4mg po daily. These medicines should be continued if they are efficacious and are tolerated by the patient. Refractory cases should be referred for specialty care.

Mixed stress and urge incontinence: Imipramine 10-25mg po q hs

Retention with overflow incontinence: Patients with significant symptoms, especially those suspected to have overflow incontinence, should have a bladder scan or catheter passed into the bladder per urethra to determine if there is significant residual urine. If there is greater than 200-300cc, consider intermittent self-catheterization or even indwelling Foley catheter if patient is debilitated and also having trouble with recurrent infections or renal insufficiency.

In males with enlarged prostate and poor flow: Decrease prostate resistance with alpha-blockers: **tamsulosin** 0.4mg po q day or **alfuzosin** 10mg po q day. If patient has urinary retention, place Foley catheter for 3-7 days and then remove and perform intermittent (self-) catheterization (*See Part 8: Procedures: Chapter 30: Bladder Catheterization*) q4-6h to keep bladder volume under 300cc. Alternatively, leave Foley catheter in place and refer to urology for further evaluation and treatment. Place patient on antibiotics if urine appears infected (WBCs or bacteria or nitrite positive). For those patients in whom it is too difficult to pass a Foley catheter, use a curved tip (coude) tip catheter or consider suprapubic catheter aspiration or placement if patient markedly distended and urology not available. *See Part 8: Procedures: Chapter 30: Suprapubic Bladder Aspiration (Tap) or Catheter Placement*. Antibiotics for chronic suppression of infection, such as **nitrofurantoin** 50mg po bid or **trimethoprim/sulfamethoxazole** 1 po q hs.

Patient Education

General: Avoid dehydration. Women tend to avoid fluids to minimize going to the bathroom and leaking, leading to significant dehydration.

Medications: Cold medications and antihistamines for sinus problems will counteract alpha-blockers and vice versa. Side effects of oxybutynin chloride and tolterodine tartrate include dry mouth, dry eyes and constipation. If patient develops blurred vision or other neurological side effects-stop medication immediately.

No Improvement/Deterioration: If other neurological symptoms such as visual disturbance, muscle weakness or sensory loss become apparent, refer patient to hospital for further evaluation

Follow-up Actions

Return Evaluation: Evaluate for effectiveness of therapy and the necessity for referral to an urologist for surgery or other treatment. Stress incontinence refractory to pelvic floor exercises may require surgical therapy including a sub-urethral sling or peri-urethral injection of bulking agent.

Evacuation/Consultation Criteria: Evacuate all unstable patients and those with neurological findings (ie, cauda equina) as soon as possible. Additionally, refer at some time all patients with overflow incontinence, those with stress incontinence that is interfering with work, those with urge incontinence who deteriorate or fail to improve, or any patient with a continuing requirement for medication.

Chapter 8: Genitourinary: Urolithiasis (Kidney or Ureteral Stones)

LTC Steve Waxman, MC, USA & LTC (P) Douglas Soderdahl, MC, USA

Introduction: Kidney stone pain is generally acknowledged as one of the worst a person can suffer. Stones in the kidney generally do not cause pain until they move into a position that obstructs the normal flow of urine. This usually happens as the stone passes into the ureter. The majority of symptomatic stones can be managed with hydration and pain control. Fever, vomiting and severe pain not controlled by oral medication requires intravenous treatment. Evacuate these patients with persistent symptoms that are unresponsive to pain management or with intractable GI symptoms or high fever beyond 24 hours. If pain management is effective, expectant management for spontaneous stone management can be extended and the decision to evacuate be made at the local level.

Subjective: Symptoms

Intense, intermittent flank or inguinal pain radiating into the scrotum or ipsilateral lower quadrant and not related to activity; nausea and vomiting; urinary frequency and burning (if stone at urethra/bladder junction); fever, patients generally cannot find a comfortable position
Focused History: *Was your pain of sudden onset? Is it colicky in nature?* (These are classic symptoms of a stone.) *Have you had a kidney stone before?* (Patients with a prior history of stones are more likely to have a recurrence.)

Objective: Signs

Fever, severe costovertebral angle (CVA) and /or abdominal tenderness which waxes and wanes, vomiting. The pain can start in the back and wrap around the flank and abdomen. The pain can sometimes radiate to the testicle in men.
Using Basic Tools:
1. Examine the patient between the lower chest and scrotum/pelvis.
2. Check for a tender liver by pushing under the anterior right ribs while the patient takes a deep breath.
3. Check for a hernia.
4. In men, examine the scrotum for epididymitis or torsion. Also, examine above the prostate on the rectal exam for any fullness on the side of symptoms.
5. Do a bimanual pelvic exam to check for adnexal tenderness.
6. Check for costovertebral angle (CVA) tenderness. Lightly thump the right and left lower ribs in the back. Increased tenderness suggests kidney pain.
7. Check for peritoneal signs. If pain increases with light tapping on the abdomen, shaking the abdomen, striking the heel of the foot, or there is significant irritation of the abdominal contents, then bowel inflammation/perforation (appendicitis, etc.) is suggested.
8. Light thumping over the right lower anterior chest wall would suggest gallbladder irritation. This, combined with increased pain on eating, especially in young, overweight women is suggestive of gallbladder disease.

Using Advanced Tools: Labs: Urine dipstick will most often show the presence of blood; however hematuria is not always present. The urine may also be infected as evidenced by a positive leukocyte esterase or nitrite. Urinalysis may reveal casts, blood. Abdominal x-ray to assess for presence of stones. Straining of the urine for stones may facilitate diagnosis of underlying condition predisposing to stone formation. While ultrasound may show hydronephrosis from obstruction, it is not a good study to identify ureteral stones. Plain films may also miss small ureteral stones and will not show obstruction. The best imaging study if available is a non-contrast CAT scan of the abdomen and pelvis.

Assessment:

Severe side pain not related to position, which waxes and wanes, without evidence of an abnormal genital exam or peritoneal signs strongly suggests urolithiasis.
Differential Diagnosis: Any disease process between the lower chest and upper thigh can be considered.
Lower lobe pneumonia or pulmonary process: Abnormal breath sounds.
Abdominal causes (*see Part 3: General Symptoms: Acute Abdominal Pain*): Liver disease; cholecystitis/cholelithiasis (gallbladder) diverticulitis including Meckel's; appendicitis; mesenteric adenitis; abdominal aortic aneurysm
Other kidney problem: Waxing and waning pain excludes pyelonephritis, cysts, tumor or ischemic injury.
Musculoskeletal pain: This includes aches due to viral illness.
Inguinal hernia: Distinguish by exam
Urologic: Epididymitis: tender epididymis; testicular torsion: tender testis; congenital ureteropelvic junction obstruction
Gynecologic: Abnormal pelvic exam (*see Part 3: General Symptoms: Gynecologic Problems*): ectopic pregnancy, pelvic inflammatory disease, torsion of ovary, ovarian cyst, tubo-ovarian abscess

Plan:
Treatment
Primary:
1. Pain control (in order of preference): **Ketorolac** 30mg IM q6h is highly effective in relieving stone pain. A parenteral narcotic such as **morphine sulfate** 2-10mg IM/IV q3-4h prn can also be used (can combine with ketorolac). Oral narcotic medicines that also contain **acetaminophen** are also helpful if patient can tolerate po medicines. *See Part 8: Procedures: Chapter 30: Pain Assessment and Control*
2. Hydration: po if tolerated and IV as required to replace volume loss (eg, nausea and vomiting) and maintain well hydrated state.
3. Antibiotics if the urine appears infected or when fever is present in a suspected urinary stone patient: *See Part 4: Organ Systems: Chapter 8: Urinary Tracy Infections: Pyelonephritis*
4. Anti-emetics as needed: **Promethazine** 25mg IM, **prochlorperazine** 5mg slow IV (or 25mg by rectal suppository) or **ondansetron** 2-4mg IV.
5. If medical evacuation delayed or not an option; steps to facilitate stone passage can be considered. Most patients benefit from increased fluid intake. Specific medications (eg, smooth muscle relaxant [anti-hypertensive meds] calcium channel blocker

(usually **nifedipine** 10mg po tid) or alpha blocker (usually **tamsulosin** 0.4mg po q day) increase likelihood of stone passage. Effect on BP must be monitored if these meds are used.

Primitive: Increase fluid intake to encourage passage of stone.

Patient Education

General: Maintain good hydration.

Diet: Increased water and citrus juice intake may prevent further stone formation.

Prevention and Hygiene: Goal to hydrate enough to produce 2L of urine per day.

Follow-up Actions

Return Evaluation: All suspected stone patients need to eventually have an abdominal film taken to assess the presence of stones.

Evacuation/Consultation Criteria: Evacuate ASAP patients with fever, persistent severe pain and persistent vomiting. Patients with active stone disease, (formation of new stones, increase in size of old stones, or the continued passage of gravel) will require further evaluation to identify underlying causes of stone disease (eg, hypercalcemia [most often due to primary hyperparathyroidism], hypercalciuria, hyperuricosuria, hypocitraturia, and hyperoxaluria).

Chapter 8: Genitourinary: Urinary Tract Infection

LTC Steve Waxman, MC, USA & LTC Douglas Soderdahl, MC, USA

Introduction: The causative organisms of cystitis, acute prostatitis and pyelonephritis are the same. The treatment of acute bacterial urinary tract infection (UTI) depends on the location of the infection and the presence of complicating factors. For the vast majority of infections, the fluoroquinolone antibiotics are highly effective. Bladder infections (cystitis) are treated for 3-7 days, kidney (pyelonephritis) for 14-21 days and prostate (prostatitis) for up to 30 days. In the male, it is practical to assume that any leukoesterase positive or culture positive bacterial urinary tract infection involves the prostate so treat for 30 days. Prostatitis and epididymitis are covered in separate sections. Urethral discharge suggests urethritis, which may be sexually transmitted. Therefore, primary treatment is different, although the fluoroquinolones are a good alternative. Urethral discharge is covered in the STD chapter.

Subjective: **Symptoms**

Burning, frequency, urgency, fever, flank pain. Nausea, vomiting.

Focused History: *Any dysuria, urgency, frequency, or supra-pubic pain?* (These are the classic symptoms of a UTI in the bladder or prostate.) *Any fevers or flank pain?* (These may indicate an infection of the kidney and/or nephrolithiasis.)

Objective: **Signs**

Using Basic Tools: Fever, flank tenderness, fatigue, vomiting, and suprapubic tenderness.

Using Advanced Tools: Labs: Urinalysis: Pyuria (leukoesterase +) and nitrite positive indicates infection (some gram-positive organisms may be nitrite negative). Nitrite + and leukoesterase negative specimen usually means the specimen is contaminated with skin flora. Gram's stain: identify and quantify WBCs, gram-positive or gram-negative rods and epithelial contamination. Ideally urine is collected for culture before the first dose of antibiotic is administered. Complete blood count (CBC) with differential, electrolytes, glucose, BUN, creatinine.

Assessment: **Differential Diagnosis**

Cystitis: Burning or frequency, and leukoesterase-positive urine in a female

Pyelonephritis: Fever or flank pain, and leukoesterase-positive urine in a female

Microhematuria without pyuria: Pyelonephritis is less likely; patient may have other reasons for microhematuria (tumor, stone, etc.).

Peri-ureteral inflammation: Inflammation around the ureter (eg, appendicitis, PID) can result in an abnormal urinalysis.

Contamination: Positive nitrite, negative leukoesterase and negative heme is likely skin contamination of the urine specimen.

Prostatitis: UTI symptoms in a male with leukoesterase-positive urine. Urine can be normal in patients with prostatitis and epididymitis. Positive nitrite or leukoesterase-positive or bacteria positive with large numbers of epithelial cells suggests contamination (ie, unable to get a good clean catch in female or uncircumcised male).

Plan:

Treatment

Cystitis: Trimethoprim 160mg-**sulfamethoxazole** 800mg (**Septra DS**) 1 tab po bid x 3 days or **nitrofurantoin** 100mg po bid x 7 days or **ciprofloxacin** 500mg po bid x 7-10 days or **levofloxacin** 500mg po q day x 7-10 days. **Nitrofurantoin** or **cephalexin** 500mg po tid x 7-10 days should be safe to treat UTIs during pregnancy. If female patients develop a yeast infection during the course of antibiotic, then treat with **fluconazole** 150mg po x 1,

Cystitis with complicating factors: If patient has history of infections every 1-2 months, consider placement on suppression until seen by urology. It may take longer to eradicate cystitis in women who are postmenopausal.

Pyelonephritis: Moderately ill (able to tolerate po meds): Fluoroquinolones (**levofloxacin** 500mg po q day or **ciprofloxin** 500mg po bid) x 2 weeks. Fluoroquinolones should not be used in pregnancy.

Alternative: Amoxicillin/clavulanate 875/125mg po q12h (or 500/125mg po tid) x 2 weeks or **cephalexin** 500mg po qid x 2 weeks. Closely follow patient's condition clinically and as available with CBC, Glu, electrolytes, BUN, Cr.

Pyelonephritis: Moderately ill (unable to tolerate po medications): **Cefotaxime** 1.0g q12h IV (up to 2.0g q4h IV) or ceftriaxone 1-2.0g IV q day. Continue IV therapy until clear clinical improvement then switch to po as described in this section.

Alternative: Ciprofloxacin (400mg IV q12h) or **levofloxacin** (750mg IV q24h). Continue IV therapy until clear clinical improvement then switch to po as described. Once patient is clinically improved, treat with quinolones x 2 weeks. Levofloxacin has a broader spectrum of coverage for UTI.

Note: Fluoroquinolones should be avoided in pregnancy due to risk of teratogenicity. If quinolones are not available, use **Septra DS** po tid until afebrile, and then bid x 2 weeks. Nitrofurantoin is not useful for deep tissue infections such as pyelonephritis.

Pyelonephritis: Severely ill: Treat 2-3 weeks with IV regimen (as previously discussed, unable to tolerate po medications). Following 2-3 weeks of IV regimen, follow with 2 weeks of po antibiotics (see previous, for patients able to tolerate po meds). Check for co-morbidities. Rule out diabetic ketoacidosis or abscess or hydronephrosis immediately (*See evacuation consultation criteria*).

Pyelonephritis with complicating factors (recurrent UTIs, post-menopausal): After initial treatment, begin and continue antibiotic suppression regimen until seen by urology: **nitrofurantoin** 50mg po q day or **Septra DS** ½ po q hs or **ciprofloxacin** 250mg po q hs or **cephalexin** 250mg po q hs.(**Note:** Septra should not be given at term pregnancy (category C).

Empiric: Failure of symptoms and urinalysis to improve suggests resistance to the antibiotic being used. Antibiotics should be changed if there is no improvement after 3-4 days. Patients with a fever can be expected to take several days to become afebrile. Recurrence of UTI within weeks of completing the initial course of antibiotics suggests an inadequate duration of treatment or reinfection. A longer course of antibiotics, possibly with the addition of 2-3 months of suppression is indicated. Urine culture data is extremely valuable in both cases.

Patient Education

General: Hydrate well to ensure urination every 2 hours. Cranberry juice is a good fluid choice. Complete all antibiotics.

Follow-up Actions

Evacuation/Consultation Criteria: Evacuate unstable patients ASAP. Patients with clinical pyelonephritis that are moderately-severely ill or have a history of an abnormal upper urinary tract will require kidney imaging initially if possible with CT scan or ultrasound to rule out obstruction. Patients who are not responding to treatment should be re-imaged after 48-72 hours to rule out renal abscess. Refer patients with pyelonephritis or patients with cystitis that does not resolve within 3 days of initiating treatment for evaluation.

Chapter 9: Podiatry: Heel Spur Syndrome (heel spur, heel bursitis, plantar fasciitis)

CDR Raymond Fritz, MSC, USNR (Ret)

Introduction: Heel spur syndrome is one of the most common foot problems seen in the special operations community. The term "heel spur syndrome" refers to any to heel pain with or without a spur that typically develops from excessive repetitive strain on the plantar fascia. The plantar fascia is loaded when weight is applied (standing), causing pain along the plantar fascia, particularly where the fascia connects to the heel tubercle. Associated pain can range from a "tolerable nuisance" to difficulty walking. Chronic conditions may last for years if not properly treated and 90% of cases in military personnel are caused by a combination of faulty foot mechanics and high level of use.

Subjective: Symptoms

Insidious onset of pain in plantar aspect of the foot near the heel frequently following a minor excessive stretch or strain of the plantar fascia. May be bilateral.

Focused History: *Do you remember hurting your heel?* (no direct trauma other than military training, usually gradual) *When does it hurt the most?* (It is the most severe in the morning or when standing up. The tight inflamed painful fascia improves as it stretches back out when weight bearing.) *Are your symptoms improved with shoes that offer better arch support?* (Most express some immediate relief with increased arch support.)

Objective: Signs

Using Basis Tools: Palpation reveals point tenderness over medial tubercle of the calcaneus at the level of the plantar fascial attachment. Pain may radiate distally causing pain and swelling in the arch and although more common in pronated foot type, can present in a high-arch foot type. Other structures may be sore due to compensatory gait changes (eg, a tight and painful Achilles tendon).

Using Advanced Tools: X-rays: A spur is seen about 60% of the time and other causes (eg, fracture, bone cyst or arthritic changes) may be seen on x-ray.

Assessment: Differential Diagnosis

Bursitis: Palpate tenderness (inflamed bursa) directly below the calcaneal tubercle. Referred pain from low back: L-4 L-5 extends to the heel as part of the area of distribution for this nerve root level.

Stress fracture: Sometimes visible on x-ray; not common in calcaneus.

Foreign body: Usually an entrance portal visible

Arthritis (Reiter's, psoriatic, ankylosing spondylitis, rheumatoid): *See Part 3: General Symptoms: Joint Problems: Joint Pain*

Nerve entrapment: Point tenderness over nerve; pain radiating into heel; positive Tinel sign*.

Tarsal tunnel syndrome: Compression of the posterior tibial nerve; positive Tinel sign*.

*Tinel sign is pain radiating distally along the course of a nerve that can often be elicited with gentler percussion.

Plan:

Treatment

Primary:

1. Conservative: Ice (not heat) massage, Achilles stretching, heel pad (foreign body, bursitis, arthritides).
    a. Ice massage: Use ice directly on heel and arch but limit to 8-10 minutes 4-6 x day; use Dixie cup technique or frozen plastic water bottle or gel pack if available.
    b. Dixie cup technique when freezer available: Fill cup with water and freeze. Keep several ice cups on hand. Tear cup down to expose ice and use as an applicator to heel area.
    c. Achilles tendon stretching: **Note:** Any limitation in ankle dorsiflexion increases force on plantar fascia.
2. Rest strap: Tape the foot to support the arch
3. Remove any splinter, glass or metal when the operational tempo permits.
4. Anti-inflammatories: **Ibuprofen** 800mg po tid with food; arthritides may need steroid injection. **Cortisone** injection for acute pain: Injection mixture: 1/2cc long acting steroid ie, **betamethasone, dexamethasone acetate**, and 1cc **bupivacaine** 0.5% plain. (*See video on electronic version*)
5. Consider a **bupivacaine** block to the posterior tibial nerve if previous training and experience.
6. Rest is mandatory to allow healing.

Alternative: Arch supports, injection (2cc of **bupivacaine** 0.5% mixed with 1/2cc of **dexamethasone acetate** or other long acting steroid could prove helpful for short mission if pain significant).

Primitive: Place soft, supportive material under boot insole arch area. (eg, eye patch, 4x4 gauze cut to fit)

Patient Education

General: Get better arch support. Avoid walking barefoot if possible. For dive ops, use boot with fin if operational mission involves movement overland once exiting water.

Medications: Gastritis side effects with NSAIDs.

Prevention: Good shoe support and arch support. Prescription orthotics may be best measure when obvious faulty foot mechanics present. Good flexibility program.

Follow-up Actions

Return Evaluation: Follow-up 1 week or check more regularly if teammate. Try 2^(nd) injection and stronger oral anti-inflammatory if not resolved. Recommend against narcotics if operational.

Evacuation/Consultation Criteria: Evacuation not normally necessary. If conservative measures fail to give any significant relief, consult podiatry or orthopedics. Custom orthotics will be the best consideration for the chronic recurrent case. Consult physical therapy for treatment modalities. Athletic trainer also great resource. Consult rheumatology if inflammatory etiology suspected (ie, Reiter's syndrome).

Note: Remember to rule out referred pain. Think mechanical – do not just treat symptoms. Flexibility program is a key factor in treatment and prevention.

Chapter 9: Podiatry: Ingrown Toenail

CDR Raymond Fritz, MSC, USNR (Ret)

Introduction: An ingrown nail occurs when the nail border or corner presses on the surrounding soft tissue. This condition is painful and often results in an infection once the skin is broken, with the offending nail corner acting like a foreign body introducing pathogens. An ingrown nail may result from improper trimming of nails, injury, tight shoes, genetic predisposition and fungal nail infections.

Subjective: Symptoms

Toe pain, especially in shoes; history of recurrent ingrown nails and infections, and previous procedures to remove the nail.

Focused History: *Is this ingrown nail a chronic recurring problem?* (This is often the case and the patient will tell you the problem and how it was previously treated.)

Objective: Signs

Using Basic Tools: Inspection and palpation: Great toe is most common site with secondary infection (ie, purulence, tenderness, erythema and edema); excessive granulation tissue may indicate chronic condition; malodorous wound may indicate gram-negative bacteria.

Using Advanced Tools: X-rays are rarely required but may be useful to rule out osteomyelitis or subungual exostosis (bony growth under the toenail) in selected cases (eg, long history of untreated or recurrent infection).

Assessment: Differential Diagnosis

One of the following conditions may exist as a secondary condition:

Subungual exostosis: Spur on the distal phalanx which pushes upward causing the nail to incurvate

Fungal nail infection: Obvious nail discoloration and thickening. Often thick fungal nails incurvate and do become ingrown

Subungual hematoma: Blood discoloration of nail. Blood oozing from under the nail

Foreign body reaction (granuloma): Proud flesh sometimes present as a result of a chronic untreated ingrown nail irritation

Paronychia: A primary infection of the nail fold or secondary to the irritation of a nail edge

Plan:

Treatment

Primary: Partial nail avulsion

1. Perform digital block using **lidocaine** 1% or **bupivacaine** 0.5% plain (no epinephrine for digits.) *See Part 5: Specialty Areas: Chapter 19: Local and Regional Anesthesia: Digital Block of the Finger or Toe*
2. Use elevator to free nail from bed along border. Also free nail from overlying soft tissue.
3. Use an English nail anvil or nail clipper to remove the offending nail border. Scissors will also work.
4. Use curette to remove infected necrotic tissue or excessive granulation tissue (proud flesh) from the nail groove.
5. Dress with povidone-iodine gauze and Kling. Coban or Elastoplast helps hold dressing in place.
6. Elevate foot and apply warm soaks or compresses tid.
7. Antibiotics for 7 days: **Dicloxacillin** 500mg po qid or **cephalexin** 500mg po qid for broader coverage. Give **erythromycin** 500mg po qid to penicillin allergic.
8. Pain control: **Ibuprofen** 800mg po tid prn pain.

Alternative: Remove nail corner with clipper, antibiotics

Primitive: Lift side of nail corner and remove with small scissors

Patient Education

General: Instructions on soaking: add few ounces of **povidone-iodine** solution to water; remove loose necrotic tissue or scab covering with washcloth while soaking to promote drainage when infected and speed the healing process. Recurrent problems must be addressed once infection resolved to prevent a future recurrence. Definitive procedures can be planned when the operational tempo permits.

Prevention and Hygiene: Cut nails straight across and choose appropriate foot wear with wide toe-box.

No Improvement/Deterioration: If problem recurs following conservative management, patient may require consult for definitive procedure.

Follow-up Actions

Return Evaluation: At 3-5 days, check for any remaining nail spicules (small, needle-shaped pieces) or signs of infection.

Evacuation/Consultation Criteria: Evacuation usually not necessary. Definitive procedure (partial nail avulsion with phenol application) will destroy the nail matrix and prevent re-growth. Consult podiatrist or dermatologist if condition is recurrent and not responding to treatment.

Chapter 9: Podiatry: Plantar Warts

CDR Raymond Fritz, MSC, USNR (Ret)

Introduction: Warts are caused by human papillomavirus and can be found anywhere on the skin when the virus is introduced through a crack in the skin of a susceptible individual. When located on the sole of the foot, these warts are called plantar warts. A plantar wart can be found as a single lesion or grouped together (referred to as a mosaic wart). Most common areas include the ball of the foot and heel, where increased pressure and irritation is common. Discrete plantar corns are sometimes mistaken for warts. Warts are often ignored until they become painful.

Subjective: Symptoms

Pain, especially if wart is on prominent plantar area. May have tried over-the-counter preparations that were successful treatments in the past. Other family or team members may have warts as well since warts are contagious.

Focused History: *How long has the lesion been present?* (Warts may be present acutely at the site of a chronic pressure callus.) *Did you ever have a wart in the past?* (Some are more susceptible to warts. Often treated in the past for the same problem.)

Objective: Signs

Using Basic Tools: Inspection: A wart has tiny dots in the center which, are small vascular elements. These dots are often black (dried blood) due to irritation, when located on the plantar aspect of the foot. Palpation: Lesions tender to palpation and squeezing especially if located on weight-bearing area; callus may form over the wart, increasing pain. Warts are painful when squeezed with side-to-side pressure.

Assessment: Differential Diagnosis

Corn/callus: Does not bleed with debridement since the corn or callus is a thickening of the stratum corneum which is the avascular layer of dead cell build up (*see Part 5: Specialty Areas: Chapter 9: Corns and Calluses*). A wart may bleed with debridement due to its vascular elements.

Pyogenic granuloma: Pyogenic granuloma bleeds easily.

Plan:

Treatment

Primary:

1. Débride overlying callus with #15 or 10 blade to allow medicine to reach wart.
2. Apply aperture (doughnut) pad to keep topical preparation isolated over the wart. 1/8" felt padding with sticky back works well. Pre-cut felt pads are available, but if material is in sheets, cut and size to fit. Moleskin is OK to cover but it will not relieve the load on a tender area. The padding and aperture prevents adjacent skin irritation. The hole matches up with the lesion, serving 2 purposes. It keeps the acid in contact with the wart tissue, protecting the good skin which is more vulnerable to acid breakdown. It takes pressure off the painful wart by redistributing pressure away from painful area.
3. Apply 60% **salicylic acid** paste (or **monochloroacetic acid**) to wart. Tape to cover and hold in place for 3 days. Any kind of tape will suffice.
4. Repeat treatment in one week.
5. Surgical curettage should be reserved for unresponsive cases and is not recommended in the field. Curettage reduces the chance of plantar scarring, when done correctly, the procedure does not involve penetration below the dermis.
6. A surgical excision of a wart using two semi-elliptical incisions is a consideration for a wart in a non-weight bearing area. Surgical excision should never be performed on weight bearing areas because of the risk of scarring and subsequent pain with ambulation.

Alternative: Liquid nitrogen (LN$_2$), **trichloroacetic acid,** many over-the-counter preparations. An application of **cantharidin**, which causes blistering, may be helpful when in non-operational mode. **Imiquimod** and **podofilox** are both prescription drugs that can be used, but expense can be an issue especially since it only works sometimes. It is better to use in select cases when primary measures fail. In operational mode the key is comfort. In present day lengthy operational ongoing active tempo coupled with spread among teammates, recommend active regular treatment until warts eliminated.

Primitive: Pad around wart to increase comfort in the field. Hold other treatment if short-term mission.

Patient Education

General: The cause of the wart is a virus. Topical re-treatment may be required. Discontinue treatment for a few days if the area becomes too sore and painful. Also discontinue if the area becomes infected. Do not pick at warts as this can spread the virus.

Medications: Use over-the-counter anti-inflammatories if pain significant.

Prevention and Hygiene: Use deck shoes or sandals in shower/pool areas to prevent spread among troops.

Follow-up Actions

Return Evaluation: Follow up weekly until resolved

Evacuation/Consultation Criteria: Evacuation not normally necessary. Consult podiatry or dermatology for resistant cases.

Chapter 9: Podiatry: Bunion (Hallux Abductor Valgus)

CDR Raymond Fritz, MSC, USNR (Ret)

Introduction: A bunion is an enlargement at the 1st metatarsal head. The great toe deviates laterally. Often there is no bump, but rather an angulation of the first metatarsal (hallux abductor valgus) that makes the head of this bone more prominent. Genetic factors, foot mechanics and poorly fitting or excessively worn shoes are commonly blamed for the development of both deformities. Pain is a result of cartilage erosion, bursitis and neuritis in the affected joints.

Subjective: Symptoms

Pain near first metatarsal head, history of a progressive deformity over time.

Focused History: *Is there pain over the prominent metatarsal head or within the great toe joint?* (Classic bunion pain is due to shoe pressure on the 1st metatarsal head rather than joint pain. Joint pain is often a result of limitation of motion, as well as, degenerative changes. If no pain, hallux valgus requires no immediate treatment in an operational environment.) *Is the pain a result of wearing certain shoes?* (usually the case for symptomatic bunions)

Objective: Signs

Using Basic Tools: Inspection: Bump, erythema and tenderness medially (tibial aspect) over the first metatarsal head; joint stiffness in more chronic cases, especially with excessive pronation (flat feet).

Using Advanced Tools: X-rays are helpful in evaluating angular relationships and joint integrity when available, but are not required.

Assessment: **Differential Diagnosis:** Diagnose by clinical presentation/appearance:

Rigid toe due to traumatic osteoarthritis (hallux rigidus or limitus): R/O if no pain or limitation with joint motion

Toe joint displacement/swelling (metatarsalgia, sesamoiditis): R/O if no pain with palpation of sesamoid or plantar aspect of met head

Local toe irritation (shoe irritation in absence of deformity): R/O if no evidence of skin irritation and no deformity visible

Plan:
Treatment
Primary:
1. Change to a wider shoe or soft sneaker if operationally permissible.
2. Use bunion pads. OTC bunion pads come in all shapes and sizes. A doughnut hole cut in felt or several layers of moleskin will work as a substitute for a bunion pad.
3. NSAIDs for pain relief. Ice massage if acute presentation
4. Arch supports and orthotics in severely pronated feet

Alternate: Inject **dexamethasone acetate** 0.25cc (or other long acting steroid) and 0.5% **bupivacaine** 0.5cc SC just medial to the metatarsal head as a one-time temporary pain relief measure during an operation. Multiple injections could weaken joint structures, causing progression of the deformity. Shoe or boot pressure can irritate the cutaneous nerve running medially along the first metatarsal head, causing severe neuritis pain and making ambulation difficult.

Primitive: Cut a hole in the boot over the bump if pain is severe.

Patient Education
General: Although these are structural deformities, changing shoe style and size may provide the most relief in an operational setting when surgery is not an option.
Activity: Limit running for 1-2 days. If pain is severe, wear open sandals for 2 days, if possible.
Medications: Ibuprofen 800mg po tid with meals
Prevention and Hygiene: Avoid tight shoes. Wear larger and wider boots, if necessary.

Follow-up Actions
Return Evaluation: 1-2 weeks
Evacuation/Consultation Criteria: Evacuation is not usually necessary. If no change with conservative measures, refer to podiatric or orthopedic surgeon.
Notes: Wider boot, shoe and running shoes are most important for pain relief. Postpone surgical correction until absolutely necessary. If deformity and symptoms are severe and conservative measures fail, elective surgery is an option.

Chapter 9: Podiatry: Corns and Calluses
CDR Raymond Fritz, MSC, USNR (Ret)

Introduction: A callus is a thickening of the outer layer of skin, in response to pressure or friction that serves as a protective mechanism to prevent skin breakdown. The hyperkeratotic change for corns and calluses is similar except a corn involves a discrete pressure spot, typically over a bone. Foot and toe deformities are subject to higher pressures and shoe irritation. A boot may rub a hammertoe at the knuckle and result in a painful corn. Corns may also develop between toes where two bones press together. Typical callus patterns are seen in certain foot types.

Subjective: **Symptoms**
Pain; history of a corn or callus in the same areas.
Focused History: *Has this happened before?* (If there is a significant foot prominence or deformity, there is usually a history of repeated callus build up. Find out if this is a recent problem that correlates to new footwear.)

Objective: **Signs**
Inspection: Thickened, dry skin over prominent bones (corn); larger patches of thickened, dry skin over friction areas from walking (calluses); tenderness, blisters, breakdown and infection after continued irritation.

Assessment: **Differential Diagnosis**
Wart: Black dots (dried blood) consistent with tiny vascular elements in warts. Warts bleed when trimmed.
Foreign body: Clinical presentation often reveals an entry point or mark

Plan:
Treatment
Primary: Trim areas with #15 blade or beaver blade. Trim with #10 blade for larger callus areas. Place felt with a doughnut-shaped hole cut in the middle (or pre-cut felt available over the counter) around area to relieve pressure and friction. Medicated pads are not recommended.
Alternative: Pad around prominent areas without trimming to protect and prevent irritation.
Primitive: Sand callus or corn gently with abrasive stone.

Patient Education
General: Daily foot inspections in the field if possible.
Prevention and Hygiene: Trim corns and calluses. Safest technique is to file areas with callus stone. Inspect shoes for frayed seams or torn liner. Check shoe fit. Mitigate source of pressure and deformities. There are many shoe and boot options available, such as depth shoes for digital deformities as well as extra widths. Orthotics address abnormal pressure areas and may eliminate chronic build up associated with certain foot types.

Follow-up Actions
Evacuation/Consultation Criteria: Evacuation not necessary. Refer to podiatrist for orthotics or surgery to correct deformities, or for other advanced foot care.

Chapter 9: Podiatry: Stress Fractures of the Foot

CDR Raymond Fritz, MSC, USNR (Ret)

Introduction: A stress fracture may affect any bone. The most common stress fracture in the foot, known in the military as a march fracture, is the 2nd metatarsal. Stress fractures are often seen in intense training programs around week 4, when bone absorption exceeds bone-building activity. Improper preparation, as well as, errors in training (warm-up, stretching, program progression) are causative factors.

Subjective: Symptoms

Pain in a specific area that persists during and after exercise; history of increased activity in a new program; or a specific event, such as a long run, which significantly exceeds previous training.

Focused History: *Does the pain lessen with activity or increase?* (Stress fractures do not usually improve with activity. Pain persists during the activity.) *Was there a recent increase in activity? Was there an increase in mileage? Was there an increase in intensity?* (Often program changes or new program demands cause bone depletion to get ahead of the bone remolding. The osteoclasts get ahead of the osteoblasts.) *When did your symptoms began in reference to the start of your new training program?* (Stress fractures are more prevalent at week 3-4 of a new activity or program.) *Did you do stretching and warm up activities?* (Check for higher incidence among given teams or units which could reflect back on the PT cadre.)

Objective: Signs

Using Basic Tools: Point tenderness with palpation. (Tibial stress fracture most common at junction of middle and lower thirds or middle and upper thirds of the bone. Tibial stress fractures/shin splints are often related to poor foot mechanics.) Significant edema in the dorsum of the foot over metatarsal fracture; compensatory antalgic gait.

Using Advanced Tools: X-rays (if available): Initially normal but repeat study at 3-4 weeks after onset will often show slight callus formation.

Assessment: Differential Diagnosis

Metatarsal stress fracture: Very specific pinpoint tenderness directly over the bone shaft dorsally

Metatarsalgia: Pain with palpation of the met head from the plantar aspect of the ball of the foot

Freiberg's neuroma: Pain with interspace palpation

Capsulitis: Pain surrounding the joint and often present with motion of the joint

Plan:

Treatment

Primary:

1. Conservative: Rest until point tenderness subsides; ice (24-48 hours) and NSAIDs (*see Part 8: Procedures: Chapter 30: Pain Assessment and Control*). Diagnosis of stress fracture mandates eliminating running until no point tenderness at site. Recurrence is high if bone is not allowed to heal completely
2. Alternate exercise: Swimming or biking in place of running to maintain cardiovascular fitness. Gradually resume a running program once pain free.
3. Identify biomechanical and structural predisposing factors (ie, tibial varum, cavus foot, flatfoot, long 2nd or short 1st metatarsal) and treat with appropriate custom foot orthotics.
4. Short term immobilization if necessary, especially with non-compliant individuals.

Alternative: Arch supports, padding to decrease weight on specific area. A metatarsal pad or doughnut cutout will decrease weight on the metatarsal when correctly placed.

Primitive: For metatarsal stress fractures, duct tape two tongue blades transversely across boot just behind the metatarsal heads, or use other substitute material to fill arch area to get some weight off the involved metatarsal head.

Patient Education

General: Do alternate activities to maintain fitness. Return to running activities progressively after time off. Start with a walking program for one week once pain free. If still symptom-free, start running short distances the second week. Slowly increase distance and speed.

Diet: One calcium carbonate tablet a day, and balanced diet with adequate calcium.

Medications: Be alert for gastritis with NSAIDs. Take the NSAIDS with food. Stay well hydrated.

Prevention: Perform proper warm up, stretching, warm down activities, wear good-fitting, high-performance athletic shoes. Change running shoes every 3-6 months depending on mileage. The mid-sole will wear out long before the outer sole.

Follow-up Actions

Return Evaluation: At 2 week intervals until released to full duty. Cannot resume full duty unless pain free. Consider immobilization

Evacuation/Consultation Criteria: Evacuation not necessary unless mission requires heavy weight-bearing or long hikes. Podiatry or orthopedic consultation recommended for stress fractures. Custom orthotics, highly recommended, especially in recurrent cases and are absolutely the best way to address abnormal foot mechanics when responsible for recurrent stress fractures.

Notes: If stress fracture incidence or any specific injury statistically increases in any one team or unit, take a closer look at the training program and cadre. Encourage troops to present early rather than suffering with the "suck it up...No pain, no gain" attitude until disabled.

Chapter 9: Podiatry: Friction Foot Blisters

CDR Raymond Fritz, MSC, USNR (Ret)

Introduction: Friction blisters are a common injury in the military. Training programs subject individuals to high intensity activities, including high-mileage running and land navigation. Footwear is often new and sometimes ill-fitting. Swim fins may also cause blisters. Hyperhidrosis (excessive sweating) of the feet may increase friction over pressure areas in the shoe. A high arch or cavus foot may be more susceptible to shoe rub and blister formation on the top of the foot, as well as, over the metatarsal head area.

Subjective: **Symptoms**

Sore feet, blister, history of high-level training or running

Focused History: *Have you had problems with blisters in the past?* (suggests ongoing problems) *Did you recently buy new shoes? Are they causing pressure and irritation?* (determines if new shoes are causing the problem) *Do you have a problem with foot perspiration?* (Increased moisture will increase friction.)

Objective: **Signs**

Inspection: Obvious blisters over involved areas.

Assessment: Diagnosis is based on clinical presentation.

Differential Diagnosis

Genetic blister disease: Inconsistent patterns; more diffuse

Epidermolysis bullosa: Inherited disease in which bullae form from slight trauma

Insect bite: Discrete area often not necessarily in a high pressure or friction area.

Burn: Not usually consistent with pressure from shoe. Sunburn and spills usually affect the top of the feet when unprotected.

Plan:

Treatment:

Primary:

1. Prevent additional and future blisters.
2. Aspirate blister with a sterile needle. Avoid penetration if non-painful and free of infection, skin is the best biological dressing. Avoid penetrating deep tissues for fear of introducing infection. If infected, best to deroof and apply topical antibiotics.
3. Cleanse with povidone-iodine and cover with moleskin.
4. Leave the "roof" of the blister in place to act as a biological dressing. This will decrease tenderness until new skin forms and matures in a few days.
5. Do not inject blister with benzoin (no longer the preferred method for blister treatment).
6. If infected, the blistered skin covering should be removed using a scalpel or scissors. Cleanse the area and apply a thin layer of **bacitracin/neomycin/polymyxin B** or **bacitracin** followed by a thin non-adherent dressing. Then apply moleskin over the dressing and adjacent skin to hold everything in place. Coban and Elastoplast also work well for holding dressings in place on the foot.
7. Avoid bulky coverings if an operator is in the field (in boots) and must continue with the mission. Topical anesthetic may help

Alternative:

Option 1: If the blister is already open as a result of repetitive irritation, the underlying skin is usually clean and red. Remove remaining loose skin, cleanse and treat open area as previously discussed. Place felt "doughnut" around blister to decrease pressure and irritation.

Option 2: Apply tincture of benzoin topically to toughen the skin and hold moleskin in place. Drain fluid with fine gauge needle (27-30). Apply an antibiotic ointment, a layer of DuoDerm over top and a doughnut pad to prevent rubbing. Blister roof may reattach to underlying skin, allowing rapid healing and return to duty.

Primitive: Pop the blister if large and painful. Cleanse if conditions permit. Place moleskin or duct tape over the area and continue with the operation.

Patient Education

General: Continue with activities if possible. If infection or deeper ulceration develops, rest feet and eliminate pressure to allow healing.

Prevention and Hygiene:

1. Make sure boots/shoe are the right size and width (fit the larger, longer foot). Try shoes on and stand to check fit. If orthotics or other shoe devices are used, remember to try shoes on with the orthotics in them before purchasing. The longest toe should be one thumb width from the end of the shoe. Try a short test run and then check your feet. Avoid wearing new boots for the first time on a field exercise.
2. Always carry extra socks in the field. Wear synthetic moisture wicking socks (ie, polypropylene) next to the skin and wool as a second layer because it retains insulating properties when wet. Fit boots with the two-layer sock system at the time of the boot purchase. Do not wear cotton socks. Cotton retains moisture and increases the coefficient of friction. Change socks often to keep them clean and dry.
3. For hyperhidrosis, apply products such as alum or Drysol (drying prevents skin softening) to the soles of the feet 3 x a week as needed.
4. Apply moleskin patches to areas that previously blistered.
5. Pad hammertoes and other prominent areas with Silipos or other padding devices. An optional method: spray clean, dry feet with AeroZoin (40% tincture of benzoin, 60% alcohol), let dry, then apply thin layer of Hydropel. Use a single sock with this method.

Follow-up Actions

Return Evaluation: Only if needed

Evacuation/Consultation Criteria: Evacuation is not necessary unless cellulitis develops. Refer to dermatology or podiatry (structural foot abnormality) for evaluation of underlying foot or skin problems.

Chapter 10: Dentistry: General Information

COL Robert Cinatl, DC, USA; COL Charles Middleton, DC, USA; COL P. Shannon Allison, DC, USA

General Information: Ensure all team members are Dental Category 1 (all treatment complete) to include removal of 3rd molars (tooth numbers 1, 16, 17, 32; aka "wisdom teeth") before deployment. Dental Category 2 (some treatment is pending, but not judged to precipitate an emergency within 12 months) is not adequate for Special Operations soldiers. Whenever possible, include the Dental Surgeon in any treatment of indigenous populations. Refer US personnel to the Dental Surgeon for definitive care if emergency care is necessary by the medic.

Figure 5-1. Anatomy of the Tooth

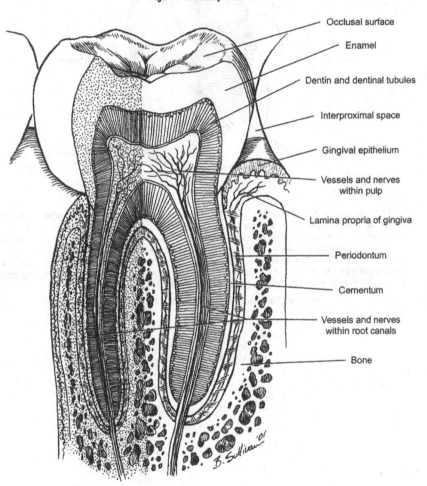

- Occlusal surface
- Enamel
- Dentin and dentinal tubules
- Interproximal space
- Gingival epithelium
- Vessels and nerves within pulp
- Lamina propria of gingiva
- Periodontum
- Cementum
- Vessels and nerves within root canals
- Bone

Anatomy:
1. Teeth have four structural components (*see Figure 5-1*):
    a. the pulp: live connective tissue with blood and lymph vessels, and nerve fibers
    b. the dentin: the bulk of the tooth, with 10,000 tubules/square millimeter, hence is sensitive when exposed
    c. the enamel: highly crystalline, covers the crown of the tooth
    d. the cementum: a thin covering over the root of the tooth that allows the fibers of the periodontal ligament (PDL) to hold the tooth to the alveolar bone
2. The crown has five surfaces (*see Figure 5-2*):
    a. the occlusal (biting) surface
    b. the lingual (tongue side) surface
    c. the facial or buccal (cheek side) surface
    d. the two surfaces that come in contact with adjacent teeth (mesial- the contacting surface nearest the midline and distal- the farthest from the midline)

Figure 5-2. Occlusal Surface of the Tooth

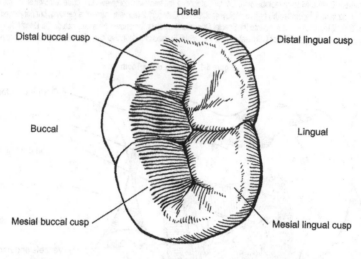

Distal

Distal buccal cusp

Distal lingual cusp

Buccal

Lingual

Mesial buccal cusp

Mesial lingual cusp

Mesial

3. North American tooth numbering, the so-called Universal System (*see Figures 5-3, 5-4 and 5-5*), is No. 1 (upper right third molar) to No. 32 (lower right third molar). The nomenclature for teeth varies around the globe. When treating in conjunction with any other nationalities, ensure the same nomenclature is used consistently. "No. 11" ("eleven") in the Universal System is the maxillary left canine, which is not the same as the FDI Two-Digit System that calls the maxillary right central incisor "No. 11" ("one-one"). Pronunciation of the FDI Two-Digit System is to say each digit individually, hence, "12" is "one-two" (not "twelve"), and in Spanish is "uno-dos" (not "doce"). No. 24, "two-four" is the upper left first premolar, and in German that tooth is "zwei-vier" not vierundzwangzig. You can name all the teeth in another language (11-85) by merely knowing the names of digits 1-8.

Figure 5-3. Universal System, North American Tooth Numbering

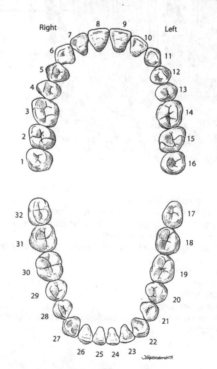

Figure 5-4. Numbering Systems for Permanent Teeth

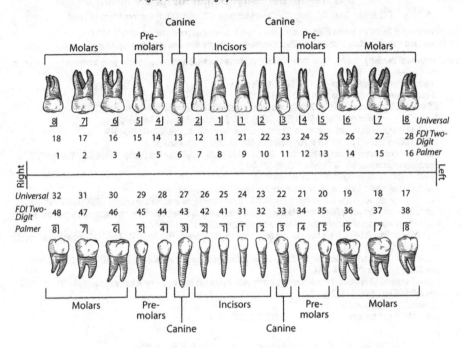

Figure 5-5. Numbering Systems for Deciduous Teeth

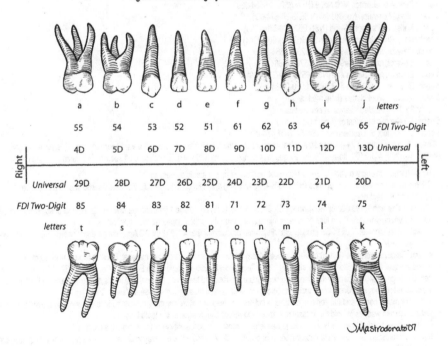

Chapter 10: Dentistry: Dental Kit for the Field

COL Robert Cinatl, DC, USA; COL Charles Middleton, DC, USA; COL P. Shannon Allison, DC, USA

Suggested Minimal Dental Kit for the Field: Always include the cold sterilization immersible set: 6530-01-530-4731: Cold Sterilization Jar with Strainer; and a sterilizing fluid, such as Cidex 28 or Wescodyne. Follow the directions of the fluid for time of immersion.

Operative/General Dentistry: You may order more of these instruments in order to have one set to treat while another set is in a chemical sterilant or autoclave.

    2 each: Syringe, cartridge, dental (NSN 6515-01-010-8761)
    25 each: 27 gauge dental needle (NSN 6515-00-181-7412)
    100 each: 0.5% **bupivacaine** with 1:200,000 **epinephrine** anesthetic 1.8 ml capsule (NSN 6505-01-189-3973)
    2 each: Combined mirror dental No. 5 (NSN 6520-00-782-2648) & handle (NSN 6520-00-541-9350)
    2 each: Combination instrument explorer No. 23 and periodontal probe No. 4 (NSN 6520-00-890-1643)
    2 each: McCalls 13S/14S periodontal scaler, (NSN 6520-00-890-2050), or equivalent
    2 each: Diamond sharpening surface for scaler (NSN 5345-01-529-6204; "DMT Diamond Diasharp Credit Card Sharpener")
    2 each: Spoon excavator No. 36/37 (NSN 6520-00-935-7184)
    2 each: Dental spatula No. 324 (NSN 6520-00-556-8000)
    2 each: Plugger, plastic filling, dental--Woodson No. 2 (NSN 6520-00-536-5405)
    1 each: Syringe, air, dental (the bulb syringe to dry a tooth, not the same as the anesthetizing syringe). (NSN 6520-00-501-8000)
    1 each: Box kit of Intermediate Restorative Material (IRM): one bottle of zinc oxide powder, one small spoon dispenser, one bottle of eugenol liquid with dropper. Listed under "cement" in the formulary. NSN 6520-01-169-1762
    20 each: Adper Prompt L-Pop single step etch and bond, order the box of twenty, Item No. 41923 from 3M Company: www.3MESPE.com, or (800) 634-2249
    1 pack: Nitinol Classic orthodontic wire, size "16 by 16", individually packaged, 10 wires/ pack, order catalog No. 297-803 from www.3MESPE.com, or (800) 634-2249
    1 pack: Transbond XT syringes of translucent dental composite, a pack has four 4 gram syringes, order catalog No. 712-036 from www.3MESPE.com, (800) 634-2249
    100 each: Cotton rolls and cotton gauze
    1 each: Mixing pad; parchment paper, dental (NSN 6520-01-257-1908)

Surgery:
    1 each: Tooth extraction forceps No.150AS - universal maxillary forceps (NSN 6520-00-180-5964)
    1 each: Tooth extraction forceps No. 23 - mandibular "cowhorn" forceps (NSN 6520-01-057-6542)
    1 each: Periosteal elevator, Molt No. 9 (NSN 6520-00-584-2699)
    1 each: Straight elevator, No. 301 (NSN 6520-00-524-3050)
    1 each: Mallet, oral surgery, Mead (NSN 6520-00-540-2050)
    1 each: No. 4 Chandler osteotome (NSN 6520-01-006-9344)
    1 each: Elevator, root, West #9L (NSN 6520-00-864-6789)
    1 each: Elevator, root, West #9R (NSN 6520-00-864-6790)
    1 each: Elevator, root, Seldin #1L (NSN 6520-00-524-5400)
    1 each: Elevator, root, Seldin #1R (NSN 6520-00-5405)
    5 each: No. 15 scalpel blades (from medical set)
    1 each: Bard Parker blade handle (from medical set)
    5 each: 3-0 chromic gut sutures (from medical set)
    1 each: Crunch tool by Leatherman (NSN 5110-01-474-0895)
    10 each: 5-inch lengths of 24-gauge soft surgical wire, pre-stretched, for Ivy loops. Order 200 yard spools from ACE Surgical Supply, Boston, MA (800) 441-3100: Item 0800090, 24 gauge, 4 ounce, approx $30 each. Stretch wire off spool before cutting to 5-inch lengths

Optional Items (beyond the Tactical Set) which must be ordered by the medic as desired:
    3% **mepivacaine** without epinephrine (NSN 6505-01-242-9149) anesthetic 1.8mL carpule (for patients who should not receive exogenous epinephrine)
    2% **lidocaine** with 1:100,000 **epinephrine** (NSN 6505-01-146-1139) anesthetic 1.8mL carpule (the standard dental anesthetic in the US).
    Topical **benzocaine** 20% (for a less noticeable injection technique) & cotton-tipped wooden applicators
    1 each: Glass ionomer (Fuji IX-GP pronounced "Fuji Nine" product number 439901 by GC America) for a longer-term restoration than the issued IRM
    1 each: Calcium hydroxide (Dycal) to place in deep decay before the actual restorative material. Dycal is two small tubes of paste, mixed in equal amounts. Stomahesive strips by ConvaTec Corp, No. 255-42, order from Edgepark Co. @ (800) 321-0591 for direct delivery; approx. $40 for pack of 15. Use to quickly secure repositioned teeth with this material that is similar to Bazooka bubblegum.
    Viscous lidocaine, in 100cc bottles: topical for oral pain, lesions, and irritated throat. Use as "swish & spit."
    Tofflemire matrix bands and the Tofflemire matrix band holder. Used to restore the interproximal surface of a tooth destroyed by decay. Wizard wooden wedges to hold the Tofflemire matrix band holder snugly against the tooth.
    Dental enamel hatchet (various types) used to cleave off enamel over soft decay in order to restore a tooth.
    Can of compressed "air" (usually a fluorocarbon propellant) to clear debris while excavating decay (the tac set provides a squeeze ball air syringe)
    Portable hand held electric dental drill with thirty to forty No. 245 excavating burs. These are expensive items and difficult to sterilize in the field.

Chapter 10: Dentistry: Oral and Dental Problems: Calculus (Tartar)

COL Robert Cinatl, DC, USA; COL Charles Middleton, DC, USA; COL P. Shannon Allison, DC, USA

Introduction: One of the most useful skills by a medic to treat an indigenous population is to remove calculus. Anesthetic is optional, hence saving time and resources. "Scaling" means removing calculus, and can cease at any time without harming the patient, unlike extractions, which must be completed once started, regardless of difficulty or time necessary. No radiographic image is required to scale calculus from teeth. The material is porous, like coral in the ocean, and harbors many species of bacteria. If a goal is to treat a number of people on the first visit to a local area, plan to scale the same limited area on all patients rather than completely scale only a few patients. Suggested: scale the lower right quadrant (teeth No. 25 to 32, as present) on all inhabitants, then on subsequent visits to the locale, treat a second quadrant, then a third, etc. Be aware that removing calculus on some teeth with very severe bone loss may cause that tooth to be lost since in some cases the tooth is stable only due to huge calculus accumulation.

Subjective: **Symptoms**
No symptoms may be expressed by the patient since the slow accumulation of this hard material allows the patient to become accustomed to its presence.

Objective: **Signs**
The material may be cream colored to black, and may have a soft layer of new plaque on the external surface.

Assessment:
Decide before beginning how many teeth will be treated on each patient if treating multiple patients of an indigenous population.

Plan: **Treatment**
Engage the calculus with the cutting edge of the scaler, not the tip of the scaler. Chip away carefully so as to not break the tip of the McCall scaler. Sharpen the scaler as often as needed to maintain an edge sharp enough to shave a fingernail. Do not use the sharp point of the scaler since it can gouge a tooth; the point is merely the joining of the two cutting surfaces. Review more information on the electronic version.

Chapter 10: Dentistry: Oral and Dental Problems: Periodontal Abscess

COL Robert Cinatl, DC, USA; COL Charles Middleton, DC, USA; COL P. Shannon Allison, DC, USA

Introduction: This acute suppurative infection occurs in the periodontal tissues alongside the root of a tooth and involves the alveolar bone, periodontal ligament and gingival tissues. Irritation from a foreign body, subgingival calculus ("tartar," hard calcific deposits on the teeth), and bacterial invasion of the periodontal tissues are common causes.

Subjective: **Symptoms**
Deep, throbbing, well-localized pain of the soft tissues surrounding the tooth. The tooth may feel elevated in its socket.

Objective: **Signs**
Redness, tenderness and swelling of the surrounding gingiva; sensitivity to percussion; mobile tooth; cervical lymphadenopathy is possible in extreme cases; fever (especially in children); purulent exudate.

Assessment: **Differential Diagnosis**
Chronic apical abscess from a necrotic pulp

Plan: **Treatment**
1. Carefully follow the terrain of the gingival sulcus (the "gutter" around the neck of the tooth) and probe with the No. 4 periodontal probe to locate the site of the infection. You may be able to drain the gingival crevice and locate any foreign body (such as a popcorn kernel).
2. (Optional if resources exist): Spread the tissues gently and irrigate with saline to remove remaining pus or debris from the abscess.
3. Anesthetize the area. Remove any foreign bodies. Scale the surface of the root with the McCall 13S/14S periodontal scaler as the definitive treatment.
4. The patient may rinse with warm saline hourly for comfort.
5. Administer antibiotic regimen if systemic conditions are present (elevated temperature, lymphadenopathy).
6. Refer US personnel for definitive care by the Dental Surgeon.

Chapter 10: Dentistry: Oral and Dental Problems: Acute Necrotizing Ulcerative Gingivitis

COL Robert Cinatl, DC, USA; COL Charles Middleton, DC, USA; COL P. Shannon Allison, DC, USA

Introduction: Acute Necrotizing Ulcerative Gingivitis is aka Vincent's Disease or "trench mouth." Necrotic gingiva that produces a remarkably foul, metallic odor. General poor diet, fatigue, stress, lack of oral hygiene, and poor health are the most important precipitating factors. This disease is not transmissible. Untreated lesions are progressively destructive of the gingival tissues and underlying bone.

Subjective: **Symptoms**
Constant gnawing pain, marked gingival sensitivity and hemorrhage, fetid odor, foul metallic taste, general malaise and anorexia.

Objective: **Signs**
Necrosis, ulcers with a grey pseudomembrane cover, cervical lymphadenitis, fever. Advanced cases involve underlying bone

Assessment: **Differential Diagnosis**
Blood dyscrasias or vitamin deficiencies (scurvy), HIV-related periodontitis.

Plan: **Treatment**

Establish good oral hygiene in acute cases by following these steps:

1. First day: Swab the teeth and gingiva thoroughly with a 1:1 aqueous solution of 3% hydrogen peroxide on a cotton-tipped applicator. Repeat. Instruct the patient to rinse his mouth at hourly intervals with this same 1:1 solution. Issue the patient one pint hydrogen peroxide. Caution patient not to use this treatment for more than two days (due to possibility of precipitating a fungal infection). Place the patient on an adequate soft diet and advise a copious fluid intake. Adequate rest, food, and fluid are critical. Analgesics may be administered. Have patient return in 24 hours.
2. Second – third day: Patient will be much more comfortable. Using a soft toothbrush soaked first in hot water, clean the patient's teeth without touching the gingiva. Maintain the hourly hydrogen peroxide mouthwash regimen and have patient brush with a soft toothbrush warmed in hot water. Have patient return in 24 hours.
3. Third – fourth day: Patient is essentially free of pain. Clean patient's teeth as before. Floss between all teeth. Discontinue hydrogen peroxide mouthwash regimen. May initiate **chlorhexidine** rinse bid for the next four to five days. Have patient brush tid-qid and floss once per day.
4. After treatment, the acute form subsides and the chronic phase ensues. Although clinical symptoms are minimal, tissue destruction continues until further corrective measures are completed. Definitive care consists of cleaning and scaling of the teeth by a dental officer, instruction in oral hygiene. In some cases, re-contouring the tissues involved in the infection is necessary by a periodontist.

Notes: Unless the patient develops systemic involvement, antibiotic therapy (including lozenges) should not be instituted. As in other oral disorders, the use of silver nitrate or other caustics is definitely contraindicated. Any case of gingivitis that does not respond well within 24-48 hours should be referred for evaluation for underlying blood dyscrasias or vitamin deficiencies.

Chapter 10: Dentistry: Oral and Dental Problems: Toothaches

COL Robert Cinatl, DC, USA; COL Charles Middleton, DC, USA; COL P. Shannon Allison, DC, USA

Introduction: Toothaches are usually associated with one of the following: caries (decay); fractures of tooth, crown, or root; or acute periapical (at the end of the root) abscess. All tooth surfaces may be affected by dental decay.

1. Dental Caries ("cavities")

Subjective: **Symptoms**

Intermittent or continuous pain, usually intense. Cold, sweet, or acid substances may worsen the pain.

Objective: **Signs**

Determining the offending tooth may be difficult. It may be grossly decayed, with the enamel missing and dentin area discolored. However, decay between the teeth can progress completely to the pulp with no observable evidence; only bitewing radiographs at the dental clinic will reveal such decay. A tooth with deep decay will be tender and sensitive to heat and cold. Tapping the tooth with the end of a dental mirror may elicit pain. When conducting a thermal test, use a normal tooth as a basis for comparison. A vital tooth will give a painful response to cold; a necrotic tooth will elicit no response to cold. However, a pulp may be almost completely necrotic yet the last remaining nerve fibers will still respond to a stimulus, thus providing a false positive; the pulp still requires removal.

Assessment: **Differential Diagnosis**

Caries in a vital tooth may be symptomatic. Caries in a non-vital ("dead") tooth produces no symptoms from decay, only from the bacteria living off the necrotic pulp. Maxillary posterior teeth: sinusitis can mimic toothache. Two tests to differentiate sinusitis from toothache:

1. The patient stands up, bends forward at the waist and holds toes for 90 seconds. If the pain migrates to an infraorbital pain, it may indicate the purulent exudate in the sinus has rolled to the lowest gravitational surface.
2. Have the patient hop eight times. If the pain is accentuated with contact of the feet on the floor, it may indicate the weight of a purulent exudate in the sinus is irritating the soft tissue lining of the sinus and mimicking tooth pain. *See Part 3: General Symptoms: ENT Problems: Sinusitis*

Plan:

Treatment

Primary: Remove caries and place a temporary restoration. Local anesthetic is necessary before excavating decay. *See Part 5: Specialty Areas: Chapter 10: Dental Procedure: Dental Anesthesia*

Alternate: For teeth that are still vital: **Eugenol (IRM liquid)** is an agent that will temporarily soothe hyperemic pulp tissue if treated indirectly (if not in direct contact with the pulp). A mix of **zinc oxide** and **eugenol** applied directly to vital pulp will kill the pulp. A dental officer must provide definitive care in the near future when a temporary restoration is placed in the field.

2. Acute Periapical Abscess: Purulent material is at the apex, or end, of the root (hence, "peri-apical").

Subjective: **Symptoms**

Repeated episodes of pain that have gradually become more continuous and intense. The accumulating pus causes increased pressure and the tooth will feel "high" to the patient; it will seem to be the first tooth to strike when the teeth are brought together. Malaise and anorexia are sometimes reported.

Objective: **Signs**

Severe tooth pain on percussion is significant. Always begin percussion testing on a tooth that appears normal, then progress to the suspected tooth. Swollen, tender gingival tissues around the tooth may or may not be present. Fever. Bright red elevation of the soft tissues somewhere in the quadrant due to burrowing of pus through alveolar bone. A draining sinus tract may be distant from the culprit tooth; radiographs are required for an accurate diagnosis.

Assessment:

Pain on percussion of posterior maxillary teeth may indicate sinusitis. Rule out sinusitis with the same tests as in Dental Caries.

Plan:

Treatment

Drainage usually provides immediate relief from pain (*see Part 5: Specialty Areas: Chapter 10: Dental Procedures: Draining a Tooth Abscess*). Consider antibiotics (*see Part 5: Specialty Areas: Chapter 10: Dental Procedures: Antibiotics*). Extracting the offending tooth should be a last resort. Evacuate for definitive care to a dental clinic.

Figure 5-6. Untreated Acute Periapical Abscess
Note: Arrows indicate possible routes of infection and pain.

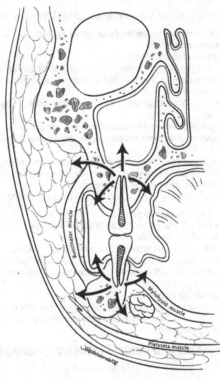

3. Untreated Acute Periapical Abscess: The typical course: accumulation of pus and destruction of bone at the apex (end of root) of the tooth, invasion of the marrow spaces and destruction of bone trabeculae, destruction of the cortex and displacement of the periosteum by suppurative material, rupture of the periosteum with resulting gingival swelling ("gum boil" or parulis) and finally spontaneous drainage by rupture of the parulis, which relieves pressure and may reduce the patient's willingness to undergo treatment since pain has "disappeared." *See Figure 5-6*

Subjective: **Symptoms**

Various presentations, depending on direction of spread of the abscess, which is usually toward the lateral aspect of the jaw, but may drain into the palate, under the tongue, or through the facial epidermis.

Objective: **Signs**

Erythema, swelling with fluctuance, and purulent drainage; fever, malaise and anorexia are common. Infection can spread through the facial spaces of the neck, and grave, possibly fatal complications (eg, Ludwig's angina) may result. If a cellulitis is present, consider IV antibiotics and rapid involvement of other treatment professionals. Protect the airway and do not waste time.

Assessment:

Rapid progression of a neoplasm may be included in the differential diagnosis, but an infection will expand much faster.

Plan: **Treatment**

a. Administer antibiotics for 7-10 days; *see Part 5: Specialty Areas: Chapter 10: Dental Procedures: Antibiotics*
b. Extract tooth after the acute symptoms subside. Positively identify the involved tooth.
c. Drain abscess surgically even with spontaneous drainage. Otherwise, the infection will recur, especially during periods of lowered resistance.
d. Evacuate for definitive care if extraction does not resolve the infection.

4. Tooth/Crown Fractures. Anterior (front) teeth are particularly susceptible to injuries that result in fracture of the crown. Cusps of posterior teeth can fracture if a large amalgam restoration is present.

Subjective: Symptoms

History of trauma or biting hard object; the patient feels a jagged tooth edge; sensitivity to heat/cold.

Objective: Signs

Visibly broken or cracked tooth.

Assessment:

Look for other injury if related to trauma, especially loss of consciousness.

Plan: Treatment

For simple fractures of the crown involving little or no dentin, smooth the rough edges of the tooth with an emery board or small flat file.

For extensive fractures of the crown involving considerable dentin but not the pulp:
   a. Isolate and dry the tooth with cotton gauze or rolls.
   b. Cover the exposed dentin using one of several methods:
      (1) Adper Prompt L-Pop: activate by squeezing the blisters toward the wand, agitate the wand vertically to mix the fluids, scrub the wand on the fracture for three seconds, then cure with a white light source (Minimag or Surefire) for one minute. Refer to the electronic version to review use of the Adper wand.
      (2) Glass ionomer cement can be used as a substitute for IRM, and has the advantage of adhering to teeth. You must order this material outside the formulary.
      (3) Cover the exposed dentin with **zinc oxide-eugenol paste (IRM)** (retention on anterior fractures is difficult). A dental officer may have an aluminum crown, which can be trimmed and contoured then filled with this paste and placed over the tooth. IRM is listed under "cement" in the formulary.
      (4) Incorporate cotton fibers into a mix of zinc oxide and eugenol (the fibers give additional strength) and place this over the involved tooth, using the adjacent teeth and the spaces between them for retention. Have the patient bite to be sure neither the bands nor the "splint" interferes with bringing the teeth together.
   c. As soon as possible, arrange for treatment by the Dental Surgeon, or an Area Support Dental Company.

Extensive fractures involving the dentin and exposed pulp:
   1. Anesthetize the tooth. *See Part 5: Specialty Areas: Chapter 10: Dental Procedures*
   2. Isolate and dry the tooth with cotton gauze or rolls.
   3. Scrub Adper Prompt L-Pop around the pulp exposure, but not on the pulp itself. Pull wisps of cotton from the end of a cotton roll, roll this into a tiny wad and place on the exposed pulp. Cover the wad and the tooth surfaces that have been prepped with the Adper Prompt L-Pop with the translucent "composite" paste, Transbond XT. Expose the paste to a white light source (Minimag or Surefire) for one minute or until hard.
   4. Glass ionomer cement is an alternate material.
   5. The efficacy of this treatment regimen depends on the size of the pulp exposure. If the exposure is larger than 1.5mm, you may be forced to perform an extraction, if no definitive treatment by a dental officer is possible.
   6. Evacuate for definitive care in a dental clinic.

Chapter 10: Dentistry: Oral and Dental Problems: Luxated (Dislocated) Tooth

COL Robert Cinatl, DC, USA; COL Charles Middleton, DC, USA; COL P. Shannon Allison, DC, USA

Introduction: A tooth traumatically moved from normal position.

Subjective: Symptoms

History of trauma, such as a high velocity blunt blow or a fall. Occupants of hatches in armored vehicles may impact the hatch during a sudden stop.

Objective: Signs

Visibly malpositioned tooth, loose in the socket, or several teeth as a segment moving together.

Assessment:

Evaluate for other injury if related to trauma, such as loss of consciousness.

Plan: Treatment

Administer local anesthetic (*see Part 5: Specialty Areas: Chapter 10: Dental Procedures*). Manually reposition tooth into normal position and instruct the patient to stabilize tooth with gentle pressure during splinting procedure. Splint to adjacent teeth with Adper Prompt L-Pop, Transbond XT and wire. Extend any splint to two teeth on the right, and two teeth on the left of all visibly dislocated or fractured teeth. Alternates to the technique in the electronic version include: heavy monofilament fishing line, an IRM/cotton fiber splint, or glass ionomer splint.

Chapter 10: Dentistry: Oral and Dental Problems: Avulsed Tooth

COL Robert Cinatl, DC, USA; COL Charles Middleton, DC, USA; COL P. Shannon Allison, DC, USA

Introduction: Tooth completely removed from socket.

Subjective: Symptoms

History of trauma—the patient may literally present with tooth in hand.

Objective: **Signs**

Visible space or empty socket. Assessment: Evaluate for other injury if related to trauma, such as loss of consciousness.

Plan: **Treatment**

1. If tooth has been saved, transport avulsed tooth in any clean liquid medium (water, saline, patient's saliva) (not milk). Do not allow the tooth to dry. Gently rinse tooth with 0.9% normal saline if available. Do not scrape off any debris or attempt to scale the tooth.
2. Administer local anesthetic. *See Part 5: Specialty Areas: Chapter 10: Dental Procedures*
3. Replace tooth into its socket. If blood clot prevents tooth placement, rinse socket with saline from a Monoject syringe, or similar device, to remove the blood clot.
4. Splint the tooth to adjacent teeth with Adper Prompt L-Pop, Transbond XT and dental wire. Alternates include: IRM/cotton fiber splint, a glass ionomer splint, or even a paper clip.
5. Provide pain relief. Use **acetaminophen** or **ibuprofen** for mild pain. Use **acetaminophen** with **codeine** for more severe pain *provided no closed head injury* is involved. *See Part 8: Procedures: Chapter 30: Pain Assessment and Control*
6. Administer antibiotic regimen. *See Part 5: Specialty Areas: Chapter 10: Antibiotics*
7. Evacuate for definitive dental care such as endodontics ("root canal"). A partially avulsed tooth that is repositioned is usually permanently retained. A completely avulsed tooth may be permanently retained if replaced in the socket with minimal handling in less than one hour. When the replacement time exceeds one hour, the long-term retention rate drops and root resorption usually occurs in the next 12-60 months.

Chapter 10: Dentistry: Oral and Dental Problems: Localized Osteitis ("Dry Socket")

COL Robert Cinatl, DC, USA; COL Charles Middleton, DC, USA; COL P. Shannon Allison, DC, USA

Introduction: Caused by loss of blood clot at the site of an extracted tooth. Increases in frequency with increasing age, smoking, and failure to rest after an extraction, thus preventing the clot to adequately organize.

Subjective: **Symptoms**

Constant moderate to severe pain; may involve entire side of mandible; occurs 3-5 days after extraction, usually of a lower molar; foul taste and odor in mouth.

Objective: **Signs**

Visible open wound without clot; no fever; no purulent exudate or other signs of systemic infection.

Assessment: **Differential Diagnosis**

Abscess, trauma, osteomyelitis.

Plan: **Treatment**

1. Irrigation of extraction site with warm saline in a Monoject syringe or similar device.
2. Cut approximately two inch strip of iodoform gauze and apply one to two drops of **eugenol** (IRM liquid). Place eugenol/gauze gently into affected socket.
3. Change medicated gauze daily until symptoms are gone (may be 1-5 days).
4. May also administer a NSAID for pain. Antibiotics are rarely indicated. Despite the level of discomfort, alveolar osteitis will heal even with no treatment.

Chapter 10: Dentistry: Oral and Dental Problems: Herpetic Lesions (Cold Sores, Fever Blisters)

COL Robert Cinatl, DC, USA; COL Charles Middleton, DC, USA; COL P. Shannon Allison, DC, USA

Introduction: A re-activated dormant virus. Predisposing factors include stress, the common cold and other upper respiratory infections, gastrointestinal disorders, nutritional deficiencies, food allergies, and traumatic injuries to the oral mucosa. In females, menstruation and pregnancy. The herpetic lesion is highly contagious. The course of each episode is 2 weeks with or without treatment.

Subjective: **Symptoms**

Intense pain, itching, burning. Children with the primary or initial episode experience greater pain, larger affected area, anorexia, dehydration.

Objective: **Signs**

Small, localized ulcerations around the lips (few blisters in mouth) with a bright red, flat or slightly raised border; later, ulcer covered by white plaque; generalized infections produce large area of fiery red, swollen, and extremely painful mucosa (*see Appendices: Color Plates: A-22.D*). Children with the primary episode have more extensive and serious oral involvement resulting in anorexia and dehydration.

Assessment: **Differential Diagnosis**

Herpes zoster recurrent episode ("shingles"), oral syphilis, burns, erythema multiforme (Stevens-Johnson syndrome).

Plan: **Treatment**

1. Prevent spread of virus to eyes, fingers, genitals, or other people.
2. Treat precipitating factors. Stress and fatigue is simply treated with rest. The disease is self-limited and spontaneously resolves, though recurrence can be prevented.
3. Antibiotics may prevent secondary infection in severe cases only.
4. Force fluids to prevent dehydration.
5. Do not use topical steroids.
6. Apply viscous **lidocaine** or other topical anesthetic for pain. Antiviral drugs may shorten the episode by one day.

Chapter 10: Dentistry: Oral and Dental Problems: Aphthous Ulcers ("Canker" Sores)

COL Robert Cinatl, DC, USA; COL Charles Middleton, DC, USA; COL P. Shannon Allison, DC, USA

Introduction: Aphthous ulcers are common manifestations of various systemic diseases such as Behçet's syndrome, HIV, autoimmune disorders, and Crohn's disease. They are not contagious or caused by an infectious agent, and will heal in two weeks without sequelae. Stress, acidic foods, and chemical sensitivities, and stretching the mucosa may trigger an attack.

Subjective: Symptoms
Burning, itching, or stinging

Objective: Signs
Macule progressing to small dull grey ulcer surrounded by reddish halo (bull's eye) on oral tissues. Lymph nodes may be swollen in the affected area.

Assessment: Differential Diagnosis
Herpetic lesions or other oral lesions; may be seen in more serious systemic and local diseases including Sutton's disease, Behçet's disease, Reiter's syndrome, leukopenias, Crohn's disease and ulcerative colitis.

Plan: Treatment
Apply viscous **lidocaine** and/or topical steroids to reduce pain. The steroids such as **triamcinolone** in Orabase gel, **fluocinonide** gel, **dexamethasone** rinses are not in the SF formulary but may be available from higher units if requested. Address underlying disorders and/or avoid triggers. Maintain healthy diet, ample fluids, and adequate rest.

Chapter 10: Dentistry: Oral and Dental Problems: Pericoronitis

COL Robert Cinatl, DC, USA; COL Charles Middleton, DC, USA; COL P. Shannon Allison, DC, USA

Introduction: Acute inflammation of tissue flaps over partially erupted teeth, especially lower 3rd molars (teeth Nos. 17 & 32, or "wisdom" teeth) caused by trauma from opposing teeth, food and debris, and bacteria.

Subjective: Symptoms
Marked pain radiating to the ear, throat and the floor of the mouth; fever; general malaise; muscle spasm in jaw.

Objective: Signs
Red, swollen, tender, possibly suppurative, gingiva localized over tooth; fever; cervical lymphadenopathy; trismus of the masticator muscles.

Assessment: Differential Diagnosis
Periapical abscess, trauma from opposing tooth.

Plan: Treatment
1. Good oral hygiene is mandatory
2. Flush between the partially exposed tooth and the overlying gingiva with a syringe.
3. Repeat this treatment at daily intervals until the inflammation subsides. Stress that oral hygiene must be maintained, brushing over the infected area several times throughout the day.
4. Prescribe an adequate soft diet.
5. Extract the opposing tooth if necessary. Do NOT attempt to extract the offending lower 3rd molar in the field—such an extraction requires the resources of a full-capability dental clinic in the event of a complicated extraction.
6. Antibiotic therapy may be indicated if the cervical nodes are swollen, or fever exists, and/or trismus of the masticator muscle exists. Extraction of the offending tooth must be arranged if the case warrants antibiotics since the subsequent episodes will only be worse.

Chapter 10: Dentistry: Oral and Dental Problems: Candidiasis (Thrush)

Candidiasis (Thrush): *See Part 5: Specialty Areas: Chapter 12: Fungal Infections: Candidiasis (Thrush) & Chapter 15: Most Common Pediatric Diseases: Mouth Problems: Thrush*

Chapter 10: Dentistry: Oral and Dental Problems: Barodontalgia

Barodontalgia: *See Part 6: Operational Environment: Chapter 21: Barodontalgia*

Chapter 10: Dentistry: Oral and Dental Problems: Injuries of the Jaw

Injuries of the Jaw: *See sections on "Jaw Dislocation" and "Jaw Fracture" at http://merckmanuals.com/home/sec08/ch117/ch117a.html*

Chapter 10: Dentistry: Oral and Dental Problems: Dislocation of the Temporomandibular Joint(s)

COL Glenn Reside, DC, USA (Ret) & COL Charles Middleton, DC, USA

Introduction. Dislocation of the temporomandibular joint (TMJ) occurs frequently, usually caused by mandibular hypermobility, but can also be caused by stress and trauma. The mandibular condyle translocates anteriorly in front of the articular eminence and becomes locked in that position (*see the electronic version*). Muscle spasm may then prevent the patient from closing the jaw into normal occlusion. Dislocation may be unilateral or bilateral and may occur spontaneously after opening the mouth widely while yawning, eating, or during a dental procedure. Dislocation of the TMJ is usually painful, is not self-reducing, and usually requires professional management.

Subjective: Symptoms
Pain in the preauricular area

Objective: Signs
Mouth locked in an open position; tender, bony prominence in preauricular area(s)

Assessment: Differential Diagnosis
Fractured mandible, or other trauma or lesion

Plan:
Treatment

Primary: Explain the procedure to the patient so he will relax. Manually reposition the mandibular condyle into the glenoid fossa by moving the dislocated mandible *inferiorly* and *anteriorly* from in front of the articular eminence, then, posteriorly behind the articular eminence, and finally, superiorly into the glenoid fossa.

1. Place yourself in the position to best control the patient's mandible and head: stand behind the patient, or stand in front of the patient.
2. Wrap your thumbs in gauze or a small towel (to avoid being bitten) and put them inside the patient's mouth on the last molar, or just lateral to the last molar. All four fingers of each hand should be placed along the inferior border of the mandible.
3. Apply firm, continuous pressure anteriorly and inferiorly, rotating the mandible down and away from the eminence. Then holding inferior pressure, move the mandible posterior to the eminence and superiorly into the fossa.
4. After the dislocation is reduced, it is imperative to maintain pressure on the chin to hold the teeth together because the patient frequently will reflexively open their mouth and dislocate again. The muscles of mastication are frequently in spasm while the mandible is dislocated and will forcefully close the mouth when the condyle is replaced into the glenoid fossa. Protect your thumbs from being bitten.

Alternate: If the muscles of mastication are in such spasm that you cannot manually manipulate the condyle, sedate the patient with a muscle relaxant such as **diazepam** 5-10mg po or **midazolam** 1-5mg IV prior to reducing the dislocation. In extremely rare cases, the patient may require general anesthesia in conjunction with the reduction. If the patient tends to reflexively open the mouth and cause repeat dislocations, apply a dressing over the top of the head and under the jaw to inhibit the motion of the mandible.

Primitive: Warm, moist heat to the sides of the face to relax the temporalis and masseter muscles and allow the patient to reduce the dislocation by himself.

Patient Education

General: Activity: Avoid trauma to the mandible. Avoid opening mouth too wide while chewing or yawning.

Diet: Cut food into small pieces. Chew a soft diet until the preauricular tenderness resolves.

Medications: Over-the-counter analgesics, such as acetaminophen 325-650mg po q6h not to exceed 4,000mg in a 24 period, or ibuprofen 200-800mg q6h not to exceed 3,200mg per 24 hour period.

Prevention and Hygiene: Avoid opening mouth wide while yawning, talking, eating, etc.

No Improvement/Deterioration: Refer to an oral-maxillofacial surgeon.

Follow-up Actions

Evacuation/Consultation Criteria: Evacuation is not usually necessary. If you are unable to achieve a proper reduction or if the patient presents on multiple occasions requiring emergent reduction, refer the patient to an oral and maxillofacial surgeon for evaluation and treatment.

Chapter 10: Dentistry: Antibiotics

COL Robert Cinatl, DC, USA; COL Charles Middleton, DC, USA; COL P. Shannon Allison, DC, USA

Dental Antibiotics. Administer antibiotics for 7-10 days duration. **Note:** Erythromycin is not indicated for dental infections

Table 5-1. Oral Dosages of Dental Antibiotics

Drug	Adults	Children
Penicillin VK Requires 500mg doses to perfuse the bone since 250mg is an insufficient dosage	Normal loading dose is 1g po, followed by 500mg q6h.	50mg/kg of body weight **per day**, divided into four equal doses for the day. Use adult doses over 12 years of age.
Clindamycin	600mg po loading dose followed by 300mg q6h.	20mg/kg of body weight per day divided into four equal doses for the day.

Chapter 10: Dentistry: Dental Procedures: Thermal Test for Pulpitis
COL Robert Cinatl, DC, USA; COL Charles Middleton, DC, USA; COL P. Shannon Allison, DC, USA

Introduction: If hot and cold are used, test a normal tooth as a basis for comparison. The application of cold to normal teeth elicits pain in most instances, but the response ceases soon after the stimulus is removed. A diseased tooth, compared to a normal tooth, varies in its reaction to the temperature test. For example, a reaction to cold could persist after the cold is removed, but the tooth responds very little to heat. Or, the reaction to heat persists after the heat source is removed, but the tooth appears to respond very little or not at all to cold. *See the electronic version.*

Perform procedure as follows:
1. Isolate the teeth to be tested from the saliva with packs of 2"x2" gauze.
2. Test an unsuspected tooth first to establish a baseline of the time elapsed until the tooth feels normal to the patient.
3. Cold test: Place a frozen carpule of dental anesthetic (if pre-prepared and available) on the tooth crown.
   Note the response and its duration. A vital tooth will give a painful response to cold that abates after the cold stimulus is removed.
4. Heat test: Heat an instrument (eg, a mouth mirror handle) and touch against the tooth. Note the response time and duration in seconds. Similar pattern to cold test.

Chapter 10: Dentistry: Dental Procedures: Dental Anesthesia: Anesthetics
COL Robert Cinatl, DC, USA; COL Charles Middleton, DC, USA; COL P. Shannon Allison, DC, USA

Introduction: (Analgesia – block pain impulses; Anesthesia – block all nerve impulses). *Refer to document at http://tinyurl.com/3w9vekh* for photographs of the proper location of the needle and syringe. Do not guess.

Table 5-2. Anesthetic Solutions

Drug	Description	Duration	Adult Max. Dose	Child Max. Dose
0.5% **bupivacaine** with 1/200,000 **epinephrine** (in the tactical set issued)	1.8mL carpule with blue lines	6-8 hours	10 carpules for healthy 70kg adult	2-3 carpules for child under age 12 (<50kg)
2% **lidocaine** with 1/100,000 **epinephrine** (must be ordered separately from the tactical set issued)	1.8mL carpule with red lines	2-4 hours	8 carpules for healthy 70kg adult	2-3 carpules for child under age 12 (<50kg); average is approximately one carpule per twenty pounds
3% **mepivacaine** without **epinephrine** (must be ordered separately from the tactical set issued)	1.8mL carpule with tan lines	½ -1 hour	6 carpules for healthy 70kg adult	1-2 carpules for child under age 12 (<50kg)

Note: Anesthetic agents with vasoconstrictors (epinephrine) should never be used in areas with limited blood supply: fingers, toes, ears, nose, and penis.

Chapter 10: Dentistry: Dental Procedures: Dental Anesthesia: Infraorbital Block
COL Robert Cinatl, DC, USA; COL Charles Middleton, DC, USA; COL P. Shannon Allison, DC, USA

Infraorbital block: (*See Figure 5-7*) Anesthesia for maxillary extraction.
A. Infiltration of anesthetic will provide adequate analgesia for most of the maxillary teeth.
B. Technique. Both facial and palatal injections (*see Figure 5-7*) must be performed. The palatal is an infiltration 3mm from the tooth, inject a few drops until the tissue blanches (not the same as the Greater Palatine block).
   (1) **Facial nerves:** Anterior teeth are serviced by the infraorbital nerve; posterior teeth by the posterior superior alveolar nerve.
      (a) Insert the needle into the mucobuccal fold directly above the tooth. Shaking the cheek and lip during needle insertion can help alleviate injection discomfort.
      (b) Advance the needle upward about one half of an inch until the needle gently contacts bone (this should approximate the root end).
      (c) Aspirate to ensure that the needle has not entered a blood vessel. Slowly deposit one carpule.

   Infiltration: A modification of the infraorbital block is to deposit anesthetic fluid at the root apex of a maxillary tooth. Retract the upper lip to provide a taut mucosa, insert the needle to the length to approximate the position of the apex, and deposit one carpule. The maxillary bone is porous and allows perfusion of anesthetic to the nerve fibers; the mandible is too dense to allow infiltration.

Figure 5-7. Infraorbital Block: Facial Injection

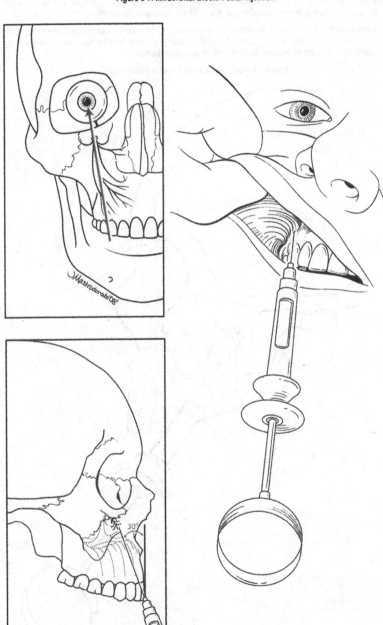

Chapter 10: Dentistry: Dental Procedures: Dental Anesthesia: Posterior Superior Alveolar Nerve Injection

COL Robert Cinatl, DC, USA; COL Charles Middleton, DC, USA; COL P. Shannon Allison, DC, USA

Posterior superior alveolar (PSA) nerve injection: (*see Figure 5-8*) Services the third molars (Nos. 1, 16), the second molars (Nos. 2, 15), and most of the first molars (Nos. 3, 14). The mesiobuccal cusp of the maxillary first molar (Nos. 3, 14) is not serviced by the PSA nerve! You must inject at the apex of the root of the mesiobuccal cusp of Nos. 3, 14 to ensure adequate anesthesia of the entire first molar.

The needle enters superior to the second molar. If perforation of the mucosa is apical to the first molar, you will contact the bone of the zygomatic buttress. Direct the needle 45° superiorly, and 45° medially in order to guide the tip of the needle around the maxillary tuberosity. Ensure to aspirate in this highly vascularized area. Deposit an entire carpule for the PSA.

Figure 5-8. Posterior Superior Alveolar Nerve Injection

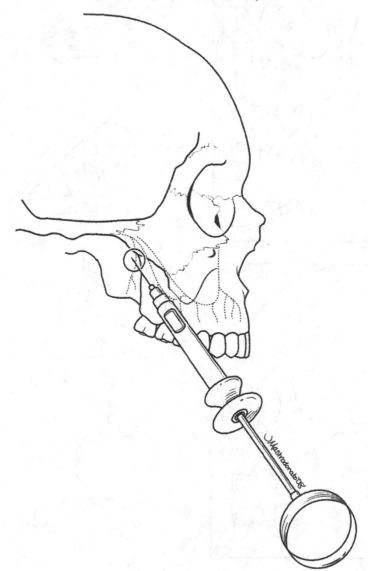

Chapter 10: Dentistry: Dental Procedures: Dental Anesthesia:
Greater Palatine Injection

COL Robert Cinatl, DC, USA; COL Charles Middleton, DC, USA; COL P. Shannon Allison, DC, USA

Greater palatine injection: (*see Figure 5-9 and the electronic version*) The palatal injection is very uncomfortable.

    A. Apply firm pressure to palatal injection site with a finger or mirror handle for 3-4 seconds. This helps to minimize needle insertion discomfort.

    B. Insert the needle halfway between the second molar and the midline of the palate. If the second molar is missing, estimate its previous location. Do not use the first molar as a substitute since the foramen of the nerve is not near the first molar.

    C. Deposit a small amount (<¼ carpule) of anesthetic solution. Do not "balloon" the tissue.

Figure 5-9. Greater Palatine Injection

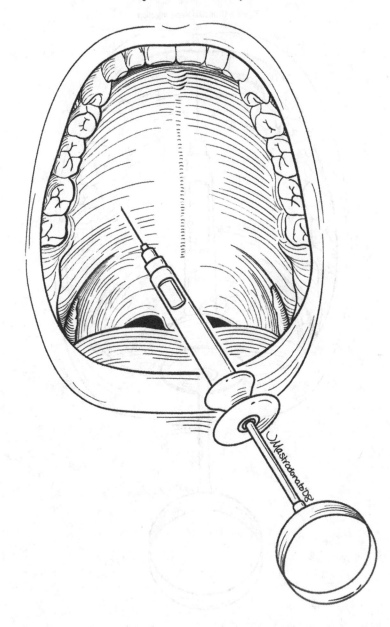

Chapter 10: Dentistry: Dental Procedures: Dental Anesthesia: Incisal Nerve Injection

COL Robert Cinatl, DC, USA; COL Charles Middleton, DC, USA; COL P. Shannon Allison, DC, USA

Incisal nerve injection: (*see Figure 5-10*) ONLY for extraction of the maxillary central incisors (teeth Nos. 8 & 9). The incisal nerve has no space in its bony canal to expand, hence the fluid of the anesthetic has no avenue to escape, and the technique is therefore extremely uncomfortable. Due to this discomfort, begin with anesthesia to the facial innervation on both sides of the midline, either both right and left infraorbital blocks, or infiltration at the apices of both central incisors. Once the facial anesthesia is complete, place two drops of anesthetic in the facial of the incisal papilla (the triangular soft tissue between Nos. 8 & 9). Those drops of fluid will blanch the tissue on the palatal side of the papilla and provide partial comfort for the final anesthetic. The third step is anesthetic fluid into the incisal papilla on the palatal (*see Figure 5-10*), which will still cause discomfort, but is rapidly successful. Advise the patient before the third step that they will still feel a "mosquito bite" but it will be very short in duration.

Figure 5-10. Incisal Nerve Injection

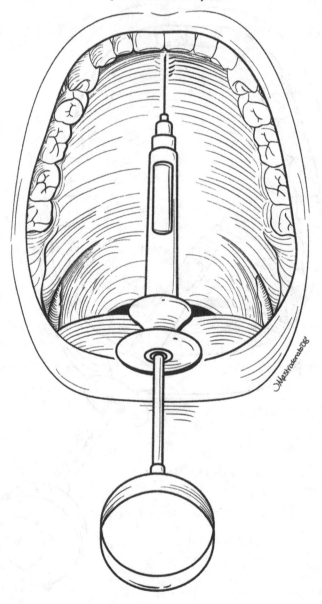

Chapter 10: Dentistry: Dental Procedures: Dental Anesthesia: Inferior Alveolar Block

COL Robert Cinatl, DC, USA; COL Charles Middleton, DC, USA; COL P. Shannon Allison, DC, USA

Inferior alveolar block: (*see Figure 5-11*) Block the inferior alveolar nerve as it enters the mandibular foramen on the medial aspect of the ramus of the mandible. This foramen is located midway between the anterior and posterior borders of the ramus and approximately one-half inch above the biting surface of the lower molars. Estimate the width of the ramus at this level by placing the thumb of your "helper" hand on the anterior surface of the ramus (intraorally) and the middle finger on the posterior surface extraorally. The inferior alveolar nerve enters the canal of the mandible midway between these two fingers.

A. Place the thumb on the biting surface of the lower molars so that the pad of the thumb will contact the anterior border of the ramus.

B. Place the barrel of the syringe on the lower bicuspids on the side opposite of the side to be anesthetized.

C. Insert the needle into the tissue of the side to be anesthetized about one-half of an inch distal from the tip of the thumb on a line horizontally bisecting the thumbnail.

D. Advance the needle to contact the medial surface of the ramus. A 1-inch soft tissue penetration will usually suffice to position the needle tip in the area of the mandibular foramen. Slowly deposit one carpule. Due to variation in anatomy, even an experienced practitioner will achieve only partial anesthesia in 20% of injections. Do not hesitate to re-anesthetize for a mandibular block in order to attain a comfortable patient.

Figure 5-11. Inferior Alveolar Block

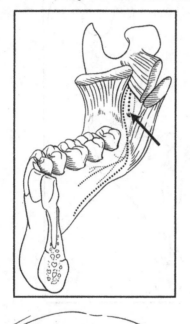

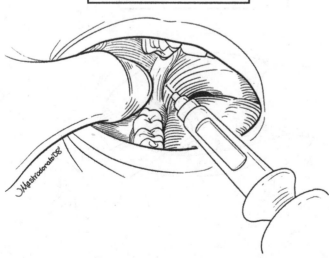

Chapter 10: Dentistry: Dental Procedures: Dental Anesthesia: Long Buccal Injection

COL Robert Cinatl, DC, USA; COL Charles Middleton, DC, USA; COL P. Shannon Allison, DC, USA

Long buccal injection: (*see Figure 5-12*) Complete anesthesia of the lower arch with a long buccal injection to anesthetize the buccal and gingival soft tissue. The nerve trunk servicing the buccal tissue branches early off the trigeminal ganglion and requires a separate injection. Insert the needle 45° distal and buccal from the most distal tooth in the arch. Inject one-half carpule.

After a 5 minute interval, evaluate the results of the injections to the inferior alveolar nerve, the buccal nerve, and the lingual nerve by checking the following symptoms:

    A. Numbness to the lower teeth and alveolar bone up to the midline.
    B. Numbness extending to the midline of the lower lip and tongue on the injected side.
    C. Numbness of the facial and lingual gingival tissue extending to the midline on the injected side.

Do not attempt extraction until the signs described are present.

Figure 5-12. Long Buccal Injection

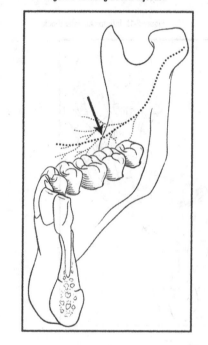

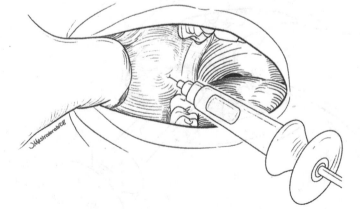

Chapter 10: Dentistry: Dental Procedures: Temporary Restorations

COL Robert Cinatl, DC, USA; COL Charles Middleton, DC, USA; COL P. Shannon Allison, DC, USA

What to Do:

1. Remove only the softest of the soft decayed material with the 36/37 "spoon" excavator. If the patient is properly anesthetized he should feel no pain.
2. Blow out the dislodged chips with the bulb air syringe.
3. Isolate the tooth with gauze packs and gently dry the cavity with cotton pellets.
4. Mix the Intermediate Restorative Material (IRM) zinc oxide powder with 2-3 drops of eugenol (IRM liquid) on a clean dry surface (parchment pad) until a thick puttylike mix is obtained. *See the electronic version*
5. Fill the cavity with the IRM putty, tamping it gently with the Woodson Plastic Instrument #2, or a moistened cotton tip applicator.
6. Have the patient bite several times to compress the putty, and to avoid a "high" restoration with the opposite teeth when the material sets hard.
7. Remove surplus filling material by lightly rubbing the tooth with a moist cotton pellet; the putty will harden within 5-10 minutes.
8. If IRM is not available, a cotton pellet slightly moistened with eugenol may be left in the cavity. Glass ionomer cement is an excellent substitute for the IRM and can be placed directly against exposed pulpal tissue.
9. Instruct the patient that the procedure is temporary and a dentist must provide definitive care.

Chapter 10: Dentistry: Dental Procedures: Tooth Extraction

COL Robert Cinatl, DC, USA; COL Charles Middleton, DC, USA; COL P. Shannon Allison, DC, USA

Introduction: View the photos and artwork on the electronic version. Avoid extractions on anyone who can be evacuated for definitive care by the Dental Surgeon. This section describes only one extraction technique.

1. Although many types of extraction forceps are manufactured, the removal of any erupted tooth can usually be accomplished with either the maxillary universal forceps, No. 150, or the mandibular cowhorn forceps, No. 23.
2. Technique after anesthetizing the surgical site:
   a. Sever the attachment of the gingival tissue to the tooth with the Molt No. 9 into the crevice between the tooth and the gingiva, around the circumference of the tooth. The tooth-tissue attachment should be severed to the level of the alveolar bone.
   b. Place the No. 301 elevator at a perpendicular to the long axis of the tooth, with the concave surface of the elevator toward the tooth to be extracted. Expand the bone with this instrument. Using slow movements, rotate the 301 clockwise or counterclockwise.
   c. Guide the beaks of the forceps under the gingiva on the facial and lingual surfaces of the tooth. Apply pressure toward the root of the tooth to force the tips of the forceps as far apically on the root as possible.
   d. Loosen teeth by slowly rocking the tooth with progressively increasing traction in a facial-lingual direction. To loosen single-rooted teeth, combine this rocking motion with rotation.
   e. When the tooth is loose, deliver it by exerting gentle traction. Follow the direction in which the tooth moves most easily and follow this path for delivery.
   f. Inspect the extracted tooth to determine if the roots have been fractured: intact root tips are blunt at the end. Fractured roots have a "crew cut" end, in which case you must decide whether to retrieve the remaining root with the 9R/9L root tip picks, or leave the tips alone. Refer to the electronic version before beginning extractions.
   g. After the extraction, compress the sides of the empty socket (this repositions the bone that has been splayed by the extraction) and place a folded dampened 2x2 gauze over the wound. Instruct the patient to maintain light biting pressure on this compress for 60 minutes. Repeat if necessary to control hemorrhage. Caution the patient NOT TO RINSE the mouth for at least 12 hours since this may disturb the clot. Tobacco use, and/or lack of rest for the first 48 hours can lead to loss of the blood clot. Good oral hygiene will decrease the chance of infection.

Chapter 10: Dentistry: Dental Procedures: Draining a Tooth Abscess

COL Robert Cinatl, DC, USA; COL Charles Middleton, DC, USA; COL P. Shannon Allison, DC, USA

Introduction Two methods may be used to accomplish adequate drainage:

1. For a "pointed" abscess, incise the fluctuant area using a stab procedure. Blunt dissection with a hemostat may help to establish drainage at the site. Suture a small drain or slice of surgical tubing in the wound to maintain drainage and leave until the drain is unproductive (may be one-five days). Local anesthetic should be used but pain control may not be easy to obtain.
2. For buccal or facial infections, the incision can be made in the vestibule or area of attached and unattached tissue next to the affected tooth, down to bone, and then dissected into the pus/exudate pocket.
3. If decay is evident, establish drainage through the tooth. Stabilize the tooth firmly with the fingers; remove the soft decay with a spoon-shaped instrument until an opening into the pulp chamber is made. Finger pressure on the gingiva near the root of the tooth may force pus out through the chamber opening. Irrigate with a Monoject syringe or equivalent. Dry with wisps of cotton and remove wisps when wet. Seal off with IRM or Transbond XT. Definitive treatment by a dental officer is required regardless of resolution of acute symptoms

Chapter 10: Dentistry: Dental Procedures: Stabilizing a Fractured Mandible with Ivy Loops

Stabilizing a Fractured Mandible with Ivy Loops: *See http://emedicine.medscape.com/article/870075*

Chapter 10: Dentistry: Civil Action Planning

COL Robert Cinatl, DC, USA; COL Charles Middleton, DC, USA; COL P. Shannon Allison, DC, USA

Security of a treatment location is the prime concern for the team, which is no surprise. The team decides who plans and monitors security; the medic will be too busy with patient care to properly perform security duty during a medical civic action. Be prepared to request your preferred location from local inhabitants even when a different location is offered—some locations may be too enthusiastically offered by locals. Never begin at the same time of day in a return visit to a location, never end at the same time during a return visit to a location. Learn 30-40 dental terms in the local language in order to clearly understand the patient.

A major contribution by a medic is treatment of dental disease for a local population. Cost of materials is very low per patient, and numerous patients can be treated in a day. The great value of dental care is that the results are not readily identifiable by an external observer—people who cooperate with us benefit, but are not immediately singled out. Issuing soccer balls, on the other hand, is highly identifiable, and a soccer ball can be confiscated by anyone. Medics are highly advised to include a Dental Surgeon for the first three missions since dental care is tutored more than learned by bookwork. Time is the most critical planning factor, more than expendable supplies. Consider treating the local security forces (police and military) before the civilian population. Repeating short visits are preferred to a single long visit in order to maximize productivity. Opsec may require that a civil action begin at 1600 rather than early morning in order to limit the period that the treatment team is stationary since sunlight is necessary even when headlamps are used. The team may need to limit a stationary treatment time to 2-3 hours--no one can argue that the sun has set. Ensure that all inhabitants in an area are afforded an equal amount of treatment to lessen civil friction upon departure of the treatment team. Close coordination with the team leader is highly advised since the team leader must be the identifiable head of the mission. One method to ensure this, and to ensure the treatment team is not overwhelmed, is to identify all patients at the beginning, with a queue established for logical patient flow. When the designated person hands out Popsicle sticks numbered 1-20, the population recognizes him as the main resource. Children receive their own Popsicle stick to avoid families overwhelming the treatment team. Additional Popsicle sticks may be issued if treatment flows well, but avoid by all means the inferred promise of treatment to too many patients.

A likely first visit would provide periodontal scaling with the McCall 13S/14S scaler on every patient's lower right quadrant only. Anesthesia would make the patients more comfortable, but ensure sufficient expendable supplies exist to treat everyone equally. One week later after healing, all treated people will note the improved health in this area, and look forward to your return. The second visit to an area would provide scaling on one other quadrant. The return visit may be only to treat other inhabitants on the same initial quadrant until all inhabitants are at the same level of care. Cooperating people may receive more care, but in order to protect them, do not move them to the front of the line. An alternate first visit would be to treat one painful problem per patient. The variety of problems, and the instruments necessary, are much greater. More time per patient may be needed. More experience in dental procedures is necessary to quickly evaluate and treat patients so that patient flow is predictable and the maximum number of people may be seen per day. Limit the options you provide until you are very proficient. Describe the options you provide if you desire to give the patient a choice. Restoration of teeth is possible with modern materials. The lifespan of many teeth can be extended by treatment by a medic, provided you are tutored over several days by a dentist (such as your Dental Surgeon) and by treating 40-100 teeth in order to see the great variety of problems and solutions. Materials to use include the Adper Prompt L-Pop and Transbond XT composite by 3M; and Fuji IX glass ionomer. Teeth that have a history of hot and cold sensitivity, but not spontaneous pain, may be candidates for simple restorations. Six sets of instruments may be necessary to assure sufficient instruments for a day long mission, with instruments properly immersed in a cold sterilization fluid in your sterilization bottle ("Cold Sterilization Jar With Strainer" 6530-01-530-4731). Access to soft decay may require use of a dental enamel hatchet, which is not a component of the tac set. Decay in the interproximal surface will require a "matrix band" (such as a Tofflemire matrix band), and Wizard wooden wedges, neither are components of the tac set. Less involved restorations are limited to the occlusal surface (chewing surface) only. Ensure that restorations are not "high" (excess restorative material), and do not expect a patient to "wear down" excess material through use—teeth do not survive, and you will be viewed as incompetent. Do not attempt to restore any tooth that exhibits apical pathology or a draining sinus tract. Ensure you are tutored in any new material; do not guess. Observe all standards of sterility and proper care. Cease treatment and pack up if you cannot provide your best care. Make no promises you cannot complete that same day. Some people will be left with pathology in place; do not attempt treatment that is beyond your scope of knowledge and experience, even though the people may sincerely ask you. Always take all garbage back to base camp.

Expendable Supplies: Plan to excess. Per patient: Ten 2x2 gauze. One needle. Three carpules of anesthetic. One Chux. One facemask. Two sets of gloves per patient. Disposable mirrors are wasteful; order sufficient No. 5 dental mirrors (the handle is a separate NSN).

Nonexpendable Supplies: your tactical set (dental module) does not provide sufficient instruments for a civic action. Plan ahead to order instruments such as No. 5 mirrors and mirror handles; and McCall 13S/14S, with a DMT Diamond Diasharp Credit Card Sharpener for each scaler. Borrow forceps, 301 elevator, Seldin 1R & 1L, No. 9R & 9L root tip picks from other tac sets. If you desire other forceps, such as 88R and 88L maxillary molar forceps, order them before deployment. If you desire a restorative material such as Fuji IX (pronounced "nine"), order the material before deployment to ensure you have it and can practice with it before treating patients.

Overall clinic: Sharps container. Biohazard bags. Spare batteries for headlamp. Numbered Popsicle sticks (20-40). Multiple medics in the same location can treat more patients. Instrument cleaning and patient records can be performed by a non-medic. Envision where the patient queue will stage, whether that location is secure for the queue, and secure from the treatment area.

Chapter 11: Sexually Transmitted Diseases: Introduction to STDs

CDR Leslie Fenton, MC, USN (Ret)

STDs are a preventable major risk to mission readiness, and prevention starts with changing sexual behaviors that put people at risk. The ability to discuss the potential adverse impact of risky behavior on mission readiness, identify and treat STDs, and provide responsible follow-up (to include mitigating risk of adverse impact on family members on redeployment) are critical skills. The Centers for Disease Control (CDC) recommends that the prevention and control of STDs be based on: 1) education and counseling; 2) identification of infected persons; 3) effective diagnosis and treatment; 4) evaluation/treatment, counseling of sex partners and 5) preexposure vaccination of persons at risk for vaccine-preventable STDs. Common symptoms of STDs include vaginal or urethral discharge, genital ulcers, arthritis, skin lesions and pelvic pain, but many infected patients will be asymptomatic, increasing the risk of complication and transmission of disease. Patients who present with symptoms or signs for a particular STD should be evaluated for all common STDs (eg, syphilis and HIV serology; if negative, repeat HIV test in 4-6 weeks). They should be informed concerning all the STDs for which they are being tested and whether testing for a common STD (eg, genital herpes) is not being performed. Specific service reporting and follow up requirements should be identified and followed. For more information, *see Part 3: General Symptoms: Gynecological Problems; Male Genital Problems; Part 5: Specialty Areas: Chapter 11: Genital Ulcers; Urethral Discharge; Chapter 11: Viral Infections: Hepatitis B (and Hepatitis D); Hepatitis C; Human Immunodeficiency Virus & Part 4: Organ Systems: Viral Infections: Molluscum Contagiosum & Warts (Including Venereal Warts/Condyloma).*

Chapter 11: Sexually Transmitted Diseases: Urethral Discharge

Maj Nicholas Conger, USAF, MC

Introduction: Gonorrhea, chlamydia, trichomonas, bacterial vaginosis and candidiasis can present as a urethral discharge syndrome. The primary focus of this section is diagnosis and management of 2 of the most common STDs, gonorrhea and chlamydia, which classically present with urethral discharges. Patients presumed to be infected with either of these diseases (based on symptoms) should receive treatment for both organisms. *Neisseria gonorrhoeae* causes gonorrhea and appears on Gram's stain as a clump of gram-negative intracellular diplococci. Asymptomatic infection can occur especially in the cervix, rectum and oropharynx. Disseminated gonorrhea presents with infectious arthritis, tenosynovitis, and a characteristic gun metal blue skin lesion surrounded by a red halo, usually on the extremities (arthritis-dermatitis syndrome). The incubation period is 2-14 days after exposure. Most nonspecific or non-gonococcal urethritis (NGU) and cervicitis is caused by *Chlamydia trachomatis*, but *Ureaplasma*, genital *Mycoplasma*, *Trichomonas* and herpes simplex are also implicated. These are some of the most common STDs in the US and a leading cause of female infertility. Infant eye and lung infections are consequent to maternal genital infection with *Chlamydia*. Incubation period is 7-12 days after exposure. A thick mucus discharge with pain on urination and genital ulcer suggests coincident infection by herpes simplex. Incubation period is 2-12 days after exposure.

Subjective: **Symptoms**
Male: Acute (<3 days): Dysuria with discharge/without discharge- usually NGU Chronic (>10 days) urethral stricture; Female: Acute (<3 days): Dysuria or frequent urination, vaginal discharge, pain with intercourse, lower pelvic pain; Chronic (>10 days): PID, infertility Either: Sub-acute (3-10 days): Painful joints, gun metal blue skin lesions (gonorrhea) tenosynovitis
Focused History: For females: *Have you had unprotected sex with a new partner in the past 6 weeks?* (incubation period 2 weeks for gonorrhea; longer for NGU) *Have you had discharge stains in your underwear?* (suggests gonorrhea) For males: *Are you having any difficulty retracting your foreskin?* (suggests phimosis with gonorrhea) *Do you have pain (burning) with urination?*

Objective: **Signs**
Using Basic Tools: Inspection: Acute (<3 days): Purulent yellow to green discharge (both gonorrhea and chlamydia), mucoid/scant discharge (more consistent with NGU), if oropharyngeal exposure, see red tonsils with exudate (gonorrhea), Sub acute (3-10 days): Infection of periurethral glands, epididymitis, if disseminated gonorrhea: red, tender swollen joints and tendon insertions, fever to 102°F. If other prominent symptoms or signs (eg, pruritus, icterus, weight. loss, genital ulcer), consider infection by other or additional organisms. For more information, *see Part 3: General Symptoms: Gynecologic Problems; Male Genital Problems; Part 4: Organ Systems: Chapter 6: Viral Infections: Molluscum Contagiosum; Warts (including Venereal Warts/Condyloma); Part 5: Specialty Areas: Chapter 11: Urethral Discharge; Genital Ulcers; Chapter 12: Viral Infections: Hepatitis B (and Hepatitis D); Hepatitis C & Human Immunodeficiency Virus.*
Using Advanced Tools: Labs: Gram's stain: Urethral discharge shows gram-negative intracellular diplococci within white blood cells (lower diagnostic sensitivity in females), or many polymorphonuclear neutrophils but no organisms (NGU), pregnancy test to guide drug selection.

Assessment: **Differential Diagnosis:** Other causes of dysuria include:
Trichomonas: Malodorous urethral/vaginal discharge in females. *See Part 3: General Symptoms: Gynecological Problems: Vaginal Trichomonas*
Vaginal candidiasis: Pruritus, white curd-like discharge in females. *See Part 3: General Symptoms: Gynecological Problems: Candida Vaginitis/Vulvitis*
Herpes simplex: Presence of mucoid discharge with skin ulcer.
Urinary tract infection: Usually includes frequency, urgency; sometimes hematuria. *See Part 4: Organ Systems: Chapter 8: Urinary Tract Infection*
Arthritis-dermatitis: Syndrome of disseminated gonorrhea may resemble meningococcemia with a gonorrhea rash on extremities (distinctive bluish lesions surrounded by erythema).

Plan:
Treatment: Always treat for both gonorrhea and chlamydia.
Primary: Ceftriaxone 125mg IM single dose **and** **azithromycin** 1g po single dose

Alternatives: Choose one from Column **A** and one from Column **B**:

Column A	Column B
cefixime 400mg po single dose	**doxycycline** 100mg po bid x 7 days
ceftriaxone 125mg IM single dose	**azithromycin** 1g po single dose
	erythromycin 500mg po qid x 7 days

Fluoroquinolones are no longer recommended due to increased resistance.

Pregnant patient: **Ceftriaxone, cefixime, azithromycin,** and **erythromycin** can be used; do not use doxycycline in pregnant or nursing females.

Test: All patients for syphilis (RPR) and HIV (rapid or ELISA test), if available.

Patient Education

General: Education and counseling based on the "Five Ps": Partners (evaluate and treat recent sexual contacts), Prevention of Pregnancy, Protection from STDs, Practices, Past History of STDs. Deployed personnel should be counseled regarding risk to family members following deployment.

No Improvement/Deterioration: Always treat patient as if co-infected with chlamydia

Medications: Avoid taking doxycycline with antacids, milk, iron pills or multivitamins. Avoid sun exposure. Do not use doxycycline in children, or nursing or pregnant mothers.

Prevention and Hygiene: Use barrier protection (latex condoms) or abstinence for duration of treatment.

Follow-up Actions

No Improvement/Deterioration: If relapse occurs, treat NGU/cervicitis for 21 days with **doxycycline** 100mg po bid. Also evaluate and treat partner. For recurrent urethritis after treatment of patient and partner, give **metronidazole** 2g po in single dose and **erythromycin** 500mg po qid for 7 days (discuss Antabuse effect of **metronidazole** and do not use during pregnancy).

Return Evaluation: Follow-up all patients should have syphilis and HIV serology; if negative, repeat HIV test in 4-6 weeks. Specific service reporting and follow up requirements should be identified and followed.

Evacuation/Consultation Criteria: Evacuation is not usually required. Consult urology, gynecology, infectious disease or preventive medicine experts as needed.

Chapter 11: Sexually Transmitted Diseases: Genital Ulcers

LCDR Timothy Whitman, MC, USN

Introduction: Genital ulcers have a wide variety of sexually transmitted causes and the presence of genital ulcers is an important factor in the sexual spread of HIV. It is important to know what ulcer causing pathogens are most prevalent in the area of exposure. **Herpes** is caused by herpes simplex (HSV) type 1 and 2, both of which can cause genital ulcers. HSV 1 is usually milder and often associated with oral sores, "fever blisters" (*see Appendices: Color Plates Figure A.22-D*), keratoconjunctivitis and encephalitis. HSV 2 causes a more severe initial episode (fever, exudative pharyngitis, toxic appearance, multiple genital lesions), and then recurs as a localized cluster of vesicles that ulcerate painfully. HSV 2 is associated with aseptic meningitis and radiculitis. Vaginal delivery in pregnant women with active genital infection poses a high risk to her newborn (disseminated HSV and death). The incubation period for HSV is 2-12 days after exposure. **Syphilis** (caused by the spirochete *Treponema pallidum*), is known as the "great imitator." Left untreated, up to 1/3 of patients will develop tertiary syphilis (CNS infection, aortic aneurysm, gummas of the skin, bone and visceral organs). Syphilis is curable in all stages but treatment may yield a Jarisch-Herxheimer reaction with fever, rigors and intensification of the lesions 2-24 hours after initiating treatment. Incubation period of primary stage syphilis is 10 days to 3 months. **Chancroid,** caused by *Hemophilus ducreyi,* (incubation period 3-7 days) is associated with an increased risk for HIV transmission and may co-exist with other causes of genital ulcers (eg, herpes infection). **Granuloma inguinale** (GI) is caused by gram-negative *Calymmatobacterium granulomatis* (incubation period 1-12 weeks) which causes beefy red granulomas that progress slowly and can cover the genitalia and heal slowly with scarring. Patients can spread lesions to other areas through autoinoculation. **Lymphogranuloma venereum** (LGV) is caused by variants of *Chlamydia trachomatis* and starts as a painless vesicle or nodule that then ulcerates and heals. Days to weeks later, regional lymph nodes become inflamed and tender. Suppuration, scarring, systemic infection, chronic elephantiasis and rectal strictures have been seen in untreated infection. **HIV-specific ulcers** come from acute HIV infection or late HIV infection. **Geographic Associations:** Herpes simplex virus and syphilis are worldwide. Chancroid is especially seen in Africa and Asia and is the most frequent kind of genital ulcer in the tropics. LGV is most prevalent in tropical and sub-tropical countries. Granuloma inguinale is most often associated with exposure in India, Australia, South Pacific, Brazil and South Africa. HIV-specific ulcers are found everywhere.

Subjective: Symptoms

Painless ulcer: Syphilis, LGV, granuloma inguinale (Donovanosis)

Painful ulcer: Herpes simplex, chancroid, phagedenic ulcer (an otherwise painless ulcer secondarily infected with bacteria)

Constitutional: Acute (1-3 days): Fever (in LGV and 1st episode HSV)

Specific: Acute (1-3 days): Generally starts as papule that ulcerates, HSV: Paresthesias can precede outbreak, syphilis: rash including palms and soles. Chronic (>1 month): LGV may be very chronic; HSV often recurs

Focused History: *When was the last time you had oral, vaginal and/or anal sex?* (various incubation periods for difference organisms) *Have you had this symptom before?* (HSV is often recurrent in same area.) *Is the sore painful? (see differential diagnosis) Did the sore start out as a painless ulcer then become more painful?* (possible phagedenic ulcer) *How long has the genital sore been present?* (HSV usually resolves in ten days; syphilis in 3-6 weeks; others can be less likely to resolve without specific therapy.)

Objective: **Signs**
  Using Basic Tools: Inspection
    HSV: Acute (1-3 days): Vesicles in clusters, 1st time may have fever; **Sub-acute (3-10 days):** Shallow painful ulcer (often multiple);
    Chronic (>1 month): In AIDS patients - huge non-healing ulcers
    Chancroid: Acute (1-3 days): Papules **Sub-acute (3-10 days):** Painful, shaggy edged, deep ulcers; suppurative regional adenopathy;
    Chronic (>1 month): Phimosis
    Granuloma Inguinale: Acute (1-3 days): Bright red, painless, satiny-surface, raised plaque, often in folds between scrotum or labia
    and thighs; **Sub acute (3-10 days):** The border of the ulcer shows rolled edge.
    LGV: Acute (1-3 days): Painless vesicle or nodule that ulcerates and heals; may have fever; **Sub-acute (3-10 days):** Groove sign
    (lymph node adheres above and below inguinal ligament); **Chronic (>1 month):** Chronic elephantiasis of genitals, rectal strictures,
    rectal fistula
    Syphilis: Acute (1-3 days): Painless ulcer with rolled border (chancre) heals without Rx in 3-6 weeks. **Chronic (>1 month):**
    Secondary syphilis: 2-4 weeks after chancre, see generalized rash including palms and soles; can also see flat genital warts, loss
    of hair, patches on the mucous membranes
    Tertiary or late (5-20 years) syphilis: Gummas (tumor like masses in skin/bone/viscera) neurologic abnormalities - "neurosyphilis":
    (posterior column findings such as slapped foot gait, loss of deep tendon reflexes, loss of position sense or hot/cold sense); also
    develop abnormal pupillary reflexes, dementia Auscultation: In late syphilis, may hear aortic regurgitation murmur. Palpation: Most
    patients with genital ulcers develop tender regional adenopathy.
  Using Advanced Tools: Labs: Gram's stain pus from bubo (enlarged fluctuant node): large numbers of small gram-negative
  coccobacilli in a "school of fish" pattern (chancroid). *See Appendices: Color Plates: Figure A-23.C.* Giemsa stain edge of tissue scraping
  from edge of ulcer: intracytoplasmic bacilli in the macrophages (Donovan bodies of granuloma inguinale); Giemsa stain of tissue scraping
  at base of the ulcer (Tzanck smear): observe for multinucleated giant cells (herpes); RPR for syphilis: may be negative during early stage,
  and should be repeated in 4-6 weeks.

Assessment: Although in the operational setting, diagnosing the cause of genital ulcers is initially based mainly on the clinical history and
inspection, it should be recognized that optimally all patients with genital ulcers should have serologic testing for syphilis (including both
nontreponemal-RPR and treponemal FTA-ABS and repeated 1 and 3 months later), HIV and a diagnostic evaluation for herpes. Whether
patients are tested for other causes (eg, chancroid, LGV, GI) depends on the geographic location and prevalence of the disease.
  Differential Diagnosis: Classic presentation (as described previously) is a useful guide but appearance of lesions vary and overlap, with
  multiple agents possibly involved at the same time and in the same lesion.
    Herpes: Multiple, shallow, tender ulcers (sensitivity 35%, specificity 94%). Note that chancroid and syphilis can present as multiple
    painful ulcers.
    Syphilis: Painless, indurated, clean-based ulcer (sensitivity 31%, specificity 98%). Helpful clues for syphilis are sexual history, prior
    healed chancre, rash on palms and soles, and absence of any skin lesions that look like targets. Both LGV and HSV can present
    this way as well.
    Chancroid: Deep, undermined, purulent ulcer (sensitivity 34%, specificity 94%)
    Granuloma inguinale: Extensive progressive lesions, granulation tissue, rolled edges
    LGV: In acute stage, small and shallow lesions May have rapid spontaneous healing so that lesions may not be observed.
    Behçet's syndrome: Recurrent symptoms with oral ulcers, conjunctivitis and uveitis.
    Erythema multiforme: May include a history of herpes or mycoplasma infection in the past, characteristic target lesions seen
    (especially on face and trunk)
    Trauma: History of trauma
    Malignancy: May be difficult to differentiate, important to consider if history of exposure to infectious etiology not present.
    Infectious exanthems: May be difficult to differentiate
    Drug reactions: Suspected by history of use of medication

Plan:
  Treatment: Herpes simplex
    Primary: Valacyclovir 1000mg po q12h x 10 days (use 500mg po q day x 5 days, for recurrence) or **famciclovir** 250mg po q8h x
    5-10 days (use 125mg bid for 3-5 days for recurrence)
    Alternative: Acyclovir 400mg po q8h x 10-14 days if initial episode, for 5 days, if recurrence
  Patient Education
    This virus can be sexually transmitted even in the absence of active lesions. Latex condoms are recommended.
    Prevention and Hygiene: Health care workers should wear gloves to handle lesions to reduce risk of local inoculation to the hand
    (herpetic whitlow).
    No Improvement/Deterioration: Resistant herpes has been described in HIV patients who have been maintained chronically on antiviral
    agents. Consider screening for HIV.
  Treatment: Syphilis
    Primary: Primary and secondary syphilis: **benzathine penicillin** 2.4mu IM in a single dose
    Neurosyphilis: **penicillin G** 2-4mu IV q4h x 10 -14 days (23% failure rate reported)
    Latent: **benzathine penicillin** 2.4mu IM q week x 3 doses
    Alternative: Primary and secondary syphilis: **doxycycline** 100mg po bid x 14 days
    Neurosyphilis: **ceftriaxone** 2g IV or IM q day x 14 days
    Latent: **doxycycline** 100mg po bid x 28 days

Treatment: Chancroid
Primary: Antibiotics: **Ceftriaxone** 250mg IM single dose; needle aspirate fluctuant nodes to avoid rupture
Alternatives: Azithromycin 1g po single dose or **erythromycin** 500mg po qid x 7 days or **ciprofloxacin** 500mg po bid x 3 days
Prevention: Treat all sexual partners dating from 2 weeks prior to onset of symptoms
Return Evaluation: Screen for HIV in 4-6 weeks
Treatment: LGV
Primary: **Azithromycin** 500mg po q day x 7 days or 1g po each week x 4 doses; drain fluctuant buboes by needle aspiration, avoid incision and drainage which can cause sinus tracts.
Alternatives: Doxycycline 100mg po bid x 21-30 days or **ceftriaxone** 1g IM q day x 14 days or **ciprofloxacin** 750mg po q day x 21 days or **erythromycin** 1000mg po bid x 21 days.
No Improvement/Deterioration: Drug resistant strains have been seen. Expect to see a treatment response by seven days but prolonged therapy is needed to avoid relapse.
Patient Education: Limit activity if possible during early week of antibiotics to decrease risk of strictures.
Treatment: Granuloma inguinale
Primary: **Azithromycin** 500mg po q day x 7 days or 1g po each week x 4 doses
Alternatives: Doxycycline 100mg po bid x 21-30 days or **ceftriaxone** 1g IM q day x 14 days or **ciprofloxacin** 750mg po q day x 21 days or **erythromycin** 1g po bid x 21 days
No Improvement/Deterioration: Drug resistant strains have been seen. Expect to see a treatment response by seven days but prolonged therapy is needed to avoid relapse.
Follow-up Actions
Return Evaluation: Refer for VDRL lab test at 6 and 12 months and expect titer to fall. If latent syphilis, another VDRL at 24 months is recommended. HIV test at 4-6 weeks.
Evacuation/Consultant Criteria: Evacuation is not usually required for any of these conditions in the acute phase. Consult urology, gynecology, infectious disease or preventive medicine experts as needed, particularly in chronic cases.
Notes: Congenital syphilis causes preterm delivery, snuffles (obstructed nasal respiration), rash, stillbirth. It can be asymptomatic initially, but manifestations can include Hutchinson's teeth, saddlenose, saber shins, deafness. Suspect this if the umbilical cord is swollen and demonstrates a red/white/blue pattern like a barber pole.

Chapter 12: Infectious Diseases: Parasitic Infections: Amebiasis

COL Glenn Wortmann, MC, USA

Introduction: Third leading parasitic cause of death in developing nations. Caused by *Entamoeba histolytica*. Transmitted through contaminated food or water. Incubation: 2-4 weeks.

Subjective: **Symptoms**
Gradual onset of bloody diarrhea with associated abdominal pain and tenderness.
Focused History: *Do you have bloody diarrhea and abdominal pain?* (Abdominal pain and bloody stools suggests amebiasis or bacterial colitis.) *Do you have a fever?* (1/3 of patients)

Objective: **Signs**
Using Basic Tools: Vital signs: Temperature over 101°F. Inspection: Bloody, loose, mucus-containing stools. Palpation: The liver may be enlarged and tender.
Using Advanced Tools: Labs: Heme positive (guaiac test) stool. O & P: Multiple examinations (minimum of 3) of stool to demonstrate *E. histolytica* trophozoites.

Assessment:
Differential Diagnosis: Diarrhea from:
Giardiasis: Stool examination for the presence of *Giardia*. *See Part 5: Specialty Areas: Chapter 12: Parasitic Infections: Giardiasis*
Viral gastroenteritis: Cannot be diagnosed using Basic or Advanced tools. *See Part 3: General Symptoms: Diarrhea, Acute*
Bacterial gastroenteritis: Cannot be diagnosed using Basic or Advanced tools. *See Part 3: General Symptoms: Diarrhea, Acute & Part 4: Organ Systems: Chapter 7: Acute Bacterial Food Poisoning*
Cryptosporidiosis: Cannot be diagnosed using Basic or Advanced tools. Requires tertiary laboratory support.
Isosporiasis: Cannot be diagnosed using Basic or Advanced tools. Requires tertiary laboratory support.
***E. coli* 0157:H7:** Cannot be diagnosed using Basic or Advanced tools. Requires tertiary laboratory support. *See Part 3: General Symptoms: Diarrhea, Acute*
Shigellosis: Cannot be diagnosed using Basic or Advanced tools. Requires tertiary laboratory support. *Part 4: Organ Systems: Chapter 7: Acute Bacterial Food Poisoning*
Inflammatory bowel disease: Cannot be diagnosed using Basic or Advanced tools. Requires tertiary laboratory support.

Plan:
Treatment
Metronidazole 750mg tid po x 10 days, followed by **paromomycin** 30mg/kg/d po in 3 divided doses x 10 days. Maintain oral fluids.
Patient Education
General: Maintain adequate oral intake of fluids to avoid volume depletion.
Activity: As tolerated.
Diet: As tolerated.
Medications: Metronidazole should not be used in the first trimester of pregnancy. Avoid alcohol to avoid an Antabuse-like effect (anxiety, vomiting, headache, etc.).

Prevention and Hygiene: Filters with pores <1 micron or boiling for 1 min. can make water safe. Good hand washing and safe food preparation.

Follow-up Actions

Return Evaluation: If diarrhea continues, consider other etiologies. Stool should be examined after treatment, as continued *E. histolytica* infection mandates re-treatment.

Consultation Criteria: Failure to improve after initiation of antibiotics.

Chapter 12: Infectious Diseases: Parasitic Infections: Ascariasis (Roundworm)

COL Glenn Wortmann, MC, USA

Introduction: The most common intestinal worm, *Ascaris* infects more than 1 billion people worldwide, who ingest eggs in contaminated food and drink. The eggs hatch in the small intestine, penetrate the intestinal wall and travel by venous circulation to the lungs. The larvae then pass into the trachea and pharynx and are swallowed. They migrate through the GI tract becoming mature worms in the small intestine. Incubation period is 4-8 weeks. *Ascaris* is also known as roundworm, and is large enough to easily see without magnification.

Subjective: **Symptoms**

Abdominal pain (obstruction of bowel or bile ducts [biliary colic] with worms); wheezing and coughing (pneumonitis [Löeffler's syndrome]); occasional liver enlargement; fever. Worms (some larger than earthworm) pass from the anus, nose and mouth and are often brought for diagnosis.

Focused History: *Have you seen a worm in your stool?* (occasionally migrate out of the intestine) *How large was the worm?* (often the size of an earthworm)

Objective: **Signs**

Using Basic Tools: Auscultation: Decreased bowel sounds. Palpation: Occasionally hepatomegaly; abdominal tenderness

Using Advanced Tools: Labs: Stool O&P (identify eggs or the adult worm); CBC (nutritional anemia)

Assessment: **Differential Diagnosis**

Worm in stool: The presence of a visible worm in the stool is usually diagnostic.

Cough/wheezes: Asthma and pneumonia can cause similar findings.

Plan:

Treatment

Primary: **Albendazole** 400mg po once

Alternative: **Mebendazole** 100mg po bid x 3 days

Patient Education

General: Wash hands thoroughly.

Activity: As tolerated

Diet: As tolerated

Medications: Occasional gastrointestinal side-effects

Prevention and Hygiene: Hand washing

No Improvement/Deterioration: Refer for evaluation

Follow-up Actions

Return Evaluation: As needed

Consultation Criteria: Failure to improve.

Chapter 12: Infectious Diseases: Parasitic Infections: Babesiosis

COL Glenn Wortmann, MC, USA

Introduction: Babesiosis is caused by *Babesia* species protozoa and is transmitted by deer tick bites. Infection is most commonly reported in the Northeastern US, but has also occurred in Europe. It is typically a mild illness in healthy people but it can be fatal, particularly in immunocompromised patients (especially splenectomized patients). Incubation period is a few days to weeks.

Subjective: **Symptoms:**

Fever following tick bite, malaise, fatigue, chills, headache and possibly, jaundice.

Focused History: *Do you recall being bitten by a tick?* (Tick bites cause babesiosis.) *Do you recall the size of the tick that bit you?* (transmitted by the small deer tick) *How long ago were you bitten by a tick?* (The incubation period is a few days to a few weeks.)

Objective: **Signs:**

Using Basic Tools: Fever, sometimes jaundice

Using Advanced Tools: Labs: Giemsa or Wright stained thin or thick blood smears may confirm the presence of *Babesia* inside red blood cells, and significant hemolytic anemia.

Assessment: **Differential Diagnosis**

Malaria: Microscopic evaluation of a stained blood smear can reveal malaria parasites, but these can appear very similar to *Babesia*, and referral to an expert microscopist is recommended. A rapid malaria dipstick test is now available, and can be used to test a blood sample for malaria. *See Part 5: Specialty Areas: Chapter 12: Parasitic Infections: Malaria*

Viral infections: Not able to be diagnosed using Basic and Advanced tools.

Other tick-borne infections (**Rocky Mountain spotted fever, relapsing fever**): *See Part 5: Specialty Areas: Chapter 12: Rickettsial Infections: Rickettsial Infections (Murine, Rickettsial Pox, Scrub Typhus, Louse-Borne Typhus, Boutonneuse Fever) & Spirochetal Infections: Relapsing Fever*

Plan:

Treatment: Most patients with mild disease recover without treatment.

Primary: **Azithromycin** 500mg po, then 250mg po q day x 6 days <u>and</u> **atovaquone** 750mg po bid x 7 days

Alternative: **Clindamycin** 600mg po tid x 10 days <u>and</u> **quinine** 650mg po tid x 10 days.

Patient Education

General: Avoid tick bites

Activity: As tolerated

Diet: As tolerated

Medications: Occasional gastrointestinal side effects.

Prevention and Hygiene: Avoid tick bites

No Improvement/Deterioration: Return for evaluation

Follow-up Actions

Return Evaluation: As needed

Consultation Criteria: Failure to improve.

Zoonotic Disease Considerations:

Agent: *Babesia microti, B. bovis, B. divergens*

Principal Animal Hosts: Cattle, wild rodents

Clinical Disease in Animals: Fever (106°F or higher), poor appetite, increased respiratory rate, muscle tremors, anemia, jaundice, weight loss

Probable Mode of Transmission: Bite of infected *Ixodes* tick

Known Distribution: Worldwide, rare; Europe (*B. divergens*)

Chapter 12: Infectious Diseases: Parasitic Infections: Clonorchiasis (Chinese liver fluke)

COL Glenn Wortmann, MC, USA

Introduction: The Chinese or oriental liver fluke, *Clonorchis sinensis*, is acquired by eating raw or undercooked freshwater fish. Clonorchiasis is endemic to the Far East.

Subjective: Symptoms

Most infections are asymptomatic, but heavy worm burdens may cause right upper quadrant pain (worms block bile and pancreatic ducts), loss of appetite and fever.

Focused History: *Do you have pain in your right upper abdomen?* (Right upper abdominal pain is typical.) *How long have you been experiencing abdominal pain?* (can be chronic) *Where have you traveled recently?* (Travel to an endemic area suggests diagnosis of clonorchiasis.)

Objective: Signs

Using Basic Tools: Palpation: Right upper quadrant tenderness, liver enlargement and jaundice (rarely).

Using Advanced Tools: Labs: Identification of *Clonorchis* eggs in the stool on O&P evaluation.

Assessment: Differential Diagnosis

Cholangitis: Cannot be diagnosed using Basic and Advanced tools. Requires ultrasound and/or CT scan. *See Part 4: Organ Systems: Acute Cholecystitis*

Cholecystitis: *See Part 4: Organ Systems: Acute Cholecystitis*

Fascioliasis: Stool examination for the presence of the parasite

Plan:

Treatment

Primary: **Praziquantel** 75mg/kg/day po tid x 1 day

Alternate: **Albendazole** 10mg/kg per day x 7 days

Patient Education

General: Avoid improperly prepared fish.

Activity: As tolerated

Diet: As tolerated

Medications: Occasional gastrointestinal side effects

Prevention and Hygiene: Avoid improperly cooked fish.

No Improvement/Deterioration: Referral for evaluation

Follow-up Actions

Return Evaluation: As needed

Consultation Criteria: Failure to improve

Zoonotic Disease Considerations:

Principal Animal Hosts: Dogs, cats, swine, rats

Clinical Disease in Animals: Possible hepatic signs

Probable Mode of Transmission: Ingestion of raw or partially cooked infected freshwater fish

Known Distribution: Asia

Chapter 12: Infectious Diseases: Parasitic Infections: Cyclosporiasis
COL Glenn Wortmann, MC, USA

Introduction: Cyclosporiasis is transmitted by fecal contamination of water or food. *Cyclospora* infections occur worldwide, and are an increasingly recognized cause of parasitic diarrhea. Transmission seems to be waterborne and more common during summer months. The incubation period averages one week.

Subjective: Symptoms
Watery diarrhea, fatigue, abdominal cramps and fever (in 25%). Diarrhea can be prolonged (up to 45 days) but is generally self-limited.
Focused History: *Are you experiencing diarrhea? If so, is it watery and non-bloody?* (typical diarrhea) *How long have you been experiencing diarrhea?* (Diarrhea lasting >1 week is typical.)

Objective: Signs
Using Basic Tools: Watery (>6 stools per day) diarrhea without blood
Using Advanced Tools: Labs: Cyclospora oocysts in O&P examination of the stool.

Assessment: Differential Diagnosis
There are many possible causes of diarrhea. Although the presence of watery diarrhea suggests cyclosporiasis, it can also be seen with *Cryptosporidia, Microsporidia* or *Isospora. See Part 3: General Symptoms: Diarrhea, Acute*

Plan:
Treatment
Most infections are self-limited. Use **trimethoprim-sulfamethoxazole DS** po bid x 7 days for chronic infections.
Patient Education
General: Oral fluids to avoid volume depletion
Activity: As tolerated
Diet: As tolerated
Medications: Trimethoprim-sulfamethoxazole can occasionally cause a rash.
Prevention and Hygiene: Avoid contaminated food and water.
No Improvement/Deterioration: Return for re-evaluation.
Follow-up Actions
Return Evaluation: Consider alternative causes of diarrhea.
Consultation Criteria: Failure to improve with conservative measures.

Chapter 12: Infectious Diseases: Parasitic Infections: Dracunculiasis (Guinea Worm Disease)
CDR John Sanders, MC, USN

Introduction: Dracunculiasis, also known as guinea worm, is caused by the nematode (roundworm) *Dracunculus medinensis*. Infection occurs from ingestion of water containing copepods (water fleas) that are infected with larvae. The larvae penetrate the intestinal wall and migrate to connective and subcutaneous tissues where they develop into adults, mate, and continue to mature. Approximately a year after infection, adult female worms, which grow to be 2-3 feet long, begin to emerge from the skin (usually 1-3 emerge simultaneously), creating a painful blister. If the emerging worms make contact with water, they expel larvae into the water, which copepods ingest. The emergence of the worms is painful and often incapacitates people for 2-3 months. The open sore also often becomes secondarily infected with bacteria. Humans are the only known host of *D. medinensis*. **Geographic Associations:** In the past, this parasite caused infection and substantial morbidity in many parts of Africa, Yemen, and India, but thanks to an intense eradication program, the parasite is now only found in 9 sub-saharan African countries, with 90% of cases reported from Ghana and the Sudan. **Seasonal Variation:** In some areas, transmission is temporally associated with rainy season, which increases the depth of "step wells," facilitating the maintenance of the parasite life cycle, but generally, transmission can occur year round. **Risk Factors:** The only significant risk factor is the ingestion of water containing infected copepods. However, women in endemic countries tend to be infected more often than men because they are often responsible for cooking, cleaning, and water gathering, which increase their opportunities for exposure.

Subjective: Symptoms
Just prior to the formation of the skin papule, which occurs 10-14 months after infection, systemic symptoms such as fever, urticaria, pruritus, dizziness, nausea, vomiting and diarrhea can occur and generally last a few days. Over days to a few weeks, the papule develops into a painful blister. The rupture of the blister and the emergence of the worm are excruciatingly painful. If the worm is not then fully extracted or breaks, a painful inflammatory reaction along the worm tract can develop. Complications of the infection include secondary bacterial infections of the exit site that can lead to systemic sepsis, tetanus, and occasional migration of the worm to sites other than skin, such as the lung, eye, or spinal cord, resulting in abscesses at these locations. Chronic problems, including arthritis and contractures, can develop due to the prolonged local inflammation, especially if the worm migrates through a joint.
Focused History: *Have you ever been to sub-saharan Africa? Did you ingest local water while traveling in Africa?*

Objective: Signs
Using Basic Tools: Inspection and Palpation: Initial signs may include low grade fever, urticaria, and mild swelling of the affected area. Subsequently, there will be the development of a tender papule, usually on the lower extremity. This papule will develop into a tender blister, measuring 2-7cm. After this blister ruptures, the end of a long, thin, white worm will be obvious emerging from the tissue. There are often multiple papules/blisters that appear at the same time.

Assessment: Differential Diagnosis

Myiasis: Larvae of certain flies can infest human tissues causing a tender furuncle containing a fly larva, which can be mistaken for a worm. However, these larvae are only a few centimeters long and are wide, rather than the 2-3 feet long, very thin guinea worm.
See Part 4: Organ Systems: Chapter 6: Superficial Fungal Infections: Myiasis

Plan:
Treatment
Primary: There is no specific therapy besides slow extraction of the worm. Supportive treatment with anti-inflammatories and analgesics should be offered. The procedure of choice is the slow extraction of the worm. The worm is so long that it cannot be pulled out at once, but requires that the patient wind the worm around a stick, extracting it a few centimeters each day. The process generally takes weeks-months to extract the entire worm. If the worm breaks, an effort should be made to remove the remaining worm. Antibiotics may be required for secondary bacterial infections. Give immunization against tetanus.
Empiric: Treatment should focus on pain relief, sterile dressings to prevent secondary infections, and antibiotics for infections if they occur.
Primitive: Slow extraction of the worm can be accomplished with primitive tools, such as a twig or match stick.
Patient Education
General: It is very important to keep the wound clean and free of infection while removing the worm. It is important to try to remove the entire worm to prevent further inflammatory reactions.
Activity: As tolerated.
Diet: As tolerated.
Prevention and Hygiene: Avoid ingestion of water containing infected copepods. The lifecycle of the worm can be broken by simply filtering the water (even through cheesecloth), using insecticide to kill the copepods, or preventing infected persons from entering the water.
No Improvement/Deterioration: Development of secondary infection (cellulitis or an abscess) or a local inflammatory reaction.
Wound Care: Extraction of the worm, local care for the wound, and sterile dressings.
Follow-up Actions
Return Evaluation: The patient should be seen regularly until the worm is fully extracted and the wound is healed.
Evacuation/Consultation Criteria: If the wound develops a severe secondary infection or a severe inflammatory reaction occurs, the patient should be evacuated to a higher level of care.
Note: There is an expectation that this infection may be eradicated from the world within the next several years.

Chapter 12: Infectious Diseases: Parasitic Infections: Enterobiasis (Pinworms)

COL Glenn Wortmann, MC, USA

Introduction: Enterobiasis is contracted by ingesting the eggs of the *Enterobius vermicularis* nematode. Pinworms inhabit the large intestines of humans. Enterobiasis occurs worldwide, particularly in temperate climates and is common among children.

Subjective: Symptoms
Perianal and perineal itching, as well as restless sleep. Females may present with vaginal itching.
Focused History: *Have you noticed itching in the perineal or perianal area?* (Pinworms often cause itching.) *Is the itching worse at night?* (Nocturnal pruritus is common.)

Objective: Signs
Using Basic Tools: Adult worms (about 1cm long) may occasionally be seen in the perianal area.
Using Advanced Tools: Labs: O&P of stool should reveal pinworm eggs. Alternatively, apply Scotch tape to the perianal region first thing in the morning and then examine the tape affixed to a slide microscopically for eggs.

Assessment: The presence of perineal/perianal itching, especially in a child, is very suggestive of pinworms.
Differential Diagnosis
Candidal dermatitis: Can cause similar complaints. Diagnosis requires scraping the rash gently with a scalpel blade, and then placing the sample on a microscope slide. After placing several drops of KOH on the sample, yeast forms can be visualized under microscopic review.

Plan:
Treatment
Primary: Albendazole 400mg po once, repeat in 2 weeks; or **mebendazole** 100mg po once, repeat in 2 weeks
Alternative: Pyrantel pamoate 11mg/kg po and repeat in 2 weeks
Patient Education
General: Treat all family members to avoid re-infection.
Activity: As tolerated
Diet: As tolerated
Medications: Occasional gastrointestinal side effects
Prevention and Hygiene: Wash bed linens and night clothes in hot water to destroy eggs.
No Improvement/Deterioration: Referral for evaluation
Follow-up Actions
Return Evaluation: As needed
Consultation Criteria: Failure to improve

Chapter 12: Infectious Diseases: Parasitic Infections: Fascioliasis
COL Glenn Wortmann, MC, USA

Introduction: *Fasciola hepatica* infections are seen in sheep- and cattle-raising areas worldwide, with most cases occurring in South America, Europe, Africa, China and Australia. Humans become infected by eating aquatic plants (especially watercress) grown in water contaminated with feces from infected animals or humans (night soil). Most human infections are mild, although heavy infections can result in extensive liver damage. Even without treatment, many patients will have no symptoms. If flukes lodge in the extrahepatic biliary ducts, right upper quadrant (RUQ) abdominal pain may occur.

Subjective: Symptoms
In moderate-to-severe infections: Diarrhea, RUQ abdominal pain (biliary colic), weakness, malaise and night sweats, fever, jaundice.
Focused History: *Have you noted a fever? Have you noticed pain in your right upper abdomen?* (typical symptoms; right upper quadrant pain occurs as worms migrate to the liver) *How long ago were you in South America, Europe, Africa, China or Australia?* (Symptoms usually occur at least 12 weeks after ingestion of the eggs.)

Objective: Signs
Using Basic Tools: Palpation: Hepatomegaly and splenomegaly
Using Advanced Tools: Labs: O & P of stool to identify *Fasciola* eggs.

Assessment: Differential Diagnosis: Travel to an endemic area is critical for considering the diagnosis.
Cholecystitis/cholangitis: *See Part 4: Organ Systems: Chapter 7: Acute Cholecystitis*
Clonorchiasis: *See Part 5: Specialty Areas: Chapter 12: Parasitic Infections: Clonorchiasis (Chinese Live Fluke)*

Plan:
Treatment
   Bithionol 30-50mg/kg per day po in 3 divided doses on alternate days for a duration of 10-15 days (available from the CDC).
   Triclabendazole 10mg/kg po for 1-2 days has been demonstrated to be a safe and effective alternative. Although it is commercially available in some countries such as Egypt, it has not been approved for sale in the United States.
Patient Education
   General: Avoid improperly prepared food (particularly aquatic plants in endemic areas).
   Medications: Bithionol can cause photosensitivity and gastrointestinal symptoms.
Follow-up Actions
   Evacuation/Consultation Criteria: Evacuate unstable patients and those unable to complete the mission. Consult infectious disease specialist or internist.

Zoonotic Disease Considerations:
   Principal Animal Hosts: Cattle, sheep, and other large ruminants
   Clinical Disease in Animals: Cattle – asymptomatic; sheep – distended painful abdomen, anemia, and sudden death
   Probable Mode of Transmission: Ingestion of contaminated greens

Chapter 12: Infectious Diseases: Parasitic Infections: Fasciolopsiasis
COL Glenn Wortmann, MC, USA

Introduction: Fasciolopsiasis is caused by the giant intestinal fluke, *Fasciolopsis buski*, found in the Far East and Southeast Asia. Humans are infected by eating raw water plants (eg, water chestnut/water bamboo) onto which the organism has attached. The parasite eggs can be found about 3 months after ingestion.

Subjective: Symptoms
Usually asymptomatic, although infection may cause diarrhea and abdominal cramping, with vomiting and anorexia.
Focused History: *Have you noticed diarrhea?* (Most infections are asymptomatic, but diarrhea may occur) *Have you eaten any raw water plants, such as water chestnuts, in the previous few months?* (typical exposure) *How long ago did you eat a water plant?* (Symptoms usually occur several months after ingestion.)

Objective: Signs
Using Basic Tools: Massive infection can cause intestinal obstruction, edema of face/legs and ascites.
Using Advanced Tools: Labs: O & P of stool: Identification of the *F. buski* eggs or large flukes in the stool.

Assessment: Differential Diagnosis
There are many potential causes of diarrhea (*see Part 3: General Symptoms: Diarrhea, Acute*). Clues to fasciolopsiasis are travel to an endemic region and diarrhea developing several months after the ingestion of raw water plants.

Plan:
Treatment
   Praziquantel 25mg/kg po tid x 1 day
Patient Education
   General: Avoid ingestion of raw water plants
   Activity: As tolerated
   Diet: As tolerated
   Medications: Occasional nausea with praziquantel

Prevention and Hygiene: Avoid foods that may be contaminated
No Improvement/Deterioration: Return for re-evaluation.
Follow-up Actions
Return Evaluation: Investigate for other possible causes of diarrhea
Consultation Criteria: Failure to improve

Zoonotic Disease Considerations:
Agent: *Fasciolopsis buski*
Principal Animal Hosts: Pigs
Clinical Disease in Animals: Usually asymptomatic, although diarrhea can occur
Probable Mode of Transmission: Ingestion
Known Distribution: Asia and the Indian subcontinent

Chapter 12: Infectious Diseases: Parasitic Infections: Filariasis (Elephantiasis)

COL Glenn Wortmann, MC, USA

Introduction: Filariasis refers to infection by one of several nematodes found in the tropics and subtropics. *See Part 4: Organ Systems: Chapter 6: Superficial Fungal Infections: Loiasis & Onchocerciasis (River Blindness).* Lymphatic-dwelling nematodes are discussed here. They are transmitted by mosquitoes and cause three similar conditions: Bancroftian filariasis (*Wuchereria bancrofti*), Malayan, or Brugian filariasis (*Brugia malayi*) and Timorean filariasis (*B. timori*). Adult worms live in the lymphatics and release microfilaria, which can take up to a year to appear in the blood after infection, thus making diagnosis difficult.

Subjective: **Symptoms**
Early symptoms can include swollen lymph nodes (especially in the groin), headache and fever. Long-standing cases may present with lymphedema (which causes swollen legs [elephantiasis], scrotum, breasts, genitalia, etc.) Tropical pulmonary eosinophilia is a complication of filarial infection associated with intermittent nocturnal asthma, fever and interstitial lung disease.
Focused History: *Have you had repeated episodes of swollen lymph nodes?* (Recurrent lymphadenitis is typical.) *How long have/did you lived in this/that area?* (Most of the chronic complications of filariasis occur in long-term residents of endemic areas.)

Objective: **Signs**
Using Basic Tools: Intermittent fever and swollen lymph nodes. Chronic infection results in the swelling associated with elephantiasis.
Using Advanced Tools: Labs: Giemsa stained thick and thin blood smears may reveal microfilariae. Diagnose by examining a blood smear for the presence of microfilariae. Most microfilariae are active at night, but many in SE Asia are best detected between 10 am and 2 pm. The presence of retrograde lymphadenitis is also helpful.

Assessment: **Differential Diagnosis**
Lymphadenitis may also be seen with acute bacterial or viral infections.

Plan:
Treatment
Primary: **Ivermectin** 200-400mcg/kg po as a single dose.
Alternate: Diethylcarbamazine citrate (DEC) 6mg/kg po daily x 2 weeks.
Note: Drugs only clear the microfilaria, not all adult worms. Relapses are common and may respond to repeated treatment.
Patient Education
General: Avoid insect bites
Activity: As tolerated
Diet: As tolerated
Medications: Occasional gastrointestinal side effects. DEC can have generalized side effects, requiring pain relief and steroids.
Prevention and Hygiene: Avoid mosquito bites through the use of permethrin treatment of uniforms and the use of DEET.
No Improvement/Deterioration: Return for evaluation
Follow-up Actions
Return Evaluation: As needed
Consultation Criteria: Failure to improve

Chapter 12: Infectious Diseases: Parasitic Infections: Giardiasis

COL Glenn Wortmann, MC, USA

Introduction: Giardiasis is a common water-borne cause of diarrhea throughout the world. It is transmitted by fecal contamination of food or water. Treating water with chlorine may not kill *Giardia* cysts, especially if the water is cold. Incubation period is 3-25 days, with an average of about one week.

Subjective: **Symptoms**
Diarrhea (often prolonged), abdominal cramps, bloating, nausea and vomiting.
Focused History: *Have you had watery diarrhea?* (common for giardiasis) *Do you taste rotten eggs when you burp?* (Sulfuric belching is often noted.) *How long have you been experiencing diarrhea?* (can extend for months)

Objective: **Signs**
Using Basic Tools: Watery diarrhea, usually non-bloody
Using Advanced Tools: Labs: Look for organism in stool O & P samples (repeat test in at least 3 stools before considering negative).

Assessment: Prolonged watery diarrhea and sulfuric belching suggest *Giardia*.
Differential Diagnosis: Other causes of watery diarrhea, such as *E. coli*, *Salmonella* and Norovirus (*see Part 3: General Symptoms: Diarrhea, Acute*); Giardiasis requires a microscope to identify the organism.

Plan:
Treatment
Primary: Tinidazole 2g po once or **nitazoxanide** 500mg po bid x 3 days
Alternative: Metronidazole 500mg po tid x 5-7 days
Note: Avoid metronidazole use in first trimester of pregnancy. Use **paromomycin** 25-35mg/kg/d po in 3 divided doses x 7 days.
Patient Education
General: Maintain oral fluids to avoid volume depletion.
Activity: As tolerated
Diet: *Giardia* infection can result in transient lactose intolerance, so patients should avoid lactose-containing foods such as milk or cheese.
Medications: Avoid alcohol use while taking metronidazole.
Prevention and Hygiene: Boiling is probably the best water treatment. Most commercial water filters will not remove *Giardia* from water. If using iodine or chlorine, treat water with iodine or chlorine for at least 20 minutes before use. Avoid fecal-oral contamination with good hygiene.
No Improvement/Deterioration: Return for re-evaluation promptly.
Follow-up Actions
Return Evaluation: Consider alternative causes of diarrhea.
Consultation Criteria: Condition not responding to treatment.
Zoonotic Disease Considerations:
Agent: *Giardia lamblia*
Principal Animal Hosts: Dogs
Clinical Disease in Animals: May be asymptomatic; chronic diarrhea, steatorrhea, weight loss
Probable Mode of Transmission: Water
Known Distribution: Worldwide; common

Chapter 12: Infectious Diseases: Parasitic Infections: Gnathostomiasis
CDR John Sanders, MC, USN

Introduction: Gnathostomiasis is caused when the nematode (roundworm), *Gnathostoma spinigerum* (or rarely by other species), migrates through cutaneous, visceral, neural, or ocular tissues resulting in inflammatory reactions in those tissues. Gnathostoma is usually a parasite of dogs, cats, and other wild mammals, and humans usually acquire the infection by eating raw or undercooked fish or poultry. This infection is usually associated with Southeast Asia (eg, Thailand and Japan) and likely due to the eating habits in those regions. However, it has recently become an increasing problem in Central and South America (eg, Mexico) probably due to the consumption of ceviche (a popular dish made of various species of saltwater or freshwater raw fish marinated in lime juice). There are also case reports from Africa and the Middle East.

Subjective: **Symptoms**
Systemic symptoms such as fever, arthralgias, myalgias, malaise, anorexia, nausea, vomiting, diarrhea, and epigastric pain may occur as soon as 24-48 hours after ingestion of the larvae and usually resolve within a week. The classic symptoms are caused by the migrating larvae causing localized swellings that typically last 1-2 weeks and are associated with edema, pain, itching and variable erythema. Localized swellings can appear anywhere on the body (most common site is the trunk), begin as early as 3-4 weeks after ingestion and be accompanied by pruritus, low-grade fever, loss of appetite and nausea. The parasite can survive for years and lesions can recur for months to years in untreated patients. *Gnathostoma* can migrate to other tissues throughout the body, including the CNS, GI or GU, lungs, and eye, causing local inflammatory reactions resulting in organ dysfunction or loss of vision. Larval penetration into the brain usually results in the sudden onset of severe radicular pain or headache as well as paresthesias in the trunk or a limb, followed by paralysis of extremities or cranial nerves. The diagnosis is based on the clinical picture and history of travel.
Focused History: *Where have you been traveling?* (ie, Southeast Asia, Central or South America) *Have you ever eaten any undercooked or raw fish? Have you ever eaten raw poultry, snakes, or frogs?*

Objective: **Signs**
Using Basic Tools: Inspection and Palpation: 1-3cm soft, mildly tender, subcutaneous nodules (usually on the trunk, but can be anywhere), often associated with urticarial plaques (hives).
Using Advanced Tools: Peripheral blood smear (eosinophilia is expected). Definitive diagnosis will require a serologic test and tissue biopsy.

Assessment: **Differential Diagnosis**
Cutaneous larva migrans (CLM): A migratory skin rash caused when the infective larvae of animal hookworms (usually *Ancylostoma braziliense*) penetrate the skin and migrate in superficial tissues. Lesions are usually itchy or painful and may be papular or vesiculobullous, but can be distinguished from gnathostomiasis since they are characteristically serpiginous (creeping in wavy lines). *See Part 5: Specialty Areas: Chapter 12: Parasitic Infections: Hookworm & Cutaneous Larva Migrans*
Strongyloidiasis: Chronic strongyloidiasis can be associated with larva currens (recurrent, itchy, urticarial or serpiginous skin lesions). These lesions typically do not have the nodular swellings of gnathostomiasis. *See Part 5: Specialty Areas: Chapter 12: Parasitic Infections: Strongyloidiasis (Cutaneous Larva Currens)*
Loiasis: Caused by the *Loa loa* worm, this disease is characterized by localized areas of angioedema known as Calabar swellings.

These are warm, itchy or painful swellings that may come and go, often recurring multiple times per year. It can be distinguished from gnathostomiasis since the worm can sometimes be visible in the eye (crossing the conjunctiva). *See Part 4: Organ Systems: Chapter 6: Superficial Fungal Infections: Loiasis*

Echinococcosis, dirofilariasis, cysticercosis, onchocerciasis, and toxocariasis: Nodular or cystic lesions of the skin can be found in each but these are not typically migratory.

Plan:
Treatment
Primary: **Ivermectin** 0.2mg/kg/d po x 2 days is considered safe and likely effective.
Alternative: Albendazole 400mg po bid x 21 days
Patient Education
General: This is likely a parasite acquired by eating raw fish, but further evaluation by specialists will be required to confirm the diagnosis.
Activity: As tolerated.
Diet: As tolerated.
Prevention and Hygiene: Avoid eating raw fish.
Follow-up Actions
Return Evaluation: As needed for recurrence of symptoms.
Evacuation/Consultation Criteria: If symptoms are confined to subcutaneous swellings and itching, definitive evaluation can be briefly delayed. However, any changes in vision or neurologic status should require immediate evacuation to a higher level of care.

Zoonotic Disease Considerations:
Agent: *Gnathostoma spinigerum*
Principal Animal Hosts: Dogs, cats, wild mammals
Clinical Disease in Animals: The adult worm normally lives in a swelling (tumor) in the wall of the stomach and usually does not cause significant illness in the normal host.
Probable Mode of Transmission: Eating uncooked food infected with the larval third stage of the helminth; such foods typically include fish, shrimp, crab, crayfish, frog, or chicken.
Known Distribution: SE Asia, Central and South America, Africa, Middle East

Chapter 12: Infectious Diseases: Parasitic Infections: Hookworm and Cutaneous Larva Migrans
COL Glenn Wortmann, MC, USA

Introduction: Several species of hookworm can infect humans, most commonly *Necator americanus* or *Ancylostoma duodenale*. An estimated one fourth of the world's population is infected, and the geographic distribution is in the tropical and subtropical zones. Eggs in feces from infected people and animals are deposited on the ground and hatch into larvae. Larvae infect by direct penetrating skin, migrating to the lungs and up to the esophagus. They are then swallowed and travel to the small intestine. Symptoms become evident weeks to months after infection. Eosinophilia is common. Cutaneous larva migrans (CLM) is a unique serpentine lesion created by a canine or feline hookworm, *A. caninum*, *A. braziliense*, which migrates through the skin but is unable to penetrate the dermis. The lesions are very pruritic; thread-like; found most commonly on the feet, hands, and buttocks; and become progressively larger with time. The larvae usually die, but may require treatment.

Subjective: **Symptoms**
"Ground itch" (an itchy, red rash at the site of larval penetration through the skin), cough, abdominal pain, diarrhea, and CLM lesions; can also be asymptomatic.
Focused History: *Have you had a rash?* (Ground itch and CLM are typical.) *Are you more fatigued?* (due to anemia)

Objective: **Signs**
Using Basic Tools: Ground itch at entry site, CLM rash (serpentine, slightly elevated, erythematous, palpable tract)
Using Advanced Tools: Labs: CBC: Anemia noted by hematocrit; eosinophilia noted on WBC. O&P of stool: Hookworm eggs may not be seen early in infection, so repeat test in one week if the initial test is negative.

Assessment: **Differential Diagnosis**
Anemia: Multiple potential causes, but the presence of iron-deficiency anemia in multiple patients in a community suggests hookworm infection.
CLC rash: Cutaneous larva currens rash of *Strongyloides* infection. Other symptoms of human hookworm are non-specific and may be confused with many diagnoses. *See Part 5: Specialty Areas: Chapter 12: Parasitic Infections: Strongyloidiasis (Cutaneous Larva Currens) & Appendices: Color Plates: Figure A-23.F*

Plan:
Treatment
Hookworm: Repeat stool O & P and re-treat as needed.
Primary: Mebendazole 100mg po bid x 3 days, or 500mg po in a single dose
Alternative: Albendazole 400mg po once or **pyrantel pamoate** 11mg/kg per day x 3 days, not to exceed 1g/day
CLM
Primary: Ivermectin 150-200mcg/kg po once
Alternative: Albendazole 400mg po q day x 3 days or topical **thiabendazole** 10% solution applied 1cm around leading edge of the CLM lesion.

Patient Education

General: Avoid contaminated soil, especially sandy beaches with shady areas. Shoes should be worn to prevent infection.

Medications: Watch for occasional gastrointestinal side effects (diarrhea and abdominal pain).

Prevention and Hygiene: Avoid contaminated soil.

No Improvement/Deterioration: Return for re-evaluation.

Follow-up Actions

Evacuation/Consultation Criteria: Evacuation not normally necessary, unless patient fails to improve.

Zoonotic Considerations

Principal Animal Hosts: Dogs, cats, sheep, swine

Clinical Disease in Animals: *Ancylostoma spp.* - anemia, unthriftiness, melena, emaciation, weakness of chronic disease

Chapter 12: Infectious Diseases: Parasitic Infections: Leishmaniasis

COL Glenn Wortmann, MC, USA

Introduction: Leishmaniasis is transmitted by a bite from an infected sandfly. Infection by *Leishmania* species protozoa can result in cutaneous, mucocutaneous or visceral disease (kala-azar). The incubation period can be long, up to 6 months after exposure. Two cutaneous types: Old World disease in Asia, Africa, Middle East; and New World disease in Central and South America. The visceral form, found in most tropical areas worldwide, is often fatal.

Subjective: Symptoms

Cutaneous: Non-healing skin lesion which is usually ulcerative. This skin sore often starts as a papule that enlarges and ulcerates. Sometimes trauma to the skin can initiate the infection at a site distant to the sandfly bite.

Visceral (kala-azar): Fever often >104°F which can be intermittent, with chills, wasting, night sweats, nonproductive cough, abdominal complaints, fatigue and an enlarged abdomen.

Focused History: *Do you remember insect/sandfly bites?* (exposure) *Did you have trauma here before this sore developed?* (typical history) *How long have you noticed your skin sore(s)?* (tend to be chronic and non-healing)

Objective: Signs

Using Basic Tools:

Cutaneous: Chronic skin lesions, usually ulcerative but can be infiltrative or papular; crust often forms over the surface and secondary bacterial infections can occur; usually on exposed portions of the body (frequently extremities and face); regional adenopathy. *See Appendices: Color Plates: Figure A-24.A*

Visceral: Fever, wasting, lymphadenopathy, skin changes, hepatosplenomegaly; late peripheral edema, renal failure and bleeding.

Using Advanced Tools:

Cutaneous: Scraping the surface of the skin ulcer with a scalpel, smear sample onto a glass slide. When stained with Giemsa stain and examined under a microscope, the amastigote form of *Leishmania* should be visible.

Visceral: A dipstick assay (Kalazar Detect rapid test) is available and can be used in a field setting. Definitive diagnosis requires a liver or bone marrow biopsy.

Assessment: Differential Diagnosis

Cutaneous (chronic skin lesion)

Sporotrichosis: Diagnosis requires a tissue biopsy and culture

Syphilis: Diagnosis requires a blood test for a RPR/FTA assay. *See Part 5: Specialty Areas: Chapter 11: Genital Ulcers*

Leprosy: Diagnosis requires a tissue biopsy and histopathological review. *See Part 4: Organ Systems: Chapter 6: Mycobacterial Infections: Leprosy (Hansen's Disease)*

Neoplasm: Diagnosis requires a tissue biopsy and histopathological review

Visceral (fever and hepatosplenomegaly)

Malaria: Diagnosis requires a blood sample for microscopy or malaria dipstick testing. *See Part 5: Specialty Areas: Chapter 12: Parasitic Infections: Malaria*

Typhoid: Diagnosis requires blood culture in a laboratory. *See Specialty Areas: Chapter 12: Bacterial Infections: Typhoid Fever*

Typhus: Diagnosis requires a blood sample for testing Rickettsial antibodies. *See Specialty Areas: Chapter 12: Rickettsial Infections*

Acute Chagas' disease: Requires a blood sample sent to a reference laboratory or a tissue sample for histopathological review. *See Specialty Areas: Chapter 12: Parasitic Infections: American Trypanosomiasis (American Chagas' Disease)*

Tuberculosis: Requires a tissue biopsy for histopathological review and culture in a reference laboratory. *See Part 5: Specialty Areas: Chapter 6: Mycobacterial Infections: Tuberculosis*

Plan:

Treatment

Primary:

Cutaneous: Usually self-limited. Old World cutaneous form may respond to **fluconazole** 200mg po q day x 42 days. **Pentavalent antimony** for very difficult cases.

Visceral: **Liposomal amphotericin B (AmBisome)** 21mg/kg given as 3mg/kg/day on 7 days over a 21-day period

Alterative: Pentavalent antimony (sodium stibogluconate [Pentostam]) from Walter Reed Army Medical Center.

Patient Education

General: Avoid sandfly bites.

Activity: As tolerated

Diet: As tolerated

Medications: As tolerated

Prevention and Hygiene: Avoid sandfly bites.

Wound Care: Keep wound clean, dry, and protected.

No Improvement/Deterioration: Return for referral to a higher level of care.

Follow-up Actions

Evacuation/Consultation Criteria: Cutaneous form requires non-urgent referral to a specialist in tropical medicine. Visceral *leishmaniasis* is potentially life threatening so patient should be transferred to infectious diseases/tropical medicine care urgently.

Note: Definitive diagnosis is made by identification of the cultured organism from biopsy of skin (cutaneous disease) or liver/spleen or bone marrow (visceral disease). Walter Reed Army Medical Center is the DoD site with comprehensive diagnostic capability for military beneficiaries.

Zoonotic Disease Considerations:

Principal Animal Hosts: Dogs, wild canids

Clinical Disease in Animals: Skin lesions, weight loss, poor appetite, lymphadenopathy, ocular lesions, renal failure, epistaxis, lameness, anemia.

Chapter 12: Infectious Diseases: Parasitic Infections: Malaria

COL Glenn Wortmann, MC, USA

Introduction: Malaria is a tremendous problem in tropical, developing countries, causing 2-3 million deaths/year. There are 4 species of malaria protozoa which infect humans: *Plasmodium vivax* (incubation period of 12 days-10 months); *P. ovale* (similar to vivax); *P. malariae* (incubation period of 1 month); and *P. falciparum* (most deadly; incubation period 5-30 days). Mosquito bite, needlestick or a blood transfusion from an infected person transmits malaria.

Subjective: Symptoms

Headache, chills, sweats, and muscle aches are common; abdominal pain and diarrhea may occur.

Focused History: *Have you had a fever?* (Fever in a patient in or returning from a malarious area must be considered to be malaria until proven otherwise.) *Do you have any other symptoms?* (Chills, low back pain and myalgias are often seen with malaria.)

Objective: Signs

Using Basic Tools: Vital signs: Temperature over 100.4°F. Cyclic fevers (occurring every other day with *P. vivax* and *P. ovale* and every 3rd day with *P. malariae*) may occur (although this is an unreliable finding). Inspection: Sweats and rigors may be seen. Palpation: Enlarged liver and spleen may occur.

Using Advanced Tools: Labs: Thick and thin blood smears stained with Giemsa. *See Appendices: Color Plates: A-25, A-26.I, A-26.L & A-26.O.* The thick smear is reported to be 30 x more sensitive than the thin smear, but the thin smear is required for species identification. Smears should be done 2-3 x a day for 48 hours to exclude the diagnosis of malaria. A new dipstick malaria rapid diagnostic assay is now available for testing a blood sample. Although it is less sensitive than microscopy, it is very useful for those who are not experienced in recognizing malaria parasites under a microscope.

Assessment: Differential Diagnosis

Fever: (*see Part 3: General Symptoms: Fever*) Other causes of fever include leptospirosis, dengue, typhoid fever (*see ID sections* on these) and bacterial meningitis (*see Part 4: Organ Systems: Meningitis*).

Plan:

Treatment

Primary:

1. *P. falciparum:*
   a. In Haiti, the Dominican Republic and Central America west of the Panama Canal, uncomplicated *P. falciparum* can be treated with **chloroquine** 1g (600mg base), then 500mg (300mg base) 6 hours later, then 500mg (300mg base) at 24 and 48 hours.
   b. In the remainder of world, *P. falciparum* has become resistant to chloroquine. In that case, treatment of uncomplicated malaria consists of **quinine sulfate** 650mg po q8h x 3-7 days plus **doxycycline** 100mg po bid x 7 days (alternative choices for treatment are listed in this section).
   c. For patients with severe malaria (parasitemia >5%, impaired consciousness, seizures, respiratory distress, substantial bleeding or shock), evacuation and therapy with IV **quinine** or **quinidine** is recommended. The drug **artesunate** has recently become available from the CDC for the treatment of severe malaria, and may prove to be a better alternative than quinine/quinidine.
2. Species other than *P. falciparum:*
   a. **Chloroquine** 1g (600mg base), then 500mg (300 mg base) 6 hours later, then 500mg (300mg base) at 24 and 48 hours.
   b. In Oceania, chloroquine resistant *P. vivax* has been reported, and therapy as per chloroquine resistant *P. falciparum* should be given.
   c. To prevent relapses with *P. vivax* and *P. ovale*, give **primaquine phosphate** 30mg base po per day x 14 days.
3. **Unknown Malaria Species:** Treat as *P. falciparum*.
4. **For children: Chloroquine** 10mg base/kg po followed by 5mg base/kg at 12, 24 and 36 hours or **mefloquine** 15mg base/kg po in a single dose. Alternative: **Quinine** 10mg salt/kg po q8h x 7 days + **clindamycin** 10mg/kg po bid x 3-7 days.
5. **Medication Contraindications:** Primaquine should not be given to pregnant women or newborn babies because of the risk of hemolysis. Doxycycline and tetracycline should not be given to pregnant women or children less than 8 years old. Chloroquine,

quinine, and quinidine are considered safe in all trimesters of pregnancy, and there is evidence that mefloquine is safe in the second and third trimesters.

Alternative: Quinine 650mg po tid + **clindamycin** 600mg po tid x 5 days. Other alternatives are **mefloquine** 1,250mg as a single dose or **Malarone (atovaquone** and **proguanil hydrochloride)** 4 tablets po q day x 3 days.

Patient Education

General: Malaria is transmitted by mosquitoes that are active from dusk to dawn, so avoid outdoor activities during that time.

Activity: As tolerated

Diet: As tolerated

Medications: Doxycycline can cause photosensitivity, so avoid the sun or use sunscreen. Primaquine can cause hemolytic anemia in patients with glucose-6-phosphate dehydrogenase (G6PD) deficiency, and is contraindicated in severe deficiency.

Prevention and Hygiene: Prophylaxis:

1. For travel to areas without chloroquine-resistant *P. falciparum*, give **chloroquine** 300mg base weekly beginning 1-2 weeks before travel and continuing 4 weeks after returning.
2. For travel to areas with chloroquine-resistant *P. falciparum*, give **mefloquine** 250mg weekly 1-2 weeks before travel, weekly during travel and continuing 4 weeks after returning. **Doxycycline** 100mg po q d beginning 1-2 days before travel, during travel and continuing 4 weeks after returning is an alternative regimen (watch for photosensitivity). Another well-tolerated option is **Malarone** 1 tab po q d beginning 1-2 days prior to travel, daily during travel, and then continuing daily for one week after returning from travel.
3. For patients with prolonged exposure to *P. vivax* and *P. ovale*, give **primaquine phosphate** 30mg base po per day for 2 weeks after returning from travel (Need to check for G6PD deficiency prior to use, as this drug can cause severe and potentially fatal anemia in patients who are G6PD-deficient.)
4. The avoidance of mosquito bites is critical, as no drug is 100% successful in preventing malaria. Use of bed nets, DEET lotion/sprays and permethrin-treated clothing will all decrease the risk of malaria.

No Improvement/Deterioration: Return for re-evaluation promptly.

Follow-up Actions

Return Evaluation: Repeat smears to assess effectiveness of treatment.

Evacuation/Consultation Criteria: The presence of severe malaria should prompt consultation with an expert in malaria. For complicated malaria (cerebral dysfunction, renal failure, very high parasitemia, ARDS) rapid evacuation to a higher echelon care facility is needed.

Chapter 12: Infectious Diseases: Parasitic Infections: Paragonimiasis

COL Glenn Wortmann, MC, USA

Introduction: The only lung fluke that infects man, *Paragonimus* is found throughout the Far East (particularly China), in West Africa and in several parts of Central and South America. It is acquired from eating raw, salted, dried, pickled or incompletely cooked freshwater crabs, crayfish and shrimp.

Subjective: **Symptoms**

Most infections are asymptomatic. Heavier infections result in chronic productive cough, chest pain (pleuritic), hemoptysis and night sweats. Extrapulmonary disease can be found in subcutaneous tissues, liver, lymph nodes, others.

Focused History *Have you had a cough? If so, has your cough been bloody?* (typical symptoms) *How long have you had a cough?* (can have chronic bronchitis)

Objective: **Signs**

Using Basic Tools: Cough, hemoptysis, tender chest, rales and decreased breath sounds.

Using Advanced Tools: Labs: Eggs in O & P of sputum (particularly in colored flecks) or feces. CXR: Increased markings and atelectasis on effected side (consolidation).

Assessment: Diagnose empirically by history of bloody cough in an endemic area.

Differential Diagnosis: Chronic cough: pneumonia, tuberculosis, lung cancer and chronic bronchitis.

Plan:

Treatment

Primary: Praziquantel 25mg/kg po tid x 3 days.

Alternative: Triclabendazole 10mg/kg po for one dose (available through the Centers for Disease Control)

Patient Education

General/ Diet/Prevention and Hygiene: Avoid improperly cooked freshwater crabs, crayfish and shrimp.

Activity: As tolerated Medications: Occasional gastrointestinal side effects.

No Improvement/Deterioration: Return for evaluation.

Follow-up Actions

Return Evaluation: As needed

Consultation Criteria: Failure to improve

Zoonotic Disease Considerations

Principal Animal Hosts: Dogs, cats, swine

Clinical Disease in Animals: Can migrate aberrantly and produce cysts in brain and spinal cord; may have neurological signs based on location of lesion.

Chapter 12: Infectious Diseases: Parasitic Infections: Schistosomiasis

COL Glenn Wortmann, MC, USA

Introduction: A blood fluke (trematode) infection found in most tropical areas, particularly Asia and South America, characterized by adult male and female worms living in the veins of a human host. Three major disease syndromes occur in schistosomiasis: dermatitis, Katayama fever (marked by fever, diffusely enlarged lymph nodes and eosinophilia) and chronic infection. Infection occurs while swimming, wading, rafting, washing etc. in contaminated fresh water. Penetration of the skin by worm larvae causes dermatitis in the first 24 hours, but the clinical symptoms of acute schistosomiasis develop 2 weeks-3 months after exposure. Chronic schistosomiasis can result in abdominal pain or liver failure (*Schistosoma mansoni, S. japonicum*) or hematuria or kidney problems (*S. hematobium*).

Subjective: **Symptoms**
> **Dermatitis:** A pruritic rash known as swimmer's itch.
> **Katayama fever:** Occurs 4-8 weeks after infection and presents with acute fever, chills, headache, sweating and cough.
> **Chronic infection:** Can result in abdominal pain with diarrhea or hematuria.
> **Focused History:** *Have you been exposed to fresh water (eg, swimming in a lake or pond)?* (typical exposure in endemic areas) *Did you notice a rash after swimming?* (Rash is caused by the organism invading the skin.) *How long ago were you exposed to fresh water?* (Fever and lymphadenopathy from schistosomiasis occur 4-8 weeks after exposure.)

Objective: **Signs**
> **Using Basic Tools:** Dermatitis: A papular rash; Katayama fever: Fever and lymphadenopathy; chronic infection; enlargement of the liver and spleen may be noted, weight loss is common; hematuria may occur.
> **Using Advanced Tools:** Labs: Diagnose by finding schistosome eggs in O & P of feces or urine. *See Appendices: Color Plates: Figure A-26.M*

Assessment: **Differential Diagnosis**
> **Fever and lymphadenopathy:** Any possible etiologies to include secondary syphilis, mononucleosis and HIV. Enlargement of liver; chronic liver diseases (Hepatitis B, hepatitis C and others)
> **Hematuria:** Kidney stones, urinary tract infections, bladder cancer and others

Plan:
> **Treatment**
>> **Praziquantel** 20mg/kg po bid x 1 day for *S. mansoni* and *S. hematobium*; 20mg/kg po tid x 1 day for *S. japonica*. If Katayama fever is present, treatment may result in initial clinical deterioration. Use steroids (**prednisolone** 40mg po q day x 5 days) in conjunction with the praziquantel. All infections should be treated to avoid the chronic complications of this parasitic illness.
> **Patient Education**
>> General: Avoid contact with fresh water in endemic areas.
>> Activity: As tolerated
>> Diet: As tolerated
>> Medications: Praziquantel is usually very well tolerated
>> Prevention and Hygiene: Avoid contact with fresh water in endemic areas.
>> No Improvement/Deterioration: Refer to clinic.
> **Follow-up Actions**
>> **Return Evaluation:** Refer to higher level of care as needed.
>> **Consultation Criteria:** Failure to improve

Zoonotic Disease Considerations:
> Agent: *Schistosoma spp.*, Schistosome cercariae (swimmer's itch)
> Principal Animal Hosts: Cattle, buffalo, swine, dogs, cats, sheep, goats (depending on species and location)
> Clinical Disease in Animals: Ruminants - hemorrhagic enteritis, anemia, emaciation
> Probable Mode of Transmission: Penetration of unbroken skin by cercariae from infected snails in water
> Known Distribution: Worldwide, depending on species and location

Chapter 12: Infectious Diseases: Parasitic Infections: Strongyloidiasis (Cutaneous Larva Currens)

COL Glenn Wortmann, MC, USA

Introduction: *Strongyloides stercoralis* is found worldwide in the warm, damp soil of the tropics and subtropics, especially in Southeast Asia. Larvae penetrate the skin and travel to the lungs, then are coughed up and swallowed where they pass into the small intestine and mature into adults. Incubation period is 2-4 weeks, but because of an autoinoculation cycle the parasite can be reactivated many years later when host is immunocompromised (steroids, chemotherapy, AIDS, advanced age). This may result in a hyperinfection syndrome that can result in overwhelming infection and death.

Subjective: **Symptoms**
> Diarrhea, abdominal pain, nausea, cough, wheezing, SOB.
> **Focused History:** *Have you noticed a rash around your anus or trunk?* (CLC) *Is the rash migrating?* (CLC migrates.) *How long have you been having symptoms?* (can last for years)

Objective: **Signs**

Using Basic Tools: CLC rash (migrating, thread-like, erythematous, pruritic, maculopapular, rapidly moving rash [several cm per hour] at the site of larval penetration, often occurs on the buttocks region from external autoinfection); rales, wheezes, SOB and epigastric tenderness.

Using Advanced Tools: Labs: O & P of stool: identify *Strongyloides* larvae in a fresh stool sample (multiple tests may be needed). *See Appendices: Color Plates: Figure A-23.B*

Assessment: **Differential Diagnosis**

Hookworm: CLC appears similar to cutaneous larva migrans rash but moves faster and may be perianal. *See Part 5: Specialty Areas: Chapter 12: Parasitic Infections: Hookworm and Cutaneous Larva Migrans*

Diarrhea: Multiple causes. *See Part 3: General Symptoms: Diarrhea, Acute*

Plan:

Treatment Repeat stool O & P and re-treat as needed.
  Primary: Ivermectin 200mcg/kg/d po x 2 days
  Alternative: Albendazole 400mg po bid x 3 days

Patient Education
  General: Avoid contaminated soil.
  Medications: Watch for occasional gastrointestinal side effects (diarrhea and abdominal pain).
  Prevention and Hygiene: Avoid exposure to contaminated soil.
  No Improvement/Deterioration: Return for re-evaluation.

Follow-up Actions
  Evacuation/Consultation Criteria: Evacuation usually not necessary, unless patient fails to improve.

Zoonotic Disease Considerations:
  Principal Animal Hosts: Dogs, cats
  Clinical Disease in Animals: Bloody-mucoid diarrhea, emaciation, reduced growth rate.

Chapter 12: Infectious Diseases: Parasitic Infections: Taeniasis (Tapeworm Infections)

COL Glenn Wortmann, MC, USA

Introduction: Tapeworms infection occurs through eating infected fish, beef, pork or other contaminated food. Adult tapeworms, ranging from several millimeters to 25 meters long, live in the intestine. Encysted larvae enter the human host through raw or undercooked beef, pork or fish, or by contact with human feces (night soil) used as fertilizer.

Subjective: **Symptoms**

Most infections are asymptomatic. Heavy infections may result in abdominal pain, weight loss, nervousness, diarrhea, and a sensation of the contracting worms leaving the anus. The larval form of pork tapeworm can migrate to multiple areas of the body, to include the brain, causing seizures or death.

Focused History: *Have you noticed worms in your stool?* (may be tapeworm, pinworm or others) *How large are the worms?* (Tapeworm segments seen in the stool are usually <1cm.)

Objective: **Signs**

Using Basic Tools: Segments of worm in stool; in cysticercosis, seizures may occur.

Using Advanced Tools: Labs: O & P of stool: Egg release is variable, so examine stool samples from several days.

Assessment: Diagnose by identifying eggs in the stool or identifying the proglottids (segments) in stool or on anal swab.

Differential Diagnosis:

Worms in stool: Ascariasis (roundworm) can also be seen in the stool, although it is typically larger.

Seizures: There are many possible causes of seizures, to include epilepsy and meningitis. The presence of seizures in a patient living in area endemic for pork tapeworm (Africa, South America, Eastern Europe, SE Asia) should prompt the consideration of cysticercosis.

Plan:

Treatment
  Primary: Praziquantel 5-10mg/kg po as a one-time dose. For the dwarf tapeworm, the dose of **praziquantel** is 25mg/kg po, and repeat in 10 days.

Patient Education
  General: Avoid improperly prepared foods
  Activity: As tolerated
  Diet: As tolerated
  Medications: Occasional gastrointestinal side-effects
  Prevention and Hygiene: Avoid improperly cooked beef, pork or fish
  No Improvement/Deterioration: Return for evaluation

Follow-up Actions
  Return Evaluation: As needed
  Consultation Criteria: Failure to improve. For the diagnosis of cysticercosis, referral to a tertiary medical center for CT or MRI scan of the head may show multiple calcified lesions.

Zoonotic Disease Considerations

Fish tapeworm disease
Agents: *Diphyllobothrium latum, D. pacificum, D. dendriticum, D. ursi, D. dalliae, D. klebanovskii*
Principal Animal Hosts: Dogs, bears, foxes, minks, cats, dogs, pigs, walruses, seals, other fish-eating mammals
Clinical Disease in Animals: In fish, the larval stages encyst in the visceral organs and muscle while the adults are found in the intestinal tract, leading to possible mechanical obstruction in fish or mammals.
Probable Mode of Transmission: Ingestion of raw or undercooked fish

Dwarf tapeworm disease
Agent: *Hymenolepis nana* (the only human tapeworm without an obligatory intermediate host)
Principal Animal Host: Humans, mice
Clinical Disease in Animals: Found in the small intestine of rats, mice and hamsters. Reduced growth or weight loss in rodents.
Probable Mode of Transmission: Ingestion of eggs in contaminated food or water; directly from fecal contaminated fingers
Known Distribution: USA, Latin America, Australia, Mediterranean countries, the Near East and India

Beef tapeworm disease
Agent: *Taenia saginata, Cysticercus bovis* (cyst form)
Principal Animal Hosts: Cattle, water buffalo
Clinical Disease in Animals: Fluid-filled vesicle in the skeletal and cardiac musculature
Probable Mode of Transmission: Ingestion of undercooked beef containing *Cysticercus bovis*
Known Distribution: Worldwide

Pork tapeworm disease
Agent: *Taenia solium, Cysticercus cellulosae* (cyst form)
Principal Animal Hosts: Swine, man
Clinical Disease in Animals: Fluid-filled vesicle in the skeletal and cardiac musculature
Probable Mode of Transmission: Ingestion of undercooked pork containing *Cysticercus cellulosae*
Known Distribution: Worldwide where swine are raised; rare in USA, Canada, UK, Scandinavia

Echinococcosis (Cystic hydrated disease)
Agent: *Echinococcus granulosus*
Principal Animal Hosts: Dogs, cattle, sheep, swine, rodents, deer
Clinical Disease in Animals: Typically asymptomatic
Probable Mode of Transmission: Ingestion of tapeworm eggs
Known Distribution: Worldwide

Dipylidiasis (Dog tapeworm)
Agent: *Dipylidium caninum*
Principal Animal Hosts: Dogs, cats, fleas
Clinical Disease in Animals: Asymptomatic, flea infestation
Probable Mode of Transmission: Ingestion of fleas
Known Distribution: Worldwide

Chapter 12: Infectious Diseases: Parasitic Infections: Trichinellosis (Trichinosis)

COL Glenn Wortmann, MC, USA

Introduction: Trichinosis develops when undercooked meat contaminated with *Trichinella spiralis* is ingested. Most infections result from eating undercooked pork, although bear or walrus meat can transmit the infection. Symptoms appear from a few to 15 days after ingestion.

Subjective: **Symptoms:**
Most infections are asymptomatic. For heavier exposures, diarrhea, fever, periorbital edema, photophobia and muscle pain occurs.
Focused History: *Have you eaten undercooked pork in the last few weeks?* (Symptoms peak 2-3 weeks after ingestion) *Are your muscles sore and weak?* (Myalgias and weakness are common.) *How long have you been having symptoms?* (Trichinosis is usually a self-limited infection, lasting for a few weeks.)

Objective: **Signs:**
Using Basic Tools: Fever. Inspection: Splinter hemorrhages under the nails and conjunctivae; upper eyelid edema. Palpation: Muscle tenderness
Using Advanced Tools: Labs: Review of peripheral blood smears will show an increased number of eosinophils.

Assessment: Fever and myalgias after recent ingestion of pork is very suggestive of trichinosis.
Differential Diagnosis: Fever and muscle tenderness as in:
Myositis: Requires a muscle biopsy and histopathological review for diagnosis
Tetanus: Is diagnosed clinically, by the presence of lockjaw and uncontrollable muscle contractions (tetany)

Plan:
Treatment
Supportive therapy with bed rest and pain medication. For severe disease, **prednisone** 50mg po q day x 10 days may be beneficial. In the rare event that a patient is known to have eaten infected meat within a week, give **mebendazole** 200-400mg po tid x 3 days, then 400-500mg po tid x 10 days. Mebendazole is only effective against intestinal worms. It does not kill muscle larvae, so it has no effect on established infections.
Patient Education
General: Avoid improperly prepared foods
Activity: As tolerated

Diet: As tolerated

Medications: Occasional gastrointestinal side effects

Prevention and Hygiene: Avoid improperly cooked pork.

No Improvement/Deterioration: Return for evaluation

Follow-up Actions

Return Evaluation: As needed

Consultation Criteria: Failure to improve. For definitive diagnosis, antibody testing (serology) for *Trichinella* is available at reference laboratories.

Zoonotic Disease Considerations:

Principal Animal Hosts: Swine, rodents, bears

Clinical Disease in Animals: Asymptomatic

Probable Mode of Transmission: Ingestion of meat containing trichinella worms encysted in striated muscle.

Known Distribution: Worldwide, especially sub-arctic

Chapter 12: Infectious Diseases: Parasitic Infections: Trichuriasis (Whipworm)

COL Glenn Wortmann, MC, USA

Introduction: Whipworm (*Trichuris trichiura*) is one of the most common human worm infections, with approximately 800 million cases occurring worldwide. It is spread by fecal-oral transmission or ingesting vegetables contaminated with whipworm eggs. Infection is generally asymptomatic, but patients with heavy worm burdens may present with anemia, bloody diarrhea, growth retardation or rectal prolapse. Children ages 5-15 are most commonly infected.

Subjective: **Symptoms**

Usually asymptomatic; may have abdominal pain, bloody diarrhea, malaise, and rectal prolapse.

Focused History: *Have you experienced bloody diarrhea? Have you had a decrease in your energy level?* (Whipworm can cause bloody diarrhea and iron deficiency anemia.)

Objective: **Signs**

Using Basic Tools: Bloody diarrhea, tender abdomen, rectal prolapse

Using Advanced Tools: Labs: CBC with low HCT; stool for O&P for characteristic lemon-shaped egg; *see Appendices: Color Plates: Figure A-26.H*

Assessment: **Differential Diagnosis:** Bloody diarrhea/anemia from:

Amebiasis: Diagnosis requires microscopic examination of stool specimens for the presence of *Entamoeba histolytica*. Antigen-detection kits for testing stool are also commercially available.

Shigellosis: Diagnosis requires stool culture

Inflammatory bowel disease: Diagnosis requires biopsy of the colonic mucosa followed by histopathological review

Plan:

Treatment

Primary: Albendazole 400mg po for one dose and repeat in 2 weeks

Alternative: Mebendazole 100mg po once and repeat in 1-2 weeks

Patient Education

Prevention: Avoid uncooked vegetables in endemic areas

Medications: For heavy infection, retreatment may be needed

Zoonotic Disease Considerations:

Principal Animal Hosts: Man, canids, and swine

Clinical Disease in Animals: Usually asymptomatic; can see melena, anemia, anorexia, unthriftiness in heavy infestations

Probable Mode of Transmission: Ingestion of embryonated eggs

Chapter 12: Infectious Diseases: Parasitic Infections: Trypanosomiasis, African (Sleeping Sickness)

COL Glenn Wortmann, MC, USA

Introduction: Transmitted by tsetse fly bites, infection with *Trypanosoma brucei* may cause either West African (*T. brucei gambiense*) or East African (*T. brucei rhodesiense*) trypanosomiasis. Sleeping sickness is endemic in 36 African countries. In the more rapidly progressive *T.b. rhodesiense* infection, the incubation period is 3 days to a few weeks. In *T.b. gambiense*, the incubation period may last several months to years.

Subjective: **Symptoms**

A painful trypanosomal chancre may develop at the site of the tsetse fly bite.

West African: Fever develops weeks to months after the bite, followed by lymphadenopathy. Personality changes, intense headache and difficulty walking eventually occur. The final phase is marked by progressive neurologic impairment ending in coma and death.

East African: The onset of symptoms usually occurs more rapidly, with fever, malaise and headache occurring within a few days to weeks. Lymph node swelling is not as common. Without treatment, death usually occurs within weeks to months.

Focused History: *Do you remember a painful insect bite?* (The tsetse fly bite is usually painful.) *Have you noticed a rash?* (A rash is common with East African disease.) *Where have you been traveling? When might have you been exposed to a tsetse fly?* (The incubation period for East African disease is usually a few days, while that for West African disease is weeks to months.)

Objective: Signs
Using Basic Tools: Inspection: fever, tachycardia, painless enlarged lymph nodes, painful chancre at bite site with surrounding edema.
Using Advanced Tools: Trypanosomes seen on examination of thick and thin peripheral blood smears; *see Appendices: Color Plates: Figure A-26.K*

Assessment: Diagnose by identifying organism on blood smear.
Differential Diagnosis:
Cutaneous leishmaniasis: Skin lesions can appear similar to trypanosomiasis. *See Part 5: Specialty Areas: Chapter 12: Parasitic Infections: Leishmaniasis*
Pyoderma: Skin lesions can appear similar to trypanosomiasis.
Rabies, meningitis, encephalitis, organic brain disease: Later stages of trypanosomiasis can result in altered mental status. *See Part 5: Specialty Areas: Chapter 12: Viral Infections: Rabies; Parasitic Infections: Malaria & Part 4: Organ Systems: Chapter 5: Meningitis*
Tuberculosis, malaria: Other common causes of fever and common to endemic area. *See Part 5: Specialty Areas: Chapter 12: Mycobacterial Infections: Tuberculosis & Parasitic Infections: Malaria*

Plan:
Treatment: Requires evacuation to a medical center with infectious disease and tropical medicine support for definitive diagnosis and treatment

Patient Education
General: Avoid tsetse fly bites by wearing protective clothing.
Activity: As tolerated
Diet: As tolerated.
Medications: Since medications have several severe side effects, they should only be given at a tertiary care center.
Prevention and Hygiene: Avoid insect bites.
Follow-up Actions
Consultation Criteria: All suspected cases should be referred for consultation.

Zoonotic Disease Considerations:
Principal Animal Hosts: Dogs, ruminants, carnivores
Clinical Disease in Animals: Intermittent fever, anemia, weight loss; may be asymptomatic.

Chapter 12: Infectious Diseases: Parasitic Infections: Trypanosomiasis, American (Chagas' Disease)
COL Glenn Wortmann, MC, USA

Introduction: Transmitted by kissing bug bite or blood transfusion. *Trypanosoma cruzi* has been isolated from many wild and domestic animals from the southern US and through all of Latin America. Incubation period is 5-14 days after bite, 30-40 days after transfusion.

Subjective: Symptoms
Acute: Fever; malaise; red, swollen site of inoculation with an enlarged draining lymph node; Romaña's sign (unilateral, painless swelling of eyelid if inoculation was via the eye) occasionally, CNS symptoms (eg, seizures) or myocarditis. Chronic: Years later: heart failure; enlargement of the esophagus or colon may cause dysphagia and/or constipation.
Focused History: *Do you recall an unusual, red, swollen insect bite or swelling around one eye?* (distinctive bite or Romaña's sign suggestive of Chagas' disease) *Did you ever live in Central or South America, Mexico, or South Texas?* (endemic to area)

Objective: Signs
Using Basic Tools: Variable fever; lymphadenopathy; Romaña's sign; hard, red, painful nodule (chagoma) at the bite site.
Using Advanced Tools: Labs: Parasites in peripheral blood smears (thick and thin) can be found during febrile periods early in the course of infection, *see Appendices: Color Plates: Figure A-26.K.*

Assessment: Differential Diagnosis
Leishmaniasis and bacterial skin infections: May have similar skin lesion (chagoma). *See Part 5: Specialty Areas: Chapter 12: Parasitic Infections: Leishmaniasis & Part 4: Organ Systems: Chapter 6: Bacterial Infections: Staphylococcal Infections*
Symptoms of chronic Chagas' disease: Congestive heart failure (eg, myocardial infarctions and hypertension)

Plan:
Treatment
Acute Chagas' disease: **Nifurtimox** or **benznidazole** from CDC in Atlanta, GA (for investigational use only) and from some hospitals in the endemic area.
Patient Education
General: Prevent insect bites (specifically kissing bugs, which are often found in thatched roofs and bite at night)
Activity: As tolerated
Diet: As tolerated
Medications: Per CDC guidelines.
Prevention and Hygiene: Avoid insect bites and infested areas; wear protective clothing.
Follow-up Actions
Evacuation/Consultation Criteria: Refer to tropical medicine/infectious disease specialist when possible.

Zoonotic Disease Considerations:
Principal Animal Hosts: Dogs, cats, rodents
Clinical Disease in Animals: Intermittent fever, anemia, weight loss; may be asymptomatic
Probable Mode of Transmission: Contaminated bite wounds or contact with fecal matter of Reduviidae family of insects (kissing bugs).
Known Distribution: Western Hemisphere; Texas, Mexico, Central and South America

Chapter 12: Infectious Diseases: Mycobacterial Infections: Nontuberculous Mycobacterial Infections

COL Duane Hospenthal, MC, USA

Introduction: Nontuberculous mycobacterial (NTM) or mycobacteria other than tuberculosis (MOTT) infectious diseases may present as: lymphadenitis (*Mycobacterium avium* complex [MAC] and *M. scrofulaceum*); skin and soft tissue infection (*M. fortuitum*, *M. abscessus*, *M. marinum*, and *M. ulcerans*); and pulmonary disease (MAC or *M. kansasii*). Lymphadenitis in children age 1-5 years is most commonly caused by *M. avium* complex. In adults, lymphadenitis is due to *M. tuberculosis* in 90% of cases. Pulmonary syndromes are usually chronic, often occurring in persons with other underlying pulmonary disease.

Subjective: Symptoms
Lymphadenitis (painless enlargement of the lymph nodes of the neck), usually unilateral; skin and soft tissue infections (edema, erythema; pulmonary infection); chronic, productive cough with fever and weight loss; accompanied by malaise, night sweats and hemoptysis.
Focused History: *Do you have any swollen areas?* (Lymphadenitis usually involves only one lymph node chain.) *Have you been in contact with any kittens?* (Cat scratch disease/bartonellosis is spread by young cats; also causes lymphadenitis.)

Objective: Signs
Using Basic Tools: Normal vital signs.
  Lymphadenitis: Enlarged, unilateral nodes of the neck (usually anterior cervical chain) that may spontaneously form sinus tracts and drain. No overlying erythema. Individual nodes are difficult to identify.
  Skin and soft tissue infection: "Swimming pool or fish tank granuloma" caused by *M. marinum* starts as a papule (usually on extremity) that slowly enlarges and ulcerates. These lesions are associated with water or fish exposure. Introduction of the organism is likely via an abrasion or puncture.
  Pulmonary disease: Presents similarly to tuberculosis. Perform PPD testing to rule out tuberculosis. See *Part 5: Specialty Areas: Chapter 12: Mycobacterial Infections: Tuberculosis*
Using Advanced Tools: CXR may reveal thin-walled cavities and more pleural thickening than tuberculosis.

Assessment: Differential Diagnosis
Cat scratch disease: Exposure to cats, pain. *See Part 5: Specialty Areas: Chapter 12: Bacterial Infections: Bartonella Infections (Cat Scratch Disease, Oroya Fever, Trench Fever)*
Lymphoma: Similar systemic symptoms (biopsy of lymph node to define pathology may be required)
Tuberculous lymphadenitis: Also called scrofula; positive PPD or TB exposure.
Other skin and soft tissue infection: Such as nocardiosis (no water exposure), sporotrichosis (exposure to soil, organic gardening materials), leishmaniasis (endemic area, sandfly exposure); (*see Part 5: Specialty Areas: Chapter 12: Parasitic Infections: Leishmaniasis*).
Other pulmonary disease: *See Part 5: Specialty Areas: Chapter 12: Mycobacterial Infections: Tuberculosis; Part 4: Organ Systems: Chapter 3: Pneumonia & Chronic Obstructive Pulmonary Disease*

Plan:
Treatment
  Primary: Lymphadenitis (due to MAC or *M. scrofulaceum*): excisional surgery without antimicrobial drugs. **Cutaneous lesions** (due to *M. marinum*): **doxycycline** 100mg po bid or **trimethoprim/sulfamethoxazole** 160/800mg po bid x 3 months. Excisional therapy is also an option.
  Other syndromes: Therapy based on site of disease, organism and susceptibility testing results.
  Alternative: A multitude of regimens exist for most of these infections.
  Consult an expert for guidance.
Patient Education
  General: NTM infections are not contagious to others.
  Activity: As tolerated.
  Diet: No limitations.
  Medications: Based on selected regimen.
  Prevention and Hygiene: Avoid swimming with unhealed wounds.
  No Improvement/Deterioration: Reevaluation and repeat culture and susceptibility testing.
Follow-up Actions
  Wound Care: Local care (clean, dry, protect, topical antibiotics) to prevent secondary bacterial infection.
  Return Evaluation: Routine follow-up required for pulmonary infections.
  Consultation Criteria: Management of chronic pulmonary infection usually requires specialty consultation. Although the acid-fast bacilli can be detected in lesion, sputum, or biopsy material, culture is required to confirm diagnosis.
  Note: Disseminated *M. avium* complex (DMAC) is another NTM disease that is virtually restricted to persons with late stage AIDS. This infection presents as a chronic febrile wasting syndrome with associated anemia and MAC bacteremia.

Chapter 12: Infectious Diseases: Mycobacterial Infections: Tuberculosis

COL Duane Hospenthal, MC, USA

Introduction: *Mycobacterium Tuberculosis, M. Bovis* and others cause tuberculosis (TB), a chronic pulmonary infection that is seen worldwide. Infection is spread by airborne particles. Clinical disease (TB) develops in only about 10% of those infected. Others have latent tuberculosis infection (LTBI), since they do not have evidence of active disease. Disease in adults usually occurs secondary to reactivation of past infection. Disease occurs more frequently in children and in adults who are immunocompromised, including secondary to HIV infection, malignancy, chronic steroid therapy, uncontrolled diabetes, malnutrition, silicosis, or who are smokers. Extrapulmonary disease occurs in approximately 15% of infected persons and can affect virtually any organ system (*see Part 4: Organ Systems: Chapter 6: Mycobacterial Infections: Cutaneous Tuberculosis*) and can disseminate throughout the body. Purified protein derivative (PPD) skin testing can be used to document TB infection (active) or screen for exposure (LTBI). Many countries immunize infants and children with Bacillus Calmette-Guérin (BCG) vaccine, which may cause falsely positive reactions to PPD testing. These reactions wane with time, so a positive reaction to PPD testing in adults should not be dismissed as a reaction to BCG given as a child.

Subjective: Symptoms

Chronic productive cough (bloody), chest pain, fever, chills, night sweats, anorexia, weight loss, fatigue.

Focused History: *Do you cough up blood?* (other causes of chronic cough not usually associated with hemoptysis) *Do your night sweats drench your bedding or bedclothes?* (Sweating in bed is normal; having "drenching" sweats is not.) *How long have you been coughing?* (A cough lasting longer than 2-3 weeks is unlikely from other bacterial or viral infections.)

Objective: Signs

Using Basic Tools: Vital signs: Normal to low-grade fever, weight loss. Percussion: Unilateral, localized dullness over the upper lung fields. Auscultation: Decreased breath sounds or rales corresponding to percussed dullness (upper lung fields)

Using Advanced Tools: CXR: consolidation or cavitary lesion in upper lung fields; PPD skin testing to document tuberculosis infection.

Note: PPD may be negative in persons with active infections.

Assessment: Differential Diagnosis

Chronic bronchitis or COPD: Chronic cough not typically associated with progressive weight loss or night sweats

Lung cancer: Usually seen in patient with smoking history

Fungal pneumonias (histoplasmosis, blastomycosis, paracoccidioidomycosis): Chronic pulmonary symptoms are rare and usually seen in smokers in endemic areas.

Plan:

Treatment

Primary: Base the selection of antimycobacterial drugs on knowledge of local resistance patterns. Usually, 4 drugs are initiated. The most common regimen is **isoniazid (INH), rifampin (RIF), pyrazinamide (PZA),** and **ethambutol (EMB)** (or **streptomycin (SM)**). In cases of sensitive TB, these drugs are given for 8 weeks, followed by a 4 month course of **INH** and **RIF** only. This course is extended to 7 months in patients with cavities or who have sputum cultures which remain positive after the end of the initial 8 weeks of therapy. Medicines may be given 2, 3 or 7 x each week. Use directly observed therapy (DOT) to assure compliance. Treat PPD positive contacts without active disease (LTBI) with **isoniazid** 300mg/day po x 9-12 months. Children under 5 years of age who are contacts of an active pulmonary case should receive **isoniazid** 10-20mg/kg (300mg maximum) po even if initial PPD is negative. If the PPD remains negative on retesting after 3 months, **INH** may be stopped.

Table 5-3. Antimycobacterial Drugs

Drug	Daily dose, mg/kg (max dose)	Twice weekly dose, mg/kg (max)	Thrice weekly dose, mg/kg (max)	Adverse reactions	Monitoring
INH	5 (300mg)	15 (900mg)	15 (900mg)	liver dysfunction, peripheral neuropath	baseline liver enzymes
RIF	10 (600mg)	10 (600mg)	10 (600mg)	drug interactions, liver dysfunction, bleeding problems	baseline CBC, liver enzymes
PZA	15-30 (2g)	50-70 (4g)	50-70 (3g)	liver dysfunction, hyperuricemia	baseline uric acid, liver enzymes
EMB	15-25 (1.6)	50 (4.0)	25-30 (2.4)	optic neuritis	baseline and monthly visual acuity and color vision testing
SM	15 (1g)	25-30 (1.5g)	25-30 (1.5g)	ototoxicity, renal toxicity	baseline and hearing and renal function testing repeat

Alternative: Alternate regimens are usually based on results of susceptibility testing.

Patient Education

General: Comply with the medication regimen to avoid developing resistant disease, and then spreading it to others.

Medications: *See Table 5-3*

Prevention and Hygiene: Isolate patient for several weeks until not contagious. Ideally, patients should remain isolated until sputum is smear negative (serially over at least 3 days). They should use a mask or cover their mouth with every cough. All contacts should be screened with PPD for active and latent infection. PPD positive contacts should get chest radiography to rule out active disease.

Follow-up Actions

Return Evaluation: Monitor patient monthly for drug toxicity.

Evacuation/Consultation Criteria: Evacuation not necessary unless clinically unstable or patient develops significant medication side effect. Consult with pulmonologist, infectious disease specialist or primary care physician prior to treatment and as necessary.

Notes: Multidrug resistant tuberculosis (MDR-TB) is defined as any *M. tuberculosis* that is resistant to both INH and RIF. XDR-TB is defined as MDR-TB that additionally is resistant to fluoroquinolones and at least one of three injectable second-line drugs (capreomycin, kanamycin, and amikacin).

PPD skin testing is done as follows:
1. Placement of PPD: inject 5IU (0.1mL) intradermally into flexor surface of LEFT forearm (so you will remember where to look for reaction).
2. Interpretation of PPD reaction:
   a. Measure diameter (in mm) of INDURATION or swelling (not redness) of reaction, when viewed in cross-section at 48-72 hours.
   b. >5mm is positive in HIV patients, and in close or household contacts of a patient with an active TB infection
   c. >10mm is positive for those personnel exposed to people at high-risk for having TB. This standard applies to medical personnel and team members
   d. >15mm is positive for personnel with no risk factors for exposure. This standard applies to most Americans.

Zoonotic Disease Considerations

Agent: *Mycobacterium bovis*

Principal Animal Hosts: Cattle

Clinical Disease in Animals: Progressive emaciation, lethargy, weakness, anorexia, low-grade fever; chronic bronchopneumonia with moist cough, progressing to tachypnea and dyspnea.

Probable Mode of Transmission: Ingestion, inhalation (occupational exposure to farmers)

Known Distribution: Worldwide; rare in N. America, western Europe, Japan, Australia, New Zealand

Chapter 12: Infectious Diseases: Fungal Infections: Introduction to Fungal Infections (Mycoses)

COL Duane Hospenthal, MC, USA

The fungal infections discussed in this subchapter, with the exception of the superficial presentations of candidiasis, are diseases that can rarely be diagnosed or treated in the field. Cryptococcosis is found worldwide but symptoms are most common in the immunosuppressed and are not acutely life-threatening. Blastomycosis, coccidioidomycosis, histoplasmosis, and paracoccidioidomycosis are endemic fungal infections that should be included in a differential diagnosis so individuals with potential infections may be removed or referred to higher echelons of care.

Chapter 12: Infectious Diseases: Fungal Infections: Blastomycosis (North American Blastomycosis, Gilchrist Disease)

COL Duane Hospenthal, MC, USA

Introduction: *Blastomyces dermatitidis* is a yeast-like fungus that causes a spectrum of disease including asymptomatic infection, acute and chronic pulmonary infection and disseminated infection of the skin, bone, GU tract, and rarely, the CNS. This infection is seen most often in central and southeast US in areas near rivers or streams. Approximately 1/2 of exposed persons will develop symptomatic disease. The incubation period is 30-45 days. Most individuals seeking care for this infection have progressive pulmonary disease or cutaneous lesions.

Subjective: Symptoms

Acute pulmonary infection produces fever, cough, and pleuritic chest pain. Chronic pulmonary disease presents with similar symptoms over a longer course. Skin lesions are typically painless or slightly tender. Chronic pulmonary disease can also include hemoptysis, weight loss, and skin lesions.

Focused History: *Have you had any recent travel/exposure to rivers or streams in the central or southeast US?* (endemic area)

Objective: Signs

Using Basic Tools: Inspection: Skin lesions are most often located on the face, scalp, neck, and extremities. These begin as red papules or nodules that enlarge and then ulcerate or become verrucous. Associated adenopathy is uncommon. Auscultation: Pulmonary infection is associated with diffuse auscultatory findings and fever.

Using Advanced Tools: Labs: Large (8-15mm), thick-walled, broad-based, budding yeast cells may be visible on Gram's stain of sputum or lesional aspirate or discharge.

Assessment: **Differential Diagnosis**

Acute pulmonary infection: Influenza, bacterial pneumonia

Chronic pulmonary infection: Tuberculosis, lung cancer, other fungal pneumonias

Skin lesions: Squamous cell carcinoma, mycosis fungoides

Plan:

Treatment

Primary: Amphotericin B 0.7-1.0mg/kg/d IV is required in life-threatening infections, all central nervous system infections, infections in immunocompromised patients and in pregnant patients. This agent should not be administered in the field. *See Part 5: Specialty Areas: Chapter 12: Fungal Infections: Candidiasis (Thrush)* **Itraconazole** can be used in all other infections at a dose of 200mg po once or twice daily, usually for 6-12 months, and as a follow on agent after patients receiving amphotericin B are clinically improved.

Alternative: Ketoconazole 400-800mg po q day or **fluconazole** 400-800mg po q day x 6-12 months.

Patient Education

General: Acute pulmonary infection may resolve untreated in 1-3 weeks. All other forms carry a high risk of death if not treated.

Activity: As tolerated.

Diet: No limitations.

Medications: See precautions listed for oral azoles (itraconazole, ketoconazole and fluconazole) and IV amphotericin B in the Candidiasis section.

Prevention and Hygiene: None necessary.

Follow-up Actions

Wound Care: Local care to prevent secondary bacterial infection.

Return Evaluation: Observe patients over a 1-2 year period for resolution of infection.

Consultation Criteria: Refer all patients to a specialist for care.

Zoonotic Disease Considerations:

Principal Animal Hosts: Dogs, cats, horses

Clinical Disease in Animals: Nonspecific, dependent on organ involvement; weight loss, coughing, anorexia, diarrhea, ocular disease, lameness, skin lesions, fever

Probable Mode of Transmission: Environmental or animal exposure

Known Distribution: Worldwide

Chapter 12: Infectious Diseases: Fungal Infections: Candidiasis (Thrush)

COL Duane Hospenthal, MC, USA

Introduction: *Candida albicans* is a yeast normally found in the mouth, intestines, and vagina. Overgrowth of this yeast can cause skin or mucosal diseases including oropharyngeal candidiasis (thrush), intertrigo (disease limited to moist skin folds), esophagitis, and vaginitis. In adults, disease commonly occurs in diabetics, the immunocompromised, and after antibiotic treatment for other disorders. Inhaled and oral corticosteroid preparations also increase risk. Disseminated, life-threatening infection can also occur in severely immunocompromised persons. Oral candidiasis (thrush) in a young adult should always raise the suspicion of immunocompromise, especially undiagnosed HIV infection.

Subjective: **Symptoms**

Oral thrush: Usually asymptomatic; may cause mouth discomfort or difficulty swallowing. Esophageal thrush: Painful or difficult swallowing. Intertrigo: Local burning-like pain, often with pruritus. Vaginal thrush: Itching, pain with intercourse and change in the odor or consistency of vaginal discharge.

Focused History: *Do you have difficulty or pain with swallowing?* (suggests esophageal or oral lesions) *Do you have diabetes? Have you recently taken antibiotics or corticosteroids?* (Hyperglycemia, antibiotic or steroid exposure may precede oral or vaginal disease.)

Objective: **Signs**

Using Basic Tools: Inspection: Oral/esophageal: white plaques, which are scraped to reveal an erythematous base and are seen on any oral mucosal surface except the tongue. Cutaneous (intertrigo or vulvar) is an erythematous, shiny rash with small "satellite" lesions at its periphery. Candidal vaginitis is associated with a curd-like vaginal discharge (*see Part 3: General Symptoms: Gynecological Problems: Candidal Vaginitis/Vulvitis*).

Using Advanced Tools: Labs: Potassium hydroxide (KOH) wet mount of scrapings or discharge reveals typical yeast, usually with pseudohyphae and/or hyphae. *See Part 8: Procedures: Chapter 32: Wet Mount and KOH Prep*

Assessment: **Differential Diagnosis**

Oropharyngeal candidiasis: Particulate debris secondary to poor oral hygiene (debris is usually easily removed)

Esophageal candidiasis: Esophagitis due to herpes simplex, cytomegalovirus, aphthous ulcers, and toxins

Candidal vaginitis: Trichomoniasis, bacterial vaginosis (can be differentiated with wet mount)

Plan:

Treatment

Primary:

Oropharyngeal candidiasis: **Nystatin** solution, 400,000-600,000units po qid as a swish and swallow x 7-14 days.

Esophageal candidiasis: **Fluconazole** 200mg/day po or IV x 14 days.

Intertrigo: **Nystatin** powder or **clotrimazole** or **miconazole** cream bid until resolved.

Candidal vaginitis: *See Part 3: General Symptoms: Gynecological Problems: Candidal Vaginitis/Vulvitis.*

Alternative: Oropharyngeal candidiasis: **Clotrimazole** troches (lozenges) 10mg 5/day x 7-14 days, or **fluconazole** 50-200mg/day po x 7-14 days, or **itraconazole** 100-200mg/day po, or **ketoconazole** 200mg/day po. Esophageal candidiasis: **Itraconazole** 100-200mg/day oral solution (give without food) x 7 days, or **amphotericin B** 0.3-0.5mg/kg/day IV in refractory cases. This should only be considered in consultation with referring physician. Use of IV amphotericin B should be avoided in the field secondary to its many toxicities, which require higher levels of supportive care and laboratory monitoring for safety. The less toxic lipid formulations of this drug also require higher levels of care for safe usage.

Primitive: Gentian violet applied topically.

Patient Education

General: This is a superficial infection that should resolve with standard therapy. It can occur in healthy people, but could indicate other disease such as diabetes or immunocompromise.

Medications: Topical antifungals have virtually no adverse effects associated with their use. The oral azoles, fluconazole, itraconazole, and ketoconazole are all well tolerated. These drugs may interact with other drugs processed through the liver, altering the levels of drugs such as oral diabetes, seizure, and anticlotting medications. Ketoconazole used long-term may affect steroid hormones, causing irregular menses in women and decreased libido or breast tissue enlargement in men. All azole antifungals may rarely cause severe liver damage. Malaise, nausea, vomiting, weight loss, and infusion site phlebitis (vein inflammation) may also occur. IV use of amphotericin B is associated with infusion-related fever, headache, chills, myalgias, and rigors. Decreased blood potassium and magnesium often complicate therapy. Use of amphotericin B can also cause anemia and kidney dysfunction.

Prevention and Hygiene: None necessary

No Improvement/Deterioration: Further evaluation is necessary if infection does not resolve within 2 weeks.

Follow-up Actions

Return Evaluation: If lesions do not resolve consider alternate treatment.

Evacuation/Consultation Criteria: Evacuation is not required for most patients. However, those with recurrent thrush, disseminated infection or who require intravenous amphotericin B therapy should be referred to the appropriate higher echelon of care.

Chapter 12: Infectious Diseases: Fungal Infections: Coccidioidomycosis (Valley Fever, Desert Rheumatism)

COL Duane Hospenthal, MC, USA

Introduction: *Coccidioides immitis* is a dimorphic fungus that causes disease ranging from self-limited pulmonary infection to chronic meningitis. Incubation period is 7-21 days. More than 60% of all infections are asymptomatic. Most symptomatic infections take the form of acute pulmonary disease. Untreated, acute infection resolves in 95% of patients. About 1% of those infected develop chronic pulmonary disease or disseminated infection to the meninges, skin, bone, or soft tissue. **Geographic Associations:** It occurs in the southwest deserts of the US and northern Mexico, and in a few pockets of Central and South America. It has frequently been reported in service members training at Ft. Irwin, California. Incidence peaks during dry periods following rains, usually in summer and fall, and is often associated with wind and dust storms. **Risk Factors:** Non-Caucasians, pregnancy and immunocompromised patients are at higher risk for dissemination and severe disease.

Subjective: **Symptoms**

Cough (usually dry), fever, pleuritic chest pain, malaise, headache, anorexia, myalgia and often rash; severe disease may present with a sepsis-like syndrome. Large joint pain may occur after asymptomatic infection, especially in white females (desert rheumatism). Meningitis presents with chronic headache, memory loss, lethargy, or confusion.

Focused History: *Have you traveled recently to the deserts of the southwest US or northern Mexico?* (endemic areas of disease)

Objective: **Signs**

Using Basic Tools: Vital signs: Fever and tachypnea; Inspection: Various rashes: Diffuse, faint erythematous rash lasting less than one week; or erythema multiforme (painless, diffuse rash consisting of rings and disks); or erythema nodosum (painful red nodules usually occurring on the shins). Auscultation: Diffuse auscultatory findings (abnormal breath sounds).

Using Advanced Tools: Ophthalmoscope: Patients with meningitis may have papilledema on funduscopy. Labs: Eosinophils may be seen on blood smear. Gram's stain or KOH of sputum for spherules (10-80μm round structures with 2-5μm round endospores inside)

Assessment: **Differential Diagnosis**

Acute pulmonary disease: Influenza, "atypical" pneumonia, histoplasmosis, blastomycosis. See respective topics in Respiratory and ID

Meningitis: Tuberculosis, syphilis, cryptococcosis (*see Part 4: Organ Systems: Chapter 5: Meningitis*); and CNS tumors. See *Part 4: Organ Systems: Chapter 6: Seizure Disorders and Epilepsy*

Plan:

Treatment

Primary: Observation is the treatment of choice for acute pulmonary infection and for asymptomatic cavitary disease in patients not at increased risk for dissemination or chronic disease. **Amphotericin B** 0.5-1.5mg/kg/d IV (until clinical response) should be used in acute life-threatening infection. This can be followed with **fluconazole** 400-800mg po q day to complete 3-6 months of therapy. Meningeal infection is treated with **fluconazole** 400-800mg po daily for life. All other forms of coccidioidomycosis are treated with long-term **fluconazole**.

Alternative: Itraconazole 200mg po bid or tid may be used in non-meningeal infections. Intrathecal **amphotericin B** is occasionally used in meningitis failing azole therapy or in the initial therapy of severe meningeal disease.

Patient Education

General: Acute pulmonary disease will likely resolve untreated in 6-8 weeks. Meningeal disease requires lifelong therapy.

Medications: *See Part 5: Specialty Areas: Chapter 12: Fungal Infections: Candidiasis (Thrush)* for adverse effects of intravenous amphotericin B and azole antifungals.

Prevention and Hygiene: No human-to-human spread. Others should avoid inhaling dust where patient was exposed.

Follow-up Actions

Return Evaluation: Patients should be evaluated frequently for progressive disease.

Evacuation/Consultation Criteria: Evacuate and refer all patients to a specialist for care.

Zoonotic Disease Considerations:

Principal Animal Hosts: Dogs; less common, horses and other livestock

Clinical Disease in Animals: Nonspecific, dependent on organ involvement; fever, lethargy, chronic cough

Probable Mode of Transmission: Environmental (aerosol) exposure

Known Distribution: Western hemisphere, similar to human disease

Chapter 12: Infectious Diseases: Fungal Infections: Histoplasmosis (Darling's Disease)

COL Duane Hospenthal, MC, USA

Introduction: *Histoplasma capsulatum* is a dimorphic fungus that can cause disease ranging from asymptomatic pulmonary infection to life-threatening disseminated infection. Acute infection occurs 3-21 days after exposure. Most infection is asymptomatic or self-limiting pulmonary disease. Severity is dependent on patient's immunity and intensity of exposure. Chronic pulmonary disease, mediastinitis and disseminated disease are rare. **Geographic Associations:** Found worldwide, this infection is most common in the central US (Mississippi and Ohio River basins). **Risk Factors:** Outbreaks may occur with the removal of debris containing contaminated bird or bat droppings. Outbreaks in military personnel have been documented after clearing barracks and bunkers. Immunocompromised persons are at higher risk to develop disseminated disease.

Subjective: **Symptoms**

Acute (days): Malaise, fever, chills, anorexia, myalgias, cough, pleuritic chest pain. **Chronic (months):** Cough

Focused History: *Have you traveled to the Midwest US recently?* (endemic in Ohio and Mississippi River valleys) *Have you been in caves or been near bird droppings lately?* (The fungus is found in debris and soil contaminated with bat or bird guano.)

Objective: **Signs**

Using Basic Tools: Inspection: Fever, weight loss; hypotension and shock in immunocompromised patient (sepsis). Auscultation: Coarse breath sounds, pleural friction rub. Palpation: Hepatomegaly and/or splenomegaly may be seen in disseminated infection.

Using Advanced Tools: CXR: Hilar or mediastinal lymphadenopathy with or without patchy infiltrates. Labs: KOH identification on smear of sputum is usually quite difficult. Organism is a small, budding yeast (2-4µm) often found inside macrophages.

Assessment: **Differential Diagnosis**

Acute pulmonary infection: Influenza. *See Part 4: Organ Systems: Chapter 3: Influenza*

Chronic pulmonary infection: Tuberculosis, other fungal infections. *See Part 5: Specialty Areas: Chapter 12: Mycobacterial Infections: Tuberculosis*

Plan:

Treatment

Primary: Therapy is not needed in asymptomatic or acute pulmonary infection unless associated with hypoxemia or symptoms longer than one month. **Itraconazole** 200-400mg po daily for 6-12 weeks can be given in those cases that do not spontaneously improve/resolve. For severe infection, including acute or chronic pulmonary disease, disseminated disease or meningitis, give **amphotericin B** 0.7-1.0mg/kg (or **lipid formulations of amphotericin B** 3-5mg/kg) IV q day for 1-2 weeks (4-6 weeks for meningitis). This therapy can be changed to **itraconazole** 200mg po bid x 12 weeks (12 months for disseminated or meningeal infections). Corticosteroids (**methylprednisolone** 0.5-1.0 mg/kg/d IV) for 1-2 weeks have been suggested in moderate to severe acute pulmonary infections.

Alternative: **Ketoconazole** 200-800mg po q day can be used as an alternative to itraconazole.

Patient Education

General: Most acute pulmonary infections resolve spontaneously in 3-4 weeks.

Medications: See precautions listed for oral azoles (itraconazole, ketoconazole) and IV amphotericin B in *Part 5: Specialty Areas: Chapter 12: Fungal Infections: Candidiasis (Thrush).*

Prevention and Hygiene: Encourage others to avoid areas where patient was exposed.

Follow-up Actions

Return Evaluation: Follow-up is required in chronic infection and during long term antifungal therapy.

Evacuation/Consultation Criteria: Evacuate all chronic and disseminated cases for referral to specialty care.

Notes: Lung granulomas, and hilar and splenic calcifications are commonly seen on CXR of persons who have had acute pulmonary histoplasmosis in the past. Outside the endemic area however, lung granulomas and hilar calcifications more commonly represent inactive tuberculosis.

Zoonotic Disease Considerations:

Principal Animal Hosts: Dogs

Clinical Disease in Animals: Nonspecific, dependent on organ involvement; emaciation, chronic cough, persistent diarrhea, fever, anemia, hepatomegaly, splenomegaly, lymphadenopathy; ulcerative lesions on skin; ocular disease

Probable Mode of Transmission: Environmental (aerosol) exposure primarily in river valleys

Known Distribution: Worldwide

Chapter 12: Infectious Diseases: Fungal Infections: Paracoccidioidomycosis (South American Blastomycosis)

COL Duane Hospenthal, MC, USA

Introduction: *Paracoccidioides brasiliensis* is a dimorphic fungus that typically causes chronic, progressive, pulmonary disease in rural male workers. It may occur in individuals who live in or have visited the forests of Central or South America and southern Mexico, and present with mucocutaneous lesions of the face. Disease may remain asymptomatic for prolonged periods (up to 15 years).

Subjective: Symptoms
Chronic, productive cough, +/- bloody sputum; shortness of breath; weight loss; painful mouth or nose ulcers; hoarseness.
Focused History: *Have you ever lived in or visited rural South America?* (exposure) *How long have you been coughing?* (usually >3 weeks)

Objective: Signs
Using Basic Tools: Vital signs: Normal. Inspection: Ulcerative lesions of the face, mouth, larynx, or pharynx. Auscultation: Rales or decreased breath sounds in the middle or lower lung fields.

Assessment: Differential Diagnosis
Pulmonary disease: Tuberculosis (usually have night sweats, no oral lesions), COPD (usually have smoking history)
Mucocutaneous disease: Leishmaniasis, leprosy, syphilis

Plan:
Treatment
Primary: Itraconazole 200mg po q day x 6 months.
Alternative: Sulfadiazine 4g po q day for weeks to months, based on clinical response, then 2g q day for 3-5 years. Other sulfa-based antibiotics can be used. **Amphotericin B** 0.7-1.0mg/kg/d IV can be used in life-threatening and unresponsive infections.
Ketoconazole 200-400mg po q day x 6-18 months has also been used.

Patient Education
General: Disease is chronic and progressive if not treated
Activity: As tolerated
Diet: No limitations
Medications: Hypersensitivity rashes and bone marrow depression can complicate use of sulfa-based drugs. (See precautions listed for oral azoles (itraconazole, ketoconazole, fluconazole) and intravenous amphotericin B in *Part 5: Specialty Areas: Chapter 12: Fungal Infections: Candidiasis (Thrush)*.
No Improvement/Deterioration: Relapse is common. Follow up if disease worsens or recurs

Follow-up Actions
Wound Care: Local care (clean, dry, protect, use topical antibiotics) to prevent secondary bacterial infection.
Return Evaluation: Patients should be seen routinely for years.
Consultation Criteria: Required for diagnosis and as clinically indicated.
Notes: Paracoccidioidomycosis has a less common juvenile form which causes acute, progressive, disseminated infection similar to acute disseminated histoplasmosis seen with AIDS and in younger individuals.

Chapter 12: Infectious Diseases: Viral Infections: Introduction to Viral Infections

CDR Timothy Burgess, MC, USN

Viruses are minute nucleic acid-containing particles with an outer protein coat that are invisible under a light microscope. Many hundreds of species of viruses live and replicate inside plants and animals. Fortunately, most human viral pathogens cause acute, self-limited illnesses for which symptomatic treatment is sufficient. A few, however, are sources of diseases including smallpox (eradicated but considered a potential bioterrorism threat), influenza, measles, and human immunodeficiency virus (HIV). Some viruses are transmitted to humans by the bites of insect vectors (eg, dengue, transmitted by *Aedes* mosquitoes) or from infected animals, eg, rabies. It is difficult to diagnose most viral infections with certainty at the time of illness. Confirmation often requires a specialized viral culture, or recognition of the viral antigen or genome (RNA or DNA) using specialized tests that are often only available in referral or research laboratories. At present there are only a few antiviral drugs, used for a limited number of infections. Therefore, most diagnosis of viral infections in the field will be on clinical grounds, and most treatment will be supportive care. Practically speaking, one of the key clinical tasks for the SOF medic regarding patients with viral infections will be considering and ruling out or treating other diseases that present similarly to viral infections, such as malaria, typhoid, etc.

Chapter 12: Infectious Diseases: Viral Infections: Adenoviruses

LTC Clinton K. Murray, MC, USA

Introduction: Adenoviruses are a family of viruses that typically result in febrile illnesses manifested by upper respiratory tract symptoms such as pharyngitis or coryza in young patients including military basic trainees. Most diseases are self-limited but can occasionally result in severe disease with associated gastrointestinal, ophthalmologic, genitourinary, and neurologic complications. There are over 50 human adenovirus subtypes. Beginning in 1971, military recruits received an oral live vaccine with adenovirus types 4 and 7 but manufacturing of this vaccine stopped in 1996. Since 1999, there have been 10 to 12% of military recruits developing adenovirus infection during basic training. This virus is very contagious and can be shed in the feces for months to years after initial infection. **Geographic Association:** The disease is present worldwide. **Seasonal Variation:** In temperate regions, disease is more frequent in the fall or winter months. In tropical regions, it occurs in wet and cooler months. **Risk Factors:** Young people, especially living in crowded conditions, training facilities and ships are at higher risk of developing disease.

Subjective: Symptoms

The primary presentation is pharyngitis and coryza often associated with conjunctivitis, bronchitis and occasionally pneumonia; eye complaints can occur; gastrointestinal symptoms can occur; nervous system abnormalities also occur. Typically symptoms persist for 2-5 days then spontaneously resolves.

Focused History: *Are you undergoing basic training or living in very close quarters?* (high risk environments for disease outbreak) *Do you have upper respiratory tract symptoms?* (usually patients have pharyngitis and runny eyes) *Do you have any close contacts that have been ill with a similar illness in the past few weeks?* (contagious illness that moves rapidly through closed communities)

Objective: Signs

Using Basic Tools: Fever up to 102°F. Inspection: Exudative tonsillitis; conjunctivitis; otitis media; keratoconjunctivitis typically bilateral with preauricular adenopathy. Auscultation: Possible rales. Palpation: Cervical adenopathy

Using Advanced Tools: Labs: Monospot to rule out mononucleosis, group A-streptococcus rapid screen to rule out strep throat; rapid influenza test to rule out influenza

Assessment: Differential Diagnosis

Group A streptococcal: More exudates, confirm with rapid strep test. *See Part 3: General Symptoms: ENT Problems: Pharyngitis, Adult*
Mononucleosis: More adenopathy, confirm with monospot. *See Part 5: Specialty Areas: Chapter 12: Viral Infections: Mononucleosis*
Other viral pneumonia: No differences clinically. *See Part 4: Organ Systems: Chapter 4: Pneumonia*
Influenza: More systemic disease, myalgias, confirm with rapid influenza test. *See Part 4: Organ Systems: Chapter 4: Influenza*
Common cold: *See Part 4: Organ Systems: Chapter 4: Common Cold (Upper Respiratory Tract Infection)*

Plan:

Treatment: Supportive care as no antiviral medications have proven effective and there is typically no need for therapy with this self-limited illness.

Patient Education

General: Apply good hand hygiene, cover mouth if cough or sneeze. For ocular disease, aggressive hand hygiene is required.
Diet: Regular with increased fluid intake.
Medications: Acetaminophen can be used for patient comfort.
Prevention and Hygiene: Vaccine currently being developed and it may be available in the near future for military basic trainees.

Follow-up Actions

Evacuation/Consultation Criteria: Evacuate any unstable patients for consultative care.

Chapter 12: Infectious Diseases: Viral Infections: Arboviral Encephalitis (TBE, JE, WN, St. Louis)

Lt Col Gregory Deye, USAF, MC

Introduction: Arthropod-borne encephalitis viruses (Arboviruses, eg, flavivirus, alphavirus, and bunyavirus) share certain characteristics of transmission to humans via an arthropod vector and the ability to infect the central nervous system. Viral life-cycles and reservoirs vary and humans and horses are commonly accidental hosts. These viruses are often geographically restricted due to the need for particular reservoirs and vectors. Suspicion of a particular diagnosis is guided by knowledge of locally endemic arboviruses as all present in a similar way. Although Japanese encephalitis (JE), West Nile (WN), tick-borne encephalitis (TBE), St. Louis encephalitis (SLE), Kunjin, and Murray Valley encephalitis (MVE) flaviviruses have all been associated with sporadic fatal meningoencephalitis in humans, typically, many hundreds of asymptomatic infections occur for each clinical case of encephalitis. Japanese encephalitis is the most common and one of the most dangerous arboviral causes of encephalitis (inflammation of the brain tissue), with over 50,000 cases reported annually. Case fatality rates range from .3-60% with wide variation due to the frequency of mild or asymptomatic infection. Permanent neurologic or psychiatric sequelae are roughly twice as common as death. An effective vaccine exists for JE and TBE and personnel deployed to areas where these diseases are endemic should receive appropriate immunization. Less common causes of arboviral encephalitis include the alphaviruses: Western equine encephalitis (WEE), Eastern equine encephalitis (EEE), Venezuelan equine encephalitis (VEE); and the California group (CG) of bunyaviruses such as La Crosse virus (LAC). There are few clinical features to distinguish the types of encephalitis, so half the cases do not have a specific pathogen isolated. Birds (JE, WN, SLE, EEE, WEE), rodents and small mammals (VEE, LAC), and other animals play prominent roles as natural reservoirs for these pathogens. Horses can serve as a warning sign of ongoing viral transmission in a specific area. The alphaviruses and some flaviviruses (JE, SLE, MVE) are associated with epidemic disease in susceptible human populations. Case fatality rates from arboviral encephalitis range from <10% (WN, WEE, SLE, TBE) to 33% (EEE). **Geographic Association:** WN virus is widely dispersed through Asia, Africa, the Middle East, and the US JE virus is distributed throughout East Asia and Oceania. TBE is found in forested areas throughout Europe and Central Asia. SLE is widely distributed in the Americas. Kunjin and MVE are restricted to Australia and New Guinea. The alphaviruses and most CG viruses are principally found in the Americas. In highly endemic areas, adults are usually immune to these arboviruses through previous asymptomatic infection. **Seasonal Variation:** These diseases are associated with periods of vector (usually mosquito) abundance, typically warm and wet times of the year in the tropics. In the US, cases of encephalitis usually peak in the late summer/early fall. **Risk Factors:** Exposure to infectious viruses in vectors or animal hosts commonly occurs in rural or suburban areas (JE, SLE, CG, WEE, EEE) but SLE and WN viruses in particular may occur in urban outbreaks. Children (especially <1year of age) are at risk for severe disease with death or neurologic sequelae with WEE, EEE, JE, and LAC, while older adults >55 years of age are at greater risk with SLE, WN, and VEE viruses.

Subjective: Symptoms

Sudden fever, headache, vomiting, and dizziness; rapid progression of mental status changes--disorientation, focal neurologic signs, seizures, stupor and coma; followed usually by recovery, or death (1-60% mortality) or severe sequelae.

Focused History: *Have you completed the full vaccination series for JE?* (significantly decreased risk of JE) *Was fever your first symptom?* (Typically, see sudden rise of fever after a period of apparent recovery from acute febrile illness, or without any prodromal symptoms.) *Have you traveled outside the country or been bitten by mosquitoes recently? If so, where?* (Look for opportunity for infection in endemic area within past several weeks.) *Have there been recent outbreaks of animal diseases in the area?* (Look for epidemics of equine encephalitis [VEE, EEE, and WEE], pig abortions [JE] and bird deaths [WN, SLE].)

Objective: Signs
Using Basic Tools: Vitals signs: Fever and respiratory insufficiency. Inspection: Transient weakness, diminished sensorium, abnormal deep tendon reflexes, sensory disturbances; limb paralysis (JE, TBE, WNV), paresis of the shoulder girdle or arms (TBE); tremors, abnormal movements, and cranial nerve abnormalities (gaze paralysis, speech disorders) (JE). Palpation: Nuchal (neck) rigidity may be present. Neurological: Use Glasgow coma scale (GCS) to track progression of mental status changes, and gauge need for medical evacuation or consultation. *See Appendices: Table A-5: Glasgow Coma Scale*
Using Advanced Tools: Definitive diagnosis may require lumbar puncture, CT, EEG and other advanced testing.

Assessment: Differential Diagnosis
Herpes simplex encephalitis: Focal, non-motor changes (personality, speech, temporal seizures)
Other Herpesviruses or HIV: *See Part 5: Specialty Areas: Chapter 12: Viral Infections: Human Immunodeficiency Virus & Infectious Mononucleosis*
Rabies, TB, Bacterial Meningitis: *See specific ID section*
Subdural hematoma and other trauma: *See http://emedicine.medscape.com/article/828005*

Plan:
Treatment: There is no drug treatment for JE or other arboviruses. Closely monitor obtunded patients (seizures, aspiration, etc.) pending evacuation.
Patient Education
    General: Arboviruses are not directly transmitted from person to person
    Activity: Bedrest.
    Diet: As tolerated.
    Medications: Analgesics for fever or pain. *See Part 8: Procedures: Chapter 30: Pain Assessment and Control*
    Prevention and Hygiene: Vaccinate at-risk personnel against JE and TBE. Decrease exposure to mosquito vectors (*see Part 5: Specialty Areas: Chapter 13: Malaria Prevention and Control*).
Follow-up Actions
    Return Evaluation: Decreasing Glasgow coma scale score, or onset of seizures or focal neurologic symptoms indicate disease progression and requirement for emergent evaluation. Onset of coma or respiratory failure necessitates intensive care for airway management and possible assisted ventilation.
    Evacuation/Consultation Criteria: Evacuate suspected cases of arboviral encephalitis early and urgently. Consult infectious disease specialists whenever this diagnosis is suspected.

Zoonotic Disease Considerations
Japanese encephalitis
Agent: Japanese encephalitis virus (flavivirus)
Principal Animal Hosts: Horses, swine, wild birds
Clinical Disease in Animals: Abortion in swine - teratogenic, hydrocephalus; stillbirth, mummification, embryonic death, and infertility (SMEDI)
Probable Mode of Transmission: Bites of mosquitoes (*Culex* spp.)
Known Distribution: Asia, Pacific islands from Japan to the Philippines

Chapter 12: Infectious Diseases: Viral Infections: Dengue Fever (Dengue Hemorrhagic Fever/Dengue Shock Syndrome)

CDR Timothy H. Burgess, MC, USN

Introduction: Dengue fever is a mosquito-borne viral infection especially prevalent in dense, urban centers in the tropics and subtropics. Many dengue infections are asymptomatic, but it may present as an acute, undifferentiated fever with headache and muscle ache (myalgia). Classically, excruciating pains in the back, muscles, and joints ('breakbone fever') occur in adults. Most patients recovery fully, but some individuals with previous exposure to dengue will develop a more severe form called dengue hemorrhagic fever/dengue shock syndrome (DHF/ DSS), with hypotension and bleeding, which in some cases can progress to shock and death. DHF/DSS is the result of leakage of plasma from capillaries, that leads effectively to temporary hypovolemia and shock. **Geographic Association:** Wet tropical and subtropical areas in most of Latin America, Asia and the Pacific Islands. **Seasonal Variation:** Outbreaks typically follow rainy seasons in tropical regions, which produce increased densities of the mosquito vector. However, year-round transmission is found in endemic regions. **Risk Factors:** Travel to dengue-endemic area, with exposure to mosquito bites, is the principle risk factor. The mosquito vectors, *Aedes* spp., bite in the daytime and are often associated with human habitations.

Subjective: Symptoms
Include sudden onset of fever, headache, and myalgias after a brief (1-2 days) prodrome of sore throat, nausea, and abdominal pain. Other symptoms: chills, malaise, prostration (similar to severe flu), retro-orbital pain, photophobia. DHF: Coincident with fever "breaking", the patient's clinical condition suddenly worsens with marked weakness, facial pallor, diaphoresis, abdominal pain, circumoral cyanosis, rash, and bleeding. Mental status changes may be seen.
Focused History: *What symptom bothers you the most?* (Severe headache, muscle pain, retro-orbital pain, photophobia are typical.) *When did you first feel sick?* (Typically, patient recalls exact time of onset of fever, headache, and prostration, usually within past several days.) *Have you traveled [to regions with known dengue] within the past 2 weeks?* (Look for travel to endemic areas to establish exposure.)

Objective: Signs

Using Basic Tools: Vitals: Fever, occasionally as high as 104°F, over 3–7 days ("saddle-back fever"); Tachycardia, or "relative bradycardia". Narrow pulse pressure (the difference between systolic BP and diastolic BP is <20mmHg), and/or hypotension, are danger signs that suggest DSS. Inspection: Flushing with conjunctival injection; prominent maculopapular, blanching rash over trunk and extremities, sparing palms and soles. Petechiae, purpura, bleeding, confusion or altered mental status are danger signs that suggest DHF/DSS. Palpation: Cervical lymphadenopathy; hepatomegaly; diffuse, abdominal tenderness without guarding.

Using Advanced Tools: Labs: Neutropenia on WBC (<2 x10⁶/mm³); blood smears x 3 to rule out malaria; serial hematocrit and platelet counts (increasing hematocrit, rising more than 20% above baseline, or a single hematocrit value of >50% and/or decreasing platelet count to <100,000/mm³ both suggest DHF). DHF: A tourniquet test may be helpful if DHF is suspected: inflate BP cuff to a point midway between systolic and diastolic blood pressures, maintain for 5 minutes, release pressure and wait 2 minutes or more, then count the number of petechiae that appear in a quarter-sized area (2.5cm diameter) on the skin distal to the cuff. More than 10 petechiae indicate vascular or platelet disorder and suggest DHF. This test is used because it is non-invasive and requires minimal tools, but it is non-specific. A positive test raises concern for DHF, but is not definitive. The hematocrit is initially elevated in DHF/DSS, and decreases with successful IV fluid resuscitation. Hematocrit often decreases even further after 48 hours, as the fluid that was lost from the bloodstream into the tissues due to the temporary capillary leakage is re-absorbed. During treatment, improved circulation (normalized pulse and blood pressure) usually correlates with normalizing (decreasing) hematocrit. Decreasing hematocrit with persistent signs of circulatory failure (tachycardia, hypotension) suggests the possibility of internal bleeding.

Assessment: Differential Diagnosis

Malaria: Rule out with serial blood smears.

Chikungunya: Virus transmitted by same type of mosquito, characterized by fever, rash, painful joints; very common in Africa, Asia, and Indian Ocean

Measles (rubeola): Coryza, respiratory symptoms, Koplik spots, discrete rash from face to trunk

Rubella: Postauricular lymph nodes in children

Meningococcal fever: Painful, palpable purpura and shock

Rickettsial or other bacterial fevers: Vesicular or petechial rashes including the palms and soles.

Other viral hemorrhagic fevers: *See Part 5: Specialty Areas: Chapter 12: Viral Infections: Yellow Fever & Part 6: Operational Environment: Chapter 25: Biological Warfare: Viral Hemorrhagic Fevers*

Plan:

Treatment

General: There is no specific treatment. Treat symptoms including fever (**acetaminophen**, 10mg/kg/dose (pediatric) up to 650mg (adult) po q6h) and pain (eg, **codeine** 15–30mg po (adults), up to q4h PRN; *see Part 8: Procedures: Chapter 30: Pain Assessment and Control* if pain does not respond to acetaminophen). AVOID aspirin and NSAIDs such as ibuprofen due to possibility of increased risk for bleeding complications.

Dengue Hemorrhagic Fever (DHF): Stabilize cardiovascular compromise with fluid replacement (monitor hematocrit and response to therapy closely ie, q2h). Anticipate approximately 10–20cc of normal saline or lactated Ringer's per kg of body weight will be required per hour (or as a bolus if the blood pressure is not palpable), and adjust fluid resuscitation based on clinical response. IV fluids should be continued for 24-48 hours, with constant monitoring and adjustment as required to maintain blood pressure and urinary output. The target is normal pulse rate and blood pressure and normalizing hematocrit. If shock does not respond to IV fluids, the use of plasma or plasma expanders may be required. IV fluid replacement should be tailored to the patient's response, and decreased when blood pressure is stabilized, to avoid over-replacement of fluid which may lead to pulmonary edema or other complications. Initiate medical evacuation as soon as possible. *See Part 7: Trauma: Chapter 27: Hypovolemic Shock*

Patient Education

General: Use universal precautions with patient. Prevent mosquito access to patient.

Activity: Bed rest

Diet: Regular, maintain fluids

Prevention and Hygiene: Use personal protection against insect bites. Avoid exposure to daytime- and dusk-biting mosquitoes, remove mosquito breeding sites. *See Part 5: Specialty Areas: Chapter 13: Preventive Medicine: Pest Control*

No Improvements/Deterioration: Return for re-evaluation.

Follow-up Actions

Patients without signs of bleeding or hypotension can be observed and re-evaluated every 1-2 days until 2 days after fever has resolved; at that point risk of DHF is minimal. Subjective worsening, any signs of bleeding or shock should prompt urgent re-evaluation and raise suspicion for DHF.

Evacuation/Consultation Criteria: Whenever possible evacuate all DHF cases early and urgently, as well as all dengue patients who cannot complete the mission. Consult infectious disease experts for all DHF patients. All patients with suspected DHF should be hospitalized. Hypovolemic shock that results from plasma leakage is an emergency; IV fluid treatment with careful monitoring is potentially lifesaving.

Chapter 12: Infectious Diseases: Viral Infections: Hantavirus

Lt Col Gregory Deye, USAF, MC

Introduction: Hantaviruses infect rodents worldwide and aerosolization of rodent excreta (especially urine) is responsible for transmitting infection. With the exception of Andes virus, there is no human-to-human transmission of Hantaviruses. Hantaviruses are usually divided into old-world Hantaviruses that generally cause hemorrhagic fever with renal syndrome (HFRS), or new-world hantaviruses that generally cause hantavirus cardiopulmonary syndrome (HCPS). There are many Hantaviruses, with the most important being the Hantaan and Seoul viruses (found in Korea, China, and far eastern Russia) which cause HFRS. Dobrava virus (found in the Balkans) also causes HFRS. Puumala virus (found in Western Europe and Scandinavia) causes a milder form of HFRS. Sin Nombre virus, mainly found in the western US, Canada and South America, causes HCPS. The incubation period is generally 1-4 weeks.

Subjective: Symptoms

HFRS: Constitutional: Acute (1-4 days): High fever, chills, myalgias, headache; Sub-acute (5-14 days): Low grade fever, apprehension; Chronic (>2 weeks): Fatigue and lethargy. Specific: Acute (1-4 days): Abdominal pains, flushed face; Sub-acute (5-14 days): Low urine output, back pain; Chronic (>2 weeks): Diuresis, renal concentrating defect.

HCPS: Constitutional: Same as HFRS. Specific: Acute (1-4 days): Dizziness, abdominal pain, diarrhea; Sub-acute (5-14 days): Dyspnea, non-productive cough, shock

Focused History: *Have you recently seen evidence of mice/rats near or in where you live or sleep? (typical exposure) Have others in your family, village or unit had similar symptoms? (Outbreaks occur in others similarly exposed.)*

Objective: Signs

Using Basic Tools:

HFRS: Acute (1-4 days): Toxic appearance, fever to 104°F, conjunctival injection, flushed face/neck/ upper torso (blanches with pressure), dermatographism (drawing on skin leaves an exaggerated mark); Sub-acute (5-14 days): Temperature up to 101°F, truncal and axillary fold petechiae, lowered blood pressure, low urine output up to day 7, profound diuresis thereafter (up to liters/day). In many cases, diuresis phase indicates the onset of recovery

HCPS: Inspection: Acute (1-4 days): Increased respiratory rate, accessory muscle use for breathing, Fever to 104°F Auscultation: Acute (1-4 days): Lungs often normal, tachycardia, and mild hypotension; Sub acute (5-14 days): Diffuse "Velcro" crackles

Using Advanced Tools:

HFRS: Urine is dilute (specific gravity 1.010) with proteinuria, hematuria, occasional red and white blood cell casts; may see elevated white blood count, thrombocytopenia, increased hematocrit (up to 55-65% in severe infection).

HCPS: Pulse oximetry may demonstrate hypoxia even if CXR is normal in HCPS. CXR may show bilateral whiteout, pleural effusion, increased vascular markings; may see elevated WBC, thrombocytopenia, increased hematocrit (up to 55-65% in severe infection).

Assessment: Differential Diagnosis

Leptospirosis: Pulmonary hemorrhage presentation of leptospirosis (as seen in Hawaii) may present similarly to HPS. Travel history, conjunctival redness and skin contact with standing fresh water all suggest leptospirosis.

Hemorrhagic fever virus: More prominent bleeding (HFRS can have bleeding, but late in course) and rash seen with some types.

Dengue: See Part 5: Specialty Areas: Chapter 12: Viral Infections: Dengue Fever *(Dengue Hemorrhagic Fever/Dengue Shock Syndrome)*

Typhus: Responds to doxycycline, presents with a rash, lowered white blood cell count and tache noire (ulcer covered with black crust) for some types. Also consider scrub typhus, plague and tularemia.

Plan:

Treatment

Primary: Avoid excess fluids; consider blood transfusion and Trendelenburg position for shock. Oxygen supplementation as required. For HFRS, **ribavirin** 2g IV loading dose, then 1g q6h x 4 days, then 500mg q8h x 6 days.

Patient Education

General: This infection has high mortality. Deaths can occur until several weeks after defervescence through circulatory collapse.

Activity: Bedrest

Diet: As tolerated

Medications: In HFRS, once patient enters the polyuric phase (about day 8), replace urine losses carefully to avoid dehydration (use careful output measurements).

Prevention and Hygiene: Minimize human-rodent contact. Protect food source, keep rodents out of sleeping places, wet down deserted dwellings (preferably with detergent or disinfectant) to avoid aerosolization and clean out before living there. Use gloves to handle dead rodents and their nests.

Follow-up Actions

Consultation Criteria: Monitor oxygenation with a pulse oximeter. Be prepared to intubate for respiratory failure. Use fluids modestly in HPS to maintain cardiac output. Most deaths occur within the first 48 hours.

Evacuation: Patient needs to be transported to hospital where dialysis (HFRS) and ventilatory support (HPS) are available. Avoid air transport once patient enters the capillary leak syndrome presentation of this illness.

Zoonotic Disease Considerations

Principal Animal Hosts: Rodents

Clinical Disease in Animals: Asymptomatic

Probable Mode of Transmission: Aerosols from rodent excretions and secretions

Known Distribution: Worldwide

Chapter 12: Infectious Diseases: Viral Infections: Hepatitis A

COL Duane Hospenthal, MC, USA

Introduction: Hepatitis A virus (HAV) infection is spread through fecal contamination of food or water, or by person-to-person contact. Infection occurs worldwide with increased incidence in developing nations. Incubation period averages 28 days. Virus is excreted in the stool of infected individuals prior to the development of symptoms. Peak infectivity occurs 2 weeks prior to the development of jaundice. Most individuals recover spontaneously and completely. No "carrier state" exists. Children can have unrecognized infection and may shed virus for several months, making them a major source of infection to others. US service members should be protected from infection with pre-deployment immunization.

Subjective: Symptoms

Abrupt onset fever, nausea, anorexia and malaise, often following several days of nonspecific upper respiratory tract symptoms. Jaundice usually develops days later along with right upper quadrant abdominal pain, dark urine, light-colored stool and pruritus.

Focused History: *When did you notice you were turning yellow?* (Jaundice develops several days after other symptoms. In chronic liver disease, jaundice may develop more slowly, usually without fever or other acute symptoms.) *Is your urine darker than usual? Are your stools lighter in color than usual?* (typical symptoms) *Is anyone else ill?* (contamination from a common source) *Have you injected drugs or had unprotected sex with a new partner?* (risk for hepatitis B and C)

Objective: Signs

Using Basic Tools: Vital signs: Low grade fever. Inspection: Jaundice of skin, sclerae, and mucous membranes under tongue. Palpation: Smooth, tender, enlarged liver edge beyond costal margin.

Using Advanced Tools: Labs: Urinalysis reveals positive urobilinogen.

Assessment:

Differential Diagnosis

Hepatitis B, D, and C: Usually will have parenteral or sexual exposure

Hepatitis E: May not be distinguishable

Mononucleosis (Epstein-Barr virus or cytomegalovirus): Usually associated with sore throat, more severe fever, malaise, and anorexia. May have positive Monospot. *See Part 5: Specialty Areas: Chapter 12: Viral Infections: Infectious Mononucleosis*

Leptospirosis: Fresh water exposure, conjunctival suffusion, myalgias, more severe fever. *See Part 5: Specialty Areas: Chapter 12: Spirochetal Infections: Leptospirosis*

Yellow fever: Myalgia, more severe fever and malaise. *See Part 5: Specialty Areas: Chapter 12: Viral Infections: Yellow Fever*

Malaria: More severe, often cyclic, fever. *See Part 5: Specialty Areas: Chapter 12: Parasitic Infections: Malaria*

Chemicals (including drugs and alcohol): History of toxic ingestion (wild mushrooms, acetaminophen), heavy alcohol use, no fever

Plan:

Treatment

Primary: Supportive care

Patient Education

General: Most persons with acute infection will recover within 3 weeks.

Activity: Bedrest

Diet: Refrain from use of all alcohol products.

Medications: Avoid medications that are cleared by the liver, including acetaminophen.

Prevention and Hygiene: Isolate infected persons up to 1 week after the onset of jaundice. Appropriate handwashing, food preparation, waste disposal (feces are highly infective), and water purification. Post-exposure immunization is recommended in exposed, unvaccinated individuals. Alternately, and in those over 40 years, under 12 months, or immunocompromised, treatment with immune globulin, 0.02mL/kg, should be given to close contacts if less than 2 weeks from last exposure. Widespread immunization of susceptible people may be effective in stopping outbreaks.

No Improvement/Deterioration: Evacuate for evaluation if suspicion of hepatic failure.

Follow-up Actions

Consultation Criteria: Refer cases of HAV infection that do not improve or that progress to encephalopathy.

Chapter 12: Infectious Diseases: Viral Infections: Hepatitis B (and Hepatitis D)

COL Duane Hospenthal, MC, USA

Introduction: Hepatitis B virus (HBV) is spread via sexual intercourse, birthing and exposure to blood and blood products. HBV can cause both acute and chronic infection. 5-10% of acutely infected adults develop chronic infection. In contrast, perinatal infection leads to chronic infection in 70-90% of individuals. Chronically infected persons are the reservoir for this infection and are at risk to develop cirrhosis and hepatocellular carcinoma (HCC). The highest incidence of chronic disease is in Asia and Africa.

Subjective: Symptoms

Acute infection: (*See Part 5: Specialty Areas: Chapter 12: Viral Infections: Hepatitis A*) 10% of acute HBV infection is symptomatic. If symptoms do occur, they develop after an incubation period averaging 75 days. Chronic infection is only rarely associated with nonspecific symptoms such as malaise and fatigue.

Focused History: (for chronic hepatitis): *Have you ever been told you had hepatitis or jaundice?* (Chronic hepatitis may occur after acute hepatitis.) *How long have you had malaise and/or fatigue?* (These symptoms for greater than a month usually denote a chronic process.)

Objective: Signs

See Part 5: Specialty Areas: Chapter 12: Viral Infections: Hepatitis A for signs of acute hepatitis.

Using Basic Tools (chronic disease): Vital signs: Normal. Inspection: Signs of chronic liver disease - telangiectasias (new blood vessel formation in the skin) over the upper chest, back and arms, reddened palms, gynecomastia, small testes

Assessment: Differential Diagnosis

Acute hepatitis: Same as listed in Hepatitis A

Chronic hepatitis: Hepatitis C, autoimmune hepatitis, hemochromatosis, chronic alcoholic liver disease, and other primary liver disorders.

Plan:

Treatment

Primary: Supportive care for acute hepatitis.

Chronic hepatitis: Referral to gastroenterology or infectious disease specialist.

Patient Education

General: Most adults recover from acute hepatitis within 4 weeks. Over 90% become immune and do not develop chronic infection.

Activity: Bedrest

Diet: Refrain from use of all alcohol products

Prevention and Hygiene: Sexual partners and children should be tested. Consider HBV immunization of close contacts if not immune. Patient should not donate blood, tissues or semen. Condom use decreases sexual transmission. Avoid sharing toothbrushes and razors.

No Improvement/Deterioration: Evacuate for evaluation of hepatic failure.

Follow-up Actions

Return Evaluation/Consultation Criteria: All patients suspected to have chronic Hepatitis B should be referred to a specialist.

Notes: Hepatitis D or Delta Hepatitis (HDV) is caused by a defective virus that only causes disease in the presence of HBV. HDV disease is similar to HBV, occurring in persons previously or concurrently infected with HBV. Found worldwide, endemic pockets occur in South America, Africa, the Middle East, and in the Pacific islands. HDV is often diagnosed when a person with known HBV infection is noted to have a flare-up of disease or a second course of acute hepatitis.

Chapter 12: Infectious Diseases: Viral Infections: Hepatitis C

COL Duane Hospenthal, MC, USA

Introduction: Hepatitis C virus (HCV) is a common cause of chronic hepatitis. This virus is transmitted by exposure to blood and blood products and less frequently, perinatally or by sexual intercourse. Acute infection (incubation period 6-7 weeks) is rarely diagnosed, but chronic disease develops in more than 60% of those infected. Persons with chronic disease are at risk to develop cirrhosis and hepatocellular carcinoma (HCC).

Subjective: **Symptoms**

Acute infection is asymptomatic or associated with nonspecific symptoms in most patients. Typical symptoms associated with Hepatitis A virus (HAV) infection are only rarely present and then usually to milder degree. Chronic infection is only rarely associated with nonspecific symptoms such as malaise and fatigue.

Focused History: *Have you ever been told you had hepatitis or jaundice?* (Chronic hepatitis may occur after acute hepatitis.) *How long have you had malaise and/or fatigue?* (These symptoms for greater than a month usually denote a chronic process.)

Objective: **Signs**

Using Basic Tools (chronic disease): Vital signs: Normal. Inspection: Jaundice may be seen in 20-30% of acutely infected individuals. Stigmata of chronic liver disease - telangiectasias (new blood vessel formation in the skin) over the upper chest, back and arms, reddened palms, gynecomastia, small testes

Assessment: **Differential Diagnosis**

Acute hepatitis: Same as listed in Hepatitis A

Chronic hepatitis: Hepatitis B, autoimmune hepatitis, hemochromatosis, chronic alcoholic liver disease, and other primary liver disorders

Plan:

Treatment

Primary: Supportive care for acute infection

Chronic hepatitis: Referral to gastroenterology or infectious disease specialist

Patient Education

General: The natural history of chronic hepatitis C is currently not clear. All patients may not need specific therapy, but some will benefit from specific (typically Interferon containing combination) therapy.

Activity: As tolerated.

Diet: Refrain from all alcohol products.

Prevention and Hygiene: Sexual partners and children should be tested. Patient should not donate blood, tissues or semen. Sexual transmission likely occurs at a very low rate. Those infected should inform all sexual partners. Use of condoms in long-term monogamous couples is not absolutely required. Avoid sharing toothbrushes and razors.

Follow-up Actions

Return Evaluation/Consultation Criteria: All patients suspected to have chronic hepatitis C should be referred to a specialist.

Note: Other diseases associated with HCV infection include cryoglobulinemia, porphyria cutanea tarda and glomerulonephritis.

Chapter 12: Infectious Diseases: Viral Infections: Hepatitis E

COL Duane Hospenthal, MC, USA

Introduction: Hepatitis E virus (HEV) causes infection that is spread through fecal contamination of water or food. Infection is endemic in India, Southeast and Central Asia, the Middle East, northern Africa and Mexico, with increased incidence in developing nations. Incubation period averages 4-5 weeks. Virus is excreted into the stool of infected individuals prior to the development of symptoms. Most individuals recover spontaneously and completely in 1-4 weeks. No "carrier state" exists.

Subjective: **Symptoms**

General: Flu-like illness with fever, nausea, anorexia and malaise. Jaundice usually develops a few days later, often accompanied by resolution of the flu-like symptoms. Pruritus may accompany jaundice. Local: Right upper quadrant abdominal pain, dark urine, light-colored stool

Focused History: *When did you notice you were turning yellow?* (In acute hepatitis E, jaundice develops several days after the other symptoms. In chronic liver disease, jaundice may develop more slowly, usually without fever or other acute symptoms.) *Is anyone else ill?* (Hepatitis E can occur in outbreaks from common source contamination.) *Is your urine darker than usual? Are your stools lighter than usual?* (typical symptoms) *Have you injected drugs or had unprotected sex with a new partner?* (Hepatitis B is associated with parenteral exposures; hepatitis E is not.)

Objective: Signs

Using Basic Tools: Vital signs: Low grade fever. Inspection: Jaundice of skin, sclerae, and mucous membranes under tongue. Palpation: Smooth, tender, liver edge beyond costal margin; may also have splenomegaly

Using Advanced Tools: Labs: Urinalysis reveals positive urobilinogen.

Assessment: **Differential Diagnosis**

Same as for Hepatitis A.

Plan:

Treatment

Primary: Supportive care

Patient Education

General: Most persons with acute infection will recover within 4 weeks.

Activity: Bedrest

Diet: Refrain from use of all alcohol products

Medications: Avoid medications that are cleared by the liver, including acetaminophen.

Prevention and Hygiene: Safe drinking water source is of the utmost importance. Handwashing, safe food preparation and waste disposal (feces are highly infective) are essential. Stool is infectious 1 week prior to symptoms and remains so as long as 2 weeks into the illness. Isolation of those infected from susceptible persons is not necessary because person-to-person transmission is low.

No Improvement/Deterioration: Evacuate for evaluation if suspicion of hepatic failure.

Follow-up Actions

Consultation Criteria: Refer cases of HEV infection that do not improve or progress to encephalopathy.

Note: The mortality rate of HEV is low (0.07% -0.6%) except for pregnant women in whom a high mortality is reported (15-25%). During outbreaks the attack rate is higher in pregnant women, highest in those in their second or third trimesters.

Chapter 12: Infectious Diseases: Viral Infections: Hepatitis* Chart

COL Duane Hospenthal, MC, USA

Table 5-4. Acute Hepatitis

Disease	Hepatitis A / Hepatitis E	Hepatitis B / Hepatitis D	Hepatitis C	Other Important Causes**	
				Other infections (eg, leptospirosis, yellow fever)	Toxins (eg, Amanita mushrooms), Drugs (eg, acetaminophen), Alcohol
Route of acquisition (common)	Oral-fecal	Blood, perinatal, sexual	Blood	Disease-specific	Ingestion
Precautions to person- avoid spread	Contact precautions***	Standard precautions****	Standard precautions	Most not spread person-to-person; disease-specific: including avoiding vectors	Not spread to-person
Prevention	Handwashing, proper food preparation and waste disposal; immunization or immune globulin prior to, or during outbreak to, or during outbreak of Hepatitis A; isolation of infected patients	Avoid unprotected sexual contact, and exposure to blood; immunization and/or immune globulin for Hepatitis B	Avoid exposure to blood	Disease-specific: including immunization (yellow fever) and chemoprophylaxis (leptospirosis)	Avoidance of the specific toxin or drug

Table 5-4. Acute Hepatitis, continued

Disease	Hepatitis A / Hepatitis E	Hepatitis B / Hepatitis D	Hepatitis C	Other Important Causes**	
				Other infections (eg, leptospirosis, yellow fever)	Toxins (eg, Amanita mushrooms), Drugs (eg, acetaminophen), Alcohol
Treatment (acute)	Supportive	Supportive*****	Supportive*****	Disease-specific; usually supportive	Supportive

*See Infectious Diseases section for detailed discussions of individual causes of hepatitis.
**Must also consider gallbladder disease with acute pain (not commonly jaundiced), pancreatic cancer with painless jaundice, and many other diseases of the liver and hepatobiliary system.
***Contact precautions include use of gloves, gowns or other barriers when in contact with patient, patient waste, clothes, or linens.
****Standard precautions include use of gloves (and other personal protective equipment, ie, gowns, masks and eyewear or face shield as indicated) when drawing blood or coming into contact with blood or other body fluids.
*****Patients with chronic infection should be referred to specialty care for assessment and specific therapy as indicated.

Chapter 12: Infectious Diseases:
Viral Infections: Human Immunodeficiency Virus

Maj Nicholas Conger, USAF, MC

Introduction: Human immunodeficiency virus (HIV), a retrovirus, is transmitted through sexual contact, needlestick/sharps, perinatally, infected blood/body fluid contact with non-intact skin or mucous membranes, breastfeeding and blood transfusion. Infected individuals may be free of signs of disease for years after infection. Acquired immune deficiency syndrome (AIDS) is the failure of the immune system seen during the late stage of HIV infection. The incubation period for HIV is several weeks (commonly) to months (less usual) after exposure. Untreated infection is eventually fatal in an average of about 10 years.

Subjective: **Symptoms**
Acute (1-30 days): Fever to 102°F, malaise, myalgias, night sweats, sore throat, gastrointestinal symptoms, maculopapular rash, oral ulcers. Sub-acute (30 days-1 year): Generalized adenopathy. Chronic (>1 year): Fevers, sweats, fatigue, weight loss, oral thrush, shingles, symptoms of opportunistic infection, including wasting syndrome, recurrent *Salmonella* infections, HIV dementia, *Pneumocystis jiroveci* pneumonia, chronic fevers, toxoplasmosis of brain, chronic diarrhea of >one month, cryptococcal meningitis and more other unusual infections, oral and esophageal candidiasis, recurrent herpes simplex eruptions, severe seborrheic dermatitis, recurrent pneumonia, tuberculosis. These malignancies are also frequently seen in AIDS: invasive cervical cancer, Kaposi's sarcoma, lymphoma.
Focused History: *Are any of your sexual partners chronically ill? Have you tested positive for HIV? Have you had unexplained weight loss, whitish curds in mouth, fevers, sweats or chronic diarrhea?* (increased risk if answer YES) *Do you ALWAYS use protection (such as condoms) during sex?* (increased risk if answer NO) *When did you last test negative for HIV?* (document to assess time period for future testing)

Objective: **Signs**
Any patient may have HIV, appearing normal at early stages, and universal precautions should be used in assessing all patients
Using Basic Tools: Inspection: Acute (1-30 days): Fever to 102°F, aphthous oral ulcers, maculopapular rash on neck and trunk. Sub-acute (30 days-1 year): Generalized adenopathy. Chronic (>1 year): Fevers as high as 104°F, cachexia, oral thrush, herpes zoster, signs of opportunistic infection. Palpation: Sub-acute (30 days-1 year): Generalized adenopathy
Using Advanced Tools: Lab: Blood smear for lymphopenia and atypical lymphocytes; rapid tests are available and increasingly reliable. These could potentially be carried by medics in future, but positives should be referred on for definitive traditional testing.

Assessment: **Differential Diagnosis** (in addition to AIDS and HIV-related illnesses)
Generalized TB: HIV patients are often co-infected with TB and may have chest x-ray findings. *See Part 5: Specialty Areas: Chapter 12: Mycobacterial Infections: Tuberculosis*
Disseminated histoplasmosis: Febrile wasting illness, unlikely to have oral thrush or shingles. *See Part 5: Specialty Areas: Chapter 12: Fungal Infections: Histoplasmosis (Darling's Disease)*
Visceral leishmaniasis: Chronic wasting, febrile illness with prominent hepatosplenomegaly (unusual for HIV alone), pancytopenia; history of travel to endemic area. *See Part 5: Specialty Areas: Chapter 12: Parasitic Infections: Leishmaniasis*
Lymphoma: May present in a disseminated form like HIV symptoms; pronounced lymphadenopathy, splenomegaly
Acute viral illness: Eg, CMV, mononucleosis, hepatitis B, and adenovirus. *See Part 5: Specialty Areas: Chapter 12: Viral Infections: Adenoviruses; Hepatitis A; Hepatitis B (and Hepatitis D); Hepatitis C; Hepatitis E & Infectious Mononucleosis*

Plan:
Treatment: There is no cure. Evacuate newly diagnosed team member with HIV with an escort (suicide watch). Safeguard his weapon. DO NOT attempt to institute treatment in the field; there is no "rush to treat" HIV. Place a PPD to identify exposure (if >5mm in HIV positive) and treatment for latent TB. Treat active opportunistic infections (*see appropriate topic*). Refer local nationals to host nation medical resources.

Patient Education

General: Reinforce that sexual partners that "appear healthy" can still carry HIV. Women should know that this can be transmitted to child when pregnant and that medication during pregnancy can significantly decrease transmission.

Diet: Maintain nourishment (AIDS patients are often severely malnourished). Replace vitamins. Note frequent lactose intolerance.

Prevention and Hygiene: Use latex condoms for sexual intercourse. Do not have unprotected sex, re-use needles, or share sharp personal hygiene items such as razors. Do not breastfeed baby if formula is available, safe, cheap, and not dependent on unsafe water supply. Avoid contact with ill persons to avoid contracting diseases.

Notes: Medics should use body fluid precautions: latex gloves and gown to handle fluids; add eye protection and mask for potential contact with blood and body fluids under pressure (needle stick, dental work, etc.). Wash skin well with soap and water if it becomes contaminated with body fluids. Feces, nasal secretions, saliva, sputum, sweat, tears, urine, and vomitus are not considered infectious unless they contain blood.

Post-exposure (antiviral) prophylaxis to HIV is a consideration if there is reason to believe that there has been a significant exposure to infectious body fluids from an HIV infected individual. Even in the case of an exposure from an HIV infected individual, the risk of becoming infected with HIV is low (<1%). That risk can be further broken down into low risk and high risk exposures and a determination of action required based on the level of exposure risk.

Low risk exposure: Solid needle, superficial injection or percutaneous exposure from a sharp, contaminated from a low risk source (eg, patient with asymptomatic HIV infection, typically the viral load <1500 copies/mL). Give (BASIC REGIMEN): **zidovudine/ lamivudine (COMBIVIR):** 1 tab po bid x 4 weeks (or until source is proven negative).

Higher risk exposures: Large splash of blood to mucous membranes (eyes, mouth) or broken skin, large bore hollow needle with presence of visible blood on the device, deep into skin, needle that was in vein or artery of source patient or exposure from a known high risk source (eg, patient with symptoms of HIV or AIDS). Give BASIC REGIMEN + **efavirenz (SUSTIVA)** 600mg po q hs.

If the source is unknown (eg, splash from inappropriately stored blood, stick from a sharps container) and the exposure occurred in a setting where it is likely that HIV infected patients are being treated (eg, medical clinic in sub-Saharan Africa, emergency room of inner city hospital), post-exposure prophylaxis should be considered.

Anti-retrovirals must be started ASAP (within 1 hour goal); not proven effective if given beyond 72 hours. Prophylactic regimens should be continued for 4 weeks or until source patient of needlestick is proven negative; Side effects (headache, malaise, nausea, vomiting) are common; if significant, stop efavirenz and try **Combivir** alone. Needlestick victim should be tested at baseline, 4 weeks, and 12 weeks after exposure; test for HepB and HCV as well.

These meds are not on medication list; medics should consider carrying at a minimum **Combivir** for prevention of exposure if use of sharp instruments (surgical procedures) on local population on missions in areas of hyperendemicity (sub-Saharan Africa).

Figure 5-13. Schematic Course of Untreated HIV

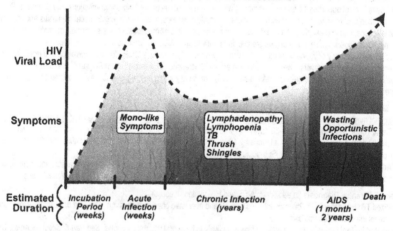

Chapter 12: Infectious Diseases: Viral Infections: Infectious Mononucleosis

Lt Col Gregory Deye, USAF, MC

Introduction: Infectious mononucleosis (IM) is caused by one of the most common human viruses, the Epstein-Barr virus (EBV), a member of the herpes virus family. In the developed world, "mono" is particularly common in young adults (ages 17-25 years), where it is transmitted by passage of infectious oral secretions or sexual contact. In developing countries, almost all children are infected by 3 years of age. EBV infects 80-90% of all persons by adulthood, but only 50% will develop clinical disease. Time from infection to appearance of symptoms is 4-6 weeks. **Risk Factors:** Transmission is facilitated by crowded conditions allowing close contact, such as among military recruits. Because of prolonged excretion of infectious virus, transmission may be maintained in susceptible communities for months.

Subjective: **Symptoms**

Acute (2-7 days): Fever, chills, malaise, anorexia, severe sore throat. **Sub-acute (1-2 weeks):** Fever, fatigue, malaise, severe sore throat, rash, swollen lymph nodes in neck. **Chronic (2 weeks to 3 months):** Fatigue, malaise. A maculopapular rash is common if the patient receives amoxicillin or ampicillin.

Focused History: *Do you have a cough?* (IM rarely has clinical pulmonary manifestations.) *How long have you felt sick? What were your first symptoms?* (Usually, a patient presents with malaise lasting several days to a week, followed by fever, sore throat, and enlarged lymph nodes in the neck.) *Has anyone you live with been sick with a similar illness in the past few months?* (indolent but contagious illness, requiring exchange of saliva)

Objective: Signs

Using Basic Tools: Vital signs: Fever to 100.4–104°F, typically peaks in afternoon. Inspection: Nontoxic appearance, swollen neck, faint measles-like rash, pharyngitis with edema or exudative tonsillitis, palatal petechiae (red spots on back of throat). Palpation: Splenic enlargement, +/- hepatomegaly; swollen cervical lymph nodes (discrete, firm to touch, tender but without fluctuance, posterior > anterior nodes often involved). Auscultation: Stridor from upper airway obstruction (rare). Percussion: Mild tenderness over liver

Using Advanced Tools: Labs: Monospot test 85% sensitive after 1 week of illness; differential reveals lymphocytosis with >10% atypical lymphocytes.

Assessment: Differential Diagnosis

Pharyngitis: Occasionally with exudate.

Other upper respiratory tract infections: Mononucleosis persists longer. *See Part 4: Organ Systems: Chapter 3: Common Cold (Upper Respiratory Tract Infections)*

Hepatitis A, B: Prolonged malaise and fatigue with jaundice typically observed later in course of illness.

Hepatomegaly: Cytomegalovirus and HIV are less likely to be associated with severe pharyngitis.

Toxoplasma and rubella: Rare causes of IM-like syndromes, but may be a significant risk to the fetus if they occur during pregnancy.

Generalized lymphadenopathy: Zoonoses (eg, brucellosis and leptospirosis) are unlikely. *See Part 5: Specialty Areas: Chapter 12: Bacterial Infections: Brucellosis & Spirochetal Infections: Leptospirosis*

Plan:

Treatment

1. Treatment is supportive, usually for relief of throat pain and fevers. Give **acetaminophen** 500-1000mg po tid-qid prn pain.
2. For impending airway obstruction, give **prednisone** 1mg/kg po q day x 3 days, then taper over a week. Alternatively, give **prednisone** 50mg po and taper off by 10mg/d over 5 days.

Patient Education

General: No heavy lifting or contact sports or parachuting for 4 weeks after onset of illness to prevent splenic rupture.

Activity: Rest during acute illness.

Diet: As tolerated. Increase fluids.

Medications: Take acetaminophen (instead of aspirin) for pain and fever to avoid risk of Reye's syndrome.

Prevention and Hygiene: Avoid close contact with others until well after secretions resolve.

No Improvements/Deterioration: Return immediately for sudden onset of severe abdominal pain, or fainting or lightheadedness after abdominal trauma.

Follow-up Actions

Return Evaluation: Examine liver and spleen carefully, for tenderness, enlargement or rupture.

Evacuation/Consultation Criteria: Consider evacuation for patient with enlarged spleen prophylactically, to avoid emergent evacuation (and poor prognosis) for a ruptured spleen. Splenic rupture occurs in 1 case per 1000 and usually occurs 4-21 days into illness. Decision about evacuation should be made depending on circumstances. Otherwise, evacuation is not typically necessary, unless patient becomes unstable or is too fatigued to complete the mission. Consult primary care physician, infectious disease specialist or pulmonologist as needed, and consult a general surgeon urgently for a suspected splenic rupture.

Chapter 12: Infectious Diseases: Viral Infections: Monkeypox

CDR Timothy Burgess, MC, USN

Introduction: Monkeypox is an acute viral febrile illness that produces a rash similar to smallpox, but clinical disease is generally milder than smallpox. The monkeypox virus is carried by rodents and is endemic in West and Central Africa with the West African strain less virulent than the Central African strain. The disease was first identified in captive monkeys (Europe in the 1950s) with infection in humans first recognized in Africa in the 1970s. **Geographic Associations:** Most human cases have occurred in Africa but an outbreak of human cases was reported in the US in 2003, which was traced to infected rodents imported from Africa. **Seasonal Variation:** There is no seasonal variation. **Risk Factors:** Primarily in persons having contact with infected animals, but limited human-to-human transmission has occurred and humans and monkeys are considered 'incidental' hosts. Most infections are asymptomatic and most patients with symptoms have a mild, self-limited illness. An invasive exposure (eg, bite) is more likely to cause systemic illness (secondary soft tissue infection, pneumonitis, ocular complications and encephalitis). In patients with significant clinical illness, fatality rates of up to 10% have been reported with most of the deaths occurring in the 2nd week of infection. There is some evidence to suggest that prior vaccination (vaccinia virus) to smallpox has a significant protective effect against the clinical manifestations of monkeypox.

Subjective: Symptoms

Rash (97%), fever (85%), chills (71%), "swollen glands" (71%), headache (65%) and myalgias (56%). The rash usually begins 1–2 days after the onset of a fever and lasts for 2-3 weeks (median 8-12 days). The fever typically lasts 1 week.

Focused History: *Have you recently been in central or western Africa?* (area with highest risk of exposure). *Have you been exposed to animals known to carry the virus?* (Most human cases are acquired from contact with small forest animals.) *Have you had chickenpox before?* (This is the most common disease in the differential diagnosis; if there is a reliable history of chickenpox in the past, it is very unlikely the current illness is chickenpox.) *Have you had a smallpox vaccination?* (Smallpox vaccination is thought to be protective against developing the major clinical manifestations of monkeypox.)

Objective: **Signs**

Using Basic Tools: Inspection: Rash consists of pustules or vesicles (possibly hemorrhagic) that are usually uniform in appearance that start on the trunk and spread peripherally to include the palms and soles (*see Appendices: Color Plates Figure A-24.B*). Palpation: Lesions are usually firm and deep-seated in the skin. Prominent swelling of regional lymph nodes, eg, in the neck, axilla, and inguinal regions may be identified.

Using Advanced Tools: Not routinely available in the field. Polymerase chain reaction (PCR) testing of material from lesions, serology testing of blood, and electron microscopy of biopsy specimens.

Assessment:

This disease is diagnosed in the field based on history (eg, risk of exposure, onset of fever followed by rash) and physical examination (typical lesions). Most patients will recover from monkeypox without definitive treatment. The World Health Organization (WHO) developed a severity scale based on the number of lesions (or "pocks"):

Benign: 5–25 lesions
Moderate: 26–100 lesions
Grave: 101–250 lesions
Plus Grave: >250 lesions

Differential Diagnosis

Smallpox: It may be difficult to distinguish a mild to moderate case of smallpox from monkeypox based on the rash alone. Lymphadenopathy is not generally a common finding in smallpox and presence of lymphadenopathy is more consistent with diagnosis of monkeypox (in monkeypox endemic area). Possibility of smallpox should always be considered, especially in patient who has not had recent travel to Africa.

Chickenpox: Rash is similar in appearance but chickenpox lesions are more shallow and lesions are seen in various stages of development. Monkeypox lesions are typically deeper and usually all lesions are at the same stage of development.

Plan:

Treatment

Primary: Supportive Care: IV fluid hydration for patients with signs of volume depletion (tachycardia, narrow pulse pressure, low BP, orthostatic pulse increase or BP drop). **Acetaminophen** 500mg po q4-6h prn fever or myalgia. If cellulitis (secondary bacterial infection) develops, it should be treated with antibiotics (eg, **amoxicillin/clavulanic acid** 875mg po bid x 7-10 days for adults or **cephalexin** 250mg po qid x 7-10 days for adults, and topical **mupirocin** ointment bid x 7-10 days. *See Part 4: Organ Systems: Chapter 6: Bacterial Infections: Erysipelas and Cellulitis*

Patient Education

General: Keep wounds clean to reduce risk of secondary skin infections

Activity: Bedrest if severely ill. During the first week of the rash, patient is infectious and should be isolated (until all scabs separate). Diet: No special diet

Prevention and Hygiene: Avoid contact with ill animals; both contact and airborne precautions should be used for any patients with a generalized rash in which either monkeypox or smallpox are considered. possible. Postexposure vaccination (vaccinia virus) to smallpox is recommended for patients known to be exposed to the monkeypox virus (outbreak or healthcare workers with direct contact to patients). Optimal time for post-exposure vaccination is within 4 days of exposure but CDC recommends vaccination for up to 14 days post exposure.

No Improvement/Deterioration: Watch for signs of dehydration and secondary skin infection.

Follow-up Actions

Return Evaluation: Follow-up in 1–2 weeks or sooner if condition worsens.

Evacuation/Consultation Criteria: This is a relatively rare disease; majority of infections are asymptomatic and most patients with benign to moderate symptoms will recover and require only supportive care. In an outbreak of monkeypox, smallpox (bioterrorism) may need to be ruled out, so upper echelon consultation should be sought, if possible. In severe cases (grave, plus grave, life-threatening symptoms), use of investigational treatment (eg, Cidofovir) may be available at upper echelon levels of care.

Zoonotic Disease Considerations

Agent: Monkeypox virus, an orthopox virus related to variola (agent of smallpox)

Principal Animal Hosts: Rodents, particularly the Giant Gambian rat. Cases have been reported in patients bitten by infected prairie dogs. Clinical Disease in Animals: Rash illness in monkeys and some rodents.

Probable Mode of Transmission: Close contact, bites

Known Distribution: West and Central Africa; rare cases have been reported elsewhere and most frequently were associated with exported animals from endemic area.

Chapter 12: Infectious Diseases: Viral Infections: Norovirus

Lt Col George Christopher, USAF, MC

Introduction: Noroviruses (Norwalk-like viruses), are the most common cause of epidemic gastroenteritis. Outbreaks with high attack rates occur among closed military populations, including crews of naval vessels, military trainees, and patients and staff of health care facilities. Outbreaks have disrupted military operations on naval vessels, and temporarily closed a British military field hospital in Bagram, Afghanistan in 2002. Noroviruses are transmitted through contaminated water; shellfish that concentrate virus during filter feeding; and foods contaminated at their source or by infected food handlers. Other possible routes include contamination of hands after touching objects or surfaces previously contaminated by stool or vomitus, inhalation of aerosols generated during projectile vomiting, or environmental aerosols generated during the cleaning of areas grossly contaminated by vomitus or stool. Incubation ranges from 12-48 hours, but may be up to 4 days in secondary cases. Illness varies from mild to severe; rare cases have been reported with clinical features of sepsis and meningoencephalitis.

Subjective: Symptoms

Abrupt onset of nausea, vomiting (possibly projectile), abdominal cramping, and watery non-bloody diarrhea. Presentation will vary with different degrees of vomiting vs. diarrhea; cases have been described without vomiting. Systemic symptoms may include fever, malaise, headache, and muscle aches. Severe presentations during the 2002 Bagram epidemic included photophobia, meningismus, and obtundation.

Focused History: *Do you have any "unsafe" food or water exposures? Do any other members of your unit, or other contacts, have similar symptoms?* (epidemic potential)

Objective: Signs

Using Basic Tools: Possibly low BP. Inspection: Poor skin turgor due to dehydration; rare cases with obtundation. Palpation: Mild diffuse abdominal tenderness; rare cases with meningeal signs.

Using Advanced Tools: Labs: Microscopic exam of feces, concentration techniques for ova & parasites (O & P), stool cultures to rule out other causes of acute gastroenteritis. Blood smears may show low peripheral white blood cell counts. Low platelet counts may be common. There may mild elevations of liver function tests, decreased serum albumin, and microscopic and dip-stick evidence of blood in the urine. Microscopic exam of stool will be negative for O & P or fecal leukocytes.

Assessment: Differential Diagnosis

Staphylococcal food poisoning (staphylococcal enterotoxin B), other causes of acute gastroenteritis. Severe cases may suggest bacterial sepsis, or rarely, meningitis, or encephalitis. If fever, chills, headache, back, abdominal and extremity pain and nausea and vomiting present with nuchal or back rigidity, the possibility of meningococcal meningitis must be considered and immediate management with IV antibiotics initiated. Depending on geographic exposure, considerations may include malaria, typhoid fever, rickettsial diseases, prodromal hemorrhagic fevers; these are less likely with epidemic pattern, short incubation, and abrupt onset of symptoms (no prodrome).

Plan:

Treatment:

Primary

Supportive care with rest and hydration. Remove from healthy personnel, if possible. Consider IM anti-emetic treatment (**promethazine** 25mg with repeat doses of 12.5mg to 25mg q4-6h). Oral tablets or rectal suppositories may not be feasible due to vomiting and diarrhea. **Loperamide** 2 tablets after first loose stool, then one after each loose stool, but not over 4 tablets per 24-hour period. Severe, atypical disease suggesting shigellosis, bacterial sepsis, meningitis, or malaria would be an indication for initial empiric therapy pending clarification of diagnosis.

Patient Education

General: Illness typically resolves within 1-5 days; full recovery is the rule, even for severe cases.

Activity: Rest until recovered. Remove from food-handling duties for up to 2 weeks.

Diet: Bowel rest; advance to clear liquids and solid food as tolerated; avoid milk/dairy products for approximately 2 weeks (may develop a transient lactose intolerance).

Medications: Side effects of promethazine may include drowsiness; rarely spastic movement disorders, high fever with muscle breakdown (neuroleptic-malignant syndrome); these rare complications are medical emergencies requiring immediate expert care.

Prevention and Hygiene: Avoid sick contacts, wash hands frequently, clean environmental surfaces grossly contaminated by vomitus or stool with a disinfectant; masks should be considered during cleaning.

No Improvement/Deterioration: Failure to promptly improve within 1-2 days suggests another diagnosis; consider evacuation for further evaluation.

Follow-up Actions

Return Evaluation: Typically not needed after recovery

Evacuation/Consultation Criteria: Norovirus infection is typically brief and self-limited; treat in place. Evacuation would be indicated only in very severe cases with uncertain diagnosis. During the Bagram epidemic, contact and airborne precautions were used during evacuation of a patient with severe disease with no secondary transmission to aircraft crew or caregivers. Report suspected cases and outbreaks to public health authorities.

Notes:

Post-Exposure Surveillance: Consider limited duty/active surveillance for 4 days for mobile mission-essential contacts performing critical tasks.

Infection Control: Standard precautions with the addition of contact precautions if there is a risk for splashes of vomitus or stool that might contaminate clothing; while caring for incontinent patients; and during institutional outbreaks. Some authorities suggest droplet precautions to prevent possible transmission by aerosols generated during projectile vomiting. Consider private rooms and cohorting patients; consider anti-emetic treatments to reduce potential transmission and environmental contamination due to vomitus and aerosols generated by vomiting.

Environmental Disinfection: After standard cleaning of surfaces contaminated by stool or vomitus, use an approved virucidal disinfectant with activity against noroviruses. Chlorine bleach in a dilution of one part bleach per 50 parts water (1000ppm) may be used; a concentration of up to 5000ppm may be necessary for heavily contaminated or difficult to clean surfaces. Quaternary ammonium disinfectants are not active against noroviruses; phenolic disinfectants may not be active at the concentrations recommended by the manufacturer.

Chapter 12: Infectious Diseases: Viral Infections: Poliovirus

CDR Timothy H. Burgess, MC, USN

Introduction: Poliovirus is an enterovirus spread through fecal or pharyngeal secretions and is the cause of paralytic poliomyelitis. The clinical syndrome of poliomyelitis is termed "acute flaccid paralysis" (AFP). The incubation period is 7-14 days following exposure to the virus. Typically, enterovirus infections are asymptomatic or minor febrile illnesses. Only about 1% of polio infections result in clinically apparent neurologic disease. **Geographic Association:** Polio is primarily a disease associated with poor sanitation and is found primarily in the developing countries of Asia and Africa. It has been eradicated from the Western hemisphere through immunization, except for rare imported cases and rare cases of vaccine-associated paralytic poliomyelitis (VAPP), a rare consequence of the live-attenuated oral polio vaccine. **Seasonal Variation:** None in the tropics. In the past, clusters of infections occurred during fall months in temperate regions. **Risk Factors:** Outbreaks occur in unvaccinated populations, typically those living in poor conditions or those objecting to immunization. While rare (<5% of symptomatic poliovirus infections), the frequency of paralytic polio increases with increasing age at time of infection. In endemic regions, 90-95% of cases occur before age 6 (median age for polio is 1 year) Secondary problems: Myelitis; peripheral neuropathy; skeletal deformity in affected limbs; post-polio syndrome.

Subjective: Symptoms

Malaise, headache, nausea, vomiting, and sore throat; uneventful recovery within several days (abortive poliomyelitis); 10-20% of symptomatic infections progress with severe muscle spasms, neck and back stiffness, and muscle tenderness lasting about 10 days with complete recovery (nonparalytic poliomyelitis); few (0.1%) of all polio patients develop paralytic poliomyelitis: asymmetric weakness or paralysis ("acute flaccid paralysis").

Focused History: *Have you completed the full polio vaccination series?* (drastically reduces chance of polio infection) *Did fever precede the limb weakness?* (Flaccid limb paralysis, especially if asymmetric, after acute febrile illness in a child or young adult is probable polio until proven otherwise.) *Have you traveled overseas or otherwise been exposed to poliovirus (including vaccine virus) recently (for troops or others from developed countries)?* (Travel to endemic area or other contact within past several weeks establishes risk for infection.) *Are there other cases like this in the area/village/household?* (Outbreaks may be focal.)

Objective: Signs

Using Basic Tools: Vitals: Fever; rarely, respiratory embarrassment leading to paralysis. Inspection: Various findings: asymmetric flaccid paralysis from lower motor neuron damage (spinal poliomyelitis); paralysis of respiratory muscles or bulbar paralysis leading to respiratory impairment; cranial nerve palsies without sensory loss or dysphagia; deep tendon reflexes diminished or lost asymmetrically. Palpation: Nuchal (neck) rigidity.

Using Advanced Tools: Not available in the field (eg, viral cultures of spinal fluid)

Assessment: Differential Diagnosis

Coxsackievirus A7 and enterovirus 71: Rare cases include asymmetric acute flaccid limb paralysis with a clinical picture that is virtually identical to polio.

Japanese encephalitis virus: See Part 5: Specialty Areas: Chapter 12: Viral Infections: Arboviral Encephalitis (TBE, JE, WN, St. Louis)

West Nile virus: Can cause asymmetric acute flaccid paralysis identical to polio. See Part 5: Specialty Areas: Chapter 12: Viral Infections: Arboviral Encephalitis (TBE, JE, WN, St. Louis)

Acute Guillain-Barré syndrome (post-infectious polyneuritis): May be clinically similar in presentation, but usually has an afebrile, symmetric paralysis, often associated with sensory loss. Important to differentiate due to potential for intervention (immunoglobulin, plasmapheresis).

Mumps: Neurological complications can include meningitis, encephalitis, Guillain-Barré syndrome, ascending polyradiculitis, transverse myelitis and facial palsy.

Tuberculous meningitis: Paralytic phase follows prodromal and meningitic phases and may progress rapidly from confusion to stupor and coma (often with hemiparesis).

Brain abscess: History of unilateral headache and unilateral neurologic signs.

Rhabdomyolysis: Patients may experience a rapid developing symmetrical quadriparesis, but have significant muscle pain and markedly elevated CPK levels.

Early disseminated Lyme disease: May include a painful radiculopathy and cranial nerve palsy as well as peripheral nerve palsies. See Part 5: Specialty Areas: Chapter 12: Spirochetal Infections: Lyme Disease

Other infections: Diphtheria and botulism may produce acute flaccid paralysis. See Part 3: General Symptoms: ENT Problems: Pharyngitis, Adult & Part 4: Organ Systems: Chapter 7: Acute Bacterial Food Poisoning

Plan:

Treatment

Supportive care is indicated, including analgesics for fever or pain such as **acetaminophen** 650mg po/PR q4h or **ibuprofen** 400mg po q6h for adults (see Part 8: Procedures: Chapter 30: Pain Assessment and Control). No specific treatment exists for these viruses.

Patient Education

General: Do not expose others to infected body fluids (enteric precautions).

Activity: Rest on firm bed with footboard and sponge rubber pads or rolls. Physical therapy with early mobilization after illness is important during convalescence; brace and lightly splint the affected limbs.

Diet: As tolerated.

Prevention and Hygiene: Provide safe drinking water. Immunize with trivalent poliovirus vaccine. Eradication of polio has been achieved in the Western hemisphere and a global campaign is underway using mass immunization to control outbreaks of disease. The US immunization practice is to use inactivated polio vaccine (IPV), while the global campaign utilizes live-attenuated oral polio vaccine (OPV). The policy difference is because of the small but definite risk of vaccine-associated paralytic polio due to OPV, about 1 case in 10 million vaccinations. In the US, because there is no wild polio transmission, the risk of polio is slightly higher from OPV than it is from no vaccine for unimmunized people. In places where there is still polio, however, the OPV is used because it is very effective, easily administered (oral not injection), and causes "secondary vaccinations" since vaccinated people shed the vaccine in their stool. Both IPV and OPV are equally effective after the complete series is administered. There is no risk of vaccine-associated polio from IPV.

No Improvements/Deterioration: Return for new, recurrent or worsening symptoms.

Follow-up Actions

Return Evaluation: Respiratory compromise or bulbar involvement requires intensive care (airway management, assisted ventilation).

Evacuation/Consultation Criteria: Evacuate patients suspected of having of polio. Consult infectious disease or preventive medicine physician for any suspected case of polio.

Notes: Post-polio syndrome has been increasingly recognized among polio survivors in the past decade. This late complication is characterized by recurrence or worsening of prior paralysis that had eventually resolved, often along with pain involving affected limbs, several years after resolution of the initial paralytic illness. The weakness is slowly progressive and may wax and wane over time. The degree of severity of initial paralysis seems to predict the likelihood of subsequent muscle weakness. Post-polio syndrome might occur in as many as 25% to 50% of polio survivors, although exact estimates are difficult and severity of post-polio symptoms may vary. The mechanism is not clear, but it does not involve new or recurrent polio infection; patients are not contagious. There is presently no specific treatment for post-polio syndrome, although "non-fatiguing exercise" may improve muscle strength.

Chapter 12: Infectious Diseases: Viral Infections: Rabies

Maj Nicholas Conger, USAF, MC

Introduction: Rabies is an, acute, viral encephalomyelitis caused by the rabies virus (a Lyssavirus). Patients may present with an encephalitic (hyperactive), paralytic (CNS symptoms late), or an atypical form, but all disease invariably leads to progressive encephalopathy and death. Illness occurs following exposure to saliva from infected animals (dogs, bats or other mammals). The incubation period is variable, and may be lengthy (usually 20-90 days). Immunization before, or after exposure BEFORE symptoms can abort the course of disease. Only one case report of successful therapy following development of symptoms in a vaccine naïve patient exists (therapy included chemical induced coma plus ribavirin and amantadine). **Geographic Association:** Rabies occurs most commonly in developing nations of Asia, possibly the UK.

Risk Factors: Dogs bites in endemic areas account for 90% of cases worldwide. Rabies can be acquired from any bite or scratch with saliva contamination from dogs or other mammals (bats, foxes, skunks, other carnivores). Awakening to find a bat within an enclosed domicile is also a specific risk for rabies. Pre-exposure prophylactic vaccination is very effective and is strongly recommended for travelers who will be in rabies enzootic areas for >30 days. This includes most SOF personnel for most deployments.

Subjective: **Symptoms**

Tingling or pain at inoculation site (45% of cases); malaise, fatigue, headache or fever for 2-7 days; progression to apprehension, agitation, hyperactivity, bizarre behavior, hallucinations, nuchal (neck) rigidity, paralysis, coma and death (99% mortality) over 7-12 days.

Focused History: *Was patient bitten or scratched by an animal? Have there been behavioral changes or increased aggressiveness or quadriparesis? How long has the patient been ill?* (Duration longer than 5 days with progression rules out intoxication and some viral encephalitides.)

Objective: **Signs**

Using Basic Tools: Vital signs: fever; rapid, shallow respirations; occasionally irregular RR and HR in later stages. Inspection: Agitated or frightened appearance is characteristic after CNS involvement with rabies. Classical spasms of pharynx or larynx during attempts to eat or drink ("hydrophobia") are seen in 50% of cases. Often ascending paralysis from bitten limb spreads to bulbar muscles and finally the onset of coma. Neurological: Use Glasgow coma scale to track progression of mental status changes, and help gauge need for medical evacuation or consultation (*see Appendices: Table A-5: Glasgow Coma Scale*). Auscultation: Late cardiac dysrhythmias coincident with myocardial involvement.

Using Advanced Tools: Confirmation of rabies diagnosis requires special clinical specimens (corneal scraping, skin biopsy, brain material) and specialized laboratory facilities for immunofluorescence or PCR unavailable in the field.

Assessment:

Rabies must be considered in any patient presenting with acute progressive encephalitis regardless of a history of an animal bite or known exposure. Exposure to rabies should be assumed in any person who has been bitten by a terrestrial mammalian carnivore (eg, dog, cat, raccoon, skunk, fox, coyote), bat, or large rodent (muskrat, beaver) in whom the presence of rabies cannot be proven to be absent (ie, by direct observation for >10 days or laboratory analysis).

Differential Diagnosis: Pathognomonic (indicative) features include hydrophobia and inspiratory spasms.

Polio: Asymmetric ascending paralysis after minor febrile illness; encephalitic symptoms are rare.

Viral encephalitides: Respiratory symptoms not as prevalent as with rabies

Intoxication (eg, tetanus, botulism, drugs): Does not generally present with progression of CNS changes

Guillain-Barré syndrome: May mimic the paralytic form of rabies infection

Plan:

Treatment: Following credible rabies exposure

1. Immediately scrub wounds or broken mucous membranes with soap or detergent and water.
2. Débride or copiously irrigate wounds with water or sterile saline (preferred) using a 19 gauge blunt needle and a 35mL syringe to provide adequate pressure (7 psi) and volume. Do not close the wound.
3. Give **human rabies immune globulin (HRIG)** and human diploid cell vaccine (HDCV) or rabies vaccine adsorbed (RVA) as follows: Unvaccinated individuals:
   a. Give **human rabies immune globulin** (HRIG) 20IU/kg body weight) once on day 0. If anatomically feasible, attempt to infiltrate the full dose into and around the site of the wound, then inject remainder of dose IM into the gluteal region using a clean needle. HRIG should not be administered in the same syringe, nor into the same anatomical site as the vaccine, or more than 7 days after the initiation of the vaccine.
   b. Give **human diploid cell vaccine (HDCV)** or **rabies vaccine adsorbed (RVA)** 1.0mL IM (deltoid area remote from site of bite in adults, anterolateral thigh area in infants and young children) beginning immediately on day 0, then repeat on day 3,7,14 and 28 for a total of 5 doses. NEVER administer rabies vaccine in the gluteal region.
   Vaccinated patients: (ie, patients that have completed 3 doses pre-exposure vaccine prior to credible exposure to rabies, which includes intradermal and IM protocols given to most SOF personnel): Give HDCV or RVA 1mL IM booster dose in deltoid immediately at presentation and again 3 days later. DO NOT GIVE HRIG to pre-exposure vaccinated individuals. Pre-exposure vaccination does not guarantee protection against rabies, but it does buy time to get to definitive treatment if bitten, and it does decrease the number of post-exposure boosters required.
4. Give tetanus prophylaxis and antibiotic treatment; see *Part 7: Trauma: Chapter 28: Human and Animal Bites*
5. Use narcotics or benzodiazepines judiciously for agitation; see *Part 8: Procedures: Chapter 30: Pain Assessment and Control*
6. If possible, isolate suspected animal source and observe 10 days for signs of rabies. It is not necessary to sever the animal's head for analysis.

Patient Education

General: Keep body fluids isolated from others (body fluid precautions).

Activity: Rest

Diet: As tolerated, but swallowing may be difficult with advanced disease.

Prevention and Hygiene: Pre-exposure prophylactic vaccination is very effective and strongly recommended for all travelers who will be in rabies enzootic areas for >30 days. Give HDCV or RVA 1.0mL IM into the deltoid on days 0,7,21 or 28, or HDCV 0.1mL intradermally on days 0, 7, 21, or 28.

Notes: 1) In the event of vaccine shortage, there are some data that lower dosages of vaccine (0.1mL) may be effective for pre-exposure prophylaxis. While this is not currently recommended, it may effectively stretch a limited vaccine supply in austere environments. This is not recommended for post-exposure prophylaxis. 2) There are reports that drugs given for antimalarial prophylaxis (eg, chloroquine, mefloquine) administered concurrently with human diploid cell vaccine (HDCV) decreases the antibody response to the vaccine. Rabies prophylaxis should be completed before any antimalarial prophylaxis begins. If this is not possible, the IM regimen (not the intradermal regimen) should be used.

Follow-up Actions

Wound Care: Usually no special care required after initial treatment.

Return Evaluation: Evaluate for progression of neurological signs.

Evacuation/Consultation Criteria: Evacuate personnel suspected of exposure to rabies or a rabid animal. Consult infectious disease or preventive medicine specialists for any suspicion of rabies.

Zoonotic Disease Considerations

Principal Animal Hosts: Wild and domestic canids, raccoons, skunks, bats

Clinical Disease in Animals: Acute neurologic dysfunction, ataxia, progressive paralysis, absent reflexes; behavioral changes: anorexia, nervousness, irritability, hyperexcitability, uncharacteristic aggressiveness (wildlife lose fear of man; nocturnal animals seen during the daytime); furious form: pronounced aggressiveness ("mad dog" syndrome), progressing to ataxia, seizures and death; dumb or paralytic form: paralysis of throat or masseter muscles, profuse salivation, inability to swallow, progressing to coma and death. Some animals are obviously infected and are ill, while others may harbor the virus without any untoward effects.

Chapter 12: Infectious Diseases: Viral Infections: Yellow Fever

CDR Timothy H. Burgess, MC, USN

Introduction: Yellow fever is a mosquito-borne viral illness that can cause a life-threatening viral hemorrhagic fever with liver, renal, cardiac and blood clotting dysfunction. As with other viral hemorrhagic fevers, fluid management based on close clinical monitoring of hemodynamic status (eg, urinary output, heart rate, BP) is critical to recovery (see *Part 6: Operational Environment: Chapter 25: Biological Warfare: Viral Hemorrhagic Fevers*). The incubation period following mosquito bite is typically 3-6 days and although 80-90% of patients recover completely; between 10-20% of infected patients will go on (after a brief remission of hours to days) to develop jaundice and hemorrhagic disease (up to 50% mortality rate) with survivors requiring several weeks or months of convalescence. **Geographic Association:** Yellow fever is not transmitted in the US but occurs in jungle environments in Africa (90% of approximately 200,000 annual cases) and in jungle and possibly urban areas in Central and South America. Travelers to these areas require immunization with booster doses required every 10 years. **Seasonal Variation:** As with other arboviral illnesses, epidemics may follow the rainy season, particularly in areas contiguous to rain forests where jungle yellow fever is enzootic (monkeys as intermediate hosts). Endemic yellow fever occurs sporadically year-round. **Risk Factors:**

Travel to endemic areas without prior vaccination to yellow fever. Occupational exposure (forest clearing and agriculture) among young adult males accounts for many of the cases of yellow fever in forest regions of tropical Latin America.

Subjective: Symptoms

Abrupt onset of fever, chills, headache, backache, vomiting for 2-3 days; in severe cases the patient's condition worsens over the next 3-10 days with coffee-ground hematemesis ("black vomit"), jaundice, and disorientation.

Focused History: *Have you ever been vaccinated against yellow fever?* (decreases risk of yellow fever to <1%) *When did you first feel sick?* (Typically, patient recalls exact time of onset of fever, headache, and prostration, usually within past week.) *Have you traveled overseas in the past 3 weeks? If so, where?* (look for travel to endemic areas)

Objective: Signs

Using Basic Tools: Vitals: Fever to 102-104°F; hypotension and relative bradycardia; occasional arrhythmias. Inspection: facial flushing with conjunctival injection, strawberry tongue (red edges with central prominent papillae); Advanced disease: Bleeding from orifices (epistaxis, hematemesis, and melena), jaundice. Palpation: Epigastric or RUQ abdominal tenderness

Using Advanced Tools: Labs: Proteinuria on urinalysis (nephritis); CBC (neutropenia typical), hematocrit and platelet count; *see Part 5: Specialty Areas: Chapter 12: Viral Infections: Dengue Fever (Dengue Hemorrhagic Fever/Dengue Shock Syndrome)*; type and cross match if bleeding; blood smear to rule out malaria.

Assessment: Sudden onset of high fever without prodromal symptoms or rash is characteristic, when accompanied by the classical triad of albuminuria, jaundice and hematemesis.

Differential Diagnosis

Rickettsial fevers: Maculopapular rash that begins at the wrists and ankles and spread to the trunk. *See Part 5: Specialty Areas: Chapter 12: Rickettsial Infections: Rickettsial Infections (Murine, Rickettsial Pox, RMSF, Scrub Typhus, Louse-Borne Typhus, Boutonneuse Fever)*

Leptospirosis: Conjunctival suffusion (permeated with blood), non-productive cough. *See Part 5: Specialty Areas: Chapter 12: Spirochetal Infections: Leptospirosis*

Dengue hemorrhagic Fever: *See Part 5: Specialty Areas: Chapter 12: Viral Infections: Dengue Fever (Dengue Hemorrhagic Fever/ Dengue Shock Syndrome)*

Other hemorrhagic fevers (Rift Valley, Lassa, Marburg or Ebola): Not usually associated with jaundice. History of travel to specific geographic areas. *See Part 6: Operational Environment: Chapter 25: Biological Warfare: Viral Hemorrhagic Fevers*

Snake bite (viper): History of snake bite may have similar consumptive coagulopathy, but usually without jaundice or proteinuria.

Severe malaria: Identification of parasite on (Giemsa stain) thick and thin blood smears. *See Part 5: Specialty Areas: Chapter 12: Parasitic Infections: Malaria*

Typhoid fever: Relative bradycardia and or pulse temperature dissociation. *See Part 5: Specialty Areas: Chapter 12: Bacterial Infections: Typhoid Fever*

Viral hepatitis: Abdominal discomfort (RUQ) may predominate, without signs of bleeding diathesis. *See Part 5: Specialty Areas: Chapter 12: Viral Infections: Hepatitis A; Hepatitis B (and Hepatitis D); Hepatitis C & Hepatitis E*

Plan:

Treatment

1. There is no specific treatment for yellow fever.
2. Supportive care: **codeine** 15–30mg po q6h prn for pain (*see Part 8: Procedures: Chapter 30: Pain Assessment and Control*). For nausea/vomiting, give **dimenhydrinate** 50mg IM q6-12h prn, or **prochlorperazine** 25mg PR bid, or 5-10mg IM q3-4 or 5-10mg po tid-qid prn.
3. Early medical evacuation of all but mildly ill patients or if any evidence of end organ damage or hemorrhagic complications.
4. If unable to evacuate and bleeding or shock occurs, begin fluid resuscitation with IV isotonic fluid bolus, followed by IV colloids (*see Part 7: Trauma: Chapter 27: Resuscitation Fluid*). Monitor vital signs, CAREFULLY insert NG tube and Foley catheter, monitor I & O, hematocrit and platelet count. Blood transfusion as required to maintain adequate tissue perfusion (*See Part 8: Procedures: Chapter 30: Blood Transfusion*).

Patient Education

General: Use universal precautions with all patients with suspected hemorrhagic fever. Prevent mosquito access to patient.

Activity: Bedrest

Diet: NPO if hemorrhagic, until stable

Medications: Avoid acetaminophen (liver damage) and aspirin (bleeding)

Prevention and Hygiene: Immunize with licensed yellow fever vaccine. Booster doses are recommended every 10 years for travel to yellow fever-endemic regions. Avoid suspected foci of yellow fever or other hemorrhagic fevers. Practice personal protective measures against mosquitoes (*see Part 5: Specialty Areas: Chapter 13: Malaria Prevention and Control*).

Follow-up Actions

Return Evaluation: Assess for onset of hemorrhagic signs, and evacuate if necessary.

Evacuation/Consultation Criteria: Urgently evacuate all suspected hemorrhagic cases (hematologic abnormalities, profound bleeding, or vascular instability). Consult infectious disease specialists for all cases of hemorrhagic yellow fever, and for any cases in team members.

Note: Serology may be performed to confirm diagnosis and for epidemiologic case definition.

Chapter 12: Infectious Diseases: Rickettsial Infections: Rickettsial Infections (Murine, Rickettsialpox, RMSF, Scrub Typhus, Louse-Borne Typhus, Boutonneuse Fever)

Lt Col Gregory Deye, USAF, MC

Introduction: Rickettsia are obligate intracellular bacteria that are transmitted to humans by arthropod vectors, often from animal reservoirs. There are many known rickettsial human pathogens, and new species continue to be discovered. These pathogens are generally grouped as Typhus Fevers, Spotted Fever Group (SFG) organisms, or Non-rickettsial intracellular organisms. The presence or absence of an eschar (tache noir) can help to differentiate SFG pathogens. Some SFG organisms can demonstrate remarkably restricted geographical range. Because clinical characteristics exhibit considerable overlap, diagnostic considerations should be directed by a knowledge of locally endemic infections (*see Table 5-5*). *Rickettsia rickettsii* is a tick-borne bacterium that causes **Rocky Mountain spotted fever** (RMSF) in the New World. Other tick-borne spotted fevers include African and Mediterranean tick fever (or **Boutonneuse fever**, *Rickettsia conorii*), Queensland tick typhus (*Rickettsia australis*). All these "spotted fevers" present similarly and are managed the same way. RMSF is fatal in 3% of cases and mortality is associated with delay in diagnosis or adequate treatment (eg, failure to treat with doxycycline). The incubation period is 3-12 days after a tick bite. *Rickettsia prowazekii* causes the severe illness **typhus** (or epidemic or louse-borne typhus), and is transmitted worldwide between humans by the body louse. In the US, contact with flying squirrels has also been associated with transmission. A milder illness may recur years after the first attack, not associated with re-infection (Brill-Zinsser disease). The incubation period is 7-14 days. **Murine typhus** is caused by *Rickettsia typhi*, which is transmitted worldwide by flies that feed on rats. The illness resembles louse borne typhus but is much milder. Murine typhus peaks in the late summer/autumn and is prevalent in the urban environment. The incubation period is 6-18 days. *Orientia tsutsugamushi* infection follows chigger bites in the Asiatic-Pacific area and causes **scrub typhus**. The dark punched-out skin ulcer at site of the bite is known as the "tache noire" (also in most spotted fevers), and is helpful to clinically suggest this infection. The incubation period is 7-21 days. **Rickettsialpox** is caused by *Rickettsia akari* and is transmitted by rodent mite and chigger bites. The vesicular rash is similar to chickenpox, and is seen in urban areas of the northeastern US and some other areas in the world (Africa, Ukraine). The incubation period is 9-14 days.

Subjective: Symptoms
Spotted fevers: Acute (1-3 days): Fever >102°F, headache, myalgias, rash (typical but not in all cases), tache noire (except RMSF, Astrakhan), mental status changes. Sub-acute (4-7 days): Same as acute. Chronic (>1 week): Continued myalgias, rash, and tache noire
Typhus group: Acute (1-3 days): Fever (can last up to 14 days), chills, myalgias, headache Sub-acute (4-7 days): Rash, ± cough Chronic (>1 week): Cough, rash
Focused History: *Have you had a recent tick bite?* (exposure) *Did you have a flu-like illness and fever a couple of days before the rash?* (c/w typhus group infection) *Have you been in the woods or traveled overseas in the last 2 weeks?* (exposure; see introduction section for geographic clues). *Do you have a dark scab-like skin sore with surrounding redness?* (the tache noire of scrub typhus and other rickettsial infections)

Objective: Signs
Using Basic Tools: Inspection
All: Fever to 104°F, terminates by day 14 (except Brill-Zinsser, which may recur), often ill-appearing
Sub-acute/Chronic: Rash
Rocky Mountain spotted fever (and other spotted fevers): Sub-acute (4-7 days): maculopapular rash that starts on extremities includes palms/soles/face, petechiae and hemorrhagic lesions can occur, digital gangrene is rare. **Chronic (>1 week):** May see late desquamation
Typhus (louse borne): **Acute (1-3 days):** Conjunctival injection **Sub-acute (4-7 days):** Small macules in axilla/trunk that spread over body and can become dark in color (hemorrhagic). Rare digital gangrene
Scrub typhus: Acute (1-3 days): Tache noire; *see Appendices: Color Plates: Figure A-21.F* **Sub-acute (4-7 days):** Spreading dull red maculopapular rash starts on trunk, spreads to extremities
Murine typhus: Sub-acute (4-7 days): Maculopapular rash that is sparse and discrete mainly trunk and extremities, can be palm/soles
Rickettsialpox: Acute (1-3 days): Tache noire; *see Appendices: Color Plates: Figure A-21.F* **Sub-acute (4-7 days):** Maculopapular rash with vesicles that crust; spares palms and soles

Assessment: This is a clinical diagnosis.
Differential Diagnosis
Typhoid fever: Usually rose spots are few and short-lived, elevated WBC
Malaria: No rash; parasites seen on blood smears.
Leptospirosis: Patients generally have more intense conjunctival redness, may see jaundice, petechial type rash
Meningococcemia: Petechial rash may progress to purpura, meningitis symptoms are common, rapid progression
Dengue: Prominent myalgias and fever (breakbone fever)
Others: Syphilis (usually no fever), drug reaction or side effect, rubeola or rubella (different rash; *see ID specific section*).

Plan:

Rocky Mountain spotted fever (and **Boutonneuse fever**): Treat early based on clinical considerations.

Treatment: Doxycycline 100mg po bid x 7 days (or at least 48 hours afebrile), or **chloramphenicol** 500mg po qid x 7 days.

Typhus

Treatment: Primary: Doxycycline 200mg po load, then 100mg po q12h x 10 days (or until 48 hours afebrile), or **tetracycline** 25mg/kg po in divided 6-8 hour doses until 48-72 hours afebrile, or **doxycycline** 200mg po x single dose.

Alternatives: Chloramphenicol adult-500-1000mg IV q6h pediatric-80mg/kg/d divided q6h. Though these agents are preferred, in situations in which they are unavailable, there are in vitro and limited clinical data to support the use of **ciprofloxacin** or **azithromycin**. Optimal dosing has not been established for these agents. Use IV fluids cautiously.

Murine typhus

Treatment: Doxycycline 100mg po q12h until 48 hours afebrile

Scrub typhus

Treatment: Doxycycline 100mg po q12h x 7 days (resistance in Thailand to tetracycline and chloramphenicol)

Rickettsialpox

Treatment: Doxycycline 100mg po q12h x 5–7 days (and until 48 hours afebrile)

Patient Education

Medications: Do not take doxycycline with iron, milk or milk products, multivitamins or antacids, and avoid the sun. Tetracyclines are often associated with mild gastritis and gastrointestinal upset. Take with food to help with this symptom. Avoid sulfa medications during this illness as they can make symptoms worse.

Prevention and Hygiene: Avoid ticks (remove attached or crawling ticks after exposure to tick infested area); control fleas, lice, rats (*see Part 5: Specialty Areas: Chapter 13: Pest Control*).

Follow-up Actions

Evacuation/Consultation Criteria: Evacuate unstable patients and those unable to complete the mission, including those with RMSF. Consult infectious disease or primary care physician for RMSF cases and as needed.

Zoonotic Disease Considerations for RMSF

Principal Animal Hosts: Rabbits, field mice, dogs
Clinical Disease in Animals: Fever, anorexia, lymphadenopathy, polyarthritis, coughing, dyspnea, abdominal pain, edema of face, or extremities
Probable Mode of Transmission: Bite of infected ticks or crushing *Dermacentor variabilis* or *andersoni* ticks on skin
Known Distribution: Western Hemisphere

Zoonotic Disease Considerations for Boutonneuse Fever

Principal Animal Hosts: Dogs, rodents
Clinical Disease in Animals: Asymptomatic or mild febrile illness
Probable Mode of Transmission: Bite of infected tick
Known Distribution: Europe, Asia, Africa

Zoonotic Disease Considerations for Typhus

Principal Animal Hosts: Flying squirrels, unclear significance for human transmission
Clinical Disease in Animals: Asymptomatic
Probable Mode of Transmission: Human louse; squirrel fleas or ticks suspected
Known Distribution: Worldwide; Eastern USA in squirrels

Zoonotic Disease Considerations for Murine Typhus

Principal Animal Hosts: Rats, cats, opossums
Clinical Disease in Animals: Asymptomatic
Probable Mode of Transmission: Infected rodent fleas; possibly cat fleas
Known Distribution: Worldwide

Zoonotic Disease Considerations for Scrub Typhus

Principal Animal Hosts: Rodents
Clinical Disease in Animals: Asymptomatic
Probable Mode of Transmission: Bite of infected larval trombiculid mites
Known Distribution: Focal areas in Asia (as far west as Pakistan and at altitudes of 10,000 ft), Australia, and East Indies.

Zoonotic Disease Considerations for Rickettsialpox

Principal Animal Hosts: Mice
Clinical Disease in Animals: Asymptomatic
Probable Mode of Transmission: Bite of infected rodent mites, *Liponyssoides* spp.
Known Distribution: Eastern USA, Africa, and Russia; rare

Chapter 12: Infectious Diseases: Rickettsial Infections: Rickettsial Infection Chart

Lt Col Gregory Deye, USAF, MC

Table 5-5. Rickettsial Chart

Antigenic Group: Typhus fevers

Disease	Agent	Predominant Symptoms*	Vector or Acquisition Mechanism	Animal Reservoir	Geographic Distribution Outside the US
Epidemic typhus, Sylvatic typhus	*Rickettsia prowazekii*	Headache, chills, fever, prostration, confusion, photophobia, vomiting, rash (generally starting on trunk)	Human body louse, squirrel flea and louse	Humans, flying squirrels (US)	Cool mountainous regions of Africa, Asia, and Central and South America
Murine typhus	*R. typhi*	As above, generally less severe	Rat flea	Rats, mice	Worldwide

Antigenic Group: Spotted fevers

Disease	Agent	Predominant Symptoms*	Vector or Acquisition Mechanism	Animal Reservoir	Geographic Distribution Outside the US
African tick-bite fever	*R. africae*	Fever, eschar(s), regional adenopathy, maculopapular or vesicular rash subtle or absent	Tick	Rodents	Sub-Saharan Africa
Aneruptive fever	*R. he!vetica*	Fever, headache, myalgia	Tick	Rodents	Old World
Australian spotted fever	*R. marmionii*	Fever, eschar, maculopapular or vesicular rash, adenopathy	Tick	Rodents	Australia
Cat flea rickettsiosis	*R. felis*	As murine typhus, generally less severe	Cat and dog fleas	Domestic cats, opossums	Europe, South America
Far Eastern spotted fever	*R. heilongjiangensis*	Fever, eschar, macular or maculopapular rash, lymphadenopathy, enlarged lymph nodes	Tick	Rodents	Far East of Russia, Northern China
Flinders Island spotted fever, Thai tick typhus	*R. honei*	Mild spotted fever, eschar and adenopathy are rare	Tick	Not defined	Australia, Thailand
Lymphangitis associated rickettsiosis	*R. sibirica* subsp. mongolotimonae	Fever, multiple eschars, regional adenopathy and lymphangitis, maculopapular rash	Tick	Rodents	Southern France, Portugal, Asia, Africa
Maculatum infection	*R. parkeri*	Fever, eschar, rash maculopapular to vesicular	Tick	Rodents	Brazil, Uruguay, USA
Mediterranean spotted fevers‡	*R. conorii*	Fever, eschar, regional adenopathy, maculopapular on extremities	Tick	Dogs, rodents	Africa, India, Europe, Middle East, Mediterranean
North Asian tick typhus	*R. sibirica*	Fever, eschar(s), regional adenopathy, maculopapular rash	Tick	Rodents	Russia, China, Mongolia
Oriental spotted fever	*R. japonica*	As Above	Tick	Rodents	Japan
Queensland tick typhus	*R. australis*	Fever, eschar, regional adenopathy, rash on extremities	Tick	Not defined	Australia, Tasmania

Table 5-5. Rickettsial Chart, continued

Antigenic Group: Spotted fevers, continued

Disease	Agent	Predominant Symptoms*	Vector or Acquisition Mechanism	Animal Reservoir	Geographic Distribution Outside the US
Rickettsialpox	R. akari	Fever, eschar, adenopathy, disseminated vesicular rash	Mite	House mice	Russia, South Africa, Korea, Turkey, Balkan Countries
Rocky Mountain spotted fever, Sao Paulo exanthematic typhus, Minas Gerais exanthematic typhus, Brazilian spotted fever	R. rickettsii	Headache, fever, abdominal pain, macular rash progressing into papular or petechial (generally starting on extremities)	Tick	Rodents	Mexico, Central, and South America
Tick-borne lymphadenopathy (TIBOLA), Dermacentor-borne necrosis and lymphadenopathy (DEBONEL)	R. slovaca	Necrosis erythema, cervical lymphadenopathy and enlarged lymph nodes, rare maculopapular rash	Tick	Lagomorphs, rodents	Europe, Asia
Unnamed rickettsiosis	R. aeschlimannii	Fever, eschar, maculopapular rash	Tick	Domestic and wild animals	Africa

Antigenic Group: Orientia

Disease	Agent	Predominant Symptoms*	Vector or Acquisition Mechanism	Animal Reservoir	Geographic Distribution Outside the US
Scrub Typhus	Orientia tsutsugamushi	Fever, headache, sweating, conjunctival injection, adenopathy, eschar, rash (starting on trunk), respiratory distress	Mite	Rodents	South, Central, Eastern, and Southeast Asia and Australia
Unnamed rickettsiosis	R. aeschlimannii	Fever, eschar, maculopapular rash	Tick	Domestic and wild animals	Africa

Antigenic Group: Coxiella

Disease	Agent	Predominant Symptoms*	Vector or Acquisition Mechanism	Animal Reservoir	Geographic Distribution Outside the US
Q fever	Coxiella burnetii	Fever, headache, chills, sweating, pneumonia, hepatitis, endocarditis	Most human infections are acquired by inhalation of infectious aerosols; tick	Goats, sheep, cattle, domestic cats, other	Worldwide

Table 5-5. Rickettsial Chart, continued

Antigenic Group: Bartonella

Disease	Agent	Predominant Symptoms*	Vector or Acquisition Mechanism	Animal Reservoir	Geographic Distribution Outside the US
Cat-scratch disease	Bartonella henselae	Fever, adenopathy, neuroretinitis, encephalitis	Cat flea	Domestic cats	Worldwide
Trench fever	B. quintana	Fever, headache, pain in shins, splenomegaly, disseminated rash	Human body louse	Humans	Worldwide
Oroya fever	B. bacilliformis	Fever, headache, anemia, shifting joint and muscle pain, nodular dermal eruption	Sand fly	Unknown	Peru, Ecuador, Colombia

Antigenic Group: Ehrlichia

Disease	Agent	Predominant Symptoms*	Vector or Acquisition Mechanism	Animal Reservoir	Geographic Distribution Outside the US
Ehrlichosis	Ehrlichia chaffeensis‡	Fever, headache, nausea, occasionally rash	Tick	Various large and small mammals, including deer and rodents	Worldwide

Antigenic Group: Anaplasma

Disease	Agent	Predominant Symptoms*	Vector or Acquisition Mechanism	Animal Reservoir	Geographic Distribution Outside the US
Anaplasmosis	Anaplasma phago-cytophilum#	Fever, headache, nausea, occasionally rash	Tick	Small mammals, and rodents	Europe, Asia, Africa

Antigenic Group: Neorickettsia

Disease	Agent	Predominant Symptoms*	Vector or Acquisition Mechanism	Animal Reservoir	Geographic Distribution Outside the US
Sennetsu fever	Neorickettsia sennetsu	Fever, chills, headache, sore throat, insomnia	Fish, fluke	Fish	Japan, Malaysia

*   This represents only a partial list of symptoms. Patients may have different symptoms or only a few of those listed.
‡   Includes 4 different subspecies that can be distinguished serologically and by PCR assay, and respectively are the etiologic agents of Boutonneuse fever and Mediterranean tick fever in Southern Europe and Africa (R. conorii subsp. conorii), Indian tick typhus in South Asia (R. conorii subsp. indica), Israeli tick typhus in Southern Europe and Middle East (R. conorii subsp. israelensis), and Astrakhan spotted fever in the North Caspian region of Russia (R. conorii subsp. caspiae).
#   Organisms antigenically related to these species are associated with ehrlichial diseases outside the CONUS.

Part 5: Specialty Areas: Chapter 12: Infectious Diseases: Rickettsial Infections: Q Fever

Lt Col Gregory Deye, USAF, MC

Introduction: Q fever is caused by *Coxiella burnetii*, intracellular bacteria that infect sheep, cattle, goats, and occasionally cats. Infected animals are often asymptomatic. Humans are infected by inhaling aerosol or contaminated dust or ingesting infected raw milk. Tick bite and blood transfusion are rare methods of infection. Because the bacteria are present in high concentration in placental material of infected animals, there is a seasonal predominance during the spring lambing/calving season. The incubation period is 4-28 days. Usually *Coxiella* causes a mild, self-limited illness in humans consisting of fever, headache, and myalgia, though occasionally more severe acute illness, including pneumonia, hepatitis or CNS infection can occur. Chronic infection, mainly endocarditis, develops in a minority of untreated patients. Q fever is a potential bio-warfare threat.

Subjective: Symptoms
Constitutional Acute (1-7 days): Sweats, chills, fever (abrupt onset), severe retro-orbital headache, myalgias, malaise.
Chronic (>3weeks): Fever continues if endocarditis develops (although rare, this is the most serious and often fatal [24%] form of chronic infection).
Specific Sub-acute (8-20 days): Non-productive cough; 1% have neurologic symptoms-weakness, meningitis, sensory loss, paresthesias
Focused History: *In the past month, have you had exposure to a pregnant animal that gave birth? Have you been within visual distance of cattle, sheep or goats? Have you ingested unpasteurized milk? Have you recently had a tick bite?* (any affirmative suggests possible exposure)

Objective: Signs
Using Basic Tools: Inspection: Acute (<1 week): Fever to 104°F Chronic (>3 weeks): If fever persists 3 weeks, r/o endocarditis (rare): check for embolic events (splinter hemorrhages, Roth spots [advanced tools], Osler's nodes), clubbed fingers. Auscultation: Acute (<1 week): Inspiratory crackles. Chronic (>3 weeks): Diastolic murmur of aortic regurgitation. Palpation: Sub-acute (8-20 days): Hepatomegaly 5%, splenomegaly, rare neurologic findings: sensory loss, cranial nerve palsies, cerebellar signs
Using Advanced Tools: CXR may show pneumonitis (diffuse inflammation), 1/3 have pleural effusions.

Assessment: Differential Diagnosis
Influenza: Febrile respiratory infection of relatively short duration without history of risk of exposure to *Coxiella burnetii. See Part 4: Organ Systems: Chapter 3: Influenza*
Salmonella: Febrile illness with gastrointestinal symptoms which can persist for weeks, food/water borne. *See Part 4: Organ Systems: Chapter 7: Acute Bacterial Food Poisoning*
Malaria: Recurrent fever; blood smears show parasite. *See Part 5: Specialty Areas: Chapter 12: Parasitic Infections: Malaria*
Hepatitis: Often less prominent fever; jaundice may be present; more prominent anorexia, malaise and fatigue. *See Part 5: Specialty Areas: Chapter 12: Viral Infections: Hepatitis A; Hepatitis B (and Hepatitis D); Hepatitis C & Hepatitis E*
Atypical pneumonia: Can mimic Q fever pneumonia; ask about relevant exposure history to lead to Q fever diagnosis. *See Part 4: Organ Systems: Chapter 3: Pneumonia*
Other diagnoses: Brucellosis, psittacosis, typhus, rickettsial infection, dengue, arboviral infection. *See these sections in ID chapter*

Plan:
Treatment
Primary:
Acute infection: **Doxycycline** 100mg po bid x 14 days. Consider a fluoroquinolone (eg, **ciprofloxacin** or **levofloxacin** 750mg po bid x 14 days) as an alternative for patients with strong history of exposure to *Coxiella burnetii* and symptoms of meningoencephalitis.
Chronic infection: Requires referral/consult with ID and prolonged therapy (>18 months); **levofloxacin** 750mg po bid and **rifampin** 300mg po bid.

Patient Education
Prevention and Hygiene: Drink pasteurized milk. Burn or bury highly infectious *Coxiella*-contaminated tissue. Risk of chronic infection is increased in exposed individuals with history of abnormal heart valves.

Zoonotic Disease Considerations
Principal Animal Hosts: Sheep, cattle, goats, occasionally cats
Clinical Disease in Animals: Usually subclinical; anorexia, abortion

Chapter 12: Infectious Diseases: Spirochetal Infections: Leptospirosis

LTC Clinton K. Murray, MC, USA

Introduction: Leptospirosis is a spirochetal infection typically acquired after exposure of mucous membranes or breaks in the skin to water contaminated with urine from infected wild and domestic animals. Presentation can range from asymptomatic illness to an influenza-like illness to severe illness resulting in death. Leptospirosis infection has an incubation period of 2-20 days. **Geographic Association:** The disease is present around the world, but the majority of the disease occurs in tropical regions. **Seasonal Variation:** Disease transmission can occur year round but is often worse in times on increased rains and warmer months. **Risk Factors:** Breaks in the skin with fresh water exposure.

Subjective: Symptoms

Presentation can range from asymptomatic illness to fulminate disease with renal, liver and lung complications resulting in death. Initial presentation typically includes fevers, myalgias and headaches. Nausea, vomiting and diarrhea can occur in 50% of cases and pulmonary presentation in up to 1/3 of cases. Although classically described as a biphasic illness, this typically occurs in less than 50% of cases.

Focused History: *Have you had a fever that resolved after one week then recurred?* (occasional pattern) *Have you recently waded, swam or bathed in freshwater?* (typical exposure in endemic area) *Do your calves or back and neck muscles ache or feel stiff?* (typical myalgias)

Objective: Signs

Using Basic Tools: Vital signs: Fever to 104°F; can be biphasic (first episode lasts 3-9 days, then 3 days without fever, then recurs); Inspection: Conjunctival effusion is frequently present. Jaundice can occur with Weil's syndrome, the most severe form of the disease. Auscultation: Respiratory distress with pulmonary involvement - tachypnea, rales. Palpation: Muscle tenderness, lymphadenopathy, (including submandibular as in pharyngitis), skin rash, edema, abdominal pain

Using Advanced Tools: Labs: Routine laboratory tests are typically nondiagnostic.

Assessment:

Differential Diagnosis: Diseases endemic to the region of infection should be sought including:

Malaria: Fevers but no conjunctival changes

Yellow fever: Jaundice, more bleeding manifestations, vaccine available

Dengue fever: Mosquito-borne febrile illness with prominent myalgias, headache; diffuse rash, petechia can be present

Meningococcus: Fever often with petechia progressing to purpura rash; +/- meningitis

Rickettsial infection: Tick-borne infection; associated with fevers and elevated liver associated enzymes

Influenza: More nasopharyngeal symptoms, cough, sore throat

Hepatitis: More anorexia, malaise, vaccine available for A and B

Other diseases to consider include **babesiosis, typhoid, brucellosis, Colorado tick fever, viral meningitis,** tularemia, **typhoid fever, influenza.** *See sections on these in ID and Respiratory chapters.*

Plan:

Treatment

Primary: Doxycycline 100mg po bid x 7 days

Alternative: Azithromycin 500mg po day 1, then 250mg for 4 more days

Severe disease: **Penicillin** 1.5 million units IV q6h x 7 days or **ceftriaxone** 1g IV q day x 7 days

Patient Education

Activity: Avoid sun exposure with doxycycline.

Diet: As tolerated

Medications: Photosensitivity with doxycycline treatment. Therapy can result in a Jarisch-Herxheimer reaction (fever, tachycardia, mild hypotension, chills, vasodilatation within 2 hours of treatment; peaking at 7-8 hours and resolving in one day). Avoid doxycycline in young children and pregnant/nursing mothers.

Prevention and Hygiene: Use doxycycline 200mg po q week prophylactically during period of exposure. Dispose of urine appropriately to avoid further transmission. Wear boots and avoid skin or mucous membrane exposure to streams, standing water and mud after rainy season.

No Improvement/Deterioration: Return for re-evaluation promptly.

Follow-up Actions

Evacuation/Consultation Criteria: Refer patients who develop complications.

Zoonotic Disease Considerations:

Principal Animal Hosts: Dogs, cattle, swine, mice, rats, horses, goats, sheep

Clinical Disease in Animals: Usually asymptomatic renal infection; animal vaccines are available

Chapter 12: Infectious Diseases: Spirochetal Infections: Lyme Disease

COL Glenn Wortmann, MC, USA

Introduction: Lyme disease is a tick-borne zoonotic infection caused by *Borrelia burgdorferi*. In the US, it is most commonly found in the Northeast. It also occurs in Europe, Scandinavia, Russia, China, Japan and Australia and is transmitted by the bite of an ixodid tick (deer tick), primarily during the summer months when ticks are most active. The incubation period after a tick bite is 3-32 days

Subjective: Symptoms

Early stage disease: Erythema migrans (circular, erythematous rash) at bite site in 75% of patients, with multiple lesions present in 50% of patients; fever, Bell's palsy, fatigue, malaise and cardiac abnormalities (dropped beats, chest pain, pericarditis).

Later stage disease: Joint stiffness, myalgias, pain and swelling; headache; polyneuropathy; CNS neurological problems (cerebellar ataxia, coma).

Focused History: *Do you recall being bitten by a tick?* (only 20-30 % recall bite) *Do you recall the size of the tick that bit you?* (Lyme disease is transmitted by the small deer tick.) *How long ago were you bitten by a tick?* (The incubation period for erythema migrans is 3-32 days.)

Objective: Signs

Using Basic Tools: Diagnostic rash of erythema migrans (EM) about 7 days after bite (*see Appendices: Color Plates: Figure A-23.E*); peripheral cranial nerve VII palsy (facial paralysis), bradycardia, fever, generalized adenopathy, swelling in large joints (particularly knees), dropped heart beats, abnormal neurological exam.

Using Advanced Tools: ECG: Pericarditis, heart block. Serology testing is available for confirmation at most hospitals but is often negative with early infection.

Assessment:
The rash of erythema migrans is diagnostic of Lyme disease.

Differential Diagnosis:

Cellulitis, arthropod bite, contact dermatitis, pityriasis rosea, tinea corporis, drug reaction: May mimic rash of erythema migrans.

Plan:
Treatment Acute infection (erythema migrans):

Primary: Amoxicillin 500mg po tid or **doxycycline** 100mg po bid x 14-21 days.

Alternate: Cefuroxime axetil 500mg po bid x 14-21 days

Neurologic infection: **Ceftriaxone** 30mg/kg IV q day x 14-21 days

Patient Education

General: Prevent tick bites, particularly in spring and early summer.

Activity: As tolerated. Avoid sun exposure while on doxycycline.

Diet: As tolerated

Medications: Occasional gastrointestinal side effects. Doxycycline should be avoided during pregnancy, breastfeeding and in children.

Prevention and Hygiene: Personal protective measures (insecticide, etc.) against ticks.

No Improvement/Deterioration: Return for evaluation.

Follow-up Actions

Consultation Criteria: Failure to improve.

Zoonotic Disease Considerations:
Principal Animal Hosts: Deer, wild rodents

Clinical Disease in Animals: Limb or joint disease, neurologic, cardiac, renal abnormalities

Chapter 12: Infectious Diseases: Spirochetal Infections: Relapsing Fever
LTC Clinton K. Murray, MC, USA

Introduction: Relapsing fever is caused by the spirochete *Borrelia recurrentis* resulting in tick-borne (TBRF) and louse-borne (LBRF) forms of the disease. TBRF is spread by the soft-bodied ticks that reside inside houses, dwellings and caves with 50% risk of infection after a bite from an infected tick. LBRF is spread by the body louse, which only feeds on humans. The disease is spread by crushing the louse between the fingers and inoculating the wound with the organism. LBRF was associated with epidemics during major wars. **Geographic Association:** TBRF occurs in every continent except Antarctica, Australia and southwest Pacific; LBRF is only endemic in Ethiopia and Sudan although epidemics can occur anywhere as it is associated with homeless shelters; times of famine and war; and movements and congregations of refugees. **Seasonal Variation:** TBRF occurs during any season but typically when exposed to the vectors' environment. LBRF occurs more frequently during periods of overcrowding especially during winter months when more clothes are worn and washed less. **Risk Factors:** Exposure to soft-bodied ticks or lice in at risk environments.

Subjective: Symptoms
There is a sudden onset of fevers (up to 105°F) with intervals of afebrile period, which recurs at least twice. LBRF first fever episode is typically 3-6 days in duration with one single milder episode. TBRF has multiple febrile episodes of 1-3 days duration. Intervals between fever episodes for TBRF and LBRF ranges from 4-14 days. The first episode ends in rigors, increase in blood pressure and fevers followed in 15-30 minutes with sweating, falling temperature, and hypotension. LBRF can be associated with epistaxis and petechiae.

Focused History: *Have you had on-and-off fevers lasting several days at a time?* (typical pattern, but may be seen with other endemic diseases) *Have you had a recent tick bite?* (exposure) *Have you been around refugee camps recently?* (typical environment for LBRF)

Objective: Signs
Using Basic Tools: Inspection: monitor for fevers with alterations in vital signs with possible bleeding episodes with LBRF. Auscultation: If myocarditis develops: S3 and bibasilar rales. Palpation: Splenomegaly occurs in the majority of LBRF and 10% of TBRF. If neurologic involvement: cranial nerve palsies VII/VIII, bilateral or unilateral Bell's palsy

Using Advanced Tools: Labs: decreased platelets and mild anemia; Giemsa or Wright's stain of a thin blood smear taken during fever may show spirochetes with darkfield exam.

Assessment:
Differential Diagnosis: Diseases endemic to the region of infection should be sought including:

Malaria: Non-falciparum malaria may have periodic fevers

Lyme disease: Classic rash with low grade temperatures

Leptospirosis: Water exposure with febrile illness

Dengue: Mosquito-borne febrile illness with prominent myalgias, headache, diffuse rash

Meningococcus: Fever often with petechia progressing to purpura rash; +/- meningitis

Rickettsial infection: Tick-borne infection; associated with fevers and elevated liver associated enzymes

Other considerations include **babesiosis, typhoid, brucellosis, Colorado tick fever, viral meningitis, tularemia, typhoid fever, influenza.**

Plan:
Treatment:
Primary: Doxycycline 100mg po bid x 10 days
Alternative: Erythromycin 500mg po qid x 10 days (use for pregnant women, children <8 years)
Patient Education
General: Doxycycline and erythromycin may cause GI upset. Relapsing fever acquired during pregnancy can lead to stillbirth or abortion.

Activity: Watch for photosensitivity while taking doxycycline. Avoid sun and use sunscreen.

Diet: Avoid taking milk products when taking doxycycline.

Medications: Start antibiotics when afebrile or near the end of a febrile period to avoid a potential Jarisch-Herxheimer reaction (fever, tachycardia, mild hypotension, chills, vasodilatation within 2 hours of treatment; peaking at 7-8 hours and resolving in 1 day). Give acetaminophen 650mg po 2 hours before antibiotics and 2 hours after with the 1st dose to modify the Jarisch-Herxheimer reaction. Avoid doxycycline in young children and pregnant/nursing mothers.

Prevention and Hygiene: Prevent tick bites (spray interior of tick-infested dwelling with insecticide). Prophylaxis following suspected exposure to tick or louse bite in endemic area: doxycycline 200mg po day one, followed by 100mg po daily x 4 days after exposure. No Improvement/Deterioration: Return promptly for re-evaluation.
Follow-up Actions
Evacuation/Consultation Criteria: Refer patients who develop complications.

Chapter 12: Infectious Diseases: Bacterial Infections: *Acinetobacter* Infections
LTC Clinton K. Murray, MC, USA

Introduction: *Acinetobacter* spp. are rod shaped, aerobic, gram-negative bacteria noted for their relative low virulence but also for their ability to develop resistance to a broad array of antimicrobial agents. *Acinetobacter* spp. have gained military notoriety because of their resistance to almost all commonly used antibiotics and because they have become one of the most prevalent bacteria infecting combat casualties' wounds during OIF and OEF. Although the vast majority of patients develop infections while receiving care in the hospital setting, community associated infections have been reported especially in Australia and southeast Asia. There are over 21 species, but the 4 commonly causing disease in humans are grouped as a complex known as *Acinetobacter baumannii-calcoaceticus* complex. **Geographic Association:** Acinetobacter is present worldwide but mostly associated with hospital environments. **Risk Factors:** Receiving treatment at tertiary care center where use of broad-spectrum antibiotics is high.

Subjective: Symptoms
The primary presentation is based upon underlying illness or injury site. Infections with *Acinetobacter* are similar to other bacteria infecting an organ system or a traumatic injury.

Focused History: *Have you recently been hospitalized especially for a prolonged period of time?* (This infection is associated with nosocomial transmission.)

Objective: Signs
Using Basic Tools: Monitor injury sites for evidence of infection including systemic fevers and purulent drainage.

Using Advanced Tools: Labs: Gram's stain can be performed but *Acinetobacter* can appear gram-positive or gram-negative. Bacterial cultures are needed to identify the bacteria and determine the ideal antibiotic necessary for therapy.

Assessment: Differential Diagnosis
The differential diagnosis includes the typical bacteria that would infect the organ system or injury site in question. Other bacteria that should be considered responsible for infections are gram-negative bacteria such as *Klebsiella pneumoniae* or *Pseudomonas aeruginosa* and the gram-positive bacteria *Staphylococcus aureus*.

Plan:
Treatment
As the tip of the spear, SOF medics are often asked to provide medical care under extreme conditions in austere environments with limited resources. This reality does not reduce the responsibility for careful cost to benefit analysis for all types of medical care. The use of broad spectrum antibiotics is without a doubt adding to the incidence of resistant organisms and every reasonable effort to limit the use of broad spectrum antibiotics should be made. It must be emphasized that broad spectrum antibiotics are NOT required for EVERY instance of injury (eg, limited extremity trauma where imminent medical evacuation is available). It is strongly recommended to obtain cultures to prove the identification of the infecting bacteria and use antibiotics based upon those results whenever possible
Patient Education
General: Apply good hand hygiene and wound care to prevent transmission to other injured or sick personnel.

Diet: Regular with increased fluid intake.

Medications: Based upon resistance panel of the bacteria culture.

Prevention and Hygiene: Good infection control procedures within hospital environments. No field expedient measures are needed
Follow-up Actions
Evacuation/Consultation Criteria: Patient should be cared for in a tertiary care facility with adequate microbiological support and infectious disease expertise.

Chapter 12: Infectious Diseases: Bacterial Infections: Anthrax

Lt Col George Christopher, USAF, MC

Introduction: Anthrax is caused by the gram-positive, nonmotile, sporulating bacillus, *Bacillus anthracis*. Anthrax is a disease of cattle, other livestock, and certain large plant-eating wild animals. Humans generally are infected through work with products such as hides, hair, or bone meal from infected animals. Clinical presentations depend on the site of entry, and include cutaneous (skin) (entry of spores into skin abrasions or unapparent lesions, or introduced by biting flies), oropharyngeal and gastrointestinal (ingestion of contaminated meat), and inhalational anthrax (inhalation of spores). Meningitis can complicate anthrax (up to 50% in inhalational cases) due to spread through the blood stream to the central nervous system. The spores of *B. anthracis* pose a biological weapons threat. They are infectious by inhalation and cause severe and often fatal disease. An accidental release of spores in 1979 from a military microbiology facility in the former Soviet Union caused the largest known epidemic of inhalational anthrax; 66 deaths occurred among people living or working downwind of the release point; animals died up to 35 miles downwind, and was a disastrous "proof of concept" that an outdoor release of aerosolized spores can produce mass casualties over a large area. The bio-terror attacks in the US in autumn 2001 using spores mailed in envelopes caused 22 cases, 11 cases each of cutaneous and inhalational disease, 5 of whom died. *See Part 6: Operational Environment: Chapter 25: Biological Warfare: Inhalational Anthrax*

Subjective: Symptoms

Cutaneous anthrax: A small red papule that enlarges and develops into a nontender skin ulcer with black scab (eschar), local swelling which may be severe; development of large blisters over swollen area, painful lymph nodes, fever, malaise, fatigue.

Oropharyngeal anthrax: Severe sore throat, severe local swelling, difficulty swallowing, difficulty breathing, swollen lymph nodes in the neck, fever, malaise, fatigue, muscle aches.

Gastrointestinal anthrax: Abdominal pain, nausea, vomiting, diarrhea, which may be bloody, abdominal swelling, fever, malaise, muscle aches

Inhalational anthrax: Fever, malaise, cough (usually non-productive), vague chest pain, drenching night sweats, nausea and/or vomiting, shortness of breath. Upper respiratory symptoms are typically absent.

Anthrax meningitis: Headache, stiff neck, decreased level of consciousness.

Focused history: *Have you handled sick animals, animal carcasses, animal hides, wools, meat, or other animal products from a non-commercial source?* (cutaneous, oropharyngeal or gastrointestinal disease) *Is anyone else in your unit ill with similar symptoms?* (For outbreaks of oropharyngeal or gastrointestinal disease, consider contaminated meat, for inhalational disease, consider biological attack until proven otherwise.) *Do you have difficulty swallowing or breathing?* (Severe local swelling in oropharyngeal anthrax can lead to upper airway obstruction; difficulty breathing may signal inhalational anthrax.)

Objective: Signs

Using Basic Tools: Fever; rapid heart rate, low blood pressure

Cutaneous anthrax: Inspection: Small papule or nodule; classically a non-tender ulcer with black scab; marked local swelling, vesicles or blisters, tender regional lymph nodes

Oropharyngeal anthrax: Inspection: Redness of throat, necrotic ulcer or scab involving the hard palate, tonsils, or throat; swelling of soft tissues of throat and neck (possible upper airway obstruction). Palpation: Enlarged lymph nodes of the neck.

Gastrointestinal anthrax: Inspection: Abdominal distention. Palpation: Diffuse abdominal tenderness, fluid wave. Percussion: Shifting dullness (massive ascites may develop). Auscultation: Decreased bowel sounds (ileus may develop)

Inhalational anthrax: Inspection: Rapid respiratory rate, respiratory distress, swelling of neck and/or chest wall. Percussion: Dullness to percussion (may develop large pleural effusions) Auscultation: rales, distant breath sounds

Anthrax meningitis: Inspection: Obtundation. Palpation: Stiff neck (meningeal signs)

Using Advanced Tools: Gram's stain of skin lesion drainage or other fluid (pleural fluid, cerebrospinal fluid, blood late in course) may show large box-car shaped bacteria. *See Appendices: Color Plate Figure A-23.A.*

Assessment: Differential Diagnosis

Cutaneous anthrax: Typhus (typically will have diffuse macular rash), ulceroglandular tularemia, vasculitic ulcer (typically without swelling), brown recluse spider bite, MRSA, cellulitis

Oropharyngeal anthrax: Pharyngitis due to Group A *streptococcus*, adenoviruses, Epstein-Barr virus; diphtheria, pharyngeal plague

Gastrointestinal anthrax: Other causes of gastroenteritis. Classically described as severe with high mortality; however, reports of 2 outbreaks suggest that most cases feature mild gastroenteritis with favorable outcome.

Inhalational anthrax: Pneumonias due to other bacteria; mediastinal disease due to TB (less acute), histoplasmosis (less acute), sarcoidosis (less acute)

Meningeal anthrax: Other causes of bacterial meningitis

Plan:
　Treatment

Table 5-6. Specific Antibiotics

	Initial Therapy	Duration of Therapy
Inhalational		
Adults	**Ciprofloxacin** 400mg IV q12 h or **doxycycline** 200mg IV x one, then 100mg IV q12h[a] AND 1-2 additional antimicrobials[b]	IV initially until clinically improved, then convert to: **ciprofloxacin** 500mg po q12h or **doxycycline** 100mg po q12h. Complete duration 60 days
Children	**Ciprofloxacin** 1-15mg/kg IV q12h or **doxycycline**: >8 yrs and >45 kg: adult dose >8 yrs and <45 kg: 2.2mg/kg IV q12h ≤8 yrs: 2.2mg/kg IV q12h 1-2 additional antimicrobials[b]	IV initially until clinically improved, then convert to: **ciprofloxacin** 10-15mg/kg po q12h or **doxycycline**: >8 yrs and >45 kg: adult dose >8 yrs and <45 kg: 2.2mg/kg IV q12h ≤8 yrs: 2.2mg/kg IV q12h Complete duration 60 days
Cutaneous		
Adults	**Ciprofloxacin** 500mg po q12h or **doxycycline** 100mg po q12h. **Amoxicillin** 500mg po tid may be considered after initial clinical improvement in cases due to susceptible strains.	60 days for cases due to bioweapons exposure (in order to prophylax possible incubating inhalational disease.) Shorter duration of therapy (10-14 days) may be considered for naturally acquired cases of cutaneous anthrax.
Children	**Ciprofloxacin** 10-15mg/kg po q12h(c) or **doxycycline**: >8 yrs and >45 kg: adult dose >8 yrs and <45 kg: 2.2mg/kg IV every 12 hours ≤8 yrs: 2.2mg/kg IV every 12 hours **Amoxicillin** 500mg/kg/daily divided in 3 doses may be considered after initial clinical improvement in cases due to susceptible strains.	60 days for cases due to bioweapons exposure (in order to prophylax possible incubating inhalational disease.) Shorter duration of therapy (10-14 days) may be considered for naturally acquired cases of cutaneous anthrax.

(a) **Doxycycline** is not recommended for cases complicated by meningoencephalitis. Therapy for pregnant women same as non-pregnant adults; therapy for immunocompromised persons same as for non-immunocompromised persons.

(b) **Clindamycin** is recommended as one of the additional antibiotics due to its potential inhibition of toxin production. **Clindamycin** and **rifampin** may be good initial "additional drug" choices. At least one of the drugs should have good CNS penetration (eg **ampicillin, rifampin, vancomycin**). Anthrax is NOT susceptible to cephalosporins or TMP-SMX and these drugs should not be used to treat anthrax.

(c) Pediatric dose of **ciprofloxacin** not to exceed one gm/day. The usual contraindications to using ciprofloxacin in pediatric patients do not apply due to the poor prognosis of inhalational anthrax. Use alternative medications for naturally acquired cases of cutaneous anthrax in pediatric and pregnant patients. Initial antibiotic treatments for inhalational anthrax may be used for oropharyngeal and gastrointestinal disease; the duration of treatment for naturally acquired cases is not well defined; consider a full 60 days, if tolerated. Shorter courses (10-14 days) may be considered for naturally acquired cutaneous anthrax. Supportive care for inhalational or oropharyngeal anthrax includes maintaining the airway. Tracheostomy is indicated for upper airway obstruction due to oropharyngeal anthrax.

Prevention:
　Pre-Exposure Prophylaxis: Immunization before deployment. The anthrax vaccine consists of a cell-free sterile filtrate from culture of a non-disease producing strain of *B. anthracis*. The vaccine has been fully FDA licensed since 1970, and has been determined by the FDA to be safe and effective for preventing anthrax due to all routes of exposure, including inhalation. Service members receive at least 3 doses of vaccine before deployment to a high-risk location. Doses are given at 0, 2, and 6 weeks, and 6, 12, and 18 months, followed by annual boosters. Approximately 30% of men and 60% of women experience mild local side effects such as redness and swelling. These typically resolve within a few days. A lump at the injection site forms in about 50% of recipients, and lasts a few weeks. Larger local reactions occur in 1-4%. Systemic side effects such as fever, muscle aches, and fatigue occur in 5-35% of recipients; these typically resolve within a week. Severe allergic reactions occur in approximately 1 in 100,000 vaccines. Multi-year studies have found no long-term adverse effects. Mild reactions typically require no treatment. Moderate to severe reactions can be treated with topical steroids, antihistamines, analgesics, or for severe local reactions, a short course of **prednisone**. Personnel who have had moderate reactions can be premedicated before their next dose, and can receive the vaccine via IM (vs. subcutaneous) injection to reduce local side effects on a case-by-case basis. For severe reactions, defer further doses pending expert referral.
　Chemoprophylaxis: Ciprofloxacin 500mg po q12h may be given prior to imminent anthrax attack. Doxycycline 100mg po q12h is an alternative. The chemoprophylaxis should be discontinued after attack if the use of anthrax has been excluded.
　Post-exposure prophylaxis following biological attack: Chemoprophylaxis following a biological weapons anthrax exposure. Immunization and prophylaxis is not necessary following contact with naturally occurring human or animal cases.

Table 5-7. Chemoprophylaxis

	Primary Option	Alternative
Adults	Ciprofloxacin 500mg po bid	Doxycycline 100mg po bid or amoxicillin 500mg po tid[c]
Pregnant Women	Ciprofloxacin 500mg po bid	Amoxicillin 500mg po tid
Children	Ciprofloxacin 10-15mg/kg po bid[d]	Doxycycline: >8 yrs and >45 kg: adult dose >8 yrs and <45 kg: 2.2mg/kg po bid ≤8 yrs: 2.2mg/kg po bid

a) Adapted from Morb Mortal Wkly Rep 2001; 50:889-893, duration of prophylaxis is 60 days in all cases.
b) Includes immunocompromised person
c) According to CDC recommendations, **amoxicillin** is suitable for post-exposure prophylaxis only after 10-14 days of fluoroquinolone or **doxycycline** treatment and then only if there are contraindications to these 2 classes of medications (eg, pregnancy, lactating mother, or intolerance of other antimicrobials)
d) **Ciprofloxacin** dose not to exceed 1g/day. The usual contraindications to using ciprofloxacin in pediatric patients do not apply due to the poor prognosis of inhalational anthrax.

Chemoprophylaxis should be withdrawn under careful observation and with access to an medical treatment facility. If fever develops following the withdrawal of chemoprophylaxis, treat for anthrax until the diagnosis is clear.

Patient Education

General: Natural cases of cutaneous anthrax respond well to treatment with survival over 95%. Gastrointestinal, oropharyngeal, inhalational, or any cases due to a biological attack are serious and should undergo expert consultation.

Activity: No restrictions for mild cutaneous disease; bed rest for other forms.

Diet: No restrictions for mild cutaneous disease; NPO for other forms

Medications: Potential side effects may include nausea, diarrhea; minimize sun exposure to avoid skin rash (doxycycline).

Prevention and Hygiene: Avoid contact with infected and dead animals, their hides, wool, or other products. Not transmitted from person-to-person transmission. Standard infection control measures are appropriate.

No Improvement/Deterioration: Skin ulcer may progress for 2-3 days even on effective therapy due to delayed effect of infection. This is normal, not a sign of treatment failure. Other forms of anthrax may progress rapidly with death within 24-48 hours.

Wound Care: Cover eschar (scab) with clean dry dressing. Do not débride or surgically disrupt eschar: may cause spread through the blood stream and formation of spores, introducing the risk of transmission.

Follow-up Actions

Consultation Criteria: Report all suspected cases to public health authorities. Refer to specialized care.

Evacuation: Evacuate all cases; use standard infection control measures. Consult with medical and command authorities before evacuating biological casualties.

Notes: Handling of remains: Consult command authority regarding transport of remains. The vegetative bacteria in the cadaver are not contagious, but may form spores and a transmission hazard if exposed to air by open wounds or procedures such as autopsies. The remains of anthrax victims may pose hazards to pathologists, medical examiners, coroners, and morticians. Post-mortem examinations should be limited. Appropriate personal protection should be used during the performance of autopsies, including gowns, caps, eye protection, and respiratory protection with either a N-95 mask or a powered air purifying respirator equipped with N-95 or higher filters. Remains should not be embalmed due to risks to mortuary personnel. Cremation or burial of un-embalmed remains in a hermetically sealed casket is advised by the Department of Health and Human Services.

Zoonotic Disease Considerations:

Naturally occurring anthrax in plant-eating wild animals and livestock may be encountered in many areas of the world where SOF operate. The natural reservoir of B. anthracis spores is the soil. Animals contract anthrax by ingesting spores from the soil during grazing. The spores enter through scrapes or abrasions in the gastrointestinal tract; the risk is increased by eating shrubs or other abrasive plant material. Animals die suddenly of septic shock and may bleed from the mouth and nose. Avoid sick or dead animals. If necessary, carcasses should be disposed by incineration or deep burial with lime. A live attenuated vaccine is available for veterinary use.

Chapter 12: Infectious Diseases: Bacterial Infections: Bartonella Infections (Cat Scratch Disease, Oroya Fever, Trench Fever)

LTC Clinton K. Murray, MC, USA

Introduction: Bartonella species are gram-negative bacteria that cause several different illnesses. B. henselae is responsible for cat scratch disease, which is associated with lymphadenopathy and variable fever following a cat scratch or bite. B. bacilliformis causes a biphasic illness known as bartonellosis, or Carrion's disease, transmitted by the bite of a sand fly resulting in a potentially life-threatening fever, Oroya fever, followed by an eruptive chronic skin phase (verruga peruana). B. quintana is spread by lice and was traditionally associated with trench fever with large outbreaks during World War I and less so during World War II but more recently presents as endocarditis. **Geographic Associations:** Cat scratch disease has a worldwide distribution. Carrion's disease is limited to certain Andean regions of Peru, Columbia and Ecuador limited by the environmental requirements of the sand fly vector. Trench fever is present in the US, and Europe with limited data from other regions of the world. **Seasonal Variation:** There is no season variability with cat scratch disease. The seasonality of Carrion's disease is associated with the presence of the vector but there can be a delay from exposure to presentation. Given the delayed presentation of trench fever after exposure to lice, there is no seasonality to presentation. **Risk Factors:** The greatest risk factor for development of disease is exposure to the respective vectors. Immunosuppression, such as HIV, is associated with greater complication with B. quintana.

Subjective: Symptoms

Cat scratch disease: Vesicles appear at the inoculation site that progress to papules over 1-3 weeks; regional tender adenopathy (2 weeks after exposure) that can occasionally suppurate; nodes subside in 2-5 months without treatment. Fever in 33%-50% of infected children. Can develop ocular manifestation, visceral organ involvement, and neurological manifestation.

Carrion's disease: Fever, which can persist up to 6 weeks; pallor; weakness; chills; muscle/joint aches. After 2-20 weeks, crops of painless, red, 2-4mm skin lesions can be seen, mainly on head and extremities.

Trench fever: Headache; fever (episodic fever of 3-5 days duration - can have fever relapses up to 10 years later); back/leg ache; shin pain; transient rash (maculopapular).

Focused History: *Have you been scratched or bitten by a cat (especially a kitten) in the last 2 weeks?* (evidence to suggest cat scratch disease exposure) *Have you traveled in the past month to Peru, Ecuador or Colombia?* (where Carrion's disease is endemic) *Have you been around anyone with lice or poor body hygiene?* (ie, trench fever exposure) *Do you have a new skin rash or sore?* (Look for the verrucous lesion of Carrion's disease and the crusted papule at the inoculation site of cat scratch.) *Do you have any swollen or sore lymph nodes?* (In cat scratch disease, you can see fluctuant, red, regional adenopathy.)

Objective: Signs

Using Basic Tools:

Cat scratch disease: Vesicle or papule at inoculation site, variable fever >101°F; Later: tender, fluctuant, regional adenopathy, which may last about 3 months. 12% have splenomegaly. *See Appendices: Color Plate Figure A-22.A.*

Carrion's disease: Most commonly see fever, pallor, malaise, hepatomegaly and lymphadenopathy. Skin lesion lesions appear 2-8 weeks after exposure and can present in 3 patterns: miliary (pinpoint papules), nodular (subdermic), and mular. The mular lesions are highly vascular, bulbous, ulcerate and can bleed easily.

Trench fever: Can range from mild influenza like illness to debilitating disease after an incubation period of 15-25 days. In addition, patients can have bone pain (particularly the shins) and a maculopapular rash. Illnesses range from a single brief episode to one that last 6 weeks in duration and can be associated with recurrent febrile episodes.

Using Advanced Tools: Labs: The Oroya fever organism can be seen on a peripheral blood smear inside red blood cells and can result in severe anemia.

Assessment: Differential Diagnosis

Cat scratch disease: Mycobacterium disease (tuberculosis, mycobacterium avium complex), malignancy. Tender lymph nodes include tularemia, *Norcardia* infection, plague, Lyme disease, anthrax.

Carrion's disease: Oroya fever can resemble other endemic infections such as typhoid fever, malaria, brucellosis. Verruga peruana skin lesions can resemble yaws, syphilis, pyogenic granulomas, Kaposi's sarcoma (KS).

Trench fever: Resembles other febrile diseases endemic to the country of origin including influenza like illnesses.

Plan:

Treatment

Cat scratch disease: Some suggest not treating mild to moderate disease but **azithromycin** 500mg po day 1, then 250mg po q day x 4 days with analgesics is effective.

Carrion's disease: Oroya fever: Chloramphenicol 500mg po/IV q6h + **penicillin** 500mg po x 14 days. Alternative is **ciprofloxacin** 500mg po q12h x 14 days.

Verruga peruana: Rifampin 10mg/kg/day po (max dose 600 mg) x 10-14 days

Trench fever: Doxycycline 100mg po q day x 14 days; alternative is **azithromycin** 500mg po q day x14 days

Patient Education

General: **Cat scratch disease:** Avoid cats, especially kittens, and clean any wounds immediately. **Carrion's disease:** Watch for late development of skin lesions

Activity: As tolerated

Diet: Regular

Prevention and Hygiene: **Cat scratch disease:** Avoid playing with unknown cats, especially kittens; **Carrion's disease:** Use personal protective measures during the nocturnal biting cycle of sand fly while in endemic areas; **Trench fever:** Control body lice; use good personal hygiene.

No Improvement/Deterioration: Return if fever persists for more than 1 week or if (cat scratch disease) lymph nodes start to drain pus

Follow-up Actions

Return Evaluation: Cat scratch disease: relieve pain in fluctuant lymph node with needle aspiration; avoid incision and drainage.

Carrion's disease: monitor for secondary bacterial infection of verruga peruana

Evacuation/Consultation Criteria: Evacuation is not usually necessary, but may be indicated for some unstable patients.

Zoonotic Disease Considerations:

Cat Scratch disease

Principal Animal Host: Cats, especially kittens.

Clinical Disease in Animals: Asymptomatic carriers

Known Distribution: Worldwide

Chapter 12: Infectious Diseases: Bacterial Infections: Brucellosis

LCDR Timothy Whitman, MC, USN

Introduction: Brucellosis is a common febrile illness in the Mideast, Mexico and South America. It is a bacterial infection acquired by ingesting raw milk, unpasteurized cheese or by direct contact with secretions or birth products of infected animals (cattle, goats, buffalo, camels, reindeer, caribou, yaks, coyotes, deer or swine). Average incubation period is 2 weeks, but can take up to several months.

Subjective: Symptoms
Acute (1-7 days): PM fever >100°F; profuse, malodorous sweating; flu-like symptoms and a peculiar taste in mouth. Sub-acute (1-2 weeks): Fever, weight loss, arthralgias and myalgias. Chronic (weeks to months): Recurrent undulant fever if not treated, arthralgias or arthritis, constipation, depression and back pain.

Focused History: *Have you had any raw milk or cheese? Have you come in contact with cattle, goats, buffalo, camels, reindeer, caribou, yaks, coyotes, deer or swine? Do you have a fever?* (up to 104°F) *How long have you had fever?* (weeks to months) *Do any of your joints hurt?* (Arthritis is usually in the knee or hip.) *Do you have back pain?* (particularly unilateral sacro-iliac symptoms)

Objective: Signs
Using Basic Tools: Vital signs: Temperatures to 104°F. Palpation: Acute (1-7 days): Generalized adenopathy. Sub-acute (1-2 weeks): Swollen/red joints, hepatomegaly (>50%), splenomegaly (30%)

Assessment: Travel history, animal exposure and consuming unpasteurized milk products.
Differential Diagnosis:
Typhoid fever: *See Part 5: Specialty Areas: Chapter 12: Bacterial Infections: Typhoid Fever*
Nonpulmonary tuberculosis: *See Part 5: Specialty Areas: Chapter 12: Mycobacterial Infections: Non-tuberculosis Mycobacterial Infections*
Non-falciparum malaria: With chronic relapses of fever. *See Part 5: Specialty Areas: Chapter 12: Parasitic Infections: Malaria*

Plan:
Treatment: Always use 2 antibiotics for 6 weeks.
Primary: Doxycycline 100mg po bid x 6 weeks with **gentamicin** 3-5mg/kg IV q day (diluted in 50-100mL of NS or D5W and infused over 30 – 60 minutes in divided doses q 8h) x 14 days. Side effects include nephrotoxicity (to include oliguria, renal damage, renal failure). Ideally dose of gentamicin is adjusted following peak and trough blood levels which will not be available in the field.
Alternate: Doxycycline 100mg po bid x 6 weeks plus **rifampin** 900mg po q day x 6 weeks (easier as all po therapy) Children <7 yrs: Do not give doxycycline. Give **trimethoprim-sulfamethoxazole** 10-12mg/kg/day of the **trimethoprim** component and 50-60mg/kg /day of the **sulfamethoxazole** component po in 2 divided doses x 6 weeks plus **rifampin** 15-20mg/kg/day (not to exceed 600mg/day) in 2 divided doses x 6 weeks.
Patient Education
Diet: Avoid untreated milk; boil milk, if pasteurization status is unknown.
Prevention and Hygiene: Handle animal carcasses carefully. Hunters should use gloves or barriers when dressing wild animals. Be careful when handling tissues and fetuses from aborted animals.
No Improvement/Deterioration: Return for persistent fever over 7 days.
Follow-up Actions
Consultation Criteria: Refer chronically febrile patients to higher level of care when available.

Zoonotic Disease Considerations
Agent: *Brucella canis, B. suis, B. abortus, B. melitensis*
Principal Animal Hosts: Dogs *(B. canis)*, swine *(B. suis)*, cattle *(B. abortus)*, goats *(B. melitensis)*
Clinical Disease in Animals: Dogs *(B. canis)* - Last trimester abortions; swine *(B. suis)* - abortion; cattle *(B. abortus)* - last half gestation abortions; goats *(B. melitensis)* - abortion.
Probable Mode of Transmission: *B. abortus* - Contact with birth products and consumption of milk products, *B. melitensis* - Consumption of milk products
Known Distribution: *B. canis* - rare, *B. suis* - northern hemisphere, *B. abortus* & *B. melitensis* – worldwide

Chapter 12: Infectious Diseases: Bacterial Infections: Cholera

CDR John Sanders, MC, USN

Introduction: Cholera is caused by a toxin produced by the bacterium *Vibrio cholerae*. A few hours to 5 days following ingestion of food or water contaminated with *Vibrio cholerae*, patients develop sudden onset of severe diarrhea, nausea, and vomiting. Although most cases are difficult to distinguish from other causes of diarrhea, severe cases (cholera gravis) are characterized by massive (500-1000mL/hour) watery diarrhea that contain flecks of mucus ("rice-water stools"). Dehydration and electrolyte imbalance can lead to death in >50% of untreated patients. **Geographic Associations:** Cholera, endemic in the developing countries of Asia and Africa, has been seen in South & Central America (1990s) and can be found across the Indian subcontinent and throughout the Middle East. **Seasonal Variation:** Can occur year round, but is often associated with outbreaks during rainy seasons, especially during floods, when people are exposed to large amounts of contaminated water. **Risk Factors:** Travel to an endemic area (a country where the disease is present) with ingestion of contaminated food and water. Ingestion of raw or undercooked shellfish (raw oysters).

Subjective: Symptoms
Days 1-2: Diarrhea may begin gradually, but often presents suddenly with frequent, voluminous watery stools. Vomiting is very common. Mild to moderate abdominal cramps are common but severe abdominal pain is rare. Fever is uncommon. Patients may present after only a few hours of illness with massive volume loss (up to 10% of body weight) and associated signs and symptoms of severe

dehydration, including orthostatic hypotension, dizziness, loss of consciousness, and severe lassitude. In addition to the severe volume loss, cholera causes severe electrolyte imbalances (low potassium, low sodium, etc.) and hypoglycemia (low blood sugar), resulting in severe muscle cramps, mental status changes, seizures, renal failure, arrhythmias, ileus, and metabolic acidosis.

Days 3-4: Diarrhea persists, but the volume and rate of stools typically begins to diminish. Vomiting also diminishes.

Days 5-6: Diarrhea and vomiting typically resolve. Total volume loss over hours to days may be up to 100% of body weight.

Focused History: *Have you traveled to an area experiencing a cholera outbreak? Have you traveled to a developing country in South or Central America, Asia, or Africa? Have you recently eaten raw or undercooked shellfish, such as raw oysters?* (It is difficult to distinguish the cause of a dehydrating diarrheal illness based on history alone, but these questions reflect the typical risk factors for cholera.)

Objective: Signs

Using Basic Tools: Inspection: Patients present with frequent, large volume, watery stools. The stools rapidly take a "rice-water" appearance and often have a mild "fishy" odor. The patients are often so dehydrated and weak that they are not able to stand without assistance, have severe lassitude, and often have mental status changes. Skin and mucous membranes may appear dry. Palpation: Due to severe dehydration, peripheral pulses are often weak and rapid. Skin turgor is decreased so that "pinched skin" will not quickly return to normal.

Using Advanced Tools: Labs: Gram's stain of stool; may show sheets of curved gram-negative rods. Culture stool.

Assessment:

World Health Organization (WHO) Assessment of severity of volume depletion among adults with diarrhea

Table 5-8. WHO Dehydration Severity

Examination	Mild dehydration	Moderate dehydration	Severe dehydration
Look at:			
Mental status	Alert	Restless, irritable	Lethargic or unconscious
Eyes	Normal	Sunken	Very sunken and dry
Tears	Present	Absent	Absent
Mouth/tongue	Moist, slightly dry	Dry	Very dry
Thirst	Increased thirst	Thirsty, drinks eagerly	Drink poorly or not able to drink
Feel:			
Skin pinch	Goes back rapidly	Goes back slowly	Goes back very slowly (tenting)
Pulse	Normal	Rapid, weak	Very fast, weak or nonpalpable
Decide degree of hydration	Mild dehydration, <5% of body weight	Moderate dehydration, from 5-10% of body weight	Severe dehydration, >10% of body weight

Differential Diagnosis

***Vibrio cholerae* non-O1 (non-agglutinating):** *Vibrio cholerae* species that can cause diarrhea, but do not usually cause severe disease and do not result in outbreaks (are not causes of "cholera"). Diagnosed by advanced microbiologic testing.

Enterotoxigenic *E. coli* (ETEC): The most common cause of travelers' diarrhea and produces a toxin very similar to the cholera toxin. It can present with severe watery diarrhea but does not usually present as an epidemic outbreak of diarrhea. Diagnosed by advanced microbiologic testing.

Rotavirus: Rotavirus is now the most common cause of dehydrating diarrhea in children worldwide and can cause similar symptoms as cholera in children. It does not usually present in large outbreaks or cause severe disease in adults. Diagnosed by advanced microbiologic testing.

Other causes of traveler's diarrhea: Bacteria, viruses, and parasites causing less severe diarrhea not usually presenting as large outbreaks. *See Part 3: General Symptoms: Diarrhea, Acute*

Plan:

Treatment

Primary: The key to successfully treating cholera is rehydration and electrolyte replacement. Oral rehydration solutions (ORS) have reduced the mortality from cholera from >50% to <1% when used appropriately. The ORS formulation currently recommended by WHO has a reduced osmolality, but most available commercial brands are adequate. ORS is as effective as IV hydration in treating mild to moderate dehydration caused by diarrhea and is the treatment of choice. Antibiotic therapy (not necessary for the treatment of cholera) reduces the volume of diarrhea by one-half and the duration of *Vibrio* excretion to about one day. **Doxycycline** 300mg po x1 is the treatment of choice. Alternative is **ciprofloxacin** 500mg po bid x 3 days. Therapy with ORS is divided into rehydration and maintenance phases. Rehydration phase: Replace fluid deficit quickly over 3-4 hours by administering ORS by spoon or syringe in frequent small amounts (≤5mL administered q 1-2 minutes) for a total of 50mL/kg in mild dehydration and 100 mL/kg in moderate dehydration. Start emergent IV rehydration with 20mL/kg of lactated Ringers in patients with severe dehydration (loss of >10% of body weight) or who are unable to drink because of vomiting or mental status changes. Maintenance phase: Give ORS in amounts to match ongoing fluid losses (1mL of ORS for each gram of diarrheal stool or 10mL/kg of ORS for each stool and 2mL/kg of ORS for each emesis). Start feeding after completion of the rehydration phase, with the goal to return the patient to an age-appropriate unrestricted diet as quickly as possible.

Empiric: Oral Rehydration Solution. Consider empiric therapy (**ciprofloxacin** and **loperamide**) for travelers' diarrhea.

Primitive: Make an ORS by mixing 8 level teaspoons of sugar and 1 level teaspoon of salt in 1 liter of clean water.

Patient Education

General: Increase oral fluid intake to maintain hydration.

Activity: Patient should be restricted from food preparation and handling. Otherwise, as tolerated.

Diet: Increase oral fluids. Advance diet as tolerated.

Prevention and Hygiene: Boil drinking water for one minute.

No Improvement/Deterioration: Consider alternative causes of diarrhea.

Follow-up Actions

Return Evaluation: As needed if failure to improve with rehydration.

Evacuation/Consultation Criteria: If unable to maintain hydration status, patient should be evacuated to a higher level of care.

Chapter 12: Infectious Diseases: Bacterial Infections: Ehrlichiosis

COL Glenn Wortmann, MC, USA

Introduction: Ehrlichiosis is a tick-borne bacterial illness. Human infection with *Ehrlichia* has only recently been appreciated, with the first case reported in 1987. Most disease occurs in the United States (10 cases/100,000 population in rural and suburban areas south of New Jersey to Kansas as well as in California), although it has been reported in Africa, Scandinavia and Western Europe. The severity of infection ranges from subclinical to fatal.

Subjective: **Symptoms**

Headache, fever, rash, myalgias.

Focused History: *Have you had a tick bite recently?* (typical exposure) *Do you have a headache and fever?* (suggests ehrlichiosis in late spring and early summer) *How long have you felt sick?* (often presents with the abrupt onset of fever, headache and myalgias)

Objective: **Signs**

Using Basic Tools: Temperature over 101°F; rash in 30% (most commonly involving the trunk; not associated with site of tick bite).

Using Advanced Tools: Serology testing of blood is available at many hospitals.

Assessment

Many infections present similarly, but fever and headache (especially in a patient with exposure to ticks) should prompt the consideration of ehrlichiosis.

Differential Diagnosis: Significant overlap of symptoms with numerous diseases (eg, various viral syndromes, Rocky Mountain spotted fever, meningitis, typhoid fever, tularemia, tick-borne encephalitis, toxic shock syndrome, babesiosis, Colorado tick fever, leptospirosis).

Plan:

Treatment

Primary: Doxycycline 100mg po bid x 7-10 days. Treatment often results in rapid clinical improvement and defervescence within 1-2 days.

Alternative: Rifampin 300mg po bid x 7-10 days (limited data on efficacy)

Patient Education:

General: Avoid tick exposure.

Activity: As tolerated.

Diet: As tolerated.

Medications: Doxycycline can cause photosensitivity, and in general, should not be given to young children or pregnant/ breastfeeding women. However, ehrlichiosis can be a fatal infection, and the risk of toxicity to young children and pregnant/breastfeeding women is generally low. If possible, consult with an ID physician to help decide the risk/benefit ratio.

Prevention and Hygiene: Avoid tick exposure.

No Improvement/Deterioration: Return for evaluation.

Follow-up Actions

Consultation Criteria: Failure to improve after initiation of antibiotics.

Chapter 12: Infectious Diseases: Bacterial Infections: Melioidosis

Lt Col George Christopher, USAF, MC

Introduction: Melioidosis is caused by *Burkholderia pseudomallei* (formerly *Pseudomonas pseudomallei*), a gram-negative aerobic bacillus found in soil and fresh water throughout the tropics. Illness follows inoculation of gross or unapparent skin lesions with contaminated soil or water, aspiration or ingestion of contaminated water, or inhalation of aerosols of contaminated soil or water. Pulmonary disease occurred among US forces during the Vietnam conflict, thought to be due to inhalation of aerosols of contaminated water generated by helicopter propeller draft in irrigated rice fields. The most common presentation is acute respiratory disease, which can vary from a mild bronchitis to severe necrotizing pneumonia. Other presentations include acute local disease of skin and soft tissue, acute septicemic disease, or chronic suppurative disease with spread to brain, liver, bone, spleen, lymph nodes, and eyes. Chronic pulmonary disease can follow acute pulmonary disease, or reactivate years after exposure, with clinical and x-ray findings similar to tuberculosis. Case fatality rate reaches 90% for acute septicemic disease, but is variable for other forms. Because of potential severe disease following exposure to aerosols, melioidosis is considered a possible biological weapons threat.

Subjective: **Symptoms**

Acute pulmonary disease: May begin abruptly, or with a vague prodrome of headache, loss of appetite, and muscle aches. Symptoms may include SOB, pleuritic or dull aching chest pain, and cough which may be nonproductive or produce purulent or bloody sputum.

Soft tissue infection: Fever, acute or subacute localized nodule with pain, redness, swelling, warmth, and discharge

Acute septicemic disease: Fever, headache, sore throat, diarrhea, rash, severe SOB.

Chronic pulmonary disease: Fever, malaise, weight loss, pleuritic chest pain, nonproductive or productive cough, hemoptysis, progressive exertional SOB. May reactivate years after exposure, similar to TB.

Chronic suppurative disease: Fever, malaise, weight loss; local symptoms depend on site, and may include localized pain, swelling, redness, discharge.

Focused History: *Have you been exposed to soil, water, or aerosols (especially generated by aircraft) in the tropics? Do you have shortness of breath?* (Dyspnea may signal severe respiratory disease with impending respiratory failure and or septicemia.) *Are other members of your unit sick with similar symptoms?* (Consider common source exposure such as aircraft draft or biological attack.)

Objective: **Signs**

Using Basic Tools: Fever, often in excess of 102°F is common.

Acute pulmonary disease: Inspection: In severe cases, rapid respirations, respiratory distress, cyanosis. Percussion: Dullness to percussion may be present, Auscultation: Findings may be minimal, but may include pulmonary rales.

Acute soft tissue infection: Inspection: Skin nodules, local redness, and tenderness; possibly purulent discharge, lymphangitic streaking with purulent discharge. Palpation: Local tenderness, enlarged tender regional lymph nodes

Acute septicemic disease: Inspection: Rapid respiratory rate, respiratory distress, cyanosis, flushing, and rash (may begin as a generalized papular rash that may progress to pustular rash). Percussion: Dullness to percussion may be present. Auscultation: Findings may be minimal, but may include pulmonary rales. Palpation: Enlarged liver and spleen may be present.

Chronic pulmonary disease: Inspection: Possibly enlarged supraclavicular lymph nodes. Percussion: Possibly dullness to percussion due to pleural effusion. Auscultation: Possibly pulmonary rales or distant breath sounds. Palpation: Possibly enlarged supraclavicular lymph nodes

Chronic suppurative disease: Inspection: Localized swelling, redness, discharge depending on site of involvement.

Using Advanced Tools: Labs: Microscopic evaluation of exudate may reveal gram-negative bacilli; methylene blue or Wright's stain will show a "safety pin" bipolar appearance. Diagnosis can be confirmed through standard cultures of sputum, blood, urine, or exudate. Serologic tests are available; however, negative or single low titers are nondiagnostic. Leukocyte count varies from normal to over 20,000 white blood cells/cubic millimeter.

Assessment: **Differential Diagnosis**

Acute pulmonary disease: Other causes of community acquired pneumonia, pneumonic plague, pneumonic tularemia

Soft tissue infection: Infections due to *Staphylococcus aureus*, commensal soil and water flora including vibrios, *Aeromonas*, *Pseudomonas*; ulceroglandular tularemia, and sporotrichosis

Acute septicemic disease: Early considerations may include meningococcemia, gonococcemia, spotted fevers, hemorrhagic fevers; later considerations may include staphylococcal endocarditis, and orthopox virus infections (smallpox, monkeypox).

Chronic pulmonary disease: Tuberculosis, non-tuberculous mycobacterial infections, histoplasmosis, blastomycosis, coccidiomycosis, other causes of chronic pneumonia

Chronic suppurative disease: Staphylococcal or other bacterial abscesses; tuberculosis; other mycobacterial or fungal infections

Plan:

Treatment

Initial therapy for all cases of mild – severe melioidosis consists of **ceftazidime** 50mg/kg, up to 2g IV per dose q6h; consider the addition of **sulfamethoxazole/trimethoprim** 40/8mg/kg, up to 1,600/320mg (2 double-strength tablets) po q12h. Duration of IV antibiotic therapy is 14 days, but may be longer for critical illness, severe pulmonary disease, deep-seated abscesses, bone, joint, or neurologic involvement. Initial treatment is followed by at least 3 months of **sulfamethoxazole/trimethoprim** 40/8mg/kg, up to 1600/320mg po q12h, with or without **doxycycline** 100mg po q12h. **Amoxicillin-clavulanate** 60mg/kg/day po in 3 divided oral doses x 20 weeks may be considered for pregnant women, children >40kg, or patients with sulfa allergy. Incision and drainage is indicated for large abscesses, but not for multiple small hepatic or splenic abscesses. Early ventilatory support may be necessary for cases of severe pulmonary disease. **Folic acid** 5mg po daily is given in both initial and extended course of therapy to prevent or reduce the antifolate activity of TMP-SMX.

Patient Education

General: This is a serious disease, but curable with prolonged treatment. Most frequent cause of relapse is non-compliance in taking medication. Evacuation for further evaluation and treatment is key.

Activity: Varies with severity of disease.

Prevention and Hygiene: Cleaning of superficial abrasions/deep wounds; minimize exposure to surface water and wet season soils and aerosols generated from them.

Diet: As tolerated.

Medications: Potential side effects include diarrhea, rash.

Prevention and Hygiene: Standard precautions. Disease is not transmitted from person-to-person.

No Improvement/Deterioration: May include progressive respiratory disease, diffuse pustular rash, septic shock.

Wound Care: Keep skin lesions clean and dry; use gauze dressings when indicated.

Follow-up Actions
    Return Evaluation: Will require long-term follow-up. Relapse is common as this is potentially a chronic disease.
    Evacuation/Consultation Criteria: Report cases to public health authorities; refer all cases for expert care. Evacuate using standard precautions; respiratory precautions if diagnosis is unclear and tuberculosis is still under consideration, droplet precautions if diagnosis is unclear and plague is still a consideration. Consult medical chain of command if diagnosis is unclear as the possibility of tuberculosis, orthopox virus infection, hemorrhagic fevers, or biological attack are operationally relevant concerns

Chapter 12: Infectious Diseases: Bacterial Infections: Plague
Lt Col George Christopher, USAF, MC

Introduction: Plague is caused by *Yersinia pestis*, a gram-negative bacillus maintained primarily in rodents in many parts of the world including the western United States, parts of South America, Africa, and Asia. *Y. pestis* is a potential biological weapons threat, and was reportedly investigated and mass-produced in the former Soviet Union biological weapons program. *See Part 6: Operational Environment: Chapter 25: Biological Warfare: Pneumonic Plague.* Rodents are the primary reservoir; domestic cats and wild carnivores can also transmit plague to humans. Plague is usually transmitted by infected fleas from rodent to human, dog or cat to human, or person to person. Animal bites or scratches, and direct contact with infected animals or their tissues can also transmit plague. Respiratory droplet transmission can occur from people or cats with pneumonic plague. Biological warfare delivery would occur by aerosol. *Y. pestis* is introduced by flea bite, carried to regional lymph nodes, and then causes intense infection and inflammation in the lymph node group. **Bubonic plague** is named for "bubo," derived from the Greek word for "groin," because most cases involve the femoral lymph nodes draining the legs. Other lymph node groups can be involved, depending on the site of the flea bite. The case fatality rate for untreated bubonic plague is approximately 60%, but less than 5% with prompt treatment. **Primary pneumonic plague** occurs after inhalation of *Y. pestis*, which may occur by respiratory droplet or aerosol transmission. An epidemic of pneumonic plague could follow an aerosol biological weapons attack. **Septicemic plague** can develop from any form of plague. The bacteria spread through the blood stream resulting in spread to the lung and other organs, septic shock, and clotting of small arteries, resulting in gangrene of the digits with or without detectable lymph node involvement. Case fatality rate for pneumonic and septicemic plague is 100% for untreated cases. **Plague meningitis** is a relatively rare (up to 6%) complication that can present one or more weeks after initial presentation of bubonic or septicemic plague. It presents especially in patients who have received less than therapeutic levels of antibiotics or an antibiotic that does not adequately cross the blood brain barrier (eg, tetracyclines).

Subjective: **Symptoms**
    Bubonic plague: Redness, swelling, severe pain and tenderness of regional lymph nodes and overlying skin/soft tissue; development of fever, malaise, fatigue, muscle aches. **Pneumonic tularemia:** Fever, cough, substernal chest tightness, pleuritic chest pain, shortness of breath, malaise, muscle ache. **Septicemic plague:** Fever, malaise, fatigue, obtundation, gangrene of fingers and/or toes.
    Plague meningitis: Symptoms are consistent with subacute bacterial meningitis.
    Focused History: *Do you have any exposures to wild animals? Is anyone else in your unit ill with similar symptoms?* (For outbreaks of pneumonic disease, consider biological attack.)

Objective: **Signs**
    Using Basic Tools: Bubonic plague: Fever, low blood pressure; focal redness, swelling, warmth and severe tenderness regional lymph nodes and overlying skin/soft tissue. A small macule or ulcer at the site of the fleabite is present in only 25% of cases; clinically apparent lymphangitis does not occur. Gangrene of digits in advanced cases. **Pneumonic plague:** Fever, low blood pressure, and respiratory distress. Physical exam may feature rales, friction rubs, changes in breath sounds and dullness to percussion suggesting consolidation or effusions. **Septicemic plague:** Fever, low blood pressure; may feature lung findings as in pneumonic plague; possibly gangrene of digits and/or ecchymoses (large bruise-like lesions on the skin). **Plague meningitis:** Signs are consistent with subacute bacterial meningitis.
    Using Advanced Tools: Labs: Gram's, Wright-Giemsa, or Wayson stains of sputum, blood, or fluid extracted from a bube, and culture.
    Rapid Diagnostic Test: A rapid diagnostic test with 100% sensitivity and specificity against laboratory isolates of *Y. pestis*, other *Yersinia* species and other bacteria capable of detecting *Y. pestis* F1 antigen within 15 minutes has been developed and field-tested. The Army and Air Force are fielding a rapid detection PCR-based environmental test (called JBAIDS). It is currently approved for environmental testing only with the exception of anthrax. The FDA (clinical use) packages for plague and tularemia are currently under review.

Assessment: **Differential Diagnosis**
    Bubonic plague: Glandular tularemia, cat scratch disease, acute regional lymphadenitis due to other bacteria; TB, lymphoma (all of these are typically less acute; less pain and with less systemic toxicity than plague). Lymphogranuloma venereum or other sexually transmitted diseases (These typically cause inguinal, not femoral lymphadenitis, and are usually less acute).
    Pneumonic tularemia: Staphylococcal, pneumococcal or other severe, rapidly progressive pneumonias; pneumonic tularemia or inhalational anthrax (especially if hilar adenopathy is prominent).
    Septicemic plague: Disseminated intravascular coagulation due to other causes of bacterial sepsis or vasculitis.
    Plague meningitis: CSF demonstrates leukocytosis with neutrophil predominance and possible gram-negative coccobacilli.

Plan:
    Procedures: Buboes may be reduced with needle aspiration to reduce pain and obtain specimen for diagnostic tests, but buboes should not be incised.
    Treatment: Supportive care includes hydration, analgesia. Buboes resolve with antibiotic treatment; needle aspiration or incision and drainage of buboes is typically not needed, but may be indicated if they become fluctuant.

Table 5-9. Plague Treatment Plan

	Primary Option	Alternative
Adults	Gentamicin 5mg/kg IM or IV once daily or 2mg/kg loading dose followed by 1.7mg/kg IM or IV tid Meningitis: Chloramphenicol 25mg/kg IV loading doses, followed by 15mg/kg IV, qid x 14 days	Doxycycline 100mg IV/po bid or 200mg IV once daily, or Ciprofloxacin 400mg IV/po bid Trimethoprim–Sulfamethoxazole (160/800mg) [Bactrim DS] po bid
Pregnant Women	Gentamicin 5mg/kg IM or IV once daily or 2mg/kg loading dose followed by 1.7mg/kg IM or IV tid	Ciprofloxacin 400mg IV or po bid Trimethoprim–Sulfamethoxazole (160/800mg) [Bactrim DS] po bid
Children	Gentamicin 2.5mg/kg IM or IV q8h (q12h for premature infants and neonates less than one week of age)	Doxycycline If > 45kg, give adult dose; if < 45kg give 2.2mg/kg IV bid (maximum, 200mg/day), or Ciprofloxacin 15mg/kg IV bid

Patient Education

General: This is a severely debilitating disease and highly lethal requiring aggressive treatment.
Activity: Bed rest
Diet: As tolerated. Keep patient well hydrated to minimize risk of gentamicin side effects.
Medications: Side effects of gentamicin include kidney and inner ear damage. Report ringing in the ears, hearing loss, dizziness (early signs of ear toxicity).
Prevention and Hygiene: Avoid contact with rodents and other wild animals, sick animals and animal carcasses. Use long sleeves and blouse trousers to minimize skin exposure to fleas; use DEET arthropod repellent and treat uniforms with permethrin as directed.
No Improvement/Deterioration: Progression can include gangrene, respiratory involvement, septic shock. Disseminated intravascular coagulation in plague causes gangrene, but bleeding is rare.
Wound Care: Buboes may be reduced with needle aspiration, but should not be incised.

Follow-up Actions

Consultation/Evacuation Criteria: Report suspected cases to public health authorities immediately. Refer to specialized care. Internationally quarantinable disease. Consult medical and command authorities before evacuating. Use standard precautions if transporting patients with bubonic plague; add droplet precautions for suspected pulmonary involvement.

Table 5-10. Post-Exposure Prophylaxis Following Biological Attack or Exposure to a Case of Pneumonic Plague

	Primary Option
Adults	Doxycycline 100mg po bid, or Ciprofloxacin 500mg po bid
Pregnant Women	Doxycycline 100mg po bid, or Ciprofloxacin 500mg po bid Trimethoprim–Sulfamethoxazole (160/800mg) [Bactrim DS] po bid
Children	Doxycycline If ≥45kg, give adult dose; if <45kg give 2.2mg/kg po bid (maximum, 200mg/day), or Ciprofloxacin 20mg/kg po bid Trimethoprim–Sulfamethoxazole po bid (4mg/kg of trimethoprim component) for prophylaxis in children

Prophylaxis should be offered to household, other face-to-face contacts, and health care workers caring for cases of pneumonic plague, health care workers who have experienced a needle-stick or other percutaneous or mucosal blood/body fluid exposure from a plague patient, and those exposed to aerosol biological attack. Prophylaxis is continued for 7 days past the last possible exposure. Prophylaxis is also considered for those at risk for flea bites while in areas experiencing epidemic bubonic plague. Prophylaxis is not typically needed after contact with a case of bubonic plague, or septicemic plague without respiratory involvement.
Notes: Hospital Infection Control: Standard infection control measures for care of patients with bubonic plague. Place pneumonic plague patients under droplet precautions, and maintain until the patient has completed 72 hours of therapy and until a favorable response to treatment is observed.

Zoonotic Disease Considerations:

Reservoirs: Rodents including rats, prairie dogs, rock squirrels.
Vectors: Fleas
Distribution: Western United States, parts of South America, Africa and Asia.
Pets: Plague has been transmitted to humans by respiratory droplets from infected cats, and can be potentially spread by bites, scratches, and fleas of infected pets. Postexposure prophylaxis should be considered to mammalian household pets exposed to cases of human pneumonic plague.

Chapter 12: Infectious Diseases: Bacterial Infections: Rat Bite Fever

COL Glenn Wortmann, MC, USA

Introduction: Caused by infection with *Streptobacillus* moniliformis or *Spirillum minor*, rat-bite fever is transmitted by the bite of a rodent and has worldwide distribution. Contaminated water and milk have been implicated in outbreaks. Incubation period is 3-10 days. The case fatality rate is as high as 25% in untreated patients.

Subjective: Symptoms
Fever, chills, headache, myalgias, arthralgias and rash
Focused History: *Do you recall being bitten by a rat?* (typical history) *How long ago were you bitten by a rat?* (incubation period is 3-10 days) *Do you have a rash?* (typical in most patients)

Objective: Signs
Using Basic Tools: Vitals signs: Fever. Inspection: The rash can be maculopapular, morbilliform or petechial, and erupts over the palms, soles and extremities. Approximately 50% of patients develop an asymmetric polyarthritis.
Using Advanced Tools: Labs: Culture of blood, joint fluid or pus may demonstrate organism.

Assessment:
Differential Diagnosis: There are numerous other potential causes of fever/rash *(see Part 3: General Symptoms: Rash with Fever)*. A history or signs of rat bite (typically that has healed spontaneously) within the past 10 days suggests the diagnosis.
Measles: *See Part 5: Specialty Areas: Chapter 15: Most Common Pediatric Diseases: Skin Problems: Viral Exanthems*
Meningococcemia: *See Part 4: Organ Systems: Chapter 6: Bacterial Infections: Meningococcemia*
Rocky Mountain spotted fever: *See Part 5: Specialty Areas: Chapter 12: Rickettsial Infections: Rickettsial Infections (Murine, Rickettsialpox, RMSF, Scrub Typhus, Louse-Borne Typhus, Boutonneuse Fever)*
Secondary syphilis: *See Part 5: Specialty Areas: Chapter 11: Genital Ulcers*

Plan:
Treatment
The presence of fever and rash after a rat bite should suggest a diagnosis of rat bite fever and treatment should be given empirically. For moderately to severely ill patients, give **penicillin** 200,000 units IV q4h x 10-14 days. For mildly ill patients, **amoxicillin** 500mg po tid x 14 days is probably adequate. For penicillin-allergic patients, give **tetracycline** 500mg po q6h x 10-14 days or **doxycycline** 100mg po q12h x 10-14 days.

Patient Education
General: Avoid rat bites.
Activity: As tolerated
Diet: As tolerated
Medications: Occasional gastrointestinal side effects. Tetracycline and doxycycline should be avoided in children and pregnant women.
Prevention and Hygiene: Avoid rat bites. Prophylaxis following a rat bite may decrease risk of developing rat bite fever. Give penicillin (2g per day in adults; 25,000 to 50,000 units per kg per day in children) po x 3 days.
No Improvement/Deterioration: Return for evaluation.

Follow-up Actions
Return Evaluation: Referral as needed. Relapses are common.
Consultation Criteria: Failure to improve.

Zoonotic Disease Considerations
Principal Animal Hosts: Rodents
Clinical Disease in Animals: Arthritis, pericarditis
Probable Mode of Transmission: Rodent bites, water-or food-borne
Known Distribution: Worldwide; rare

Chapter 12: Infectious Diseases: Bacterial Infections: Acute Rheumatic Fever

LCDR Timothy Whitman, MC, USN

Introduction: Acute rheumatic fever (ARF) develops between 2-4 weeks as a delayed non-infectious response to a typically self-limited but untreated streptococcal pharyngitis (1-3% persons). A majority of the 470,000 new cases of rheumatic fever and 233,000 deaths each year due to ARF or rheumatic heart disease occur in developing countries. Certain group A strep strains are more likely to cause ARF. Peak incidence is from 5-20 years of age. Recurrences are common (50%).

Subjective: Symptoms
Fever; migratory polyarthralgias (eg, knees, ankles, elbows or wrists); rash which can wax and wane over months; subcutaneous nodules and chorea. If carditis is present, patient may have palpitations, chest pain, or SOB and other symptoms of congestive heart failure (CHF).
Focused History: *Have you had a sore throat in the last few weeks?* (ARF follows a strep throat infection.) *Have you taken your temperature or do you feel hot?* (expect to document a temperature >100°F) *Have you felt sick for a long time?* (ARF may present with chronic signs such as Sydenham's chorea and the rash of erythema marginatum, as described in this section.)

Objective: Signs
Using Basic Tools: Vital signs: Fever to 102°F (up to 21 days); rapid respiratory rate (if carditis); Inspection: Erythema marginatum rash (irregularly edged, transient, lacy, macular rash [pink rimmed with internal blanching] found on the trunk and extremities) which

waxes and wanes for months; chorea (short, abrupt, non-purposeful movements, which often disappear during sleep and grimacing). Palpation: Migratory large joint inflammation (arthritis); 10% have subcutaneous nodules on extensor elbows and forearms which last up to 4 weeks. Auscultation: If carditis: bibasilar rales, aortic insufficiency or mitral regurgitation murmurs, pericardial friction rub, S3 gallop.

Using Advanced Tools: If carditis, CXR may show cardiomegaly. ECG may show prolonged PR interval but can also show essentially any degree of heart block.

Assessment:

Polyarthritis is often the main presenting symptom and suspicion of ARF should be considered in children or young adults who present with signs of arthritis and/or carditis, even without a history of pharyngitis. Diagnosis is based on clinical observation and application of the Jones criteria for diagnosis: 2 major criteria, or 1 major and 2 minor criteria and evidence for prior streptococcal infections (prior scarlet fever, + throat culture)

Major Criteria: Carditis, polyarthritis, subcutaneous nodules, and chorea, erythema marginatum rash

Minor Criteria: Fever, arthralgias, prior rheumatic fever, heart block seen on ECG

Differential Diagnosis

Gonococcal arthritis: Sexual exposure; dysuria; urethral discharge; characteristic gun metal blue skin lesion

Subacute bacterial endocarditis: Typically few joints involved; may see embolic skin lesions; diagnosis made by blood cultures (if available)

Lyme disease: Fever less frequent; fewer joints involved; history of tick bite

Reiter's syndrome: Fever is unusual; prior history of sexually transmitted disease or acute diarrheal illness; characteristic skin lesions (painless, superficial erosions) in genital area /soles of feet

Myocarditis (viral or other causes): Classic joint symptoms or the erythema marginatum rash less likely

Pericarditis (from other causes): Typically without history of pharyngitis 2-4 weeks prior to symptoms. May see diffuse ST segment elevations. *See Part 4: Organ Systems: Chapter 11: Pericarditis*

Plan:

Treatment

Primary: **Benzathine penicillin** 1.2MU IM (600,000 U in children) X 1 or **penicillin** V 250mg po qid x 10 days

Salicylates: **Aspirin** 4-8g per day divided into qid dosing x 3-4 weeks. *See Part 4: Organ Systems: Chapter 11: Congestive Heart Failure (Pulmonary Edema)* for discussion and management of congestive heart failure.

Alternative: Erythromycin 40mg/kg po q day (max dose of 1000mg q day) divided into qid dosing x 10 days for patients allergic to **penicillin**. Other NSAIDs may be used in place of aspirin.

Patient Education

General: This can be a relapsing condition.

Activity: Patients with arthritis or carditis should be on bedrest for 2 weeks (up to 8 weeks if cardiac failure present).

Diet: Regular

Medications: Expect tinnitus with high dose aspirin

Follow-up Actions

Secondary prophylaxis with **benzathine penicillin** 1.2MU IM q3-4 weeks until age 18, or for 5 years after acute episode. Alternate for patients allergic to penicillin is **erythromycin** 250mg po bid. If carditis (eg, CHF) or valve involvement, prophylaxis is given until age 25 or 10 years after last ARF episode.

Evacuation/Consultation: Patients with evidence of carditis (eg, CHF) or valve disease should be referred for further evaluation and management.

Chapter 12: Infectious Diseases: Bacterial Infections: Streptococcal Infections, Life-Threatening

LCDR Timothy Whitman, MC, USN

Introduction: Streptococci are gram-positive bacteria. Some species are pathogenic in humans, responsible for illnesses ranging in severity from mild upper respiratory infections to life-threatening necrotizing fasciitis. Fulminant necrotizing fasciitis due to group A streptococcus may begin at a site of trivial trauma (for example a paper cut, abrasion on a cinder block), with rapid progression over 24-72 hours and 20-70% mortality even with ICU care. This is a deep-seated, fast moving infection that destroys fascia, fat, muscle and other tissue but may spare the skin. It often involves the extremities. Streptococcal infection of muscle (myositis) often is from blood infection, not associated with trauma. It may involve a single muscle group and be associated with compartment syndrome (*see Part 8: Procedures: Chapter: 30: Compartment Syndrome*). For other streptococcal infections (*see Part 3: General Symptoms: ENT Problems: Pharyngitis, Adult & Part 5: Specialty Areas: Chapter 15: Most Common Pediatric Diseases: Throat Problems, Pharyngitis*. Group B Streptococcal Infection: *See Part 3: General Symptoms: Obstetric Problems: Preterm Labor & Part 4: Organ Systems: Chapter 6: Bacterial Infections: Erysipelas and Cellulitis & Impetigo*

Subjective: Symptoms

Initial flu-like symptoms with fever to 104°F, abrupt onset of extreme pain which often precedes other signs and symptoms (eg, tenderness and erythema) at site of initial infection. Pain typically is in an extremity but may mimic appendicitis, PID, cholecystitis or pericarditis.

Focused History: *On a scale 1-10, how severe is the pain in the affected area?* (Great pain accompanying mild skin changes suggests a deeper infection.) *Have you had any trauma in this area recently?* (risk factor) Have you had any blisters? (suggests a deep tissue infection if no local injury such as frostbite or burns)

Objective: **Signs**

Using Basic Tools: Vital signs: Acute (<24 hr): Fever as high as 105°F, SBP <110, increased heart rate, Inspection: Ill-appearing abrupt onset red/swollen affected area, confusion/mental status changes common. Sub-acute (1-7 days): Continuation of acute signs, red swollen area spreads locally, color turns to blue/purple with bullae, may see gangrene by day 4-5. Chronic (>7 days): Earlier signs continue, clear demarcation at site of involvement. Palpation: Acute (<24 hr): Tenderness >inflammatory change, area warm to touch; may see capillary leak syndrome with generalized edema (the "Michelin man" look) In myositis, find changes consistent with compartment syndrome of affected area. Sub-acute/Chronic: Continuation of earlier signs, other physical findings related to multi-organ system failure in severe cases. *See Part 4: Organ Systems: Chapter 3: Acute Respiratory Distress Syndrome*

Using Advanced Tools: Lab: Gram's stain (blood, throat, wound and debrided tissue) for gram-positive cocci in chains. *See Appendices: Color Plates: Figure A-26.E.* BUN, Cr: (Renal dysfunction is present in virtually all severely ill patients by 48 to 72 hrs). CXR: Look for signs of ARDS development

Assessment: **Differential Diagnosis:**

Necrotizing fasciitis (due to other organisms): Infection may be polymicrobial (eg, *Clostridia*; crepitus on physical exam or gas on x-ray) *See Part 3: General Symptoms: Male Genital Problems: Genital Inflammation*

Cellulitis or lymphangitis (due to other organisms): Deep streptococcal infection is much more painful and purpuric. ARDS (or multi-organ failure due to other cause); *see Part 4: Organ Systems: Chapter 3: Acute Respiratory Distress Syndrome*

Plan:

Treatment of Presumed Severe Streptococcal Infection

1. If medical evacuation possible:
   a. Start empiric antibiotic therapy and continue through medical evacuation: **Penicillin** 24MU/day IV (4MU q4h) and **clindamycin** 900mg IV q8h. (**Clindamycin** decreases streptococcal toxin production.) Alternative: **Clindamycin** 900mg IV q8h plus one of the following: **ticarcillin-clavulanate** 3.1g q4h or **piperacillin-tazobactam** 4.5g q6h through medical evacuation.
   b. Oxygen, IV fluids (LR or NS) and other treatment; *see Part 4: Organ Systems: Chapter 3: Acute Respiratory Distress Syndrome.*
   c. Evacuate (urgent) for surgical and intensive care support.
2. If evacuation is delayed or not possible:
   a. Give antibiotics as above and continue therapy for 14 days.
   b. Aggressively débride deep-seated infection. External findings are often the "tip of the iceberg" regarding tissue involvement. *See Part 8: Procedures: Chapter 30: Wound Debridement*
   c. Oxygen, IV fluids (LR or NS) *See Part 4: Organ Systems: Chapter 3: Acute Respiratory Distress Syndrome & Part 7: Trauma: Chapter 27: Hypovolemic Shock*
   d. Intravenous **immunoglobulin** (IVIG) 150mg/kg/day x 5 days given early may decrease mortality.

Patient Education

General: The infection control recommendation for this is contact isolation and if in the lungs, respiratory droplet precautions.

Prevention: Secondary cases are rare, but consider streptococcal prophylaxis (penicillin V potassium 250mg po qid x 10 days) of close contacts.

Follow-up Actions

Evacuation/Consultation Criteria: Evacuate suspected cases immediately. Consult infectious disease specialist early.

Zoonotic Disease Considerations

Agent: Group A *Streptococcus* spp.

Principal Animal Hosts: Cattle, swine, and horses

Clinical Disease in Animals: Meningitis and arthritis in swine; mastitis in cattle and horses; respiratory disease and strangles in horses

Probable Mode of Transmission: Direct contact; ingestion of raw milk

Known Distribution: Worldwide

Chapter 12: Infectious Diseases: Bacterial Infections: Tetanus

LCDR Timothy Whitman, MC, USN

Introduction: *Clostridium tetani* bacteria are introduced into the body through contaminated open wounds, burns, frostbite, needles, or unclean cutting/dressing of the umbilical cord. About one million cases per year occur worldwide, especially in tropical and developing countries (50% cases are neonatal). Tetanus has a case fatality rate of 10-90%. The incubation period is 3-30 days, depending on the dose and the distance of inoculation from the central nervous system. The tetanus toxin (tetanospasmin) causes acute central nervous system intoxication. There are 4 subtypes described for tetanus: generalized, localized, cephalic and neonatal. All personnel should have current immunization status for tetanus verified prior to deployment. *See Part 5: Specialty Areas: Chapter 13: Immunization Chart*

Subjective: **Symptoms**

Neonatal cases: Weakness, irritability, trouble nursing, unable to suck

Specific: Acute (1-7days): Pain at wound site, local muscle spasticity. Sub-acute (7-14 days): Trismus (lockjaw), painful tetanic spasm, glottic or respiratory muscle spasm, urinary retention, constipation, rigid abdominal wall muscles, trouble swallowing. Chronic (>2 weeks): Slow recovery phase (4 weeks)

Focused History: *Have you received a tetanus immunization? If so, when was the last one?* (If within 5-10 years, then tetanus is very unlikely. Also if mother of baby had tetanus vaccination, then neonatal tetanus is unlikely.) *Have you recently had a potentially contaminated wound?* (typical exposure) *Does loud noise/coughing/people touching you/gusts of air trigger painful muscle spasms?* (typical stimuli for spasms)

Objective: **Signs**

Using Basic Tools: Inspection: Acute (1-7 days): Afebrile; localized muscle spasticity, localized pain at inoculation site; neonatal cases: unable to nurse, with stiff muscles or spasms. Sub-acute (7-14 days): Afebrile, tetanic spasm (stimulus induced) trismus (lockjaw), opisthotonos (arched back spasm), glottic/respiratory muscle spasm, cyanosis/asphyxia, profuse sweating. Palpation: Sub-acute (7-14 days): Abdominal muscle wall rigidity. Percussion: Acute (1-7 days): Brisk local deep tendon reflexes.

Assessment: Diagnose from the history and physical findings/clinical observation.

Differential Diagnosis

Meningoencephalitis: Usually associated with fever; true seizures and mental status changes not seen in tetanus.

Strychnine poisoning: Mimics tetanus; abdominal wall muscle rigidity more often seen in tetanus; ask about an ingestion history

Hypocalcemic tetany: Involves extremities; rare to see lockjaw; tapping on facial nerve (over parotid) can induce facial muscle spasm in low calcium states (Chvostek's sign)

Generalized seizures: Associated with loss of consciousness; no trismus

Phenothiazine toxicity: Drug history; can see torticollis (not in tetanus); relieved with diphenhydramine (not in tetanus)

Plan:

Treatment

Primary:

1. Maintain airway (ET tube can stimulate spasm so may need early tracheostomy for respiratory difficulty)
2. Medications:
   a. **Tetanus (human) immune globulin (HTIG, Hyper-Tet)** 500IU IM or injected directly into wound
   b. **Tetanus immunization** 0.5mL IM at site away from HTIG administration. *See Table 5-11*
   c. Narcotic analgesia with **acetaminophen** with **codeine** 1-2 tabs po q4h prn pain
   d. **Diazepam** titrated for effect 5-10mg IV q2-4h to control muscle spasms. **Lorazepam** 1mg IM q1h may be used to control muscle spasms while awaiting IV access and ability to give diazepam.
   e. **Metronidazole** 30mg/kg/day (not >4G/day) IV divided in q6h dosing for 7-10 days (average about 500mg q6h). Can also be given 1gm per rectum q8h. **Alternate Antibiotic: Penicillin G** 4 million units IV q6h x 10 days or **doxycycline** 100mg IV q12 h x 10 days
3. Nursing care: Keep patient in a quiet, darkened room; avoid unnecessary touching; use Foley catheter for urinary retention.

Patient Education

Activity: Bedrest

Diet: High calorie, initially use tube or IV feeding.

Prevention and Hygiene: Use topical antibiotics to umbilical stump. Clean all wounds thoroughly. Maintain current tetanus immunization status (*see Table 5-11*):

Table 5-11. Tetanus Immunization Chart

Tetanus Immunization Status	Minor clean wound	Major clean wound	Contaminated wound
Fully immunized recent Td* booster	—	—	—
Fully immunized Td booster 5-10 years ago	—	Tdap*	Tdap*
Fully immunized no booster >10 years	Tdap*	Tdap*	Tdap*
Unknown, none, or incomplete immunization	Tdap*	Tdap* and TIG** (250 U)	Tdap* and TIG** (500 U)

*Tdap is Tetanus, Diphtheria and Pertussis vaccine; ** TIG is Tetanus Immune Globulin

Note: Tetanus vaccination of mother gives her protection and protects the newborn in the first few weeks of life.

Follow-up Actions

Wound Care: If needed, débride the wound to avoid secondary infection. *See Part 8: Procedures: Chapter 30: Wound Debridement*

Return Evaluation: Those with natural tetanus do not develop immunity (not enough toxin exposure). They need to be re-vaccinated at 4-6 weeks then 1 month later.

Evacuation/Consultation Criteria: The level of care needed requires transfer to hospital.

Chapter 12: Infectious Diseases: Bacterial Infections: Tularemia

Lt Col George Christopher, USAF, MC

Introduction: Tularemia is caused by *Francisella tularensis*, an aerobic catalase-positive, gram-negative coccobacillus. *F. tularensis* is maintained in numerous mammalian (including rabbits, hares, rodents) and tick reservoirs, and survives in contaminated dusts. Transmission is by ticks and deerflies; also mosquitoes (in Sweden, Finland, and the former Soviet Union), direct contact with infected animals, inhalation of aerosols generated by skinning/processing infected animals, inhalation of environmental aerosols of contaminated dust, and ingestion of contaminated food or water. Because of its low infective dose, stability in aerosols, and disease severity, *F. tularensis* is a Category A biological weapons threat. *See Part 6: Operational Environment: Chapter 25: Biological Warfare.* Clinical syndromes vary with portal of entry.

Ulceroglandular, pharyngeal, and oculoglandular tularemia feature local disease at the portal of entry with regional involvement of the lymph nodes draining the portal of entry. Glandular tularemia features inflammation of regional lymph nodes without an apparent skin lesion at the portal of entry. Pneumonia may complicate inhalation of organisms, or spread of organisms from another site to the lung through the bloodstream. Typhoidal tularemia, a vague febrile illness without specific findings, can follow infection through any portal of entry.

Subjective: Symptoms

Ulceroglandular tularemia: Focal redness, swelling, pain and tenderness of skin/soft tissue; development of a tender skin ulcer with scab, painful lymph nodes, fever, fatigue, and muscle aches

Glandular tularemia: Painful, enlarged regional lymph nodes, fever, fatigue, and muscle ache

Pharyngeal tularemia: Severe sore throat, swollen cervical lymph nodes, fever, fatigue, and muscle aches

Oculoglandular tularemia: Acute eye pain and conjunctival drainage, blurred vision, swollen, painful pre-auricular or pre-parotid adenopathy, fever, malaise, and myalgias

Pneumonic tularemia: Fever, cough (usually non-productive), substernal chest tightness, pleuritic chest pain, malaise, and myalgias

Typhoidal tularemia: Fever, malaise, fatigue, vague abdominal pain, and myalgias. Meningitis rarely may complicate typhoidal form of the disease.

Focused History: *Do you have any "unsafe" food or water exposures, tick bites, exposures to wild animals or tick-infested areas? Is anyone else in your unit ill with similar symptoms?* (For outbreaks of pharyngeal or typhoidal disease, consider contaminated food or water; for outbreaks of pneumonic or typhoidal disease, consider environmental aerosols or biological attack.) *Do you have eye pain or impaired vision?* (Oculoglandular disease may rarely result in corneal ulceration.)

Objective: Signs
Using Basic Tools:

Ulceroglandular tularemia: Fever, focal redness, edema, warmth, and tenderness of skin/soft tissue; tender skin ulcer with central eschar and rolled-up margins, lymphangitic streaking, tender regional adenopathy

Glandular tularemia: Fever, tender regional lymphadenopathy

Pharyngeal tularemia: Fever, severe erythema, posterior pharyngeal or tonsillar exudate, possibly pharyngeal ulcers and/or membrane mimicking diphtheria; cervical and/or preauricular lymphadenopathy

Oculoglandular tularemia: Fever, conjunctival erythema and discharge; possibly small conjunctival papules or ulcers; tender pre auricular or pre-parotid adenopathy

Pneumonic tularemia: Fever, physical exam may otherwise be normal, or may feature rales, friction rubs; changes to percussion suggesting consolidation or effusions.

Typhoidal tularemia: Exam may be normal, or disclose tender, enlarged liver or spleen.

All forms: May feature secondary skin rashes, which may be diffuse maculopapular or vesiculopapular rashes, erythema nodosum, erythema multiforme, or urticaria

Using Advanced Tools: Labs: *F. tularensis* is a laboratory hazard; notify lab if tularemia is suspected. Cultures of blood, pleural fluid, wound exudate, and tissue (biopsy or deep scraping of ulcers; lymph nodes; superficial swab of ulcer acceptable alternative if biopsy, deep scraping not available).

Assessment: Differential Diagnosis

Ulceroglandular tularemia: Typhus, cutaneous anthrax, bubonic plague (typically no ulcer or eschar present), vasculitic ulcer.

Glandular tularemia: Cat scratch disease, bubonic plague (typically more pain and systemic toxicity). A "lymphangitic" presentation can mimic skin disease due to streptococci, sporotrichosis (typically less acute), nontuberculous mycobacterial infection (typically less acute). Acute regional adenitis due to other bacteria; TB, lymphoma (typically less acute).

Pharyngeal tularemia: Pharyngitis due to Group A streptococcus, adenoviruses, Epstein-Barr virus; diphtheria, pharyngeal plague or anthrax

Oculoglandular tularemia: Other causes of oculoglandular syndrome-adenoviruses, enteroviruses, cat scratch disease

Pneumonic tularemia: Pneumococcal or other severe community-acquired pneumonias; pneumonic plague or inhalational anthrax (especially if hilar adenopathy is prominent)

Typhoidal tularemia: Typhoid fever, Q fever, rickettsial infections, cytomegalovirus, Epstein-Barr virus, viral hepatitis, other causes of nonspecific febrile diseases. Symptoms of meningitis may rarely complicate typhoidal form.

Table 5-12. Tularemia Treatment Plan

	Primary Option	Alternative
Adults	Gentamicin 5mg/kg IM or IV once daily	Doxycycline 100mg IV or po bid or 20mg IV once daily, or Ciprofloxacin 400mg IV or 500-750mg po bid
Pregnant Women	Gentamicin 5mg/kg IM or IV once daily	Doxycycline 100mg IV or po bid, or Ciprofloxacin 400mg IV or 500-750 mg po bid
Children	Gentamicin 2.5mg/kg IM or IV tid (bid for premature infants or neonates under one week of age).	Doxycycline: If ≥45 kg, give adult dose; if <45 kg give 2.2mg/kg IV or po bid (maximum, 200mg/day), or Ciprofloxacin 15mg/kg IV or po bid

Plan:

Treatment

Chloramphenicol 25mg/kg IV, then 15mg/kg (to a max of 4g/day) qid x 14 days should be added to other antibiotic therapy if meningitis is suspected.

Doxycycline or **ciprofloxacin** may be given po or IV depending on the intensity of exposure or severity of illness; IV is recommended for biological warfare casualties. Duration of therapy is 10 days for gentamicin and ciprofloxacin, and 14-21 days for doxycycline.

Patient Education

General: This is a debilitating disease requiring evacuation for further care.

Activity: Most patients will require bed rest due to debilitation.

Diet: As tolerated.

Medications: Side effects of gentamicin may include kidney and inner ear damage. Report ringing in the ears, hearing loss, dizziness (early signs of ear toxicity).

Prevention and Hygiene: Avoid contact with rodents and other wild animals, sick animals, and animal carcasses. Use water only from approved sources. Use long sleeves and blouse trousers to minimize skin exposure to fleas; use DEET arthropod repellent and treat uniforms with permethrin as directed; not transmitted person-to-person.

No Improvement/Deterioration: Progressive malaise and fatigue. This disease requires referral for hospitalization.

Follow-up Actions

Evacuation/Consultation Criteria: Report suspected cases to public health authorities. Refer to specialized care if available. Evacuate using standard infection control measures. Consult medical and command authorities before evacuating biological casualties.

Table 5-13. Tularemia Treatment: Post-Exposure Prophylaxis Following Biological Attack
Recommended duration of prophylaxis is 14 days.

	Primary Option	Alternative
Adults	**Doxycycline** 100mg po bid, or **Ciprofloxacin** 500mg po bid	**Chloramphenicol** 25mg/kg po qid
Pregnant Women	**Doxycycline** 100mg po bid, or **Ciprofloxacin** 500mg po bid	**Chloramphenicol** 25mg/kg po qid
Children	**Doxycycline** If >45 kg, give adult dose; if <45 kg give 2.2mg/kg po bid (maximum, 200mg/day), or **Ciprofloxacin** 20mg/kg po bid	**Chloramphenicol** 25mg/kg po qid

Notes: Not transmitted from person-to-person transmission; standard infection control measures are appropriate; use additional measures if diagnosis is unclear and other items in differential diagnosis have not been excluded (eg, droplet precautions if pneumonic plague is still a consideration).

Zoonotic Disease Considerations

Reservoirs: Numerous mammals, usually rabbits, hares, and rodents including squirrels, muskrats, voles, and mice

Vectors: Ticks, biting flies. Mosquitoes in Sweden, Finland, former Soviet Union

Distribution: Temperate regions Northern Hemisphere

Chapter 12: Infectious Diseases: Bacterial Infections: Typhoid Fever

CDR John Sanders, MC, USN

Introduction: Typhoid fever is caused by infection with the bacteria *Salmonella typhi*. Typhoid fever is a nonspecific febrile illness, which can last several weeks and can be complicated by intestinal perforation and sepsis. Food (especially undercooked meat and eggs) and water contaminated by feces or urine from patients or chronic carriers is implicated in transmission. The incubation period is 1-3 weeks after exposure. Mortality had been >15% in pre-antibiotic era but now less than 1.5% with appropriate treatment. Relapse of symptoms can occur in 1-6% of patients, usually presenting 2-3 weeks after initial resolution of fever. **Geographic Associations:** Worldwide distribution, most common in developing countries with poor hygiene. **Seasonal Variation:** Incidence tends to increase in warmer months, but may occur year round. **Risk Factors:** Travel to developing country with ingestion of local food/water.

Subjective: **Symptoms**

1st week: Fever (rising "stepladder" pattern), abdominal pain, cough, weakness, myalgias, anorexia

2nd-4th weeks: Continued fever, weakness, myalgias, anorexia, and diarrhea or constipation; if increasing abdominal pain, lower GI bleed, consider intestinal perforation.

>4 weeks: Slow resolution of symptoms; if fevers persist, consider metastatic focus of infection (endocarditis, renal abscess, osteomyelitis, etc.)

Focused History: *How long have you felt feverish?* (Fever gradually builds and lasts for 3 weeks.) *Have you noticed any red to pink spots on your abdomen or chest?* (Transient rose spots are seen in 10-50% of patients.) *Have you recently traveled in a developing country?* (very common cause of fever in endemic areas) *Did you eat the local food or drink local water while traveling? Have you noticed blood in your stool?* (may require surgical evaluation for intestinal perforation)

Objective: **Signs**

Using Basic Tools: Acute (3-7 days) Vital signs: Stepladder temperatures to 104°F (usually in afternoon/night), relative bradycardia in 25%. Inspection: Moderately ill appearing; rose spots (2-3mm pink to red macules on chest/abdomen that fade with pressure) in fair skinned persons; furry tongue (thick white to brown coating that spares edges). Palpation: Abdominal distension; mild, diffuse abdominal tenderness. **Sub-acute** (1-3 weeks): Palpation: Splenomegaly (50%). Percussion: Liver can be slightly enlarged 2-3cm below costal margin. **Using Advanced Tools:** Labs: Urine (<40%), blood (40-80%), and stool (30-40%) cultures will confirm diagnosis. Other clues from stool include fecal leukocytes (may suggest an invasive gastroenteritis). Blood smear may demonstrate low WBC, anemia (low RBC count), and thrombocytopenia (low platelet count). Liver enzymes may be mildly elevated (AST/ALT <300IU/mL). Many countries rely on non specific serologic test, the Widal test, but this is not recommended. More specific serologic assays are in development.

Differential Diagnosis (*See relevant sections in Part 5: Specialty Areas: Chapter 12*)

Non-typhoidal Salmonella (paratyphoid fever or other Salmonella infection): Infections are sometimes considered milder, without rose spots, but difficult to distinguish without culture results.

Tuberculosis: Generally chronic, lower grade fever; night sweats; cough; hemoptysis; abnormal CXR

Hepatitis: More often see jaundice, dark urine, gastrointestinal symptoms, malaise and fatigue

Leptospirosis: Remarkable conjunctival injection; has similar fever pattern; history of exposure to contaminated fresh water

Malaria: Thick and thin blood smears will help detect the malaria parasite.

Amebic liver abscess: May see more tenderness in hepatic region

Brucellosis: Chronic febrile illness with relative bradycardia, splenomegaly; animal exposure, occupation may help differentiate

Q Fever: Exhibit similar S/S and lab markers ie, abdominal pain, cough and pneumonia, frontal headache and high fever, relative bradycardia, thrombocytopenia

Paratyphoid fever: Presents in a similar way but is often thought to be milder, and is caused by *Salmonella paratyphi*.

Plan:

Treatment

Primary: Ciprofloxacin 500mg po or IV q12h x 10 days. Some resistance has been seen and this should be used with caution in Asia. **Alternatives: Ceftriaxone** 2gm IV or IM q day x 14 days (recent study suggests that a 5 day course may be as effective) or **azithromycin** 1g load po on day 1, then 500mg po days 2-6. Pediatric dosing: **Ceftriaxone** 100mg/kg/day (max 4g) IV or IM q day x 10-14 days or **ciprofloxacin** 30mg/kg/day (max of 1gm) po or IV q12h x 10 days or **azithromycin** 10mg/kg/day (max 500mg) load po on day 1, then 5mg/kg/day po on days 2-6. **Note:** For delirium or shock, give steroids before first dose of antibiotic: **dexamethasone** load 3mg/kg IV, then 1mg/kg IV q6h x 48 hrs.

Empiric: Appropriate antibiotics should be started empirically pending diagnosis.

Patient Education

General: Most patients treated with antibiotics respond within a few days, but the entire course of antibiotics needs to be completed.

Activity: The patient should be provided ample opportunity for rest (Quarters or Limited Duty) until symptoms resolve.

Diet: Vigorous oral rehydration, 3-4 liters first day, then follow and replace losses. Maintain nutrition/electrolytes.

Prevention and Hygiene: Immunize with live attenuated oral ty21a vaccine (boost q 5 years) or the typhoid polysaccharide Vi vaccine (boost q 2 years) pre-deployment. Practice hand washing, fly control, water treatment. *Salmonella typhi* is killed by heating food or water to 135°F, iodination or chlorination. Avoid fresh, uncooked vegetables and fruits unless you can peel or carefully wash them yourself. Excretion of the bacteria in the stool for more than 12 months after the acute infection (chronic carriage) occurs in from 1-6% (higher in patients with gall stones) and represents an infectious risk to others. Individuals with history of infection should be restricted from food preparation or handling duties until documentation of negative stool culture post-treatment.

No Improvement/Deterioration: Patient should be advised to watch for the following: 1. Failure of fever to resolve within 72 hours of antibiotics or return of fever after completing treatment. 2. Increasing abdominal pain. 3. Blood in stool.

Follow-up Actions

Return Evaluation: Patient should return if symptoms do not begin to resolve in 72 hours after initiating treatment or symptoms return after the completion of treatment. If relapse, re-treat with alternative antibiotic (consider 10-14 days of ceftriaxone). Consider non-GI source of infection such as endocarditis, visceral or renal abscesses, or osteomyelitis.

Evacuation/Consultation Criteria: Send to higher level of care where more diagnostic tools available when stable.

Note: Multidrug resistance has been increasingly reported around the world, making empiric use of ampicillin, trimethoprim sulfamethoxazole, or chloramphenicol unreliable.

Chapter 13: Preventive Medicine: Introduction

LTC (P) Robert Mott, MC, USA

Introduction: Preventive medicine (PM) procedures minimize disease and non-battle injuries (DNBI) during war and contingency operations. PM measures should be integrated into all missions and training exercises. Areas of responsibility include: medical readiness, health promotion, personal protective measures against arthropods, hearing and vision protection, acquisition and treatment of potable water; acquisition, handling and preparation of food; monitoring and implementing vector (insect and rodent) control programs; monitoring the construction and maintenance of personal hygiene (washing) facilities, as well as solid and liquid waste disposal systems. Vision protection is not addressed in this chapter because of job series specificity of vision standards and safety eyewear requirements. Both are addressed in USACHPPM Tech Guide 006.

Chapter 13: Preventive Medicine: Immunization Chart

LTC (P) Robert Mott, MC, USA

Note: For more detailed product information (including contraindications) and current guidelines, refer to vaccine package inserts; Advisory Committee on Immunization Practices (ACIP) guidelines - http://www.cdc.gov/vaccines/recs/acip/default.htm; MILVAX - www.vaccines.army.mil; AR 40-562/BUMED INST 6230.15A/AFJI 48-110/CG COMDTINST M6230.4F; Service regulations; and COCOM guidance.

Table 5-14. Immunizations Quick Reference Guide

Vaccine	Initial dosage/route	Booster Dose	Comments
Anthrax	0.5mL SC at 0, 2, 4 weeks, then 6, 12, and 18 months	0.5mL SC annually	Annual booster
Hepatitis A	1.0mL IM at 0, and 6-12 months (HAVRIX, VAQTA)	None currently required	None
Hepatitis B	1.0mL IM at 0, 1, and 6 months	None currently required	None
Hepatitis A + B	1.0mL IM at 0, 1, and 6 months (TWINRIX)	None currently required	None
Human Papillomavirus (HPV)	0.5mL IM at 0, 2, and 6 months (GARDASIL)	None currently required	Females age 9-26 years
Influenza (2 types of vaccine used)	a. Inactivated : 0.5mL IM annually in October (FLUZONE, FLUARIX)	None currently required	Annual
	b. Live attenuated: Refrigerated Form: (0.1mL per nostril) Frozen Form: (0.25mL per nostril) (FluMist)	None currently required	Annual
Japanese B Encephalitis	1.0mL SC at 0, 7, and 30 days (JE-VAX)	One additional dose (1.0mL SC) after 2-3 years if risk exposure persists.	By geographic area only
Measles, Mumps, Rubella	0.5mL SC at 0 and 30 days (MMR-II)	None currently required	Required if born after 1956 and no serological evidence of previous exposure
Meningococcal (2 types of vaccine used)	a. Conjugate (preferred) 0.5mL IM single dose (Menactra)	None currently required	Serotypes A, C, Y W-135
	b. Polysaccharide 0.5mL SC single dose (Menomune)	0.5mL SC every 3-5 years for people at high risk	Serotypes A, C, Y W-135
Polio (IPV)	0.5mL SC at 0, 1-2 months, and 6-12 months (IPOL)	0.5mL SC for travel to highly endemic areas	Single IPV dose meets readiness requirement for travel
Rabies (Pre-exposure)	1.0mL IM at 0, 7, and 21-28 days (IMOVAX, RabAvert)	None currently required except animal/lab workers at high risk	See Rabies chapter for post-exposure vaccination and treatment with RIG
Smallpox	Bifurcated needle with one drop of vaccine is pressed into the skin of the upper arm 3 times for primary series, 15 times for revaccinations	None currently required	Live virus can spread to other locations on body and other people
Tetanus Diphtheria (Td) Acellular Pertussis (Tdap)	Td 0.5mL IM at 0, 1-2, and 8-14 months	Tdap, 0.5mL IM every 10 yrs or as prophylaxis after severe/dirty wounds (Tdap Adacel)	Required if no documentation of previous immunization
Typhoid (2 types of vaccine used)	a. Injectable Vaccine 0.5mL IM (Typhim Vi): b. Oral vaccine: one capsule every other day for a total of four capsules (Vivotif)	Boost with same vaccine if possible a. Typhim Vi 0.5mL IM every 2 years b. Oral vaccine: repeat 4 dose	For capsules, do not lengthen interval. Swallow with cool drink 1 hr before meal. Do not take within 24 hours of taking mefloquine or antibiotics
Varicella	0.5mL SC at 0, and 1-2 months	None currently required	Required if no serological evidence of previous exposure
Yellow Fever	0.5mL SC	0.5mL SC every 10 years	None

Chapter 13: Preventive Medicine: Surveillance for Illness and Injury

LTC (P) Robert Mott, MC, USA

Medics must compile daily sick call logs and review them for possible disease outbreaks or biological warfare exposures. This tool can also be used to educate host nation personnel in preventive medicine and disease surveillance. It is important to calculate rates (new cases divided by the number of people at risk during a specific time period) in order to compare trends over time. The information gathered must be forwarded to your next higher headquarters. Automated systems, like JMeWS, should be used IAW service and theater policies. When automated systems are not available, the following DNBI report form (*See Joint Staff Memorandum MCM-0006-02*) should be used for disease non-battle injury (DNBI) surveillance and reporting.

Figure 5-14. DNBI Report

Line 1   Unit/Command:_____   Location:_____

Line 2   Strength: a. Male: _____   b. Female: _____   c. Total: _____

Line 3   Reporting Period: a. DD/MM/YY: _____ (Sunday 0001HR) through (Saturday 2359HR)

Line 4   Prepared by: a. Name: _____   b. Phone: _____   c. E-Mail: _____

Category	Initial visits this period (a)	Total to date (b)	Rate: column (a) divided by total strength (line 2c) (c)	Days of light duty (d)	Lost Work Days (e)	Admits to Hospital (f)
Line 5 Stress Reactions (Combat/Operational)						
Line 6 Dermatologic						
Line 7 GI, Infectious						
Line 8 Gynecologic						
Line 9 Heat/Cold Injuries						
Line 10 Injury, Recreational/Sports						
Line 11 Injury, MVA						
Line 12 Injury, Work/Training						
Line 13 Injury, Other						
Line 14 Ophthalmologic						
Line 15 Psychiatric, Mental Disorder						
Line 16 Respiratory						
Line 17 STDs						
Line 18 Fever, Unexplained						
Line 19 All Other, Medical/Surgical						
Line 20 TOTAL DNBI						
Line 21 Dental						

Problems Identified: _____

Corrective Actions: _____

Chapter 13: Preventive Medicine: Malaria Prevention and Control

LTC (P) Robert Mott, MC, USA

1. Identify the type(s) of malaria, malaria drug resistance, geographic areas at risk and the seasons of the year for risk. Consult Armed Forces Medical Intelligence Center (AFMIC), US Centers for Disease Control and Prevention, or other sources.
2. Design a prevention and control program that includes:
   a. Prophylactic drugs (See Part 5: Specialty Areas: Chapter 12: Parasitic Infections: Malaria)
   b. DoD Arthropod Repellent System (DEET for skin and permethrin for uniforms and netting). Ensure personnel are properly supplied with these products and know how to use them (See Tech Guide No. 36).
   Note: These measures are also important for other arthropod-borne diseases, such as Dengue, that do not have prophylactic medications.

Table 5-15. DoD Arthropod Repellant System Items

Item	National Stock Number (NSN)
33% DEET Lotion	NSN 6840-01-284-3982
DEET lotion with sunscreen	NSN 6840-01-288-2188
Camouflage face paint with DEET	NSN 6840-01-493-7334
Permethrin IDA Kit	NSN 6840-01-345-0237
Permethrin Aerosol Spray	NSN 6840-01-278-1336

c. Permethrin-treated bed netting

Table 5-16. Permethrin-Treated Bed Netting Items

Item	National Stock Number (NSN)
Light Weight Pop-Up Bed Net (Green)	NSN 3740-01-516-4415
Light Weight Pop-Up Bed Net (Brown)	NSN 3740-01-518-7310

d. Command emphasis on compliance with medications and personal protective measures.

Figure 5-15. Maximum Malaria Protection

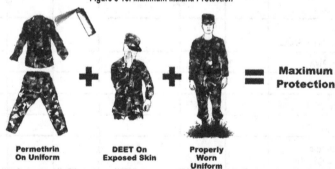

Permethrin On Uniform + DEET On Exposed Skin + Properly Worn Uniform = Maximum Protection

3. Discourage use of non-approved repellents. They are less effective and can be dangerous.
4. Administer prophylactic drugs to those who do not have contraindications, comply with pre-deployment dosing requirements, and advise patients of possible side effects. Provide alternative drug prophylaxis for those unable to take the first line regimen. Consider directly observed therapy (DOT). Determine need for terminal prophylaxis with primaquine (must know patient's G6PD status).
5. Make certain that all personnel know the symptoms of malaria and seek care for all febrile illnesses.
6. Know how and where to obtain a reliable malaria diagnosis (FDA approved rapid tests, expert microscopy).
7. Ensure that all infected patients are protected from biting mosquitoes to prevent transmitting malaria to others
8. Implement a vector control program (see Part 5: Specialty Areas: Chapter 13: Pest Control).

Chapter 13: Preventive Medicine: Field Sanitation (see FM 4-25.12)

LTC (P) Robert Mott, MC, USA

1. **General:**
   a. Factors that create a high risk for food-borne diseases: poor food inspection and sanitation, use of human and animal waste for fertilizer, poor personal hygiene habits, inadequate refrigeration, and lack of eradication programs for food-borne diseases such as hepatitis A and brucellosis.
   b. Food transportation, storage, preparation and service have direct bearing on success or failure of a mission. Dining Facility sanitation

is a chronic operational problem. The prospect of disease outbreaks, particularly dysentery and food poisoning must be recognized as a constant threat to unit health.

c. Potentially Hazardous Foods (PHFs): All food that contains milk, milk products, eggs, meat, poultry, fish, shellfish, or other ingredients in a form capable of supporting rapid growth of infectious or toxic microorganisms. PHFs are typically high in protein and have a water content greater than 85% and a pH greater than 4.5.

d. Factors that most often cause food-borne disease outbreaks:
  (1) Failure to keep PHF cold (below 40°F internal temp)
  (2) Failure to keep PHF hot (above 145°F internal temp)
  (3) Preparing foods a day or more before being served
  (4) Sick employees who practice poor personal hygiene to handle food

e. Food contamination can be classified into three categories:
  (1) Biological: contamination by pathogenic microorganisms (protozoa, bacteria, fungus, virus) or unacceptable levels of spoilage. This category is the major threat to personnel.
  (2) Chemical: contamination with chemical warfare agents, industrial chemicals, and/or other adulterating chemicals (zinc, copper, cadmium, pesticides, etc.).
  (3) Physical: contamination by arthropods, debris, radioactive particles, etc.

f. Bacteria that multiply at temperatures between 60°F and 125°F cause most food-borne illnesses. Maintain the internal temperature of cooked foods that will be served hot at 145°F or above. Maintain the internal temperatures of foods served cold at 40°F or below to control any bacteria that may be present in the food,

g. High food temperatures (160°F to 212°F) reached in boiling, baking, frying, and roasting will kill most bacteria that can cause food borne illness. Prompt refrigeration to 40°F or below in containers less than 2 inches deep inhibits growth of most (but not all) of these bacteria. Freezing at 0°F or below essentially stops bacteria growth, but will not kill bacteria that are already present.

h. Thorough reheating to an internal temperature of 165°F or above will kill bacteria that may have grown during storage. Foods that have been improperly stored or otherwise mishandled cannot be made safe by reheating.

i. Everything that touches food during preparation and serving must be clean to avoid introducing illness-causing bacteria.

2. **Procurement of Food:**
  a. Order of preference for food acquisition
    (1) US Military rations brought with unit or previously cached.
    (2) Local food procured from sources approved by supporting Veterinary and Environmental Science Officers.
    (3) Local food procured from unapproved sources.
  b. Guidelines for the use of food procured from unapproved sources:
    (1) Avoid local street vendors. Poor hygiene increases risk of contaminated food (ie, fecal-oral contamination).
    (2) All ice is contaminated. Freezing will not kill disease-causing organisms. Anything with ice in it or on it should be considered contaminated (ie, alcohol in the drink does not make the ice in it safe).
    (3) Semi-perishable rations (canned and dried products) are relatively safe and should be chosen over fresh food. Protect canned and dried foods from extreme heating and freezing. Do not use swollen or leaking cans.
    (4) Do not procure moldy grain or grain contaminated with insect larvae.
    (5) Wash raw fresh fruits and vegetables in potable water and disinfect with one of these methods:
      (a) Dip in boiling water for 15 seconds. Place small amounts of produce in net bags, completely submerge items for 15 seconds, remove and allow cooling. Not recommended for leafy vegetables.
      (b) Disinfect with chlorine. Immerse for at least 15 minutes in a 100ppm solution of chlorine or 30 minutes in a 50ppm solution. Rinse the produce thoroughly with potable water before cooking or eating. Break apart "head" produce such as lettuce, cabbage or celery before disinfection.

Table 5-17. Disinfection

Bleach: (Clorox)		70% Calcium Hypochlorite	
50 ppm =	4.84 oz in 32 gallons	50 ppm =	0.32 oz in 32 gallons
100 ppm =	9.68 oz in 32 gallons	100 ppm =	0.64 oz in 32 gallons
200 ppm =	1 tablespoon per gallon		

  (6) Always cook eggs to prevent salmonellosis. Blood and meat spots are acceptable, but cracked and rotten eggs are not acceptable and should be discarded.
  (7) Boil unpasteurized dairy products for at least 15 seconds to prevent tuberculosis, brucellosis, Q fever, etc. Avoid cheese, butter and ice cream made from unpasteurized milk, which can carry these diseases.
  (8) Cook all seafood to prevent hepatitis, tapeworms, flukes, cholera, etc.
    (a) Avoid shellfish - cooking does not degrade some toxins (red tide).
    (b) Certain saltwater fish have heat stable toxins that are not destroyed during cooking. Do not eat any species that the native population does not eat.
    (c) Avoid large predatory reef fish, like barracuda, grouper, snapper, jack, mackerel, and triggerfish, which may accumulate toxins (ciguatera).
  (9) Eat carcass or muscle meat rather than visceral meat (liver, heart, kidney, etc.). Muscle flesh is less likely to be contaminated. Fresh meat from healthy animals is safe if cooked thoroughly.

(a)   Be aware of geographic areas where toxins may occur in seafood.

(b)   Perform an antemortem examination (before slaughtering), use correct field slaughter methods and perform a postmortem examination (after slaughtering). *See Part 5: Specialty Areas: Chapter 14: Antemortem Exam & Postmortem Exam*

(c)   Color of meat should be red to slightly-red brown. Do not consume green or brown beef if possible. Avoid meat with off odors, such as sour or sweet, fruity smells. Cook meat until it is WELL DONE- do not eat rare, medium, or bloody meat. Sausages and meat products should be well cooked.

3.   **Food Storage and Preservation**

a.   Protect canned and dried foods from extreme heat and freezing.

b.   Store and preserve perishables (eg, meat, poultry, fish) by refrigerating at or below 40°F. Because refrigeration or potable ice is often not available, slaughter what you need, cook thoroughly and then consume immediately. Meat can be preserved by methods other than refrigeration if time and resources are available (eg, smoking, curing, making jerky or pemmican, salting, and pickling). *See Part 5: Specialty Areas: Chapter 14: Food Storage and Restoration*

c.   Semi-perishable foods such as potatoes and onions should be stored in a dry place off the ground, allowing air to circulate around them, retarding decay and spoilage.

d.   Store staple products (flour, sugar, etc.) in metal cans with tight-fitting lids.

e.   Do not store acidic foods or beverages such as tomatoes or citric juices in galvanized cans. This will prevent zinc poisoning.

4.   **Preparing and Serving Food:**

a.   Use pesticides according to the directions on the container. Limit residual sprays to crack and crevice treatment only. Protect all foods and food contact surfaces when applying pesticides.

b.   Coordinate food preparation and consumption to eliminate unnecessary lapses of time.

c.   Leftover food presents a problem. Produce the least amount of leftovers by planning meals. Discard items held at unsafe temperatures (40°F to 145°F) for 3 or more hours. Never save PHF foods such as creamed beef, casseroles or gravies.

d.   Meat may contain disease-producing agents that cannot be detected by inspection. Follow cooking procedures strictly to ensure heat penetrates to the center of the meat and that all the meat is cooked to at least 165°F. This applies to poultry, pork, beef and any stuffing or other foods containing these meats.

5.   **Cleaning and Disinfecting:**

a.   Cooking utensils and mess kits should be cleaned, disinfected, and properly stored after each use (*see Figure 5-16*). They must be scraped free of food particles, washed in hot (120°F-130°F) soapy water, rinsed in boiling water, sanitized for at least 10 seconds in another container of boiling water, and allowed to air dry. They must be stored in a clean, covered container that is protected from dust and vermin.

b.   When it is impossible to heat the water, utensils must be washed in soapy water, rinsed in 2 cans of clear water, then immersed in the 4th container of chlorine sanitizing solution for at least 30 seconds. Chemical sanitizing solutions are prepared in the following order of preference:

(1)   Use Disinfectant, Food Service, (NSN: 6840-00-810-6396) as specified on the label.

(2)   Use 1 level mess kit spoonful of calcium hypochlorite for every 10 gallons of water (250ppm solution).

(3)   Use 1 canteen cup of 5% liquid bleach in 32 gallons of water (250ppm solution).

c.   If mess kits become soiled or contaminated between meals, they should be rewashed prior to use as described previously. A pre-wash of boiling water should be available for use prior to all meals.

Figure 5-16. Mess Wash Setup

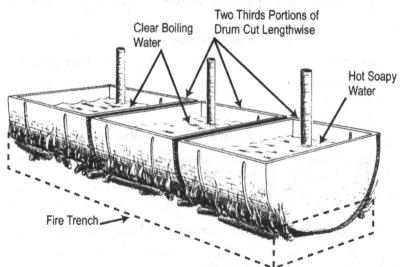

5-100

Chapter 13: Preventive Medicine: Waste Disposal (*see TM Med 593*)

LTC (P) Robert Mott, MC, USA

1. **General:**
   a. Proper waste disposal is necessary to prevent disease during real world contingencies and training exercises. Liquid and solid wastes produced under field conditions can amount to 100 pounds per person per day, especially when shower facilities are available. Without proper waste disposal methods, a camp will soon become an ideal breeding ground for flies, mosquitoes, rats, mice and other pests that spread diseases such as plague, dysentery, typhoid, dengue fever, and other vector-borne diseases.
   b. Types of waste: Human (feces and urine), animal, garbage, kitchen and bath liquid waste, rubbish, hazardous waste.
   c. Select disposal methods compatible with location, military situation and regulations.

2. **Human Waste Disposal:**
   a. Under field conditions, bury human waste when feasible.
   b. Devices most commonly used for various field situations are as follows:
      (1)   Cat Hole Latrine (for patrols); *see Figure 5-17*

Figure 5-17. Cat Hole Latrine

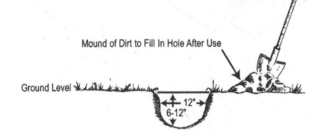

Mound of Dirt to Fill In Hole After Use

Ground Level

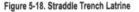

12"

6-12"

      (2)   Straddle Trench Latrine (1-3 day bivouac site); *see Figure 5-18*

Figure 5-18. Straddle Trench Latrine

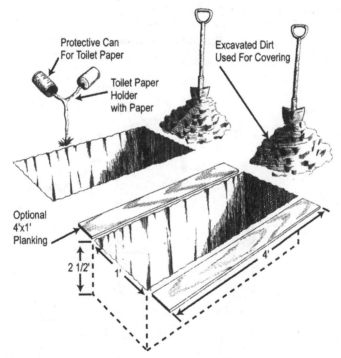

Protective Can
For Toilet Paper

Toilet Paper
Holder
with Paper

Excavated Dirt
Used For Covering

Optional
4'x1'
Planking

2 1/2'

1'

4'

(3) Deep Pit Latrine (temporary camp); *see Figure 5-19*

Figure 5-19. Deep Pit Latrine

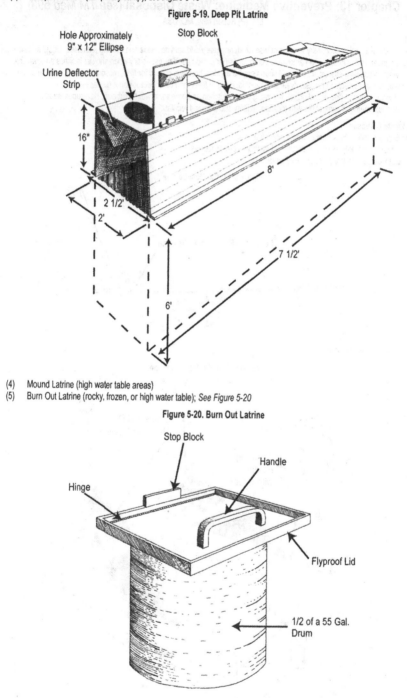

(4) Mound Latrine (high water table areas)
(5) Burn Out Latrine (rocky, frozen, or high water table); *See Figure 5-20*

Figure 5-20. Burn Out Latrine

(6) Pail Latrine (rocky, frozen, or high water table); see Figure 5-21

Figure 5-21. Pail Latrine

(7) Urine Soakage Pits (overnight or longer)
a. Through urinal; see Figure 5-22

Figure 5-22. Trough Urinal

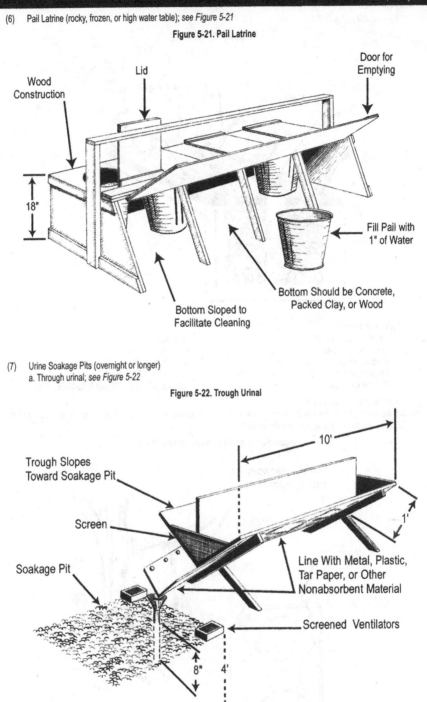

b. Pipe urinal; *see Figure 5-23*

Figure 5-23. Pipe Urinal

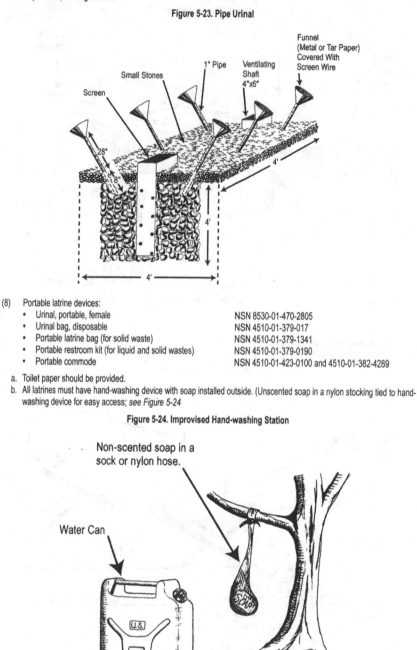

(8) Portable latrine devices:
- Urinal, portable, female   NSN 8530-01-470-2805
- Urinal bag, disposable   NSN 4510-01-379-017
- Portable latrine bag (for solid waste)   NSN 4510-01-379-1341
- Portable restroom kit (for liquid and solid wastes)   NSN 4510-01-379-0190
- Portable commode   NSN 4510-01-423-0100 and 4510-01-382-4289

a. Toilet paper should be provided.
b. All latrines must have hand-washing device with soap installed outside. (Unscented soap in a nylon stocking tied to hand-washing device for easy access; *see Figure 5-24*

Figure 5-24. Improvised Hand-washing Station

Non-scented soap in a
sock or nylon hose.

Water Can

c. Latrine Maintenance: Conduct the following procedures routinely:
- Inspect and spray for insects at least 2 x a week.
- Latrine seats and boxes should be scrubbed with soap and water and sanitized with a disinfectant on a daily basis.
- Ensure that the latrine box remains insect proof (fly-tight) at all times.

d. Pail Latrine: Clean daily. Dispose by burning (using 1 part gasoline and 4 parts diesel fuel) or hauling and burying (rinse pail with water and empty rinse water in the disposal site). If available, dispose of waste at a sewage treatment plant. Emptying and hauling containers of waste must be closely supervised to prevent careless spillage. Use plastic bag liners to reduce risk of accidental spillage. The filled bags are tied at the top then are disposed of by burning or burial.

e. Constructing and Closing Urinals: Construct 1 per 20 men. Locate urine pits so the urine will not drain into the pit latrine unless the ground is porous enough to absorb the extra liquid. The urine soakage pit is the best means of urine disposal in the field. When a urine soakage pit is closed or abandoned it should be sprayed with residual pesticide and mounded over with 2 feet of compacted soil. Mark the site with a sign that labeled: CLOSED SOAKAGE PIT, date and unit (security permitting).

f. Closing Latrines: Close a latrine when it is filled to within 1 foot of the ground surface or when it is abandoned. Spray the contents of the pit, the sidewalls and the ground surface surrounding the pit with a residual pesticide. Fill the pit up to the ground surface with successive 3 inch layers of earth. Pack each layer down and spray it with pesticide before adding the next layer of dirt. Mound the latrine pit over with at least 1 foot of dirt and spray it again. Indicate the location of the latrine with a sign marked: CLOSED LATRINE, date and unit (security permitting)

3. Liquid Waste (Kitchen, Bath):

a. Most common ways used to dispose of kitchen or bath liquid waste are: soakage pits, soakage trenches, evaporation beds, and grease traps.

b. Use soakage pits for all water facilities (ie, under water trailer faucets, Lyster bags, and hand washing devices).

c. Rules for construction, maintenance, and closing of liquid waste disposal devices:

  1. Do not dig pit or trench into ground water table to avoid contamination.
  2. Place one site adjacent to the mess kit laundry to avoid spillage.
  3. Dig drainage ditches around each pit/trench to prevent surface water runoff from flowing into the soakage pits or trenches.
  4. Police the soakage pit/trench area, as needed.
  5. Use an approved residual pesticide on the pit/trench contents and the surrounding ground area to control insects.
  6. When the pit/trench becomes clogged, close it by covering it with 1 foot of compacted dirt and mark it with a sign indicating the type of pit, date closed, and unit (security permitting).

4. Garbage and Rubbish (Refuse) Disposal:

a. Burial or incineration

b. Collect personnel refuse in: 32 gallon galvanized can with cover, 55 gallon drum with improvised cover, or in plastic bags (rubbish only).

c. Incinerate combustible refuse when tactical situation and local policy permits. Incinerate refuse in a barrel or inclined plane incinerator. Burial methods depend on the amount of refuse to be buried-small amounts (1-2 barrels) can be buried using a pit, but large amounts will need to be placed in a sanitary landfill on the local economy.

5. Regulated Medical Waste (RMW):

a. Classification

  (1) Regulated medical waste (RMW) is waste generated by medical, veterinary, and dental treatment facilities, which are capable of causing disease, and may pose a health risk. These wastes are defined in US Army MEDCOM Reg 40-35 and include cultures and stocks of infectious agents; pathological waste (tissues, organs, body parts, teeth); human blood/blood products; isolation waste from patient rooms; sharps (syringes, scalpels, blades); human body fluids (semen, vaginal secretions, cerebrospinal fluids, pleural fluids) and contaminated animal carcasses, body parts, and bedding used in animal research.

  (2) Identify diseases unique to a specific theater. The theater surgeon should designate whether non-bloody wastes from these diseases require management as RMW. The decision is based on the nature of the disease, prevalence, method of transmission, and other risks.

  (3) Whole bodies are not considered RMW. Quartermaster units will manage human bodies according to Joint Publication (JP) 4-06.

  (4) Animal body parts, carcasses, and bedding (not contaminated by medical research) are not considered RMW, and may be incinerated or placed in landfill.

  (5) Personnel handling blood-soaked clothing or equipment (such as body armor) should adhere to the handling guidance provided in paragraph 5b below. To render items non-infectious, wash blood-soaked items with soap and hot water. Adhere to the cleaning guidance provided on clothing/equipment labels, or consult with Quartermaster personnel for detailed laundering instructions. Logistics personnel will evaluate item serviceability and make the final decision regarding disposition of government-issued clothing and equipment.

b. Handling

  (1) Use standard precautions when handling wastes generated as a result of treating patients or animals. Personal protective equipment includes protective gloves (latex, butyl rubber, or other types impermeable to blood), masks/safety goggles/safety glasses, and other equipment that will prevent personnel from contracting communicable illnesses from patients or their wastes. Exposed skin should be washed with soap and water.

  (2) Personnel should wear both skin protection and respiratory protection when burning or incinerating medical waste, and should avoid standing in the resulting smoke plume. An air-purifying respirator (cartridge or canister) with a high-efficiency particulate air (HEPA) filter is recommended. Commercial respirators approved by the National Institute for Occupational Safety and Health with a P100 or N100 rating are preferred. The M40 protective mask should only be used until commercial respirators are obtained. Paper surgical masks do not protect from hazards inherent in the burning of waste and should not be substituted for an air-purifying respirator. Respiratory protection is only needed for those personnel remaining in the immediate vicinity of the burning process. Personnel tasked to incinerate medical waste must be medically cleared to wear a respirator, properly fit-tested on an approved respirator, and enrolled in a medical surveillance program. **Note:** Burning RMW or any other waste is not authorized for CONUS field training exercises

c. Collection, Segregation, and Storage

(1) Contact the supporting Medical Logistics unit or Class VIII manager for medical waste storage containers. Collect RMW at the point of generation in red bags (or other color specified for the theater). Sharps will be collected in puncture-resistant, leak-resistant, and uniquely colored or marked containers. If proper sharps containers are not available, use any rigid plastic or metal containers (such as coffee cans or plastic drink bottles) for collection. These nonstandard containers should be placed into red bags or proper sharps containers as soon as possible for disposal.

(2) All bags or receptacles used to segregate, transport, or store RMW will be clearly marked with the universal biohazard symbol and the word "BIOHAZARD" in English and any other language suitable for the region.

(3) Never mix RMW with regular trash or Hazardous Waste, unless required for the burning process. Medical personnel should also take care to ensure clothing and bandages placed into red bags do not contain ammunition or other unexploded ordnance.

(4) Store RMW in secure, ventilated areas that offer protection from the sun, rain, scavengers, and pests. Collection in a covered cargo trailer facilitates the transport of the waste from the medical facility.

(5) Medical waste (other than sharps containers) should not be stored above 40°F (4.4°C) for longer than 5 days.

d. Transporting RMW in the Field Environment:

(1) RMW is considered a Hazardous Material for transportation purposes and must comply with the requirements of 49 CFR 100-185 and DOD 4500.9-R. RMW transported by military aircraft must comply with the AFMAN 24-204(I).

(2) Transport RMW in military, government, or contractor vehicles. Use of privately owned vehicles is not authorized.

(3) The RMW must be secured to prevent excessive movement and will not be transported alongside items intended for consumption.

(4) A spill kit must be readily available to decontaminate any surfaces in the event of a leak or spill and shall include: appropriate PPE, a disinfectant, absorbent material, and equipment used to gather spill residues. The kit may be assembled at the local level or purchased commercially.

(5) If RMW must be transported across public roads, the driver must receive training according to 49 CFR 177.

(6) Vehicles used to transport RMW must be cleaned and disinfected prior to use for any other purpose.

e. Treatment and Disposal

(1) On installations in the US and overseas, commercial contractors will be used for RMW disposal (DLA/DRMS does not manage medical waste). All RMW generated during field exercises should be backhauled to garrison. During contingency operations, RMW may be incinerated, burned, sterilized, or buried according to guidance provided in the combatant command's operations order. Incineration and burn activities should be conducted as far downwind as possible (at least 450 feet) from troop locations and living areas.

(2) Incineration: Use of a commercial incinerator capable of subjecting the waste to a minimum burn temperature of 1500°F (816°C) for at least 1 hour is the preferred method of destruction. Incinerator operators must be trained on proper operating and maintenance procedures, safety measures (to include PPE use), emergency response, and local environmental requirements. Incinerator bottom ash and air pollution control ash (if applicable) should be tested for HW properties prior to disposal in a solid waste landfill. Aerosol cans, gas cylinders, and batteries should never be incinerated. Seek approval from the local commander prior to operating field expedient devices such as the inclined-plane incinerator with vapor burner (described in FM 4-25.12).

(3) Burning in barrels: Burning RMW in barrels or pits is permissible if approved by appropriate command personnel and local officials, and conform to regulatory policies for the region. Whenever possible, avoid burning when wind and other conditions could cause smoke to blow in the direction of personnel at the base camp. Only personnel involved in the actual burning need to wear respiratory protection. To ignite the burn, mix one part gasoline with five parts JP-8. Use a stick or pole to light the fuel from a distance of at least 3 feet. Mixing medical waste with regular solid waste (approximately 50/50 mixture) will help ensure the hottest and cleanest burn possible. The remaining ash may be buried in a solid waste landfill. Aerosol cans, gas cylinders, and batteries should never be burned.

(4) Sterilization: Steam sterilization is another alternative to treatment of RMW. Ensure the waste is secured in autoclave bags (regular plastic bags may melt) prior to placement in the sterilizer. Autoclave indicator tape, if available, will demonstrate when sterilization is complete. Guidelines for minimum operational temperatures and detention times are: 250°F for 90 minutes at 15 pounds per square inch (psi) gauge pressure, 272°F for 45 minutes at 27 psi gauge pressure, or 320°F for 16 minutes at 80 psi gauge pressure. After the RMW is sterilized and cooled, the waste may be managed as general trash. Ensure care is taken when handling the waste to minimize needle sticks. STERILIZERS USED TO AUTOCLAVE MEDICAL WASTE MUST NEVER BE USED TO STERILIZE OTHER MEDICAL ITEMS (such as medical instruments or dressings). Permanently and indelibly mark medical waste incinerators as "For Medical Waste Only—Do Not Use for Sterilization" or words to that effect. Have a contingency plan in place to manage waste that was intended for sterilization if the steam sterilizer becomes nonfunctional.

(5) Retrograding: Retrograding waste back to the rear where facilities are available may be feasible if burning, incineration, or sterilization is not possible. International agreements govern the retrograde of medical waste, and any such movement must be coordinated through the combatant command.

(6) Burial: The last resort is burying untreated medical waste in a sanitary landfill. This method should be employed only during contingency operations in areas with low water tables. Care must be taken to bury RMW below the scavenger depth of 8 feet. A layer of lime may be placed over the waste prior to burial to accelerate decomposition and provide a measure of chemical disinfection. Because the Army will most likely have to retrieve this waste later, medical waste burial sites must be marked and grid locations reported through the chain of command.

(7) Alternative technologies: Alternative technologies may also be used to treat and dispose of RMW. If connected to a functional domestic wastewater treatment plant, bulk blood or blood products may be poured into clinical sinks. See Table 5-18 for more information.

Table 5-18. Treatment and Disposal Methods for Regulated Medical Waste

Type of RMW	Method of treatment	Method of disposal
Microbiological	Steam sterilization [1] Chemical disinfection Incineration	Municipal landfill Municipal landfill Municipal landfill
Pathological	Incineration [2] Cremation [2] Chemical sterilization [3] Steam sterilization [3]	Municipal landfill Burial Domestic wastewater treatment plant Domestic wastewater treatment plan
Bulk blood & suction canister waste	Steam sterilization [4] Incineration [4]	Domestic wastewater treatment plant Municipal landfill
Sharps and sharps containers	Steam sterilization Incineration	Municipal landfill Municipal landfill

Notes:

[1]. Preferred method for cultures and stocks because they can be treated at point of generation.

[2]. Anatomical pathology waste (that is, large body parts) must be treated either by incineration or cremation prior to disposal.

[3]. This only applies to placentas, small organs and small body parts that may be steam sterilized or chemically sterilized, ground, and discharged to a domestic wastewater treatment plant.

[4]. Bulk blood or suction canister waste known to be infectious must be treated by incineration or steam sterilization before disposal.

Chapter 13: Preventive Medicine: Field Water Purification
(see FM 21-10/MCRP 4-11.1D)

LTC (P) Robert Mott, MC, USA

1. Treat and disinfect all sources of water other than US Military Installation or Quartermaster produced or approved water in the field.
2. Minimize the possibility of water-borne illness by selecting proper sources.
3. Water consumed by personnel will come from four possible sources. These sources are prioritized in the order in which they should be chosen for use:
   a. Fixed Facility (closed pipe system with treatment)
   b. Water Production Points (portable units, ie, (ROWPU - [Reverse Osmosis Water Purification Unit])
   c. Bottled water
   d. Emergency (raw water from the five natural sources) from:
      (1) Surface water (lakes, rivers, streams)
      (2) Ground water (wells, springs)
      (3) Rain water
      (4) Ice
      (5) Snow
4. Easy access to large quantities of water will usually make surface water the best emergency source. When selecting a water source for a Special Operations unit, consider certain factors:
   a. Military Situation: *Does the site provide cover and concealment? Is the site accessible to Soldiers? Can water be extracted with available equipment? Can the source be used without interference from the enemy? Is the water source accessible under all weather conditions? Is the site a safe distance from targets?*
   b. Quantity of Water: *Is there enough water in the source to sustain the troops for the desired time? Can enough water be acquired quickly?*
   c. Quality of the Water: A detailed site survey is critical in selecting a quality water source. Check the site for possible sources of pollution: dead fish, frogs, or other animals; excessive algae growth; oil slicks or sludge deposits; and the conditions of vegetation around the site. Dead or mottled vegetation may indicate chemical agent contamination. If possible, reconnoiter for a distance of two miles upstream of the source to locate any possible sources of contamination. Locate any bivouac site at least 100 feet downstream of the water point. Avoid using stagnant or swampy areas as water sources.
5. Water Treatment:
   a. During deployments personnel will utilize the following prioritization and standards for water treatment of the four types of water sources:
      (1) Fixed Facility: Chlorinate to a minimum of 2ppm prior to consumption. If individual containers (2 quarts or less) are to be used for transport/storage of water, treat with iodine tabs (2 tabs/quart) or chlorinate to 2ppm prior to consumption. If bulk containers (>5 gallons) are to be used for storage/transportation of water, chlorinate to 2ppm. This water source is preferable to all others.
      (2) Water Production Points: Chlorinate to 2ppm prior to consumption.
      (3) Bottled Water: Carbonated bottled water needs no further treatment. If the containers are broken down and the water is placed in other containers (not the originals), then treat the water with iodine (2 tabs/quart) or chlorine (2ppm). This source is preferred when approved fixed facilities are not available.
      (4) Emergency Water: Select the least contaminated raw water source available. Filter water with a KATADYN or SWEETWATER filter system (both systems are GSA approved and can be purchased through your logistics channels) or through any system with

an absolute pore size of 0.2 microns or smaller. USACHPPM has a database on their website with test results for COTS filters and treatment systems. Treat water with iodine (2 tabs/quart) or chlorine (2ppm) prior to consumption. Seawater must not be utilized for consumption.

b. Determination of Chlorine Residual: The N, N-diethyl-p-phenylene-diamine (DPD) chlorine residual determination kit has been placed in the updated field chlorination kits. The new kit consists of a color comparator with color comparisons for measuring 1, 1.5, 2, 3, 5, and 10mg/L chlorine residual.

c. Use the following guidelines for treating water:

  (1) Individual Canteen (1 or 2 Quart)

  (2) Iodine Tabs - NSN 6850-00-985-7166. Use 2 tabs per quart.

  (3) Chlorine - Chlorination kit: NSN 6850-00-270-6225

    (a) Locate water source. Fill canteen with cleanest water available.

    (b) Prepare a solution by pouring the contents of one (1) ampule of calcium hypochlorite into 1/2 canteen cup of water. Thoroughly mix the solution.

    (c) Add 1 canteen capful (NBC WATER CAP) per quart.

    (d) Shake the canteen to mix. Wait five (5) minutes (contact time). Loosen cap to allow water to seep around the threads of the neck and cap of the canteen. Re-tighten cap. Wait an additional twenty-five (25) minutes before using the water.

    (e) In cold weather, wait 40 minutes before using the water.

  (4) Chlorine - Bleach:

    (a) Locate water source. Fill canteen with cleanest water available.

    (b) Use 2-3 drops of household bleach per quart

    (c) Follow directions in steps 4 and 5.

  (5) Boiling (least preferred):

    (a) Locate water source. Use cleanest water available.

    (b) Bring water to a roiling boil for 3-5 minutes. This will kill most organisms that are known to cause intestinal diseases.

    (c) In areas where Giardia, Entamoeba histolytica or viral hepatitis are known to be present, boil water for thirty (30) minutes to ensure destruction of the microorganisms.

    (d) In emergency situations, boil water for a minimum of 15-30 seconds.

    (e) High altitudes may require additional boiling.

    (f) Allow water to cool before dispensing or drinking.

    (g) Boiling provides no residual protection against recontamination and should only be used as a last resort. Water can become re-contaminated if not protected properly after decontamination.

  (6) Other Chemical treatments:

    (a) Povidone-iodine solution 10%, NOT THE SCRUB SOLUTION): 16 drops per liter gives 8ppm iodine. Contact time is 20 minutes minimum or 90 minutes for cold, turbid water.

    (b) Chlor-Floc tablets: 1 tablet per liter of water makes 8.4ppm chlorine. Contact time is 15 minutes minimum or 60-90 minutes for cold, turbid water. These tablets have a flocculation material to clear turbid water. After treatment, the water must be strained before drinking, ie, through a T-shirt.

6. Depending on the nature and extent of the operation, determine the need to conduct area mosquito control operations, to include control or elimination of breeding sites, use of larvicides and use of sprays.

Chapter 13: Preventive Medicine: Pest Control

LTC (P) Robert Mott, MC, USA

1. **Note:** Pests that require a blood meal are attracted to humans or animals by carbon dioxide emitted from the body.

2. Identify and eliminate breeding sites for mosquitoes and other insects by improving drainage, disposing of refuse properly and applying appropriate chemicals.

3. Clear dense vegetation or other harborages inhabited by pests from living areas.

4. Use chemical pesticides properly. Follow the instructions on the label.

  a. Ensure that the chemical pesticides you are using are effective against the vectors you want to control.

  b. Mix chemical pesticides in proper concentrations and dispense in sufficient density to control the desired pest.

  c. Spray approved pesticides into areas of heavy vegetation that cannot be cleared.

  d. Apply approved bait pesticides in areas where rodents are suspected to frequent. Trap rodents when feasible, since it is a safer alternative to chemical pesticides.

  e. Dispense chemical pesticides using proper personal protective measures. Wear eye protection, rubber gloves and facemask respirator when handling pesticides.

  f. Ensure that chemical pesticides used inside living areas are labeled safe for such use.

  g. Ensure all chemical pesticides are always stored in safe, secured areas.

  h. Properly dispose of all empty pesticide containers and materials contaminated with pesticides according to product labels.

5. Remove food sources. Avoid eating in sleeping areas. Even small amounts of food attract insects and rodents.

6. Do not have pets near living areas. They harbor fleas, ticks and other insects and can attract mosquitoes and other pests.

7. Use personal protective measures, to include respiratory protection, when entering areas suspected of housing rodents or birds.

Chapter 13: Preventive Medicine: Rabies Control

LTC (P) Robert Mott, MC, US

1. Assess the rabies threat in the deployment area and initiate a control program, if needed.

2. Identify personnel at risk and vaccinate them pre-deployment.

3. Maintain and review current guidelines for pre- and post-exposure rabies management (*see Part 5: Specialty Areas: Chapter 12: Viral Infections: Rabies*). Know where to obtain post-exposure vaccine and Rabies Immune Globulin (RIG).
4. Identify rabies testing laboratory (if available) and domestic and wild animal control resources in the deployment area.
5. Immunize pets and domestic animals.
6. Impound stray animals.
7. Work with animal control personnel to reduce the wild animal reservoir if necessary and feasible.
8. Identify, evaluate, treat and report human exposures.
9. Conduct surveillance for human cases and cases in domestic and wild animals.
10. Advise the command on the rabies threat and recommend preventive countermeasures.
11. Inform at-risk personnel about the transmission, prevention and clinical aspects of rabies. Stress the importance of reporting animal bites or other suspicious animal contact.

Chapter 13: Preventive Medicine: Landfill Management

LTC (P) Robert Mott, MC, US

Note: In the US, military personnel must abide by EPA standards for landfills even on deployments. Consult land managers or custodians for guidance as needed.

1. Suggestions for a host nation landfill operation:
   a. Identify a large area of land that will not be used for many years after the landfill is closed.
   b. Use a dump truck and a bucket loader if available
   c. Find an area close to the site to store excavated dirt while the landfill is constructed.
   d. The pit will need to be lined will a nonporous membrane (such as clay) to prevent pollutants from leaching into the water table and contaminating the water.
   e. Size: Use 1 acre per year per 10,000 people as an estimate. High water tables or rocky soil will limit pit depth.

2. Pit Operations:
   a. The pit must be accessible to vehicles (dump trucks) and so allow them to enter the pit. The bucket loader must cover the refuse throughout the day and at the end of the day.
   b. Dispose of refuse in 10 feet wide sub-compartments in the landfill and cover them as the landfill is filled.
   c. Do not fill the sub-compartments with more than 6 feet of trash. Cover at the end of every day or when full.
   d. Use a windscreen on the downwind side of the landfill to catch debris.

Chapter 13: Preventive Medicine: Hearing Protection

LTC (P) Robert Mott, MC, US

1. Plan for Noise:
   a. Ensure that hearing conservation is part of the unit SOP.
   b. Ensure all service members are medically fitted for hearing protectors and are issued multiple sets. Ensure all service members have annual hearing test/screening.
   c. Train unit to do mission while wearing hearing protectors.
   d. Identify existing noise in your unit. If necessary, request PVNTMED assistance in identifying sources. Post **Noise Hazard** signs in noise hazardous areas and on noise hazardous equipment.
   e. Control noise sources. Isolate by distance; that is, keep troops away from noise, if possible. Isolate by barrier; for example, use sandbags. Use organic equipment controls; for example, keep mufflers and engine covers in good repair.

2. Enforce Individual Protective Measures:
   a. Ensure that service members wear earplugs or other hearing protective devices. Clean hearing protectors regularly.
   b. Do not remove inserts from aircraft or tracked vehicle helmets.
   c. Avoid unnecessary exposure. Limit necessary exposure to short, infrequent, mission-essential times.

Chapter 14: Veterinary Medicine: Antemortem Exam

LTC Joseph G. Williamson, VC, USA

When: Antemortem exam is the inspection of a live animal prior to slaughtering it for food purposes. Accept only those animals that are healthy, free of harmful diseases and chemicals and capable of being converted into wholesome products for consumption. This screening process only removes obviously diseased animals. A postmortem exam should be conducted prior to consuming any tissue or organ system.
See Part 5: Specialty Areas: Chapter 14: Postmortem Exam

What You Need: Gloves and a stethoscope

What To Do: Observe the animal at rest and in motion. You may see lameness, pain, neuromuscular deficits and/or systemic disease states in a moving animal that are not apparent in an animal at rest. Look for abnormal conditions such as continuous scratching/rubbing, emaciation or depression.

Examination Specifics:
Lameness: Reject if limbs are deformed or have gross swelling around joints. Do not use a limb if it is damaged or broken. You may consume the rest of the carcass if it is normal.
Emaciation: Reject animal if in poor state of nutrition, as evidenced by extreme thinness.

Organ Systems Analysis:
Respiratory: Reject if animal has difficulty breathing, severe coughing or excessive muco-purulent discharges.

Digestive: Reject if animal fails to eat, drink, or defecate.

Urinary: Reject if posture is abnormal when urinating, if animal strains to urinate or if urine has an unnatural color (hematuria).

Reproductive: Reject animals with foul discharges from vulva, mammaries or prepuce; or with retained placentas/fetal membranes.

CNS: Reject all animals that show depression or disinterest in environment, are "downer" animals (prefer to stay down on the ground), that will not respond to stimuli, have abnormal gaits or movements, or are hypersensitive to normal stimuli.

Mucous membranes: Reject if mucous membranes are pale, "muddy" or yellow-colored.

Skin and hair coat: Reject if skin is yellow-colored or has diffuse discolorations (red or black) or lesions. Consider rejecting animals that have obvious hair loss indicative of systemic disease.

What Not To Do:

1. Do not accept animal if diffuse lesions are found. If lesions are localized, they may be trimmed and the carcass retained for consumption.
2. Do not consume an animal from an unknown source unless the carcass passes the antemortem and postmortem examinations and is cleared for consumption.

Chapter 14: Veterinary Medicine: Humane Slaughter and Field Dressing

LTC Joseph G. Williamson, VC, USA

When: It may become necessary to capture, dress, and slaughter game in order to eat and continue the mission. The following guide is one of many ways to humanely slaughter and dress animals in a field environment. Pistols are recommended as the round will be easier to aim on the animal's head and will be less likely to exit the animal and ricochet. Perform an antemortem exam prior to slaughtering the animal, and a post-mortem exam after. *See Food Preservation section* to process meat that is not immediately consumed.

What You Need: Knife, firearm, rope, gloves

What To Do:

1. **Humane Kill** (*see Figure 5-25*): The following diagrams illustrate the proper position for a firearm to humanely kill/stun various livestock species. Natural tendency is to place barrel perpendicular to animal's head which places bullet too low. Incline barrel so it tends more toward the animal's nose (more horizontal) and aim toward where the skull attaches to the spine. Be sure to aim along the center of the head. Note in example "B", shooting from the back of the head, that such a method may be better used for animals with horns which can be restrained. There is more likelihood to miss from the back of the head if the head cannot be restrained (ie, does not have horns to hold) and the animal is moving its head.

Figure 5-25. Humane Kill

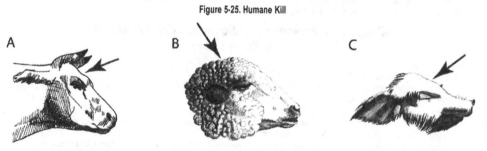

2. **Procedures for Field Dressing:**
   a. After killing the animal, bleed it promptly by cutting its throat at point A (*see Figure 5-26*). If the head is to be salvaged, then insert knife at point B, cutting deeply until blood flows freely.

Figure 5-26. Field Dressing Procedure: Cutting Throat

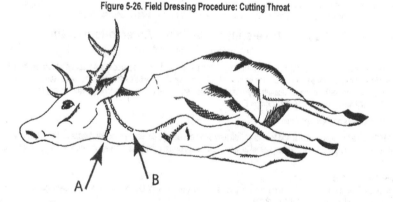

   b. Remove genitals or udder (*see Figure 5-27*). Prop the carcass belly up using rocks or brush for support. Cut circular area shown in illustration. Remove musk glands at points A and B to prevent tainting the meat.

Figure 5-27. Field Dressing Procedure: Removal of Genitals/Udder

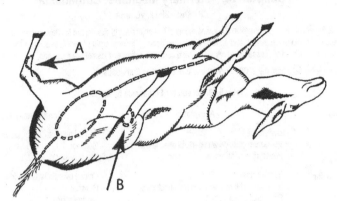

c. Split hide from tail to throat (*see Figure 5-28*) by **carefully** inserting the knife under the skin, but do not perforate the paunch or intestines. Cut around the anus and free the bung so it may be removed with the intestines. Cut around the diaphragm to free it from rib cage.

Figure 5-28. Field Dressing Procedure: Splitting Hide from Tail to Throat

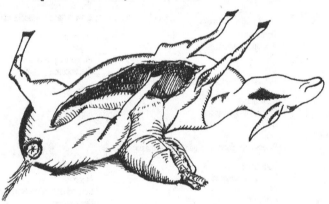

d. Reach forward to cut the vessels, gullet and windpipe. Free the gullet and viscera and remove them from the animal. If skinning the animal, it is best to peel the hide off. Using a knife can perforate and contaminate the meat.

3. **Skinning** (*see Figure 5-29*): Make circumferential cuts around each limb above the elbow; connect them to midline cut and PEEL, DO NOT CUT OR SCRAPE away hide.

Figure 5-29. Skinning

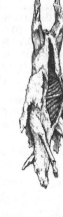

4. **Preparation:**
    a. **Pork:** After slaughter, ensure animal is bled out completely before scalding or boiling off the hair.
    b. **Poultry:** There are several methods of slaughter:
        (1) wringing the neck
        (2) dislocating the neck or
        (3) beheading
        Bleed out animal completely before boiling. Boil the bird to remove skin contaminants and ease the removal of the feathers. Then eviscerate by opening the abdominal cavity and removing organs. The carcass is ready for cooking and consumption.

What Not To Do:
    1. Do not slaughter sick or debilitated animals for consumption.
    2. Do not use a blade to skin the carcass; PEEL the hide from the body.
    3. Do not consume meat until it is well cooked.

Chapter 14: Veterinary Medicine: Euthanasia

CPT Kristin Bloink, VC, USA

What: Euthanasia is the act of killing an animal in a humane manner. The objectives of this act are to alleviate pain and suffering, minimize fear and anxiety before consciousness is lost, and achieve a pain-free death. The ideal order of events to achieve these objectives is loss of consciousness, loss of motor function, cessation of respiratory and cardiac function and loss of brain function.

What You Need: See Table 5-19 from the 2000 Report of the AVMA Panel on Euthanasia

Table 5-19. Acceptable Euthanasia by Species

Species	Acceptable	Conditionally Acceptable
Equine	Barbiturates Potassium chloride with general anesthesia Penetrating captive bolt	Chloral hydrate IV with sedation Gunshot Electrocution
Bovine, caprine, ovine	Barbiturates Potassium chloride with general anesthesia Penetrating captive bolt	Chloral hydrate IV with sedation Gunshot Electrocution
Swine	Barbiturates CO_2 Potassium chloride with general anesthesia Penetrating captive bolt	Inhalant anesthetics CO Chloral hydrate IV with sedation Gunshot Electrocution Blow to head (<3 weeks of age)
Canine	Barbiturates Inhalant anesthetics CO_2 CO Potassium chloride with general anesthesia	Nitrogen Argon Penetrating captive bolt Electrocution
Feline	Barbiturates Inhalant anesthetics CO_2 CO Potassium chloride with general anesthesia	Nitrogen Argon
Rabbit	Barbiturates Inhalant anesthetics CO_2 CO	Nitrogen Argon Cervical dislocation (<1kg body weight) Decapitation
Zoo animals	Potassium chloride with general anesthesia Barbiturates Inhalant anesthetics CO_2 CO Potassium chloride with general anesthesia	Penetrating captive bolt Nitrogen Argon Penetrating captive bolt Gunshot

What To Do: In most environments where military operations are taking place, IV barbiturates, CO, or gunshot techniques will be the most readily available euthanasia methods.

Barbiturates: Ideally delivered IV. The most common agents are **pentobarbital sodium** with or without **phenytoin sodium**.

CO: Use commercial compressed gas, not vehicle exhaust. Create a sealed chamber to protect operators/bystanders and to achieve at least a 6% CO concentration.

Gunshot: Select the appropriate firearm for the situation with the goal being penetration and destruction of brain tissue without emergence from the contralateral side of the head. The differences in brain position and skull conformation between species must be considered. *See Figure 5-25*

Equine: Target is the crossover point where the lines between the corner of each eye and the base of the opposite ear cross on the forehead

Bovine/Caprine/Ovine: *See Part 5: Specialty Areas: Chapter 14: Humane Slaughter and Field Dressing*

Swine: *See Part 5: Specialty Areas: Chapter 14: Humane Slaughter and Field Dressing*

Definitively confirm death by listening for cessation of heart function

What Not To Do:
1. Do not neglect human psychological responses by animal owners, bystanders and euthanasia staff.
2. Do not allow consumption of any portion of the carcass by humans or animals if chemical agents are used in the euthanasia process

Chapter 14: Veterinary Medicine: Postmortem Exam

LTC Joseph G. Williamson, VC, USA

When: Upon completion of a thorough Antemortem Exam, examine animal carcasses immediately after slaughter and evisceration for possible lesions that indicate unsuitability of meat for consumption. Examine all parts of the carcass. The following guidelines are for any species that may be consumed in the field environment. Avoid introducing external contamination to the carcass.

What You Need: Gloves, sharp knife

What To Do: Examine:
1. **General:** Condemn animals with gross contamination of interior surfaces or organ systems and/or discoloration of peritoneal or pleural cavities. Generalized abscesses, emaciation, and jaundiced organs or tissues are reasons for condemnation. <u>Localized lesions are acceptable but generalized conditions are not</u>. Consider acute disease processes vs. chronic processes. Lymphadenopathy indicates disease or inflammation in the area drained by the enlarged nodes. Local adenopathy may indicate a local process only (condemn only affected area), while more extensive adenopathy probably implies widespread disease process.
2. **Head:** Inspect for swelling or firm masses along jaw or face. Palpate and examine lymph nodes of the head and neck for gross swellings or lesions.
3. **Viscera:** Palpate and examine the lymph nodes. Inspect and palpate all surfaces for abnormalities, discoloration, masses and parasites; examine the heart, lungs and diaphragm as well. Slice open organs and examine for parasites, infection, or disease states, such as tumors. **Note:** Examine viscera away from the carcass to avoid contamination.
4. **Joints and Skeletal Muscles:** Bruises and localized lesions may be removed and the rest of the carcass consumed. For arthritic and swollen joints, remove affected limb, and then consume carcass if arthritis is not due to systemic disease such as septicemia or caseous (cheese-like) lymphadenitis. Do not consume broken or mangled limbs.
5. **Neoplasia, Tumors or Abnormal Growths:** Condemn organ system and/or carcass if spread throughout.
6. **Off Odors:** Condemn carcass with strong odors of urine, ketones (a fruity smell) or pungent sexual odors.

What Not To Do:
1. Do not consume organs that appear discolored.
2. Do not consume the liver if it appears spotty, discolored, or friable (crumbly).
Note: Systemic illness and internal disease states may not be evident on antemortem exam; therefore postmortem exam is a necessity when an animal is from an unknown or non-approved source. When in doubt, do not consume and do not cure, smoke or otherwise preserve the meat.

Chapter 14: Veterinary Medicine: Food Storage and Preservation

LTC Joseph G. Williamson, VC, USA

When: The easiest way to avoid food-borne illnesses in a field environment is to immediately consume well-cleaned and cooked foodstuffs. When excess food must be stored and preserved for future use, follow these rules: preserve and store only wholesome foods that were initially safe to eat; use only potable water and spices when curing or preserving food; cold storage/freezing is the best method if available; periodic re-examination of stored products is essential to ensure wholesomeness and prevent consumption of contaminated or deteriorated food (moldy, infested, stale). Avoid food- and water-borne diseases through continuous use of these guidelines.

What You Need: Knife, meat, potable water, salt, 1% salt solution (brine), string, green hardwoods, building, saltpeter **(potassium nitrate)**, spices, fire source, hay, salt box and/or brine pan, boiling pot.

What To Do:
1. **Curing:** Although it may be done alone, curing should be done in association with smoking. Various spices, salts, sugars and brines can be used.
   a. Raw meat should be clean, edible and sliced against the grain into manageable pieces (step one of beef prep for smoking). Salt the meat in a dry, sheltered area secure from rodents and insects. Always CURE before SMOKING.
   b. Use coarse salt, not table salt. Additional spices may be added to the salt for flavor. If using brine, then the solution should be 1% salt (one pound of salt to 9 pints water). Use clean plastic, glass or earthenware containers, not wood or metal containers to hold brine solutions.
   c. Construct a salt box large enough to hold all of the meat. Cover the bottom of the box with salt. Rub salt into meat thoroughly and place in box. Separate pieces of meat to avoid contact. Cover with salt. Repeat this procedure in two days and again in two days. DO NOT REUSE salt or brine; discard after each use and begin with fresh salt or brine.
   d. On day six, remove from salt box. Dry the meat by pacing a layer of green pine straw, hay, grasses, etc. on the floor and cover hay with salt. Place meat on salt-covered hay; cover again with salt then top with hay. Ensure that the area is free of rodents and insects.
   e. Wash salt-cured meat before eating.
2. **Smoking:** There are several acceptable procedures for smoking meat and different step by step processes. The one outlined here has the elements that are common to all methods.
   a. Smokehouse: Use any well-sealed building with a vented roof and a floor that can have a fire pit. Fire pit should be centered, roughly 2 feet deep. The diameter depends on the building size and how much meat is to be smoked.
   b. Firewood: Use green wood from deciduous trees (ones that shed leaves in winter). Conifers such as pines and firs give an odd taste to meat and should not be used. Let fire burn down to coals and then stoke it with green wood to produce "cold smoke" (less than 85°F). Avoid flames during the smoking process.

    c. Rafters: Rafters should also be green wood and run the length of the smokehouse. Suspend meat from rope or twine 4-5 feet from top of fire pit. Allow even smoking and avoid contact spoilage by ensuring that all meat hangs free.

    d. Time: Smoke meat for 4-5 days, depending on size of house, size and number of pieces of meat to smoke.

    e. Meat Preparation: Prepare meat following these guidelines: BEEF - Remove large bones and joints. Trim fat and save for pemmican (a meat and fat sausage). Cut across the grain into manageable pieces and secure with a string. The hole for string should be centralized enough to prevent meat ripping during smoking. Hang meat and prepare smoking record (*see preservation records and recommendations below*). PORK - Use hot water to remove hair from skin of animal. **DO NOT** remove layered fat or the bones, except ball and socket joints. Do not scrape the fat that oozes during the smoking process (rendered fat).

    f. Smoked meat should be edible for up to one year depending on climate, condition of meat prior to smoking, insect, and rodent control. Souring or the appearance of holes or moisture patches does not condemn the meat. Open up the sour area. If it clears up in 24 hours then it is still edible, if not then discard. If in doubt, throw it out.

3. **Jerky:** Light and nutritious. Use only red meat.

    a. Trim fat from meat and cut meat WITH the grain of muscle into 12-inch long strips no more than 1 inch thick and ½ inch wide.

    b. Pack meat into salt for 10-12 days. Completely cover each strip with salt and do not allow strips to touch.

    c. Smoke meat after salting.

    d. Meat may also be dried over slow coals or sun-dried (sprinkle with pepper and hang about 20 feet into air above insect line).

    e. Wash before eating if salt cured.

4. **Pemmican:** Two basic ingredients: lean meat that is not salt cured and rendered fat.

    a. Use 6 lbs. of beef to make one pound of pemmican. Dry, pound and shred the meat.

    b. Prepare a casing, such as intestine, by cleaning (strip out contents and boil) and tying one end.

    c. Place shredded beef lightly into casing, DO NOT PACK.

    d. Render fat by boiling cut up or ground up (preferred) fat. The fat will separate into tallow, the liquefied oil from fat, and (cracklings), the fat residue. Cracklings can be eaten.

    e. Pour hot tallow into casing which heats the meat and fills the casing. The mixture in the casing should be 60% tallow and 40% meat. Tie casing closed and seal it by pouring tallow on tied ends.

    f. Allow pemmican to harden. Should last for approximately 5 years.

5. **Salting and Pickling:** Dry salt meat or immerse in a salt solution. Follow guidelines in Curing Section. Use 10:1 table salt to saltpeter (potassium nitrate) for both. For pickling, mix 50 pounds of salt and 5 pounds of saltpeter with 20 gallons of water.

6. **Canning and Other Methods:** These procedures are effective but require resources and equipment not readily available in a field environment.

7. **Preservation Records:** Record the steps taken during meat preservation. Records should have the following information at a minimum: meat type, date, source of meat, weight and cut of meat, total time cured (preserved), wood used and/or type and amount of salt/seasoning/brine used.

What Not To Do:

Do not use meat that is unfit for consumption based on ante- or postmortem exams. Use only potable water.

Chapter 14: Veterinary Medicine: Animal Restraint and Physical Exam

LTC Joseph Williamson, VC, USA & CPT Kristin Bloink, VC, USA

When: Physical exams are an important part of animal care and ownership. If utilizing animals for the carrying of equipment, as a food source, or treating them as part of an exercise, examinations should be conducted in a thorough way using the SOAP format. Handle animals with caution when you examine or treat them. Insist that owners restrain livestock. Do not attempt restraint without assistance. Apply only the restraint necessary to perform required tasks.

Table 5-20. Signs of Displeasure and Defense Mechanisms By Species

All species exhibit different signs of displeasure and defense mechanisms:

Species	Signs	Defense
Equine	Ears back Head bobbing Vocalizations	Kicking back with hindlimbs Rising up with forelimbs Biting
Bovine, caprine, ovine	Alert posture Charging Snorting	Lateral kick with hindlimbs Charging/goring

Table 5-20. Signs of Displeasure and Defense Mechanisms By Species, continued

Species	Signs	Defense
Porcine	Vocalizations Charging	Biting Charging
Camelid	Ears back Chewing Tail up Vocalizations	Spitting Biting Kicking in all directions with all limbs Charging
Canine	Vocalizations Growling/Barking Hair raised on back Ears erect	Biting Clawing
Feline	Vocalizations Growling/Hissing Back arched Hair raised on back Ears erect Tail whipping	Biting Scratching

What You Need: Rope, twitch, nose lead, stethoscope, pen, paper, leather gloves, exam gloves, light source, rectal thermometer (large animal style preferred)

What To Do:

1. **Restraint:** Allow owner and/or indigenous persons to handle and restrain the animals as much as possible. This is probably the most difficult part of the examination and may be the most dangerous. Use the following to assist the locals in restraining the animal.

    a. **Halter:** Fasten a rope loop around the animal's neck with a bowline knot to make a temporary rope halter. Pull a bight of the standing end through the loop from rear to front and place over the animal's nose. Pull tight when in use.

Figure 5-30. Halter Restraint

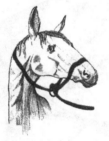

    b. **Twitch:** For horses. A twitch is a small loop of rope or smooth chain twisted around the upper lip of the horse to divert attention from work being done elsewhere on the horse. Twist the rope or chain with a stick or rod to tighten the twitch, but avoid circulatory compromise. Too much force will harm the horse's lip.

Figure 5-31. Twitch Restraint

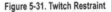

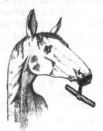

    c. **Casting a cow (Burley method):** You will need approximately 40 feet of rope, with the center of the rope over the withers and wrapped as shown in the diagram.

Figure 5-32. Casting a Cow (Burley Method)

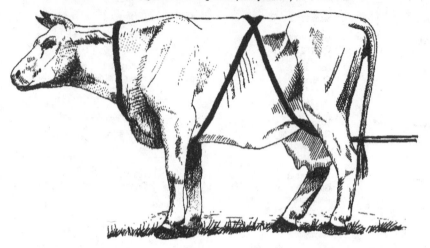

While maintaining control of the head, pull tightly on the ends of the rope and the cow will fall. To tie the rear legs, keep both ropes taut and slide the uppermost rope along the undersurface of the rear leg to the fetlock. Then carry the end around the leg and above the hock, across the cannon bone and back around the fetlock. Secure leg with several of these figure 8s

Restraining the legs: Tie all four feet together to restrain the animal after it has been cast (dropped). Tie a rope to one leg below the fetlock. Tie the other legs to this one alternately, first a front leg, then a rear one and repeat.

Figure 5-33. Restraining the Legs

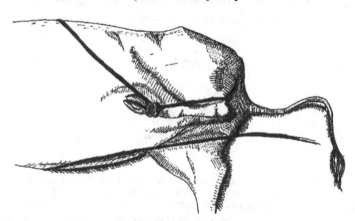

d. **Cattle tail restraint:** Bend the tail of the cow toward the side or back of the animal to distract the cow. Stand to the side of cow to avoid being kicked. Secure tail base with both hands to avoid damaging the tail and bend.

e. **Camelid restraint:** Trained animals will know how to kush (lie down with feet/legs folded underneath); this position prevents kicking. In untrained animals, a rope can be brought behind the hindlimbs at the level of the fetlock to cause the hindlimbs to buckle. Once the animal is down, the ends of the rope are brought medial to the stifles and tied in front of the hump(s). Some camels are halter trained while others can be controlled with pressure on a wooden peg through the nostril (regional differences) for control of the head.

f. **Porcine restraint:** A hog snare may be used to catch pigs by the upper jaw. The animal is cornered then the loop of the snare is placed around the upper jaw of the pig, behind the canines. The snare is then tightened. Smaller pigs may be restrained by manually holding them off the ground by grasping both frontlimbs or both hindlimbs.

2. **Examination:** Once an animal is sufficiently and securely restrained, begin the physical exam. General observations and clinical signs are similar to those found in humans. Follow the SOAP approach, just as when examining a human patient. Remember: the diseases and injuries of animals can be similar to those in humans, but seek advice from appropriate veterinary providers or the Merck Veterinary Manual, if available. One can only diagnose and treat based on his level of knowledge and understanding of veterinary medicine.

Table 5-21. Normal Physiological Values by Species

Species	Rectal Temp °F	Heart Rate	Resp. Rate	Feces (lbs/day)	Urine (mL/kg/ day)	WBC x 1000	HCT%
Horse	100.5	23-70	12	30-50	3-18	6-12	39-52
Cow	100.5	60-70	30	30-100	17-45	4-12	24-48
Sheep	103	60-120	19	2-6.5	10-14	4-12	24-50
Goat	104	70-135	15-20		10-14	6-16	24-48
Pig	102	58-86	15-18	1-6.5	5-30	11-22	32-50
Dog	101.5	100-130	22	0-1.5	20-100	6-18	37-55
Cat	101.5	110-140	26		10-200	8-15	24-45
Rabbit	102.5	123-304	55			6-10	36-48
Camel	95-105	35-60	8-16		2-6	7-15	22-32

2. **Animal care and management:**
   a. Have enough clean, potable water available to the animals. Maintain a clean source and keep it free of feces and foreign material. Many animals will not drink contaminated or soiled water.
   b. Have food or forage readily available. Allow animals to graze land and pastures. Keep feed clean, palatable and free of pests.
   c. Shelter animals when possible.
   d. CONTINUOUS monitoring of the animals for signs of disease and/or parasites will prevent disease transmission within the herd and to humans. A zoonosis is a disease transmissible between animals and man. Many zoonoses are threats in the field environment and precautions need to be taken to minimize them. Monitor and cull sick or debilitated animals. Review the Preventive Medicine chapter and individual infectious disease sections for specifics on zoonoses and how to prevent them.

What Not To Do:
   1. Do not attempt to restrain animals by yourself.
   2. Do not abuse animals. Abuse is unethical, unnecessary and may jeopardize the relationship with native personnel.
   3. Do not alienate local medical and veterinary personnel. Work with them and assist them.

Chapter 14: Veterinary Medicine: Large Animal Obstetrics

LTC Joseph G. Williamson, VC, USA

Introduction: Many millions of animals have been born without assistance and forced extraction may do more harm than good. If the female is giving birth naturally, leave her alone. Do not assist. When to intervene is dependent on the state of parturition, the presentation of the fetus, duration of labor and history of underlying disease processes. The owner will usually be more able to perform intervention if it is necessary. This outline will provide only the basics of "normal" parturition and guidelines for observation and minimal intervention. We will use the cow model throughout.

Subjective: **Symptoms**

Prior to parturition a normal animal will walk with difficulty, often looking back at her flanks. The udder may swell and become distended with milk, the tailhead ligament will relax and her vulva may swell and begin to discharge mucus or fluid. Restlessness and seeking a quiet isolated area is common. Some may demonstrate an aversion to food and human contact. Pasture animals such as sheep may separate from the herd and lamb on their own. NOT all animals will lie down for childbirth. Duration of labor varies considerably between species (15 minutes for horse; up to 7 hours for a pig litter), and is longer in animals giving birth for the 1st time. The farmer should know pregnancy status of animals and their due date. He/she may also be of assistance in controlling the animal and giving medical history.

Objective: **Signs**

No tools or special equipment are required for a normal birth. Use of rectal thermometer is contraindicated. Animal will present with an enlarged abdomen and a drop in body temperature 1-2° below normal 12-24 hours before birth (*see Part 5: Specialty Areas: Chapter 14: Physical Exam and Restraint*). In cattle, fetal membranes filled with fluid are visible outside the cow. Forelimbs and head emerge first from vagina, followed by rest of animal. Anterior presentation with front feet first is the norm, but posterior presentation may occur and not be a cause for alarm. Placenta and afterbirth will follow. Problem/difficult births can include posterior presentation, head or limb deviations and complications arising from multiple births.

Assessment: **Differential Diagnosis**

Tumor, bloat, pseudopregnancy

Plan:
Treatment
1. The owner/farmer should be in control of the animal at all times.
2. Minimize exposure to fetal fluids or tissues.
3. Allow fetal membranes to burst naturally during labor.
4. Occasionally the membranes will need to be ruptured after prolonged, non-progressive labor. Use a blunt, sterile instrument to make an opening in the membranes without harming the fetus.
5. If a complication arises, including labor for an extended period of time with little or no result, then the farmer may attempt intervention.
6. Veterinary assistance is needed for complicated deliveries.
7. To assist in extracting a fetus that is partially exposed with visible head, forelimbs or shoulder, GENTLY provide traction on the fetus downward and toward the hind limbs of the mother. If difficulty occurs, consult with any available veterinary professionals.
8. After the delivery, ensure the young are being cleaned and cared for by the mother and that they have risen and attempted to move about.
9. Do not attempt to remove fetal membranes after birth as this may tear uterine tissue. Allow them to be expelled naturally.
10. Examine offspring for abnormalities and/or deformities. Turn over to farmer.

Chapter 14: Veterinary Medicine: IV Fluid Infusion
LTC Joseph G. Williamson, VC, USA

When: An animal needs intravenous (IV) medication or fluid resuscitation

What You Need: IV catheters, IV administration sets, alcohol or povidone/iodine swabs and appropriate medication/fluids.

What To Do:
1. Inspect and prepare the equipment for an IV infusion.
2. Select the IV site. Sites differ according to species:
   a. Equine: Jugular vein. Avoid the upper 1/3 of the vein to minimize the risk of perforating the carotid artery.
   b. Bovine, caprine or ovine: Jugular vein. Alternate sites: Tail vein or the milk vein in females
   c. Feline: Jugular vein. Alternate site: Cephalic vein
   d. Canine: *See Part 5: Specialty Areas: Chapter 14: Canine: Placement of an IV Catheter*
3. Prep the IV site. Shave the IV site if possible and wipe with povidone/iodine or alcohol swabs.
4. Administer the IV. Follow the same procedure steps as with humans.
5. Secure the IV. Ensure that the animal cannot pull out the IV and injure self.
6. Record the procedure.

What Not To Do:
1. Do not allow air to enter the blood stream.
2. Do not allow blood to infiltrate the IV.
3. Do not allow the animal to pull out the IV.

Chapter 14: Veterinary Medicine: Animal Diseases: Bloat in Bovine
LTC Joseph G. Williamson, VC, USA

Introduction: Bloat is an over-distention of the rumen and reticulum in cattle. Frothy bloat is cause by switching rapidly from poor to rich diets or by diets high in grain or legumes. Free gas bloat is generally due to failure to eructate (belch) free gas because of a physical obstruction. Swollen, gas-filled distention of the abdominal organs may prevent normal respiration.

Subjective: **Symptoms**
Owner complaints about animals: difficulty breathing and frothing about the mouth, standing with legs splayed, refusing to eat, or drink.

Objective: **Signs**
Distention of the left flank, tympanic gas-filled or froth-filled abdominal cavity, dyspnea, tachycardia. Collapse and death may result if problem persists.

Assessment: **Differential Diagnosis**
Peritonitis, ascites, pregnancy.

Plan: **Treatment**
Primary: Insert oral stomach tube only with appropriate veterinary supervision and gastric lavage with anti-frothing agents such as vegetable oil.
Alternative: Trocarization: Insert a 14 gauge needle or trocar into gas-filled rumen (rumenotomy), expose the stomach and suture it to body wall if animal is down or condition life-threatening. These procedures should be done by trained veterinary personnel.

Chapter 14: Veterinary Medicine: Animal Diseases: Milk Fever/Parturient Paresis (bovine/caprine/ovine)
CPT Kristin Bloink, VC, USA

Introduction: Milk fever is a common condition in cows, sheep and goats around parturition. Sheep and goats are susceptible 6 weeks prior to and 10 weeks post parturition. Cows are most susceptible during the first 72 hours following parturition. It is hypocalcemia caused by inadequate calcium stores and/or inadequate calcium in the diet. This is an acute, life-threatening condition.

Subjective: **Symptoms**

Owner complains that the animal is excitable, confused, restless, and often not milking well. In advanced stages, the animal may be down and even paralyzed.

Objective: **Signs**

Using Basic Tools: Ataxia, tremors involving triceps and ears, head bobbing, down flaccid animal. "S" shaped curve to neck in recumbent animals. Tachycardia (rate up to 120bpm). Constipation, loss of anal sphincter tone. Signs of bloat, rumen distention, due to GI stasis. Poor milk production.

Assessment:

Differential Diagnosis: Toxic mastitis, toxic metritis (uterine infection), calving paralysis (damage to sciatic and other lumbar roots during calving), pregnancy toxemia (prepartum sheep and goats)

Plan:

Treatment

Goal is to replace calcium as soon as possible to avoid nerve and muscle damage and death. Initiate IV if possible. Give **calcium gluconate** (may contain phosphorous and magnesium as well) IV, SQ or intraperitoneally (IV preferred). Dose is 1g calcium/100 lbs of body weight. Give slowly over 10-20 minutes while monitoring heart rate. Slow or stop therapy if dysrhythmias or severe bradycardia (<30/bpm) occurs. Restart therapy when cardiac changes resolve. Results: 75% of animals will show resolution of signs within 2 hours. Animals without a marked response in 4-8 hours should be retreated. 25-30% of animals will relapse within 24-48 hours and will require re-treatment.

Prevention and Hygiene:

Good nutrition but avoidance of diets high in alfalfa or clover late in gestation. Avoid movement or other stressful events during the last 8 weeks of gestation. Reduce heavy parasite burdens.

Chapter 14: Veterinary Medicine: Animal Diseases: Foot Rot in Caprine

LTC Joseph G. Williamson, VC, USA

Introduction: Foot rot is a significant problem in sheep and goats, occurring most commonly on pastures during times of persistent moisture. Susceptibility to the disease varies by species and environment. Morbidity can be up to 75% within a flock, from either the primary or a secondary infection.

Subjective: **Symptoms**

Owner complains about animals: slow weight gains or weight loss, reluctance to move about, fetid odors emanating from the feet, lameness. Systemic signs may also be reported.

Objective: **Signs**

Using Basic Tools:

Benign: No clinical signs. Other animals in herd affected

Intermediate: Mild to moderate signs, +/- fever (normal temp is 103-104°F), foot odor may be present, mild lameness

Virulent Form: Systemic signs of fever/anorexia, lameness, fetid odor, swelling of soft tissue, sloughing of the foot, inflammation of deep tissues, secondary infections.

Using Advanced Tools: Labs: Bacterial cultures may identify organism.

Assessment: **Differential Diagnosis**

Other bacterial or fungal infections, trauma, bluetongue (inflammation of mouth and nose; sometimes accompanied by lameness), ulcerative dermatosis

Plan: **Treatment**

Treat infected animals. Observe other animals in flock for signs of infection.

1. Trim (débride) all exposed and necrotic tissues. This is critical for proper treatment of tissues.
2. Apply local disinfectant (**5% formalin, 10% ZnSO4, or 5% CuSO4**)
3. Administer antibiotics (infected animals): **Penicillin** 50-70,000u/kg IM and **dihydrostreptomycin** at 22,500-32,000u/lb.
4. Move animal to dry pasture or ground.

Prevention and Hygiene: Cull (remove from herd) or destroy recurrent carriers to protect rest of animals.

Chapter 14: Veterinary Medicine: Animal Diseases: Lameness in Equine

LTC Joseph G. Williamson, VC, USA

Introduction: Lameness is a general term associated with pain in one or more legs due to injury, illness or conformational abnormalities. Lameness resulting from injury and infection will be discussed here. Conformational injuries, fractures and the majority of the soft tissue malfunctions require extensive treatment and/or diagnostic tests that are beyond the capabilities of the medic in the field. Systematically conduct a physical examination. Begin by examining the hoof and work your way up to the shoulder or pelvis. Look for lesions, injuries, swelling and bounding pulses. Use hoof testers (special pliers used to squeeze soft tissue) to apply light pressure to all parts of the hoof, to include the wall, frog and sole. Check for sores, abscesses and painful conditions not readily seen on exam.

Subjective: **Symptoms**

Owner complains of animal being lame (not bearing weight on the affected limb or carrying it in an unnatural or awkward position). Subtle lameness may only be detected at the trot or on hard-packed surfaces. Owner may report foul odor from hoof; obvious injury, swelling or lesions; animal constantly shifting weight or standing with hind limbs under its body to take weight off the front limbs.

Objective: **Signs**

Using Basic Tools: Fetid odor from hoof, bounding digital pulses, swelling of joints or leg, hot hoof walls, tenderness elicited with hoof testers (or substitute), abnormal or stilted gait, bowed or swollen tendon and tendon sheaths.

Assessment: **Differential Diagnosis**

Thrush: Fetid odor with moist exudative dermatitis of the underside of the hoof. Laminitis, conformational abnormalities, bowed tendons, traumatic injury, fractures.

Plan:

Treatment

Once identified as the cause of the lameness, trim the affected tissue if possible.

Treat thrush with antiseptics, such as **iodine** or **copper sulfate**

Treat laminitis with pain relievers: **Phenylbutazone** 4.4-8.8mg/kg/day divided bid or tid slowly IV or po, tapering off over 5 days. (po is treatment of choice) or **flunixin meglumine** 1.1mg/kg once daily up to tid, po/IM or IV (with endotoxemia).

For fractures and severe dislocations, consult with veterinarian and owner for disposition options.

Prevention

Maintain proper hygiene and foot care by keeping feet trimmed and picked clean. A farrier should perform proper trimming, padding and shoeing of hoof.

Chapter 14: Veterinary Medicine: Animal Diseases: Skin Diseases in Swine

CPT Kristin Bloink, VC, USA

Introduction: Skin infections are common in swine, especially in those pigs raised in crowded, unclean environments. *Erysipelothrix rhusiopathiae* is a very common bacterium that affects the skin of pigs, commonly leads to septicemia and a 75% mortality rate. This bacteria and condition is <u>zoonotic</u> and can easily spread to humans through direct skin contact with affected pigs. This condition is usually acute, but if left untreated can progress to a chronic state with non-suppurative arthritis and/or vegetative endocarditis in pigs and humans.

Subjective: **Symptoms**

Owner complains that the animal(s) are dull, feverish, and anorexic. Skin lesions are often not readily apparent until about the 3 days after clinical signs develop. The lesions have a characteristic red raised diamond shape.

Objective: **Signs**

Using Basic Tools: Fever with associated listlessness, dry feces and increased water consumption. Red raised diamond shaped skin lesions are almost definitive for diagnosis of the disease. A stiff gait or signs of congestive heart failure are often apparent in chronically affected animals.

Assessment: **Differential Diagnosis**

Lice, swine pox, flea/fly bites, sarcoptic mange, zinc deficiency, dermatophytoses, early hog cholera, sunburn, pityriasis rosea

Plan:

Treatment

Procaine Penicillin G 40,000IU/kg IM once daily x 4 days; treating all affected animals and decontaminating environment (bleach water)

Prevention: Good hygiene of both pigs and housing; Good nutrition. A vaccine (**bacterin**) exists but only provides coverage for 6 months to 1 year.

Chapter 14: Veterinary Medicine: Animal Diseases: Acute Mastitis

LTC Joseph G. Williamson, VC, USA

Introduction: Mastitis is the most costly disease to the dairy industry in the US and in most countries of the world. Many bacteria, including *Staphylococcus, Streptococcus* and *Coliforms* can cause it. These pathogens cause inflammation of the gland after traumatic injury or exposure to chemical irritants. It is usually a herd health problem. Good hygiene and sanitation are necessary, or treatment will fail.

Subjective: **Symptoms**

Owner complains that the animal is reluctant to be milked, has swollen milk glands, will not eat, is generally depressed, will not rise move around (walking may cause discomfort to the gland).

Objective: **Signs**

Using Basic Tools:

Peracute*: Swollen, hot, tender milk glands; abnormal secretions; fever

Acute: Mild systemic signs; gland changes as with peracute

Sub-acute: No systemic changes, mild gland changes

*Peracute: Very acute or violent

Assessment: **Differential Diagnosis**

Tumor, cellulitis, stone in milk duct, trauma

The California Mastitis Test can be used as a diagnostic test when coupled with clinical signs. Perform the test by stripping milk from each quarter (4 quarters per udder), mixing it with the reagent in the kit and observing for clumped or stringy milk.

Plan:

Treatment

1. Strip (milk) affected quarters dry, bid during therapy. Continue until condition resolved.
2. DO NOT consume milk.
3. C & S is critical prior to treatment with antibiotics. Only treat with antibiotics labeled "FOR VETERINARY USE ONLY" and if applies, "MAMMARY INFUSION." Medics will have to shop for these. For Streptococcal species: **Procaine Penicillin G** Intramammary Infusion for lactating animals at 100,000 units per gland for 3 days. For Staphylococcal species: Dry treatment (not milking) is best; results disappointing if treated during lactation. Mammary infusion with pre-mixed antibiotics. For other species - base treatment on C & S. Infuse paste antibiotics into the milk glands. The paste is in a pre-measured plastic infusion syringe. Gently push the tip into teat duct and infuse antibiotics.
4. If paste antibiotics are unavailable, apply hot compresses as often as possible during peracute and acute phases.
5. Give IV antibiotics, only under the supervision of a veterinarian, if animal has signs of systemic infection (fever, lassitude, poor appetite, etc.).

Chapter 14: Veterinary Medicine: Animal Diseases: Diarrhea in Porcine

LTC Joseph G. Williamson, VC, USA

Introduction: Diarrhea, or scours, is a common and highly contagious problem in pigs. It may be attributed to many agents: Enterogenic *E. coli*, *Treponema hyodysenteriae*, *Salmonella*, Rotavirus or others. The disease may affect individuals or the whole herd but is not a zoonotic threat. Herd health and condition is a vital tool in assessing diarrhea in the pigs. Sporadic death or deaths only in newborns may suggest the diagnosis. Diarrhea will be found in the pens and on the ground. Diarrhea storms, with sudden deaths or high death rates, are not uncommon.

Subjective: Symptoms

Animal owner complains of unthrifty pigs (dry skin, thin, dirty/covered with feces), diarrhea, anorexia and weakness and sudden death.

Objective: Signs

Using Basic Tools: Diarrhea (pale yellow, watery to mucopurulent with flecks of mucosa), fever, lethargy, anorexia, conjunctivitis, failure to grow; weight loss and sudden death. Remember, with multiple etiological agents, signs may be varied or even subclinical.

Assessment:

Definitive diagnosis requires lab support. Tissue samples gathered postmortem should be analyzed in a competent lab. Necropsy lesions and findings may also be helpful in diagnosis.

Differential Diagnosis: Many agents associated with a variety of diseases can cause diarrhea in pigs.

Plan:

Treatment

Segregate, isolate and treat all affected pigs. Provide fluids: Fresh water or oral rehydration salts. Antibiotics have limited value and probably should not be used. Provide high quality nutritious feed. In some cases, eradication and depopulation will be warranted. Local government must direct this action. "All-in and All-out" practices when replenishing stock: remove all pigs, sanitize stalls and premises and replenish with new animals from one source all at the same time.

Prevention: Report large outbreaks to appropriate agencies. Improve the sanitation of the farm. Vaccines exist for some of the disease agents. Coordinate vaccination programs through the local veterinarian and the appropriate ministries.

Chapter 14: Veterinary Medicine: Animal Diseases: Conjunctivitis (Pinkeye)

LTC Joseph G. Williamson, VC, USA

Introduction: Pinkeye is a common ocular disturbance that may be associated with irritation or trauma to the eye caused by *Moraxella bovis*. Transmission through a herd is usually by dust, droplets, or by flies or other insects.

Subjective: Symptoms

Owner complains that animals have conjunctivitis and discharge from the affected eye.

Objective: Signs

Conjunctivitis, central corneal ulceration-opacity (opacity begins on the periphery and migrates centrally), mucopurulent discharge (yellow green color, viscous discharge), edematous eyelids, periorbital edema. May have underlying trauma or irritation

Assessment: Differential Diagnosis

Corneal ulcer or traumatic injury

Plan:

Treatment

Administer antibiotics (**penicillin, nitrofurazone, tetracycline** or **gentamicin**) as ophthalmic ointments or by subconjunctival injection. Apply topical ocular anesthetic (**tetracaine** will suffice). Direct a 25 gauge needle into sub-conjunctiva and slowly administer treatment.

Prevention: Isolate affected animals. Maintain hygiene and insect control.

Chapter 14: Veterinary Medicine: Equine Procedures: Castrate a Stallion

LTC William Bosworth, VC, ARNG

What: Castration makes a male horse less aggressive, less dangerous, and prevents fighting, and makes the animal easier to handle as it matures.

When: Castration of mature stallions should be reserved for when there are no mules, geldings, or mares available to ride and there is no other alternative. It is best to castrate the male animal shortly after birth, as young animals will heal quickly from the procedure. However, some animals, such as draft, or working, animals are castrated after puberty near their mature weight to develop male characteristics and strength that would not be present if they were castrated early in life. It is best to castrate during the dry season when the fly population is lower. Castrating older animals requires training by a skilled worker to ensure that the animal is not put under undo distress and to ensure that the procedure is done properly. The optimal time to castrate horses, donkeys, or mules is at 2 months of age. Castrating older equines (up to 2-3 years of age and older) requires the supervision and skills of a veterinarian. Complications increase when stallions are castrated older than 2-3 years of age. Castration of fractious or unmanageable adult stallions may have minimal or no immediate effect on improving the animal's attitude and his tolerance to being handled. The animal's attitude and manageability may improve after several months or years.

Safety Note: Horses of any age are dangerous to handle, and can easily kill or severely injure a person during handling, restraint, anesthesia, and recovery while conducting this procedure, especially if that person has not worked with horses. Maintain situational awareness at all times!

What You Need: Clean, hot water with disinfectant, syringes and needles, scalpel, sharp knife, or razor blade, clamping device, sterilization with boiling water, antiseptic (povidone-iodine), **tetanus antitoxin** (if never vaccinated) or **toxoid** (if previously vaccinated), **lidocaine**, **ketamine**, **xylazine**, or other general anesthetic for colts and stallions over 2 months of age, injectable antibiotics, such as **cefazolin**, **cephalexin**, absorbable suture (size 0)

What To Do:
1. Restrain the horse securely using physical and/or chemical restraint.
2. Check the scrotum for any abnormal swelling. Suspect a hernia if swelling is noted; this horse should not be castrated.
3. Procedure can be done with the horse lying down or standing.
4. Field anesthesia and physical restraint:
   a. **Xylazine** 2mg/kg IM, or **xylazine** 0.5-1mg/kg plus **butorphanol** 0.025mg/kg IM
   b. Wait 10-20 minutes to take effect (head drops to knees) before giving **ketamine**
   c. If adequate sedation does not occur, re-dose with 1/2 the **xylazine** or add **butorphanol** (if not already given)
   d. Once the horse is adequately sedated, induce with **ketamine** 2mg/kg IV. Do not inject into the carotid artery!!**
   e. Protect the horse's head as the induction dose takes effect to prevent injury. Use lead ropes attached to a halter to control the horse's head as he goes down.
   f. Use ropes to restrain the topside rear leg in flexion to prevent kicking.
   g. Provide any other physical restraint necessary to prevent injury to the veterinarian, medic, or other assistants.
5. Inject 10mL **lidocaine** in the skin of the scrotum where each incision is to be made
6. Inject 10mL **lidocaine** through the skin into each spermatic cord
7. Make an incision through the skin of the scrotum where the local anesthetic was placed. Cut through to the testis, but not through the tunica (white covering).
8. Repeat for second testis
9. Remove the testes from the scrotum and cut through the tunica to free the testes
10. Ligate the spermatic cord with absorbable suture 2-3 times to control bleeding.
11. Clamp the cord distal to the ligatures and cut through the cord with a scalpel.
12. Repeat for second testis
13. Place antiseptic on incise
14. Leave the incisions open for a few days to allow for drainage of pus or serum.
15. **Cefazolin** 11mg/kg may be given IM or IV to prevent infection
16. Observe for bleeding. A few drops of blood is normal.
17. The horse should recover to a standing position within an hour. He will be sedated for the next 6-8 hours. He will be ready to ride once the incisions are healed, usually 7-10 days.
18. Open the incision if it becomes infected or swollen and treat as an abscess. You may need to repeat the sedation and field anesthesia procedure described previously to open the incision and drain the abscess. **Cephalexin** 25mg/kg may be given po bid to qid x 7 days or 2 days after signs of infection resolves.
19. Give **tetanus antitoxin** (if never vaccinated) at the time of castration, or **toxoid** (if previously vaccinated at least 3 weeks prior to the procedure). Follow label directions for dose and route.

What Not To Do:
1. Do not use a Burdizzo tool or rubber rings to castrate horses, donkeys or mules.
2. Do not castrate a stallion with a scrotal hernia!
3. Do not close the incisions!
4. Do not leave any testicular or epididymis tissue (will continue to act as an un-castrated stallion)!
5. Do not use acepromazine on any male equine.
6. **Do not inject any drugs into the carotid artery! Carotid injections will result in a horse that rears up and over onto its back and head, resulting in a fractured skull, death of the horse, and serious injury or death of anyone near the horse. To ensure that you are in the jugular vein, remove the needle from the syringe, stick the needle into the jugular vein, and observe the blood flow. If the blood pulses from the needle, you are in the carotid. Remove the needle, place direct pressure on the carotid artery for 5 minutes, and try again. Once you are in the jugular vein, place the syringe back on the needle, and inject the drug.

Chapter 14: Veterinary Medicine: Equine Procedures: Colic in Equine

LTC Joseph G. Williamson, VC, USA

Introduction: Colic is a nonspecific term describing sporadic abdominal pain and discomfort in the equine. Horses may suffer from a myriad of gastrointestinal problems, including intestinal impaction or strangulation, which falls under the general term of colic. Signs can vary from mild discomfort to shock and death. The severity of clinical signs is not necessarily associated with the seriousness of the disease.

Subjective: Symptoms
Owner complaints about animal: Restlessness, poor appetite. Inquire about duration of signs and progression (clue to severity), fecal output (indicates obstruction), history of colic in this animal and diet.

Objective: Signs
Auscultate for bowel sounds in all 4 quadrants of the abdomen. Check mucous membranes and hydration status. Examine feces for blood or mucus. Only a veterinarian should do rectal exam.

Mild: Animal seems uncomfortable, frequent urination, looking at flank, mild sweating.

Moderate: Increased heart and respiratory rates, restlessness (getting up and down), kicking at flank, diminished stool output, increased sweating

Severe: Increased heart and respiratory rates, extreme anxiety and restlessness (rolling on the ground), profuse sweating, muddy colored mucous membranes, signs of shock

Note: Clinical signs may not directly relate to actual severity of disease. Horses, as in humans, have varying thresholds for pain and therefore the clinical signs may be misleading. Consult a veterinarian (if available) for all colic cases.

Assessment: Differential Diagnosis
Trauma to abdomen, gas, GI tract worm infection, pregnancy with/without complications (ask owner about animal's mating history).

Plan:
Treatment
1. Walk the horse. Walking may relieve gas and aid in the movement of obstructions or stool into colon and out of the animal. It will also keep the horse from injury by keeping it up and moving.
2. Provide fresh clean water.
3. Laxatives and wetting agents are useful. Administer orally or through a naso-gastric tube: mineral oil 2-4 liters q12h, bran mashes (mash food to soften it before giving to horse with sore gums), water. Naso-gastric intubation should only be attempted by experienced personnel.
4. Analgesics may be given if signs warrant. However, they may mask a deteriorating condition so use with caution and under veterinary supervision. Analgesics: **Flunixin meglumine**: 1.1mg/kg IV q12h, **Xylazine**: 0.1-1.0mg/kg as necessary IM or IV, **Butorphanol**: 0.02-0.05mg/kg IM or IV as necessary.

Owner Education
Manage the herd properly to reduce the likelihood of colic. Offer a high-roughage diet and elevate hay bins to prevent sand impactions. Provide a good de-worming program that ensures pasture rotation and varying de-wormers. Give plenty of fresh, clean water.

Chapter 14: Veterinary Medicine: Equine Procedures: Float Equine Teeth

LTC William Bosworth, VC, ARNG

What: "Floating" equine teeth is the removal of the sharp points of teeth to allow a horse to eat with normal occlusion and without pain. (While floating teeth is usually associated with equines, geriatric ruminants [cattle, sheep, and goats] can develop sharp points on their molars that will affect their ability to masticate their food.) The techniques described for horses can be used for ruminants, ensuring that the appropriate sized instruments are used for the sheep and goat. A horse in a grazing environment will wear their teeth down in a normal pattern. Stabled horses that eat grain will cause the teeth to wear abnormally, allowing sharp points to develop. The equine mandible is narrower than the maxilla causing sharp points to form on the lingual surface of the lower arcade and the buccal surface of the upper arcade. These sharp points, when long enough, will cause pain to the horse when it eats, injuring the buccal and lingual surfaces. Many horses can be floated without sedation or anesthesia depending on the temperament of the animal and the skill of equine dentist. The goal is to balance the animal's teeth and achieve 70% or greater occlusion of the molars and premolars.

When: Float the teeth when: sharp points when the teeth are palpated, weight loss with adequate diet, and a horse that attempts to eat, but has food that falls out of its mouth. This spillage is called "quidding."

What You Need: Rasp or float; bucket, warm water, **chlorhexidine** solution, 60mL syringe with catheter tip, speculum or gag, chemical restraint (**xylazine** 100mg/mL).

What To Do:
1. Perform chemical restraint, if needed, place gag or speculum
   a. **Xylazine** 2mg/kg IM, or
   b. **Xylazine** 0.5-1mg/kg plus **butorphanol** 0.025mg/kg IM
2. Insert the float over the sharp points of the upper arcade (buccal surface) at approximately 60° angle.
3. Perform long, smooth strokes with the float or rasp to remove the sharp points.
4. Keep checking for smoothness until all the points are removed.
5. Repeat for other side of upper arcade.
6. Remove the lingual sharp points on the lower arcade in a similar fashion.
7. Flush with warm water and **chlorhexidine** solution to clean blood and enamel particles removed by the float as needed during the procedure.

What Not To Do:
1. Do not file without an even rhythm.
2. Do not use an improper float angle.
3. Do not fail to file the points at the back of the mouth.

Chapter 14: Veterinary Medicine: Pack Animal Harnessing

LTC William Bosworth, VC, ARNG

What: Pack animals can be the most reliable mode of transportation in mountainous terrain or remote areas with poor roads that are, or can become, impassable to military vehicles and tractor-trailers. The SOF medic must know how to pack an animal safely without causing harm to the animal or to himself.

When: The use of pack animals is dictated by terrain and the environment. Pack animals can allow SOF to blend into the environment and/or provide new supplies without alerting enemy forces, and to move supplies and equipment by foot more efficiently. Properly conditioned animals and personnel trained in handling pack trains can move 20-30 miles per day in mountainous terrain transporting 150-300 pounds per animal. Properly fitting the pack saddle and harness, and balancing the load are extremely important to successful pack animal operations. Many animals are suited for pack animal operations, and the type available for use by SOF depends on the region of the world where SOF is operating. This section will focus on horses, mules, and donkeys.

What You Need:
1. Grooming equipment
2. Pack saddles (sawbuck, Bradshaw, Decker, hybrids)
3. Saddle harness:
   a. Rigging
   b. Cinches
   c. Breast collar
   d. Breaching
   e. Crupper
4. Halter
5. Saddle pack pad
6. Saddle cover
7. Canvas tarp to lash over the top of a load
8. Lash rope and cinch
9. Sling rope
10. Panniers (cargo containers that hang from the pack saddle)

What To Do:
1. Groom the animal to remove any debris that can cause saddle sores
2. Treat any saddle sores found during grooming
3. Place the saddle pad square on the back, forward of final placement, and slide rearward into position (helps to prevent sores), and should be positioned over the withers
4. Place enough saddle pads to keep the saddle off the withers when the saddle has settled after being loaded.
5. Use pads that are thicker over the withers as the pads tend to slip rearward.
6. Allow 4-6 inches of exposed padding at the front and rear of the saddle.
7. The forward edge of the saddle should be 2-3 inches to the rear of the shoulder blades.
8. Fasten the front cinch first, ensuring that the latigos and cinches are not twisted. The front cinch should be a hand's width to the rear of the front leg.
9. Place the breast collar just above the point of the shoulder. Adjust the connector straps to the same length so that the breast collar is snug when the front leg is fully extended.
10. Adjust the breeching by placing the spider on the rump and adjust the back straps to rest on the highest point of the shoulder. Keep both straps the same length to keep the ring centered.
11. Adjust the hip straps so the breeching is halfway between the base of the tail and bottom of the hindquarters.
12. Slide the crupper under the tail and attach it, if used. Ensure the crupper is snug under the tail, but not too tight.
13. Adjust the connecting straps so that the breeching is snug, not too tight to hinder the animal's gait, nor too loose.
14. Connect the quarter straps to the front cinch ring. The upper quarter strap should be snug, and the lower quarter strap should have a 1-inch sag.
15. Pull the animal's tail out of the breeching.
16. Tighten the front cinch, allowing one finger to pass easily between the cinch and the animal's chest.
17. Tighten the rear cinch to allow the whole hand to slip under it. Center the rear cinch on the animal's belly. The cinch rings should be the same distance from the rigging.
18. Fasten the cinch:
    a. Run the latigo through the cinch ring (towards the packer) and back up through the rigging ring (towards the animal).
    b. Form a half-Windsor knot by bringing the running end of the latigo around the portion running through the rigging ring, then up through the rear of the rigging ring, and down through the loop that was just formed
    c. Form a quick release by passing the running end of the latigo up through the loop just formed.
19. Once the saddle is in position, and the breast collar, breeching, and cinches are snug, the packer needs to "untrack" the animal before packing the load by walking it around for approximately 30 seconds.

20. Tie up the animal and tighten the cinches again, if needed, and load the animal.
21. After the saddle and rigging is fitted to an animal, use it on the same animal throughout the entire movement to save time refitting the packsaddles each time the unit moves.
22. Unsaddle the animal in the reverse sequence.
23. Store the saddle

What Not To Do:
1. Do not approach the animal from the rear. Approach the animal from the front, at a 30° angle, with your body between the animal's head and shoulder region.
2. Do not approach without warning or by surprising the animal. Approach the animal while speaking to it in a calm voice. Initiate physical contact with the animal by touching the neck or shoulder first. Avoid sudden movements. Stay alert for a kick. Stay aware at all times to avoid injury. Just because an animal has never kicked does not mean that it will never kick.
3. Do not coil the lead rope around your hand. Hold loose bights of the rope.
4. Do not overload the animal; balance the load.
5. Do not use in cheap equipment or improper size equipment for your animals.

Chapter 14: Veterinary Medicine: Canine: Introduction to the Care of Military Working Dogs
MAJ Steve Baty, VC, USA

Military working dogs (MWD) are now frequently employed by SOF; this was not the case prior to OEF/OIF. As such, it is necessary for SOF medical personnel to have some knowledge of and familiarity with anatomy, physiology and conditions of the MWD. Conventional veterinary assets are limited in numbers and availability, depending on location, and it may well depend on the SOF medic to preserve life, limb and eyesight of these extremely valuable animals.

This section of the SOF Medical Handbook only touches on a few topics regarding MWDs. It is imperative that SOF medics seek out veterinary personnel within their units or at local installation veterinary treatment facilities to obtain basic canine first aid training. In general, however, the treatment and care a medic would provide to a human patient/casualty can be applied to the canine patient in emergent scenarios or when access to veterinary assets is denied or very limited. The most significant condition specific to the dog, and not generally seen in human patients, is gastric dilatation-volvulus (GDV). As the name implies, this condition consists of an enlargement of the stomach followed by twisting. This condition is extremely emergent and will quickly lead to the death of a dog if not treated immediately. Due to likely inaccessibility to veterinary surgical facilities in a deployed environment, it is highly recommended that all MWDs have prophylactic gastropexies (surgical attachment of the stomach to the body wall, which prevents torsion/volvulus) performed at least one month prior to deployment.

The other common condition encountered in MWDs is heat injury. Though heat injury is also seen in humans and generally treated the same, a dog will continue to work until it collapses if the handler is not cognizant of signs indicative of heat injury nor takes measures to mitigate/prevent it. Heat injury is a preventable condition, but once it strikes, can easily lead to death of a MWD due to its inability to sweat. For traumatic injuries such as penetrating projectiles, burns and blast, treat the dog as you would a human patient. However, it will be very important that the dog be quickly evacuated to a veterinary surgical facility. Medical personnel within units with MWDs must ensure that they know where veterinary assets are located in their operational area, know the medical and surgical capacity of veterinary assets, have radio/telephone contact information for those same units, and should ideally have created some rapport with supporting veterinary personnel prior to requiring emergency care. Contacting veterinary personnel as soon as practical will help the SOF medic apply the appropriate treatment to a canine patient in a timely manner.

Chapter 14: Veterinary Medicine: Canine: Gastric Dilatation/Volvulus
MAJ Steve Baty, VC, USA

Introduction: GDV is an acute life-threatening medical emergency condition, which is a leading cause of death among MWDs. GDV is characterized by acute distension of the stomach (gastric dilatation) with fluid or gas and gastric obstruction due to twisting of the stomach (gastric volvulus). The main predisposing factors for GDV appears to be large and giant canine breeds which are typically utilized as MWDs, increased age, nervous or fearful temperament, and speed of eating. Precipitating factors for GDV in predisposed dogs include single feedings of large volumes of food compared to multiple feedings of smaller amounts, management practice of feeding from an elevated food bowl, and stressful events within eight hours prior to feeding.

Subjective: **Symptoms**
Handler reports MWD appears lethargic, depressed, bloated, painful, weak, hypersalivation, and episodes of non-productive retching (many times described by handlers as trying to vomit).
Focused History: *When did you first notice something different with your MWD?* (GDV has an acute onset.) *Has your MWD had any access to a rubber ball or tennis ball?* (Suspect possible gastric foreign body if handler reports missing ball) *Current age of your dog?* (increase risk of GDV with age greater than 7 years) *When was the dog's last meal; what did it eat; how much did it eat?* (increased risk of GDV with single, large feeding) *Has the dog tried to vomit, but nothing comes out?* (non-productive retching is consistent with GDV)

Objective: **Signs**
The physical exam reveals painful/uncomfortable, distended abdomen caudal to the last rib (lack of a "waist"), splenomegaly, weak peripheral pulses, tachycardia, prolonged capillary refill time, pale mucous membranes, and dyspnea. (Normal vital signs for a canine patient are heart rate 70-120/min, respiratory rate 16-24/min, temperature 100-102°F, mucous membranes pink, and capillary refill time <2 sec.)

Assessment: Differential Diagnosis

Simple gastric dilatation without volvulus is commonly seen secondary to overeating. The stomach which is distended with ingesta is not malpositioned. Ascites can present as a non-painful abdominal distension with a chronic history. Splenic torsion without GDV is usually presented as a painful non-distended abdomen.

Plan:

Diagnostic Tests: The diagnosis is usually based upon history, clinical signs, and physical exam. A right lateral and dorsal-ventral abdominal radiograph may facilitate diagnosis if readily available and the dog's condition allows.

Treatment

Primary:

1. Seek veterinary medical care immediately as this is a surgical emergency. Even if the dog cannot be quickly evacuated to a veterinary facility, you should be in contact with a veterinarian during this emergency.
2. Place 2 large-bore IV catheters (18 gauge preferred) in front limbs or jugular veins. **Note:** Do NOT place catheters in rear limbs. Administer 90mL/kg crystalloid fluids or 20mL/kg 6% hetastarch followed by crystalloid fluids.
3. Re-assess heart rate and pulse quality q10 minutes and adjust fluid therapy as indicated.
4. Perform non-surgical, temporary gastric decompression with trocar by percutaneous placement of a large bore IV catheter (12-16 gauge, 2") caudal to the last rib in the area of maximum distension. "Ping" the area first to ensure the trocar is placed in the gas cap of the stomach and not into fluid or some other organ such as the spleen. To ping, place a stethoscope over the uppermost portion of the abdomen and then percuss the area immediately adjacent to the stethoscope diaphragm. If placement is over the gas cap, a resonant "ping" will be heard; if not, a dull thud will be heard. Pass the large bore IV catheter directly into the gas cap to release a foul-smelling gas along with a small amount of fluid. Surgical decompression and gastropexy is still required upon completion of temporary gastric decompression.
5. Administer IV antibiotics such as **cefazolin** 22mg/kg.
6. Obtain blood sample for blood gas analyses, CBC, and biochemical panel when available.
7. Transport to a veterinary surgical facility for surgical gastric decompression and gastropexy.

Alternative:

1. Non-surgical gastric decompression will be indicated if transport to veterinary surgical facility is delayed (>60minutes). Temporary gastric decompression can be performed by trocarization or passage of an orogastric tube.
2. Trocarization can be performed multiple times if dilatation continues/recurs and gas can be repeatedly released.
3. Pass the orogastric tube using a 1/4" to 3/8" (approximately 20-32 French) internal diameter. Prior to inserting into the mouth, hold the tube with the tip midway between the last rib and xiphoid process and stretch the tube to the tip of the nose, placing a piece of tape at that point. Liberally lubricate the last 4-6 inches of the tube. Pass the tube into the stomach without forcing tube (to prevent perforating esophagus or stomach). Placing the MWD in different positions, including holding the dog upright, may help passage of tube. Successful orogastric tube placement usually results in food and/or fluid filling the tube.
4. Passage of an orogastric tube generally requires some form of chemically-induced sedation/anesthesia except in very moribund dogs.
5. Surgical decompression and gastropexy is still required upon completion of temporary gastric decompression.
6. Transport as soon as possible to a veterinary surgical facility for surgical gastric decompression and gastropexy.

Handler Education

General: GDV is a medical emergency with fair prognosis with surgery and poor prognosis without surgery.

Activity: The handler should restrict activity during the recovery time.

Diet: The handler should feed post operatively per veterinarian's instructions.

Prevention: The handler should continue to feed morning and night as compared to a single feeding.

Wound Care: The ventral midline abdominal incision should be monitored daily by handler and cleaned as indicated.

Follow-up Actions

Return Evaluation: The handler should be informed to follow the instructions of the attending veterinarian.

Evacuation/Consultation Criteria: Evacuate immediately for surgical correction. Consult a veterinarian early and other appropriate specialties as needed.

Chapter 14: Veterinary Medicine: Canine: Heat Injury

MAJ Steve Baty, VC, USA

Introduction: MWDs are susceptible to heat injury since they cannot sweat like humans. Etiologies for heat injury include those that are non-exertional such as forced confinement; exertional such as exercise in hot/humid environment, and combinations of both. The result is that the dog's evaporative cooling ability is hindered, and it cannot dissipate its extra heat by panting. It occurs most frequently in hot, humid weather with a poorly acclimated animal or one that has a concurrent health problem. A common scenario involves a dog being transported in a vehicle that lacks air conditioning on a hot day while caught in traffic. Dogs worked in high temperature environments are most at risk; however, dogs can suffer heat injury in any situation where they are poorly hydrated, are working hard and ventilation/air circulation is poor. Heat injuries range from relatively mild forms where the dog pants very fast, have mild tachycardia and a rectal temperature under 106°F to heat stroke where the dog may collapse, be obtunded and in shock.

Subjective: Symptoms

Handler reports MWD has uncontrolled panting, has increased/louder breathing sounds, inability to work well, is weak and/or distressed. He could also report the dog collapsed.

Focused History: *Has your dog ever had prior heat injury?* (Previous bouts of heat injury predispose a dog to subsequent episodes.) *How long were you working the dog and what were the ambient conditions like?* (Working the dog in hot/humid conditions with no rest sets the scene for heat injury.) *Were you giving your dog access to water while working?* (Inadequately hydrated dog is more prone to heat injury.)

Objective: **Signs**

The physical examination reveals uncontrolled panting (tachypnea), increased/loud breathing sounds (dyspnea), the dog is distressed (or possibly dull with severe heat injury), weak peripheral pulses, tachycardia (above 120bpm), possibly dark mucous membranes (with severe injury), prolonged capillary refill time, shock. Rectal temperature is at or above 106°F.

Assessment: **Differential Diagnosis**

Upper respiratory obstruction due to mass effect (eg, foreign object, food or tumor) can cause respiratory distress, but many times it would also lead to heat injury due to degradation in the dog's ability to dissipate heat. Rupture of a splenic tumor (hemangiosarcoma) could cause a dog to become weak, pant and eventually collapse, but rectal temperature generally would not be elevated to 106°F or above.

Plan

Diagnostic Tests:

The diagnosis is based upon history, clinical signs, and physical exam, especially rectal temperature.

Treatment: The goals of treatment include reduction of body temperature to less than 103.5°F and improve pulse quality and circulation. External cooling should continue until the temperature is ≤103°F. Restart external cooling if subsequent monitoring indicates the MWD's temperature is increasing again. Excessive cooling may cause hypothermia, which is just as dangerous as the hyperthermia. Pulse and body temperature should be assessed q5-10 minutes until treatment is discontinued and the dog maintains a temperature below 103°F for 20 minutes.

1. Allow the dog to pant effectively by loosening the collar and muzzle as much possible without compromising MWD restraint or personnel safety. Do NOT remove the muzzle.
2. Circulate air around the dog with electric fans (where available) and make sure the people restraining and aiding the dog do not impede air-flow with their bodies.
3. Apply rubbing alcohol to feet and convex/outer surface of ears where heat exchange is high. Allow the alcohol to evaporate then apply more if needed. Do not soak the entire dog with alcohol as this may excessively cool the dog or cause toxicity due to absorption thru the skin.
4. Apply ice packs in axillae (armpits) and groin. These areas have thin fur and lots of blood vessels and the cooled blood will circulate into the rest of the body.
5. Water soaking. A FLOW of cool, but NOT cold water should be used. Water soaking is the easiest, safest, and most appropriate method for MWD handlers to cool a dog with suspected heat injury when veterinary personnel are not readily available.
6. Water Intake: When the MWD's respiration has slowed enough that panting can be controlled, small amounts (1/2 to 1 cup) of water may be offered by mouth q10 minutes until therapy is completed.
7. In animals with severe heat injury, monitor and provide therapy as previously described, and add IV fluids. As soon as possible after initiating evaluation and cooling therapy (and preferably after collecting lab samples when availability exists), place a peripheral IV catheter and administer lactated Ringer's solution at ROOM TEMPERATURE rapidly: 10-15mL/pound body weight over <u>10-15 minutes. Monitor pulse rate and quality during fluid therapy.</u> If the dog is still distressed and pulse quality is not good after the 1st fluid bolus, a 2nd fluid bolus may be initiated.

Handler Education

General: Heat injury can be a medical emergency with good prognosis with quick intervention and poor prognosis if the injury is severe prior to institution of appropriate therapy, or of therapy is delayed or inadequate.

Activity: Frequently rest a dog when working in hot environments or when the dog is required to work hard. Follow the veterinarian's instructions for activity following therapy for heat injury. Affected dogs may require a number of days of convalescence prior to returning to work.

Diet: Feed post therapy per veterinarian's instructions.

Prevention: Frequently rest the dog during work as mentioned previously. Always ensure the dog has access to water and is kept in a relatively cool environment when possible (eg, air conditioned room/vehicle, shaded area).

Follow-up Actions

Return Evaluation: The handler should be informed to follow the instructions of the attending veterinarian.

Evacuation/Consultation Criteria: Consult a veterinarian early and other appropriate specialties as needed. Treatment for heat injury can be accomplished at unit level and should be when veterinary assistance is not immediately available.

Chapter 14: Veterinary Medicine: Canine: Administer a Subcutaneous or Intramuscular Injection

MAJ Steve Baty, VC, USA

What: Administer a subcutaneous (SC) or intramuscular (IM) injection to a military working dog.

When: Subcutaneous and intramuscular injections are sometimes required for proper administration of medication or fluids.

What You Need: A 22 gauge needle, 5/8" to 1" long, is normally used for subcutaneous and intramuscular injection.

What To Do:

Subcutaneous Injections

Select the injection site. The main area for subcutaneous injections is the dorsal aspect of the trunk between the left and right shoulder blades over the spine; this area is best for large volumes. However, for injections of small volumes (5mL or less), SC injections can be made most anywhere on the dog where skin is loose, generally along the back and sides.

Intramuscular Injections

Select the injection site

1. Caudal thigh – Landmarks: Grip the back muscles of the thigh with your non-dominant hand and feel the groove in the back of the femur bone on the outside of the thigh. This is where the sciatic nerve lives. Do NOT place the needle near this groove or you risk damaging the nerve.
2. Lumbar – Landmarks: Feel the ridges on the spine and the hip bone (wing of the top of the pelvis) with the index finger and thumb of your non-injecting hand. Insert the needle between these 2 places into the thick muscle of the lower back. Aspirate the syringe to ensure you are not in a vessel prior to proceeding with the injection.

Figure 5-34. Military Working Dogs: Subcutaneous and Intramuscular Injection Sites

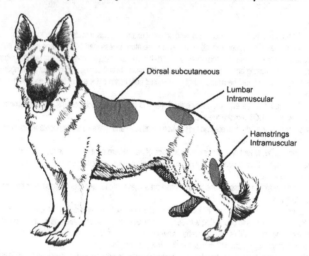

Dorsal subcutaneous

Lumbar Intramuscular

Hamstrings Intramuscular

What Not To Do: Do not try to give an injection without proper restraint of the dog. The MWD must be properly restrained during injection to avoid possible bite injury to surrounding personnel. Do not inject into a blood vessel.

Chapter 14: Veterinary Medicine: Canine: Placement of an IV Catheter

MAJ Steve Baty, VC, USA

What: Placement of an intravenous catheter in a military working dog.

When: Intravenous access is required for infusion of fluids, blood, or medications.

What You Need: Necessary materials and equipment include: Intravenous catheter with cap, various sizes of needles and syringes, a bag or bottle of sterile saline, adhesive tape, 70% isopropyl alcohol wipes, chlorhexidine or povidone-iodine surgical scrub, gauze sponges, roll gauze or self-adhesive conforming wrap, E-collar, and the dog's health record.

Figure 5-35. Military Working Dogs: Intravenous Catheter Sites

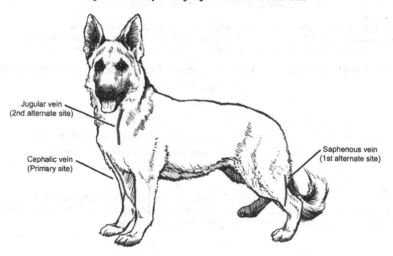

Jugular vein
(2nd alternate site)

Saphenous vein
(1st alternate site)

Cephalic vein
(Primary site)

What To Do:

1. **Select the site for catheter placement.**
   a. The cephalic vein (down the top center of the forearm) is the primary site.
   b. The lateral saphenous vein (runs along the outside of the ankle) is the alternate site.
   c. The jugular vein (run along the trachea) is the second alternate site.
2. **Have an assistant position the dog.**
   a. For cephalic IV catheter placement:
      (1) Have an assistant place and restrain the dog facing up and resting on his chest and stomach near one end of a table or other flat surface.
      (2) Direct the assistant to restrain the dog's head by wrapping his arm, farthest from the dog, around the dog's neck and cradling the dog's muzzle in his or her elbow.
      (3) Have the assistant wrap his fingers around the back of the dog's elbow and push the dog's leg slightly forward to stabilize it.
   b. For lateral saphenous IV catheter placement:
      (1) Have an assistant place and restrain the dog down on one side.
      (2) Direct the assistant to press one forearm across the dog's neck with that hand holding the forelegs and to place one finger between the front feet to achieve a more secure grip.
      (3) Have the assistant press the other arm across the dog's flank and hold the lower rear leg.
3. **Prepare the site for catheter placement.**
      (1) Clip the hair around the catheter site.
      (2) Perform a quick surgical preparation of the area with alcohol wipes, and if available, gauze soaked in dilute povidone-iodine or chlorhexidine scrub.
4. **Hold off the selected vein for 5-10 seconds before proceeding to puncture the vein.**
   a. Cephalic vein.
      (1) Direct the assistant to place the thumb of the hand holding the foreleg on the inside of the leg and rotate it slightly to the outside, applying pressure across the top of the foreleg, being careful not to over-rotate the vein.
      (2) Minimize the vein moving side-to-side by placing the thumb of the hand not holding the catheter along side the vein to stabilize it. Wrap the fingers of the same hand under the dog's leg to stabilize the leg.
   b. Lateral saphenous vein.
      (1) Steady the "up" leg by holding it with the fingers on the inside and the thumb laid alongside the vein to help prevent it rolling side-to-side.
      (2) Apply a tourniquet or have a third person apply pressure by placing their thumb over the back portion of the leg at the knee joint.
      (3) Wrap fingers over the knee cap and, while maintaining pressure, rotate the hand in a forward direction (ie, toward the dog's head).
5. **Secure the catheter to the leg with adhesive tape.**
   a. Wrap the tape around the leg, ensuring that the tape is not so tight as to cut off circulation
   b. Fold the end of the tape over making a courtesy tab.
6. **Wrap the catheter against the leg with roll gauze or self-adhesive conforming wrap.**
7. **If necessary and available, apply an E-collar to the working dog to prevent self-removal of catheter.**

Figure 5-36. Military Working Dog Wearing E-collar

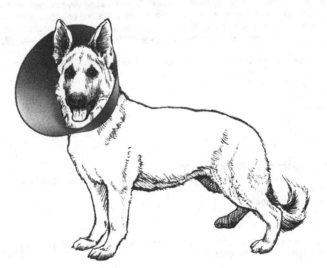

What Not To Do: The military working dog should not be left unattended as self-removal of catheter is very common. The catheter tape should not be applied so tight as to cut off circulation to the distal extremities.

Chapter 15: Pediatrics: Newborn Resuscitation

Maj William Lefkowitz, USAF, MC

When: Newborn resuscitation is straightforward but frightening if you have never been exposed to it. You will need to be able to recognize sick and/or premature infants. For stabilization of sick and premature infants, you will need to be able to give glucose, water and antibiotics, regulate temperature, and provide respiratory support. The more preterm the infant is, the more you need to worry about immature lungs (*see "respiratory distress syndrome" below*), evaporative water losses (leading to dehydration and cooling), low blood sugar and inability to feed. Infants are drowning victims. While in the uterus, they breathe through their placentas. Sometime between labor and delivery, they get cut off from oxygen. Fortunately, infants are great at protecting themselves from hypoxia. Sometimes they just need a little help. Wear gloves!

Estimating Gestation:

1. Term infant (38 wks): Typically 7 lbs (3kg), 20 inches long. Scrotum very wrinkled in males; in females, the labia majora covering labia minora. Ears are firm and nipples have a small mound of tissue (0.5-1cm) underneath them.
2. Preterm infant (32 weeks): typically 3.5 lbs (1.5kg), 16.5 inches (42cm). Scrotum smooth, labia major and minora equally prominent, ears are soft/floppy, nipples are flat, and skin is delicate/thin appearing. May have lots of thin body hair (lanugo) or cheesy coating (vernix).
3. Very preterm infant (<28 weeks): <2.5lbs (<1kg), <15 inches (38cm). Very thin skin, lots of visible veins under skin, ears pressed flat against head. Scrotum flat, no labia majora, bottom of feet smooth.

Normal vital signs:

Temperature: 98°F

Heart rate: 100-180 bpm, typically 130-150

Respiratory rate: 30-60 per minute. Hands and feet may be blue for up to 48 hours. Whatever is not blue should be warm (forearm and shins). If not, consider that the baby might be dehydrated.

Pulse ox (if you have a finger-unit that fits over an entire hand or foot), 80s for the first 10 minutes, but should be 96-100% on room air by 30 minutes of life.

Blood glucose > 40mg/dL in the first day of life, and >50mg/dL thereafter.

Activity:

Baby should be moving and reactive to the environment. Extra movements (clenching fingers, grasping, eye movement) are reassuring that the baby has reserve energy. A sick baby will stop responding to their environment. If you pick up their arm, it will drop back to the table. Breathing will be eerily regular. The most ill infants will be breathing 30 times a minute, have the tone of a water-balloon, not respond when stimulated, and be pale and cool, with very delayed capillary refill. These babies typically need fluid and positive pressure ventilation.

Respirations: There are 3 classic conditions affecting newborn respiration in the immediate newborn period. Initially the baby's lungs are filled with fluid and this is reabsorbed into the body after birth, with the help of deep breathing and adrenalin. For the first 20-30 minutes, the lungs will typically sound "wet" (crackles). If the baby is tachypneic (respiratory rate >60/min) or has labored breathing (retractions, grunting, gasping – even if <60 times a minute) watch for these conditions:

Transient tachypnea of the newborn: Breath rate between 100-120 times/minute, starting at birth or within a few hours. There are minimal retractions and there is typically good air-flow bilaterally. Babies will appear very comfortable and still respond to the environment. Saturations are typically in the high 90s on room air, minimal supplemental oxygen is needed. Anticipate this will last for hours to a couple of days. Avoid feeding by mouth when the respiratory rate is >70 or the breathing looks labored, since the baby may aspirate. You will need to balance that with making sure the blood sugars are adequate (>40mg/dL). Prognosis is very good for full uneventful recovery.

Respiratory distress syndrome: Babies born prematurely may not have the ability to keep their lungs from collapsing (missing surfactant, weak ribs). In order of increasing severity you may see:

1. Faster respiratory rate (60-80s)
2. Mild retractions
3. Nasal flaring
4. Grunting
5. Desaturations
6. Severe retractions
7. Poor perfusion
8. Slower respiratory rates (<60) with loud grunting
9. Very regular respirations in an infant that no longer responds to stimulation (Normal respirations vary over time with stimulation and activity.)
10. Very pale or very cyanotic
11. Apnea or irregular gasping
12. Death

What You Need: For an acute resuscitation you will need (in order of importance) a towel, a suction device, a way to administer positive pressure, string. A stethoscope and a thermometer are also useful.

What To Do:

A healthy baby will need minimal intervention during birth. It will be crying and moving and can be placed right on mother's chest as you dry it off. The cord can be allowed to stop pulsing as the placenta delivers. It is important to be as clean as possible, particularly around the umbilical cord. Tie the cord off about ½ inch from the abdominal surface and cut the rest away. Keep the baby warm and dry, allowing frequent breast feeding. Anticipate only about 1 or 2 urines or stools during the 1st day. Keep the umbilical stump dry; it will fall off after about 10 days. Standard newborn therapies: **Erythromycin** ointment ribbon in each eye to prevent eye infections. Give **Vitamin K** 1mg IM within an hour after birth to prevent hemorrhagic disease of the newborn. *See Part 3: General Symptoms: Obstetric Problems: Vaginal Delivery.*

There may be minimal signs of difficulty at birth that progress in severity over the first 36 hours. The mainstay of field expedient treatment is supplemental oxygen, if available, IV fluids and monitoring blood sugar. However, you may need to intermittently provide positive pressure or mouth-to-mouth-and-nose to re-expand the lung after it has collapsed. Babies are at risk for pneumothorax during this disease and treatment. Feeding during respiratory distress is not advised given the risk of aspiration. Placing the baby on their abdomen and on an incline with their head elevated will make their own breathing efforts much more effective. If you have a pulse-ox, target saturations in the low 90s and consider intervening (breaths) if the saturations fall below the low 80s on supplemental oxygen. If the baby can survive for 48 hours, they will typically start to improve. First you may notice the urine output start to increase, then the baby becomes more active and saturations will improve. Finally, the respirations will often stay increased (possibly >100 breaths/minute) for the next week or 10 days. If the baby can recover from this, there are typically no long-term problems. If you can get the baby to a place where you can intubate - ventilate, give surfactant and give long term IV fluids, do so.

Pneumothorax: Babies are at risk since their fragile lungs are atelectatic in utero and get pulled open by ribs and respiratory effort after birth. If you suspect one, *see the "troubleshooting" section.*

Resuscitation of newborn: Listed below are the 3 steps to resuscitating a baby. Each step is therapeutic (it fixes something) and diagnostic (it tells you something). The critical vital sign during newborn resuscitation is the HEART RATE. You can sometimes tell heart rate by feeling the base of the umbilical cord, by laying your hand across the chest or by listening with a stethoscope.

When the baby is delivered, if the baby is crying (or at least moving) you can just put the baby up on mom's chest without tying off the cord and wait for the cord to stop pulsing (sometimes takes minutes), while performing Step 1. If mom is sick or the baby is not moving at all, you will need to tie off the umbilical cord with some clean string. Suture used as a tie may be too sharp and cut through the jelly. You can use the tie-string of a face mask, if you have one. First just tie the cord about a foot away from the baby (you can trim this up later). Cut on the mother's side of the tied cord, otherwise the baby will bleed to death. If you can tie 2 ties an inch apart and cut between them, it will prevent this problem. At some point in the future you can tie about an inch from the baby's belly. Make sure you cinch it tight.

Step 1: Warm, Dry and Stimulate.

Therapeutic: A wet baby soon becomes a cold baby unless dried and placed near a heat source (mom's chest, if available). Optimal temperature is about 98°F. Stimulation is best accomplished by rubbing the baby with a towel or cloth during the act of drying. Use caution not to rub too hard; the skin is delicate and can be rubbed off. This act of stimulating gets the baby's adrenalin flowing and helps it transition to the outside world.

Diagnostic: The baby is "hibernating" if the heart rate is less than 100 beats per minute (bpm) after stimulation and drying. To count heart rate, you can count for 6 seconds and multiply by 10, or recall that about 2 beats per second is just over 100 (120) per minute. If the heart rate is >100 bpm, but the baby still looks sick (is not breathing or is very blue) you may need to move on to Step 2 anyway.

Step 2: Positive Pressure

Therapeutic: Lung stretch is a vagolytic and, if done adequately, will rapidly bring the heart rate to over 100 bpm. Often the baby will start breathing and crying soon after a few rescue breaths. Positive pressure is the MOST IMPORTANT tool you have for newborn resuscitation. It is unlikely that you will have a bag/mask small enough for a newborn, so you will most likely need to give mouth to mouth-and-nose breaths. Before you administer the breaths, you will need to make sure the baby's airway is opened. Position the head so the baby's face is straight up. This will sometimes be hard because of the big head. A small roll (<1 inch thick) under the shoulders sometimes helps). Suction out the mouth and nose. If you have a bulb syringe, that's OK. If you only have endotracheal tubes, take the smallest one you can find (or a small length of tubing) and suck out the mouth like drinking from a straw. Make sure you do not get any fluid in your mouth. Alternatively, you can use the sleeve of a large bore IV catheter attached to a large syringe and use it to suck out the throat. If you do not have anything to suction with, then just move on. Put your mouth over the baby's mouth and nose and blow. You want to breathe short and fast; a rate of about 60 per minute (one per second). Note that you will not need to breathe out your whole lung volume, just a puff until you see chest rise. The pitfall here is poor head position, with the baby's chin tucked forward pinching off the airway. Obviously, if you have a bag/mask small enough for a baby, that would be preferable.

Diagnostic: If after about 30 seconds of good positive pressure there is no response, the baby is diagnosed as having shock.

Step 3: Treat Shock and Troubleshoot.

Therapeutic: In the field it will be rare to have a baby recover after treating for shock, so it is probably better to jump to the troubleshooting section. If you can, intubate (3.5mm ETT at about 9cm at the lip in a term infant, 3.0mm ETT at 7.5cm at the lip in a preterm infant) and ventilate with 100% oxygen. But if you feel you need to treat shock, here is what you will need (assuming you cannot place an IV):

1. Vascular access: You can place an IV in the umbilical cord, in the largest vessel (the vein), pointing towards the baby. Use caution since injecting air into this vessel will kill the baby. The IV will probably not stay in place unless it is held. If you cut across the umbilical cord you will see 3 vessels; 1 vein and 2 arteries. The vein should be wide open and you can put a catheter into the vein directly. Make sure to tie a string around the base of the cord to pinch it off if the cord starts to bleed. Use plenty of gauze as the cord will be a slippery mess.
2. Saline or lactated Ringers solution bolus, IV over 5-10 minutes. About 30mL for each dose given to a term sized baby, 15mL for a small premature infant. You can consider blood from the placenta, but beware that the blood clots quickly and you will need to give it through a filter to avoid giving clots to the baby.

3. **Epinephrine.** The IV dose of 1:10,000 concentration is 0.1mL/kg, or about 0.5mL for a term baby, 0.2mL for a premature baby. Endotracheal tube dosing is 1mL/kg, or about 3mL for a term baby and 1mL for a premature baby. The IV doses should be flushed quickly or followed by a saline or LR bolus. The ETT dose needs no flush. Just squirt the dose down the ETT and bag it in. If you have 1:1,000 **epinephrine** in a vial, put 1mL of 1:1000 epinephrine in 9mL of normal saline, this will give a 1:10,000 concentration and from here you can draw off your dose.

TROUBLESHOOTING:

The classic reason to get this far in a baby resuscitation is that you have not really stretched open the lungs. Reposition the head and suction out the mouth. If the baby was born through meconium (baby poop), then it may have a plug of mucus in the trachea. If you can intubate and suction out the trachea, do. Finally, tension pneumothorax is a good reason to be unable to expand the lungs. On the side of the baby you suspect the pneumothorax, roll the baby to that side up. Just below the level of the nipple, in the anterior axillary line, place an IV catheter through the ribs into the pleural space (at about a 90° angle). If it works, you will hear the rush of air and the baby will improve. If the stomach is significantly inflated, this may also cause respiratory embarrassment, thus deflating the stomach (OG tube if you have one) can help.

Summary:

1. Warm, dry, stimulate
2. Check heart rate. If <100 start positive pressure
3. If positive pressure does not work, troubleshoot or treat shock.

That's it. Now if the baby's heart rate is over 100 (and assuming the baby is moving and/or breathing at this point) there are a number of things to consider simultaneously.

Fluid management: Typical fluid management in the first 2 days of life is D10W until the baby is feeding, though any fluid with glucose is acceptable. You may have to be inventive. If you have no vascular access, consider dripping the fluids in to the mouth/stomach (or letting the baby drink from a syringe). Obviously, if mom is available and the baby is able, allowing the baby to breastfeed will simplify management. If you happen to have formula, this can be used too. Do not expect the baby to eat too well. In the first few days, a teaspoon (5mL) is not unusual, but an ounce or two is better (every 3-4 hours). If you have no formula and no mother, consider feeding D10W. If you don't have D10W readily available, remember it is 10g glucose in 100mL of fluid. 20mL of D50 has 10g of dextrose. Add 20mL D50 to 80mL of fluid to get 100mL of D10W. A sugar packet from the US has 4g of sugar. Mix one sugar packet in 40mL of water to make D10W. Preferably, mix in water, but if you must, mix in saline. I have mixed sugar packets in water and fed to a baby by filling a disposable glove and punching a small hole in one of the fingers and letting the baby suck from that.

If you need to give IV fluids, a typical minimum rate for a term infant is about 10mL/hour. Typical for a preterm infant is 5mL/hour, but may be as high as 10mL/hour (eg, hot/dry environment or infant has a fever.) Use caution when giving more fluids than this because it is possible to induce congestive heart failure in the small infant by giving too much fluid. Never give a baby "one liter – wide open" even if they are dehydrated. Give 30mL aliquots and reassess after each one.

Babies that are very big (>10lb, >4kg) or very small (<6lb, <2.5kg) will often have problems maintaining a normal blood sugar. Jitteriness is a typical sign of hypoglycemia. Typical dose glucose to correct for hypoglycemia is 200mg/kg (<40mg/dL). 1mL of D50% has 500mg of glucose. A typical 3kg term infant needs at least 600mg of glucose (1.5mL has 750mg, given IV or po). For a preterm infant give 0.7mL (350mg) D50% (IV or po).

Antibiotics for newborns with indications of infection include: **ampicillin** and **cefotaxime**.

Term: **Ampicillin** 300mg IV or IM q12h and **cefotaxime** 150mg IV or IM q12h
Preterm: **Ampicillin** 150mg IV or IM q12h and **cefotaxime** 75mg IV or IM q12h
Actual dosing: <7 days old, <2 kg: **ampicillin** 50mg/kg/dose q12hr, **cefotaxime** 50mg/kd/dose q12hr <7 days old, >2kg: **ampicillin** 50mg/kg/dose q8h, **cefotaxime** 50mg/kg/dose q8h. Antibiotic therapy should be continued until clear signs of clinical resolution of infection (eg, normal vital signs and infant looks well; typically treatment is 7-10 days depending on severity of illness).

What Not To Do

1. Do not fail to re-evaluate and monitor (eg, heart rate) or fail to recognize risk of respiratory arrest (especially in pre-term infants).
2. Do not inject air into the umbilical vessels
3. Do not tie the umbilical cord loosely. Do not cut the umbilical cord on the infant side of the tie.

Chapter 15: Pediatrics: Infant and Child Assessment and Resuscitation

Lt Col Michael Meyer, USAF, MC

Introduction: Children are not small adults. A child's response (emotional, physical, or physiological) is dependent upon the age of the child and the stage of development. In general, children do not follow directions well, small children do not trust strangers, and besides natural language/communication barriers associated with different cultures, children do not have sophisticated methods of communication. A child's anatomy is somewhat different than an adult and their normal vital signs are often very different, but gradually become more adult-like as they grow. Most acute pediatric medical problems are typically related to infectious etiologies and malnutrition. Once you get past the physical and emotional differences, the physiology of disease is fairly similar, however. Knowing the weight of a child is especially important; appropriate equipment is based on the size of the child and medication dosages and IV fluid administration rates are weight-based calculations. Because they are smaller than adults, blood volume is smaller, fluid targets and expected urine output is lower and medication doses are smaller. Heart rate and respiratory rate is higher and blood pressure and volume of each breath is lower. In general, basic lab values are the same as adults (though hematocrits are typically in the 30s until adolescence, and creatinine is lower because of less muscle mass). Airway anatomy is different until about 8 years of age (the narrowest part of the trachea is the sub-glottic area, not the vocal cords). Diseases of childhood that typically kill children are rarely seen in adults (congenital heart disease and metabolic disorders).

Subjective: **Symptoms**

Infants and children do not localize disease well. Strep throat, for example, can present as a stomach ache. There is no substitute for a complete, thorough exam. In general, the child's caretaker acts as the surrogate for the child, but you may find that if you speak with the caretaker their concerns may be very different than your instinctive concerns of the child's state of health or symptoms. For example, parents might bring a child with an overwhelming late-stage cancer to your aid station and the real reason for the visit might be not be a cure, but simply a request for pain medications to make sleep more tolerable.

Focused History: It is typical for children to have unusual behaviors and responses. Therefore, it is important to ask *"how is this different than usual?"* Try not to discount a parent's observations. It is important to attempt to answer the questions: Who? What? (observations, chief complaint, symptoms, etc.) Why? (seeking medical care, how is this different) Where? (location of injury, site of pain or discomfort, etc.) When? (onset of symptoms, timing of symptoms, events surrounding injury, frequency between episodes, etc.) What helps or make things worse?

Objective: **Signs**

Using Basic Tools: Physical Examination: The severity of the underlying condition dictates the extent of the history taking and physical examination performed. You have time for a complete assessment if the child is not critically ill, but if the child is moribund you need to rapidly obtain a focused history, perform a rapid physical examination, make an assessment and simultaneously begin interventions. Some of the most sensitive observations/findings are a child's ability to recognize a parent, following parental instructions or for a parent to calm/sooth a child's discomfort. By systems: to avoid agitation, if possible, examine infant/child while parent is holding. Children sense anxiety, if you feel nervous, so will they. Show child the equipment before use; allow them to use it on you – stethoscope, otoscope, etc. Distract children by talking to them or giving them something to play with – lights, pens and tape for example. When assessing tenderness, distraction is the key. Examine quiet things early (heart, lungs, auscultation of abdomen). Examine annoying or painful things last – ears, throat, and areas of injury. The exam may not be linear, you may need to be creative and examine things as the opportunity presents. Obtain a set of vital signs. Remember to use an appropriately sized BP cuff for children; using too large of a cuff will underestimate the BP. **Note:** Normal pediatric vital signs (HR, BP, RR) are standardized based on the height, weight and age of "typical" Western children; so there may be some variability of "normal" when caring for children in other parts of the world. Based on the concept that children cannot tell you what is irritating them, observation is the key to success. Watch for response to environment: if child stops responding to noises or touching, it might suggest severe compromise and impending arrest. Vacant stare might mean severe illness/meningitis. Peritonitis, cellulitis, broken bones can lead to avoidance of movement/contact. Decreased interaction may be related to decreased cerebral perfusion. Remember to use distraction techniques while palpating for tenderness.

Assessment:

Table 5-22. Normal Vital Signs by Age (all numbers are approximate, based on several sources)

Heart Rates		Respiratory Rates	
Newborn	100-180	Newborn	30-60
<1 year	80-180	0-1 years	24-40
1-3 years	70-150	1-3 years	22-30
4-8years	60-130	4-9 years	18-24
9+ years	60-100	10-18 years	14-22

Systolic Blood Pressure:
Minimum: Newborn – 2 months = 50mmHg, 2 months to 15 years = 70 + (2 x age in years)
Maximum: up to 15 years of age ~ 100 + (2 x age in years)

Maintenance fluid requirements (If NPO):
<10kg, 4mL/kg/hr or 100mL/kg/day
10-20kg, above plus 2mL/kg/hr or 50mL/kg/day
>20kg, above plus 1mL/kg/hr or 25mL/kg/day
   • Example, a 23kg child would get 10kgx4mL/kg/hr plus 10kgx2mL/kg/hr plus 3kgx1mL/kg/hr or 40+20+3 or 63mL/hr.
   Note: A typical "70kg" adult would get 10x4 + 10x2 + 50x1 or 110mL/hr
Infants and young children (<4 yo) need a continuous dextrose infusion due to poor glycogen stores.
D5 ½ NS with 20meq/L KCl is adequate for basic electrolyte needs if NPO.

Urine output: Typically 1-3mL/kg/hr (or 25-75mL/kg/day)

Weight:
2-8 years, 50th %ile in kg is about 8 + (age x 2) (ex: 6 year old is 8 + (6*2) or 20kg.
9-14 years, 50th %ile in kg is about (age x 3.4) (ex: 12 year old is 12 x 3.4) or 41kg

Length:
2-14 years, 50th%ile in cm is about 75 + (age x 6.2) (ex: 12 year old is 75 + (12*6.2) or 150cm
Girls reach 50%ile height of 165cm at about 15 years old
Boys reach 50%ile height of 175cm at about 16 years old

Plan:

Resuscitation and Stabilization

Rapid Emergency Assessment: "The ABCs"

Airway

- Need to determine patent vs. not patent (open vs. obstructed)
- If patent, then move onto next phase of assessment
- If obstructed:
  a. Reposition with a head tilt or jaw thrust maneuver
  b. Use oropharyngeal or nasopharyngeal airway device
  c. Begin artificial ventilation

Endotracheal Intubation

- Positioning: For a child, a "pad" (folded towel, shirt) should be placed under the head to cause slight cervical spine flexion and gentle extension at the atlantooccipital joint. For infant, a "pad" may need to be placed under the shoulders to achieve appropriate "sniffing" position. **Note:** If suspected cervical spinal injury, the head/neck should be kept in neutral position using in-line traction. However, the most recent guidelines recognize that cervical spine injuries in children are a rare injury, if unsuccessful at obtaining an airway in a neutral position, then it may be necessary to intubate the child using conventional techniques.
- Airway Tools (if available): ETT, stylet, laryngoscope blades and handles, suction catheter, end tidal CO_2 detector, bag-valve-mask (BVM), supplemental oxygen.
- Endotracheal tube (ETT) size, location formulas
  a. Newborn:
    1. ETT internal diameter formula = gestational age/10. Example: slightly preterm infant (35 weeks (38-41 weeks is term)) = 3.5 ETT.
    2. Depth at lip = 6cm+wt in kg. (3kg = 9cm at lip).
  b. Infant/Child:
    1. ETT internal diameter formula = (age+16)/4. Example: 6 yo = (6+16)/4 = 5.5 ETT.
    2. Depth at the lip = 3x internal diameter (ex: 6 year old = 5.5 x 3 = 16.5cm at the lip).
    3. Un-cuffed ETT preferred if <8 years old.
  c. Always have range of ETT size available, usually ½ size larger/smaller.
    1. Special Considerations:
      - The narrowest portion of the pediatric airway (age <8 yo) is in the subglottic area, unlike adults where the vocal cords are the narrowest portion.
      - Placement of too large of ETT may damage the cricoid ring and lead to subglottic stenosis and difficulty extubating successfully.
      - Usually will attempt to ventilate with slight leak around ETT to minimize risk of traumatizing airway.
      - Utilize "cricoid pressure" to compress the esophagus and decrease risk of aspiration event.

Breathing: BVM or mouth-to-mouth or mouth-to-mouth-and-nose for infant
- Newborn
  a. 40-60 per minute, target chest rise, may need as little as 15mL/breath (5mL/kg)
  b. 3:1 ratio chest compressions to breaths ("1 and 2 and 3 and breathe and") if chest compressions given. Always synchronized. 3 compressions and 1 breath every 2 seconds = 120 events/minute
- Infant/Child
  a. 30 per minute infant, 20 per minute young child, 12 per minute older child. Target chest rise.
  b. 15:2 ratio, with compressions about 100/min. Once intubated, no longer needs to be synchronous.

Circulation:
- Exam findings seen in shock: Tachycardia, delayed capillary refill, cold extremities, weak or absent distal pulses, poor urine output, altered mental status.
  a. Typical findings in pediatric compensated shock, likely to be normotensive.
  b. Decompensated shock = Hypotension.
  c. Hypotension is a late finding in pediatric shock.
- Tachycardia is the earliest sign in shock. Pediatric patients maintain cardiac output by increasing heart rate (remember Cardiac Output = Heart Rate x Stroke Volume) since the pediatric heart can only minimally increase stroke volume. Children increase systemic vascular resistance (delayed cap refill, cold extremities, poor pulses) to maintain blood pressure.
- Pediatric shock is classically a "cold shock", so the child has decreased cardiac output, poor contractility, high SVR and is usually hypovolemic. Adult shock is classically "warm" shock where patient is vasodilated and needs vasopressor therapy early as part of resuscitation.
- #1 cause of shock worldwide is hypovolemic shock
  a. Acute gastroenteritis with diarrhea (cholera)
  b. Acute hemorrhage (trauma)
  c. Burns
  d. Sepsis
- Hypotension:
  a. Newborn: systolic <50mmHg.
  b. Infant, child: <70 + (2 x age in years) (ex: 6 year old = systolic 70 + (6x2) = 82mmHg).
  c. Cuff should cover about 2/3 of the upper arm length. Cuff pressures are prone to inaccuracy.

- Therapy
  a. Volume Replacement:
    1. In mild cases, oral rehydration can be very successful (see below)
    2. In severe cases, IV therapy may be mandatory.
    3. NS/LR 20mL/kg over 5-15 minutes IV or IO. 10mL/kg in newborn or if concerned about congestive failure.
    4. After 3rd bolus, consider using blood rather than NS or LR.

CPR Algorithms:

- Uninterrupted, deep and fast chest compressions are the key to successful CPR. Establish airway control, provide supplemental oxygen and start CPR. "Adequate" chest compressions should produce a palpable pulse. Check rhythm, shock if needed, resume CPR and give meds at same time that CPR is restarted. Continue CPR for 5 cycles of 15 compressions and 2 breaths after intervention prior to rechecking rhythm (30 seconds in a newborn). On reassessment, if rhythm changes, simply change to the algorithm for the new rhythm.
- **Epinephrine** dosing: **Epi** (1:10,000), 0.1mL/kg IV/IO every 3-5 minutes. If no IV/IO access, then give 1.0mL/kg ETT (or 0.1mL/kg of 1:1,000 epi). Must provide 5 cycles of CPR after medications given to allow for cardiac output and circulation of drug. Once you start giving epi, make it someone's job to repeat the epi every 3-5 minutes until the code is done. That way it will not be overlooked. No evidence to support using higher doses of epinephrine than the recommended dose.

Pulseless:

- **Asystole or PEA:** Resume CPR and give **epi** every 3-5 minutes. Recheck rhythm every 5 cycles of CPR.
  a. Underlying causes – <u>h</u>ypovolemia, <u>h</u>ypoxia, <u>h</u>ypo/hyperkalemia, <u>h</u>ypoglycemia, <u>h</u>ypothermia, <u>h</u>ydrogen ion (acidosis), <u>t</u>oxins, <u>t</u>amponade (cardiac), <u>t</u>ension pneumo, <u>t</u>hrombosis, <u>t</u>rauma.
- VF/VT without pulse:
  a. Defibrillate with 2J/kg x1, resume CPR for 5 cycles.
  b. Recheck rhythm. If still VF/VT, shock with 4J/kg, resume CPR and give **epi**.
  c. Recheck rhythm every 5 CPR cycles. If still VF/VT, shock again with 4J/kg.
  d. Resume CPR and consider **lidocaine** 1mg/kg IV/IO, magnesium (for Torsades) 25mg/kg IV/IO (max 2g). CPR x 5 cycles and recheck.
  e. If still in VF/VT, keep shocking with 4J/kg every 5 CPR cycles and repeating epi every 3-5 minutes.

Tachycardia with Poor Perfusion:

- Sinus Tachycardia: usually <220/min infant, <180/min child. P-wave normal, variable RR interval →treat H&Ts (*See asystole/PEA*)
- SVT: p-waves absent/abnormal intervals, RR interval not variable, usually >220/min infant, >180/min child
  a. Consider vagal maneuvers (ice to face, blow through pencil, etc) if hemodynamically stable
  b. Consider **adenosine** if IV/IO access available (0.1mg/kg – max 6mg, then double 2nd dose – rapid flush).
  c. If neither available or works (when poorly perfused) perform synchronized cardioversion (0.5-1J/kg then 2J/kg). Sedate if possible, do not delay cardioversion though.
  d. Consider **procainamide** 15mg/kg IV over 30 minutes if other methods unsuccessful. VT: synchronized cardioversion (0.5-1J/kg then 2J/kg). Consider **procainamide**.

Bradycardia with Poor Perfusion:

- HR <100 in newborns, HR <60 infants and children
- Control ventilation: BVM or mouth-to-mouth-and-nose if needed.
  a. If bradycardia and poor perfusion persists: CPR, **epinephrine** every 3-5 minutes. Consider **atropine** 0.02mg/kg (0.1mg minimum, 1.0mg max for child). Consider cardiac pacing.

Oral rehydration therapy (ORT):

From **Rehydrate.org:**

- Wash your hands with soap and water before preparing solution.
- Prepare a solution, in a clean pot, by mixing:

Eight level teaspoons of sugar and one level teaspoon of salt in 1L of clean water	- or -	1 packet of Oral Rehydration Salts (ORS) with 1L of clean drinking or boiled water (after cooled)

- Stir the mixture till all the contents dissolve.
- Wash your hands and the infant or child's hands with soap and water before feeding solution.
- Give the sick child as much of the solution as it needs, in small amounts frequently.
- Give child alternately other fluids - such as breast milk and juices.
- Continue to give solids if child is four months or older.
- If the child still needs ORS after 24 hours, make a fresh solution.
- ORS does not stop diarrhea. It prevents the body from drying up. The diarrhea will stop by itself.
- If child vomits, wait 10 minutes and give ORS again. Usually vomiting will stop.
- If diarrhea increases and /or vomiting persist, take child over to a health clinic.

Emergency considerations (starting points) for infant or child in shock

- Always consider: pulse-ox, temperature (hypothermia), and glucose check
- Intraosseous line: preferred sites in children
  a. Proximal tibia, 2cm below and 2cm medial to the tibial tuberosity on flat part of bone
  b. Distal femur 3cm above lateral condyle in the midline
  c. Distal tibia, 2cm above medial malleolus (more effective in older children)
  d. Anterosuperior iliac spine, perpendicular to the long axis of body

- Hypovolemia – treat with about 20mL/kg NS/LR by IV/IO until improved; consider giving blood after 3rd bolus. Consider that blood volume in an infant/child is approximately 75mL/kg
- Adrenal insufficiency – congenital adrenal hyperplasia presents in the first weeks of life in an infant with male appearing or ambiguous appearing genitals. Treat with **hydrocortisone**, 1mg/kg IV q6 hours (consider 3/kg initial dose)
- Metabolic disorders – typically presents with altered mental status, may be after starting new foods, or more typically after being unable to eat due to other illness. Make NPO, treat with maintenance IV glucose
  a. Hypoglycemia (<60) treat with 0.5mg/kg IV/oro-gastric/po glucose and recheck in 15 minutes
  b. Hyperglycemia (diabetic ketoacidosis, pH <7.3, bicarb <15) (Type I diabetes typically presents at around 5 years of age and at adolescence, typically at times of illness). Rehydrate and treat with **insulin** (0.1unit/kg SC or IV). Rapid re-correction may lead to cerebral edema. Watch for precipitously falling potassium as acidosis corrects
- Severe cyanosis
  a. Newborn period: pulmonary hypertension (treat with oxygen, volume), pneumothorax
  b. Infant/child – presenting with respiratory distress, consider pulmonary etiology first (pneumonia, asthma, pneumothorax). Then consider heart lesions.
- Heart lesions
  a. Ductal dependent lesions present in the first weeks of life with sudden severe cyanosis (pulmonary atresia, tricuspid atresia) or shock (coarctation of the aorta). Treat with volume and, ideally, prostaglandin if available (0.1mcg/kg/min PGE1 – causes apnea, fever, flushing, hypotension)
  b. Transposition of the aorta/pulmonary artery: most common cyanotic lesion discovered at birth because cyanosis is so profound. Treat with intravascular volume and oxygen, prostaglandin in available.
  c. Tetralogy of Fallot: most common cyanotic heart disease in infants (loud murmur – ventricular septal defect and pulmonary stenosis)
     1. "Tet spell" (hypercyanotic spell)– not enough blood getting to lungs (murmur may decrease during a spell): treatment →oxygen, decrease agitation (**morphine** 0.1mg/kg SC/IM), knee-chest position (kneeling – increases systemic vascular resistance and forces blood to lungs)
     2. Consider: glucose – **propranolol** (0.2mg/kg IV slow push) – **bicarbonate** (1meq/kg IV) – **phenylephrine** (0.02mg/kg IV)
  d. Ventricular Septal Defect: most common non-cyanotic heart disease (loud murmur)
     1. Presents in first weeks to months with gradually worsening feeding difficulty as too much blood flows through lungs. May eventually develop enough lung dysfunction to be cyanotic. If long-standing, may develop pulmonary hypertension leading to hypercyanotic spells that look like tet-spells. Avoid excess oxygen if you know about a VSD as it will lead to further over circulation of blood to the lungs.
- Trauma – consider smaller blood volume than adult (about 75mL/kg) and relatively larger internal organs that may rupture and bleed. Larger head relative to body means higher risk of cervical spine injury with trauma. Blunt trauma may not visibly injure ribs since they are more cartilaginous than adults.
- Burns – intubation for >25% BSA burns given need for pulmonary toilet. 100% oxygen to counter CO, if inhaled. BSA calculation where different than adult – head (infant 18%, child = 13%, adolescent = 9%), whole arm (not hand) = 8%, chest = 13%, back = 13%. Whole leg (thigh and leg, not foot) (infant = 10%, child = 14%, adolescent = 16%). *See Part 7: Trauma: Chapter 29: Burns (Thermal, Scald or Chemical)*
  a. "Parkland formula" = maintenance fluids + 4mL/kg/day per %BSA (ex: 50%BSA = 200mL/kg/day (or ~8mL/kg/hr). If hypotensive or UOP<1mL/kg/hr give 20mL/kg NS/LR. If UOP >3mL/kg/hr drop to about 2/3's of formula rate.

Resuscitation guidelines from PALS, © 2006 AHA.

Table 5-23. Commonly Used Pediatric Drugs and Dosages

Source: Emergency War Surgery 3rd Revision, Borden Institute, 2004, p. 33.7

Drug Name	Dosage
Phenobarbital	2–3mg/kg IV
Diazepam	0.25mg/kg IV
Midazolam HCl	0.1mg/kg IV (max 5 mg)
Atropine	0.1–0.5mg IV
Phenytoin	15–20mg/kg, administered at 0.5 to 1.5mL/kg/min as a loading dose, then 4–7mg/kg/d for maintenance.
Mannitol	0.5–1.0g/kg IV
Succinylcholine chloride	2mg/kg IV for <10kg, and 1mg/kg IV for >10kg
Ampicillin	25–50mg/kg IV q8h (q12–18h in newborns)
Gentamicin	2.5mg/kg IV q8h (q12–18h in newborns)
Metronidazole	10mg/kg IV
Acetaminophen	15mg/kg po

Table 5-24. Pediatric Medical/Surgical Equipment Sizes by Age and Weight

Source: Emergency War Surgery 3rd Revision, Borden Institute, 2004, p. 33.7

AGE, WEIGHT (kg)	AIRWAY/BREATHING							CIRCULATION			SUPPLEMENTAL EQUIPMENT		
	O₂ Mask	Oral Airway	Bag-valve	Laryngo-scope	ET Tube	Stylet	Suction	BP Cuff	IV Cath	NG Tube	Chest Tube	Urinary Cath	C-collar
Premie 3 kg	Premie Newborn	Infant	Infant	0 Straight	2.5–3.0 No Cuff	6 F	6–8 F	Premie Newborn	24-gauge	12 F	10–14 F	5 F Feeding	—
0–6 mo 3.5 kg	Newborn	Infant Small	Infant	1 Straight	3.0–3.5 No Cuff	6 F	8 F	Newborn Infant	22-gauge	12 F	12–18 F	5–8 F Feeding	—
6–12 mo 7 kg	Pediatric	Small	Pediatric	1 Straight	3.5–4.0 No Cuff	6 F	8–10 F	Infant Child	22-gauge	12 F	14–20 F	8 F	Small
1–3 y 10–12 kg	Pediatric	Small	Pediatric	1 Straight	4.0–4.5 No Cuff	6 F	10 F	Child	20–22-gauge	12 F	14–24 F	10 F	Small
4–7 y 16–18 kg	Pediatric	Medium	Pediatric	2 Straight or Curved	5.0–5.5 No Cuff	14 F	14 F	Child	20-gauge	12 F	20–32 F	10–12 F	Small
8–10 y 24–30 kg	Adult	Medium Large	Pediatric Adult	2–3 Straight or Curved	5.5–6.5 Cuffed	14 F	14 F	Child Adult	18–20-gauge	12 F	28–38 F	12 F	Medium

Chapter 15: Pediatrics: Common Pediatric Symptoms: Fever

LTC Douglas Lougee, MC, USA

Introduction: Fever is the most common reason why a parent seeks medical care for their child. In most cases, it is the body's reaction to a viral, bacterial, fungal, or parasitic infection. Occasionally, fever may result from a non-infectious cause such as auto-immune disorders (rheumatoid arthritis, rheumatic fever) or a malignancy. Most children with fever will have uncomplicated, self-limited infections, but some will have serious or life-threatening febrile diseases distinguished by careful examination. The evaluation of fever depends on child's age, concurrent symptoms and geographic location. Some febrile diseases only happen in certain regions, usually related to vector presence (malaria, dengue). Others tend to be present in developing countries (TB, typhoid fever). Likewise, infectious disease epidemics occur in distinct geographic patterns. A complete travel history is vital to diagnosis. The infectious diseases that cause fevers follow distinct seasonal variation. In temperate areas, respiratory infections are common during the colder part of the year. In tropical areas, wet and dry cycles contribute to vectors that spread infectious diseases. **Risk Factors:** Age is the most important. The very young, (ie, neonates, infants and toddlers) are relatively immune-compromised and more susceptible to infectious diseases. Vaccines may decrease this susceptibility and vaccine history may provide useful information to help suggest most likely diagnosis. Other factors that affect immune system such as HIV, cancer and malnutrition, animal, insect and ill human contacts are also important.

Subjective: **Symptoms**
Focus on symptoms that may help determine infectious syndrome: Respiratory (cough, runny nose, sore throat, earache, rapid breathing); Gastrointestinal (vomiting, diarrhea, belly pain); Urinary (dysuria, foul-smelling urine); Skin (rashes or abscesses); Bone and Joint (decreased use of a limb, bone pain, limp, refusal to stand or bear weight); CNS (irritability, stiff neck, vomiting, seizures, mental status changes); Systemic (chills, poor feeding, decreased activity, decreased fluid intake or urine output.)
Focused History: *How high is your child's temperature?* (Fever is temperature >100.4°F, but many parents do not have access to a thermometer. Most parents are accurate in noting if fever is present by touch, although they will not be able to report fever height.) *Is the fever constant?* (recurrent fever with some malaria, relapsing fever, leptospirosis) Other Symptoms: *Have you noticed* [select: *rash, headache, diarrhea, swollen lymph nodes, localized pain, stiff neck, cough*]? (identify affected systems) *Do you know other persons with similar symptoms?* (suggests contagious illness or point source outbreak)

Objective: **Signs**
Using Basic Tools: Vital signs: Heart rate and respiratory rate increase with fever. General appearance/mental status: playful, active, interactive, fussy, irritable, lethargic, non-responsive to parent, responsive to only pain, comatose. Fontanel: bulging, normal or sunken. Eyes: conjunctivitis, sunken or dry. Ears: Bulging tympanic membrane with purulent effusion and redness (otitis media). Skin: rashes, petechiae, purpura, abscess, cellulitis, capillary refill time. Nose: mucus. Oral/Pharynx: specific findings (Koplik spots (measles), lesions consistent with herpes or enteroviral infection, swollen red tonsils, palatal petechiae, exudates. Face: tenderness over sinuses, periorbital or buccal cellulitis. Neck: stiffness or lymphadenopathy, adenitis. Lungs: respiratory rate, crackles, retractions, decreased air entry. Cardiovascular: heart rate and murmurs, quality of pulses. Abdomen: soft, tender, rigidity, rebound tenderness. Extremities: decreased range of motion, redness, swelling, and effusion of joints, limping, or irritability when a limb is manipulated.
Using Advanced Tools: Labs: Testing may be used to confirm clinical diagnosis based on history and physical. Blood, urine and CSF cultures are indicated for all febrile neonates and should be strongly considered in young infants that appear seriously ill. In malarious areas or if travel history indicates, blood smears or rapid detection kits may be used to confirm diagnosis. Non-specific tests such as a complete blood count, erythrocyte sedimentation rate, or c-reactive protein may assist with determining severity of illness. Radiology may be helpful, particularly to confirm pneumonia.

Assessment:
Fever is a sign, not a diagnosis, identify the underlying cause. Identify children with possible serious conditions: neonates, young infants, children with immune-compromising conditions, children with suspected CNS, or serious systemic, skin, bone, joint, gastrointestinal or respiratory infections. Measure and support hydration and nutritional requirements. Persistent fevers may have a non-infectious cause (eg, malignancy or auto-immune disorder).

Plan:
Treatment
Empiric therapy is indicated if severe infection is suspected (bacterial, fungal, viral, or parasitic). When the diagnosis becomes clear, more specific therapy should be initiated. All febrile neonates should be treated with empiric antibiotics, (eg, **ampicillin** 50mg/kg IM or IV q6h plus **cefotaxime** 50mg/kg q12h for age 0-1 wk, q8h for age 1-4 wks) until sustained clinical improvement is verified. If unable to obtain specific testing, broad empiric antimicrobials are continued or changed according to clinical response. Supportive care must be provided (eg, IV fluids, respiratory support, and nutritional therapy). Antimicrobials are not indicated for the majority of older infants and children with mild-moderate non-specific febrile illness and can mask or delay the diagnosis of important infections (eg, meningitis, infectious endocarditis, or osteomyelitis). Most of these children will have self-limited viral infections for which specific antimicrobial medication are not effective. In cases when malaria is suspected, empiric treatment for malaria should be strongly considered while awaiting confirmation of diagnosis. Drinking fluids is extremely important and increased fluid intake is critical to prevent serious dehydration. Antipyretics (eg, **acetaminophen** 10mg/kg po q4-6h, not to exceed 5 doses in 24 hours) may be used to relieve the discomfort from fever.

Patient Education
Fever is not the "enemy"; what is causing the fever is what is important. Most children with fever will have a minor illness that will go away in just a few days and the fevers will rise and fall until the illness is gone. Drinking fluids is extremely important and care must be given to offer an increased amount of fluids. Kids with fever tend not to eat as much as usual, but this is not harmful to the child for a few days. If child is breastfeeding, the mother should be encouraged to feed more frequently. Oral Rehydration Solution should be offered for cases where fluid loss is due to diarrhea or vomiting.

Follow-up Care
Follow up if there is no improvement within 2 days or if child seems worse, develops new symptoms or is not taking sufficient fluids.
Note: There are many cultural beliefs treatments for febrile children. Most of these are harmless and can be used to enhance relationship with the child's caretakers. Cultural beliefs that are harmful to child should be diplomatically discouraged.

Chapter 15: Pediatrics: Common Pediatric Symptoms: Diarrhea and Dehydration
LTC Douglas Lougee, MC, USA

Introduction: Diarrhea is defined as an increase in water in stool and is the 2nd leading cause of death in children world-wide. Diarrhea kills children in 3 main clinical scenarios: 1) acute dehydration, 2) chronic diarrhea with malnutrition and 3) dysentery (blood and mucus in diarrhea). Children with diarrhea must be assessed for these scenarios and treated to correct the fluid, electrolyte and nutritional problems that result from diarrhea. Dehydration in children is most commonly associated with diarrhea but can also be the result of fever, intractable vomiting and uncontrolled metabolic disorders (eg, diabetes). **Geographic Association:** Present everywhere. **Seasonal Variation:** In temperate areas, epidemics of rotavirus diarrhea are common during winter months, but other types of diarrhea are common year round. In tropical areas, seasonal variation may be present according to wet or dry season.

Subjective: Symptoms
Copious watery diarrhea. If able, patients who are dehydrated will complain of thirst, weakness, lethargy.
Focused History: *How many stools has your child had?* (helps define problem as diarrhea as well as severity) *How often?* (define severity) *What do they look like?* (Watery, loose, or pure liquid helps define severity of fluid loss.) *Is blood present?* (Blood may indicate an invasive infection such as: bacillary dysentery caused by *Salmonella, Shigella, E. coli* 0157:H7, or *Campylobacter*; amoebic dysentery caused by *Entamoeba histolytica* or other invasive process.) *Is child thirsty? How much and what type of fluids is the child drinking?* (assess hydration) *How long has your child had diarrhea?* (Chronic is defined as >2 weeks, chronic is more likely to be parasitic or caused by a non-infectious process and is associated with malnutrition and increased risk for death.) *What has the child been eating?* (assess nutritional status as well as possible sources of infection) *When was last urination?* (Assess hydration; infants should be urinating at least q4h and children at least q6h while awake.) *Are there any other symptoms?* (Fever, vomiting, cough etc: vomiting is common with intestinal illnesses and may be an impediment to maintaining normal hydration; infections such as malaria may also cause diarrhea.) *Do any others in your family or village have diarrhea?* (helps assess infectious potential)

Objective: Signs
Focus on looking for signs of dehydration and malnutrition:
Using Basic Tools: Vital signs: Heart and respiratory rates may be elevated, check for fever. Obtain weight without clothing. Accurate length or height will help determine nutritional status. General appearance: note if playful, interactive, irritable, lethargic, or comatose. Look for sunken fontanel in infants. Eyes: dry or sunken. Mouth: dry mucous membranes. Skin: check capillary refill time (should be less than 2 seconds) check skin turgor by pinching skin on abdomen between umbilicus and xiphoid process: positive sign is when skin does not flatten out immediately—indicator of severe dehydration. Look for diaper rash. Abdomen: listen for bowel sounds, look for distention and feel for tenderness. Pulses: quality, compare peripheral and central pulses to note difference, absent or diminished peripheral pulses indicate shock or impending shock.
Using Advanced Tools: Acute diarrhea: Consider checking electrolytes if severely dehydrated. If febrile and ill, consider CBC and blood cultures. If suspect dysentery, stool culture and fecal leukocytes. In austere circumstances, proceed with empiric therapy without labs. Chronic diarrhea: stool ova and parasites, stool culture, CBC. When children are dehydrated, urine output will decrease to <1mL/kg/hr. **(Note:** Diabetes may cause an osmolar diuresis despite significant dehydration). Specific gravity of urine 1.030 or higher: (Note: Babies <6 months old may not be able to concentrate urine and have a normal specific gravity even when dehydrated); BUN and CR will increase due to decreased renal perfusion.

Assessment:
Classify child according to hydration status and estimate acute weight loss: no or mild dehydration (0-4% weight loss) will have no or mild signs of dehydration. Moderate dehydration (5-8% weight loss) will have some signs such as dry mouth, dry sunken eyes, tachycardia, irritability, sunken fontanel, child will have increased thirst. Severe dehydration >8% weight loss: any of the moderate plus lethargy, coma, diminished peripheral pulses, decreased skin turgor. Assess for chronic diarrhea, malnutrition and dysentery (blood and mucus in stools).
Differential Diagnosis: Most cases of acute diarrhea are infectious: viral such as rotavirus, Norwalk agent or many others, bacterial such as entero-toxigenic *E. coli* (ETEC) or *Vibrio cholera*. Acute dysenteric diarrhea may be from *Shigella, Salmonella, Campylobacter* or entero-hemorrhagic *E. coli* (EHEC also known as E. coli 0157:H7). Chronic diarrhea is either infectious (*Giardia lamblia*, amebic dysentery) or secretory from autoimmune or malabsorption (gluten enteropathy, cystic fibrosis, milk protein allergy, inadequate caloric intake also can lead to malabsorption and diarrhea). When dehydration is not due to diarrhea, the differential includes any condition that significantly affects or compromises circulation resulting in decreased mental status (eg, blood loss, sepsis, heart failure).

Plan:
Treatment
1. Fluid Replacement: Treat mild to moderate dehydration with Oral Rehydration Therapy (ORT), severe with IV/IO isotonic fluids. ORT: Use the World Health Organization (WHO) Oral Rehydration Solution (ORS) packets; one packet mixed in 1 liter clean H_2O. In developed countries, may substitute a commercially available pre-mixed oral rehydration solution (eg, Pedialyte). Mild dehydration: Continue all normal foods and liquids including clean water and breastfeeding. Offer ORS for each diarrheal stool. Moderate: Give 50-100mL ORS/kg child's weight over 2-4 hours in clinic. Mix the ORS and have parent give to child with cup or cup and spoon; if child vomiting, give ORS more slowly. Reassess child periodically during rehydration period—including a weight after rehydrated and observe for urine output. Severe: Obtain IV or IO access and give isotonic solution (normal saline or lactated Ringers) in one of two ways: 1) bolus 20mL/kg as quickly as possible and reassess. Repeat until child no longer showing

signs of shock or 2) WHO protocol: give 100mL/kg over 6 hours, with 30mL/kg given over first hour if an infant and first 30 minutes if 1-5 years old. If IV or IO is not available, may use nasogastric tube (NGT) and administer ORS at 20mL/kg for 6 hours (120mL/kg total); slow down infusion if child vomits.

2. Nutrition: Children with diarrhea should continue all normal foods and liquids as long as not sugary or fatty. Fruits, vegetables, starches and meats are good. If vomiting, may need to wait a few hours until resolves prior to feeding, but prolonged bowel rest is harmful and contraindicated for most children. Children with malnutrition should be admitted to a feeding program.

3. Medications (for diarrhea): Almost all cases of diarrhea are self-limited, but medications may be indicated in some circumstances. Children in developing countries with diarrhea should receive **zinc sulfate** 20mg po daily x 10 days. This shortens the course of diarrhea and decreases future diarrheal episodes in the following 3 months. Antibiotics may be indicated for acute dysentery but when possible; cultures should be obtained first. Antibiotic treatment of EHEC may be harmful. In austere circumstances, empiric treatment of acute bloody diarrhea which is usually caused by *Shigella* may be indicated if child is ill appearing. Antibiotic choices for *Shigella* include: **Trimethoprim-sulfamethoxazole** (base dose on TMX portion) 10mg/kg/day po divided bid x 3-5 days or **ceftriaxone** 50mg/kg IM daily x 2-5 days or **ciprofloxacin** 20mg/kg po daily divided bid x 3-5 days. The primary treatment for cholera is hydration, but antibiotics may shorten the course of illness, **azithromycin** 20mg/kg (max of 1 gram) po in a single dose. *Giardia* and amebic dysentery can be treated with **metronidazole** 15mg/kg po x 5 days. Anti-motility agents such as loperamide are not indicated in children.

Patient Education

General: Most cases of diarrhea in children are caused by infections that will go away without treatment in a few days; however dehydration can be life-threatening, so care must be given to ensure child takes enough fluids. Dehydration for which the cause is not diarrhea requires further evaluation to determine the underlying mechanism of fluid imbalance.

Activity: No restrictions.

Diet: Continue all usual foods as long as not sugary or fatty. Avoid sugary drinks such as soda or fruit juices.

Medications: Medications are usually not necessary, but in certain specific cases may be required. All of the antibiotics can cause allergic reactions or stomach upset on occasion.

Prevention and Hygiene: Use only potable water (boiled or treated) to drink and cook with. Wash hands frequently; keep flies out of cooking areas.

No Improvement/Deterioration: Return if child has increasing diarrhea, vomiting, is unable to drink, weak, blood in stools, high fevers or if not better in 3 days.

Follow-Up Actions:

Return for worsening or non-improvement. Consult preventive medicine for epidemics of diarrheal disease.

Notes: Suspect cholera if acute onset severe, watery diarrhea in children older than 5 years old. *See Part 5: Specialty Areas: Chapter 12: Bacterial Infections: Cholera*

Chapter 15: Pediatrics: Common Pediatric Symptoms: Cough and Respiratory Infection
LTC Douglas Lougee, MC, USA

Introduction: Upper airway infections are the most common cause of cough in children. Acute lower respiratory infections (pneumonia, pertussis and bronchiolitis) are the leading cause of death in children worldwide. Asthma, croup, sinusitis are also relatively common. The primary task is to distinguish between the many children with self-limited colds and the few with more serious conditions. An assessment and treatment plan used in developing countries is provided in the World Health Organization (WHO) Integrated Management of Childhood Illness (IMCI) protocol.

Subjective: Symptoms

Cough (dry hacking, dog barking, whooping, deep productive or non- productive), sneezing, runny nose, fever, chills, malaise, vomiting, wt loss. **Focused History:** *Does the child seem in good health except for the cough?* (may indicate severity of any underlying process) *What does the cough sound like?* (A dog-like bark in 6 months to 5 year old suggests croup; staccato followed by whooping suggests pertussis. **Note:** Young infants may not have classic "whoop" of pertussis, but may stop eating, vomit, turn blue and stop breathing.) *How long has child had the cough?* (>14 days, consider asthma, sinusitis, TB, or other chronic infection) *Is cough productive?* (found in asthma, pneumonia or common cold). *What sets off the child's cough? Does it happen with running, playing or laughing?* (suggests asthma) *Does the child have other symptoms?* (runny nose [cold, sinusitis]; fever [colds, pneumonia, croup]; vomiting [pneumonia or asthma]; respiratory distress with retractions and/or fast breathing [pneumonia, asthma, bronchiolitis]; stridor [croup or foreign body] poor feeding, decreased urine production [respiratory distress/shock/dehydration]; poor growth or weight loss [chronic condition]; ear pain [otitis media]) *Is there a family history of asthma, allergies or eczema?* (often present with asthma) *Do adults or other children have cough?* (eg, adults with chronic cough [TB]; multiple young children with similar symptoms [acute respiratory infections]) *Is child exposed to common irritants?* (eg, wood or tobacco smoke)

Objective: Signs

Using Basic Tools: Vital signs: Temperature/parental report of fever, respiratory rate, heart rate. Tachypnea in infants <6 months RR>60; 6-12 months RR>50; 12-60 months, RR >40 (count respiratory rate for one minute when child quiet) EENT: rhinorrhea, bulging tympanic membranes (otitis media), stridor, dry mucous membranes. Chest: retractions (suprasternal-upper airway obstruction-croup or foreign body) intracostal and subcostal-respiratory distress from lower airway problem (asthma, bronchiolitis, pneumonia). Lungs: wheezing, crackles, diminished air entry (asthma, bronchiolitis, pneumonia) **Note:** Distinguish between transmitted upper airway congestion and true crackles by auscultation of the child's nose and chest. Sounds heard from both nose and chest are upper airway noise, not true crackles. Heart: tachycardia from shock, dehydration or respiratory distress. Capillary refill: shock, dehydration. Abdomen: subcostal retractions/abdominal breathing

Using Advanced Tools: CXR, Pulse Oximetry, Pulmonary Function Testing in children over 6-8 years old.

Assessment:

Distinguish between self-limited viral upper respiratory infections (colds) and more serious conditions (pneumonia, pertussis, asthma and bronchiolitis).

Differential Diagnosis

Uncomplicated acute viral upper airway infection (eg, cold): Self limited, short duration with typical associated symptoms of viral URI.

Complicated acute upper airway infection (eg, croup): May have history of similar episodes that include symptoms of URI with barking cough and stridor consistent with some degree of upper airway obstruction

Acute lower respiratory infection (pneumonia, bronchiolitis, or pertussis): Acutely ill appearance, tachypnea, nasal flaring, rales, rhonchi, fever of acute onset (pneumonia), acute onset of expiratory wheezing (bronchiolitis), paroxysmal cough ending with a high-pitched inspiratory "whoop" (pertussis).

Aspiration: Foreign body, gastric contents. Rule out with a normal auscultation of the throat and lungs, ie, lack of high pitched breath sounds or stridor. Rule out aspiration of gastric contents with a finding of a normal chest radiograph.

Allergic or sensitization response: Asthma, allergic rhinitis.

Chronic lung disease: Cystic fibrosis may include history of meconium ileus, failure to thrive, recurrent respiratory infections or other gastrointestinal or hepatic dysfunction.

Other lung disease (eg, TB): History of exposure to household contacts.

Other non-pulmonary disease (gastroesophageal reflux, medication, congestive heart failure): May include other symptoms that point to underlying cause.

Plan:

Treatment

Uncomplicated acute upper respiratory infection (a cold): Reassurance. For children >5 years, may use OTC decongestants: **pseudoephedrine** 1mg/kg/dose (max of 60mg) po up to q6h prn congestion may be used but not necessary. Steam, clean water to clean nose. Many culturally appropriate home remedies such as honey and lemon juice are probably as effective as any medicine. (Honey is not recommended for children less than 1 year old.) Antitussives such as dextromethorphan have not been shown to be effective for young children.

Croup: *See Part 5: Specialty Areas: Chapter 15: Most Common Pediatric Diseases: Throat Problems: Croup*

Acute lower respiratory infection (pneumonia): If fever and tachypnea, abnormal lung exam or respiratory distress, consider empiric antibiotic therapy antibiotic. Give **penicillin G** 100,000units/kg/dose (max of 24 million units per day) IV/IM q6h or **ampicillin** 50mg/kg/dose (max of 12g per day) IV/IM q6-8h or **ceftriaxone** 50mg/kg/dose (max 4g per day IM or IV daily. IM/IV therapy can be discontinued and switched to po with clinical improvement such as decrease in fever. Oral antibiotics include **amoxicillin** 50-100mg/kg/day divided bid x 7-10 days or **azithromycin** 10mg/kg/dose po on day one followed by 5mg/kg/dose po on the following 4 days. Hospitalize if serious respiratory distress

Bronchiolitis: Acute lower respiratory wheezing illness in infants. Supportive treatment: IV fluids. If dehydrated, give a maintenance IV fluid such as D5 ½ NS running at 4mL/hr for each kilogram of body weight (this formula works for infants up to 10 kg). Will need to add **K+** 20 milliequivalents per liter to maintenance fluid if infant is not taking anything by mouth for more than a few hours. Supplemental oxygen by mask or nasal cannula if hypoxic or severe distress. Hospitalize or close follow up. Consider empiric antibiotics as listed under pneumonia if febrile, ill appearing or if x-ray shows a specific lobe of lung to be opacified (whiter than usual).

Pertussis: Azithromycin 10mg/kg/dose (max 500mg) po daily x 5 days or **erythromycin** 10mg/kg/dose (max 500mg/dose) po qid x 14 days. Treat family members. Young infants will need to be hospitalized for close observation and frequently need supportive care as described in bronchiolitis.

Asthma: *See Part 5: Specialty Areas: Chapter 15: Serious Pediatric Diseases: Asthma*

Sinusitis: Give **amoxicillin** 20-40mg/kg/dose po bid x 10-14 days.

Foreign object, congestive heart failure or TB: Needs advanced care

Patient Education

1. Colds do not need medicines and will go away on their own. Young children get colds frequently. This is normal. Wipe their nose and drive on!

2. Avoiding irritants such as wood and cigarette smoke inside the home may decrease respiratory illnesses in children.

3. Washing hands frequently helps prevent the spread of respiratory problems.

Follow Up Actions

If children have cold symptoms (runny nose and cough) for more than 14 days in a row, and get high fevers, stop drinking, or have trouble breathing, the parent needs to bring to medical attention.

Part 5: Specialty Areas: Chapter 15: Pediatrics: Common Pediatric Symptoms: Acute Pain in the Child

LTC Kathleen Dunn Farr, MC, USA

Introduction: It is a myth that children do not feel pain in the same way that adults do. Infants and children experience pain from acute injury, illness, and diagnostic and therapeutic procedures. The expression of pain varies with the developmental age of the child. It is your responsibility to adequately assess and control pain in your patients; this requires acute observation on your part. It is possible to provide appropriate analgesia without masking symptoms, altering mental status, or interfering with patient evaluation. Do NOT withhold required pain meds in patients you are evaluating for possible surgical intervention. Do not under-medicate your pediatric patient. When children are properly dosed and monitored, excessive sedation, respiratory depression, and addiction are rare complications. To manage pain effectively, you must routinely assess for pain, minimize the number of painful procedures, decrease anxiety using non-pharmacologic interventions, and administer appropriate analgesics before, during, and after diagnostic and therapeutic procedures/surgery. Patients often require a lower total dose of analgesics when pain is treated early and effectively. **Risk Factors:** Some cultures encourage a stoic acceptance of pain. Children who are severely malnourished, emotionally traumatized, or depressed may not exhibit typical signs of pain. Children under age 7 years and those with developmental disabilities may have difficulty verbalizing symptoms of pain. Remain alert to the possibility that these children are in pain.

Subjective: Symptoms

Children age 18-24 months use words such as "boo-boo," "owie" and "hurt" to express pain. Children are usually unable to localize pain before age 5 years.

Focused History: Ask your patient or their caretaker about the location, quality, duration, and intensity of pain. Ask how well the child is able to tolerate the pain. Correlate the history with observation of behavior, especially in younger children who may have difficulty verbalizing symptoms.

Objective: Signs

Using Basic Tools: Vital signs: Physiologic signs: increased heart rate, respiratory rate, and BP; decreased oxygen saturation. (These are the least reliable method of pain assessment and changes in vital signs may reflect a stress reaction to the situation or the exam, rather than the level of acute pain.) Behavioral signs: crying, grimace, irritable or restless, hold their body rigid. May complain of nightmares or difficulty falling or staying asleep. Parents may notice a change in sleep-wake cycles, decreased appetite, or decreased activity level.

Infants: Whimper or cry continuously or intensely, clench fists, refuse to eat.

Toddlers: Refuse to crawl or walk, become frustrated easily, act aggressively.

Preschool children: Refuse to move, not want the area touched, hesitate to admit pain if they view it as a punishment or fear the treatment.

School-age children: Have a flat-faced expression, withdraw emotionally.

Teens: May be angry, withdrawn or uncooperative

Assessment:

Assess patients using self-report (age-dependent) facilitated by using scales such as the Wong-Baker "FACES" Pain Rating Scale and the 10cm Visual Analog Scale; children as young as 4 years of age may be able to report their level of pain using the FACES Scale. Routinely assess vital signs and the presence and severity of pain. Treat in a friendly, calm environment, avoid hypothermia and noise/light stimulation in infants. Provide distractions such as colorful pictures, toys, or pinwheels, use a soothing voice; distract child by singing or telling a story. Allow caretaker to hold the child or sit nearby; encourage caretaker to rock or soothe the child with a rhythmic motion. Gently massage the child's uninjured back, scalp or extremity.

Plan:

Treatment

Primary: Ask patients about recent analgesic use. Consider the type of analgesia, dose, timing, and route of administration when formulating a plan for alleviating pain. Base the dose on body weight, physiologic development, and the clinical situation. In patients >6 months of age, multi-drug therapy, such as acetaminophen in conjunction with codeine, may reduce the amount of opioid required. Administer NSAIDS or oral opiates for mild to moderate pain. Use regional blocks or IV opiates for severe pain or immediate pain control. Avoid IM administration, which is painful and has variable absorption.

Topical anesthetic

LET (lidocaine 4%, epinephrine 0.1%, tetracaine 0.5%)
1. Use for suturing simple uncontaminated lacerations of head, neck, extremities or trunk (<5cm in length)
2. Do not use in areas supplied by end arteries (digits, genitalia, ear, or nose) or on mucous membranes
3. Place 1-3mL of liquid-saturated cotton ball or gel into wound; cover with occlusive dressing for 20-30 minutes prior to procedure

Injectable local anesthetic: Do NOT use formulations with epinephrine on digits, genitalia, ear, nose, or mucous membranes
1. **Bupivacaine** 0.25-0.75% (with or without epinephrine) 3mg/kg SQ
2. **Lidocaine** 0.5-2.0% without epinephrine up to 4.5mg/kg/dose (up to 300mg total) SQ
3. **Lidocaine** 0.5-2.0% with **epinephrine** up to 7mg/kg/dose (up to 500mg total no more frequently than q2h) SQ

NSAIDS
1. **Acetaminophen** 10-15mg/kg/dose po q6-8h
2. **Ibuprofen** (for children >6 months) 5-10mg/kg/dose po q6-8h
3. **Naproxen** (for children >2 years) 5-7mg/kg/dose po q8-12h
4. **Ketorolac** (for children >50kg) 10mg po q6h or 0.5mg/kg/dose IV q6h

Opioids
1. **Fentanyl** 1-2 mcg/kg/dose IV (over 3-5 minutes) q30-60 min PRN; **Fentanyl Oralet** (po formulation) 5-15mcg/kg/dose (maximum 400mcg/dose). **Note:** Avoid fentanyl in infants <4 months of age; po formulation is contraindicated in children <10kg.
2. **Morphine sulfate**
   a. Neonate: 0.05-0.2mg/kg/dose IV (slow push) q4h PRN
   b. Infant and child:
      0.2-0.5mg/kg/dose po q4-6h
      0.1-0.2mg/kg/dose IV q2-4h PRN
3. **Codeine** (for children >3 years of age) 0.5-1.0mg/kg/dose po q4-6h

Alternative: (adjuncts in addition to analgesics in infants): Sucrose solution. Adjunct for pain associated with minor procedures in infants <6 months of age. Administer 1-2mL of 25% sucrose solution po (drip half the amount in each cheek) or allow infant to suck solution from a bottle nipple or pacifier no more than 2 minutes before start of procedure. Administer no more than twice per hour.

Empiric: Skin-to-skin contact, breastfeeding, and swaddling may comfort infants and young children.

Primitive: Place a warm wrap or ice pack on an injured area to reduce pain from inflammation. Apply ice for 2-3 minutes to numb skin prior to minor procedures.

Patient Education

General: Discuss the indications, dose, and duration of outpatient analgesics with child's caretaker

Activity: Adequate sleep helps children cope with the effects of injury and illness. Time clinical interventions and control the child's environment to the extent possible to optimize sleep-wake cycles.

Diet: As appropriate for age; anticipate constipation when prescribing opiates

Medications (side effects): Opiates can cause itching, nausea and constipation

Prevention and Hygiene: Teach parents how to comfort their child

No Improvement/Deterioration: Return for further evaluation if child experiences severe or uncontrollable pain

Follow-up Actions

Return Evaluation: Return for further evaluation if child experiences severe or uncontrollable pain.

Evacuation/Consultation Criteria: Seek further assistance if you cannot control pain with available medications

Notes: Anxiolytics or sedatives alone do not provide analgesia and may interfere with a child's ability to express pain. Meperidine hydrochloride (Demerol) is not an opioid of choice for pain control because of nausea. Avoid aspirin in children <16 years of age due to risk for Reye syndrome.

Chapter 15: Pediatrics: Most Common Pediatric Diseases:
Eye Problems: Red Eye Without Trauma

LT John Hyatt, MC, USNR; Mary Ellen Hoehn, MD; LTC Robert W. Enzenauer, MC, USA (Ret)

Introduction: The differential diagnosis of non-traumatic red eye in older children is similar to that in the adult but evaluation of young children and infants requires certain additional considerations including neonatal infection. Examination might also reveal signs of ocular misalignment or intraocular disease. Ophthalmia neonatorum (newborn conjunctivitis) is common in developing countries, especially where rates of *Gonorrhea* and *Chlamydia* infections are high. If red eye is associated with trauma, *see Part 3: General Symptoms: Eye Problems: Eye Injury*

Subjective: Symptoms

Fever, eye pain, loss of vision, redness, discharge, foreign-body sensation, increased light sensitivity.

Focused History: *What kind of discharge has there been from the eye?* (Mucoid or watery discharge may indicate viral or chlamydial infection; purulent discharge may indicate bacterial infection.) *Do other nearby children or household members have similar symptoms?* (If so, this may indicate a contagious viral conjunctivitis.) *Are prophylactic eyedrops used on newborns in this area to prevent eye infections early in life? If so, what type?* (Silver nitrate drops used in newborns can cause a self-limited conjunctivitis lasting 2-3 days.) *Is the eye redness in child less than one month old?* (If so, systemic antibiotics likely necessary.)

Objective: Signs

Using Basic Tools: Vital signs: Fever would be consistent with systemic infection. Inspection: Examine extraocular muscles. A limitation of movement could indicate cranial nerve palsy. Misalignment ("lazy eye" or "wall eye") when focusing on an object should also be noted, though correction of "lazy eye" is beyond the scope of this manual. Palpation: An enlarged pre-auricular lymph node is common in viral, chlamydial, and herpetic conjunctivitis. Flashlight/Penlight: Though mild lid edema often occurs with conjunctivitis, consider preseptal or orbital cellulitis if there is marked edema of the lids preventing the child or the examiner from easily opening the eyes. Conjunctival injection would be expected in conjunctivitis, but can also be noted in corneal abrasions, corneal ulcers, or orbital cellulitis. In children old enough to be verbal and literate, check visual acuity with a Snellen chart (if available) or other printed material. Eye discharge and corneal involvement may decrease acuity.

Using Advanced Tools: Fluorescein strip and UV light: Observe for staining indicating a defect of the corneal epithelium. Multiple fine circular (punctate) defects can be seen in viral conjunctivitis. A dendritic pattern will usually be seen in herpetic conjunctivitis. A defect with surrounding corneal clouding (infiltrate) suggests corneal ulcer and merits more aggressive treatment. If any defect stains with fluorescein, examine closely for any foreign bodies. Ophthalmoscope: At a distance of a few feet, look directly at the child's eyes through the ophthalmoscope. You should note a symmetric red reflex. A whitish reflex (leukocoria) could indicate a congenital problem inside the eye (cataract, parasitic infection, retinal abnormality) or a tumor, and would merit more specialized evaluation as ground conditions and availability of medical evacuation allow. Topical anesthesia: One drop **proparacaine** or **tetracaine** 0.5%. These will often bring prompt, if temporary, relief of problems involving the corneal epithelium. Do not give bottles of anesthetic drops to patients as frequent, prolonged use will cause serious damage to the cornea.

Assessment:

Differential Diagnosis

Infectious causes:

Conjunctivitis in first month of life (ophthalmia neonatorum): *Gonorrhea* is usually associated with copious purulent discharge from the eye. Gram's stain of a conjunctival scraping may show gram-negative diplococci.

Chlamydia causes a discharge that is more watery or mucoid.

In older infants/children:

Viral conjunctivitis (adenovirus): Watery or mucoid discharge; may have punctate epithelial defects and/or swollen pre-auricular lymph node.

Bacterial conjunctivitis: Purulent discharge; in mild cases may be difficult to distinguish from viral

Herpes simplex virus keratitis: Dendritic figure on fluorescein staining.

Non-infectious/unrecognized minor trauma:

Corneal abrasion or ulcer: Noted on fluorescein exam

Conjunctival foreign body: Locate and remove any foreign material, may have associated corneal abrasion.

Diagnostic Tests:
For a child less than one month of age with red eye or eye discharge, perform Gram's stain of conjunctiva, if possible. Irrigate away any thick discharge. Instill a drop of **proparacaine** or **tetracaine**. Swab or gently scrape the conjunctiva inside the lower lid with a swab or sterile, blunt edge to collect sample for staining.

Plan:

Treatment

Conjunctivitis in first month of life: If gram-negative diplococci seen on stain or suspicious for *Gonorrhea*, treat with **ceftriaxone** 25-50mg/kg IV or IM as a single dose. Treatment must be systemic to treat simultaneous systemic gonococcal infection. Evacuate if develops signs of systemic illness. Lavage lids with saline to remove discharge tid-qid and apply **bacitracin** ointment qid x 2 weeks. Also give **erythromycin** 50mg/kg/day po in 4 divided doses x 10-14 days to treat unrecognized Chlamydia infection. Gram's stain cannot rule out *Chlamydia* infection, which can be associated with pneumonia in newborns, so all cases of conjunctivitis in children less than 1 month old should receive oral **erythromycin** and topical **bacitracin** per the previous regimen, regardless of the results of the results of the Gram's stain of conjunctival scraping.

Conjunctivitis in older children: Can be difficult to distinguish between viral and bacterial conjunctivitis. Most topical ophthalmic antimicrobials other than sulfacetamide are satisfactory. Any one of the following ophthalmic drops could be used 1-2 drops qid in the affected eye(s) for 5 days (assuming no known allergy): **Ciprofloxacin, trimethoprim sulfate, polymixin B sulfate, neomycin/polymixin B/gramicidin. Tobramycin** and **gentamycin** ophthalmic drops could be used 1-2 drops in the affected eye(s) 6-8 x a day x 5 days. Alternatively, a thin strip of **erythromycin** ophthalmic ointment could be used 6 x a day x 5 days.

Herpes simplex keratitis: Dendritic staining on cornea most likely means vision threatening infection and evacuation ASAP to an eye doctor. Patient will need topical antiviral ophthalmic solution and possibly **acyclovir** IV if next level of care can provide.

Suspected preseptal or orbital cellulitis: *See Part 3: General Symptoms: Eye Problems: Orbital/Periorbital Inflammation.* However, oral **levofloxacin** should be avoided in pediatric patients. For preseptal cellulitis in a child over 5 years, give **amoxicillin/clavulanate** 20-40mg/kg/day po divided into 3 doses x 10 days. If less than age 5, give **ceftriaxone** 100mg/kg/day IV divided into 2 doses x 10 days. If orbital cellulitis suspected, give **ampicillin/sulbactam** 100-200mg/kg/day IV divided into 4doses for at least 3 days (not to exceed 4g/day) followed by oral antibiotics for preseptal cellulitis for 1 week. Since this serious infection can result in blindness, evacuation to a hospital is recommended, if possible.

Corneal erosion (abrasion and ulcer): *See Part 3: General Symptoms: Eye Problems: Eye Injury*

Foreign body: *See Part 3: General Symptoms: Eye Problems: Eye Injury*

Patient Education

General: Discuss the level of injury with the patient but do not give prognosis in diseases that should be managed at a higher level of care.

Activity: As tolerated

Diet: As tolerated. Erythromycin elixir can be mixed with formula/milk.

Prevention and Hygiene: One drop of 2.5% povidone-iodine solution in each eye at birth can greatly reduce neonatal eye infections. In older children, hand washing and encouraging parents to keep them away from school/social gatherings for 2 weeks can reduce spread of viral conjunctivitis to other children.

Follow-up Actions

Return Evaluation: Follow patients closely on daily basis for signs of improvement or worsening

Evacuation/Consultation Criteria: Evacuate as indicated in treatment. Evacuate any patient not showing improvement within 24-48 hours. Consult with an ophthalmologist if available prior to using steroids in the eye.

Chapter 15: Pediatrics: Most Common Pediatric Diseases: Eye Problems: Tearing/Nasolacrimal Duct Obstruction

CPT Steven Roy Ballard, MC, USA; Mary Ellen Hoehn, MD; LTC Robert W. Enzenauer, MC, USA (Ret)

Introduction: Excessive tearing in the pediatric population in the absence of infection is primarily a nonemergent problem. It can result from chronic problems such as congenitally obstructed tear ducts, congenital glaucoma, eyelid/eyelash disorders; or more acute irritative disorders including: tear duct infections, conjunctivitis, foreign bodies, or allergies. Close inspection for signs of infection or compromised visual acuity are imperative and, along with a good history, will help delineate congenital problems from more acute diagnoses.

Subjective: **Symptoms**

Wet looking eyes, tears overflowing onto cheeks, crusting, mucopurulent material in lashes, reflux of purulent material from tear ducts, redness, swelling, irritation, pain, fever.

Focused History: *Has the child been tearing?* (Since infancy suggests congenital problem. Acute onset suggests foreign body or infection.) *Have you had prior episodes or recent ear, nose, throat infections?* (suggests tear duct infection) *Is there any pain?* (suggests signs of infection or foreign body) *Is there any discharge?* (mucoid or mucopurulent discharge also suggests signs of infection or obstruction) *Any fevers, chills, redness, or swelling?* (also suggests infectious etiology)

Objective: **Signs**

Using Basic Tools: Vital signs: Fevers suggest signs of infection. Visual acuity: Test each eye separately. Use reading material if available and child able to read. Use penlight to assess if child can fix and follow on your light. Inspection: Use penlight examination to: Examine skin for any signs of redness or swelling, particularly on nasal aspect of eyelids, and evaluate for tearing. Inspect lashes for any mucus, purulent material, or ingrowing lashes rubbing onto front of eye. Evert upper lids and look for any foreign bodies, if suspected. Examine conjunctiva for any injection or discharge. Assess for any corneal enlargement (asymmetry or larger than 12mm) or haziness (suggests congenital glaucoma). Palpation: Palpate just inferonasally to medial side of lower lid and evaluate for any purulent reflux from lower tear duct that would suggest infection. Gently palpate both closed eyes to grossly assess firmness of eye. (A firm eye in the presence of enlarged or hazy cornea could suggest congenital glaucoma.) Assess for any tenderness of the skin where there is redness or swelling.

Using Advanced Tools: Application of 1 drop of topical anesthetic (**proparacaine** or **tetracaine** 0.5%) in affected eye with pain relief suggests foreign body or ocular surface irritant. Application of 1 drop of fluorescein solution with significant retention after 5-10 minutes suggests tear duct obstruction. Failure of dye to appear in nasal passage of affected side after blowing nose 10-15 minutes later helps confirm obstruction. Labs: Gram's stain/culture of purulent secretions from punctum. Usually shows multiple strains and is not helpful in management, unless child is acutely ill.

Assessment:

Differential Diagnosis

Nasolacrimal duct obstruction: Congenital problem as a result of imperforate membrane usually at distal end of nasolacrimal duct. Inability for tears to drain leads to overflowing tears, mucopurulent material on eyelashes, and reflux of material from puncta. May or may not have concurrent evidence of infection.

Congenital glaucoma: Rare. Associated with increased intraocular pressure. Symptoms of overproduction of tears, wet nose, potentially decreased vision. Noted absence of any purulent discharge. Exam demonstrates firm globe on gentle palpation and enlarged or hazy corneas. Photophobia is often a prominent additional feature in addition to tearing.

Eyelash or eyelid disorder: In-turning of eyelids causing lashes to rub on ocular surface or poor punctal position resulting in failure of tear pump to function properly (could be secondary to prior scarring or trauma to lids). Could result in corneal abrasion that stains with use of fluorescein.

Conjunctivitis: Allergic, viral, or bacterial irritation of conjunctiva. Acute onset red eye with or without purulence. Not associated with reflux from punctum or poor drainage.

Foreign body: Often under upper lid, causing hypersecretion of tears due to eye irritation. Diagnosis based on exposure history or presence of foreign body seen on examination. May have linear corneal abrasions that stain with use of fluorescein.

Dacryocystitis (tear duct infection): Most commonly caused by nasolacrimal duct obstruction. May be mild in nature or severe with subsequent febrile illness or preseptal cellulitis. Associated with nasal swelling, purulent material expressed from punctum on examination.

Mucocele: Bluish swelling inferonasally to lower lid secondary to obstructed lacrimal sac swelling causing retention of accumulated secretions.

Lacrimal duct mass: Rare

Plan:

Treatment

Nasolacrimal duct obstruction:
1. Digital pressure to canalicular system. Teach parent to:
   a. Place finger over inner corner of eye
   b. Milk tear duct by firmly pressing and slide finger downwards alongside nose
   c. Repeat a few times each sitting qid
2. **Erythromycin** ophthalmic ointment (0.5%) 0.5 inch strip applied to lower lid of affected eye bid if purulent discharge is noted.
3. In many cultures, breast milk is recommended to be instilled into a baby's eyes to treat possible infectious drainage. There is good reasoning to support this folk treatment, since human breast milk and colostrum contains secretory IgA that can be expected to reduce bacteria and viruses.
4. If acute dacryocystitis is present, a systemic antibiotic will be needed.
5. Most cases open spontaneously by 1 year of age or with conservative treatment. If severe recurrent infections are present, surgical probing of the duct and tube placement may be needed at a higher level of care.

Congenital glaucoma: Definitive treatment is surgical at higher level of care.

Eyelash/Eyelid disorder: Remove offending eyelash (temporizing treatment). Definitive treatment is surgical at higher level of care. If corneal abrasion present, *see Part 5: Specialty Areas: Chapter 15: Most Common Pediatric Diseases: Eye Problems: Red Eye without Trauma.*

Conjunctivitis: *See Part 5: Specialty Areas: Chapter 15: Most Common Pediatric Diseases: Eye Problems: Red Eye without Trauma* for differential diagnosis and proper treatment.

Dacryocystitis: Treatment depends on severity of infection.
1. All antibiotic treatment should be administered for a minimum of 10-14 days depending on severity. For mild: afebrile and systemically well child, give **amoxicillin/clavulanate** 20-40mg/kg/day divided dose po tid or **cefaclor** 20-40mg/kg/day divided dose po tid. For severe: febrile and acutely ill, give **cefuroxime** 50-100mg/kg/day divided dose IV tid. May be switched to po antibiotics after signs of acute illness have resolved.
2. Digital pressure as described for nasolacrimal duct obstruction qid. Warm compresses qid.
3. Pain medication **acetaminophen** 10-15mg/kg po q6h prn (with or without **codeine** 0.5 -1mg/kg/day po q6h prn, not to exceed 60mg/day).
4. Surgical correction may be required as documented under nasolacrimal duct obstruction
5. Follow up if signs of worsening infection.

Mucocele: Digital massage as documented previously. Permanent treatment requires probing and surgical elimination of associated nasolacrimal duct obstruction.

Lacrimal duct mass: If solid or vascular tumor of nasolacrimal duct is suspected, patient should be transported to higher level of care for ophthalmologic consultation.

Patient Education

General: Discuss limited nature of some causes as noted, but do not give prognosis in diseases that require management at higher level of care.

Activity: As tolerated; limited if placed on IV antibiotics

Diet: Regular as tolerated

Medications:

1. Proparacaine/Tetracaine 0.5% Drops: Corneal Toxicity- Use for diagnostic purposes only. Do not dispense for patient's home use.
2. Erythromycin 0.5% Ophthalmic Ointment: Topically well tolerated; Potential eye irritation, GI upset
3. Amoxicillin/clavulanate: GI upset, rash, allergic hypersensitive
4. Cefaclor or cefuroxime: GI upset, rash, allergic hypersensitivity
5. Acetaminophen: Rash, allergic hypersensitivity
6. Codeine: GI upset, drowsiness, confusion, rash, allergic hypersensitivity

Prevention and Hygiene: Hand washing, limit contact with eye secretions, encourage parents to keep child away from school/other social settings to reduce spread in cases of viral/bacterial illness.

No Improvement/Deterioration: Signs of infection, fevers, chills, progressing redness, swelling, pain, or vision changes despite initial interventions warrants return evaluation and transport to higher level of care for ophthalmologic consultation/treatment.

Follow-up Actions

Return Evaluation: Follow any patient with signs of infection closely on daily basis for signs of improvement or deterioration.

Evacuation/Consultation Criteria: Evacuate as indicated in treatment plans. Evacuate any patient with signs of infection not improving within 24-48 hours. Ophthalmologic consultation is warranted for any patient with potential mass or vision threatening diagnosis.

Chapter 15: Pediatrics: Most Common Pediatric Diseases: Ear Problems: Otitis Media
COL Woodson Scott Jones, MC, USA

Introduction: Acute otitis media (AOM) is an infection of the middle ear space caused by a bacterial or viral infection. Though it is the most common infection for which children are prescribed antibiotics, there is growing evidence that it does not always need to be treated. The usual pathogens are *Streptococcus pneumoniae*, *Haemophilus influenzae*, and *Moraxella catarrhalis*. In countries where there is wide use of antibiotics, there is growing resistance of these organisms to the most commonly used antibiotics. **Seasonal Variations:** Most commonly occurs in the wintertime and early spring given it is commonly a complication of a viral upper respiratory infection (URI). When a child does develop AOM during an URI, it typically occurs between days 3–5 of symptoms. **Risk Factors:** Underlying anatomical defect (ie, cleft palate), particular ethnic groups (ie, American Indian, Eskimos), tobacco exposure, bottle feeding (as opposed to breast feeding) and daycare attendance.

Subjective: **Symptoms**

Ear pain, tugging on ear.

Focused History: *Is your child complaining of ear pain or tugging/pulling on ears more than usual?* (The presence of ear pain is the best clinical symptom for AOM. However, ~40% of children may not have ear pain. Ear pain may be caused by other things [*see Part 3: General Symptoms: ENT Problems: Ear Pain*]. An infant with only "tugging" on the ears and no other symptoms is unlikely to have AOM.) *Has your child been awakening at night, had a decreased appetite, and/or less active?* (These can be the more subtle symptoms associated with AOM in preverbal children) *Has your child had a fever?* (Fever is another sign of infection but less than half of children with AOM have fevers and high fevers from AOM alone are very uncommon.) *Has your child had a cough, runny nose or congestion?* (Most cases of AOM are associated with URI symptoms.) *Has there been any discharge from the ears?* (Discharge from the external canal may be from a ruptured ear drum. However, it may also represent an external otitis [*see Part 3: General Symptoms: ENT Problems: Ear Pain*].) *Has your child had ear infections before or did anyone in the family have lots of ear problems?* (Past ear infections and an "otitis prone" family history increase the child's risk for disease. One should also assess for other risk factors listed, particularly in children with recurrent ear infections.)

Objective: **Signs**

Using Advanced Tools: Inspection with otoscope to view the tympanic membrane (TM). It is helpful in children to pull the soft cartilage of the outer ear up and back to get a better view of the eardrum. It is also optimal to assess mobility of the TM by performing pneumatic otoscopy, using a bulb attached to the otoscope to assess eardrum mobility. However, this is a skill that takes practice on normal ears in cooperative patients. It is also helpful for parents to restrain the younger child because motion while examining ear causes pain to the child and impedes gaining an adequate examination. Bulging TM: The single best confirmatory finding in AOM is bulging of the TM. The ear may look like a "doughnut" or "bagel" due to the bulging eardrum with middle "dimple" created by the fixed location of the middle ear bone. Marked redness of TM: Many providers mistake a pink or red ear as a sign of infection. However, crying, fevers, and stimulation of the ear canal with the otoscope may result in the eardrum appearing red. However, if the ear looks remarkable red, this may be a sign of infection. Opaque TM: Purulent fluid behind the TM can make the ear appear non-translucent and sometimes yellow. Bubbles or air-fluid levels may be seen. However, these findings may be associated with uninfected fluid behind the TM which is referred to as otitis media with effusion (OME). This does not respond to antibiotics. Blister on TM: Children may have blisters on their TM usually associated with more pain and a bulging TM underneath. Purulent Discharge: Sometimes the TM will rupture resulting in purulent discharge coming out of the ear canal. This can be difficult to distinguish from an outer ear infection (external otitis) but usually in not associated with tenderness of with movement of the external ear as found in an external otitis. **Pitfalls:** If a child has high fevers and is ill appearing, he/she may have another serious bacterial infection along with AOM. A child may present with a protuberant outer ear that is associated with mastoiditis (*see Part 3: General Symptoms: ENT Problems: Ear Pain*). A child with chronic foul smelling drainage may have a cholesteatoma. This will require referral to a specialist.

Assessment:

Differential Diagnosis

AOM: Clinical and physical findings would include child with a bulging TM, a child with opaque fluid behind the TM or a very red TM along with other associated symptoms such as ear pain, fussiness, poor feeding, or night awakenings.

Otitis media with effusion (OME): Child has fluid behind a non-bulging TM without signs of ear pain or remarkable redness.

Otitis externa: Swollen ear canal usually with discharge associated with pain with movement of the auricle.

Dental carries: Can present with ear pain, examine oral cavity for possible dental cause of pain.

Pharyngitis: Can present with ear pain, can examine the tonsils to ensure they are not red and swollen.

Plan

Treatment

Primary:

1. Give antibiotics based on risk factors:
   a. To children that: have not received antibiotics within the past month, give **amoxicillin** 40mg/kg/dose po bid x 10 days. Alternatives for the penicillin-allergic patient include: **azithromycin** 10mg/kg po q day x 3 days or **trimethoprim/ sulfamethoxazole** 10mg/kg/24hrs (based on TMP component of TMP-SMX) divided po bid x10 days.
   b. To children with risk of infection caused by amoxicillin-resistant bacteria (eg, have received antibiotics within the past month, higher temperature [>102.2°F], and/or severe otalgia), consider giving **amoxicillin/clavulanate** 40mg/kg/ dose (based upon amoxicillin component) po bid x 10 days. Other alternatives include: **cefixime** 8mg/kg po q day x 10 days and **cefuroxime** 15mg/kg/dose po bid x 10 days. **Ceftriaxone** 50mg/kg IM x 1 dose is equivalent to an oral 10 day course of medication. However, in austere environments **ceftriaxone** should be utilized for more ill appearing children with acute otitis media and high fevers or other more serious infections.
   c. In addition to oral antibiotic therapy; children with purulent drainage from a presumed ruptured TM should also receive a topical otic antibiotic such as **neomycin/polymixin B/hydrocortisone** otic solution (3 drops in ear canal tid followed by massage of tragus to ensure penetration into ear canal).
2. Control pain: The mainstay of pain management is **ibuprofen** 10mg/kg/dose po q6h or **acetaminophen** 15mg/kg/dose po q4-6h prn. Topical otic drops that contain **benzocaine** (eg, **Auralgan** or **Americaine** otic) 4-5 drops in external auditory canal q2-3h prn pain may provide additional relief.

Primitive: Children over 2 years of age with AOM and who do not have fevers, are well appearing, do not have recurrent ear infections, and do not have medical conditions that put them at more risk for severe disease (compromised immune status), may be watched with close follow-up without antibiotic therapy. If they get worse or are not improving within 48 hours, treatment should be initiated. If the medic has limited resources, the non-ill appearing child over 2 years of age with AOM alone may be treated with pain management alone with acetaminophen or ibuprofen. There is no evidence that homeopathic remedies, warm compresses or decongestants are helpful.

Patient Education

General: Classic history of URI which worsens with fever or increased irritability. Tobacco exposure increases risk for AOM.

Diet: Breast feeding may decrease incidence.

Follow-up Actions

Return Evaluation: Patient should improve within 48 hours. If clinical symptoms are not improving, should be re-evaluated and antibiotics changed from a primary to a secondary antibiotic. The fluid may remain behind the ear for several weeks so clinical symptoms should be followed rather than the presence or absence of fluid. Children who have speech or language concerns should have their AOM followed up in 4-6 weeks and until resolution of the fluid behind the TM. Children with uninfected fluid behind their TM for greater than 3 months should be referred to higher echelon of care if available. Recurrent AOM is described as 3 or more distinct episodes within a 6 month period or 4 AOM different episodes within a year. An infection that was initially treated with amoxicillin and subsequently needed a secondary agent would count as one ear infection. Children with recurrent AOM should be referred to a higher echelon of care if available.

Chapter 15: Pediatrics: Most Common Pediatric Diseases: Mouth Problems: Thrush

CPT Jeffrey Savage, MC, USA

Introduction: Thrush (oropharyngeal candidiasis) is a fungal infection that occurs when there is overgrowth of the *Candida* fungus. Thrush is common in healthy infants and is usually a self-limited process. However, treatment is advised, especially in the presence of candidal diaper rash. Infants usually acquire the infection from their mothers at delivery and remain colonized. Thrush is rare after 12 months of age and may indicate an immunocompromised state (such as HIV). Thrush can be seen after a child has been on antibiotics for a prolonged period of time. Thrush is also more common in infants whose mothers are diabetic. *Candida* and oral candidiasis are found throughout the world and occurs year-round. **Risk factors:** Age <12 months, mother with vulvovaginal candidiasis, neutrophil defects, immunodeficiency (HIV).

Subjective: Symptoms

Thrush may be asymptomatic but may cause pain, and infants can exhibit fussiness and poor feeding. Parents will usually complain of seeing white patches in the mouth that they are unable to remove.

Focused History: *Is the child feeding well?* (Infant with thrush will often feed poorly.) *If bottlefeeding, are bottles, nipples, pacifiers being washed/boiled?* (*Candida* can be spread to other children if these are shared and/or not cleaned properly and infants may become re-infected if nipples, pacifiers, and teething toys are not cleaned or sterilized properly.) *Does the mother have cracking or irritation of the nipples or pain with breastfeeding?* (This may indicate that mother has *Candida* affecting the nipples and the need for her to be treated as well.) *What medications is the child taking?* (Thrush may be associated with use of broad spectrum antibiotics or chronic inhaled steroids as used in treatment of asthma.)

Objective: Signs

Using Basic Tools: Inspection: Utilizing a flashlight or otoscope (advanced kit), inspect the entire mucosa of the infant's mouth. Look for white, cheesy plaques with an erythematous base on the gingival mucosa, tongue, palate and buccal mucosa. Plaques are difficult to remove. Removal of plaques may cause small areas of bleeding; this is diagnostic. Angular cheilitis (painful fissuring at the corners of the mouth) may be present.

Using Advanced Tools: Scrapings of the buccal mucosa will reveal budding yeast when observed with a microscope.

Assessment:

Plaques may resemble milk or formula remaining in the mouth and differentiating this from thrush may be somewhat difficult if an infant has just fed. Milk can easily be removed from the mucosal surface using a tongue depressor or finger, whereas plaques will be difficult to remove. Plaques may resemble lesions associated with other types of disease processes such as herpes (these lesions are usually isolated to one area of the mucosa and appear as ulcers instead of plaques).

Differential Diagnosis

Candida esophagitis: Patient will have odynophagia (pain on swallowing), complain of discomfort in discrete area in mid-sternum, most likely associated with underlying immune deficiency (eg, HIV). May or may not have concomitant oropharyngeal candidiasis.

Chronic mucocutaneous candidiasis: Rare polyglandular autoimmune syndrome causing severe recurrent thrush, vaginitis, onychomycosis and chronic skin lesions. May also have symptoms of hypothyroidism and adrenal insufficiency.

Plan:

Treatment

Primary: Nystatin oral suspension 1mL (100,000 units) to each side of the mouth qid x 7-10 days. Mothers of breastfed infants need to be treated as well. The typical treatment regimen is application of **nystatin cream** to the mother's nipples and areolae bid-qid x 7-10 days. If bottle feeding, nipples need to either be boiled or washed in a mixture of equal parts vinegar and water daily; teething toys and pacifiers should also be washed or boiled.

Alternatives: If available in the local area, gentian violet may be used. The technique is to paint the entire oral mucosa with the gentian violet (0.5-1%). This usually only requires one application and is often used in refractory cases.

Empiric: Nystatin oral suspension as discussed previously. If mothers are breast feeding, they should be treated empirically with nystatin cream.

Primitive: Various cultures may have their own ways of treating thrush and if nystatin is not available, these may be tried. However, treatment is needed and nystatin is the medication of choice.

Patient Education:

General: Parents and caretakers should be informed that thrush is very common and has no relationship to cleanliness or illness (usually) in infants. There should be no restrictions on activity or changes to diet

Prevention and Hygiene: Tell parents or caretakers that re-infection often occurs because nipples, pacifiers, or teething toys are not cleaned or sterilized properly. Boil nipples, toys, and pacifiers for several minutes or wash in a mixture of equal parts vinegar and water daily. Parents need to be warned that they need to rinse boiled toys, nipples, and pacifiers in cool water and/or let them cool prior to giving them to the child.

No improvement/Deterioration: If thrush worsens, infants may exhibit increased fussiness and have decreased feeding. Because of the risk for dehydration, this necessitates prompt evaluation and treatment

Follow-up Actions:

Return Evaluation: If refractory to treatment; as noted previously, this may lead to decreased po intake and the risk of dehydration which may necessitate rehydration therapy. Non-response to treatment may indicate immune/endocrine abnormalities which would necessitate further evaluation.

Consultation Criteria: Failure to respond to treatment.

Chapter 15: Pediatrics: Most Common Pediatric Diseases: Mouth Problems: Mouth Problems

CPT Jeffrey Savage, MC, USA

Introduction: Mouth problems are a common complaint in pediatrics and the number of diseases that cause them is large. They may be a structural/developmental problem, be part of a disease process that is isolated to the oral mucosa, or just one manifestation of a disease process that affects the entire body. In many cases, problems such as lesions are viral in etiology and only symptomatic treatment is necessary. Others may be manifestations of fungal disease (*see Part 5: Specialty Areas: Chapter 15: Most Common Pediatric Diseases: Mouth Problems: Thrush*). Yet others may be indicative of nutritional deficiencies. Some of these processes, especially when associated with dental problems or nutritional deficiencies, are population health problems and the SOF medic may not have the resources initially to provide individualized treatment for these patients.

Subjective: Symptoms

Complaints of pain, especially with eating, difficulty swallowing, fever, malaise, intolerance of certain foods

Focused History: *How long has this problem or these lesions been present?* (Lesions of recent in onset [within the last week] are more likely to have an infectious etiology.) *Is the child eating?* (Oral structural defects or lesions can compromise nutritional status or may be the result of a nutritional deficiency.) *Does anyone else in the household have similar lesions or symptoms?* (may indicate spread of a viral process or may indicate a nutritional problem within the family) *Does the child have any other symptoms?* (Fever, weakness, other rash or lesion may suggest specific diagnosis.)

Objective: Signs

Using Basic Tools: Inspection: Perform a focused examination of the oral mucosa, tongue, oropharynx and the neck (cervical lymph nodes drain the oropharynx). Inspect the teeth for evidence of caries or receding gums. Note the location of the lesions (lips, gingival mucosa, buccal mucosa, hard palate, soft palate). Note the color of size of the lesions. Does the child have any other findings on examination?

Assessment/Plan:
Differential Diagnosis and Plan
Common Mouth Problems

Ankyloglossia or "tongue tie": A condition in which there is an abnormally short lingual frenulum. This may affect feeding in young infants and may impair speech development. If the child is able to extend the tongue to moisten the lower lip, there is generally no intervention needed. If the child's nutritional status is suffering because of this, refer the child for surgical intervention.

Epstein pearls: These are small, hard, white, nodular lesions usually seen on the hard palate or on the alveolar ridges, typically in newborns. They are benign and need no intervention.

Neonatal teeth: Usually a single or both central lower incisors are seen. These can affect feeding and are an aspiration risk and therefore need to be removed. They are usually loose and can generally be easily removed with forceps

Eruption cyst: Bluish or translucent dome-shaped soft tissue mass overlying the location of an erupting tooth. No treatment is needed, as the cyst will resolve with eruption of the tooth.

Aphthous ulcer or 'canker sore': Painful, small, indented area surrounded by a red border. They may be singular or multiple. They are for the most part benign and will go away without treatment. However, recurrence of multiple lesions should prompt investigation into immune deficiency and referral for further evaluation. Cause is unknown. Topical pain medications such as those found in over-the-counter oral pain relievers can be used. A 1:1:1 mixture of **diphenhydramine**, **aluminum** and **magnesium hydroxide (Maalox)**, and viscous lidocaine (often called "triple mix") can be helpful for pain and is used as a mouth rinse. Any one of these ingredients can be used alone or in combination and will provide some relief. The ingredients in this mix should only be used in older children and adults and should not be swallowed. Treatment of pain with **acetaminophen**, **ibuprofen**, or other medication is appropriate.

Mucocele: These are usually painless, smooth-surfaced, bluish or translucent, and usually <1cm in diameter. They are caused by collection of mucus in an obstructed excretory duct. When on the floor of the mouth, they are called ranulae. Mucoceles are generally benign but may affect eating. Treatment options include incision and drainage (this could be done by the medic if necessary) and surgical excision. Some may rupture on their own without intervention, although recurrence is likely.

Dental caries: Dental caries will be a common finding among children in developing nations. Poor oral hygiene is the usual cause and unfortunately, this is population-level problem for which the medic will have limited to no resources. However, in cases in which dental carries or other dental problem has led to an abscess, the medic should intervene with treatment using antibiotics and refer to a dentist if possible. Follow-up with patient as needed to check progress. Follow-up at the end of treatment is warranted as well. Give **clindamycin** 30mg/kg/day divided po tid x 7-10 days. *See Part 5: Specialty Areas: Chapter 10: Toothaches: Dental Caries*

Geographic tongue: Depressed lesions on the tongue, usually pink or red, with elevated white or yellow borders surrounding these areas. Caused by desquamation of the filiform papillae. The migrating or geographic pattern is caused by the continually changing areas that are affected. There is no known cause. This is benign and no intervention is needed.

Fissured tongue: Central deep anterior-posterior fissure in the central portion of the tongue from which smaller fissures radiate. This is a normal variant in 5% of the population. Common in Down syndrome. No intervention needed.

Gingival overgrowth: May be hereditary, infiltrative (leukemia), secondary to medications (phenytoin, nifedipine), or inflammatory. The gingiva will appear enlarged and fibrous and may bleed. In all circumstances, meticulous attention to dental hygiene is needed and unfortunately may be difficult to achieve. If gingiva are particularly edematous and hemorrhagic, leukemia should be suspected and these children referred for further evaluation and treatment if possible. If thought to be drug-induced, discontinuation of the offending drug, if possible, will help. HIV infection should also be in the differential when gingival overgrowth is seen. There is usually a brightly erythematous band of gingival that may easily bleed. In contrast to other forms of gingivitis, that caused by HIV infection does not improve with improved oral hygiene.

Viral Infections

Herpangina: Characterized by an acute onset of fever and the appearance of gray-white vesicles, which form ulcers on the posterior palate, uvula, and tonsillar pillars. It is usually caused by *Coxsackie* virus A. It is usually benign and symptoms disappear within 4-5 days. However, the child may have dysphagia, abdominal pain, vomiting, and anorexia. Treat pain with **acetaminophen** (10-15mg/kg/dose po q4-6h prn) or **ibuprofen** (10mg/kg/dose po q6h prn). "Triple mix'" or one of its components can be used in older children and adults as a swish-and-spit mouthwash. Do not use in young children who would risk swallowing the mixture.

Hand-foot-mouth disease: A viral illness also caused by a Coxsackie virus which causes vesicular lesions or red papules on the tongue, oral mucosa, hands, and feet. It may be associated with mild fever, sore throat, and malaise. Like herpangina, it is benign and usually needs no treatment. However, it too may result in dysphagia and anorexia. Treatment of pain is indicated.

Gingivostomatitis: Caused by *Herpes* simplex virus. Single or multiple groupings of small vesicles on the lips, tongue, or gingival mucosa, and occasionally extending to the pharynx. With primary infections, especially in young children, there may be fever, irritability, and drooling. Cervical lymphadenopathy may be present. The lesions are usually present for 7-14 days. Treatment of pain is indicated. Treatment is generally otherwise supportive. Topical medications have been shown to be minimally effective. Use of systemic antivirals for oral lesions in children is not well-studied, but the following is the recommended dosing regimen: **Acyclovir** 1200mg/24 hours po divided q8h x 7-10 days. Max dose in children 80mg/kg/24 hours.

Nutritional Problems: This is a list of the deficient nutrient/vitamin and subsequent findings. Note that problems with nutritional deficiencies are generally population-based problems, which will require resources often beyond the capabilities of the SOF medic. Note that angular cheilosis, pain, decreased taste, and poor dentition with loose teeth are common themes with nutritional deficiencies. A first step to helping with nutritional deficiencies is to identify what the particular deficiencies are and why they exist within the population. An evaluation of the local diet is needed. Although the medic may be limited in dealing with these issues individually, the information gathered concerning micronutrient deficiencies can help public health officers treat these effectively.

Vitamin A: Gingival hypertrophy and inflammation, increased risk of carries, desquamation of oral mucosa, delayed wound healing.
Vitamin B2 (Riboflavin): Angular cheilosis (cracking, dryness and erythema of the skin at the lateral aspects of the lips), shiny red lips, sore tongue
Vitamin B3 (Niacin): Angular cheilosis, mucositis (inflammation and desquamation of the oral mucosa), ulcerative gingivitis. Tongue may be painful and swollen.
Vitamin B6 (Pyridoxine): Angular cheilosis
Vitamin B9 (Folic Acid): Angular cheilosis, mucositis, mouth pain, inflamed gingiva
Vitamin B12 (Cyanocobalamin): Angular cheilosis, mucositis, sore or burning mouth, halitosis, loss or distortion of taste, gingivitis, predilection for apthous ulcers.
Vitamin C: Scurvy (red, swollen gingival with increased tooth mobility), malformed teeth, increased risk of candidiasis
Vitamin D: Poor dentition with loose teeth secondary to incomplete mineralization of teeth and alveolar bone
Vitamin K: Increased risk of bleeding gums.
Zinc: Associated with diminished taste
Calcium: Poor dentition with loose teeth secondary to incomplete mineralization of teeth and alveolar bone
Iron: Angular cheilosis, pallor of lips and oral mucosa
Phosphorus: Incomplete mineralization of teeth and alveolar bone leading to loose teeth and increased risk of carries

Patient Education:
General: The etiology of many soft tissue oral lesions in children is viral and these require supportive treatment only. Good oral hygiene is the key to improvement for problems with teeth and gingiva.
Diet: Avoid spicy or hot foods which may aggravate lesions and cause increased pain.
Activity: Generally unlimited

Follow-up Actions
No Improvement or Deterioration: Report any worsening pain, oral intolerance, difficulty swallowing or chewing, other systemic symptoms.
Evacuation Criteria: Severe (life-threatening) malnutrition or suspicion of immunodeficiency (eg, HIV), as resources and operational conditions permit.

Chapter 15: Pediatrics: Most Common Pediatric Diseases: Throat Problems: Croup
COL Ted Cieslak, MC, USA

Introduction: Viral croup is an Inflammation of the larynx (laryngotracheobronchitis) that typically affects younger children in the fall and early winter months and is usually caused by parainfluenza virus. Croup is a generally mild, self-limited condition, but it must be separated from epiglottitis (*see Part 5: Specialty Areas: Chapter 15: Serious Pediatric Diseases: Epiglottitis*), which is a true medical emergency. Croup is far more common than epiglottitis.

Subjective: **Symptoms**
Typically presents with a prodrome of upper respiratory tract symptoms followed by the development of a barking cough (often said to resemble the "bark" of a seal). The presence of this cough and absence of drooling, dysphagia, and true respiratory distress (as opposed to simply noisy breathing) favor the diagnosis of viral croup over epiglottitis. In croup, as opposed to epiglottis, the "bark" truly is worse than the "bite". In other words, the child may be breathing and coughing rather loudly, but generally looks otherwise quite well and may be playful and alert between coughing spells.
Focused History: *Is the child eating and acting relatively normal?* (Patients with croup do not typically appear clinically ill as compared with patients with epiglottitis who more often appear and act "sick".)

Objective: **Signs**
Using Basic Tools: Inspiratory stridor (as opposed to the expiratory wheezing seen in asthma and other conditions) and chest retractions may be present. Occasionally patient will have tachypnea. Cyanosis should prompt one to consider other diagnoses, especially epiglottitis. Pulse oximetry may be useful to confirm acceptable oxygen saturation.
Using Advanced Tools: No lab studies are necessary. A lateral neck x-ray, if available, may prove useful in ruling out epiglottitis. While viral cultures of the nasopharynx may yield the causative viruses, they require days of incubation (by which time the child is usually better) and are unlikely to be available in a field setting.

Assessment: Croup is a clinical diagnosis.
Differential Diagnosis
Epiglottitis: May also cause inspiratory stridor, but patients with epiglottitis appear much sicker. They are often agitated until the disease progresses to obtundation, which is an ominous sign. They often have higher degrees of fever (although this fact may not be of help in the individual patient), refuse to eat (in fact, are unable to swallow), and demonstrate true respiratory distress, as evidenced by cyanosis, retractions, and air hunger.
Bacterial tracheitis: A rare, but serious, entity that presents a clinical picture similar to epiglottitis.
Aspirated foreign body: Classic (though infrequently observed) presentation is sudden onset of coughing, wheezing, and decreased breath sounds with a history of a choking episode. May progress to stridor, dyspnea, and cyanosis. Chronic cases may have fever or hemoptysis. Less than 20% of aspirated foreign bodies are radio-opaque; a normal CXR does not rule out the diagnosis.

Plan
Treatment:
Supportive care and oral hydration are adequate for the vast majority of children with viral croup. As agitation makes cough and stridor worse, avoid handling the child unnecessarily. Oxygen may be beneficial in the worst cases. Nebulized **racemic epinephrine** (0.5mL of a 2.25% solution diluted with 1.5-3.5mL of sterile water; give via nebulizer over 15 minutes PRN no more frequently than q2h)

may result in short-term improvement, but children given this must be closely monitored for several hours due to a potential rebound effect. **Dexamethasone** (0.6mg/kg po or IM one time dose) may be beneficial.

Alternative: Budesonide (inhalation suspension) 2mg inhaled once via nebulizer

Primitive: Exposure to cool night air or exposure to mist (such as in bathroom) may ease croup symptoms and comfort parents.

Patient Education

General: Reassure parent that disease usually resolves without complications but to return for reevaluation if symptoms continue or get worse.

No Improvement/Deterioration: Patient should be reevaluated if condition worsens especially for signs of difficulty breathing or indications of upper airway obstruction (eg, rule out epiglottitis).

Follow-up Actions

Return Evaluation: Return for reevaluation if symptoms do not improve, worsen or if new symptoms develop.

Chapter 15: Pediatrics: Most Common Pediatric Diseases: Throat Problems: Pharyngitis
COL Ted Cieslak, MC, USA

Introduction: Most cases of pharyngitis are viral (90%) and self-limited. With a few notable exceptions, the clinician is concerned only with those cases caused by group A beta-hemolytic streptococci (GABHS). The goals of diagnosis and treatment of GABHS are prevention of rheumatic fever and of peritonsillar and retropharyngeal abscesses, as well as symptomatic improvement and decreased contagion. Potential complications include: suppurative (eg, peritonsillar abscess) and non-suppurative (eg, acute rheumatic fever and post-streptococcal glomerulonephritis).

Subjective: **Symptoms**

Sore throat, swelling and tenderness along the neck beneath the ears, rash.

Focused History: *Does your throat hurt? Have you felt warm?* (suggests fever) *Do you have pain or difficulty on swallowing?*

Objective: **Signs**

Using Basic Tools: Inspection: Enlarged and inflamed tonsils, peritonsillar swelling and erythema, palatal petechiae, swollen cervical nodes. Palpation: Tender cervical nodes.

Using Advanced Tools: Throat culture where available is beneficial in diagnosing the relatively small minority of pharyngitis patients who require therapy.

Assessment:

It may not be possible to accurately differentiate GABHS from viral pharyngitis on clinical grounds. Tonsillar exudate, petechiae on palate, peritonsillar swelling, tender cervical adenitis, and a "sandpaper" rash on the skin are findings that increase the likelihood of a diagnosis of GABHS, while rhinorrhea and congestion are more consistent with a viral etiology.

Differential Diagnosis:

GABHS pharyngitis: Typically, patients with GABHS have fever, significant odynophagia, tender cervical lymph nodes.

Viral pharyngitis: Patents with a viral etiology for their pharyngitis often have rhinorrhea and coryza.

Infectious mononucleosis: Patients with mononucleosis typically have widespread lymphadenopathy and may have tender splenomegaly. *See Part 5: Specialty Areas: Chapter 12: Viral Infections: Infectious Mononucleosis.*

Diphtheria: Although virtually eliminated in the US, diphtheria occurs in parts of the developing world. Patients with diphtheria are typically quite ill with severe odynophagia and dysphagia. Grey "pseudomembranes" can be found on the tonsils. *See Part 3: General Symptoms: ENT Problems: Pharyngitis, Adult*

Gonococcal pharyngitis: May occur in victims of sexual abuse and among those engaging in oral sex with infected individuals.

Plan:

Treatment

Primary: Most cases of pharyngitis are viral in origin and require NO specific therapy. Cases suspected to be caused by GABHS should be treated with **penicillin V** (25-50mg/kg/day po divided bid x 10 days) or **benzathine penicillin** (300,000- 1,200,000 units IM x 1). **Erythromycin** may be substituted in those with penicillin allergy. Treatment is especially important in areas where the incidence of rheumatic fever is high and in patients with prior history of rheumatic fever or "heart disease". Keep in mind that cases of "weak heart" or other cardiac conditions in children in the developing world can often be traced to previous episodes of rheumatic fever. In such cases, error on the side of overdiagnosis and therapy of GABHS is warranted.

Empiric: Treat pain with **acetaminophen** or **ibuprofen**.

Patient Education

General: Most (90%) cases of pharyngitis are benign and self-limited.

Activity: As tolerated.

Diet: As tolerated. Encourage liquid intake.

Medications: Diarrhea is common with antibiotic administration; allergic reactions occasionally occur.

Prevention & Hygiene: Patients should avoid sharing utensils, cups, and personal hygiene items.

No Improvement/Deterioration: Caretakers should be alert for difficulty in swallowing or breathing which may portend the development of a neck abscess, as well as joint pain and swelling, which may be signs of rheumatic fever.

Follow-up Actions

Return Evaluation: Generally unnecessary unless complications develop.

Consultation Criteria: Patients who cannot swallow or who develop airway compromise constitute potential surgical emergencies. Patients with joint findings, shortness of breath, fatigue, and other potential cardiac findings should be referred for cardiac evaluation.

Chapter 15: Pediatrics: Most Common Pediatric Diseases: Genital Problems: Diaper Rash
LTC Douglas Lougee, MC, USA

Introduction: Diaper rash (aka "nappy" rash) is the most common cause of primary irritant dermatitis seen in infants and is most frequently the result of irritation from urine and stool. Two other common causes are superficial infection by *Candida* yeast or bacteria (*Staphylococcus aureus* or *Streptococcus pyogenes*). Poor families in developing countries may not be as concerned with diaper rash as parents in developed world. Many parents in poor countries do not use diapers or if they do, they may use rags that are only changed with stool, not urine.

Subjective: Symptoms
Rash noted in diaper area.
Focused History: *Is infant taking any medications?* (increased risk of rash caused by yeasts) *Is infant having diarrhea?* (increased irritation and risk for rash) *Does anyone else in the family have a rash?* (may indicate other causes eg, scabies)

Objective: Signs
Using Basic Tools: Red, irritated rash that spares the deep part of creases (irritant diaper rash). Red rash with confluence in deep creases and with surrounding "islands" of redness (*Candida* yeast). Bullae (large blisters) or diffuse pustules and/or crusting (bacterial). Check mouth for yeast (thrush).
Using Advanced Tools: If suspect bacterial infection, consider skin culture (swab area and send for culture and sensitivities).

Assessment: Irritant, yeast or bacterial diaper rash or mixed picture.
Differential Diagnosis:
Irritant dermatitis: Erythema and thickening of skin in perineal area with history of contact with urine and feces.
Superficial yeast infection (*Candida*): Very frequently accompanies irritant dermatitis.
Superficial bacterial infection:
Streptococcal perianal cellulitis: Pain with defecation (possibly causing constipation), perianal erythema and tenderness, painful rectal examination. The child is most frequently afebrile and otherwise well.
Scabies: Acute pruritic dermatitis that extends to the abdomen or other areas of the skin; will likely have family members with similar symptoms. *See Part 4: Organ Systems: Bug Bites and Stings: Scabies*

Plan: Treatment
Irritant dermatitis: Apply **zinc oxide cream** or paste liberally to buttocks several times a day until redness gone.
Superficial candidal yeast infection: Apply **nystatin** or **clotrimazole** cream to rash tid-qid (eg, with each diaper change) until rash is gone.
Superficial bacterial infection: Anti-staphylococcal or anti-strep antibiotics. Apply **mupirocin** ointment tid. Give **clindamycin** 10-30mg/kg/day po in divided doses q6h if severe or large bullae. Treat until rash has resolved (typically **7** days).
Streptococcal perianal cellulitis: Give **penicillin** 25-50mg/kg/day po divided bid. Use **clindamycin** if penicillin allergic. In severe cases, give **clindamycin** 25-50mg/kg/day divided q6h until improvement, and then change to oral medication.
Patient Education
General: Change diapers frequently with frequent opportunities for "air drying" of area. Avoid rubber or plastic pants.
No Improvement/Deterioration: Return if rash does not show improvement, worsens or new skin lesions develop.
Follow-up Actions
Return Evaluation: Patients with bacterial infections (eg, perianal cellulitis) should be closely followed to insure resolution of infection. Patients should return if symptoms do not resolve or new symptoms develop.
Evacuation/Consultation Criteria: Seek medical consultation for patients with evidence of systemic infections (eg, appears acutely ill, febrile, bullae, significant lymphadenopathy or other systemic signs) or for cases that do not respond to therapy.

Chapter 15: Pediatrics: Most Common Pediatric Diseases: Skin Problems: Viral Exanthems
MAJ Paul Kwon, MC, USA

Introduction: There are myriad causes of rash and fever in young children; most of these are viral (Scarlet fever is caused by a bacterium, *Streptococcus pyogenes*, while the cause of Kawasaki's disease remains unknown.) Treatment is usually supportive, although specific therapeutic and infection control measures should be instituted in some cases. For simplicity and comparison, some of the most common causes of acute febrile rash in children are presented in table format.

Table 5-25. Childhood Viral Exanthems

Illness	Prodrome	Appearance	Labs	Treatment
Measles (Rubeola virus)	High fever with rash. Cough, runny nose, conjunctivitis. White spots ("Koplik's spots") may be seen on the buccal mucosa prior to rash.	After fever: very prominent maculo-papular maculopapular red rash with confluence. Starts from head and migrates to trunk and extremities. Unlike the case in roseola, children with measles often appear quite ill.	CBC: Lymphopenia	**Acetaminophen** (10-15mg/kg po q4h prn, not to exceed 5 doses/24 hrs) for fever; avoid opioids and salicylates. Treat secondary bacterial infections. Vaccination and immune globulin if given within 6 days of exposure. Maintain hydration. Isolation: highly contagious; airborne precautions are warranted.
Chickenpox (Varicella-Zoster virus)	Symptoms occur 10-20 days after exposure and includes 1-3 days of fever, as well as respiratory symptoms, and/or headache	After fever: red macules + tiny vesicles (described as "dew drops on a rose petal"). The rash progresses to pustules and then crusts over w/out a scar (will see different stages throughout body). Centrifugal distribution (begins on trunk and spreads to extremities); accompanied by intense pruritus.	CBC: Leukocytosis may indicate a secondary bacterial infection.	**Acetaminophen** for fever; **diphenhydramine** (5mg/kg/day po in 4 divided doses prn; do not exceed 300mg/ day) for itching; good hygiene and possible anti-staphylococcal antibiotics. Isolation: highly contagious; airborne precautions are warranted; once crusts appear is not contagious. Avoid aspirin products
Rubella (Rubella virus)	Known for its teratogenic effects. Patients can transmit the disease 5 days before and up until 5 days after the rash. In young children, it may only involve a rash up to 14 days. Other signs include swollen postauricular and occipital lymph nodes, fever, sore throat, myalgia, ocular pain. For congenital transmission, a "blueberry muffin" rash may appear at birth with multiple organ defects.	Maculopapular non-confluent small pink rash starting from head then spreading to rest of body (may fade from previously involved areas as it progresses) May have pruritus. Rash may be difficult to detect. More noticeable after hot shower.	None needed	Hydration. **Acetaminophen** as needed for fever or pain. Isolation: droplet precautions.
Scarlet Fever (Group A strep)	High fevers preceding rash and history of sore throat.	Pink-red flush with pinhead spots (like a sunburn with goose pimples). Blanches with pressure. Starts on chest then to extremities. Sometimes not on palms, soles of feet and face.	Throat culture for Group A strep.	**Penicillin** V K 50mg/ kg/d po divided q8h x 10 days If allergic to penicillin, **erythromycin** 30-50mg/kg/d po divided q6h x 10 days

Table 5-25. Childhood Viral Exanthems, continued

Illness	Prodrome	Appearance	Labs	Treatment
Roseola (Human herpesvirus 6)	Fever may reach as high as 105.8°F and last up to 8 days but usually 5 days. Watch for febrile seizures. The common age group is 6 months to 3 years of age. The infant could have mild lethargy, injected pharynx with exudates, tonsils, and tympanic membranes. May be accompanied by conjunctivitis, diarrhea and vomiting.	Rash typically appears after fever recedes-a small discrete rose-pink maculopapular rash begins on chest, abdomen, then generalizes. Children often appear remarkably well given the degree of their fever.	None needed	**Acetaminophen** and sponge baths for fevers to prevent febrile seizures. Hydration.
Erythema Infectiosum ("Fifth" Disease) (Parvovirus B19)	Many infections are clinically silent; symptomatic children have a prodrome consisting of slight fever, headache, and rhinorrhea.	Rash typically begins as an erythema or flushing of the face, giving rise to the hallmark "slapped cheek" appearance. Many children then develop a diffuse macular rash, which becomes lacy and reticulated as central clearing occurs. Some children will develop arthralgias, which often last for 2-4 weeks.	None needed in most cases; children with chronic hemolytic conditions (eg, thalassemia, Hb SS) may develop acute aplastic crisis; CBC is warranted where such concern exists.	**Acetaminophen** for fever or pain. Hydration
Hand, Foot and Mouth Disease (Coxsackie A viruses)	Begins with sore throat and low grade fever that lasts 1-2 days. Children often have difficulty feeding and can be quite irritable.	Vesicles occur inside the mouth and throat, on the lips, fingers, hands, and feet. May look like chicken pox and may break if handled	None needed	**Acetaminophen** for fever or pain. Hydration
Kawasaki's Disease (etiology unknown)	Begins with high fever (>102.2°F). A diagnosis can be made when this fever is present for 5 days and patient exhibits 4 of the 5 "CRASH" findings and no other explanation exists (see box on right):	Conjunctivitis Rash (nonspecific; may be found on trunk, genitals, and extremities) Adenopathy (usually cervical lymph nodes >1.5 cm) Strawberry tongue & cracked, red, dry lips Hands and feet may be swollen (desquamation or peeling of hands is late sign)	CBC: Leukocytosis; often marked thrombocytosis, along with elevated ESR and CRP.	High dose **aspirin** (80-100mg/kg/day po divided qid) should be given in the acute phase; dose may be lowered (3-5mg/kg/day po qAM) when platelets have stabilized. IV **immune globulin** (2 g/kg given as one dose over 8-12 hours) should be started ASAP.
Pityriasis Rosea (etiology unknown)	Fever and malaise occasionally precede rash, although most children have a minimal prodrome. The hallmark finding, however, is a "herald patch", which is typically large (1-10cm), oval, and precedes the generalized exanthem.	A symmetric exanthem (often described as present in a "Christmas tree" distribution on the back) occurs 5-10 days after the herald patch. Lesions are usually slightly raised, less than 1 cm in diameter, and finely scaled.	None needed	None needed; pruritus may be treated by standard means.

Chapter 15: Pediatrics: Serious Pediatric Diseases: Epiglottitis
COL Ted Cieslak, MC, USA

Introduction: Epiglottitis is an acute life-threatening infection usually affecting toddlers and typically caused by the gram-negative bacterium *Haemophilus influenzae* type b (Hib). While croup is far more common than epiglottitis, especially in developed nations where immunization against Hib is practiced, the consequences of a delay in diagnosis and therapy of epiglottitis can be catastrophic. Potential complications include: acute airway compromise, asphyxia and sepsis. In the developing world, where immunization is not available, epiglottitis remains a serious cause of morbidity among toddlers and young children. Immunization against Hib prevents virtually all cases of epiglottitis.

Subjective: Symptoms
Typically presents in dramatic fashion with sudden onset of fever, dysphagia, drooling, muffled voice, chest retractions, cyanosis and stridor. As opposed to the child with croup, who typically appears rather well between spasms of cough and stridor, the child with epiglottitis usually appears toxic and apprehensive. They often shun movement and prefer to remain still in a "tripod" position with the neck in hyperextension and the mouth open in an attempt to maintain a patent airway.
Focused History: *How long has patient been ill?* (Epiglottitis typically presents acutely.) *Is the child acting normally?* (Patients with epiglottitis typically appear and act ill.) *Has the child been eating?* (Patients with epiglottitis are often unable to swallow.)

Objective: Signs
Using Basic Tools: Inspection: Stridor with chest retractions and cyanosis. Fever can be variable, but is often quite high. In an austere setting, do not attempt direct visualization of the pharynx. Pulse oximetry may be useful to determine adequate oxygen saturation (>92%).
Using Advanced Tools: Examination of the epiglottis should be done only by an experienced airway specialist under controlled conditions, optimally in the operating room. Definitive diagnosis of epiglottitis is a cherry-red and swollen epiglottis on direct inspection. Lateral neck films, if available, may demonstrate the "thumb sign" of a markedly swollen epiglottis. CBC will often reveal an elevated WBC count with a left shift. Blood cultures may yield *H. influenzae*. Patient's airway MUST BE secure before you attempt lab studies or x-ray.

Assessment:
Epiglottitis is a true medical emergency. Presumptive diagnosis in the field is based on history and symptoms and therapy must be instituted immediately. Diagnosis should not be delayed while attempting to obtain neck x-rays.
Differential Diagnosis
Croup: May include inspiratory stridor, but patients with croup usually do not appear toxic, are often younger and have less fever. Patients with epiglottitis typically refuse to eat (in fact, are unable to swallow), and demonstrate true respiratory distress, as evidenced by cyanosis, retractions, and air hunger. In croup, the "bark" (barking cough) is worse than the bite. *See Part 5: Specialty Areas: Chapter 15: Most Common Pediatric Diseases: Throat Problems: Croup*
Bacterial tracheitis: Rare but serious condition that can be clinically similar to epiglottitis.

Plan:
Treatment
Primary: Keep patient calm. Allow them to assume a position of comfort (often sitting up in a "tripod" position). Avoid agitation and unnecessary movement. Oxygen should be provided by whatever means possible. Emergent endotracheal intubation is often warranted and ideally, should be performed under general anesthesia. Antibiotics should be started promptly: **Ceftriaxone** (100mg/kg/d IV divided q12h x 7 days) is an ideal choice. IV fluids should also be administered
Alternative: Other antibiotics effective against Hib include: **Cefotaxime** (200mg/kg/d IV divided q6h), **ampicillin** (300-400mg/kg/d IV divided q4-6h), and **chloramphenicol** (100mg/kg/d IV divided q6h). If IV therapy is not possible, IM is preferred to po therapy. Oral medications should not be forced down the throat of a child with epiglottitis.
Primitive: If the patient deteriorates (suffers from airway obstruction) and an operating room is not readily available, attempt to establish an airway by any means possible: bag and mask ventilation (air can often be "forced" past a markedly swollen epiglottis with a tight mask seal and forceful bagging), intubation, transtracheal ventilation (with a large bore angiocatheter attached to a 3mm endotracheal tube adapter and resuscitation bag). Emergent tracheostomy may be required.

Patient Education
General: This is a true medical emergency and patient should be watched closely for evidence of airway compromise.
Activity: Keep the patient quiet in whatever position they find most comfortable.
Diet: Patients may be unwilling or unable to eat or drink. Provide IV hydration as required.
Medications: Watch for adverse side effects of antibiotic therapy (ie, allergic reactions, pseudomembranous colitis, blood dyscrasias, nephrotoxicity).
No Improvement/Deterioration: Protection of patient's airway is the most important consideration. Early planning to insure adequate advanced airway procedures (eg, endotracheal intubation under general anesthesia) is warranted.
Follow-up Actions
Return Evaluation: Return if symptoms persist, worsen or new symptoms occur.
Evacuation/Consultation Criteria: Monitor closely and plan ahead. Patients may require endotracheal intubation under general anesthesia.

Chapter 15: Pediatrics: Serious Pediatric Diseases: Asthma
LTC Daniel P. Hsu, MC, USA

Introduction: Asthma is a chronic disease of the airways that is characterized by reversible airway obstruction, inflammation and hyperactivity. The clinical course of asthma is characterized by recurrent exacerbations of respiratory distress (cough, wheeze, shortness of breath) with periods of normal respiratory function in between. Although common triggers for asthma exacerbations are known, the severity of an acute attack is highly variable. The timing of an attack is often unpredictable. The approach to asthma treatment includes the acute treatment of exacerbations, as well as the long term control of asthma. Asthma can be categorized as mild intermittent, mild persistent, moderate persistent, or severe persistent based upon symptoms and risk for a severe exacerbation. Asthma is seen worldwide. The highest prevalence occurs in the Western Europe, North America, Central America and South America. Asthma exacerbations can occur year round, with increased prevalence during the winter (cold/flu season) as well as spring/fall (common allergy season). **Risk Factors:** Asthma, allergic rhinitis, and eczema are frequent co-morbidities. Patients with food allergies may also have a higher risk for asthma. Family history of asthma, allergies, or eczema increase the risk for asthma. Exposure to environmental irritants (second hand smoke, pollutants) increases the risk for an asthma exacerbation. Other potential triggers for an asthma exacerbation include strong emotions, extremes of temperature (hot or cold), exercise, and strong perfumes/chemicals, certain drugs such as aspirin, and food allergy exposure.

Subjective: Symptoms

Acute asthma exacerbations present with increased work of breathing, wheezing, coughing, chest pain or tightness, shortness of breath. Increase work of breathing is noted by an increased respiratory rate, retractions(suprasternal, intercostal), grunting, or nasal flaring. Table 5-26 can be used as a guide to normal respiratory rates in children.

Table 5-26. Normal Respiratory Rate in Children

Age	Breaths/minute
< 2 mo	< 60
2-12 mo	< 50
1-5 yo	< 40
6-8 yo	< 30

Chronic symptoms of asthma include intermittent symptoms of coughing, wheezing, exercise intolerance. Nocturnal symptoms are frequently worse, with cough and night awakenings. Frequent use of bronchodilators (>1-2 times/ month) is a warning sign that chronic asthma symptoms are not well controlled. Pre-treatment with bronchodilator prior to exercise is not counted when determining frequent use. **Focused History: For acute exacerbations:** *When the symptoms started, which medications were tried and were they helpful? Is the child disoriented or tiring out?* (This will indicate the severity of the exacerbation.) **For chronic asthma:** *How frequently do they have symptoms?* (both daytime and nocturnal) *Is there something that appears to trigger asthma symptoms* (Identifying triggers may assist with treatment and possible avoidance.)

Objective: Signs

Using Basic Tools: The most common physical findings during an asthma exacerbation include coughing, wheezing, increased work of breathing. In severe cases, cyanosis of the extremities or lips may be seen. Inspection: Respiratory Rate, accessory muscle use, cyanosis of the lips or extremities. Auscultation: Wheezing, crackles, decreased breath sounds, prolonged expiratory phase. Be aware that lack of wheezing can give one a false sense of security. Patients who have poor air exchange may not wheeze. If there are other signs of respiratory distress without wheezing, the patient is having a severe asthma exacerbation. Heart rate is generally increased during an asthma exacerbation. Pulse oximetry can be performed, however normal pulse oximeter readings do not rule out a severe exacerbation. Many patients with moderate to severe asthma exacerbations have normal pulse oximeter readings.
Using Advanced Tools: Peak flow may be helpful in the acute setting. Simple spirometry is helpful in the chronic setting to show evidence of airway obstruction. However, many children with asthma will have normal spirometric values. CXR may show hyperinflation. It is useful to help rule out evaluate for other causes of symptoms such as pneumonia and/or pneumothorax.

Assessment:

Differential Diagnosis: The differential diagnosis for an acute asthma exacerbation includes **pneumonia, pneumothorax,** foreign body aspiration, croup. **Pneumonia** will often have unilateral decrease in breath sounds, and is more often associated with fever. Crackles are generally audible and wheezing is uncommon. Dullness to percussion, egophony, tactile, or fremitus indicate a process other than asthma (eg, pleural effusion). However, pneumonia can trigger an exacerbation of asthma, particularly viral or atypical pneumonias. **Pneumothorax** and foreign body aspiration typically have asymmetric breath sounds. Pneumothorax will not present with wheezing. Decreased breath sounds on the side of the pneumothorax are typical. Tracheal deviation is not a common finding in childhood tension pneumothorax, and should not be relied upon for the diagnosis. **Foreign body aspiration** will also have decreased breath sounds on the side where the foreign body is trapped. The other side should be clear, unless there is bilateral foreign body aspiration. High index of suspicion should be present based on the age of the patient. Foreign body aspiration is most common in the 3-5 year age group. It is also more common on the right side. **Croup** has a very distinct "barky" cough. Lung sounds are generally clear. Stridor is frequently audible with croup. The differential diagnosis for chronic asthma includes **cystic fibrosis, ciliary dyskinesia, chronic sinusitis, GERD, recurrent aspiration, tracheoesophageal fistula, immunodeficiency, foreign body aspiration, laryngomalacia, tracheomalacia, bronchomalacia, vocal cord dysfunction,** and **airway anomalies.** The approach to a patient with a chronic cough or wheezing often requires several visits to determine the etiology. Response to bronchodilator or inhaled corticosteroids is a helpful tool in the evaluation. Cough or wheezing that is not responsive to bronchodilator makes the diagnosis of asthma less likely. Response to inhaled corticosteroids takes 3-4 wks. A patient with recurrent respiratory symptoms, cough, pneumonia, sinusitis, or otitis media should be evaluated for **cystic fibrosis** or **ciliary dyskinesia.** Chronic cough, particularly at night, is often the lone manifestation of **chronic sinusitis,** which requires 3-4 wks of antibiotics for treatment. GERD is a common cause of cough, typically nocturnal. A history of food avoidance or spitting up is common clues to diagnosing GERD. Empiric trials with medications to treat GERD may assist with the diagnosis. **Recurrent aspiration** and **immunodeficiency** often present with recurrent pneumonias. **Immunodeficiency** can present with frequent infections in other body areas, and may also present with failure to thrive. **Laryngomalacia** and **vocal cord dysfunction** present with inspiratory stridor, which may mimic wheezing. Stridor may be transmitted to the lungs, however the noise will be loudest when listening over the neck.

Tracheomalacia and **bronchomalacia** may present as wheezing in infants. Wheezing is in the setting of no respiratory distress. It is louder when the infant is placed supine, and crying. Prone or upright positioning improves the wheezing noise. Bronchodilators exacerbate wheezing or result in no change of symptoms. **Airway anomalies** such as a vascular ring or sling can cause wheezing that is unresponsive to bronchodilators.

Plan:
Treatment
Primary: Albuterol 2.5mg via nebulizer. This may be repeated q15-20 minutes.

Levalbuterol may be utilized as an alternative nebulizer medication at a dose of 1.25mg. Children who are unable to utilize the mouthpiece should have a tight fitting facemask to deliver the nebulized medication. Flow rate must be set to at least 6-8L/min. Any pressurized room air or oxygen source can be utilized for the delivery of nebulized medication. Electronic compressor machines are also available for nebulized medication delivery. An alternative that has equally efficacious results in acute asthma is to deliver **albuterol** or **levalbuterol** 2-4 puffs with the appropriate size spacer. The face mask spacer must fit tightly to the face and should cover the nose and mouth regions. The bottom of the mask should reach the chin. At 5-6 years of age, the mouthpiece spacer should be considered. Use of the mouthpiece spacer requires the ability to follow instructions for deep inspiration during treatment followed by breath holding for 5-10 seconds. Subcutaneous **epinephrine**, (0.01mg/kg/dose, max 0.5mg/dose), or **terbutaline** (0.01mg/kg/dose, max 0.4mg/dose) may be used as an adjunct to the inhaled bronchodilators or instead of inhaled bronchodilator when none are available. **Prednisone/prednisolone:** 2mg/kg/day(max 60mg), should be given in 1 daily dose. Standard length of therapy is 5 days, however may be given for 10-14 days depending on length of symptoms. Supplemental oxygen is a bronchodilator, and can be used if available.

Alternative: Nebulized ipratropium (250mcg for <4yrs, 500mcg for >4 yrs) or ipratropium HFA 2 puffs. **Ipratropium** can be delivered up to q4h. Ipratropium is not as good as albuterol for bronchodilatation.

Primitive: Use **albuterol/levalbuterol** MDI therapy.

Patient Education
General: Asthma is a chronic recurrent condition characterized by varying severity of exacerbations. A patient with mild chronic symptoms can still have a severe exacerbation. The acute management involves use of bronchodilators, but it should be emphasized long term control is achieved with daily use of inhaled corticosteroids. Triggers for asthma should be identified and avoidance/treatment should be instituted.

Activity: Activity should be limited during an acute exacerbation. However, if chronic symptoms are well controlled, there is no recommendation to limit activity.

Diet: No special dietary requirements.

Medications: Side effects of bronchodilator therapy include tachycardia, jitteriness, and nausea. Inhaled corticosteroids may increase the risk of thrush, so the patient should rinse the mouth following use.

No Improvement/Deterioration: During an acute exacerbation, if initial bronchodilator therapy is ineffective, subcutaneous epinephrine or terbutaline. The patient should be brought to the nearest medical facility.

Follow-up Actions
Return Evaluation: Patients with asthma are generally reevaluated every few months.

Evacuation/Consultation Criteria: In an acute exacerbation, if the patient does not seem to respond to bronchodilator after 3 doses in 1 hour, or if the patient needs bronchodilator more than every 4 hours, higher level care should be sought.

Note: Do not be fooled by lack of wheezing on exam. It can be a sign that the patient is experiencing a severe exacerbation. If there are other signs of respiratory distress or increased work of breathing, the patient requires emergency care.

Chapter 15: Pediatrics: Serious Pediatric Diseases: Acute Abdominal Pain
LTC Kathleen Dunn Farr, MC, USA

Introduction: There are many causes of acute abdominal pain in children. The primary goal in the management of acute abdominal pain in the child is to determine whether the condition is life-threatening. Life-threatening disorders that require surgical intervention include appendicitis, intestinal obstruction, volvulus, perforated viscus, mesenteric ischemia, and peritonitis. Do not belabor the diagnosis; the critical decision point is whether the child needs intervention at a higher level of care for a life-threatening condition. When in doubt, resuscitate, stabilize, and evacuate for evaluation by a medical officer. Young children do not always present with typical symptoms of surgical abdomen and may deteriorate rapidly. If the condition is not life-threatening, determine whether the patient requires treatment or has a self-limiting condition. **Risk Factors:** Children are at higher risk for injury from blunt abdominal trauma because of underdeveloped abdominal musculature, proportionally larger solid organs, and pliable ribs. In children under age 8 years, assume intraabdominal or intrathoracic injury with trauma until proven otherwise. Because the omentum is less developed in children, appendicitis is more likely to progress rapidly to perforation and peritonitis. **Note:** *See Part 3: General Symptoms: Acute Abdominal Pain; Part 4: Organ Systems: Chapter 7: Appendicitis & Part 5: Specialty Areas: Chapter 15: Pain in the Child*

Subjective: **Symptoms**
Focused History: Ask about the location, onset, character, severity, duration, and radiation of the pain, and aggravating/mitigating factors. In the acute surgical abdomen, pain usually precedes vomiting, while the opposite is true in medical conditions. Remember that young children have difficulty localizing pain and parents may be poor historians. *Where is the pain?* (With upper abdominal pain, focus on the stomach, duodenum, liver, or pancreas; with periumbilical pain, focus on the small intestine, proximal colon, and appendix; and with lower abdominal pain, focus on the distal colon and GU tract.) *What is the pain like?* (Visceral [deep organ] pain tends to be dull, poorly localized, midline, and often associated with nausea. Parietal [peritoneal] pain is usually sharp, intense, discrete, and well localized. Coughing and moving can aggravate this pain. Referred pain is felt at a point distant from its source. Non-specific abdominal pain [functional] is usually vague, central, and colicky [comes and goes]).

Table 5-27. Character and Possible Causes of Acute Abdominal Pain in Children

Character of Pain	Possible Cause
Colicky/intermittent pain that becomes steady	Appendicitis; strangulating intestinal obstruction; mesenteric ischemia
Cramping	Gastroenteritis
Sharp, constant pain made worse by movement	Peritonitis
Acute, sharp, constricting, "takes the breath away"	Renal or biliary colic
Dull waves with vomiting	Intestinal obstruction
Dull ache	Appendicitis; diverticulitis; pyelonephritis
Burning pain that gets better after eating	Gastroesophageal reflux disease (GERD)
Pain that starts after eating certain kinds of food	Food allergies

Have you had the pain before? (Recurrent problems include sickle cell disease, ulcer disease, gallstone colic, diverticulitis) *Was the onset sudden?* (If yes, consider perforated ulcer, renal stone, ruptured ectopic pregnancy, torsion of ovary or testis. Most other causes are more gradual in onset.) *How severe is the pain?* (Severe pain is more common with perforated viscus, kidney stone, peritonitis, or pancreatitis. Pain out of proportion to physical findings is typical of intussusception and mesenteric ischemia. Infants [usually age 2-8 weeks of age] with colic will cry or scream for up to 3 hours per day, usually in the evening. *Does the pain travel to any other part of the body?* Right scapula (gallbladder pain); left shoulder region (ruptured spleen, pancreatitis]); pubis or vagina (renal pain); back (ruptured aortic aneurysm); shoulder pain (referred subdiaphragmatic process, pneumonia) *What relieves the pain?* Antacids (peptic ulcer disease); lying as quietly as possible (peritonitis); relief with bowel movement (colonic source, constipation); relief after vomiting (proximal source) *What other symptoms occur with the pain?*
-Fever, chills (food poisoning; peritonitis; **Note:** Appendicitis seldom begins with fever – it usually begins with pain alone or pain with vomiting.)
-Vomiting
  • Vomiting that starts before pain or diarrhea (gastroenteritis; urinary tract infection [UTI])
  • Delayed vomiting, lack of bowel movement and gas (acute intestinal obstruction; longer delay with distal obstruction)
  • Dark green or yellow (intestinal obstruction; volvulus or incarcerated inguinal hernia in neonate; **Note:** Bilious vomiting in a neonate is always a surgical emergency.)
  • Bloody or coffee ground (upper GI bleed; nose bleed)
  • Projectile, non-bilious (pyloric stenosis – usually presents at 3-5 weeks of age)
-Change in stool pattern
  • Diarrhea (viral or bacterial gastroenteritis or food poisoning; unusual early in appendicitis)
  • Bloody diarrhea (inflammatory bowel disease; infectious enterocolitis; intussusception – peak incidence at 6-11 months)
  • Constipation (acute constipation usually organic, eg, intestinal obstruction; chronic constipation usually functional, often due to low fiber diet)
-Respiratory symptoms
  • Difficulty breathing (asthma associated with GERD; pneumonia; severe infection/peritonitis/impending collapse)
  • Cough, shortness of breath, chest pain (GERD; pneumonia; upper respiratory infection [URI] may precede mesenteric adenitis or sickle cell crisis)
  • Upper respiratory symptoms (streptococcal pharyngitis)
-GU symptoms
  • Scrotal or groin pain (inguinal hernia; testicular torsion; hair tourniquet) **Note:** Child may be embarrassed to mention the location of this pain
  • Urinary frequency, dysuria, urgency, +/- flank pain (urinary tract infection; pyelonephritis)
  • Amenorrhea (ectopic pregnancy)
  • Vaginal discharge (pelvic inflammatory disease [PID]; salpingitis)
-Other symptoms
  • Weight loss or poor weight gain (consistent with serious disease rather than benign abdominal pain)
  • Polyuria, polydipsia (diabetes mellitus)
  • Jaundice (hepatitis; parasites)
Have you had any recent trauma? (Traumatic pancreatitis -- especially after collision with bicycle handlebars; ruptured organs; duodenal hematoma.)
Is the child taking any medications? (Erythromycin and tetracycline may cause abdominal discomfort; Corticosteroids or immunosuppressants may mask inflammatory response and pain in peritonitis. Anticoagulants increase risk of bleeding and hematoma.)
Is there a history of substance use/abuse? (Alcohol predisposes to pancreatitis.)
Is the child sexually active? (Multiple sexual partners predispose to PID.)
Is there a significant past medical history? (Premature birth [higher risk for inguinal hernia], abdominal surgery [risk for adhesions and intestinal obstruction], Sickle cell anemia [may present with acute abdominal pain; crisis triggered by infection], HIV infection [predisposes to infection and adverse drug effects], Diabetes [diabetic ketoacidosis may present with abdominal pain], IUD placement [PID; ectopic pregnancy.]
Is there a significant family history? (Inflammatory bowel disease; migraines – associated with functional abdominal pain.)

Objective: Signs

Using Basic Tools: Inspection: Vital signs: Fever more common in patients with surgical abdomen. Kussmaul's respirations common with diabetic ketoacidosis. Toxicity (serious illness more likely in ill-looking, anxious, pale, sweating, listless, or lethargic child). Activity (child with peritonitis remains very still and resists movement; child with visceral pain often writhes during acute cramps but may feel well enough to walk between cramps). Skin: Pallor (shock; along with jaundice, suggests sickle cell crisis), Rash (purpura and arthritis suggest Henoch-Schonlein purpura), Jaundice (hemolysis or liver disease) Abdominal exam: Ask patient to distend his abdomen, flatten it, and then indicate with one finger where it hurts, hemorrhage/bruising (consider child abuse in patients with bruises in protected areas), distension (consider bowel obstruction when present with tympany to percussion and high-pitched bowel sounds in rushes). Auscultation: Change in bowel sounds (*see distension*), silent abdomen (with child who does not want to move) (ileus; peritonitis). Palpation: Begin gently, away from the area of greatest pain, Tenderness (infection, inflammation), Rebound/guarding (child may bend at waist and refuse to stand up straight; test by having patient jump up and down or have caretaker bounce child on his or her knee), Masses (neoplasm; "olive" in pyloric stenosis). Rectal (use a small finger): Check for imperforate anus, anal fissure, tenderness, masses, and blood or melena in the stool. Rectal bleeding may occur with abdominal pain (peptic ulcer disease; intussusception; volvulus) or without (polyps; arteriovenous malformations; tumors). Pelvic/GU: Examine external genitalia (penile and scrotal abnormalities; testicular torsion; hair tourniquet). Check for discharge (PID), masses (neoplasm; ovarian cyst), hernias (incarcerated inguinal hernia), adnexal/cervical motion tenderness (PID, ovarian torsion) Percussion: Use gentle percussion to test for rebound tenderness. Use deeper palpation to check for organomegaly. Hepatomegaly or splenomegaly (parasitic infection), Tympany (*see distention*), Flank pain (kidney infection).
Using Advanced Tools: Labs: CBC (elevated WBC suggests inflammation or infection; decreased hemoglobin suggests blood loss or sickle cell disease), urinalysis (rule out UTI, calculi, ketones), pregnancy test (ectopic pregnancy), stool ova and parasites (worm bolus with obstruction). Plain abdominal radiographs: check for air fluid levels (intestinal obstruction); free air (perforation of abdominal viscus); calcification (gallstones, kidney stones); soft tissue mass; abundant feces (constipation), Chest radiograph (pneumonia).

Figure 5-37. Location of Abdominal Pain and Possible Causes
Adapted from: Acute Abdominal Pain: Acute Abdomen and Surgical Gastroenterology: Merck Manual Professional

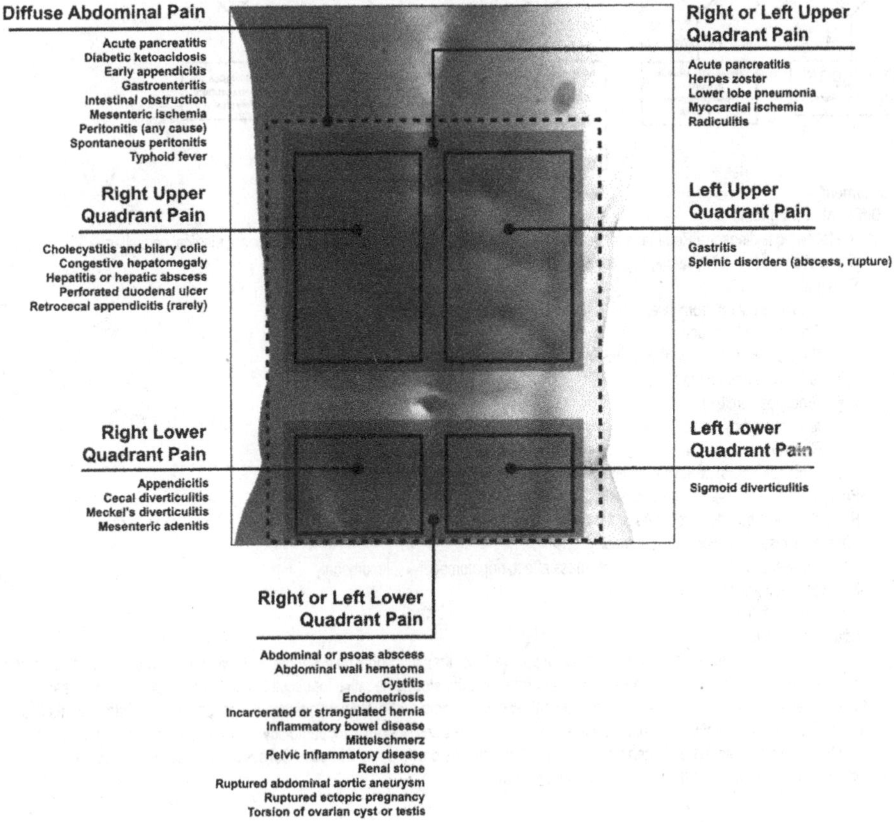

Diffuse Abdominal Pain
Acute pancreatitis
Diabetic ketoacidosis
Early appendicitis
Gastroenteritis
Intestinal obstruction
Mesenteric ischemia
Peritonitis (any cause)
Spontaneous peritonitis
Typhoid fever

Right or Left Upper Quadrant Pain
Acute pancreatitis
Herpes zoster
Lower lobe pneumonia
Myocardial ischemia
Radiculitis

Right Upper Quadrant Pain
Cholecystitis and bilary colic
Congestive hepatomegaly
Hepatitis or hepatic abscess
Perforated duodenal ulcer
Retrocecal appendicitis (rarely)

Left Upper Quadrant Pain
Gastritis
Splenic disorders (abscess, rupture)

Right Lower Quadrant Pain
Appendicitis
Cecal diverticulitis
Meckel's diverticulitis
Mesenteric adenitis

Left Lower Quadrant Pain
Sigmoid diverticulitis

Right or Left Lower Quadrant Pain
Abdominal or psoas abscess
Abdominal wall hematoma
Cystitis
Endometriosis
Incarcerated or strangulated hernia
Inflammatory bowel disease
Mittelschmerz
Pelvic inflammatory disease
Renal stone
Ruptured abdominal aortic aneurysm
Ruptured ectopic pregnancy
Torsion of ovarian cyst or testis

Figure 5-38. Evaluation of Acute Abdominal Pain in Children
Adapted from Leung AKC, Sigalet, DL. Acute Abdominal Pain in Children. American Family Physician, Vol 67, No 11, June 1, 2003: 2321-2326

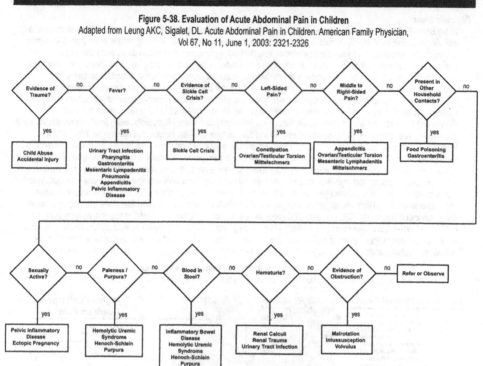

Assessment

Differential Diagnosis

The following findings are Red Flags for serious injury or illness. Consult a surgeon or appropriate medical consultant.

-Signs of shock (eg, tachycardia, hypotension, sweating, altered mental status)

-Pain that:
- Awakens patient from sleep
- Continues >12 hours
- Progresses in severity or changes in pattern (diffuse to localized)
- Is accompanied by fainting
- Precedes vomiting
- Is worsened by breathing or a change in body position
- Radiates

-Persistent (>24 hours) or severe vomiting, especially bilious, dark, or blood-tinged

-Prolonged (>24 hours), severe or bloody diarrhea

-Rigid abdomen, guarding, rebound or localized tenderness

-Abdominal distention with diffuse tympany

-Absent bowel sounds -Localized fullness, mass effect, hepatomegaly, splenomegaly

-Significant abdominal trauma

-Involuntary weight loss

-Unexplained fever

In children age 4-18 years with chronic abdominal pain (>2 months), functional pain is more likely when there are no alarm symptoms or signs ("red flags"), the physical examination is normal, and the stool is negative for occult blood. If the diagnosis is not clear after the initial evaluation and the child is stable, repeat the physical exam q4-6h. Be cautious about diagnosing viral gastroenteritis in an infant <6 weeks old; vomiting and diarrhea are more likely to be signs of significant pathology in this age group. An infant with colic may have a tight distended abdomen while crying, often with legs drawn up as if in pain. Colic is not associated with vomiting, diarrhea, fever, or weight loss, and physical exam is normal.

Table 5-28. Differential Diagnosis of Acute Abdominal Pain by Predominant Age
From Leung AKC, Sigalet, DL. Acute Abdominal Pain in Children. American Family Physician,
Vol 67, No 11, June 1, 2003: 2321-2326

Birth to one year	2-5 years	6-11 years	12-18 years
Infantile colic	Gastroenteritis	Gastroenteritis	Appendicitis
Gastroenteritis	Appendicitis	Appendicitis	Gastroenteritis
Constipation	Constipation	Constipation	Constipation
Urinary tract infection	Urinary tract infection	Functional pain	Dysmenorrhea
Intussusception	Intussusception	Urinary tract infection	Mittelschmerz
Intussusception	Volvulus	Trauma	Pelvic inflammatory disease
Volvulus	Trauma	Pharyngitis	Threatened abortion
Incarcerated hernia	Pharyngitis	Pneumonia	Ectopic pregnancy
Hirschsprung's disease	Sickle cell crisis	Sickle cell crisis	Ovarian/testicular torsion
	Henoch-Schönlein purpura	Henoch-Schönlein purpura	
	Mesenteric lymphadenitis	Mesenteric lymphadenitis	

Plan:
Treatment

Primary: Treatment depends on suspected cause of abdominal pain. Life-threatening disorders that require rapid diagnosis and evacuation for surgical intervention include appendicitis, intestinal obstruction, volvulus, perforated viscus, mesenteric ischemia, and peritonitis. If you cannot evacuate a child with symptoms of a surgical abdomen, start IV hydration, monitor hydration status (consider a Foley catheter), begin broad spectrum IV antibiotic coverage, insert a nasogastric tube with intermittent suction, treat fevers over 104°F with oral or rectal **acetaminophen**, and observe closely. Do not perform exploratory surgery without a diagnosis.
In severely ill children:

1. Start fluid resuscitation or rehydration with normal saline or lactated Ringer's solution (consider interosseous route if unable to obtain IV access)
2. Monitor hydration status (consider placing a Foley catheter); maintain urine output of 1.0cc/kg/hr in children (0.5cc/kg/hr in adults)
3. Place on NPO and insert nasogastric tube with intermittent suction.
4. Initiate pain control: Moderate doses of IV analgesics do not mask peritoneal signs and may enable you to perform a better and more thorough examination, thus facilitating diagnosis (*see Part 5: Specialty Areas: Chapter 15: Pain in the Child*).
5. Start antibiotics: If you suspect intestinal perforation, begin IV antibiotics with gram-positive, gram-negative, and anaerobic coverage (eg, **ampicillin** 200-400mg/kg/24hr divided q4-6h IV, **gentamycin** 7.5mg/kg/24hr divided q8h IV, and **metronidazole** 30mg/kg/24hr divided q6h IV. **Note:** Check Harriet Lane Handbook or other pediatric reference for neonatal dose.
6. Start IV acid suppression therapy (preferably proton pump inhibitor, eg, **esomeprazole** 10mg/day (children 1-11 years or <20kg) or 20mg/day (children > = 20kg) po or IV; **Note:** Switch to po medication when possible; doses for pediatric patients are not well established.
7. Treat fevers over 104°F with oral or rectal acetaminophen
8. Observe closely
9. Avoid antiemetics and antidiarrheal medications unless you suspect a specific, benign etiology

Empiric: Lying face down may relieve gas pain. To reduce a non-incarcerated inguinal hernia, administer pain meds, place child in Trendelenburg position, and apply ice packs to the inguinal area. Umbilical hernias rarely incarcerate and usually close spontaneously by age 12 months. Begin acid suppression therapy in patients with GERD and recurrent cough and wheezing.
Primitive: There are no effective medications for treatment of colic; swaddle or rock the infant. For constipation, sit in warm water to relax anus. Eating yogurt (with lactobacillus) helps treat infectious diarrhea and may prevent antibiotic-related diarrhea.
Patient Education

General: See Red Flags for serious injury or illness. Colic in infants usually resolves by 12 weeks of age. Encourage parents to share responsibility for care of a screaming infant ("time out") before they become overwhelmed.

Activity: As tolerated

Diet: With diarrhea, avoid milk, fruit juices, heavily carbonated beverages, coffee, and sports drink. With vomiting, encourage intake of small amounts (5-15mL) of clear liquid every 10-20 minutes. If you suspect GERD, thicken milk with cereal to decrease the frequency of vomiting. Increase fiber and fluid intake in patients with functional constipation.

No Improvement/Deterioration: See Red Flags for serious injury or illness

Follow-up Actions

Return Evaluation: See Red Flags for serious injury or illness

Evacuation/Consultation Criteria: See Red Flags for serious injury or illness.

Chapter 15: Pediatrics: Serious Pediatric Diseases: Meningitis
CPT Jeffrey Savage, MC, USA

Introduction: Infections of the central nervous system are frequently encountered in the pediatric age group and are the most common cause of fever associated with signs of CNS involvement. Viral meningitis is seen most frequently, followed by bacterial meningitis and then fungal and parasitic involvement (the last 2 are rare). Meningitis, especially if bacterial in origin, is associated with a high rate of complications and possible long-term morbidity. However, if detected and treated early, these effects can be minimized. Bacterial meningitis may present acutely with symptoms evolving rapidly over 1-24 hours. However, it is more common for meningitis to be preceded by several days of fever accompanied by upper respiratory infection or gastrointestinal symptoms followed by non-specific signs of CNS involvement such as irritability or lethargy. The bacteria that cause meningitis are different according to the age of the child and dictate the medications used. In the neonate, Group B streptococcus, gram-negative enteric organisms, *Staphylococcus aureus*, *Listeria monocytogenes* and *enterococci* are common. In older infants and children, *Haemophilus influenza* type b, *Streptococcus pneumoniae*, *Neisseria meningitidis* and *Salmonella* species are most common. Two thirds of cases of meningitis are caused by viruses, the most common of which are enteroviruses, mumps, and herpes simplex virus. **Geographic Association:** Although cases of meningitis occur throughout the world, there is an area of Sub-Saharan Africa known as the meningitis belt that runs through several countries to include Ethiopia, Chad, Niger, Nigeria, Burkina Faso, Mali, Guinea, among others. **Seasonal Variation:** Viral meningitis is more commonly seen in the spring and summer months, while bacterial meningitis occurs more often in the fall and winter months. However, either may occur any time of the year. **Risk Factors:** Living in large groups in close quarters (dorm, barracks or large extended family living space); travel or living in areas where meningitis is common (*see geographic association*); close, intimate contact with persons who have meningitis or with individuals in populations where meningitis is relatively common.

Subjective: **Symptoms**

Fever (may be the only sign in an infant), headache, nausea, anorexia/poor feeding, irritability, vomiting generalized malaise, sensitivity to light or sound, neck pain and/or rigidity, seizures, coma, and focal sensory and motor deficits.

Focused History: *Has the child been exposed to family, friends with similar symptoms? Ask about fever in the mother during labor, labs that mother have had during pregnancy* (was she positive for group B streptococcus, Chlamydia, or gonorrhea), *if the infant was ill or needed antibiotics shortly after birth.*

Objective: **Signs**

Using Basic Tools: Vital signs: Fever (may be the only sign in infants); temperature instability and hypothermia; signs of shock like increased pulse and decreased BP. Inspection: Nuchal rigidity (neck stiffness); Kernig's sign: leg or back pain when a supine patient's hip is held in 90° of flexion and the leg is passively extended at the knee. Brudzinski's sign: knee flexion and complaint of back pain when the supine patient's neck is flexed. Kernig's sign and Brudzinski's sign are not present in infants. Signs of shock (eg, mottled skin color, slow capillary refill); increased head circumference in infants/toddlers; cranial nerve palsies. Skin with exanthem, purpura or petechiae Palpation: Infants may have a bulging or tense anterior fontanelle.

Using Advanced Tools: Labs: WBC count, blood culture. Will need lumbar puncture and cerebrospinal fluid (CSF) analysis and culture when at higher level of care.

Assessment:

Differential Diagnosis

Although ideally, definitive diagnosis would be made by evaluation and culture of the CSF in a field setting, diagnosis will have to be made based on clinical suspicion (signs and symptoms). In all of these situations, the child needs to be started on the antibiotics listed in this section and referred for hospitalization if, possible.

Bacterial meningitis: If clinical suspicion, start antibiotics immediately for bacterial meningitis.

Viral meningitis: Difficult to impossible to differentiate without CSF analysis and will most likely require management as for bacterial meningitis.

Sepsis: Difficult to impossible to differentiate from bacterial meningitis clinically as meningeal signs may be absent in bacterial meningitis in infants. History (ie, others with similar symptoms during a known epidemic, eg, cholera) may suggest the cause of sepsis. Will most likely require management as for bacterial meningitis.

Plan:

Treatment

Primary: Start antibiotic therapy if clinical signs and/or symptoms. The diagnostic tests are not necessary prior to beginning treatment. Patients with suspected bacterial meningitis should be referred for hospital admission for the initial 24-48 hours to monitor hemodynamic stability, neurologic status, urine output, and electrolytes. Initial antibiotics based on age of patient and assuming a term infant weighing greater than 2kg: This is a life-threatening illness and IV antibiotic therapy may be required for 14 days or longer.

Neonate (a baby 28 days old or less): Give **ampicillin** and **gentamicin** or **cefotaxime** in the following doses:

Ampicillin:

<7 days old, give 75-150mg/kg/24hr IV/IM divided q8h

>7 days old, give 100-200mg/kg/24 hr IV/IM divided q6h

Gentamicin (assuming >34 weeks gestation)

<7 days old, give 4mg/kg/dose IV/IM q24h

>7 days old, give 4mg/kg/dose IV/IM q12-18h

Cefotaxime

< 7 days old: give 100-150mg/kg/24 hr divided q8h to 12h IV

>7 days old: 150-200mg/kg/24 hr divided q6-8h IV

Infants (1-3 months old): Give **ampicillin** and **cefotaxime** or **ceftriaxone** in the following doses:

Ampicillin 200-400mg/kg/24 hr divided q4-6h IV/IM

Cefotaxime 200mg/kg/24 hr divided 6h IV or IM

Ceftriaxone 100mg/kg/24 hr divided q12h IV or IM

Older Infants and Children: Give **ampicillin** and **ceftriaxone**, then switch to single best antibiotic when culture and sensitivity results are available. Use the same dosing as for infants 1-3 months.

Dexamethasone has been shown in some instances to have a favorable effect on outcome. 0.6mg/kg/24 hr IV divided q6h x 2 days (with or just before the 1st dose of antibiotics)

Alternative: Essentially all infants and young children who have suspected meningitis are started on empiric antibiotic therapy. It is difficult in infants and young children to distinguish viral from bacterial meningitis. If antibiotics are not available, the patient should be referred for treatment, if possible

Empiric: Empiric treatment is with the antibiotics listed previously.

Primitive: Ask how local healthcare providers usually treat meningitis. If in a situation where the medic's assets are limited, utilize the assets available in the local area.

Patient Education

General: Parents need to know that meningitis can be a devastating disease with significant sequelae, most commonly hearing loss.

Activity: no specific limits on activity

Diet: no restrictions on diet

Medications: Because recommended medications are given IV initially, patients are usually in a setting in which they can be closely observed during administration. Allergic reactions can occur with these medications and (among other things) can be manifested by rash (urticaria), itching, breathing difficulties, and swelling of the eyelids, lips, and tongue.

Prevention: Educate parents about the need for contact precautions (hand washing, refraining from drinking or eating from the same cup/plate, avoiding contact with bodily fluids, etc.).

No Improvement/Deterioration: Patients should be referred for hospital admission. Educate parent regarding signs of deterioration to include lethargy, worsening mental status, seizures, continued fever.

Follow-up Actions:

Follow up for neurologic sequelae. There is also a risk of hearing impairment as a result of meningitis.

Chapter 16: Human Nutritional Disorders: Vitamin & Mineral Facts

MAJ Victor Yu, Major, SP, USA (Ret)

Table 5-29. Vitamin/Mineral Functions

Vitamin/Mineral Name	Functions	Tolerable Upper Intake for 19-70yrs	Estimated Average Requirements for 19-50yrs
B1 Thiamine	Helps the body cells change carbohydrates into energy. It is also essential for heart function and healthy nerve cells	ND	1mg/d
B2 Riboflavin	Works with the other B vitamins. It is important for body growth and the production of red blood cells	ND	1.1mg/d
B3 Niacin	A B vitamin that helps to maintain healthy skin and nerves. It is also has cholesterol-lowering effects.	35mg/d	12mg/d
B6 Pyridoxine	Helps form red blood cells and maintain brain function. The more protein a person eats, the more vitamin B6 is needed to help the body use the protein.	100mg/d	1.1mg/d
B12 Cyanocobalamin	Like the other B vitamins, is important for metabolism. It also helps form red blood cells and maintain the central nervous system	ND	2mcg/d
C Ascorbic acid	An antioxidant that promotes healthy teeth and gums. It helps the body absorb iron and maintain healthy tissue. It also promotes wound healing	200mg/d	75mg/d

Table 5-29. Vitamin/Mineral Functions, continued

Vitamin/Mineral Name	Functions	Tolerable Upper Intake for 19-70yrs	Estimated Average Requirements for 19-50yrs
Folate Folic acid	Works with vitamin B12 to help form red blood cells. It is necessary for the production of DNA, which controls tissue growth and cell function. Any woman who is pregnant should be sure to get enough folate. Low levels of folate are linked to birth defects such as spina bifida. Many foods are now fortified with folic acid.	1,000mcg/d	320mcg/d
A Retinoids and Carotenoids	Helps in the formation and maintenance of healthy teeth, bones, soft tissue, mucous membranes, and skin.	3,000mcg/d	625mcg/d
D Calciferol	Also known as the "sunshine vitamin," since it is made by the body after being in the sun. 10-15 minutes of sunshine three times per week is enough to produce the body's requirement of vitamin D. This vitamin promotes the body's absorption of calcium, which is essential for the normal development and maintenance of healthy teeth and bones. It also helps maintain proper blood levels of calcium and phosphorus	50mcg/d	Not Available
E Tocopherol	An antioxidant, it plays a role in the formation of red blood cells and helps the body use vitamin K	1,000mg/d	12mg/d
K Phytonadione	Is necessary for blood to stick together (coagulate). Some studies suggest that it helps promote strong bones in the elderly.	ND	Not Available
Calcium	Essential role in blood clotting, muscle contraction, nerve transmission, and bone and tooth formation	2.5gm/d	Not Available
Chromium	Helps to maintain normal blood glucose levels	ND	Not Available
Copper	Component of enzymes in iron metabolism	10,000mcg/d	Not Available
Fluoride	Inhibits the initiation and progression of dental caries and stimulates new bone formation	10mg/d	Not Available
Iodine	Component of the thyroid hormones; and prevents goiter and cretinism	1,100mcg/d	Not Available
Iron	Component of hemoglobin and numerous enzymes; prevents microcytic hypochromic anemia	45mg/d	Not Available
Magnesium	Cofactor for enzyme systems	350mg/d. This amount represents intake from a pharmacological agent only and does not include intake from food and water.	Not Available
Phosphorus	Maintenance of pH, storage and transfer of energy and nucleotide synthesis. Needed for transfer of nerve impulses. Involved in calcium balance.	4gm/d	580mg/d
Zinc	Component of multiple enzymes and proteins; involved in the regulation of gene expression	40mg/d	9.4mg/d

Table 5-30. Vitamin/Mineral Sources

Vitamin Name	Dietary Sources	Deficiency	Treatment\Dietary Reference Intake (DRI)*
B1 Thiamine	Whole and enriched grains, dried beans, peas, sunflower seeds, pork	Dry beriberi-peripheral neuropathy in legs. Cerebral beriberi-dementia, Wernicke-Korsakoff syndrome. Wet beriberi - heart failure	The usual treatment daily dose for adults is 50-100mg IV or IM x 7 -14 days. Subsequently, a dose of 10mg per day po until the patient is fully recovered. Adjust dosage for children. Improvement should be apparent within 6-24 hours by reduced restlessness; the disappearance of cyanosis, reduction in heart rate, respiratory rate, and cardiac size, and clearing of pulmonary congestion. DRI=1.2mg/day
B2 Riboflavin	Milk, mushrooms, spinach, enriched grains, liver	Inflammation of mouth and tongue, cracks at corners of the mouth	DRI=1.3mg/day
B3 Niacin	Bran, enriched grains, peanuts, mushrooms, tuna, salmon, chicken, beef	Pellagra-thickened skin, swollen tongue, bloody diarrhea, psychosis	Administration of niacin will reverse the neurological symptoms and signs. 10-20mg per day in the presence of adequate amounts of dietary protein is sufficient. DRI=16 mg/day
B6 Pyridoxine	Animal protein foods, sunflower seeds, spinach, broccoli, bananas	Headache, anemia, convulsions, nausea, vomiting, flaky skin, sore tongue	DRI=1.3mg/day
B12 Cyanocobalamin	Animal foods, especially organ meats, oysters, clams. Note: Not found in plants!	Macrocytic anemia, poor nerve function	DRI=2.4mcg/day
C Ascorbic acid	Citrus fruits such as oranges and strawberries; broccoli, greens	Scurvy-bleeding and bruising around hair follicles on the lower legs, splinter hemorrhages, bleeding gums, loose teeth	Infantile scurvy - 50mg of ascorbic acid qid x 1 week then 50mg tid x 1 month, supplemented fruits and vegetables such as orange, strawberry, Brussels sprouts, and broccoli. Adult scurvy - 250mg qid until asymptomatic. Ascorbic acid of 300-500mg per day in divided doses po for several months in chronic scurvy. DRI=90mg/day
Folate Folic Acid	Green leafy vegetables, fortified cereals, organ meats, sunflower seeds, oranges	Diarrhea, poor growth, depression. Megaloblastic anemia which must be differentiated from B12 deficiency	DRI= 400mcg/day
A Retinoids and Carotenoids	Fortified milk, fortified breakfast cereals. Yellow-orange pigmented fruit such as cantaloupe and papaya; sweet potatoes and carrots. Dark leafy vegetables (spinach, broccoli, etc.). Organ meats such as liver.	Night blindness, xerophthalmia, poor growth, dry skin	Oleovitamin A, 15-25 thousand units once or twice a day po. If absorption defect is present, give same dosage IM. Be aware that the minimum toxic dose in adults is about 75-100 thousand units daily. DRI=900mcg/day
D Calciferol	Fortified milk, fish oils, sardines and salmon. Note: Most people get vitamin D from exposure to sunlight.	Rickets (children)-bowed bones, painful walking, tetany; Osteomalacia (adults)-bowed bones, fractures	Treatment can only protect against further deformities. Diet high in calcium and phosphorus, 25-100 thousand units vitamin D daily. Treat contributing disease if present. DRI=5mcg/day

Table 5-30. Vitamin/Mineral Sources, continued

Vitamin Name	Dietary Sources	Deficiency	Treatment\Dietary Reference Intake (DRI)*
E Tocopherol	Vegetable oils, margarine, green vegetables, nuts, wheat germ and whole grains	Hemolysis of red blood cells, nerve destruction	DRI= 15mg/day of tocopherol equivalents
K Phytonadione	Liver, green leafy vegetables, GI flora can produce from diet	Hemorrhage, bruising	RDA is 60-80micrograms
Calcium	Milk and dairy products, canned fish such as sardine, tofu	High risk for osteoporosis	DRI=1000mg/day
Chromium	Egg yolks, whole grains, pork, nuts, mushrooms	Peripheral neuropathy	DRI=35mcg/day
Copper	Organ meats, whole grains, beans, nuts	Anemia, low white blood cell count, poor growth	DRI=900mcg/day
Fluoride	Seaweed, tea, toothpaste, fluoridated water	Increased risk of dental caries	DRI=4mg/day
Iodine	Iodized salt, saltwater fish and shellfish	Goiter; poor growth in infancy when mother is iodine deficient during pregnancy	Iodine therapy 5 drops daily saturated solution of potassium iodine or 5-10 drops of a strong iodine solution in a glass of water. Continue until gland returns to normal size, then place patient on maintenance dose 1-2 drops daily or use iodized table salt. Encourage local government to iodize salt. DRI=150mcg/day
Iron	Red meats, seafood, broccoli, bran enriched products. Note: Plant foods are not good sources of iron!	Low blood iron; small, pale red blood cells; low blood hemoglobin values	DRI is 8mg for men and 18mg for women
Magnesium	Wheat bran, nuts, legumes, green vegetables	Weakness, muscle pain, poor heart function	DRI=400mg/day
Phosphorus	Dairy products, meats, poultry, fish	Possibly poor bone maintenance	DRI=700mg/day
Zinc	Seafood, meats, greens, whole grains	Skin rash, diarrhea, decreased appetite and sense of taste, hair loss, poor growth and development, poor wound healing	DRI=11mg/day

*DRI: Dietary Reference Intake. Values given here are for males 19-30 years old.

Chapter 17: Toxicology: Introduction to General Poisoning
COL Clifford Cloonan, MC, USA (Ret)

Introduction: Almost anything in sufficient quantity can be toxic, even substances that are essential to life such as water and oxygen. A poison is any substance that even in small quantities produces harmful physiologic or psychological effects. Poisonings are responsible for 10% of all emergency department visits, 9% of all ambulance patient transports, and 5-10% of all medical admissions to hospitals. They are the 3rd leading cause of accidental death in the US. **Risk Factors:** Approximately 80% of all accidental poisonings occur in children ages 1-4, who typically ingest household products. Few of these incidents are fatal. Adolescents and young adults are at highest risk for intentional poisonings (drug abuse/suicide). The majority of poisoning deaths occurs in individuals age 20-49, and are usually intentional. **Geographic**

Associations: Local health care providers can describe what toxins/drugs are commonly used in a specific culture for the purpose of committing suicide and to achieve altered mental status. Poisons enter the body through a variety of different routes - ingestion, inhalation, injection, and surface or dermal absorption. The toxic effects of ingested poisons may be immediate when inhaled or injected, or delayed when absorbed through the skin or ingested. Because most substances are absorbed through the small intestine, it may take several hours for the poison to enter the bloodstream. Alcohol, which is absorbed in the stomach, is a notable exception. Early management of ingested poisons focuses on removing the toxin from the stomach and chemically binding the toxin to prevent absorption in the small intestine. Alterations in mental status are common in poisonings, but there are many other causes of altered mental status that should ALWAYS be considered. In particular, do NOT assume that altered mental status is due to alcohol or drug intoxication even when the patient has clearly been drinking. Use the mnemonic AEIOUTIPS to recall other causes of altered mental status: A - Alcohol and other toxins/drugs, E - Endocrine (hypothyroidism); I - Insulin, too much (hypoglycemia), or Insulin, too little (hyperglycemia); O - Opiates (heroin, morphine, etc.) and Oxygen, too little (hypoxia); U - Uremia (kidney failure); T - Trauma (head injury, shock)/Temperature (hyper/hypothermia); I - Infection (meningitis, encephalitis); P - Psychiatric (pseudocoma); S - Space-occupying lesion (epidural/subdural hematoma), Stroke, Subarachnoid hemorrhage, Shock. When treating a poisoned/intoxicated patient, the medic should protect himself. If the patient has been poisoned by a hazardous material, this substance may also pose a risk to the medic. Patients who are intoxicated may behave irrationally or violently.

Table 5-31. Symptoms of Poisoning: Acute, Sub-acute and Chronic

	Acute (<2 hrs)	Sub-acute (2-48 hrs)	Chronic (>48 hrs)
Constitutional	Nausea/vomiting are common	Signs/symptoms of organ failure	Death or recovery+/- symptoms of chronic organ system damage

Location: Three organ systems are most likely to produce immediate morbidity and mortality:

	Acute (<2 hrs)	Sub-acute (2-48 hrs)	Chronic (>48 hrs)
Respiratory	Difficulty breathing, shortness of breath	Shortness of breath on exertion	Recovery or chronic shortness of breath, chronic cough, etc...
Cardiovascular	Fainting/near fainting, palpitations, chest pain	Postural hypotension, shortness of breath on exertion	Recovery or symptoms of CHF
CNS	Hallucinations, difficulty concentrating, headaches, visual disturbances	Numbness/tingling/painful sensations, visual disturbances	Recovery or symptoms of learning disabilities, chronic pain, long term visual disturbances

Subjective: Symptoms

Focused History: An accurate history is the most important component of the workup. If poisoning was a suicide attempt or involved the use of illicit drugs, history from patient is often inaccurate or intentionally misleading. Obtain history from friends/family members and obtain description of the scene from persons who initially found the patient. Determine which drugs (legal and illicit) or toxins to which the patient may have had access. In the event of ingestion, determine what was ingested, when it was ingested, and whether the patient vomited. *Has the patient been depressed? Is there a prior history of suicide attempts and/or psychiatric therapy? Was a suicide note written?* (If patient is awake/responsive, inquire as to whether the patient is suicidal and whether patient has taken any substance for the purpose of harming or killing him/herself. Positive answers significantly increase the likelihood that patient's current state is the result of a suicide attempt.) *If so, what was taken and when? What medications is the patient taking and what medications are available in the house? Are there any empty pill bottles, spilled pills, and/or empty/open containers of poisonous substances near the patient or out of normal location? If yes, how much of the substance or pills are missing?* (Knowledge of what was taken and in what quantities will dictate treatment based upon drug/substance category.) *Does the patient have a history of drug and/or alcohol abuse? If so, what drugs do they typically abuse?* (History of drug abuse increases likelihood that current state is the result of drug abuse overdose and knowledge of common drug(s) of abuse can be used to tailor management.) *What is the patient's occupation and/or hobbies and are toxic chemicals/ substances used, if so, which ones?* (Exposure to toxic substances may occur in the course of work/hobbies. Information about these substances can often be obtained from the manufacturer's Material Safety Data Sheet that comes with/on potentially toxic/hazardous materials. This is an important source of information about properties and hazards of chemicals.)

Objective: Signs

Focus of the initial physical examination should be on ruling out life/limb/sight threatening conditions. In poisonings these involve the respiratory, cardiovascular, and central nervous systems.

Using Basic Tools: Inspection: Should reveal spontaneous conversation, gait, posture, general appearance, affect (depressed, agitated, happy) and appearance of the skin (needle track marks or other evidence of drug use, evidence of trauma, discoloration). Vital signs can indicate type and severity of systemic effects. Monitor cardiac function. Perform a basic neuro examination with a focus on mental status (assess for agitation, mania, depression, etc., as well as basic orientation) and eyes (pupil size, equality, and reactivity, nystagmus, visual acuity, and extraocular muscles). Observe gait if possible and perform tests of cerebellar function (ie, finger-to-nose, rapidly alternating hand movements, heel-to-shin, Romberg). Pulse oximetry (**Warning:** Pulse oximetry may be normal in carbon monoxide poisoning, cyanide poisoning initially, methemoglobinemia, and other conditions causing inadequate oxygenation of the tissues). The presence of a normal pulse oximetry reading does not always indicate adequate oxygenation.

Table 5-32. Signs of Acute, Sub-acute and Chronic Poisoning

Signs	Acute (<2 hrs)	Sub-acute (2-48 hrs)	Chronic (>48 hrs)
Respiratory	Dyspnea, wheezing, stridor, apnea, hypo/hyperventilation	Shortness of breath on exertion	Recovery or COPD, restrictive lung disease, emphysema, etc.
Cardiovascular	Hypo/hypertension, tachy/ bradyarrhythmias	Signs of ischemia/infarction, postural hypotension, early CHF	Recovery or signs of chronic CV disease, ie, CHF, cardiomyopathy, recurrent tachy/bradyarrhythmias
CNS	Stroke, seizures, altered mental status to include coma, agitation/ somnolence/depression	Paralysis, seizures, persistent altered mental status	Recovery or persisting paralysis, recurrent seizures, mental retardation, persistent vegetative state

Using Advanced Tools: ECG (arrhythmias). Labs: Urinalysis, blood glucose. Drug testing is generally not available in field environments.

Assessment:
Differential Diagnosis: *See AEIOU-TIPS discussion in Introduction.*

Plan:
   Treatment
   1. Secure airway. If patient is hypoxic and/or hypoventilating, apply oxygen and assist respirations.
   2. Start an IV in all presumed poisoned patients for drug access. Fluid resuscitate as needed to support blood pressure.
   3. Treat arrhythmias per ACLS.
   4. Decontamination procedures: Decontaminate skin and mucous membranes as required with mild soap and water. Remove patient from any further exposure to toxic vapors/fumes. Gastric lavage, and/or **activated charcoal** to minimize toxins in the GI tract, consider costs/benefits of **syrup of ipecac** (if within 20 minutes of ingestion).
   Note: Inducing diarrhea is NOT effective and is likely to make the patient worse (dehydration, fluid/electrolyte imbalance). Currently the use of any treatment other than activated charcoal for decontamination is discouraged except when the substance ingested is known and there is a specific antidote or decontaminant. In general, conservative treatment is recommended over aggressive intervention. The routine use of syrup of ipecac or gastric lavage is inappropriate as the risks, although small, usually outweigh any potential benefits.
   Gastric lavage: may provide opportunity for immediate recovery of a portion of gastric contents.
      1. Administration:
         a. Use large-bore orogastric tube rather than a smaller nasogastric tube (Size 36-40 French for adults, size 24-28 French for children).
         b. Never insert large orogastric tubes nasally (may fracture/amputate nasal turbinate and/or cause serious bleeding).
      2. Complications: Agitation, tracheal intubation, esophageal perforation, aspiration pneumonitis, pediatric fluid and electrolyte imbalances.
      3. Contraindications: Altered levels of consciousness (relative contraindication if the airway is protected), low-viscosity hydrocarbons or caustic agent ingestion.
   Activated charcoal
      1. Administration
         a. Administering 20-30 minutes before gastric lavage may double the effectiveness of lavage.
         b. Do not administer until after vomiting, if ipecac has already been given.
         c. Form slurry of 1-2g/kg body weight (30-100g for adults, 15-30g for children), and administered orally or by gastric tube.
      2. Indication/Contradictions:
         a. Safe and effective treatment in most toxic ingestion
         b. Do not use for strong acid, strong alkali.
         c. Not effective for cyanide, iron or alcohol
   Syrup of ipecac: The routine use of **syrup of ipecac** is no longer recommended because in most cases the risks outweigh the benefits.
      1. Administration:
         a. In patients 1-12 years old, give 15mL followed by 2-3 glasses of water.
         b. In patients over 12 years, give 30mL followed by 2-3 glasses of water.
         c. May be repeated in 20 minutes if vomiting does not occur.
      2. Contraindications: Patient <1 year old, altered level of consciousness (aspiration), ingestion of caustic substances, loss of gag reflex, seizures, pregnancy, acute myocardial infarction, ingestion of: acids, alkalis, ammonia, petroleum distillates, non-toxic agents, rapidly acting central nervous system agents, or hydrocarbons.
      Complications: Mallory-Weiss tear of the esophagus, causing bleeding; pneumomediastinum (air trapped in chest cavity outside the lungs); diaphragmatic or gastric rupture; and/or aspiration pneumonitis. Effective in some cases if administered within 20 minutes of ingestion.

Patient Education

Prevention and Hygiene: In cases of toddler poisonings, educate mother/father regarding "poison proofing" of home. Remove all cleaning products and other toxins from children's reach; apply locks to cabinet doors, etc.

Follow-up Actions

Evacuation/Consultation Criteria: Evacuate if patient unstable. If there is any question as to the severity of the poisoning or whether the patient may have been committing an act of self-harm, consult emergency medicine/toxicology if patient unstable or serious poisoning suspected, and psychiatry if poisoning is felt to have been an act of self-harm.

Chapter 17: Toxicology: Carbon Monoxide Poisoning

LCDR Robert J. Lueken, MC, USN

Introduction: Carbon monoxide (CO) poisoning is one of the most common causes of death from poisoning worldwide. A colorless, odorless, toxic gas, CO is found in the smoke or fumes from fire, camping stoves, portable heaters, automobiles or other internal combustion engines that burn carbon-containing fuels. Depending on the level of CO in the air and the amount of exposure time, signs and symptoms of CO poisoning may develop within minutes to days. Diving gas may become contaminated with CO and can result in severe poisoning at increased partial pressures (ie, depth of dive), even with brief exposures. There are more than 15,000 cases of CO poisoning seen in emergency departments throughout the US each year and although most cases are non-fatal, it is thought that many cases go unrecognized because the symptoms can be the same as an upper respiratory infection (URI) or flu-like illness. Breathing CO results in the formation of carboxyhemoglobin (COHb), which causes a relative hypoxemia. Compared to oxygen, CO is much more readily absorbed by hemoglobin (Hgb) and the half-life of CO in the blood is approximately 5 hours with normal breathing. When a victim is removed from exposure to high levels of CO, elevated blood levels of CO will normalize after about a day. Symptoms may still be present once CO levels are normal because of cellular damage, caused by CO, through complex chemical reactions. The poisoning effects of CO on brain, cardiac and skeletal muscles can be seen in individuals with blood levels as low as 5% COHb and can result from prolonged exposure to low levels or acute exposure to high levels of CO. Serious symptoms are more often seen with COHb levels of 10% or higher; however, levels do not necessarily correlate with the severity of symptoms. **Geographic Associations:** Carbon monoxide poisoning is predominantly seen in the developing regions of the world because of poor education and the lack of primary prevention (CO detectors, clean burning fuels, adequate ventilation). **Seasonal Variation:** Warm weather exposures such as those seen following Hurricane Katrina, with dozens of cases attributed to indoor generator use, must be considered following natural disasters. Most CO poisoning is seen in the cold or winter months due to (1) malfunctioning heaters using gasoline, kerosene or propane; (2) inadequate ventilation (furnaces, fireplaces, firefighting); (3) automobile exhaust (intentional or accidental). **Risk Factors:** Coronary disease (greater risk of myocardial ischemia due to hypoxemia); neonates (fetal COHb has a longer half-life than adult COHb); smokers (baseline levels as high as 7-10% COHb); vehicle occupant (exhaust exposure results in inhaled fumes while idling or during transit); occupational exposure (eg, smoke or paint thinner fumes); intentional (inhalation of exhaust or methylene chloride fumes known as "huffing"). Although pregnancy is protective to the mother (because fetal hemoglobin has a greater affinity than adult hemoglobin for CO), the fetus has an increased risk of poisoning. CO levels in the fetus are 10-15% higher than in the mother and remain elevated longer because the half-life of COHb in the fetus is 7-9 hours. CO at levels that do not cause significant effects to the mother still may adversely affect the fetus and have been associated with an increased risk of premature labor in the 3rd trimester of pregnancy.

Subjective: **Symptoms**

Headache, dizziness, nausea & vomiting, change in mental status (from confusion to coma and death), decreased coordination, weakness. **Focused History:** *Is anyone else sick?* (Bad diving mixtures can affect dive-buddy or all divers suddenly. Entire households, classrooms or a busload of children may be exposed and may have variable symptoms.) *What were you doing before and at the time symptoms began?* (Onset may be minutes to days following exposure.) *Did anything reduce the symptoms or cause them to resolve?* (Removal from the source usually decreases symptoms over time; half-life of CO is approximately 5 hours on room air.) *Have you had these symptoms before?* (Repeated exposure to the same environment with symptoms that subsequently improve may be an indicator of a specific environmental exposure.) *Are animals sick or dying?* (Animals may become sick or die before humans are affected.) *Did you notice a bad taste while diving compressed gas/air?* (Bad tasting gas or diving mix suggests contaminated supply.) *Do you recall odor of smoke or fumes?* (Although CO is odorless, the odor of fumes or smoke may provide clues.)

Objective: **Signs**

Using Basic Tools: Signs that would be expected in hypoxia from any other cause. Early: Abnormal vital signs (tachycardia [pulse may vary, but hypoxemia usually results in fast heart rate], tachypnea). Altered mental status: Disorientation to person, place, time or situation; confusion or difficulty with concentration. Late: Cherry-red skin is a late finding and usually associated with death. Palpation: Neuro exam with frequent reassessment to define neuro deficit and monitor recovery. Non-reproducible headache: Bilateral frontal headache that is not made worse with palpation. Blood: May appear like an arterial sample on initial draw. Pulse oximetry will be normal because COHb absorbs light almost identical to OHb.

Using Advanced Tools: ECG: May show ST segment depression or T-wave inversion suggesting hypoxia leading to myocardial ischemia. Cardiac dysrhythmias related to myocardial irritation from hypoxia, ischemia or infarction.

Assessment

History (risk of exposure) and symptoms (headache, nausea, mild confusion) should prompt early treatment. More serious signs and symptoms, such as skin changes, focal neurologic deficits, altered mental status, hypoxia and coma, should prompt early evaluation for other serious life threats such as:

Differential Diagnosis

Altitude illness: HAPE, HACE (if above ~10,000 ft) *See Part 6: Operational Environment: Chapter 22: High Altitude Cerebral Edema & High Altitude Pulmonary Edema*

Decompression illness: Arterial gas embolism (if diving or flying). *See Part 6: Operational Environment: Chapter 20: Decompression Injuries: Pulmonary Over Inflation Syndrome (including Arterial Gas Embolism) & Chapter 21: Decompression Sickness*

Other medical causes:

A: **Alcohol:** History or suspicious smell of ETOH.

E: **Electrolytes, Exposure:** Abnormal i-STAT or hyperthermia, hypothermia.

I: **Insulin:** Obtain finger-stick glucose reading looking for hyperglycemia or hypoglycemia.

O: **Oxygen:** Ensure adequate $SaO_2\%$; evaluate for stroke or myocardial infarction

U: **Uremia:** Check kidney function with I-STAT & urinalysis

T: **Trauma, Toxins:** Ensure no head trauma, drugs, overdoses, poisons such as CN.

I: **Infection:** Bacteria, viruses, protozoan, rickettsia, prions

P: **Psychiatric:** History of psychosis, delirium or dementia.

S: **Sepsis:** Look for fever, tachycardia, elevated WBC count

Plan:

Treatment

Permanent disabling neurologic damage may be prevented if appropriate treatment is performed early in the illness.

1. Remove patient from the source
2. Oxygen 15L/min by non-rebreather mask, tight fitting aviator mask or endotracheal intubation. Half-life of COHb is reduced from approximately 5 hours to 1½ hours. Partial hyperbaric treatment using Gamow bag if available may be useful
   Advanced: If high suspicion for CO poisoning with significant neurological deficits, carboxyhemoglobin of 20%.
   Hyperbaric Oxygen: Treatment Table 5 or 6 (*see Part 6: Operational Environment: Chapter 20: Dive Treatment Table 5 Depth/Time Profile; Dive Treatment Table 6 Depth/Time Profile & Dive Treatment Table 6A Depth/Time Profile*) (Half-life of COHb reduced from 5 hours to 23 minutes, normalizes cell chemistry)
   Note: Half-life of fetal COHb is longer and fetus is still at risk long after levels normalize in the mother. In the 2nd or 3rd trimesters; current recommendations are to treat women with symptomatic exposure to CO or measured levels of COHb >20% with early administration of normal oxygen and hyperbaric oxygen. Hyperbaric treatment is thought to provide earlier reduction of CO levels in the fetus and may prevent adverse outcomes in the fetus that would result from untreated exposure.
3. IV or po fluids as clinically indicated to maintain adequate hydration.
4. Give **acetaminophen** 500mg po q4-6h and **oxymetazoline** nasal spray one puff q12h as needed for relief of headache discomfort /nasal congestion.

Empiric: Removal from the source and administer the antidote: Oxygen

Primitive: Medical oxygen may be replaced by diving oxygen.

Patient Education

General: If treated remotely, patient needs to be reevaluated by physicians on return home to determine if additional treatment needs to be administered. Subsequent hyperbaric treatments may be beneficial.

Activity: As condition permits.

Diet: As condition permits, based on neurologic status

Prevention and Hygiene: Determine original contamination source, prevent further exposure to the victim and others exposed to similar threat.

No Improvement/Deterioration: If persistent or worsening symptoms, patient should seek medical attention ASAP to be evaluated for worsening illness or other possible conditions.

Follow-up Actions

Return Evaluation: ASAP evaluation by physician/DMO/Flight Surgeon on return to base/home

Evacuation/Consultation Criteria: Early consultation with a Diving/Hyperbaric Medical Officer or Flight Surgeon to facilitate transfer for hyperbaric oxygen therapy.

Note: Locate the nearest hyperbaric oxygen chamber. 24 hour on-call experts available: Divers Alert Network (DAN) at Duke University at 919-684-8111 or collect: 919-684-4DAN.

Chapter 17: Toxicology: Venomous Snake Bites
COL Warner Anderson, MC, USA

Introduction: Venomous snakes cause injuries and deaths in all temperate and tropical climates. They are a particular problem in Australia, which has 40% of the world's neurotoxic snakes and about 23% of all venomous snakes. In North America, poisonous snakes cause 14-20 deaths/year. The risk of death is greatest in the very young, very old, those with cardiovascular and respiratory problems, and multiple bites. Only about 1/5 of snakebites in the US are by venomous snakes and not all these bites result in envenomation. Rattlesnakes do not inject venom in 20% of bites. The typical victim of a pit viper is a young male 11-19 years old, bitten on the hand while trying to handle the snake. Alcohol use is often a factor. Because snakes are less active during winter, the peak snakebite season in temperate climates is April-October. In the US, the majority of poisonous snake bites are by pit vipers (*Crotalidae*), specifically rattlesnakes, copperheads and cottonmouth snakes. Eastern and western diamondback rattlesnakes, although causing only about 10% of all snake bites in the U.S., are responsible for 95% of all snakebite deaths in the US. The other poisonous species of snakes in North America (not pit vipers) are the Eastern and Texas coral snakes. They are members of the *Elapidae* family, along with cobras, kraits, and mambas. Sea snakes belong to the *Hydrophidae* family.

Subjective: **Symptoms**

Variable depending on type of snake, amount of venom injected, age of victim and other factors.

Table 5-33. Snake Bite: Acute, Sub-acute and Chronic Symptoms

	Acute (2 hrs)	Sub-acute (2-48 hrs)	Chronic (>48 hrs)
Constitutional	*Crotalidae*: Rapid onset of severe pain at bite site, severe HA, marked thirst. *Elapidae/ Hydrophidae*: Little/no immediate pain at bite site	*Crotalidae*: Persistent severe pain, HA, thirst, dizziness, chills, nausea. *Elapidae*: Excessive perspiration *Hydrophidae*: Muscle aches/pains/ stiffness and pain on passive movement of arm, thigh, neck, trunk muscles	Either improving, or organ system failure (renal, respiratory, cardiovascular), disseminated hemorrhage, pruritus, fever, myalgia, arthritis suggests serum sickness secondary to antivenin admin.
Respiratory	If anaphylaxis: Difficulty breathing, shortness of breath. *Elapidae/Hydrophidae*: Severe envenomation may cause respiratory paralysis/arrest	Onset of anaphylaxis may be delayed >2 hr. so consider if SOB/ bronchospasm occur. *Elapidae/ Hydrophidae*: Respiratory paralysis/arrest possible	*Elapidae/Hydrophidae*: Respiratory paralysis may be prolonged (up to 7 days)
Cardiovascular	If anaphylaxis: Fainting/near-fainting, shock symptoms, severe envenomation may cause arrest	Palpitations, shock symptoms	Usually no long term effects
GI	Nausea/Vomiting	Nausea/Vomiting	Usually no long term effects
Neuro	*Elapidae/Hydrophidae*: Blurred vision	*Elapidae/Hydrophidae*: Paresthesias (numbness of lips/ soles of feet)	*Elapidae/Hydrophidae*: Recovery or possible long-term numbness, burning/ tingling sensation

Focused History: *Can you identify the snake?* (give appropriate antivenin) *When was your last tetanus immunization? Do you have allergies to horses/horse serum?* (check before giving serum derived from horses)

Objective: Signs
Rapid onset suggests a more severe envenomation.
Using Basic Tools:

Table 5-34. Snake Bite: Acute, Sub-acute and Chronic Signs

	Acute (2 hrs)	Sub-acute (2-48 hrs)	Chronic (>48 hrs)
Respiratory	If anaphylaxis: Bronchospasm/ respiratory arrest *Elapidae/ Hydrophidae*: May produce early respiratory paralysis/arrest but usually delayed	*Elapidae/Hydrophidae*: Respiratory paralysis/arrest, death	*Elapidae/Hydrophidae*: Respiratory paralysis/arrest can last up to a week. Death, if it occurs, tends to occur early
Cardiovascular	Anaphylaxis may cause hypotension/shock. *Crotalidae*: Diffuse bleeding, hypotension, shock. *Elapidae*: Arrhythmias, cardiac arrest	Hypotension, shock, diffuse ecchymosis	Usually no long term complications
GI	All: Vomiting	*Elapidae/Hydrophidae*: Diarrhea	Usually no long term complications
Neuro	*Elapidae/Hydrophidae*: Difficulty focusing; paralysis of eye muscles, eyelids; difficulty opening mouth, speaking, swallowing, paralysis of the jaw and tongue	*Elapidae/Hydrophidae*: Muscular incoordination, twitching, muscle paralysis(include respiratory muscles); altered mental status, coma	Range of motion, weakness, numbness, burning/tingling sensation
Renal	Usually no early renal problems	*Crotalidae*: Gross hematuria. *Hydrophidae*: Reddish-brown urine	*Crotalidae*: Renal failure or recovery
Soft Tissue	*Crotalidae*: Usually two fang punctures at site of bite, rapid onset of swelling	*Crotalidae*: Significant swelling, tissue necrosis, petechiae, ecchymosis, bullae–local & possibly diffuse	*Crotalidae*: Usually no long term morbidity, but compartment syndrome, tissue necrosis, ROM may occur

Using Advanced Tools: Labs: Hematocrit, PT/PTT, urinalysis and 12-lead ECG to assess renal and cardiac complications. Blood transfusion: type and crossmatch as required.

Assessment

Differential Diagnosis: Non-venomous snake bite; venomous bite from animal other than a snake; other sources of intoxication.

Plan:

Treatment

Rapid transport to hospital-level care, delay progress of envenomation and alleviate early symptoms.

Primary:

1. Ensure airway is patent and adequate – if not, secure airway. If hypoxic and/or hypoventilating, apply O$_2$ and assist respirations, prevent aspiration (lay the patient on side), intubate or LMA as required.
2. Start an IV in an unbitten extremity in all snake bite patients. Fluid resuscitation to support blood pressure and maintain urine output. Water or oral rehydration solutions may be given as tolerated but otherwise keep patient NPO. No alcohol! Be prepared for shock.
3. Monitor vital signs with pulse oximetry and cardiac monitoring if available. Treat arrhythmias per ACLS guidelines.
   Note: Muscle breakdown may release significant potassium, so consider hyperkalemia if arrhythmias occur.
4. Limit the systemic spread of the venom using these methods:
   a. Keep the patient as calm and inactive as possible. Reassure. Give **benzodiazepine** (eg, **diazepam** 5mg po) as needed and manage pain.
   b. Gently clean around the bite site to remove any venom from the skin, and for general wound care.
   c. Immobilize the bitten limb in a dependant position.
   d. Suctioning the bite site (not with mouth) within minutes after bite is reasonable if remote from hospital care. Do not incise over the puncture site. The use of suction is controversial but all agree: never use the mouth to apply suction.
   e. Do not apply tourniquets, ligatures, or constricting bands unless the snake is primarily neurotoxic (Australian elapid, sea snake, krait, cobra or other neurotoxic species). Neurotoxic bites only: apply a constricting band approximately 1 in. wide 2-4 inches above the bite and loose enough to admit a finger. Alternatively, wrap the bitten extremity with an elastic bandage or place it in an air splint for compression. Monitor distal pulses. Another method: Place a thick pad over the area of the bite and hold it in place with a tight wrap, wrapping from distal to proximal. If more than 30 minutes after the bite, do not apply a constricting band. Do NOT treat pit viper bites with these methods. Always check for a pulse after applying – this is not a tourniquet!
   f. Measure the circumference of a bitten extremity 10cm proximal to the bite. Track this measurement and pulses over time.
5. Remove all jewelry from bitten extremity.
6. Consider Foley catheter; record urine output and monitor fluid balance. Check urine for myoglobin (positive for blood on urine dipstick but no RBCs on microscopic exam) and blood. Avoid overhydration (rales, wheezing, orthopnea, respiratory distress, and distended jugular veins). Cautiously hydrate to maintain urine output >30-50cc/hr (adults). Give adult victims with myoglobinuria and decreased urine output 25g of **mannitol** and 100mEq (generally two ampules) **sodium bicarbonate** added to 1L 5% dextrose and infused over 4 hours to prevent myoglobinuric nephropathy.
7. Treat pain with **acetaminophen** 500–1000mg po q4 -6h (not to exceed 4g/day) and opiates as required. *See Part 8: Procedures: Chapter 30: Pain Assessment and Control.* Avoid NSAIDs, which interfere with platelet function
8. Treat nausea/vomiting with **prochlorperazine** 10mg (give slowly if administering by IV - this can cause/worsen hypotension).
9. Give tetanus toxoid.
10. Do not cauterize, incise, or amputate the bite site. Do not apply electric shock or pack bitten limb in ice. These "remedies" are urban legends.
11. If the snake can be safely killed, bring in for identification (*see Figure 5-39*). Avoid handling the snake. Be sure it is dead. **Warning:** dead snakes reflexively bite!
12. Give antivenin, which is the only proven therapy for snakebite, only if it is specific for the snake involved (monovalent), or if the envenomation is severe (polyvalent). See (and follow) package insert for antivenin-specific instructions. The administration of any type of antivenin has a risk of allergic reaction and serum sickness that can be life-threatening. Do not administer antivenin unless the specific criteria for administration are met. Remember: death from snakebite is rare and snake bite without envenomation is common. Inappropriate administration of antivenin can kill a patient who would otherwise have survived without permanent sequelae. In the US even when the offending snake is venomous, and envenomation has occurred (eg copperhead), antivenin administration is often not necessary.
13. Be prepared to treat anaphylaxis after giving antivenin with **epinephrine** 0.3cc 1:1000 IM and **diphenhydramine** 50mg IM. If patient rapidly becomes hypotensive and/or develops acute severe respiratory distress, it may necessary to give 1mg (10cc) 1:10000 **epinephrine** slowly by IV. May also give H2 blocker such as **cimetidine**, and corticosteroid such as **methylprednisolone**.

Notes:

1. Snake bites on the extremities can produce extensive swelling that may (but rarely does) lead to the development of a compartment syndrome (pain on passive stretching and active flexing of the involved muscle groups, distal paresthesias, pulselessness, tense overlying tissues). Doing a fasciotomy in a patient with a venom-induced bleeding disorder and local tissue necrosis may cause significant, even life-threatening, bleeding and/or infection. An aggressive surgical approach is more likely to cause harm than good, so delay fasciotomy (*see Part 8: Procedures: Chapter 30: Compartment Syndrome*) as long as feasible.
2. Early, prophylactic, broad-spectrum antibiotic therapy with **ceftriaxone** 1g IV or IM for one dose is reasonable but not generally recommended. Treat infection, if it develops as appropriate.

Note: Redness, swelling, pain, and increased warmth in the surrounding tissue occur in both envenomation and infection. Infection will be a late event.

Alternate: Support the airway, maintain adequate oxygen, ventilation, urine output and blood pressure until specific, neutralizing, antivenin can be administered. There is no good evidence for any first aid measures aside from those described previously.

Primitive: Maintaining airway and urine output will save most patients. An overly aggressive surgical approach and resorting to unproven therapies will cause more harm than good.

Empiric: In the proper circumstances, assume snake bite with envenomation and observe patient for 4-6 hours for development of signs/symptoms. If no signs/symptoms after 6 hours, consider bite w/o envenomation.

Patient Education

General: Do not handle snakes, especially after drinking alcohol. However, you can eat them after they are beheaded, skinned, gutted, washed and well-cooked.

Activity: Limit activity after bite. May return to activity as tolerated after resolution of symptoms.

Diet: Initially, NPO except for water. Regular diet as tolerated later.

Wound Care: Cleanse wound gently, remove any venom that may be present on the skin. Débride wound in 48-72 hrs if indicated – avoid early, excessive debridement. Watch for infection, which is difficult to distinguish from envenomation in the early stages.

No Improvement/Deterioration: Return for reassessment for cold or pulseless limb, changes in mental status, or development of blood in urine and/or decreasing urinary output.

Follow-up Actions

Return Evaluation: If antivenin has already been given, give more. Administering an inadequate amount of antivenin is a common mistake. Watch closely for sudden anaphylactic shock.

Evacuation/Consultation Criteria: Evacuate snakebite victims for intensive care if possible. Consult with emergency medicine physician if available.

Notes:

Snake identification:

Pit vipers: "pit" located below each nostril; triangular-shaped head; elliptical, not round, pupils; hollow fangs; single, not double row of scales on the ventral (belly) side distal to the anal plate; rattlesnakes usually have a rattle.

Coral snakes in US: Encircling colored bands of black, red and yellow/white, with the latter bands touching ("red on yellow, kill a fellow; red on black, venom lack"); no long fangs; small mouth makes it difficult for them to bite anything larger than finger.

Figure 5-39. General Characteristics of Venomous and Non-venomous Snakes

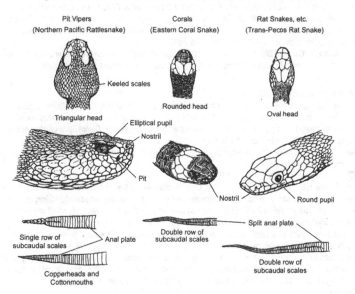

Chapter 18: Mental Health: Operational Stress

LTC Michael Doyle, MC, USA

Introduction: In a deployed/operational setting, service members who present for evaluation of emotional or psychological symptoms (or are brought in by the chain of command) do so because of an impairment in duty performance, concerns for safety, or both. Always think SAFETY. Have the chain-of-command secure the Service Member's weapon and send the service member with an escort if there is any concern for safety. Most service members presenting with signs and symptoms of an emotional or psychological disturbance do not have a mental disorder, but rather, are struggling with the stress of military operations and combat (by definition outside of normal experience).

Battle fatigue (BF) is a condition of service members who are expressing a normal response to the abnormal stress of combat who are functionally impaired to the extent that they require specific medical evaluation and disposition. **Combat and Operational Stress Reaction** is the term applied to service members who present psychologically or emotionally disturbed in non-combat situations. **Combat**

Neuropsychiatric (NP) Triage, as defined in FM 8-15, is the process used to identify the small number of patients with actual mental disorders from the larger number of patients with battle fatigue. NP Triage sorts cases based on where they can be best treated: **Duty:** returned to duty (RTD); **Rest:** provided rest, replenishment, restoration and reassurance in a location safer than the small unit; **Hold:** held for further observation; or **Refer:** referred to a higher echelon of care. This classification guides treatment planning depending on the tactical situation as well as the severity of symptoms. Combat Stress Control in a Theater of Operations includes the management of BF, NP and substance abuse cases (including those with physical injury) based on how far forward they can be managed and treated to maximize rapid RTD.

Subjective: Symptoms

Anxiety, nervousness, fear, panic, terror, sadness, guilt, depression, anger, insomnia, hallucinations, delusions, hyper-alertness, agitation, inattention, carelessness, erratic actions, outbursts, or physical exhaustion, immobility, panic running, loss of skills, or loss of memory; loss of confidence, hope, or faith; somatic complaints: muteness, blindness, deafness, paralysis or weakness; thoughts of hurting oneself or someone else.

Focused History: *How long have you had these feelings?* (longer than few days suggest mental disorder) *Can you fight? Can you do your job?* (ask the same of a supervisor – Light Battle Fatigue if affirmative) *Do you have any thoughts of wanting to hurt yourself or anyone else? Have you ever had those thoughts in the past?* (Always ask: suggests instability and a danger to the unit)

Objective: Signs

Using Basic Tools: Usually no signs except for perhaps tachycardia. Repeat the exam to ensure nothing was missed.

Assessment:

Differential Diagnosis: Undetected physical trauma - Always be concerned with a hidden injury missed in the primary or even secondary survey! With almost any mental disorder; consider the following:

Major depressive, bipolar, or schizophreniform disorders: Severe, long-lasting conditions that will not resolve without definitive psychiatric care, unlike battle fatigue, which will largely resolve within 72 hours with restoration of confidence, reassurance, replenishment, and rest.

Brief psychotic, acute stress, or conversion disorders: Temporary disturbances that may last weeks to months. Sometimes difficult to differentiate from battle fatigue. Degree of impairment/severity of symptoms coupled with prompt resolution suggests battle fatigue. Management principles for battle fatigue can provide support and symptom relief.

Post-Traumatic Stress Disorder (PTSD): Also a long-lasting disorder that appears after some trauma; not likely to occur in acute settings or immediately post-event unless there is some history of prior trauma. PTSD has symptoms similar to those of battle fatigue; history is crucial, as is time course of illness. Someone with PTSD may also suffer BF in an acutely stressful event.

Substance intoxication: History will distinguish this from battle fatigue. Assess the whole unit: substance abuse may indicate increased susceptibility to battle fatigue for individuals and units.

Mild traumatic brain injury (mTBI): Recent history of fall, "getting bell rung", or concussive blast or blasts, evaluate for mTBI. *See Part 7: Trauma: Chapter 26: Mild Traumatic Brain Injury/Concussion: Assessment and Management*

Plan:

Treatment guided by the acronym PIES:

Proximity: Treat service member as close to the unit as tactically and symptomatically possible. A violent, out-of-control patient cannot likely be treated at the battalion aid station if the battalion is actively engaged in combat, whereas one who is physically exhausted may be treated in his platoon area during a lull in the fighting. **Immediacy:** Do not delay initiation of treatment; treat as soon as symptoms are identified and tactically feasible.

Expectancy: "This will get better. You will return to your unit." Positively convey the expectation that this condition will improve and that the service member will not be evacuated.

Simplicity: Keep treatment simple. Provide the "Four Rs":

1. **Rest:** Provide place and time for adequate rest. Consider **diazepam** 2-5mg po tid or **lorazepam** 1-2mg po tid or IM. For cases of severe agitation, a neuroleptic: **haloperidol** 2-5mg IM or po or **chlorpromazine** 50-100mg po or IM q6-8h prn may be useful. **Diphenhydramine** 25-50mg po or IM may be given to enhance the therapeutic effect and reduce the risk of adverse reactions (dystonia) associated with administration of haloperidol or chlorpromazine.
2. **Reassurance:** Reassure service member that this condition will improve with rest and he will soon return to his unit
3. **Replenishment:** Food, water, hygiene
4. **Restoration** (of confidence): Often service members will have lost confidence in themselves, their equipment or their leadership. Work to restore confidence by keeping the service member in his military role—do not emphasize a "patient" role. Assign simple tasks and duties such as rehearsing battle drills, checking weapons, etc.

Patient Education

Prevention: Combat resiliency, or the ability to ward off the impairing features of combat and operational stress, is best attained through tough, realistic training, physical stamina, high morale and esprit, strong unit cohesion, and unity of effort. This is a leadership and command responsibility, but medics play an important role in assessing a unit's health along these lines. Battlemind training (www.battlemind.org) emphasizes combat resiliency and must be a part of any deployment.

Follow-up Actions

Evacuation/Consultation Criteria: At any level of care, the provider must make a determination to REST, HOLD, DUTY (RTD), or REFER battle fatigue casualties. This decision is based on the severity of symptoms and the tactical situation. Using the treatment principles above, 80% of service members presenting with impairment from psychological or emotional disturbances can be returned to duty within 72 hours. Another 10% may benefit from holding and treating for up to a week. The remaining 10% likely have mental disorders and will need referral higher for definitive care. The SOF medic's role in those cases is to ensure safety and stability for transport.

Note: Although specific to battle fatigue, these assessments and treatment principles can effectively be applied to non-combat situations such as Peace and Peace Enforcement operations, Stability and Support Operations, routine deployments and exercises.

Chapter 18: Mental Health: Anxiety Disorders

Anxiety Disorders: *See Part 3: General Symptoms: Anxiety*

Chapter 18: Mental Health: Acute Suicide Prevention

LTC Michael Doyle, MC, USA

Introduction: Suicide is a leading cause of non-combat death in the US Armed Forces. Suicidal Service Members present a challenge to command and medical personnel. Suicide attempts and completed suicides are very disruptive to units that experience them. Many suicides can be prevented through awareness of warning signs and early intervention. The vast majority of military suicides are committed by 17-25 year old white males, E-1 to E-4, with relationship problems. Suicide may be attempted by healthy personnel with an abnormal reaction to operational or relationship stress, or by someone with a mental disorder. The intent of this chapter is to address acute suicidality and enable the SOF medic to respond in that crisis situation.

Risk Factors:
- Depression and other mental disorders, or a substance-abuse disorder (often in combination with other mental disorders). More than 90% of people who die by suicide have these risk factors.
- Stressful life events, in combination with other risk factors, such as depression. However, suicide and suicidal behavior are not normal responses to stress; many people have these risk factors but are not suicidal.
- Prior suicide attempt
- Family history of mental disorder or substance abuse
- Family history of suicide
- Family violence, including physical or sexual abuse
- Firearms in the home, the method used in more than half of suicides
- Incarceration
- Exposure to the suicidal behavior of others, such as family members, peers, or media figures

Subjective: Symptoms

Overly stressed, sad, anxious, frustrated, worthless, hopeless, helpless, or guilty; thoughts of self-harm, harm to others, death or being better off dead; relationship problems

Focused History: *Have you had thoughts of hurting yourself or anyone else? Are you having thoughts now? If so, do you have a plan? Have you ever attempted suicide in the past or have you ever intentionally injured yourself? Have you been using alcohol or drugs? Do you have access to a gun? How is your relationship with your wife/girlfriend/ husband/boyfriend/significant other? Have you been giving away personal effects?* (Ask peers and supervisors if they have observed this.)

Objective: Signs

Using Basic Tools: Increasing agitation, interpersonal conflicts, anger, frustration and irritability; change in mood to sadness, new appearance of depression, social isolation and withdrawal; giving away personal effects; increased impulsivity or a history of impulsive or violent behaviors.

Assessment:

In assessing the potentially suicidal patient, the most significant determination is level of dangerousness. What is the risk of self-harm or suicide? (Err on the side of caution) The young active duty Service Member with significant relationship problems, access to a weapon and alcohol, and a prior history of violence is at substantial risk of attempting or completing suicide if he is considering this as an option. Anyone presenting with suicidal ideation with a plan or an inability to consider options other than suicide is at risk and must be assessed as a danger to himself or herself.

Differential Diagnosis: Presence of a mental disorder or personality disorder, self-mutilation and self-injurious behavior.

Plan:

Treatment - Suicidal Ideation and Attempted Suicide

1. Secure the individual's weapons and ammunition. Protect patient and others, including health care staff.
2. Monitor/accompany the suicidal individual at all times.
3. Treat injuries or medical conditions.
4. If imminently dangerous to self or others, hospitalize or place under 24-hour watch. Otherwise, manage with a "buddy watch" until the crisis has settled.
5. Identify the stressor that has precipitated this event. A chaplain can often be very helpful in settling down home-front crises.
6. Involve the chain-of-command in disposition plans.
7. If discharging a service member to his unit's custody, always have the service member contract verbally or in writing to return immediately if the thoughts of harm recur.
8. After a serious attempt or completed suicide, ask a chaplain or mental health professional to meet with the patient's ship, squad or section mates to address feelings of guilt, remorse or anger. Do not forget the medical personnel involved.
9. Remain vigilant for suicide clusters in units known for low morale, frequent or high rates of AWOL/UA, poor leadership, or other discipline problems.

Patient Education

Prevention: Closely follow service members who report suicidal ideation, even if ideation is not accompanied by intent. Let the service member know that you care and can help. Enlist the support of the chain of command.

Follow-up Actions

Evacuation/Consultation Criteria: Personnel who attempt suicide usually require evacuation. Consult mental health professionals at any point in your evaluation of a service member who presents with indications of increased risk for dangerous behavior or acts.

Chapter 18: Mental Health: Substance Abuse
LTC Michael Doyle, MC, USA

Introduction: Opiates, including codeine and oxycodone preparations, and benzodiazepines are the two categories of drugs for which life-threatening intoxication can be reversed. Barbiturate overdose is frequently fatal. Alcohol can infrequently be fatal. Alcohol, benzodiazepines, and barbiturates (found in medications like Fiorinal and Fioricet used in the treatment of migraine headaches) can cause life-threatening withdrawal after chronic use. Opiate withdrawal is uncomfortable, but not life-threatening. The focus of this chapter is on the management of the sequelae of abuse which may emerge in the deployed setting.

Subjective, Objective, Assessment and Plan:

Differential Diagnosis: Intoxicated patients should always be monitored for overt and covert overdose. *See Table 5-35* for Subjective and Objective symptoms and signs of intoxication with and withdrawal from common classes of abused substances. At times, severe withdrawal states may present as delirium or as psychosis (primarily in alcohol withdrawal, and this is rare). It is not uncommon to see signs of withdrawal from a substance (alcohol, illicit or prescribed drugs) in service members early in the course of an operation, once access to the substance is denied. Similarly, indigenous people and host nation personnel may present for care with signs and symptoms of withdrawal or intoxication.

Procedures

Essential: Supportive measures, IV hydration;

Recommended: Monitoring (Vitals at a minimum), *see Table 5-35*

Table 5-35. Substance Abuse: Intoxication and Withdrawal Signs and Symptoms

Intoxication	T	P	R	BP	Motor	Eyes	Complaints	Mental Status
Opiates	↓	↓	↓	↓	slowed	miotic pupils pinpoint in overdose	euphoria when high, N/V and constipation later	slurred speech, "nodding off", unresponsive in OD
Rx: **Naloxone**, 0.8mg/70kg slowly administered by IV.								
Benzodiazepine	NC	NC	↓	↓ (-)	ataxia uncoordination	NC to sluggish, nystagmus	Talkative, sedation with ↑ dose	irritability, emotional dis-inhibition, confusion and stupor; in severe OD, coma and death

Rx:
1. Intoxication: **Flumazenil**, 0.2mg IV over 15 seconds; repeated after 45 secs and again each subsequent minute until sedation reversed/relieved to a maximum of 1.0mg total dose given.
2. Overdose: **Flumazenil**, 0.2mg IV over 30 seconds. 0.3mg given after 30 secs if no response and up to 0.5mg each subsequent 30 second interval to a cumulative dose of 3.0mg. In rare cases for the recurrent sedation, may require additional titration up to a cumulative dose of 5.0mg.

	T	P	R	BP	Motor	Eyes	Complaints	Mental Status
Barbiturates	NC	NC	↓ ↓	↓	ataxia uncoordination	NC to sluggish, nystagmus	Talkative, slow speech and thinking	dis-inhibition, confusion, inattention, slurred speech; in OD, coma and death
Rx: Very little beyond supportive measures of ventilation, hydration and nutrition support can be provided.								
Stimulants	↑ to ↑↑	↑↑	NC to↑	↑↑	hyperreflexia	NC	Chest pain, restlessness	irritable, rapid speech, restless, poor concentration, psychotic signs & symptoms

Rx: Severe intoxication or overdose can be life-threatening (eg, >100mg methylphenidate). Emesis or lavage can be effective even late; reduce external stimuli, sedate with **chlorpromazine** 50mg IM or po q30 minutes as needed

Table 5-35. Substance Abuse: Intoxication and Withdrawal Signs and Symptoms, continued

Withdrawal	T	P	R	BP	Motor	Eyes	Complaints	Mental Status
Alcohol 12-72 hours after last drink	↑	↑↑	↑	↑↑	fine tremor, restless,	visual acuity	N/V, fatigue, anxiety, insomnia	agitated, irritable, hallucinations and delusions, illusions, confusion, seizures
Rx: Treat those with autonomic evidence of withdrawal (pulse, temp, BP or visible tremors) with **diazepam** 5-10mg po tid-qid on the first day of withdrawal. Do not give a dose once the patient begins to feel groggy or sleepy. Continue to assess and monitor vitals and treat on days 2 and 3 if T, P, BP are still elevated.								
Benzodiazepine 24-48 hours after last dose	↑	↑↑	↑	↑↑	fine tremor, restless, seizure	visual acuity	N/V, fatigue, anxiety, insomnia	agitated, irritable, hallucinations and delusions, illusions, confusion, seizures
Rx: Treat those with autonomic evidence of withdrawal (pulse, temp, BP or visible tremors) with **diazepam** 5-10mg po tid-qid on the first day of withdrawal. Do not give a dose once the patient begins to feel groggy or sleepy. Continue to assess and monitor vitals and treat on days 2 and 3 if T, P, BP are still elevated.								
Barbiturate onset at 24 hours, may last up to 14 days	↑	↑↑	↑	↑↑	fine tremor, restless	visual acuity	N/V, fatigue, anxiety, insomnia	agitated, irritable, hallucinations and delusions, illusions, confusion, seizures
Rx: Give **phenobarbital** 120mg po every 1 to 2 hours until 3 of the following 5 signs are present: 1) nystagmus, 2) drowsiness, 3) ataxia, 4) slurred speech, and 5) emotional lability. Then give no more. Phenobarbital has a long half-life and will self-taper.								
Opiates Symptoms peak at 48 hours	↑	↑	↑	↑	Restless	mydriasis, twitching and "kicking the habit"	drug craving, bone, back & muscle pain, insomnia, N/V and diarrhea	anxious, sad, irritable, with yawning, rhinorrhea, lacrimation, "gooseflesh" ("cold turkey")

Rx: Not life-threatening, only uncomfortable. Treat with **ibuprofen** 800mg po tid and **clonidine** 0.1-0.3mg po tid or qid, not to exceed more than 1mg total dose/day. Follow for signs of hypotension after each dose/day.

Chapter 18: Mental Health: Mood Disorders

Mood Disorders: *See Part 3: General Symptoms; Depression and Mania*

Chapter 18: Mental Health: Psychosis versus Delirium
LTC Michael Doyle, MC, USA

Introduction: Delirium represents a disturbance in consciousness accompanied by a change in cognitive function that develops acutely. Someone who is delirious has impairments in awareness, alertness, memory and executive functioning (ie, difficulty buttoning a shirt) and may be hallucinating. Psychosis is not a specific disorder, but rather describes a degree of severity in certain mental disorders. Someone with psychosis or a psychotic disorder has gross or obvious impairment in perceiving reality. The individual misperceives external cues and responds often to internal stimuli. He appears cognitively impaired, behaviorally disturbed, or both. Psychotic disorders are generally not amenable to treatment in a theater of operations. The most important consideration here is distinguishing psychosis (which is largely idiopathic) from delirium (which is a manifestation of a life-threatening medical condition that may be reversible). Always maintain a high index of suspicion for a physical or CNS injury!

Subjective: Symptoms
Patient often unaware of symptoms; in delirium, history of recent injury, illness. Paranoia: Unreasonable suspiciousness; feelings of persecution, being singled out or watched; includes feelings of grandiosity. Hallucinations: False sensory perceptions not associated with real external stimuli; delirious patients often have tactile and visual hallucinations; psychotic patients more often have auditory hallucinations. Delusions: False belief, based on incorrect inference about external reality; not consistent with patient's intelligence and cultural background; cannot be corrected with reasoning.
Focused History: (This may have to be obtained from a battle-buddy.): *How long has this been going on?* (Delirium has a rapid onset of hours to days; psychosis takes days to weeks.) *Do the symptoms change at night?* (Delirium is often worse at night; psychosis is not so variable.) *What medications is the patient taking?* (Anticholinergics, stimulants, anti-malarial drugs, and anti-parasitic medications have been associated with delirium.)

Objective: **Signs**

Using Basic Tools: Autonomic instability (delirium) versus normal vital signs (psychosis), assess for head trauma or occult injury (differential); diffuse hyperreflexia (delirium).

Mental Status Exam:

1. Alertness: Diminished (delirium); normal or increased (psychosis); not responsive to external stimuli (both)
2. Orientation: Disoriented to person, place, time, situation or all (delirium); oriented (psychosis) but answers may be contrived and bizarre
3. Activity: Agitated, especially in evenings (delirium); catatonia—purposeless movements or rigid posturing with waxy flexibility (psychosis)
4. Speech: Slurred words or difficult to comprehend (delirium); disorganized and uses made up words called neologisms (psychosis)
5. Thought Content: Delusions, paranoid ideation, simplified thinking (psychosis)
6. Thought Processes: Difficult to follow because of loose associations or flight of ideas; thoughts often derail or stop abruptly (psychosis)
7. Mood: Disorganized (psychosis)
8. Affect: Inappropriate to situation or stated mood; often blunted or flat (psychosis)
9. Cognition: Impaired memory, attention tasks (both)
10. Judgment: Impaired (both)

Using Advanced Tools: Labs: Evidence of medical illness in delirium; increased WBC, decreased HCT, etc.

Assessment:

Differential Diagnosis

Delirium: Orientation is generally impaired; identify underlying medical problem and treat it.
Psychosis: Orientation generally preserved; identify underlying medical problem and treat it.
Substance abuse: Alcohol withdrawal, PCP, amphetamine, cocaine intoxication appear psychotic
Seizure disorder: Temporal lobe epilepsy (often with herpes encephalitis) can appear psychotic.
Head injury: May cause delirium; obtain history from other unit members.
Mental Disorders principally associated with psychosis:
Schizophreniform disorder and schizophrenia: Ages 15-25 men, 20-35 women
Bipolar disorder, manic with psychotic features: 3rd and 4th decade, sometimes earlier
Major depressive disorder, severe with psychotic features: More common in an older population
Brief psychotic disorder: May or may not have an identifiable precipitant; begins and resolves within 30 days, often with supportive measures alone.
Identify the presence of a mental disorder first; do not worry too much about what type it is.

Plan:

Treatment

1. Secure the individual's weapons and ammo.
2. Calm the patient to protect him and others around him. Psychotic and delirious patients may pose a danger to self or others simply through agitation, reckless behavior or inappropriate activities. For both use:
   a. Benzodiazepines: **Diazepam** 5-10mg po or IM q8-12h prn agitation or **lorazepam** 2mg po, IM or IV q6-8h prn agitation.
   b. Neuroleptics: **Haloperidol** 2-5mg IM or po or **chlorpromazine** 50-100mg po or IM q6-8h prn agitation. Also consider giving **diphenhydramine** 25-50mg po or IM coincident with the haloperidol or chlorpromazine for reduction of risk of adverse reactions (dystonia).
   c. AVOID USE OF DIPHENHYDRAMINE, CHLOROPROMAZINE OR OTHER MEDICATIONS WITH ANTI-CHOLINERGIC SIDE EFFECTS IF YOU SUSPECT DELIRIUM. THESE WILL WORSEN THE DELIRIUM!
   d. If medication fails to settle down an agitated patient, consider restraint with sheets, wrapped around patient on litter. Pharmacological or physical restraint may be necessary to better evaluate and treat a delirious patient.
3. Consider IV hydration for those unable to care for self.
4. Place on watch. Protect patient and others, including health care staff.

Follow-up Actions

Evacuation/Consultation Criteria: Evacuate US service members suffering from a psychotic or delirious disorder. Host nation service members and persons should be given behavioral redirection and managed with a goal of maintaining safety for all parties.

Chapter 18: Mental Health: Recovering Human Remains: How to Prepare Yourself, Your Buddies, and the Unit

LTC Michael Doyle, MC, USA

The Mission: May include collecting the bodies of fellow Service Members so that the Mortuary Affairs specialists can return them to the United States for identification and burial. It may include collecting bodies of guerilla forces working with and killed alongside U.S. forces. The mission may require gathering and possibly burying the bodies of enemy or civilian dead to safeguard public health. The numbers of dead may be small and very personal, or they may be vast. The dead may include young men and women, elderly people, small children or infants, for whom we feel an innate empathy. Being exposed to children who have died can be especially distressing, particularly for individuals who have children of their own.

What To Expect: While in many cultures, death is viewed with stoicism, seeing mutilated bodies evokes horror in most human beings. Nonetheless, honoring the dead is customary in most societies; burials further serve public health needs. In many cases, dead bodies may be wasted by starvation, dehydration and disease (eg, Rwanda refugees or some POW and concentration camp victims). They may have been crushed and dug out from under rubble (eg, the Beirut barracks bombing or earthquake victims). They may be badly mutilated by fire, impact, blast or projectiles (eg, the victims of the air crash at Gander, Newfoundland; the civilians killed by collateral damage and fire near the Commandancia in Panama City, or the Iraqi army dead north of Kuwait). They may be victims of deliberate atrocity (eg, the Shiites of south Iraq or any side in Bosnia). Often however, the dead are victims of the horrors and destruction of war. Many who are exposed to death on this scale develop a protective "shell". Survivor reactions may include grief, anger, shock, gratitude or ingratitude, numbness or indifference. Such reactions may seem appropriate or inappropriate to you, and may affect your own reactions to the dead. In situations where the cause of death leaves few signs on the bodies (eg, the mass suicide with cyanide at Jonestown, Guyana) caregivers often have more difficulty adapting because it is harder to form the "shell." The degree of decomposition of the bodies will be determined by the temperature, climate and length of time since death. Bodies will emit a strong odor of decomposition. Workers may have to touch the remains, move them and perhaps hear the sounds of autopsies being performed or other burial activities. These sensations may interfere with work, and create disturbing memories. In body handling situations, many personnel naturally tend towards what is aptly called "graveyard humor." This is a normal human reaction or "safety valve" for very uncomfortable feelings. Other feelings may occur, including sorrow, regret, repulsion, disgust, anger and futility. SOF personnel will be exposed to death of comrades, of guerilla forces enlisted by the SOF, of civilians and of enemy forces. Anticipating and planning for these occurrences is important to forming a protective shell while ensuring any remains are handled in the safest manner considering all physical, emotional, and cultural issues.

When: Personnel may have to perform these services after any death, natural, or traumatic.

What You Need: Body bags, shovels, reporting forms, pens or pencils, bags for personal effects, labels, gloves, visual barriers/screens, deodorants

What To Do: Guidelines for How to Work with Human Remains
BEFORE
1. Learn the history, cultural background, and circumstances of the disaster or tragedy. How did it come to happen? Try to understand it the way a historian or neutral investigating commission would. It is important to demonstrate your understanding and acceptance of local customs and beliefs. When recruiting, training, and fighting next to indigenous soldiers, we must be able to assure them that their remains will be handled according to their local customs and religious beliefs (to include returning remains to family members, if possible) in a timely manner.
2. Know the culture in which you are working. Videos and photographs of the area of operation and of the victims, television news networks, and magazines may be may provide critical information of the event. If pictures of the current situation are not available, library archives may exist of similar tragedies. Share this information and discuss with team members.
3. Understand the importance and value of the recovery and disposition of human remains. Providing the deceased a respectful and dignified burial under difficult circumstances (ie, hasty and/ or mass burials may be only option), providing survivors the knowledge that their loved ones have died and received a dignified burial while providing a safer environment for the living are challenging but important goals. Concentrate on the overall mission (not on each individual) to maintain effectiveness when seeing or working with mass casualties. SOF personnel should be prepared to recover remains in an efficient and humane manner while honoring the commitment to the indigenous population. If working closely with indigenous forces, have a plan for handling their deceased. If there are outside interests in the remains of indigenous personnel that compromise this commitment to the indigenous population, the ultimate decision on disposition lies with the commander on the ground, with due consideration to the local commitment, customs, and religious beliefs.

DURING
1. Personnel who examine personal effects for identification and other purposes must not be those who have initially seen or handled the body.
2. It is a criminal act to take souvenirs or otherwise desecrate human remains.
3. Conduct funeral ceremonies consistent with the cultural norms of the society in which the recovery occurs; these may be Western rite funerals, but in many cases, these services will not. Consult with Unit chaplains and/or local clergy as they may also conduct rites or ceremonies.
4. Limit exposure to the bodies. Have screens, partitions, covers, body bags, or barriers so that people do not see the bodies unless it is necessary. Wear gloves if the job calls for touching the bodies. Mask odors with disinfectants, air-fresheners, or deodorants. (Using other scents such as perfume or aftershave lotions are of limited value in the presence of the bodies.)
5. When the mission allows, schedule frequent short breaks away from working with or around bodies.
6. Drink plenty of fluids, continue to eat well, and maintain good hygiene. To the extent possible, the command should ensure facilities for washing hands, clothing and taking hot showers after each shift. (If water is rationed, the command should make clear what can be provided and how it should be used and conserved.)
7. Hold team debriefings frequently to share thoughts and feelings with teammates.
8. Have a mental health/stress control team or chaplain lead a Critical Event Debriefing after a particularly bad event or at the end of the operation.
9. Plan individual and team activities to relax and think about things other than the tragedy. Be aware of and take steps to resolve feelings of frustration and guilt that often accompany the management of a mass casualty. DO WHAT CAN BE DONE WITH RESOURCES AVAILABLE, ONE STEP AT A TIME.
10. Stay physically fit.
11. Keep the unit Family Readiness Group fully informed about what is happening, and make sure family members and significant others are included in and supported by it.
12. Take special care of new unit members, and those with recent changes or special problems back home. If the stress caused by working with dead bodies begins to interfere with performance or ability to relax, TAKE ACTION. Do not ignore the stress. Seek out a buddy or someone to talk with about new or unusual feelings. Other people are likely to be feeling the same things. Do NOT withdraw. The unit chaplain, medic or a combat stress control/mental health team member can often help.
13. Help your buddy, coworkers, subordinate or superior if he or she shows signs of distress. Give support and encouragement, and try to get the other person to talk through the problems or feelings they are having. This will improve each person's ability to cope with the situation.

AFTER
1. Take an active part in an end-of-tour debriefing and pre-homecoming information briefing in the unit prior to leaving the operational area
2. Follow through with Family Support Group activities which recognize and honor what the unit has done and share the experience (and the praise for a hard job well done) with the families.
3. Do not be surprised if being at home brings back upsetting memories from the operation. It may be hard to talk about the memories from the operation, especially with those who were not there. This is very common, but try to talk to them anyway, and talk with teammates from the operation (best option). Do not hesitate to talk with a chaplain or with the community mental health or stress control team.

What Not To Do: Do not keep these emotions inside. Do not withdraw. Do not desecrate or take souvenirs from the bodies.

Chapter 19: Anesthesia: Inhalation Anesthesia: Drawover Method
MAJ James R. Reed, AN, USA

What: Maintenance of general anesthesia using volatile anesthetic agents after intravenous induction of anesthesia.

When: In cases where local or regional anesthesia are not appropriate due to extent of injury or required surgical procedure and TIVA, is not available. When choosing between TIVA or drawover anesthesia, the provider should select the technique with which they are most competent. For IV induction, see examples for induction of general anesthesia (TIVA); give IV medications as described for induction and follow with drawover anesthesia as described in this section.

Background: Drawover anesthesia is a simple and reliable method to deliver anesthesia using inhalation anesthetics (volatile agents) that provide all the components of anesthesia (amnesia, analgesia, autonomic stability, and muscle relaxation). The operator must be prepared to provide positive pressure ventilation to support ventilation throughout the period of anesthesia and as required during recovery. The Ohmeda Universal Portable Anesthesia Complete (UPAC) is a multi-agent, temperature compensated, drawover anesthesia device that the US Military has been employing since 1990. The British made famous the concept of drawover anesthesia in combat during the Falkland Islands War, subsequently the UPAC has been safely used extensively in the GWOT. The UPAC is lightweight (>10 lbs), does not require compressed gases or power to operate, and is free of complex flowmeters and electronics. It is ideal for austere sites. Using this system, the carrier gas is drawn through the vaporizer by the patient's spontaneous respirations or by a self-inflating bag placed between the patient and vaporizer in the circuit. Agent is picked up in the vaporizer with the carrier gas and is delivered to the patient. A one way valve placed at the distal end of the circuit prevents the patient from re-breathing exhaled gases that include agent and carbon dioxide.

THE KEY TO ANY SAFE AND SUCCESSFUL ANESTHETIC IS PERPETUAL VIGILANCE AND PRUDENT TITRATION OF MEDICATIONS TO EFFECT.

Fundamental Principles:
1. Verify level of expertise in airway management and proper setup, checkout, and use of the UPAC.
2. Vigilance is maintained during titration of volatile anesthetics (the key to maintenance of patient safety).
3. Measured efficacy of volatile anesthetics is expressed as Minimum Alveolar Concentration (MAC):
     0.3–0.5 MAC: awareness and amnesia (50% of these patients able to respond to verbal commands)
     1 MAC: 50% of patients do not move to surgical stimuli
     1:3 MAC: 95% of patients do not move to surgical stimuli

Common inhalation agent MACs:
- Halothane: 0.75%.
- Sevoflurane: 1.75%.
- Isoflurane: 1.15%.
- Enflurane: 1.65%.

MAC in the pediatric patient is increased and decreased in the elderly - remember to titrate to effect.

What You Need:
1. Normal monitoring capability (BP cuff, pulse oximeter, ECG and stethoscope). Peripheral nerve stimulator is desirable if infusing muscle relaxants.
2. Bag-Valve-Mask or other device capable of delivering positive-pressure ventilations in addition to the UPAC.
3. Suction, endotracheal tube and other airway adjuncts, laryngoscope and blades, Easy Cap CO_2 detector, tape, NG tube for stomach decompression
4. Established IV access and infuse maintenance fluids. Medications will be infused through this line, so it is imperative to have a patent line.
5. Properly assembled and checked UPAC. *See Figure 5-40 below* and check out procedure.
6. Anesthetic Agent. Isoflurane or Sevoflurane are most common in US Military inventory. When using Sevoflurane, use the Enflurane dial on the UPAC as they have similar vapor pressures (Sevoflurane 200mmHg and Enflurane 175mmHg) and will be similar in physical characteristics regarding MAC.
7. 25mm corrugated tubing to use as a scavenger tube to vent waste anesthetic gases outside away from the work area.

Figure 5-40. Portable Anesthesia System (PAC) Schematic

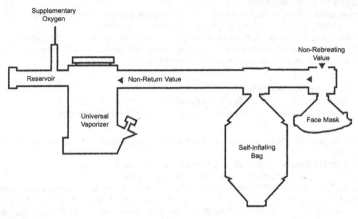

UPAC pre-procedure checkout:

Visual Check:

1. Inspect the flexible hoses for any damage, cuts, dry rot, or splits.
2. Examine the breathing assembly for damage.
3. Check all components for security of attachment.
4. Examine vaporizer for any signs of damage, if found do not use vaporizer, consider TIVA.

Internal Leak Test:

1. Turn ON the vaporizer.
2. Squeeze the self-inflating bag and hold it in this condition.
3. Cap the air inlet and supplemental oxygen nipple and then release the self-inflating bag.
4. If bag does not re-inflate, then there are no significant leaks.

External Leak Test:

1. Cap the face mask port and expiratory valve port.
2. Attempt to squeeze the self inflating bag.
3. If the bag cannot be totally squeezed, then there are no significant leaks.

What To Do:

1. Assemble medications, equipment, and perform pre-procedure checks.
2. Perform a thorough assessment of the patient and determine a safe course of anesthesia. Consider local, regional, or TIVA.
3. Apply monitors and pre-oxygenate patient.
4. Induce patient with IV agents (*see examples in Part 5: Specialty Areas: Chapter 19: Total Intravenous Anesthesia for IV induction*) and secure the patient's airway. A mask anesthetic can be done using OPA, NPA and/or manual airway stabilization techniques otherwise perform intubation using RSI technique. If patient has not fasted for 8 hours or has a history of or potential for reflux of stomach contents, then cricoid pressure should be applied until the airway is definitively secured.
5. After the airway is secured and while the patient is completely obtunded, turn the vaporizer on and begin the anesthetic. Remember if the patient is not breathing or you are not breathing for the patient, no anesthesia is being delivered. Titrate the agent to the desired effect during the procedure maintaining vigilance to patient's vital signs and respiratory status. In severely traumatized or ill patients who demonstrate intravascular fluid volume deficiency or shock, great care must be taken when using volatile anesthetic agents. This is due to their significant depressant effect on the cardiovascular system - mainly patient afterload which affects the patient's ability to maintain adequate blood pressures.
6. A balanced anesthetic technique can be performed using muscle relaxants and opioids to decrease the amount of volatile agent delivered. Great care must also be exercised when employing these agents as they have deleterious effects on the patient's respiratory status. IF MUSCLE RELAXANTS ARE EMPLOYED, YOU MUST BREATHE FOR THE PATIENT!!
7. As the procedure draws to a close and patient is to be extubated, titrate back the amount of volatile anesthetic agent delivered eventually turning it off. Ensure neuromuscular blockade has been reversed and the patient begins to breathe spontaneously. Assist patient ventilations in order to exhale the anesthetic agent. **Important:** Patients experience prolonged Excitatory Stage of Anesthesia (Stage II) using volatile drawover anesthesia. This is a potentially dangerous time as premature extubation can lead to catastrophic laryngospasm, an inability to ventilate the patient, or negative pressure pulmonary edema. The patient must be following commands in addition to a sustained head lift before extubation is performed. Enlist the help of others to maintain patient control and ensure patient safety.

Chapter 19: Anesthesia: Total Intravenous Anesthesia

MAJ Leland Bradley Morgans, AN, USA & MAJ James Reed, AN, USA

What: Induction and maintenance of general anesthesia using only the infusion of intravenous anesthetic medications.

Fundamental tenets of TIVA are:

1. The combination of medications selected for infusion must provide all the components of anesthesia: amnesia (hypnosis), analgesia,

autonomic stability, and if required, areflexia (complete muscle relaxation). *Table 5-36* lists examples of combinations that have been successfully used in the field environment.

2. Continuous infusion techniques provide more precise control over the pharmacological effects of the medications being administered, avoiding the autonomic "peaks and valleys" seen with intermittent bolus administration.

3. Vigilant titration, based on observed and anticipated patient response, is essential. Successful use of this technique allows for small increases in the anesthetic effect when necessary, as well as aggressive, but methodical downward titration of the infusion rates throughout the course of the anesthetic, resulting in a smooth emergence.

When:
As an alternative to inhalation anesthetics when:

1. Inhalation agents or their delivery devices (vaporizers) are unavailable
2. A patient requires high concentrations of oxygen and minimal drug-induced cardiovascular depression.

What You Need:

1. Normal monitoring capability (BP cuff, pulse oximeter, ECG and stethoscope). Peripheral nerve stimulator is desirable if infusing muscle relaxants.
2. Bag-Valve-Mask or other device capable of delivering positive-pressure ventilations
3. Endotracheal tube or other devices to assist in maintaining or securing the airway.
4. Established IV access and infuse maintenance fluids. Medications will be infused through this line, so it is imperative to have a patent line.
5. Infusion assisting devices, such as a Dial-A-Flow IV rate control clamp. Electronic infusion pumps are ideal but likely not available.
6. Intravenous anesthetic medications (*see Table 5-36*). These recommended dosages are designed for healthy adult patients requiring acute surgical intervention. Do not confuse these dosages with those used for long term sedation/analgesia in critical care/intensive care situations. These dosages are not recommended for the pediatric population.

Table 5-36. Dosing Guidelines for IV Agents

Drug	Loading Dose	Incremental Dose	Infusion Dose
Amnestic Agents			
Propofol	1.0-2.5mg/kg	0.25-1.0mg/kg	75-200mcg/kg/min
Midazolam	50-150mcg/kg	5-10mcg/kg	0.25-1mcg/kg/min
Analgesics			
Fentanyl	2.0-4.0mcg/kg	0.25-1.0mcg/kg	0.02-0.1mcg/kg/min
Ketamine	0.5-2.0mg/kg	0.5-1.0mg/kg	10-40mcg/kg/min
Muscle Relaxants*	**Intubating Dose**		
Vecuronium	0.08-0.1mg/kg	0.01-0.015mg/kg	0.8-1.2mcg/kg/min
Succinylcholine	1-2mg/kg	20mg boluses	0.25-0.5mg/kg/min

*These drugs paralyze the patient requiring the provider to secure the airway and provide respirations.

What To Do:

1. Conduct pre-operative system check (*see Table 5-37*).
2. Induce general anesthesia with selected medications (*see loading doses listed on Table 5-36*).
3. Secure the airway and ensure adequate oxygenation and ventilation of the patient.
4. Initiate maintenance infusions of selected medications (*see Table 5-36*).
5. Monitor the patient vigilantly and titrate infusions. If a patient has not responded to surgical stimulation during the previous 10-15 minutes, and a substantial increase in the level of surgical stress is not imminent:
   a. Reduce the infusion rate by 20%.
   b. If the patient subsequently begins to respond to surgical stimulation: Increase the infusion rate to a setting between the original rate and the reduced rate (or approximately a 10% reduction from the original setting) and administer a bolus equivalent to the amount of drug the infusion will provide during the next 5-minute period.
6. General considerations when employing continuous infusion techniques:
   a. Using a powered infusion pump will ensure continuous infusion, providing optimal control and ideal effect-site concentration.
   b. Use small-bore tubing for the medication infusion and place as close to the IV cannulation site as possible.
   c. Check carrier fluid and connections often. Empty carrier IVs will result in emergence from anesthesia or overdose.
   d. Limit the use of muscle relaxants: determine titration of infusion rates based on the usual clinical signs of anesthetic depth (lack of movement, stable blood pressure and heart rate, regular respiratory rate and rhythm). Overzealously using muscle relaxants blinds the practitioner to some of these signs, necessitating the delivery of positive-pressure ventilations throughout the procedure.
   e. Force downward titration: This is the most critical consideration when rapid post-surgical recovery is required. Review section 5.b.

What Not To Do:

Contraindications: Other than allergic reaction to the selected medication, there are no absolute contraindications to this technique.

Complications:

1. Compatibility concerns: All drugs being infused through a single access line MUST be compatible. This compatibility applies to not only the anesthetic agents, but also other medications (antibiotics) that might be administered during the course of an anesthetic.
2. False sense of security: Practice vigilant downward titration to avoid overdosing the patient but provide adequate levels of anesthesia at the same time. Remain constantly aware of your patient's vital signs.
3. Awareness: Avoid overuse of muscle relaxants, which can mask the purposeful movement usually associated with inadequate depth of anesthesia. With inadequate levels of anesthesia, patients may recall what happened in surgery.

Table 5-37. Pre-And Intraoperative System Checks For Continuous Infusion

Preoperative checks	Intraoperative checks
1. Medication infusion lines piggybacked into established IV line.	1. Medication lines remain connected to carrier fluid.
2. Medication infusion lines are primed and purged of air.	2. Carrier fluid is present and flowing.
3. Clips and clamps have been removed from medication infusion lines.	3. Pump alarms remain active.
4. If electrical infusion devices are available: Functional and in the "ON" position. Dosage settings are correct. Connected to a reliable electrical supply.	4. Drug supply in reservoir is adequate.

It is important to note that when using **ketamine** in these infusions, patients will demonstrate excessive amounts of oral secretions. **Midazolam** 2mg for adult patients should be given if possible to offset **ketamine** induced delirium.

Table 5-38. Examples of Techniques Used In The Field

Example 1.

Continuous infusion of **midazolam, ketamine,** and **vecuronium.**

Induction: **midazolam** (2mg), followed by **ketamine** (2mg/kg) and **vecuronium** 0.1mg/kg. Following intubation, initiate infusion of the same medications at the following rates:

- Midazolam (50mcg/kg/hr)
- Ketamine (1mg/kg/hr)
- Vecuronium (60mcg/kg/hr)

Obtain this infusion mixture by adding midazolam 5mg, ketamine 100mg and vecuronium 6mg to a 50mL bag of 0.9% normal saline and infuse at the rates mentioned previously. Determine the infusion rate to deliver this concentration by using the formula:

$$\frac{\text{Patient's weight (kg)}}{2} = \text{mL to be infused per hour}$$

(eg, a patient weighing 70kg would require an infusion rate of 35mL/hr).

Sample Calculations:

1. **Midazolam** infusion of 50mcg/kg/hr, means 50mcg x 70kg or 3500mcg/hr is required.
2. Using the formula:

$$\frac{\text{Patient's weight (kg)}}{2} = \text{mL to be infused per hour or } 70/2 = 35\text{mL/hr to be infused for this patient}$$

Therefore, 3500mcg/hr required divided by 35mL/hr (determined infusion rate) yields a concentration requirement of 100mcg/mL.

3. Adding 5mg of **midazolam** to 50mL of 0.9% normal saline yields a concentration of 100mcg/mL

Similar calculations yield requirements for 100mg of **ketamine** and 6mg of **vecuronium.**

Example 2.

Continuous infusion of **propofol** and **ketamine**

Induction: Propofol (2mg/kg) followed by ketamine 1mg/kg and vecuronium 0.1mg/kg.

Following intubation, initiate an infusion of propofol and ketamine. This combination requires two separate infusion bags, as the propofol infusion is deliberately titrated downward more aggressively than the ketamine. Infusion rates are as follows:

- Ketamine (1.5mg/kg/hr)
- Propofol (12mg/kg/hr) for the first 30 minutes, then (9mg/kg/hr) for 30 minutes, lastly (6mg/kg/hr).

Prepare the two infusions as follows:

Ketamine 150mg in a 50mL bag of 0.9% normal saline, yielding a concentration of 3mg/mL. Infuse at the rates mentioned previously. Determine the infusion rate to deliver this concentration by using the formula:

$$\frac{\text{Patient's weight (kg)}}{2} = \text{mL to be infused per hour}$$

Sample Calculations: For a patient weighing 80 kg:

1. Ketamine infusion of 1.5mg/kg/hr, means 1.5mg x 80 kg or 120mg/hr is required.
2. Using the formula:

$$\frac{\text{Patient's weight (kg)}}{2} = \text{mL to be infused per hour or } 80/2 = 40\text{mL/hr to be infused for this patient}$$

Therefore, 120mg/hr required divided by 40mL/hr (determined infusion rate) yields a 3 mg/mL concentration required.

3. Adding 150mg of ketamine to 50mL of 0.9% normal saline yields a concentration of 3mg/mL

Propofol can be mixed in a 50:50 solution using 0.9% normal saline. The resulting concentration (5mg/mL) allows for easy titration. To prepare the mixture, add 1000mg of propofol to a 100mL bag of 0.9% normal saline. This results in 1000mg in 200mL and creates enough propofol for most procedures under one hour in duration. With the 80kg patient, the first 30 minutes would require approximately 100mL of the solution:

    12mg/kg/hr X 80kg = 960mg/hr
    960mg/hr divided by 5mg/mL (concentration) = 192mg/hr
    192mg/hr divided by .5 (first 30 minutes) = 96mL.

The second 30 minutes would require approximately 75mL of the solution, with the subsequent infusion rate being approximately 50mL/hr. Discontinuing both infusions 15-20 minutes prior to the end of surgery results in a smooth emergence.

Example 3.

Continuous infusion of **propofol, fentanyl, ketamine (PFK)**

Induction: **Propofol** (2mg/kg) followed by **fentanyl** 100mcg and **vecuronium** 0.1mg/kg.

Following intubation, initiate an infusion of propofol at the following rates:

1. Propofol (12mg/kg/hr) for the first 30 minutes, then (9mg/kg/hr) for 30 minutes, then (6mg/kg/hr) thereafter. These rates are starting points, you must be vigilant with heart rate and blood pressure. You may have to reduce the infusion rate if the patients vital signs will not tolerate your initial drip rates.
2. Propofol can be mixed in a 50:50 solution using 0.9% normal saline. The infusion technique is described in Example 2.
3. Fentanyl 2mcg/cc is added to the mixture
4. Ketamine 2mg/cc is also added to the mixture

You will need to stop the infusion approximately 15 minutes before the end of surgery.

Pediatric patients may receive the propofol infusion as well with just **ketamine** 2mg/mL. However pediatric patients require more judicious monitoring of vital signs especially respirations and blood pressure. Therefore, sedation of the pediatric patient for must procedures is more prudent. You may sedate children with IM dose of ketamine 4mg/kg. This will stun the child and allow for IV access and performance of the procedure.

Chapter 19: Anesthesia: Local/Regional Anesthesia: Introduction

MAJ James Reed, AN, USA & MAJ Leland Bradley Morgans, AN, USA

Introduction: Regional techniques utilizing local anesthetics may be used for surgical, diagnostic, or therapeutic procedures or for providing relief of acute or chronic pain. Techniques range from subcutaneous infiltration of a small, specified area to a major regional plexus blockade.

Local Infiltration of an Area

When:

Whenever good operative conditions can be obtained with a moderate volume of local anesthetic or to perform a minor surgical procedure such as suturing a wound or excising a small tumor.

What You Need:

Sterile barrier (towels or drapes), an antiseptic prepping solution (povidone-iodine or alcohol), appropriate size syringe, 25 or 27 gauge needle, local anesthetic (see Table 5-39). **Note:** A 50:50 ratio of **lidocaine** and **bupivacaine** offers the luxury of a fast onset and long duration.

What to Do:

1. Assemble equipment.
2. Prep area and establish a sterile field with the chosen barrier.
3. Use the smallest possible gauge needle to minimize pain. With the bevel of the needle facing down and parallel to the skin, quickly insert the needle up to the hub. Begin infiltrating the desired area while withdrawing the needle. Slowly inject the medication. Perform subsequent needle insertions from this anesthetized area.
4. Injections should be systematic and delivered in a triangular geometric pattern to ensure an adequate block. Should deeper tissue levels need anesthetizing, utilize a systematic approach again, anesthetizing progressively deeper layers.
5. Adding the vasoconstrictor epinephrine delays the systemic absorption of the anesthetic, which prolongs the duration of the block and allows for the safe administration of a larger dose of local anesthetic.

Table 5-39. Infiltration Anesthetics

Drug	Concentration (%)	Plain Solutions Maximum Dose (milligrams)	Duration (minutes)	Epinephrine Containing Solutions Maximum Dose (milligrams)	Duration (minutes)
Lidocaine	0.5-1.0	300	30-60	500	120-360
Prilocaine	0.5-1.0	500	30-90	600	60-120
Bupivacaine	0.25-0.5	175	120-240	225	180-240

Pediatric infiltration: 0.25% **bupivacaine with 1:200,000 epinephrine** allows safe calculation of a maximum dosage. The maximum dose in mL equals the patient's kilogram weight. For example, a 10kg child could receive a maximum of 10mL of this solution. This solution is used for infiltration only, never digital blocks.

What Not To Do:
Contraindications: There are no specific contraindications to this technique.
1. Avoid local anesthetics in patients reporting allergies to them.
2. Avoid using vasoconstrictors with these blocks in the fingers or toes.
Complications: Tissue ischemia and necrosis - large volumes of local anesthetics and high concentrations of epinephrine can lead to ischemia and necrosis of wound edges. Should epinephrine be utilized, a concentration of 1:200,000 affords the maximum vasoconstrictive property sought for these procedures.

Chapter 19: Anesthesia: Local/Regional Anesthesia: Digital Block of the Finger or Toe
MAJ James Reed, AN, USA & MAJ Leland Bradley Morgans, AN, USA

When:
Whenever good operative conditions can be obtained with a moderate volume of local anesthetic. To perform a surgical procedure on the area.

What You Need:
An antiseptic prepping solution (povidone-iodine or alcohol), appropriate sized syringe, 25 or 27 gauge needle, local anesthetic.

Table 5-40. Anesthetics for Digital Blocks

Drug	Concentration (%)	Plain Solutions Maximum Dose (milligrams)	Duration (minutes)
Lidocaine	0.5-1.0	300	30-60
Prilocaine	0.5-1.0	500	30-90
Bupivacaine	0.25-0.5	175	120-240

What To Do:
1. Assemble equipment
2. Prep area
3. Each digit is supplied with 2 pairs of nerves: dorsal and palmar in the hand, and dorsal and plantar in the foot.
4. Insert the needle in the dorsal aspect of the digit at the level of the metacarpal (metatarsal) head. *See Figures 5-41 to 5-46.*
5. Advancing the needle in the palmar (plantar) direction, inject 1-2mL of local anesthetic on each side of the digit.
6. Slowly inject the medication with the smallest possible gauge needle to minimize pain.
7. Repeat steps 4-7 for the palm

What Not To Do:
Contraindications:
1. Avoid local anesthetics in patients reporting allergies to them.
2. Avoid using epinephrine with any type of digital block.
Complications: Tissue ischemia and necrosis. Large volumes of local anesthetics can lead to mechanical compression and ischemia. Deposit the anesthetic only on the lateral aspects of the digits to be anesthetized. Avoid total circumferential administration.

Figure 5-41. Web Space Block (Hand/Finger)

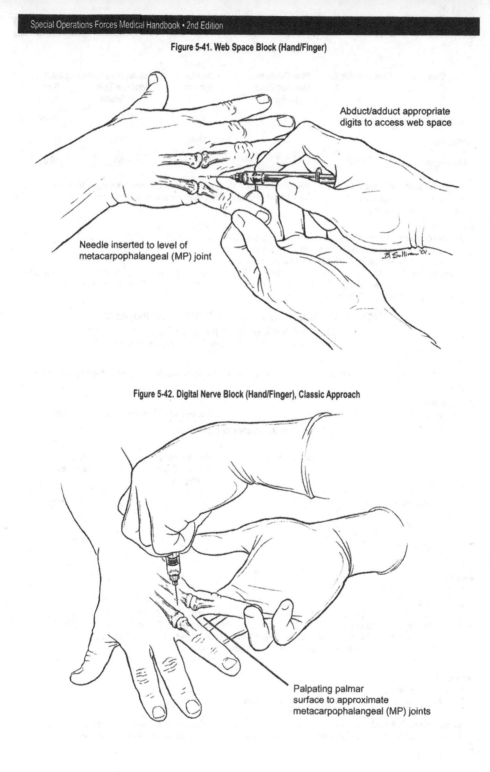

Abduct/adduct appropriate
digits to access web space

Needle inserted to level of
metacarpophalangeal (MP) joint

B. Sullivan '01.

Figure 5-42. Digital Nerve Block (Hand/Finger), Classic Approach

Palpating palmar
surface to approximate
metacarpophalangeal (MP) joints

Figure 5-43. Digital Nerve Block (Hand/Finger), Metacarpal Approach

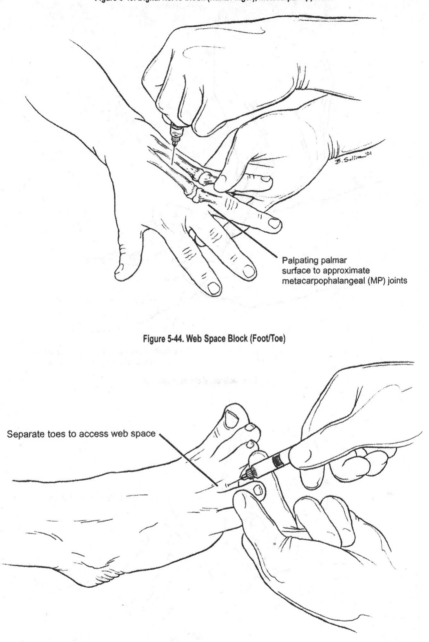

Palpating palmar
surface to approximate
metacarpophalangeal (MP) joints

Figure 5-44. Web Space Block (Foot/Toe)

Separate toes to access web space

Figure 5-45. Digital Block (Foot/Toe)

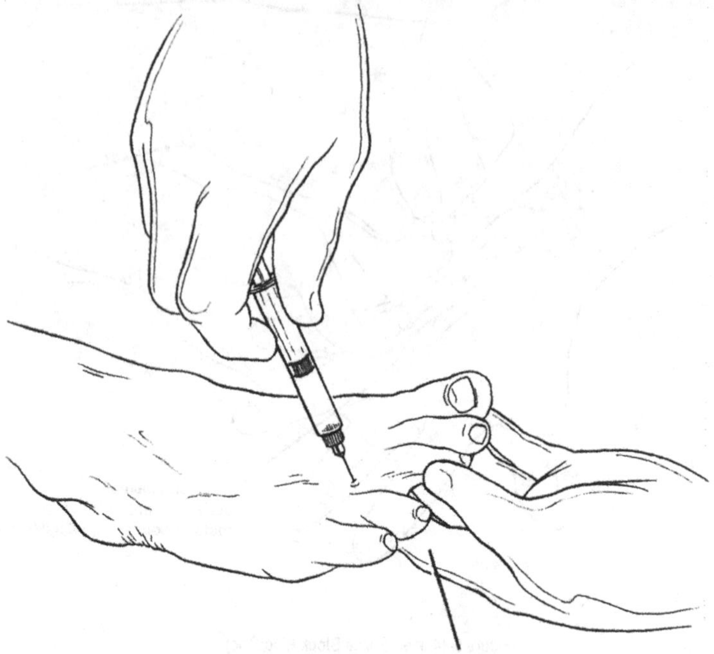

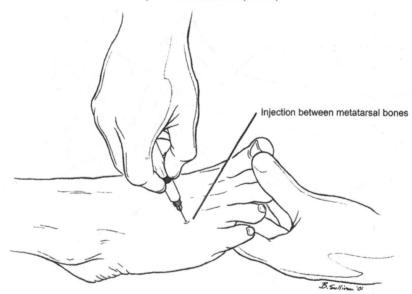

Palpation of plantar surface to approximate
metatarsophalangeal (MP) joints

Figure 5-46. Metatarsal Block (Foot/Toe)

Injection between metatarsal bones

B. Sullivan '01

Chapter 19: Anesthesia: Local/Regional Anesthesia:
Standard Approach To Blocks
MAJ James Reed, AN, USA & MAJ Leland Bradley Morgans, AN, USA

A. For the rest of this section, the following equipment will be referred to as **Standard Equipment** in the *What you Need* paragraph:
1. An antiseptic prepping solution (povidone-iodine or alcohol)
2. Appropriate sized syringe, 25 or 27 gauge needle
3. Local anesthetic

B. For the rest of this section, the following rationale will be referred to as **Standard Contraindications** in the *What Not To Do* paragraph, unless otherwise indicated: Local anesthetics should be avoided in patients reporting allergies to them.

C. For the rest of this section, the following rationale will be referred to as **Standard Complications** in the *What Not To Do* paragraph, unless otherwise indicated: Tissue ischemia and necrosis. Large volumes of local anesthetics can lead to mechanical compression and ischemia.

Chapter 19: Anesthesia: Local/Regional Anesthesia:
Nerve Blockade of the Hand and Wrist
MAJ James Reed, AN, USA & MAJ Leland Bradley Morgans, AN, USA

When: This blockade is particularly valuable when you need to maintain some motor function during surgery. Blockade will produce sensory loss in their hand, and motor loss in the intrinsic muscles of the hand, but not loss of the extension or flexion of the hand or wrist. If complete sensory and motor blockade is required, brachial plexus blockade is a more acceptable alternative.

What You Need: Standard Equipment: In order to achieve analgesia of the entire hand and wrist the ulnar, both the median and radial nerves must be blocked.

Figure 5-47. Dermatomes of Cutaneous Innervation of the Hand

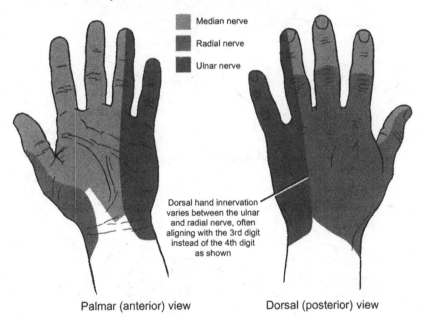

Median nerve
Radial nerve
Ulnar nerve

Dorsal hand innervation varies between the ulnar and radial nerve, often aligning with the 3rd digit instead of the 4th digit as shown

Palmar (anterior) view   Dorsal (posterior) view

Chapter 19: Anesthesia: Local/Regional Anesthesia:
Nerve Blockade of the Hand and Wrist: Ulnar Nerve Block at the Wrist

MAJ James Reed, AN, USA & MAJ Leland Bradley Morgans, AN, USA

What To Do:
1. Assemble equipment
2. Prep area
3. Block the palmar branch by inserting a 25 or 27 gauge needle at 90° to the skin, lateral to the flexor carpi ulnaris tendon and medial to the ulnar artery. This artery can be palpated with the wrist in flexion.
4. At 1-1.5cm in depth, slowly inject up to 5mL of local anesthetic solution.
5. Withdraw the needle to the subcutaneous tissue and redirect the needle laterally around the ulnar aspect of the flexor carpi ulnaris, injecting an additional 5mL of local anesthetic solution as you proceed. This will block the dorsal branch of the ulnar nerve laterally.

What Not To Do: See Standard Approach To Blocks B & C

Contraindications: Ulnar nerve blocks should be avoided when significant paresthesia can be elicited easily by palpating the nerve.

Figure 5-48. Ulnar Nerve Block (at the Wrist), Ventral Approach

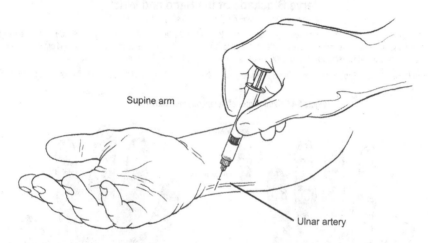

Supine arm

Ulnar artery

Figure 5-49. Ulnar Nerve Block (at the Wrist), Medial Approach

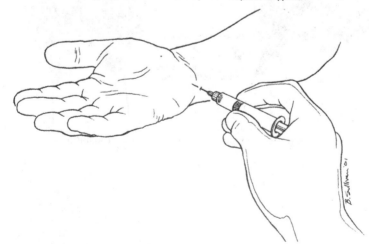

Chapter 19: Anesthesia: Local/Regional Anesthesia:
Nerve Blockade of the Hand and Wrist: Median Nerve Block at the Wrist

MAJ James Reed, AN, USA & MAJ Leland Bradley Morgans, AN, USA

What To Do:
1. Assemble equipment
2. Prep area
3. Have the patient flex their wrist against resistance to identify the palmaris longus tendon. If present, insert a 25 or 27 gauge needle just lateral to the tendon. If the palmaris longus is absent, insert the needle 1 cm medial to the ulnar border of flexor carpi radialis tendon. Insert the needle past the flexor reticulum, which is indicated by increased resistance. Then slowly advanced the needle an additional 2-3 millimeters.
4. If paresthesia is elicited, then slowly inject 5mL of local anesthetic solution. In the event of resistance to injection or pain (could be due to intraneural injection) stop and withdraw the needle 2 millimeters before continuing
5. Withdraw the needle to the subcutaneous level while injecting an additional 2-3mL of local anesthetic solution.

What Not To Do: See Standard Approach To Blocks B & C

Contraindications: Do not use a median nerve block in the presence of carpal tunnel syndrome.

Figure 5-50. Median Nerve Block at the Wrist

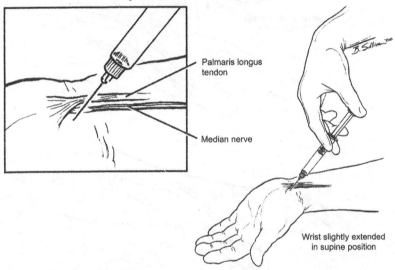

Palmaris longus tendon

Median nerve

Wrist slightly extended in supine position

Chapter 19: Anesthesia: Local/Regional Anesthesia:
Nerve Blockade of the Hand and Wrist: Radial Nerve Block at the Wrist

MAJ James Reed, AN, USA & MAJ Leland Bradley Morgans, AN, USA

What To Do:
1. Assemble equipment
2. Prep area
3. Extend the thumb against resistance, revealing the "anatomical snuff box," which is the area just above the styloid process of the radius.
4. Insert a 25 or 27 gauge needle close to the tendon of extensor pollicis longus over the styloid process of the radius. Direct it subcutaneously across the dorsum of the wrist towards the ulnar border. Inject 5-7mL of local anesthetic solution as the needle is advanced.
5. Withdraw the needle to the insertion point and redirect it across the tendon of the flexor pollicis brevis and inject and additional 2-3mL of solution subcutaneously.

What Not To Do: See Standard Approach To Blocks B & C

Figure 5-51. Radial Nerve Block at the Wrist

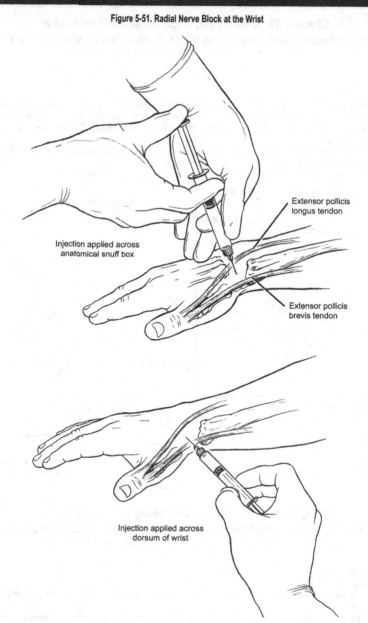

Injection applied across
anatomical snuff box

Extensor pollicis
longus tendon

Extensor pollicis
brevis tendon

Injection applied across
dorsum of wrist

Chapter 19: Anesthesia: Local/Regional Anesthesia:
Nerve Blockade of the Foot and Ankle

MAJ James Reed, AN, USA & MAJ Leland Bradley Morgans, AN, USA

When: Surgery of the toes and distal foot. The term "ankle block" denotes the location at which the local anesthetic solution is applied. This block is not suitable for surgery of the ankle. Rarely will all 5 nerves require blockade. Surgery of the medial foot requires blockade of the superficial, deep peroneal, saphenous, and tibial nerves, but not the sural nerve. Surgery of the lateral aspect of the foot requires blockade of all but the saphenous nerve.

What You Need: Standard Equipment: Complete ankle blockade is accomplished by injecting and blocking all five nerves that supply the foot. The nervous supply to the foot is made of 5 terminals: superficial n., deep peroneal n., saphenous n., sural n., and tibial n.

What Not To Do: See Standard Approach To Blocks B & C

Figure 5-52. Dermatomes of Cutaneous Innervation of the Foot

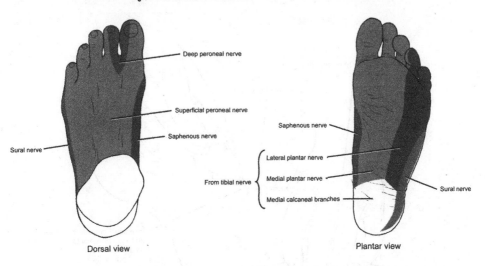

Dorsal view   Plantar view

Chapter 19: Anesthesia: Local/Regional Anesthesia: Nerve Blockade of the Foot and Ankle: Superficial Peroneal and Saphenous Nerve Blocks

MAJ James Reed, AN, USA & MAJ Leland Bradley Morgans, AN, USA

What To Do:

1. Assemble equipment
2. Prep area
3. These 2 nerves can be anesthetized by injecting a "ring" of local anesthetic solution in the subcutaneous tissue.
4. Locate the upper aspect of the medial malleolus and inject a 10mL ring of local anesthetic solution while advancing the needle toward the medial border of the lateral malleolus.

Figure 5-53. Superficial Peroneal Nerve Block

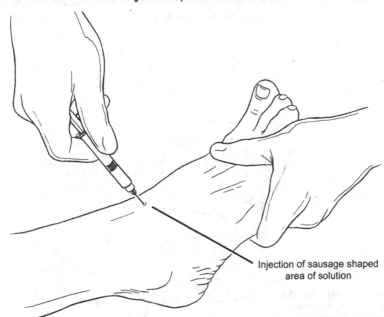

Injection of sausage shaped area of solution

Figure 5-54. Saphenous Nerve Block

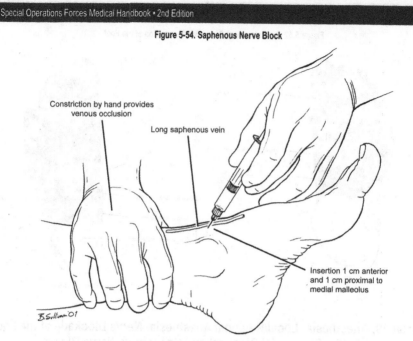

Constriction by hand provides venous occlusion

Long saphenous vein

Insertion 1 cm anterior and 1 cm proximal to medial malleolus

B. Sullivan '01

Chapter 19: Anesthesia: Local/Regional Anesthesia: Nerve Blockade of the Foot and Ankle: Sural Nerve Block

MAJ James Reed, AN, USA & MAJ Leland Bradley Morgans, AN, USA

What To Do:
1. Assemble equipment
2. Prep area
3. Rotate the leg medially to gain access to the lateral posterior aspect of the foot.
4. Inject 5mL of local anesthetic solution on the lateral side of the foot between the Achilles tendon and the posterior lateral malleolus.

Figure 5-55. Sural Nerve Block

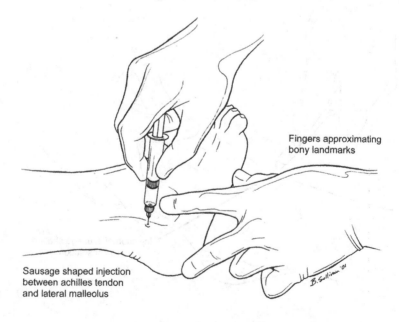

Fingers approximating bony landmarks

Sausage shaped injection between achilles tendon and lateral malleolus

B. Sullivan '01

Chapter 19: Anesthesia: Local/Regional Anesthesia:
Nerve Blockade of the Foot and Ankle: Deep Peroneal Nerve Block
MAJ James Reed, AN, USA & MAJ Leland Bradley Morgans, AN, USA

What To Do:
1. Assemble equipment
2. Prep area
3. On the dorsal surface of the foot, locate the dorsalis pedis artery and the extensor hallucis longus tendon (tendon to the great toe).
4. Insert the needle between the dorsalis pedis a. and the extensor hallucis longus. If a paresthesia of the great or second toe is obtained, inject 5mL of local anesthetic solution.
5. If a paresthesia is not obtained, advance the needle until bone is contacted and inject the 5mL of local anesthetic solution in a fan-like manner while withdrawing the needle.

Figure 5-56. Deep Peroneal Nerve Block

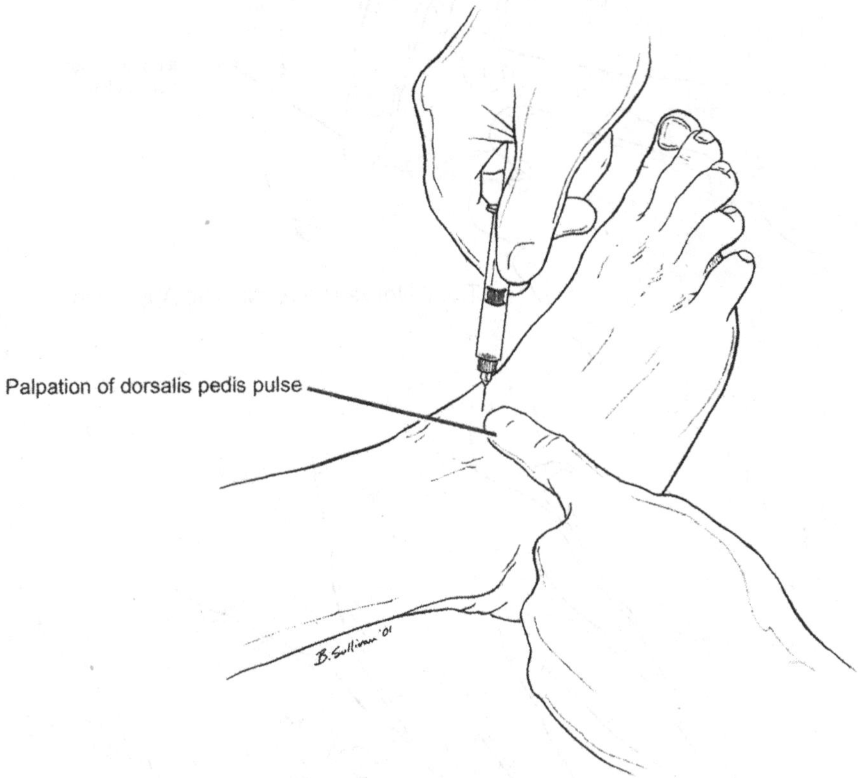

Palpation of dorsalis pedis pulse

B. Sullivan '01

Chapter 19: Anesthesia: Local/Regional Anesthesia:
Nerve Blockade of the Foot and Ankle: Tibial Nerve Block
MAJ James Reed, AN, USA & MAJ Leland Bradley Morgans, AN, USA

What To Do:
1. Assemble equipment
2. Prep area
3. Rotate the leg laterally to gain access to the medial posterior aspect of the foot.
4. Locate the posterior tibial artery. The tibial nerve lies posterior and lateral to the tibial artery.
5. Insert the needle toward the artery, anterior to the Achilles tendon and posterior to the medial malleolus, injecting 5mL of local anesthetic solution in a fan-like manner while withdrawing the needle.

Figure 5-57. Tibial Nerve Block, Classic and Sustentaculum Tali Approaches

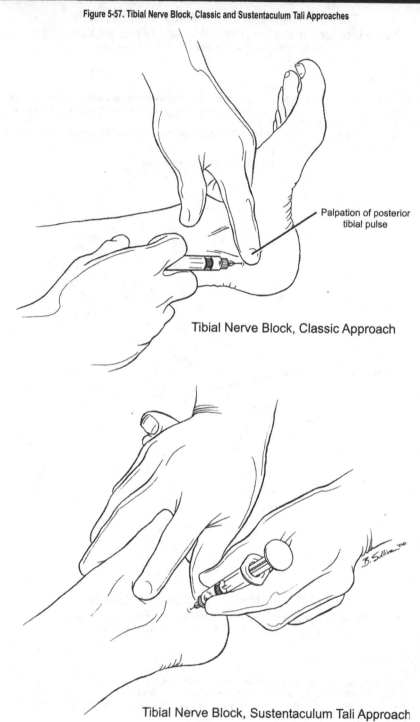

Palpation of posterior tibial pulse

Tibial Nerve Block, Classic Approach

Tibial Nerve Block, Sustentaculum Tali Approach

Chapter 19: Anesthesia: Local/Regional Anesthesia: Axillary Blockade

MAJ James Reed, AN, USA & MAJ Leland Bradley Morgans, AN, USA

Achieve regional anesthesia for surgery below the elbow by brachial plexus blockade using the axillary approach. The nervous and vascular structures of the upper arm are encased within a perivascular sheath, a tubular structure surrounding the nerves and vessels. Introducing local anesthetic solution into this sheath at the axillary level affords excellent blockade below the elbow, and many times, satisfactory anesthesia of the elbow itself.

When: For any surgical procedure of the forearm or hand; upon surgeon request or in high-risk patients where a general anesthetic would be deleterious.

What You Need: Equipment: 22 gauge needle, 60cc syringe, tourniquet, sterile gloves, anesthetic agent(s), **epinephrine**, **bicarb**, razor, prep solution and resuscitation equipment (including oxygen). local anesthetic (*see Table 5-41*)

1. Total of 50-60mL needed: 40mL to fill the plexus sheath and an additional 10-20mL are needed for ring block and musculocutaneous nerve.
2. Add 1:200,000 **epinephrine** as a marker to assist in detecting accidental intravascular injection (add 0.25cc of 1:1000 **epinephrine** to each 50mL of local for a 1:200,000 solution).
3. Combinations: Combining a fast onset local anesthetic with another of long duration is done at times to take advantage of both of these desirable characteristics. Remember to not exceed maximum dosage levels.
4. Add **NaHCO3**, 1mEq per 10mL of local anesthetic solution for all agents (except bupivacaine, where 0.1mEq is added) to accelerate the onset of block. Choice of local anesthetic solution and the appropriate concentration depends on nerves to be blocked, desired onset time and desired duration of action.

Table 5-41. Regional Anesthetics

Drug	Concentration	Onset (min)	Duration (w/epi)	Max Dose-w/epi
Chloroprocaine	2-3%	10-20 min	60-120 min	1000mg-14mg/kg
Lidocaine	0.5-1.5%	15-30 min	150-180 min	500mg-7mg/kg
Mepivacaine	1-1.5%	15-30 min	180-240 min	500mg-7mg/kg
Bupivacaine	0.25-0.5%	20-30 min	180-360 min	225mg-3mg/kg
Tetracaine	0.2-0.25%	10-20 min	240-360 min	200mg

Note: Add **epinephrine** 1:200,000 to all mixtures

What To Do:
1. Basic set up for general anesthesia; *see Part 5: Specialty Areas: Chapter 19: Total Intravenous Anesthesia*
2. Prepare patient with appropriate premedications and monitors. *See Part 5: Specialty Areas: Chapter 19: Total Intravenous Anesthesia.*
3. Patient position: Supine, with head turned away from side to be blocked and the arm abducted ~90°. The forearm is flexed to 90° and externally rotated so the dorsum of the hand lies on the table and the forearm is parallel to the long axis of the patient's body. Do not place the hand of the arm to be blocked under the head. This hyperabduction obliterates the brachial artery pulse.
4. Paresthesia technique
   a. Use the index finger of the non-dominant hand to palpate the axillary artery as high up into the axilla as possible.
   b. Prep the area with razor if needed and with povidone-iodine swabs. Place a skin wheal over the artery proximal to the index finger.
   c. Look for paresthesias by inserting the needle through the skin wheal and directing it slightly above or below the arterial pulsation (attempting to stimulate the median, ulnar or radial nerve).
   d. Angle the needle to almost the same plane as the sheath. When the patient reports a paresthesia, aspirate, then inject 2-3mL of local anesthesia as a test. The paresthesia should fade. If so, continue to inject, aspirating the syringe every 5mL to check for intravascular injection, until a volume of 40cc has been injected.
   e. Intense burning associated with the injection of a small volume indicates possible intraneural injection. STOP INJECTING.
   f. Use the remaining 10mL to block the musculocutaneous, intercostobrachiales and medial cutaneous nerves. Prep the areas as in 4b.
   g. Musculocutaneous nerve: Insert the needle into the body of the coracobrachialis muscle until it touches the humerus, withdraw 2-3mm, then inject 5mL of the remaining anesthetic solution into the muscle.
   h. Intercostobrachiales and medial brachial cutaneous n.: Subcutaneously direct the needle inferiorly and superiorly to the insertion site for the musculocutaneous block and inject the remaining 5-10mL solution as a ring block.
5. After placing the block, bring the arm to the side and massage the axilla for a few minutes to spread the anesthetic. Maintain pressure over auxiliary injection site to decrease bleeding and keep agent high in axilla.

6. Continually assess the patient for signs of systemic absorption of the anesthetic and possible toxic reaction. Elevated vital signs of excitement are seen at lower blood levels of anesthetic, progressing to CNS depression as blood levels rise. Warning signs include: Patient reporting metallic taste in mouth or circumoral paresthesias, tinnitus, drowsiness/dizziness/disorientation, visual disturbance, slurred speech, generalized twitching and tremors.

7. Always be prepared to provide airway and cardiovascular support whenever administering brachial plexus blockade.

8. Assess the block - "Push, pull, pinch, pinch" (support patient's arm during these maneuvers!)

PUSH: The patient attempts to extend the arm. Inability to do so implies block of the radial n.

PULL: Attempt to flex the arm at the elbow; inability to do so implies musculocutaneous n. block.

PINCH: The hand at the base of the thenar eminence (prominence at the base of the thumb); sensory loss implies median n. block.

PINCH: The base of the little finger; sensory loss implies ulnar n. block. Inability to spread fingers against resistance implies ulnar n. block.

9. Apply tourniquet above level of surgery prior to the operation.

What Not To Do:

Contraindications: Uncooperative patient/refusal, bleeding disorders, infection at injection site or allergies to local anesthetics.

Complications: Toxic systemic absorption/intravascular injection that can lead to cardiovascular collapse. Hematoma at injection site from axillary artery puncture. Accidental injection of agent into the nerves.

Chapter 19: Anesthesia: Local Anesthetics/Regional Anesthesia: Intravenous Regional Anesthesia (Bier Block)

MAJ Leland Bradley Morgans, AN, USA

<u>Intravenous Regional Anesthesia (Bier block):</u> Achieve regional anesthesia for surgery of the arm.

When: This technique is beneficial for short surgical procedures of the arm and allow for quick return of function and sensation of the extremity. This technique provides a simple approach for anesthesia of the arm compared to the axillary block.

What You Need: Lidocaine 0.5% without epinephrine, 2 heparin locks, pneumatic tourniquet (manual BP cuff), Esmarch wrap (rubber bandage), forceps clamp, 50mL syringe, monitoring equipment for BP, ECG, HR and pulse oximetry. Emergency airway equipment and a benzodiazepine such as **diazepam** or **midazolam** are also required in case of local anesthetic toxicity seizures.

What To Do:

1. Place an IV heparin lock in the non-surgical arm for access to provide sedation if needed, IV fluids, or quick treatment of local anesthetic toxicity seizures.

2. Test the pneumatic BP cuff prior to procedure for leaks and proper function.

3. Place IV catheter with heparin lock in injured extremity as distal as possible. The hand is preferred.

4. Place pneumatic tourniquet/BP cuff proximal to site of surgery

5. Elevate extremity and exsanguinate by wrapping with rubber bandage (Esmarch)

6. Inflate pneumatic tourniquet and clamp at 2.5x systolic BP or 300mmHg. Clamp tubing with forceps between cuff and release valve for added safety.

7. Release rubber bandage, leaving exsanguinated extremity with inflated tourniquet

8. Inject **lidocaine** 0.5% 50mL via indwelling IV catheter. Onset of anesthesia takes 5-10 minutes, so you should test for sensation before starting procedure.

9. Consider narcotics PRIOR to deflation as local anesthetic washes out and pain will return

Chapter 20: Dive Medicine: Submersion Induced Pulmonary Edema
MAJ Robert Price, MC, USA

Introduction: Submersion induced pulmonary edema (SIPE) is an important phenomenon in special operations divers, especially when the training or their mission involves surface swims in cold water. The condition is most commonly encountered during high intensity training schools (BUDS, BRC/ARS, MCD, etc). SIPE is a condition of stress failure of the pulmonary capillary bed. The mechanisms for this failure are likely related to exertion and vascular volume changes of immersion. Immersion causes peripheral vasoconstriction, which in turn increases central vascular volume. The increased hydrostatic pressure and reduction in the effect of gravity first causes fluid to accumulate in the interstitial tissues of the lungs and then into the alveoli themselves. The increased cardiac output associated with intense exertion elevates the pulmonary pressures and coupled with increased vascular volume overwhelms the pulmonary circulatory system resulting in interstitial pulmonary edema and subsequent shortness of breath, fatigue, and coughing up pink frothy sputum. Investigations into the nature of SIPE have shown this to be a non-infectious and non-inflammatory, but potentially life-threatening if unrecognized. Contributing factors include cold water immersion, over hydration pre-dive, heavy exercise, and negative pressure breathing, all of which increase central blood volume.

Subjective: Symptoms
Coughing, bloody sputum, visible shortness of breath out of proportion to level of exertion
Focused History: *Have you felt short of breath?* (Shortness of breath out of proportion to perceived level of exertion is important.) *Have you been coughing up bloody sputum?* (This symptom can support SIPE, pneumonia, or AGE.) *Did you feel the symptoms at depth? Did you have a controlled ascent?* (Panic from dyspnea at depth can result in uncontrolled ascent with increased risk of AGE.) *Have you had fevers, chills, or any cold symptoms?* (These symptoms would be more supportive of pneumonia.)

Objective: Signs
Using Basic Tools: Rales and rhonchi on lung auscultation, brief period of confusion and ataxia preceding unconsciousness, which is often the 1st sign. Hypoxia can be assessed with a pulse oximeter.
Using Advanced Tools: CXR may show unilateral or bilateral diffuse airspace opacities, which resolve quickly (within 24-48hrs) with supportive treatment (unlike pneumonia).

Assessment:
Differential Diagnosis:
Arterial gas embolism (AGE): History of rapid or uncontrolled ascent following breathing compressed gas. *See Part 6: Operational Environment: Chapter 20: Decompression Injuries: Pulmonary Over Inflation Syndrome (including Arterial Gas Embolism)*
Sea water aspiration: History of near drowning or other consistent with aspiration of sea water
Carbon monoxide poisoning: History consistent with increased risk of CO poisoning (eg, bad gas mix, proximity to exhaust fumes). *See Part 5: Specialty Areas: Chapter 17: Carbon Monoxide Poisoning*
Decompression sickness: History of diving consistent with risk for DCS. *See Part 6: Operational Environment: Chapter 20: Decompression Injuries: Decompression Sickness (Caisson Disease, the "Bends")*
Trauma: History or physical signs of trauma
Shock and other causes of hypoxia: History or physical signs to indicate increased risk of shock
Pneumonia: History of symptoms and signs to suggest URI or pneumonia prior to submersion. *See Part 4: Organ Systems: Chapter 3: Pneumonia*

Plan:
Treatment: Remove patient from the water, start oxygen and bronchodilators (eg, **albuterol** inhaler 2-3 puffs q4-6h). Primary: Perform ABCs of resuscitation. Place patient on 100% oxygen, maintain oxygen until full recovery, and then slowly wean. Monitor for 24-48 hours for residual symptoms. If patient was breathing compressed gas, treat for an AGE until proven otherwise. Evaluate to ensure no underlying cardiac problems. Patient may benefit symptomatically from diuretics (eg, **furosemide** 20-40mg IV x 1). Symptoms usually resolve spontaneously upon removal from the water but cases requiring intubation have been reported.
Primitive: Perform artificial respiration if patient in respiratory arrest.
Patient Education
General: Educate divers on SIPE. Avoid excessive fluid loading and rapid deep breathing. Have diving regulator checked for appropriate function.
Diet: Normal
Prevention and Hygiene: Educate divers on contributing factors such as over hydration, over exertion and encourage adequate thermal protection to mitigate the effects of vasoconstriction.
No Improvement/Deterioration: Consult Diving Medical Officer (DMO); treat as AGE and/or cardiopulmonary decompression sickness (chokes).
Follow-up Actions
Return Evaluation: Monitor closely for 24-48 hours for full improvement. If symptoms and CXR do not improve, treat empirically for pneumonia.
Consultation Criteria: Any residual symptoms need to be evaluated by a DMO.

Chapter 20: Dive Medicine: Barotrauma: Barotrauma to Ears
MAJ Robert Price, MC, USA

Introduction: The volume of a gas changes inversely to air pressure; gas expands as pressure drops and compresses as pressure rises. An enclosed, gas-filled cavity in the body is susceptible to injury from the expansion or compression of the gas if it is not able to equalize to the outside pressure. The middle ear is the most frequently injured body part. There are 3 types of ear barotraumas: external ear barotrauma (pinna to tympanic membrane [TM]); middle ear barotrauma (TM to cochlea) and inner ear barotrauma (round or oval window rupture, perilymph fistula). **Note:** All tables in this chapter refer to the Treatment Tables in the US Navy Diving Manual and are included at the end of this chapter. All references to paragraphs within the Treatment Tables refer to paragraphs in the Navy Diving Manual, Revision 6.

Subjective: Symptoms

Sudden loss of balance, nausea and vomiting, tinnitus, and hearing loss are seen in all 3 of conditions listed:

External ear barotrauma: Diving with ear plugs, tight fitting diving hood, cerumen impaction or some other object in the external ear canal (EAC) creates a confined space between the object and TM. This space is compressed with increasing depth, creating a vacuum, tugging the sensitive TM and creating pain. Divers feel pain during descent, typically at shallow depths.

Middle ear barotrauma: Pain, usually on descent (squeeze) but may be on ascent (reverse squeeze); caused by the eustachian tube (ET) failing to equalize pressure. ET dysfunction is often secondary to upper respiratory infection or allergies. If a diver continues deeper despite the pain, blood may fill the middle ear cavity and cause temporary conductive hearing loss and give a feeling of fullness in the ear, continued pressure may result in TM rupture. If the TM ruptures, the pain will stop but nausea and vomiting may ensue as cold water enters the middle ear and causes vertigo. The dive should be immediately aborted after a TM rupture. Alternatively, a prolonged vacuum in the middle ear will be relieved with a serous effusion seeping from lining tissues. Symptoms of a serous effusion are mild pain, popping sensations in the ear and temporary conductive hearing loss.

Inner ear barotrauma: Often associated with, and usually secondary to middle ear barotrauma. Following a forceful Valsalva, the diver may have roaring tinnitus and sensorineural hearing loss. If the vestibular symptoms are present for less than 1 minute, the vertigo is considered transient. Vertigo underwater is a life-threatening situation and the injured diver needs immediate assistance to the surface. If the vertigo lasts for more than 1 minute, the vertigo is considered persistent.

Objective: Signs

Using Basic Tools: 512Hz Tuning fork

Using Advanced Tools: Otoscope with insufflation bulb

External ear barotrauma: Inflammation of the TM unrelieved by Valsalva, edema or blood in the EAC, very tender in EAC and on tragus, severe cases have TM irritation and/or rupture, cerumen impaction is sometimes seen.

Middle ear barotrauma: TM redness, hemorrhage or rupture; blood behind TM; middle ear barotrauma graded on Teed Classification; serous effusions are typically amber-colored fluid and sometimes have bubbles behind the TM.

Table 6-1. Teed Classification

Grade	Clinical Description	Expected Healing Time
Teed 0	Symptoms without otoscopic signs	May dive same day
Teed 1	Diffuse redness and retractions of the TM	1-2 days
Teed 2	Grade 1 plus slight hemorrhage within the TM	1-4 days
Teed 3	Grade 1 plus gross hemorrhage with the TM	3-7 days
Teed 4	Dark and slightly bulging TM due to free blood in the middle ear; a fluid level may be visualized behind the TM.	5-12 days
Teed 5	Free hemorrhage into the middle ear with TM perforation; Perforation must be totally healed before diving again.	7-15 days

Inner ear barotrauma: Nausea, vomiting, ataxia, vertigo, tinnitus, sensorineural hearing loss (high frequency loss more common than low), positive fistula test*. TM rupture due to middle ear barotrauma may also be seen.

*Fistula test: Pressurize inner ear using insufflation bulb on otoscope, and evaluate for vertigo to test for round window or oval window rupture. The insufflation bulb can also be used to test for an intact TM.

Assessment:

Differential Diagnosis

External ear barotrauma: Swimmer's ear

Middle ear barotrauma: Viral/bacterial ear infection, upper respiratory infection, allergies, or anatomical causes of eustachian tube dysfunction

Inner ear barotrauma: Tertiary syphilis, Ménière's disease, arterial gas embolism, inner ear decompression sickness

Plan:

Treatment

External ear barotrauma: Avoid plugs and hoods while diving. Remove from dive status until ear is healed. Keep ear dry. Clean ear of any obstructions. If infection sets in, treat as external otitis (swimmer's ear) with **Cortisporin** otic drops 3-4 drops in affected ear bid x 7 days. To prevent external otitis, a weak acid such as 2% acetic acid and aluminum acetate (Domeboro solution) should be used after showers, swimming, or diving.

Middle ear barotrauma: Remove from dive status until asymptomatic. Use nasal decongestants (eg, **oxymetazoline**) for no more than 5 days or systemic decongestants. The <u>ONLY</u> topical ear drop solution that is safe to use in the setting of perforation is an otic suspension of **ciprofloxacin HCl** and **hydrocortisone** (Cipro HC Otic) 3-4 drops in affected ear bid x 7 days. All other ear drop solutions (Cortisporin) are <u>TOXIC</u> to the mucosa lining the middle ear space and should be avoided in the setting of possible perforation. Avoid exertion and all swimming while TM is healing. Consider empiric use of systemic antibiotics for Teed 3 or higher injury.

Inner ear barotrauma: Remove patient from water and continuously monitor until evaluated by Diving Medical Officer (DMO) or ENT physician (within 72 hrs). Maintain strict bed rest with head slightly elevated. Avoid straining or Valsalva. Do not allow flying until injury is fully healed. Obtain immediate consult with ENT if diver has persistent vertigo and ataxia. A round window or oval window rupture causes permanent disqualification from military diving.

Patient Education

General: Pressure can greatly effect the sensitive tissues in the ear. Time away from pressure is usually enough to allow the ears to heal.

Diet: Normal

Medications: Topical decongestants like oxymetazoline should be not used for more than 5 days continuously due to rebound effect. Do not use topical eardrops when there is a chance the TM is ruptured.

Prevention and Hygiene: Avoid diving hoods, equalize ears often, and avoid forceful Valsalva

No Improvement/Deterioration: Consult ENT or DMO

Follow-up Actions

Return evaluation: Weekly until healed.

Consultation Criteria: Patients with persistent vertigo, loss or significant decrease in hearing, non-healing TM rupture, large TM rupture, or foreign body stuck in EAC should be referred to ENT.

Chapter 20: Dive Medicine: Barotrauma: Other
(Dental, Sinus, GI, Skin, and Face Mask)

MAJ Robert Price, MC, USA

Introduction: The volume of a gas changes inversely to air pressure; gas expands as pressure drops and compresses as pressure rises. An enclosed, gas-filled cavity in the body is susceptible to injury from the expansion or compression of the gas if it cannot equalize to the outside pressure. Middle ear injuries are the most frequent but several other areas are subject to barotrauma, primarily on descent. Dental fillings or caries that have air trapped in the teeth can cause pain called dental barotrauma. The lining of the sinuses can be pulled off the bone allowing the cavity to fill with blood. In very rare circumstances, the bone forming the sinus may fracture. Large amounts of gas in the intestines may expand on ascent and cause intestinal pain (GI distension). Poorly fitting dry suits can have air trapped in folds and wrinkles that will compress at depth, sucking skin in to fill the vacuum (skin barotrauma/suit squeeze). If a diver does not equalize the vacuum in the facemask during descent, a mask squeeze may result.

Subjective: **Symptoms**

Dental barotrauma (barodontalgia): Pain in the teeth can occur on the descent or ascent. A tooth with thin cementum could possibly implode on the descent or explode on the ascent. Often patient cannot point out exact tooth. History typically includes recent fillings or poor dental health.

Sinus barotrauma: Usually occurs in maxillary and frontal sinuses and presents with pain over affected sinus or in maxillary teeth. Blood may be seen in the mask. Pressure on ascent can occur (reverse squeeze), usually secondary to mucosal polyps or plugs (**Note:** Use of topical decongestant prior to diving may increase risk of reverse squeeze.) Ascending or descending to decrease sinus pressure relieves pain. Predisposing conditions include sinusitis, upper respiratory infections, mucosal polyps, deviated septum, nasal polyps, smoking, persistent use of topical decongestants, and allergies.

GI distention: Flatulence and diffuse pain in abdomen (usually mild) present on ascent. History often includes pre-dive carbonated drinks and gas-producing foods.

Skin barotrauma: Pain and bruising on skin in areas of fold from a poorly fitting dry suit

Facemask squeeze: Pain in area of mask, headache, transient blurring vision. History may include diving with goggles instead of mask.

Focused history: *Did you have any tooth pain during your dive? Did you have any pain or pressure in your face on the descent or ascent?* (Symptoms will pertain to the body areas described previously for the various forms of barotrauma.)

Objective: **Signs**

Using Basic Tools:

Sinus barotrauma: Pain over sinus with percussion. Transient, bloody nasal discharge or blood in mask, transillumination of sinus can occasionally reveal fluid in the sinus

GI distention: Tympanic sound on abdominal percussion possible

Skin barotrauma: Bruising on skin typically at folds in the ill-fitting dry suit

Facemask squeeze: Redness or bruising in area of mask seal; peri-orbital bruising/petechiae; conjunctival and scleral hemorrhages

Using Advanced Tools:

Dental barotrauma: Air in tooth chamber on x-ray.

Assessment:

Differential Diagnosis

Dental barotrauma: Sinus barotrauma, tooth abscess

Sinus barotrauma: Sinus infection, dental barotrauma

GI distension: Gastritis, acute abdominal disorders

Skin barotrauma: Rash, bleeding disorders, jellyfish stings

Facemask squeeze: Facial trauma, jellyfish stings

Plan:

Treatment

Primary:

Dental barotrauma: Analgesics. Re-fill the tooth ensuring no air remains in chamber.

Sinus barotrauma: Stop dive and surface slowly, topical and systemic pain relief, as necessary. If bleeding does not stop, pack turbinates with gauze coated in antibiotic ointment in the opening of the affected sinus. If packing material is left in more than one hour, an antibiotic (eg, **amoxicillin/clavulanate** 250mg po q8h) while packing remains in place will decrease risk of colonization by staphylococcus and risk of toxic shock syndrome.

GI distention: Ascend slowly from dive

Skin barotrauma: Analgesics as necessary

Facemask squeeze: Analgesics as necessary

Patient Education

General: Educate patient on the cause of injury. Prevention is possible with all of these injuries.

Dental barotrauma: Practice good oral hygiene. Ensure fillings have no trapped gas pocket.

Sinus barotrauma: Explain how sinuses can become blocked and force blood vessels to leak while under increasing pressure. Avoid diving with URIs, mucosal polyps or allergic symptoms.

GI distension: Encourage flatulence prn on ascent.

Skin barotrauma: Ensure dry suit fits properly.

Facemask squeeze: Equalize mask.

Diet: Normal

Medications: Over-the-counter analgesics as needed. Acetaminophen 500mg po q4-6h prn pain (avoid aspirin and 1st generation NSAIDS if persistent bleeding is present), topical and systemic decongestants prn.

Prevention and hygiene: Do not dive until all symptoms have resolved.

No Improvement/Deterioration: Consult Diving Medical Officer.

Follow-up Actions

Return Evaluation: As needed.

Consultation Criteria: Dental barotrauma requires dental consult prior to returning to diving.

Chapter 20: Dive Medicine: Decompression Injuries: Decompression Sickness (Caisson Disease, the "Bends")

MAJ Robert Price, MC, USA

Introduction: While breathing air under pressure (ie, underwater), nitrogen is dissolved into body tissues. Increased pressure and prolonged exposure saturates these tissues with nitrogen. When the body is decompressed, the nitrogen comes out of solution to form bubbles in the vasculature or tissues. When the body is decompressed too fast in relation to the nitrogen load (based on time and depth of dive; listed extensively in the Navy Diving Tables), too many bubbles can form. These bubbles may precipitate out into the vascular system, skin, lungs, ears and other tissues causing a variety of symptoms that are categorized into Type I (mild) and Type II (severe) Decompression Sickness (DCS). Any neurological symptom is classified as Type II DCS. Spinal symptoms (neurological) are common in DCS associated with diving. Cerebral symptoms are common from rapid decompression at high altitudes (ie, pilot ejecting at altitude). Some authors estimate that 30% of people with typical Type I pains can have accompanying Type II symptoms. Most symptoms of DCS occur within the first 24 hours of surfacing. When the caregiver is not sure if the DCS is Type I or II, treat as Type II DCS. The term decompression illness (DCI) includes both DCS and pulmonary over inflation syndromes (POIS), which is discussed in the next section.

Subjective: **Symptoms**

DCS (Type I): Skin itching and rashes; skin marbling or red/purple patches (cutis marmorata - treat as Type II); limb swelling; peau d'orange (skin is dimpled like an orange); most joint and/or muscle pain (classically a deep dull ache)

DCS (Type II): Any Type I symptom can be present plus: various neurological symptoms: numbness, tingling, tremors, paralysis, paresthesia, mental status changes, fatigue, amnesia or bizarre behavior, lightheadedness, poor coordination or incontinence; inner ear symptoms (staggers): ringing in ears, vertigo, hearing loss, dizziness, nausea, or vomiting; cardiopulmonary symptoms (chokes): chest pain (worse with inspiration), tachypnea, cough, irritability, or loss of consciousness; pain in the hip, abdomen, thorax, pelvis or spine. Onset of symptoms must be >10min after surfacing, otherwise treat as an arterial gas embolism (AGE).

Focused History: A thorough dive history is essential to determine if the diver had adequate time and depth to make it possible that their symptoms are due to DCS. *How long was your dive? What was your deepest depth?* (identify risk of decompression sickness) *What kind of dive gear were you using? Did you have any problems during your dive? When did your symptoms begin? Did you have any other dives in the previous 12 hours?* (increased risk of decompression sickness) *If so, what was your surface interval? Did you exceed your dive table?* (identify missed decompression requirement from previous dive and increased risk of decompression sickness)

Objective: **Signs**

Using Basic Tools: Perform a complete dive history and neurological exam per the example in the appendix. Numbness, pain, weakness or paralysis of limbs, diminished or absent reflexes, decreased cognitive function, poor coordination, ataxia, hearing loss, vomiting, tachypnea, coughing; unconsciousness. Auscultate: For crackles in lung fields.

Using Advanced Tools: CXR to rule out pneumothorax.

Assessment

Differential Diagnosis:

Arterial gas embolism: History of uncontrolled ascent with symptoms. Neurological symptoms occurring within 10 minutes of surfacing should be treated as AGE. *See Part 6: Operational Environment: Chapter 20: Decompression Injuries: Pulmonary Over Inflation Syndrome (including Arterial Gas Embolism)*

Myocardial infarction: *See Part 4: Organ Systems: Chapter 1: Acute Coronary Syndrome (Acute Myocardial Infarction and Unstable Angina)*

Trauma: Physical exam may shows signs of trauma, decompression sickness and or arterial gas embolism may also be present.

Pulmonary embolus: *See Part 6: Operational Environment: Chapter 30: Decompression Injuries: Pulmonary Over Inflation Syndrome (including Arterial Gas Embolism) & Part 4: Organ Systems: Chapter 3: Deep Vein Thrombosis and Pulmonary Embolism*

Others (eg, musculoskeletal injuries): History of pain prior to diving. Prior history of injury with swelling and decreased circulation may increase subsequent risk of decompression injury.

Plan:

Treatment

Primary

1. 100% oxygen immediately.
2. Hyperbaric oxygen (HBO) recompression therapy ASAP. *See Figures 6-1, 6-3, 6-4 and 6-5 in this chapter.* For an unconscious diver, *see Figure 6-2.*
3. Complete neurological exam prior to recompression if symptoms allow. Otherwise, perform exam at depth.
4. Pregnancy test for all women of childbearing age. If patient is pregnant, benefit of recompression treatment needs to outweigh risks to unborn child (possible: retrolental fibroplasia, in utero death, birth defects).
5. If transportation to HBO chamber is necessary, transport supine and fly below 1,000 ft or pressurize the cabin to below 1,000 ft. If transporting on land, avoid mountain areas if possible (exacerbates DCS symptoms). Use fluid instead of air in bulbs on Foley, ET tube, etc. to reduce risk of rupture with pressure changes.
6. Ensure patient remains well hydrated. Fully conscious patients may be given fluids by mouth. 1-2L of water, juice or non carbonated drink, over the course of a Treatment Table 5 or 6, is usually sufficient. Stuporous or unconscious patients should always be given IV fluids (normal saline at a rate of 75-125cc/hr). If the patient is obviously dehydrated, an initial 1L bolus of normal saline may be given (for an otherwise healthy patient). No Ringer's lactate until patient is urinating. Keep fluids running so urine is clear and >30cc/hour. Catheterize patients unable to urinate. Keep patient warm and have them avoid exertion during recompression.
7. Surface if ACLS is needed and can be administered. Operational chambers are not usually equipped or approved for ACLS treatment. Follow algorithm at end of this section (*See Figure 6-1*) for no improvement or deterioration. If it appears that the patient has died in the chamber, a qualified medical person who may examine and pronounce someone dead must be consulted prior to aborting the recompression treatment. If treatment is aborted, chamber should surface as early as possible at a rate that ensures inside tender is not at risk for DCS.

Alternate: Submarine escape pod may be used if no hyperbaric chamber is available. 100% oxygen.

Primitive: 100% oxygen. In-water recompression (extremely risky; follow "In Water Recompression" instructions in Navy Diving Manual, Revision 6, page 20-11).

Patient Education

General: Recompression and hyperbaric oxygen is the treatment of choice for DCS. It is strongly recommended that pregnant women should not dive. Patient should not fly for at least 72 hours following successful recompression treatment.

Diet: Continue taking in clear fluids. Urine should be clear and of adequate volume (30cc/hr). Eat solid foods as tolerated.

Prevention and Hygiene: Follow decompression tables, stay fit, avoid alcohol, avoid trauma, and limit medications. Patient should remain at recompression chamber facility for 6 hours, and be within one hour of chamber for 24 hours following recompression treatment in case further treatment is needed.

No Improvement/Deterioration: Return for immediate reevaluation.

Follow-up Actions:

All patients with decompression injury or arterial gas embolism should be evaluated by a diving medical officer prior to returning to diving duty to verify resolution of signs and symptoms and to rule out predisposing factors that may have increased patients risk for DCS or AGE. In general, patients with Type II DCS or AGE should not return to diving for at least 4 weeks. Patients with Type I DCS should not return to diving for 7-14 days after treatment depending upon the severity of the symptoms and time to relief of symptoms during treatment.

Return Evaluation: If residual symptoms are present, additional recompression treatments may be performed AFTER consult and approval from a Diving Medical Officer (DMO). Patients should be evaluated by a Diving Medical Officer prior to return to diving duty to assess potential underlying

Consultation Criteria: DMO should be consulted immediately after a dive injury is identified. Any residual symptoms should be discussed with a DMO and appropriate medical specialist (ie, neurologist).

Evacuation: As soon as patient is stable. Comply with warnings about altitude.

Figure 6-1. Treatment of Arterial Gas Embolism or Decompression Sickness

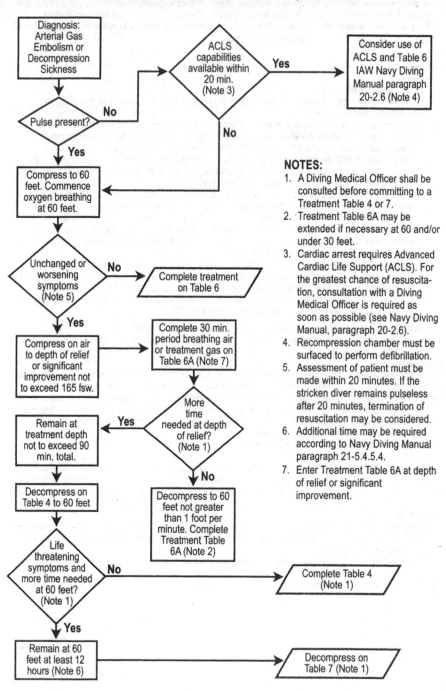

NOTES:

1. A Diving Medical Officer shall be consulted before committing to a Treatment Table 4 or 7.
2. Treatment Table 6A may be extended if necessary at 60 and/or under 30 feet.
3. Cardiac arrest requires Advanced Cardiac Life Support (ACLS). For the greatest chance of resuscitation, consultation with a Diving Medical Officer is required as soon as possible (see Navy Diving Manual, paragraph 20-2.6).
4. Recompression chamber must be surfaced to perform defibrillation.
5. Assessment of patient must be made within 20 minutes. If the stricken diver remains pulseless after 20 minutes, termination of resuscitation may be considered.
6. Additional time may be required according to Navy Diving Manual paragraph 21-5.4.5.4.
7. Enter Treatment Table 6A at depth of relief or significant improvement.

Chapter 20: Dive Medicine: Decompression Injuries:
Pulmonary Over inflation Syndrome (including Arterial Gas Embolism)
MAJ Robert Price, MC, USA

Introduction: Pulmonary Over Inflation Syndrome (POIS) or pulmonary barotrauma results typically from gas expanding in the lung as a diver ascends from depth without exhaling. The expanding gas ruptures lung and vascular tissues. Gas can then enter the pleural space (pneumothorax), mediastinum (mediastinal/subcutaneous emphysema), pulmonary venous system (creating emboli) and other tissues. The pulmonary venous emboli return to the left heart, enter the arterial system (arterial gas embolism [AGE]), travel anywhere in the body, block blood flow and cause ischemia. The central nervous system (CNS) and the heart are most susceptible to serious injury from localized hypoxia due to an AGE. As a basic rule, any diver who has obtained a breath of compressed gas at depth from any source, whether diving apparatus or diving bell, and who surfaces unconscious or loses consciousness within 10 minutes of surfacing, must be assumed to be suffering from an AGE.

Subjective: Symptoms
Symptoms: Sudden onset CNS symptoms are most common and include: dizziness, limb weakness or paralysis, hemiparesis, numbness, mental status changes, loss of consciousness, confusion, tingling, poor coordination, ataxia, difficulty speaking, visual disturbances, convulsions, personality changes, urinary retention, abdominal complaints of nausea and/or vomiting. Virtually any CNS symptom may be associated with an AGE. Symptoms of other POIS conditions may also be seen.
Focused History: *How long after surfacing did the symptoms start?* (AGE symptoms usually manifest while surfacing or within 10 minutes of surfacing from a dive.)

Objective: Signs
Using Basic Tools: Follow the neurological examination checklist from the US Navy Diving Manual in Handbook Appendix. Neurological: Numb to: Light/deep touch, pain/temperature, proprioception, vibration, 2-point tactile discrimination; decreased strength or paralysis, including hemiparesis or hemiplegia; diminished reflexes; decreased mental functioning, decreased coordination, abnormal gait. Cardio-pulmonary symptoms: Tracheal deviation, respiratory distress; blood in sputum, ECG changes (4-5%), cardiac arrest, crackles in lungs, decreased breath sounds, tympanic areas in thorax.
Using Advanced Tools: CXR if available to assess for POIS (pneumothorax, air in mediastinum or other tissues). Refer for CT if CXR is unremarkable and clinical picture indicates injury.

Assessment: A history consistent with increased risk of AGE and neurological symptoms is AGE until proven otherwise.
Differential Diagnosis:
Hypoxia: If low level of hypoxia, symptoms may progress over longer period of time with fatigue and confusion, cyanosis, more include visual changes.
Oxygen toxicity: Convulsions, tunnel vision, twitching of facial muscles
Decompression sickness: Focal or general neurological findings, which typically begin later (eg, >10 min and up to hours after a dive).
Non-dive related causes: Hypoglycemia; seizure, near drowning; myocardial infarction. May have specific medical history to suggest increased risk or diagnosis.

Plan
Treatment: See Treatment Tables (*see Figure 6-3, 6-4 and 6-5*) and Unconscious Diver Algorithm (*see Figure 6-2*) at the end of this chapter
Mediastinal/subcutaneous emphysema (POIS without AGE)
1. 100% oxygen.
2. Initial and serial neurological exams to rule out any neurologic changes suggesting AGE.
3. CXR to rule out pneumothorax.
4. If symptoms are severe, recompression to shallowest depth of relief (usually 5-10 ft).
Pneumothorax (POIS without AGE)
1. 100% oxygen as necessary.
2. Initial and serial neurological exams to rule out any neurologic changes suggesting AGE.
3. CXR to determine size and extent of pneumothorax.
4. Severe cases may require decompression by thoracentesis and/or thoracostomy.
5. Hyperbaric oxygen (HBO) recompression is generally not appropriate, and if AGE is suspected, ensure a thoracostomy is performed prior to recompression.
Arterial Gas Embolism (AGE)
Primary:
1. 100% oxygen immediately. Do not let the patient sit up prior to recompression.
2. Hyperbaric oxygen (HBO) recompression therapy as soon as possible.
3. If transportation to HBO chamber is necessary, transport supine, and fly below 1,000 ft or pressurize the cabin to below 1,000 ft. Use fluid, as opposed to air, in bulbs on Foley, ET tube, etc. to reduce risk of rupture with pressure changes.

4. Hydrate patient. Fully conscious patients may be given po fluids: 2L of water, juice or non-carbonated drink, over the course of a Treatment Table 6 (*See Figure 6-4*), is usually sufficient. Stuporous or unconscious patients should always be given IV fluids (normal saline at a rate of 75-125cc/hour). If the patient is dehydrated, give a 1L bolus of normal saline. Keep fluids running so urine is clear and at least 30cc/hour. Ringer's lactate can be used after patient is producing urine. Catheterize patients unable to urinate.

5. Be prepared to immediately treat clinically diagnosed pneumothorax with needle thoracentesis or chest tube while at depth or while surfacing. *See Part 8: Procedures: Chapter 30: Thoracostomy, Needle and Chest Tube*

6. Adjunctive treatment: **Lidocaine** has been shown to be useful in the treatment of AGE. If it is to be used clinically, evidence suggests that an appropriate end-point is attainment of a serum concentration suitable for an anti arrhythmic effect. An initial IV dose of 1mg/kg followed by a continuous infusion of 2-4mg/minute, will typically produce therapeutic serum concentrations. If an IV infusion is not established, IM administration of 4-5mg/kg will typically produce a therapeutic plasma concentration 15 minutes after dosing, lasting for around 90 minutes. Doses greater than those noted previously may be associated with major side effects, including paresthesias, ataxia, and seizures.

Alternative: Submarine escape pod may be used for recompression if no chamber is around, 100% Oxygen

Primitive: In-water recompression (extremely risky; follow "In Water Recompression" instructions in Navy Diving Manual Revision 6, page 20-11), 100% Oxygen

Patient Education

General: An AGE stops blood flow to tissues and organs distal to the blockage. By going back down to pressure, the gas bubbles causing the blockage will shrink to alleviate the AGE. Placing the patient on 100% oxygen will also enhance nitrogen re-absorption and decrease the resulting inflammatory cascade. Rapid recompression is essential to minimize neurological damage.

Activity: Lay supine during travel and recompression to minimize neurological damage.

Diet: Drink fluids to remain hydrated (if able).

Prevention and Hygiene: Avoid diving until cleared by a Diving Medical Officer (DMO).

No Improvement/Deterioration: Neurological symptoms can get worse and AGE can lead to death. Recompression as soon as possible is the best treatment to prevent permanent damage. Return daily for 3 days for assessment of possible residual symptoms.

Follow-up Actions

Return Evaluation: Assess possible residual symptoms daily for 3 days with a comprehensive neuro exam. If residual symptoms are present, additional HBO therapy may be indicated (contact DMO). Physical rehabilitation may be beneficial and neurological follow-up is required. All patients with decompression injury or AGE should be evaluated by a DMO prior to returning to diving duty to verify resolution of signs and symptoms and to rule out predisposing factors that may have increased patients risk for DCS or AGE. In general, patients with Type II DCS or AGE should not return to diving for at least 4 weeks.

Evacuation Consultation Criteria: A DMO should be consulted as soon as possible. Evacuation should be considered as soon as patient is stable. See above for specific transportation requirements for specific injuries.

Chapter 20: Dive Medicine: Decompression Injuries: Treatment Algorithm for Unconscious Divers

MAJ Robert Price, MC, USA

Figure 6-2. Treatment Algorithm for Unconscious Divers

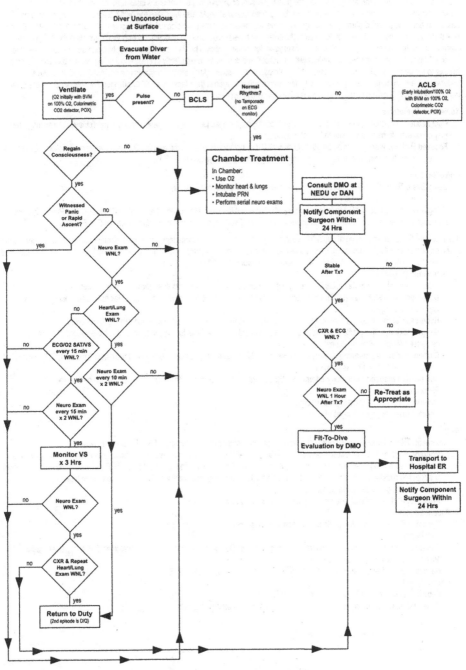

24 Hour Hotlines: NEDU (850) 230-3100; DAN (919) 684-8111

Chapter 20: Dive Medicine: Gas Problems: Hypoxia, including Shallow Water Blackout
MAJ Robert Price, MC, USA

Introduction: Hypoxia is the most common cause of unconsciousness in diving operations. As a diver depletes the residual gas from his tanks or from his lungs (breath hold diving), the partial pressure of oxygen in the diver drops insidiously, causing hypoxia and unconsciousness. The increased ambient pressure during descent and at depth also increases the partial pressure of oxygen and other gases. At depth, the elevated partial pressure of oxygen delays the onset of the physiological, hypercapnia-induced drive to breathe. By the time that "oxygen hunger" induces him to surface, the diver may have stayed too long at depth. He may then have insufficient oxygen to sustain him during ascent as the partial pressure of oxygen decreases quickly. The diver can become hypoxic and unconscious under the surface. This phenomenon is called a "shallow water blackout" and is seen more frequently in breath-hold diving. Most individuals become hypoxic to the point of helplessness at a ppO_2 of 0.11 atmospheres absolute (AtA) and unconscious at a ppO_2 of 0.10. Divers with an underwater breathing apparatus are trained to surface with residual oxygen in their tanks to avoid this danger. For special operations divers, inadequate purging in closed circuit oxygen rebreathers can cause hypoxia.

Subjective: Symptoms
Light-headedness, confusion, tingling, or numbness, confusion, impaired judgment, and vision changes (particularly color vision). There may be no symptoms or signs prior to loss of consciousness.

Focused History: *Were you doing breath hold diving? Did symptoms develop on the ascent? Did your dive rig malfunction?* (Symptoms on the ascent while doing breath holds or technical diving can suggest hypoxia or DCS.)

Objective: Signs
Using Basic Tools: Brief period of confusion and ataxia preceding unconsciousness, which is often the first sign. Hypoxia can be assessed with a pulse oximeter.

Using Advanced Tools: CXR can help determine whether or not there is a Pulmonary Over Inflation Syndrome. *See Part 6: Operational Environment: Chapter 20: Decompression Injuries: Pulmonary Over Inflation Syndrome (including Arterial Gas Embolism)*

Assessment: Symptoms occurring at depth (ie, without ascent from maximum bottom dept) are more consistent with hypoxia, oxygen toxicity or carbon dioxide toxicity (hypercapnia). Unless dive buddy is able to confirm controlled ascent and patient remains conscious, a presumptive diagnosis of arterial gas embolism (AGE) must be made and appropriate treatment initiated.

Differential Diagnosis
AGE: History of uncontrolled ascent or any symptoms occurring with <10 minutes of surfacing must be treated as an AGE.

Decompression sickness (DCS): Dive profile consistent with risk for decompression sickness. May have additional symptoms and signs to suggest DCS

Hypercapnia: Headache, increased heart rate, dizziness, fatigue, rapid breathing, visual and hearing dysfunctions

Oxygen toxicity: Dive profile or diving mixture consistent with increased risk for oxygen toxicity. May have noticed onset of decreased peripheral vision (tunnel vision)

Carbon monoxide poisoning: History of increased risk of exposure (eg, gas tanks being filled near engine exhaust, CO_2 found in divers' air space). Diver's gas analysis

Submersion induced pulmonary edema (SIPE): *See Part 6: Operational Environment: Chapter 20: Submersion Induced Pulmonary Edema*

Trauma: History or physical signs of trauma

Shock: History or physical signs of shock

Plan:
Treatment: Treat all unconscious divers (who were breathing compressed gas) for an AGE until proven otherwise.

Primary: Perform ABCs of resuscitation. Place patient on 100% oxygen, maintain oxygen until full recovery, and then slowly wean. Monitor for 24 hours for residual symptoms. If patient was breathing compressed gas, treat for an AGE until proven otherwise (ie, diver is witnessed passing out secondary to holding breath too long and responds quickly and completely to oxygen treatment). Secure diver's breathing source and tanks for testing.

Primitive: Perform artificial respiration if patient in respiratory arrest

Patient Education
General: Educate divers on hypoxia and shallow water blackout

Diet: Normal

Prevention and Hygiene: Educate and train in diving practices. Do not hyperventilate before a breath hold dive; hyperventilating drives carbon dioxide level even lower.

No Improvement/Deterioration: Consult Diving Medical Officer (DMO); treat as AGE

Follow-up Actions
Return Evaluation: Monitor for 24 hours for full improvement.

Consultation Criteria: Any residual symptoms need to be evaluated by a DMO.

Chapter 20: Dive Medicine: Gas Problems: Oxygen Toxicity

MAJ Robert Price, MC, USA

Introduction: Depth provides circumstances in which oxygen may become toxic to the body. As a diver descends in water, the partial pressure of oxygen (ppO$_2$) increases. The US Navy Diving Manual limits the ppO$_2$ during diving operations based the depth and duration of dives. Exceeding these limits risks an oxygen toxicity injury for the diver. Oxygen toxicity affects various tissues in the body, most notably the pulmonary system and the central nervous system (CNS).

Subjective: Symptoms

Pulmonary: Non-productive cough and difficulty breathing, usually exacerbated on inspiration, progressing to substernal burning and severe pain on inspiration.

CNS: Symptoms and signs are combined in the mnemonic under objective signs.

Focused History: *Did you have any visual changes? Did you hear any ringing in your ears? Are you nauseated? Did you have any tingling or twitching? Are you dizzy?*

Objective: Signs

Using Basic Tools: Pulmonary: Dyspnea, non-productive cough, diminished air exchange (cannot blow out a match or candle 12-14 inches away). CNS: "VENTID-C" is the mnemonic for oxygen toxicity. There is no specific order in which these signs and symptoms appear. The 1st sign may be convulsions. Only one sign may present or several of the signs may present: V- Visual disturbances (blurred or tunnel vision), E- Ears (tinnitus), N- Nausea, T- Twitching/tingling (often seen around the eyes and mouth), I- Irritability, D- Dizziness, C- Convulsions (tonic-clonic), often without warning.

Using Advanced Tools: CXR may reveal thickening of alveolar and interlobular septa and lung edema.

Assessment:

Differential Diagnosis: Decompression sickness (DCS), Arterial Gas Embolism, Pulmonary DCS ("Chokes"), Pulmonary Over Inflation Syndrome. *See Part 6: Operational Environment: Chapter 20: Decompression Injuries: Decompression Sickness (Caisson Disease, the "Bends") & Pulmonary Over Inflation Syndrome (including Arterial Gas Embolism)*

Plan:

Treatment

Pulmonary: Wean patient from oxygen source while maintaining normal respiratory function (pulse ox above 92%.)

CNS: Remove patient from oxygen source and return to room air at sea level. If convulsions occur at depth, slowly bring patient to surface with regulator in mouth while compressing the abdomen.

Patient Education

General: Oxygen can be toxic during long or prolonged exposure and at high partial pressures. When diving with oxygen rigs, a diver needs to stay within the limits established in the Navy Diving Manual.

Diet: Normal

Prevention and Hygiene: Do not return to diving for at least 24 hours and until Diving Medical Officer (DMO) has cleared the diver.

No Improvement/Deterioration: Consult DMO, pulmonologist or neurologist.

Follow-up Actions

Return Evaluation: Follow patient daily to ensure improvement.

Consultation Criteria: If breathing or neurological problems persist, consult DMO, pulmonologist or neurologist.

Note: A diver should never be on 100% oxygen for more than 4 hours (240 minutes) at any depth in any 24-hour period during normal diving operations.

Table 6-2. Single Depth Oxygen Exposure Limits
(from US Navy Diving Manual, Revision 6)

Depth	Maximum Oxygen Time
25 FSW	240 minutes
30 FSW	80 minutes
35 FSW	25 minutes
40 FSW	15 minutes
50 FSW	5 minutes

Table 6-3. Excursion Limits
(from US Navy Diving Manual, Revision 6)

Depth	Maximum Oxygen Time
21-40 FSW	15 minutes
41-50 FSW	5 minutes

Note: CNS oxygen toxicity has not been recorded at levels less than 1.6ATA, ie, if a diver has a reliable max depth of <20fsw, his symptoms are NOT from O$_2$ toxicity.

Chapter 20: Dive Medicine: Gas Problems: Carbon Dioxide Poisoning
MAJ Robert Price, MC, USA

Introduction: Carbon dioxide (CO_2), a colorless, odorless, tasteless gas, is a normal component of the atmosphere that can be toxic in high concentrations. A diver may experience CO_2 poisoning (hypercapnia) even without a deficiency of oxygen. Hypercapnia often results from improperly venting expired CO_2 in chamber or hard hat diving operations. Difficulties with rebreather (closed circuit or semi closed circuit) rigs like the MK 16 and MK 25, which use chemicals to remove CO_2 from the breathing supply, can also lead to hypercapnia. Skip breathing (voluntary hypoventilation) while diving also causes CO_2 to build up in the blood stream. Increased work rates and shivering due to cold water increase CO_2 generation and the chances of CO_2 poisoning. Patients usually recover within 15 minutes by breathing fresh air, but headache, nausea, and dizziness may persist after treatment.

Subjective: Symptoms
Headache, dizziness, confusion, euphoria, unconsciousness. **Note:** A diver may experience no signs or symptoms other than sudden unconsciousness.
Focused History: *Have you been diving with a rebreather? In a chamber/hard hat?* (common causes)

Objective: Signs
Using Basic Tools: Increased rate and depth of respirations, shortness of breath, increased pulse rate. Neuro exam including mini mental status exam (*see Appendices: Table A-6. Mini-Mental Status Exam*): decreased mental status (usually obvious during history questions), decreased balance, decreased strength, numbness in the extremities and unconsciousness; diver may become unconscious underwater and drown.

Assessment:
Differential Diagnosis
Hypoxia: More pronounced fatigue and confusion, more frequent cyanosis, more visual changes
Oxygen toxicity: Convulsions, tunnel vision, twitching of facial muscles
Pulmonary Over Inflation Syndrome (POIS), including Arterial Gas Embolism: Often specific and/or catastrophic neurological findings within 10 minutes of surfacing; pneumothorax, subcutaneous emphysema. *See Part 6: Operational Environment: Chapter 20: Decompression Injuries: Pulmonary Over Inflation (including Arterial Gas Embolism)*
Decompression sickness: Focal or general neurological findings, which typically begin hours after a dive

Plan:
Treatment
1. Treat for AGE or hypoxia if these conditions are suspected or cannot be ruled out. See respective sections in this chapter.
2. Otherwise, have patient rest and breathe fresh air with deep inspirations for about 30 minutes. Significant recovery should quickly occur with the possibility of some residual headache, nausea and dizziness.
3. If patient has not made significant improvement in 30 minutes, consider immediate evacuation and reconsider differential diagnoses.

Patient Education
General: Symptoms should resolve quickly by taking deep breaths of fresh air.
Activity: Rest until all symptoms resolve.
Diet: Drink plenty of replacement fluids.
Prevention and Hygiene: Change CO_2 absorbent material in LAR V prior to each dive. Work slowly in water, especially if water is very cold. Avoid skip breathing. Ventilate frequently if in a chamber or diving surface-supplied rigs.
No Improvement/Deterioration: Return promptly for reevaluation.

Follow-up Actions
Return Evaluation: See one day after treatment to ensure there are no residual symptoms.
Evacuation/Consultation Criteria: Evacuate if patient does not respond to treatment within 30 minutes. Consult a Diving Medical Officer at the earliest opportunity after beginning therapy to confirm diagnosis and treatment plan.

Chapter 20: Dive Medicine: Marine Hazards: Dangerous Marine Life: Venomous Animals
MAJ Robert Price, MC, USA

Introduction: There are a variety of creatures encountered in the water that injure through venom. Some of the venoms are mild and easily treated. Others are very toxic and extremely life-threatening. Divers are often unaware of the type of animal that bit or injured them. The medical caregiver must be prepared for a variety of signs and symptoms. This section does not address all the many creatures that can envenomate humans, but does include the noteworthy ones. Medical personnel routinely covering dives should have a text on dangerous marine life that includes animals that can envenomate.

Subjective: **Symptoms/***Objective* **Signs:** Discussed under each animal species.
Focused History: *Did you see what stung you? What treatment has been provided for you?* (Answers will guide your treatment depending on the animal species involved.)
Highly toxic fish (stonefish, zebrafish, and scorpionfish): Stings by these fish can kill, and are usually accidental--a diver steps on the fish or handles it. These fish carry venom in their spines much like other venomous fish, but their venom is much more toxic. Initial local symptoms: severe pain followed by numbness and/or hypersensitivity around the wound site lasting for days. Generalized reactions include respiratory failure and cardiovascular collapse. There is an antivenin for stonefish toxin that seems

to be somewhat effective for zebrafish and scorpionfish toxins.

Other venomous fish: Most fish envenomate through fin spines, while a diver is stepping on or handling the fish. Venom will continue to flow into the injury while the spine sheath is still in the patient. The venom is usually heat labile and may decompose in hot water (about 115°F). Initial local symptoms: severe pain followed by numbness and/or hypersensitivity around the wound site lasting for hours. General symptoms may include nausea, vomiting, sweating, mild fever, respiratory distress and collapse. Serious anaphylactic reactions are possible.

Stingrays: Stingrays are common in tropical and temperate areas. They hide in the ocean floor sand with eyes and tail exposed. Most attacks from stingrays occur from swimmers or divers stepping on them. The tail will whip up in self-defense and impale the diver/swimmer's leg with a barbed spine. The wound area has a blue rim and is typically swollen, painful, and pale. Generalized reactions can include fainting, nausea, vomiting, frequent urination and salivation, sweating, respiratory difficulty, and cardiovascular collapse. Symptoms may take months to resolve. Secondary infections and necrotic lesions often develop. The toxin is heat labile (113°F). No antivenin is available.

Coelenterates: Hazardous coelenterates include Portuguese man-of-war, sea wasp or box jellyfish, Irukandji (*Carukia barnesi*), sea nettle, sea blubber, sea anemone, and rosy anemone. The most common stinging injury is the jellyfish sting, occurring worldwide. Most jellyfish stings result only in local skin irritation and modest pain. However, a box jellyfish (sea wasp) sting can result in death within 10 minutes from cardiovascular collapse, respiratory failure and paralysis. Antivenin is available for box jellyfish toxin. The Portuguese man-of-war is rarely fatal but does cause similar generalized symptoms as the box jellyfish that resolve after about a day. Stings from the man-of-war look like a red string of beads. Irukandji syndrome causes local skin symptoms, severe nausea and vomiting, severe abdominal pain and muscle spasm, catecholamine release that can cause cardiopulmonary failure.

Coral: This porous, rock-like formation found in water often has sharp edges. Usually cuts from coral are self-limiting and have only a mild skin reaction. Unfortunately, they usually take a long while to heal. Some coral can sting (coelenterate family). One of the deadliest poisons known was found recently in coral (genus *Palythoa*). If it is introduced into a deep cut in the body, it may be fatal. No antidote is known. Divers should wear dive suits to protect them from coral cuts, especially in surging waves.

Octopi: The octopus is an underwater chameleon, changing colors often in the water trying to conceal itself from its enemies. Most species of octopi found in the US are harmless to humans. Octopi can envenomate by biting and injecting venom from salivary glands. An octopus bite consists of two small punctures, surrounded by swollen, red and painful tissue. Bleeding may be severe due to anticoagulant effects of the venom. The blue ringed octopus found in Australian and Indo-Pacific waters is often deadly. It injects a neuromuscular blocker called maculotoxin that may cause paralysis, vomiting, respiratory difficulty, visual disturbances and cardiovascular collapse. (similar to the tetrodotoxin of the puffer fish). No antivenin is available. Paralysis may last 4-12 hours (with mechanical ventilation).

Sea urchins: These round, spiny creatures carry venom in the long spines. Divers and bathers step on these animals, impaling their feet on the long spines, which typically break off. The venom may cause pain, numbness, generalized weakness, paresthesias, nausea, and vomiting. Cardiac dysrhythmias have been reported. The toxin is heat labile. Immersion of affected area in water above 115°F is recommended. Allergic reactions can accompany these injuries.

Cone shells: The cone shell is widely distributed throughout the world. The shell is a symmetrical spiral with a distinctive head. Venom is contained in darts inside the proboscis, which extrudes out of the narrow end but can reach most of the shell. A stinging or burning sensation begins at the site of the sting, followed by numbness and tingling that spread from the wound to the rest of the body. Involvement of the mouth and lips is severe. Generalized symptoms include muscular paralysis, difficulty swallowing or talking, visual disturbances and respiratory distress. A cone shell sting should be viewed as severe as snakebite. Cone shell victims will probably experience paralysis or paresis of skeletal muscle with or without myalgia. Symptoms develop within minutes and can last up to 24 hours. No antivenin is available and mortality reaches 25%.

Sea snakes: Sea snakes are air-breathing reptiles that swim underwater for great distances (over 100 miles from land). They inhabit the Pacific and Indian Oceans and the Red Sea. There are some unsubstantiated reports of sea snakes in the Caribbean Sea (reportedly coming through the Panama Canal). The neurotoxin venom of a sea snake is 2-10 times more potent than that of a cobra. Bites are usually not painful, and only about 25% cause envenomization. There is a latent period of 10 minutes to several hours after the bite before generalized symptoms develop: muscle aches and stiffness, thick tongue sensation, progressive paralysis, nausea, vomiting, difficulty with speech and swallowing, respiratory distress and failure, and smoky colored urine from myoglobinuria (which may progress to kidney failure). The venom is heat-stable and antivenin is available.

Assessment:
Differential Diagnosis: See the above list of animals that envenomate

Plan:
Treatment/Procedures
Venomous Fish, Highly Toxic Fish, Stingrays

1. Lay patient supine, reassure and observe for shock.
2. Irrigate wound with cold saline or salt water to rinse remaining toxin. Minor surgery may be required to open wound.
3. Evacuate urgently to medical treatment facility for administration of antivenin if available and intensive care support if needed. Envenomizations should not be treated in the field if the patient can be evacuated.
4. Soak wound in water as hot as patient can tolerate (<122°F) for 30-90 minutes. Use hot compresses if wound is on the face.
5. Give **diazepam** 5mg IM for muscle spasms.
6. Manage pain (see *Part 8: Procedures: Chapter 30: Pain Assessment and Control*). Do NOT use narcotics in cases of RESPIRATORY DISTRESS or FAILURE. **Lidocaine** injected into the affected area may be used in the wound for pain

relief, but NEVER use epinephrine.

7. Explore the wound and clean out any remaining spines or barbs.
8. Immobilize the affected extremity.
9. Administer **tetanus** and antibiotic prophylaxis (**tetracycline** 250mg po bid x 10 days, and **neomycin** or **bacitracin** topically bid until lesion heals).
10. Consider x-ray to look for any remaining sheaths or barbs.

Coelenterates

1. Apply vinegar or a 3-10% solution of **acetic acid** (or carbonated beverage) to sting site to neutralize stingers.
2. Gently remove any remaining tentacles with a towel or cloth.
3. For box jellyfish stings, administer antivenin slowly: 1 container (vial) IV and 3 containers IM route. Treat sensitivity reactions to the antivenin with epinephrine, along with corticosteroids and antihistamines (see Part 7: Trauma: Chapter 27: Anaphylactic Shock).
   Treat hypotension with volume expanders and pressor medication, if available.
4. Evacuate victims of box jellyfish and Portuguese man-of-war stings immediately.
5. Use topical and/or local anesthetic agents (eg, **lidocaine**).

Coral

1. Control bleeding.
2. Promptly clean with soap and water or an antiseptic solution and débride the wound. Remove all foreign particles.
3. Cover with a clean dressing.
4. Administer **tetanus** prophylaxis.
5. Topical antibiotic ointment.
6. Manage pain (see Part 8: Procedures: Chapter 27: Pain Assessment and Control). Do NOT use narcotics in cases of RESPIRATORY DISTRESS or FAILURE.
7. Evacuate to medical treatment facility if symptoms are severe.

Octopi

1. Control local bleeding with pressure
2. Clean and débride wound. Cover with clean dressing.
3. If blue-ringed octopus is suspected:
   a. Apply pressure bandage and immobilize the bitten extremity. Place extremity lower than the heart.
   b. Be prepared to administer CPR and ventilate patient
   c. Immediately evacuate patient to medical treatment facility for intensive care.
4. Administer **tetanus** prophylaxis.

Sea Urchins

1. Remove all protruding spine fragments from wound, if possible. Do not break large pieces off in the wound.
2. Bathe wound in vinegar, then soak wound in as hot water as can be tolerated (no more than 122°F).
3. Clean and débride wound and apply topical antibiotic ointment.
4. Surgical removal is often necessary for deep spines. If necessary, evacuate patient to medical treatment facility to have this performed. X-rays can identify broken spines.
5. Treat allergic reactions and bronchospasms with SC **epinephrine** and antihistamines. See Part 7: Trauma: Chapter 27: Anaphylactic Shock
6. Administer **tetanus** prophylaxis.

Cone Shells

1. Place patient supine.
2. Apply pressure bandage to wound and place injury site at a level below the heart. Keep the patient from moving.
3. Immediately transport patient to medical treatment facility for intensive care. Be prepared to ventilate patient and administer CPR. Treat symptoms with supportive care as they present.
4. Avoid any analgesics that cause respiratory depression (narcotics)
5. Administer **tetanus** prophylaxis

Sea Snakes

1. Keep victim still.
2. Apply pressure dressing to bite site and place bite in a position below the heart.
3. Incise wound and apply suction if within 2 minutes of time of bite.
4. Transport patient immediately to medical treatment facility for antivenin treatment and intensive care.
5. Place IV and administer a bolus of 1L normal saline. Continue IV at a rate of 125mL/hr to keep urine output at least 30 cc/hour. Watch patient's urine looking for smoky color (indicating myoglobinuria, renal failure).
6. Be prepared to ventilate patient and perform CPR.
7. Observe patient for at least 12 hours after a bite due to possible latent effects.
8. Administer **tetanus** prophylaxis.

Patient Education

General: Keep the patient calm and reassure him that he has probably been envenomated and will receive further treatment.
Activity: Ensure the patient rests and remains calm.
Diet: Keep patient hydrated with IV NS and keep him NPO until you are sure surgery will not be required.
Medications: Antivenins have a high incidence of serum sickness. Antihistamines (eg, hydroxyzine 50-100mg po/IM q4-6h prn

pruritus) and NSAIDs (eg, ibuprofen 600mg po tid-qid prn fever and arthralgias) will provide symptomatic relief. If more severe symptoms (eg, temp >101.3°F, severe arthralgia, severe rash), steroids (prednisone 1-2mg/kg/day po x 3-4 days or methylprednisolone 1mg/kg/day IV q day in 1 or 2 divided doses x 3-4 days) may be useful. If at all possible, administer antivenin in a medical treatment facility in order to treat the serum sickness appropriately with intensive care support.

Prevention and Hygiene: Avoid these types of marine animals.

Wound Care: Keep dressing clean and dry. Antibiotic ointment will help prevent secondary wound infections

Follow-up Actions

Return Evaluation: Monitor patients until all symptoms resolve.

Evacuation/Consultation Criteria: Refer to each individual treatment plan for evacuation guidance. Consult an emergency medicine specialist, an internist or a Diving Medical Officer (DMO) for unstable patients after envenomization. Refer recovered divers to a DMO for clearance to return to diving duty.

Note: Antivenins are available from Commonwealth Serum Lab; 45 Poplar Rd, Parkville; Melbourne, Victoria, Australia. Telephone: 011-61-3-389-1911. Telex: AA-32789.

Chapter 20: Dive Medicine: Marine Hazards: Dangerous Marine Life: Biting Animals

MAJ Robert Price, MC, USA

Introduction: Diving in open water puts a diver in an environment with numerous dangerous sea creatures. Many of these creatures are predatory and can cause significant harm to humans. This section will only deal with the marine predators that injure by biting. Other marine life may injure humans through venom (see Part 6: Operational Environment: Chapter 20: Marine Hazards: Dangerous Marine Life: Venomous Animals), electrical shock, pinching and other means. Preparedness and avoidance is the best way to prevent encounters with dangerous marine life. Signs, symptoms, assessment and treatment are all very similar for the various animals listed.

Sharks: Attacks are rare but severe. Some species (great white, tiger, white-tip, bull sharks and others) are more aggressive towards divers. Injuries range from bumps or scratches caused by contact with rough skin to large bite wounds. Treat all sharks with respect and avoid them, because they are fast, strong and potentially aggressive.

Killer whales (orcas): Killer whales are mammals that usually travel in pods of 3-40 whales. These carnivores are at the very top of the food chain in the ocean. They have great intelligence, size, speed, interlocking teeth, and powerful jaws. Even though there are no recorded attacks on humans, there is potential that any animal this big could strike or bite an irritating diver.

Barracudas: Barracudas are predatory fish found in the tropics that can grow to 10 feet in length. Most are much smaller (3-5 feet). The barracuda is a fast swimmer with extremely sharp teeth but attacks are usually less severe than those of sharks. It rarely attacks divers, but is known to attack surface swimmers or limbs dangling from boats, and is attracted to bright objects.

Moray eels: Commonly found in holes and crevices near the ocean floor in tropical and subtropical waters, the moray eel resembles a large sea snake (up to 10 feet long) in shape and movements. Its face appears more like a dog with sharp teeth. Once it bites, it may be very difficult to dislodge. The moray eel will usually bite when a diver comes too close or sticks a hand into its hole or crevice. Mild envenomization may occur with certain species. Supportive care is all that is needed for this venom.

Sea lions: These mammals can be very aggressive with divers. Large male sea lions have a reputation for nipping divers during the mating season. Divers often mistakenly assume these animals as friendly and try to approach sea lions, provoking a bite. These bites resemble dog bites and are not usually severe.

Crocodiles: Many experts feel crocodiles are more dangerous than sharks. The saltwater and Nile crocodiles can grow up to 30 feet long. Crocodiles are fast, strong and aggressive reptiles. They are territorial and often found near river estuaries and brackish water. Treat any crocodile over 3 feet long as dangerous. Divers should immediately exit any area inhabited by a crocodile.

Hippopotamuses: The hippopotamus is the number one killer of men in Africa (not counting the mosquito). It is unpredictable and made irritable by people. Its canine teeth can be up to 20 inches long and are capable of chopping boats and the people in them in half. They are very territorial and protective of their calves. Most attacks occur when victims get between the hippo and deep water. Avoid dive operations in any area where large populations of hippo are known to populate.

Subjective: Symptoms

Severe pain in area of bite or injury; confusion and shock may set in very quickly. Infection may set in 3-7 days after wounding, with pain, redness, swelling, warmth and fever.

Focused History: What bit you? What treatment has already been provided for you?

Objective: Signs

Evaluate as a trauma patient.

Using Basic Tools: Airway damage extending from mouth to lungs: tachypnea, labored breathing, spitting blood, sucking chest wound. Hemorrhagic shock: fast heart rate, pallor, hypotension. Tissue loss, deformed body parts at bite site.

Assessment:

Differential Diagnosis: Other animal bites, blast trauma, other lacerating or penetrating trauma.

Plan:

Treatment: Treat per trauma protocol in this Handbook.

Airway, Breathing, Circulation

1. Control bleeding: apply compression dressings, elevate and apply direct pressure. Use pressure points, tourniquet as needed.
2. Ensure airway is well established and administer 100% O_2. Provide O_2 as required to maintain >93% O_2 sat.
3. Infuse 1-2L Ringer's lactate or normal saline by IV for severe blood loss. Monitor vital signs.
4. Treat severe pain with **morphine** 5mg IV. Add 1-2mg doses IV. See Part 8: Procedures: Chapter 30: Pain Assessment and Control

5. Evacuate to medical treatment facility as soon as possible if trauma is severe.
6. Send any severed limbs with the patient in saline-moistened gauze on ice.
7. Cleanse and débride wounds in a clean environment. Explore wounds thoroughly, as shark teeth may not appear on x-ray.
8. Splint any extremities that look deformed or that have possible fractures. X-ray when possible
9. Monitor pulses and urine function for possible compartment syndrome and/or myoglobinuria from crush injuries.
10. Administer tetanus prophylaxis. *See Part 5: Specialty Areas: Chapter 12: Bacterial Infections: Tetanus*
11. Culture wounds for aerobes and anaerobes before starting broad-spectrum antibiotics.
12. If patient has unexplained neurological symptoms, consider decompression sickness and arterial gas embolism.

Patient Education

General: Reassure patient

Activity: Rest until all injuries are identified and treated.

Diet: Keep patient NPO since he will possibly undergo surgery very shortly

Medications: Watch for respiratory suppression with morphine.

Prevention and Hygiene: Do not swim with or challenge dangerous marine life. Avoid crocodiles on land. Do not wear shiny objects while diving. Do not panic in the water. Only as a last resort if bitten, hit snout, gills or eyes to drive attacker away.

Wound Care: Keep wounds clean, dry and covered.

Follow-up Actions

Return Evaluation: Patients should not be allowed back into the water until cleared by a Diving Medical Officer (DMO).

Evacuation/Consultation Criteria: Evacuate those with severe wounds, which require surgery. Consult a general surgeon in these cases. Consult a DMO for other diving injuries (eg, decompression sickness).

Chapter 20: Dive Medicine: Underwater Blast/Explosion/Sound Injury
MAJ Robert Price, MC, USA

Introduction: Underwater explosions create shock waves that move out in all directions at the speed of sound. Water is non-compressible, therefore it transmits the shock wave a greater distance and with more intensity than an explosion in air (this is the concept used by depth charges against submarines).

Unlike air explosions, shrapnel and debris injuries are minimal because water quickly dampens any particles propelled away from the explosion. The shock wave generated by the explosions can bounce off of the surface, ocean floor, boat hulls or sea walls and strike divers in the water with a compounding impact.

Factors affecting the intensity of an underwater explosion: size of the charge, distance from the blast, protective clothing, depth of the diver (deeper is worse), depth of ocean floor (shallow depths reflect blast more intensely) and firmness of reflective surfaces near explosion (firmer surfaces reflect blast waves better, therefore are worse for the diver). Shock waves cause implosions of gas-filled cavities in the body, tearing of tissues at gas-liquid interfaces, and emboli. *See Part 7: Trauma: Chapter 29: Blast Injuries*

Subjective: Symptoms

May be unable to talk; complaints may include chest pain, cough, pain with breathing, spitting blood, severe abdominal pain, confusion, headache, seeing "floaters" or "stars", ear pain, loss of hearing, and ringing of ears.

Focused History: *Do you have chest pain? Are you short of breath? Are you having any changes in your vision? Do you hear any ringing in your ears?* (All can occur for a number of other causes. However, with history of exposure to underwater blast these are indications of blast injury.)

Objective: Signs

Decompression sickness or arterial gas embolism may occur secondary to a rapidly aborted dive, or because the trauma of the explosion may suddenly move the diver into more shallow water.

Using Basic Tools: General: Fracture or dislocation of any body part; swollen extremities (possible heart failure). HEENT: Subcutaneous emphysema ("crackling" with palpation of the skin) over the neck (leak in the respiratory tract, such as pneumothorax); ruptured tympanic membrane (TM), tender or collapsed sinuses, blood in nose and ears, nystagmus, dizziness, vertigo, and loss of balance; distended neck veins (heart failure or cardiac tamponade). Chest: Hemoptysis, obvious discomfort with deep inspiration, rales and friction rubs upon auscultation, cough, and respiratory failure; decreased or absent breath sounds (simple, or tension pneumothorax, hemothorax); subcutaneous emphysema. GI tract: Blood in stool; rigid abdomen; rebound tenderness (probably due to intestinal rupture/hemorrhage). CNS: Mental status changes (delirium, confusion, unresponsiveness), and paralysis of any part of the body (stroke from emboli).

Using Advanced Tools: X-rays: CXR: Pneumothorax; patchy or diffuse infiltrates (pulmonary contusion) a few hours after the blast injury. Cervical spine: assess for fractures, dislocations and other abnormalities.

Assessment:

Differential Diagnosis: All of the following may be possible blast related injuries. See appropriate sections in this book or other sources for additional details.

Arterial gas embolism (AGE): *See Part 6: Operational Environment: Chapter 20: Decompression Injuries: Pulmonary Over Inflation Syndrome (including Arterial Gas Embolism)*

Decompression sickness (DCS): *See Part 6: Operational Environment: Chapter 20: Decompression Injuries: Decompression Sickness (Caisson Disease, the "Bends")*

Lungs: Pulmonary contusions, pneumothorax, tension pneumothorax, hemothorax, alveolar rupture.

Gastrointestinal: Intestinal hemorrhage, intestinal perforation, paralytic ileus, acute abdomen

Heart: Cardiac contusion, congestive heart failure, tamponade

Brain and nervous system: Brain injury/contusion, paralysis, stroke and C-spine injury.

Ears and sinuses: Ruptured TMs, conductive hearing loss, ruptured sinuses and inner ear barotraumas including round window and oval window ruptures.

Body: Fractured bones, joint dislocations.

Plan:

Treatment

1. Treat as major trauma patient. Immobilize the head and neck with a cervical collar until head/neck trauma is ruled out.
2. Secure the airway. Intubate if there is a doubt that the patient will be able to maintain his own airway. Place on 100% O_2 initially and then wean down over the next 12 hours (except CNS injury). Provide O_2 as required to maintain >95% O_2 sat.
3. Perform needle decompression in 2nd intercostal space in the mid-clavicular line if any type of pneumothorax develops followed by a thoracostomy when appropriate, or go directly to an open thoracostomy if clinical circumstances are conducive. *See Part 8: Procedures: Chapter 30: Thoracostomy, Needle and Chest Tube*

Chapter 20: Dive Medicine: "Caustic Cocktail" Chemical Burn

MAJ Robert Price, MC, USA

Introduction: Closed-circuit (no respiratory gases escape the breathing apparatus) and semi closed-circuit diving rigs use carbon dioxide (CO_2) absorbent chemicals to remove or scrub CO_2 from breathing gases. If water mixes with this solid substance (ie, water may leak into the chemical canister), an alkaline solution forms. Inhaling or swallowing this solution causes chemical burns of the pharynx and trachea.

Subjective: **Symptoms**

Burning in mouth and throat, possible headache, choking and gagging with a foul taste in mouth; in severe cases burning may extend all the way down into the lungs. History may include water getting into the rebreather rig. Disassembling the rig may find water in the CO_2 canister.

Focused History: *Did you hear any gurgling in your rig during the dive? Did your mouth start burning after you inhaled water from your rebreather rig?* (typical history)

Objective: **Sign**

Using Basic Tools: Rapid respiratory rate; choking and gagging; red, irritated and burned mucosa; pharynx may swell, compromising airway; lungs may develop rales.

Assessment:

Differential Diagnosis

Laryngospasms secondary to inhalation of saltwater: There will not be any burning or redness with this event.

Plan:

Treatment

1. Place patient in an upright position in the water and remove mouth from caustic source.
2. Repeatedly rinse mouth with fresh water. When foul or sour taste is gone, have the diver swallow several mouthfuls. If only seawater is available, only rinse mouth. Do not have the patient swallow any of the seawater.
3. If the injury is severe and extends down to the lungs, secure the airway and apply 100% O_2. Provide O_2 as required to maintain >95% O_2 sat. Patient may require intubation and mechanical ventilation, as well as immediate evacuation. *See Part 8: Procedures: Chapter 30: Initial Airway Management and Ventilatory Support & Intubation*

Patient Education

General: Remain calm and do not hyperventilate, which may worsen symptoms.

Activity: Rest until symptoms are gone and medic ensures there is no pulmonary or airway involvement.

Diet: Avoid eating until foul or sour taste is gone and pulmonary involvement is ruled out.

Prevention and Hygiene: Avoid getting water into CO_2 scrubber canister. Review and follow emergency procedures for the use of specific underwater breathing apparatus (UBA).

Wound Care: Rinse burned areas with water.

Follow-up Actions

Return Evaluation: If no hospitalization is needed, follow-up daily until symptoms are completely resolved.

Evacuation/Consultation Criteria: If respiration becomes labored or airway starts to swell, secure airway immediately and apply 100% O_2. Evacuate immediately and consult a Diving Medical Officer or pulmonologist.

Chapter 20: Dive Medicine: Dive Treatment Table 5 Depth/Time Profile

1. Descent rate - 20 ft/min.
2. Ascent rate - Not to exceed 1ft/min. Do not compensate for slower ascent rates. Compensate for faster rates by halting the ascent.
3. Time on oxygen begins on arrival at 60 feet.
4. If oxygen breathing must be interrupted because of CNS Oxygen Toxicity, allow 15 minutes after the reaction has entirely subsided and resume schedule at point of interruption. If symptoms of CNS toxicity develop again, interrupt breathing for another 15 minutes. If CNS symptoms develop 3rd time, contact a diving medical officer (DMO) as soon as possible to modify oxygen breathing periods to meet requirements. (See Paragraph 21-5.5.6.1 of the Navy Diving Manual, Revision 6)
5. Treatment Table may be extended two oxygen-breathing periods at the 30-foot stop. No air break required between oxygen breathing periods or prior to ascent.
6. Tender breathes 100 percent O_2 during ascent from the 30-foot stop to the surface. If the tender had a previous hyperbaric exposure in the previous 12 hours, an additional 20 minutes of oxygen breathing is required prior to ascent.

Figure 6-3. Dive Treatment Table 5

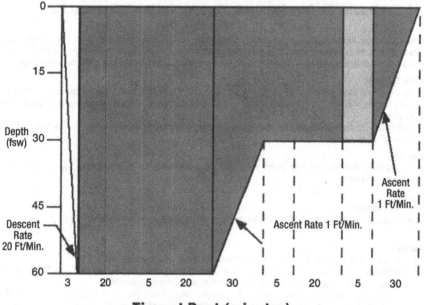

Time at Dept (minutes)

Total Elapsed Time:
135 Minutes
2 Hours 15 Minutes
(Not Including Descent Time)

Part 6: Operational Environment: Chapter 20: Dive Medicine:
Dive Table 6 Depth/Time Profile

1. Descent rate - 20ft/min.
2. Ascent rate - Not to exceed 1ft/min. Do not compensate for slower ascent rates. Compensate for faster rates by halting the ascent.
3. Time on oxygen begins on arrival at 60 feet.
4. If oxygen breathing must be interrupted because of CNS Oxygen Toxicity, allow 15 minutes after the reaction has entirely subsided and resume schedule at point of interruption. If symptoms of CNS toxicity develop again, interrupt breathing for another 15 minutes. If CNS symptoms develop 3rd time, contact a diving medical officer (DMO) as soon as possible to modify oxygen breathing periods to meet requirements. (see Paragraph 21-5.5.6.1 of the Navy Diving Manual, Revision 6)
5. Table 6 can be lengthened up to 2 additional 25 minute periods at 60 feet (20 minutes on oxygen and 5 minutes on air), or up to 2 additional 75 minute periods at 30 feet (15 minutes on air and 60 minutes on oxygen), or both.
6. Tender breathes 100 percent O_2 during the last 30 min. at 30 fsw and during ascent to the surface for an unmodified table or where there has been only a single extension at 30 or 60 feet. If there has been more than one extension, the O_2 breathing at 30 feet is increased to 60 minutes. If the tender had a hyperbaric exposure within the past 12 hours, an additional 60-minute O_2 period is taken at 30 feet.

Figure 6-4. Dive Treatment Table 6

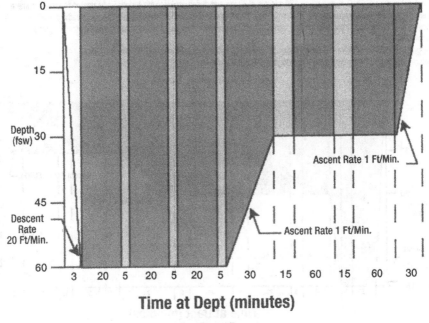

Time at Dept (minutes)

Total Elapsed Time:
285 Minutes
4 Hours 45 Minutes
(Not Including Descent Time)

Chapter 20: Dive Medicine: Dive Treatment Table 6A Depth/Time Profile

1. Descent rate - 20ft/min.
2. Ascent rate - 165 fsw to 60 fsw not to exceed 3ft/min, 60 fsw and shallower, not to exceed 1ft/min. Do not compensate for slower ascent rates. Compensate for faster rates by halting the ascent.
3. Time at treatment depth does not include compression time.
4. Table begins with initial compression to depth of 60 fsw. If initial treatment was at 60 feet, up to 20 minutes may be spent at 60 feet before compression to 165 fsw. Contact a Diving Medical Officer.
5. If a chamber is equipped with a high O_2 treatment gas, it may be administered at 165 fsw and shallower, not to exceed 2.8 ata O_2 in accordance with paragraph 21-5-7 of the Navy Diving Manual, Revision 6. Treatment gas is administered for 25 minutes interrupted by 5 minutes of air. Treatment gas is breathed during ascent from the treatment depth to 60 fsw.
6. Deeper than 60 feet, if treatment gas must be interrupted because of CNS oxygen toxicity, allow 15 minutes after the reaction has entirely subsided before resuming treatment gas. The time off treatment gas is counted as part of the time at treatment depth. If at 60 feet or shallower and oxygen breathing must be interrupted because of CNS oxygen toxicity, allow 15 minutes after the reaction has entirely subsided and resume schedule at point of interruption. f CNS symptoms develop 3rd time, contact a diving medical officer (DMO) as soon as possible to modify oxygen breathing periods to meet requirements. (See Paragraph 21-5.5.6.1.1 of the Navy Diving Manual, Revision 6)
7. Table 6A can be lengthened up to 2 additional 25 minute periods at 60 feet (20 minutes on oxygen and 5 minutes on air), or up to 2 additional 75 minute periods at 30 feet (60 minutes on oxygen and 15 minutes on air), or both.
8. Tenders breathes 100% O_2 during the last 60 minutes at 30 fsw and during ascent to the surface for an unmodified table or where there has been only a single extension at 30 or 60 fsw. If there has been more than one extension, the O_2 breathing at 30 fsw is increased to 90 minutes. If the tender had a hyperbaric exposure within the past 12 hours, an additional 60 minute O_2 breathing period is taken at 30 fsw.
9. If significant improvement is not obtained within 30 minutes at 165 feet, consult with a Diving Medical Officer before switching to Treatment Table 4. See the Navy Diving Manual, Revision 6

Figure 6-5. Dive Treatment Table 6A

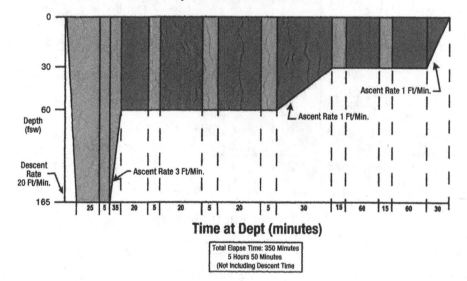

Time at Dept (minutes)

Total Elapse Time: 350 Minutes
5 Hours 50 Minutes
(Not Including Descent Time

Chapter 21: Aerospace Medicine: Cerebral Hypoxia
LTC John Albano, MC, USA

Introduction: Oxygen makes up approximately 21% of the air we breathe. As ambient atmospheric pressure decreases with increased altitude, the partial pressure of oxygen in that air also decreases. This results in decreased oxygenation of the blood and tissue hypoxia (eg, cerebral hypoxia). Healthy individuals can adapt to ambient pressures of 10,000 feet above mean sea level (MSL) for prolonged periods without hypoxic effects. However, virtually everyone who ascends to >8,000 feet without acclimatization will experience a decreased level of performance. Rapid decompression at extreme altitudes may result in death. **Risk Factor:** Underlying pulmonary disease (acute or chronic). *See Part 6: Operational Environment: Chapters 20 & 22*

Subjective: Symptoms
The effects of mild to moderate cerebral hypoxia are variable from person to person, but consistent in an individual across exposures; impaired judgment, thinking, and vision (particularly color vision); paresthesias, especially of the face and hands, are common.
Focused History: *When did symptoms start?* (Acute onset with change in altitude is typical.) *Have you had a fever or other signs of illness prior to this flight?* (Pulmonary disease is risk factor, or may suggest alternate diagnosis.) *Have you been diving or breathing compressed air in the last 48 hours?* (may suggest decompression sickness [DCS]) *Have you been flying? If so, do you know the cabin altitude of the flight?* (>10,000 feet is typical) *Are you taking any drugs or medications of any kind?* (consider substance abuse, drug reaction or allergic reaction)

Objective: Signs
Using Basic Tools: Lack of fine motor control; personality changes (eg, withdrawn, violent, or highly flamboyant activity); inattentiveness or absence periods; respiratory rate and pulse may increase; seizure activity is possible.

Assessment: Resolution of signs and symptoms with return to lower altitudes or treatment with oxygen confirms the diagnosis.
Differential Diagnosis:
Decompression sickness (DCS): Unlikely for single ascent if <18,000 feet MSL and negative history of breathing compressed air (eg, diving) within last 48 hours. *See Part 6: Operational Environment: Chapter 20: Decompression Injuries: Decompression Sickness (Caisson Disease, the "Bends")*
Substance abuse: Rule out if no history or other evidence/suspicion of taking drugs, medications, alcohol or "nutritional supplements"
Allergic or idiopathic reaction to prescription or OTC medications, including nutritional supplements: May rule out if not taking any of these substances
Atypical seizure activity: Must be considered if positive history of seizure disorder or history of head trauma involving loss of consciousness within the last 10 years

Plan:
Treatment
Primary: Supplemental oxygen under pressure via well fitted mask
Alternative: Increase oxygen concentration of inspired air by any other means (non re-breather, nasal canula, etc.)
Primitive: Increase ambient pressure by decreasing altitude or adjusting cabin altitude

Patient Education
General: Effects of hypoxia are experienced only while exposed to a hypoxic environment. Patients should not have residual effects when the hypoxic exposure ends. Patient will likely be affected in similar manner by future exposure to similar altitudes. Prevention: Early recognition of the symptoms of hypoxia allows early intervention and avoids performance decrement. Use pre mission altitude chamber testing to determine individual team member's response to the hypobaric environment.
Follow-up Actions
Return Evaluation: If symptoms or signs consider altitude induced DCS. Evaluation by neurologist is indicated at earliest opportunity.
Consultation Criteria: Consultation with Aerospace Medicine specialist, Diving Medicine specialist, Flight Surgeon, or Aeromedical PA is not required in uncomplicated cases (ie, complete resolution of signs and symptoms with return to normoxic conditions).
Notes: Hypoxia is a particular danger for HALO and HAHO missions where any impairment in judgment and thinking, can quickly lead to death or serious injury. The effects of hypoxia may present subacutely in personnel living and working at high altitude. An acute hypoxic event without complications or sequelae is not grounds for restriction or special duty status.

Chapter 21: Aerospace Medicine: Barodontalgia
LTC John Albano, MC, USA

Introduction: Dental decay can produce small pockets of gas in or around teeth and pockets of gas may also be present beneath dental amalgam or crowns. When ambient air pressure changes, the pressure differential in the trapped pocket of gas cannot be equalized and the increased pressure causes severe pain. This rare condition almost always occurs on ascent. Barodontalgia may also develop during diving operations. *See Part 6: Operational Environment: Chapter 20: Barotrauma* **Risk Factors:** Dental pathology (eg, active caries, pulpitis, periapical abscess), recently placed amalgam restorations or crowns. *See Part 5: Specialty Areas: Chapter 10*

Subjective: Symptoms
Acute onset of sharp, stabbing pain in a single tooth on ascent. This pain can be quite severe and will increase in severity with continued ascent. Symptoms abate with return to original altitude.
Focused History: *When did symptoms start?* (Acute onset associated with change in altitude [ie, pressure] is typical.) *Did you have a fever or other signs of illness prior to this flight?* (may suggest barodontalgia or other alternate diagnosis) *Have you had any dental*

problems or dental procedures recently? (typical exposure history; body slowly absorbs free gas, so older dental procedures less problematic)

Objective: Signs
Using Basic Tools: Obvious dental lesions help make the diagnosis. Percussion of the involved tooth should exacerbate symptoms

Assessment: Differential Diagnosis
Barosinusitis: May be present as pain in area of maxillary teeth; look for other signs and symptoms of maxillary sinus involvement.
Acute pulpitis or periapical abscess of the tooth: Unrelated to pressure changes
Acute infectious sinusitis: Rule out by absence of history or signs (eg, purulent nasal discharge) of sinusitis. *See Part 3: General Symptoms: ENT Problems: Sinusitis*

Plan: Treatment
Primary: Return to level of embarkation, (ie, increase ambient pressure by descent or increase cabin pressure), if possible.
Alternative: Analgesics as required. Consider fracture of tooth or removal/replacement of restoration if symptoms are unrelenting in an operational setting that precludes descent.
Patient Education
General: Whenever possible, do not fly while suffering from acute dental disease.
Prevention: Good dental hygiene and regular check-ups with dentist. Wait 24 hours after any dental treatment involving manipulation of the teeth or gums before hypobaric exposure.
Follow-up Actions
Return Evaluation: Dental exam for diagnosis and treatment of underlying pathology.
Consultation Criteria: Severe cases, if symptoms not relieved upon descent, or when underlying pathology is suspected.
Note: Barodontalgia temporarily limits special duty involving flight operations until cleared by a Flight Surgeon.

Chapter 21: Aerospace Medicine: Barosinusitis
LTC John Albano, MC, USA

Introduction: The paranasal sinuses are mucous membrane-lined air cavities in the cranial bone that communicate with the nasal cavity. They have a fixed volume, containing air, mucus, and water vapor. The pressure within the sinuses is normally equal to ambient air pressure and equalizes as ambient pressure changes. When intrasinus pressure cannot be equalized, pain will result. This is more likely to occur on descent from altitude and often due to malformations or swelling of the sinus outflow tract. The negative pressure differential results in a sinus "squeeze." Upper respiratory tract infections (RTIs), smoking, and untreated seasonal allergic conditions increase the risk of developing barosinusitis during flight. Barosinusitis (ie, "sinus squeeze") is also seen with diving. *See Part 6: Operational Environment: Chapter 20: Barotrauma*

Subjective: Symptoms
Acute onset of sharp, stabbing sinus pain on descent is classic. This pain can be quite severe and will increase in severity with continued descent. Symptoms will abate with decreasing ambient pressure resulting from return to altitude. Patients will bleed into the sinus in severe cases, thereby relieving the pressure differential and significantly reducing the pain. Symptoms of sinus congestion and facial pressure similar to that with an upper RTI will then result.
Focused History: *When did symptoms start?* (Acute onset associated with change in altitude is a key factor in differentiating from infectious etiology.) *Have you had a fever or other signs of illness prior to this flight?* (History of recent illness may provide information to support specific diagnosis.) *Have you had any dental problems or dental treatments recently?* (Consistent with barodontalgia but maxillary tooth pain can occur with any sinusitis.)

Objective: Signs
Using Basic Tools: The patient appears to be in obvious distress. Some redness and swelling of the face in the affected area may be noted though not to the degree one would expect with purulent sinusitis. Increased lacrimation is also possible. Bloody/mucoid nasal discharge may be seen from affected sinus in severe cases. Transillumination of the sinus may suggest a fluid level. Often there is tenderness to palpation over the affected sinuses.
Using Advanced Tools: X-ray: Sinus series x-rays (looking for air/fluid levels) are helpful if available.

Assessment: Differential Diagnosis
Barodontalgia: Pain caused by air trapped under a crown or amalgam or within a tooth cavity; may be suggested by maxillary sinus symptoms present on ascent
Pulpitis or periapical abscess of the tooth: If maxillary sinus symptoms associated with a diseased tooth are present on ascent
Acute infectious sinusitis: If history and symptoms sinusitis (eg, purulent discharge) are present. *See Part 3: General Symptoms: ENT Problems*

Plan: Treatment
Primary: Return to an altitude that is less than where symptoms first began (ie, decrease ambient pressure by ascent or decrease cabin pressure), if possible. Spray nasopharynx with topical nasal decongestant spray, **oxymetazoline** 2-3 puffs x 1. Slowly descend while frequently using modified Valsalva maneuver (ie, pinch nose and exhale against closed nostrils) as needed to equalize pressure in sinuses.
Alternative: Land; use oral decongestants (eg, **pseudoephedrine** 30-60mg po) and analgesics (eg, **acetaminophen** 325mg po). If symptoms persist after 2 hours, consult ENT.
Primitive: Modified Valsalva maneuver.

Patient Education

General: A sinus "squeeze" is easier to prevent than to treat. Use modified Valsalva maneuver to equalize pressure in sinuses frequently during descent; do not wait until pain develops to attempt to equalize.

Prevention: Whenever possible, do not fly while suffering from a RTI. Use oral decongestants (eg, pseudoephedrine) prior to and during flight to decrease the risk of barosinusitis in a patient who must fly with a RTI. Correct altered anatomy (eg, narrow sinus ostia; deviated nasal septum) to improve aeration of sinuses. Control allergic rhinitis manifestations.

Follow-up Actions

Return Evaluation: Patient should be followed and nasal decongestants (po or topical) should be used for several days following an episode of barosinusitis. If sinus bleeding occurs, treat as acute sinusitis. *See Part 3: General Symptoms: ENT: Sinusitis*

Consultation Criteria: No consultation is necessary in uncomplicated cases. Consult dentist if dental condition is suspected; consult ENT specialist, if possible, for sinus bleeds.

Notes: An uncomplicated sinus squeeze that quickly resolves is not a restriction to special duty status. Patients with an underlying upper RTI, sinus problem or barosinusitis with secondary sinus bleed, should be temporarily restricted from special duty involving flying or diving operations until cleared by a Flight Surgeon or DMO.

Chapter 21: Aerospace Medicine: Barotitis
LTC John Albano, MC, USA

Introduction: The middle ear is an air filled bony cavity that houses the stapes, incus, and malleus, and communicates with the posterior oropharynx via the cartilaginous eustachian tube. The middle ear has a fixed volume containing air and water vapor. The pressure within the middle ear is normally equal to the ambient pressure and equalizes through the eustachian tube as ambient pressure changes. If pressure in the middle ear cannot be equalized due to malformations or swelling of the eustachian tube, it will cause inflammation (ie, barotitis media). Barotitis externa can result if a foreign body (eg, ear plug, cerumen plug) blocks the external auditory canal (EAC). Both conditions are more likely to occur with descent, but a reverse "squeeze" can occur on ascent with similar symptoms. Barotitis may develop during both flying and diving (*see Part 6: Operational Environment: Chapter 20: Barotrauma*). Upper respiratory tract infections (RTIs) and untreated seasonal allergic conditions greatly increase the risk of developing an ear "block" during flight. Smoking may also be a contributory factor.

Subjective: **Symptoms**

Acute onset of sharp, stabbing pain in the ear on descent is classic. This pain can be quite severe and will increase in severity with continued descent. Symptoms will abate with return to altitude. In severe cases, patients will rupture the tympanic membrane (TM), thereby relieving the pressure differential and significantly reducing the pain. Hearing loss will then result. Vertigo may be associated with barotitis media or with TM rupture from either condition.

Focused History: *When did symptoms start?* (Acute onset associated with change in altitude is a key factor in differentiating from infectious etiology.) *Have you had a fever or other signs of illness prior to this flight?* (History of recent illness can illuminate risk factors and/or provide clues to make differential diagnosis.)

Objective: **Signs**

Using Basic Tools: The patient appears to be in obvious distress. The Weber test (512Hz tuning fork) lateralizes to the affected ear if only one ear is affected. If both ears are affected, the Weber test is equivocal.

Using Advanced Tools: Otoscopic exam will reveal blocked EAC in barotitis externa and retracted TM in barotitis media. Blood may be visualized behind the TM in severe cases of barotitis media.

Assessment: **Differential Diagnosis**

Acute otitis media: Bulging, red TM with poor temporal correlation of symptoms to altitude changes

Acute trauma to the EAC or TM: Insect or arthropod bite, usually visualized on otoscopic exam

Other barotrauma to the ear: Cochlear tear and/or round window rupture may be present if there is blood behind TM, vertigo, or no relief of symptoms upon return to original altitude.

Plan:

Treatment

Primary: Return to level of embarkation (ie, decrease ambient pressure by ascent or decrease cabin pressure for "squeeze" and the opposite for "reverse squeeze"), if possible. Spray nasopharynx with decongestant spray (eg, **oxymetazoline**) to decrease swelling of eustachian tube in barotitis media. Remove EAC obstruction in barotitis externa. Slowly descend (for "squeeze") while using modified Valsalva maneuver (ie, pinch nose and exhale against closed nostrils) to equalize pressure in sinuses.

Alternative: Use a Politzer bag, a device similar in appearance to an Ambu bag (and often carried on medical evacuation aircraft), to force air into the nasopharynx while the patient swallows. This will probably be more effective than the modified Valsalva maneuver. Myringotomy may be necessary in extreme cases of barotitis media.

Primitive: Modified Valsalva maneuver

Patient Education

General: It is easier to prevent an ear "block" than to treat one. Use modified Valsalva maneuver to equalize pressure in middle ear frequently during descent; do not wait until pain develops to attempt to equalize.

Prevention: Whenever possible, do not fly while suffering from an upper respiratory infection. Use oral decongestants (eg, pseudoephedrine 30-60mg po q6h) prior to and during flight decrease risk of barotitis in patients with URI. Control allergic rhinitis manifestations.

Follow-up Actions

Return Evaluation: Patient should be followed and decongestants (oral or nasal) should be used for several days following an episode of barotitis. If large hemorrhagic bullae are present in the EAC in barotitis externa, evacuation of blood with a syringe and sterile needle should be performed; small hemorrhages do not require treatment. Manage TM rupture like that from any other cause; empiric antibiotic treatment is not recommended. *See Part 3: General Symptoms: ENT Problems: Ear Pain*

Consultation Criteria: Consult ENT specialist for TM rupture, suspected middle/inner ear barotrauma, or after myringotomy

Notes: An uncomplicated ear squeeze may not require restriction of special duty status. An underlying upper RTI or other ear problem or barotitis with secondary bleed or inner/middle ear trauma, however, should temporarily restrict affected personnel from special duty involving flying or diving operations until cleared by a FS or DMO.

Chapter 21: Aerospace Medicine: Decompression Sickness
LTC John Albano, MC, USA

Introduction: Nitrogen makes up approximately 80% of the atmosphere. An inert gas, it saturates all tissues of the body. Nitrogen will expand because of decreased atmospheric pressure at altitudes above 18,000 feet above mean sea level (MSL), forming bubbles in body tissues. The tissue affected by these bubbles generally determines the severity of decompression syndrome (DCS). Type I DCS is limited to musculoskeletal pain, pruritus (with or without a macular patch type rash) and is considered clinically as mild. Type II DCS affects the cardiovascular, pulmonary; central nervous system and is clinically considered serious. DCS may be associated with exposure to low ambient pressures during flight operations or ascent from diving operations. *See Part 6: Operational Environments: Chapter 20: Decompression Injuries*

Subjective: **Symptoms**

Type I

"Bends": musculoskeletal (primarily joint) pain

"Creeps" or "itches": pruritus or feeling of insects crawling on the skin

Type II

Cardiovascular: weakness, sweating; unconsciousness

"Chokes": shortness of breath, chest pain, non-productive cough

Neurologic DCS: Any neurologic symptom is possible, including paralysis, paresis, paresthesia, loss of consciousness, headache, fatigue, seizure, and personality changes.

Focused History: *Do you have* [each of the symptoms listed]? (Answers provide insight to which body tissues are affected, thus how severe DCS may be.) *Are you taking any drugs, medications or "nutritional supplements" of any kind?* (Affirmative answer opens the possibility of allergic or idiopathic drug reaction.) *Have you flown over 18,000 feet, or been diving in the past 24 hours?* (typical exposure)

Objective: **Signs**

Using Basic Tools: Complete a basic cardiopulmonary, neurological and symptom directed physical examination. Specifically look for tenderness to palpation, hyperesthesia or hypoesthesia, paresthesia, visual field defects, spotty motor or sensory deficits, disorientation, generalized cutaneous hyperemia, cyanosis, tachypnea, tachycardia, hypotension, hemoconcentration, and decreased urinary output. Diffuse mottling of skin (particularly after hypobaric exposure) may indicate arterial gas embolism. Involvement of more than one joint is indicative of more serious DCS. Perform and document positive and negative findings for a complete neurologic examination.

Assessment: **Differential Diagnosis**

Acute hypoxia: Suggested by immediate, complete resolution of symptoms with supplemental oxygen

Reaction to medications: Identify medications being taken (including nutritional supplements)

Seizure disorder: Indicated by history of seizure disorder or head trauma involving loss of consciousness within last 10 years

Arterial gas embolism (AGE): Occurs in aerospace medicine as a consequence of catastrophic decompression of aircraft with loss of consciousness or sudden death less than15 minutes following event. *See Part 6: Operational Environment: Chapter 20: Decompression Injuries: Pulmonary Over Inflation Syndrome (including Arterial Gas Embolism)*

Plan:

Treatment

Primary: 100% oxygen via fitted mask and evacuate for hyperbaric oxygen recompression therapy. Restrict air evacuation to no higher than 1,000 feet above point of embarkation.

Alternative: Portable or transport hyperbaric chamber

Primitive: Return to sea level and 100% oxygen

Patient Education

General: DCS is a very serious condition. The threat of death or permanent neurologic injury is out of proportion to the usually mild symptoms. Pre-existing acute musculoskeletal injuries may increase the risk of joint "bends" and experience in divers suggests moderate to strenuous exercise and dehydration increases the risk of developing DCS.

Prevention and Hygiene: Allow at least 24 hours between diving operations and flying or other high altitude operations. Avoid strenuous physical activity before high altitude operations.

Follow-up Actions

Return Evaluation: Non flight-rated personnel involved in flight operations can return to duty 72 hours after successful treatment of minimal symptoms (one treatment with no recurrence of symptoms) of "pain only" Type I DCS. Service specific regulations for flight rated personnel should be followed. All patients with other than minimal ("pain only" or pruritus) symptoms should be referred to medical specialists to determine medical fitness.

Consultation Criteria: Consultation with a Diving Medical Officer (DMO), Aerospace medical specialist, or Flight Surgeon to begin medical evaluation process. Consultation with neurologist is indicated for any suspected neurologic DCS case.

Notes: DCS is a danger in any flying operation that requires ascent to 18,000 feet MSL or above. Rapid return to lower altitudes in HALO missions mitigates the threat to some degree, but evaluation by flight surgeon or diving medical officer should be accomplished as soon as operationally possible. Neurologic DCS is life-threatening and should be treated as a medical emergency. Consider any episode of DCS as grounds for temporary restriction of special duty status until cleared by competent medical authority.

Chapter 22: High Altitude Illnesses: Acute Mountain Sickness
COL Paul Rock, MC, USA (Ret)

Introduction: Acute mountain sickness (AMS) is a short-lived (days to a week) illness that occurs in people from low altitude (less than 5,000 ft) who travel rapidly to higher areas (usually more than 8,000-9,000 ft) and remain there for more than several hours. It is caused by the decreased amount of oxygen available in the low pressure atmosphere at high altitude (see *Part 6: Operational Environment: Chapter 21: Cerebral Hypoxia*). Symptoms of AMS usually go away as a person's body adapts to lower oxygen levels over a week to 10 days (altitude acclimatization). It is difficult to predict who will be more susceptible to AMS in military aged adults. Individuals who have had AMS before are likely to have it again when they go to altitude. A rapid ascent and higher final altitude make AMS more likely to occur in anyone. AMS can be expected in 40-50% of un-acclimatized individuals who ascend to 14,000 ft and the adverse effect on physical and mental performance should be considered during operational planning. Heavy physical exercise during ascent or when first arriving at high altitude increases the risk of developing AMS. Patients with symptoms of AMS can develop life-threatening altitude illnesses such as high altitude cerebral edema (HACE) and high altitude pulmonary edema (HAPE)

Subjective: Symptoms
Similar to an alcoholic "hangover"- headache (often severe), nausea (with or without vomiting), fatigue, decreased appetite and disturbed sleep. Symptoms begin within 3-24 hours after ascending to a higher elevation and are most severe in the first 24 to 48 hours.

Focused History: *When did symptoms begin?* (typically start within 24 hours <u>after</u> traveling to higher altitude) *Did you have these symptoms or an illness <u>before</u> going to higher altitude?* (Viral illness or other preexisting condition) *Have you taken any medications, drugs or alcohol?* (Intoxication with these substances can cause symptoms similar to AMS.) *Have you been in a tent, cave or vehicle with a stove or motor running?* (Carbon monoxide poisoning can cause similar symptoms.) *Do you have a cough or difficulty breathing?* (suggests HAPE) *How is your coordination? Have you been stumbling or falling?* (suggests HACE)

Objective: Signs
Using Basic Tools: Patient appears 'sick'; decreased urination; poor balance (truncal ataxia) when carrying backpack; mild swelling (edema) in the hands, feet and/or face ("puffy" around the eyes.)

Using Advanced Tools: Blood oxygen levels measured by pulse oximeter will be lower with AMS or other altitude illnesses.

Assessment: Diagnosis is made on basis of history.
Differential Diagnosis
Early HACE: Significant ataxia (cannot do "heel-to-toe walk"); swelling of optic nerve (papilledema). *See Part 6: Operational Environment: Chapter 22: High Altitude Cerebral Edema*

Coexistent HAPE: Cough; rales; frothy, pink, or blood-tinged sputum. *See Part 6: Operational Environment: Chapter 22: High Altitude Pulmonary Edema*

Other causes of headache (migraine, cluster, or tension headache; viral syndrome; meningitis; head trauma; etc.): Symptoms before ascending to altitude - stiff neck, fever or increased white cell count; history of head trauma.

Intoxication: History of ingesting medications, recreational drugs, alcohol. *See Part 5: Specialty Areas: Chapter 17: Introduction to General Poisoning & Part 5: Specialty Areas: Chapter 19: Mental Health: Substance Abuse*

Carbon monoxide poisoning: History of exposure to combustion fumes, occasional cherry-red skin color. *See Part 5: Specialty Areas: Chapter 17: Carbon Monoxide Poisoning*

Hypothermia: Lack of headache and nausea, decreased body temperature. *See Part 6: Operational Environment: Chapter 23: Hypothermia and Cold Water Immersion.*

Hyperthermia and/or dehydration: History of decreased fluid intake, elevated body temperature or tenting of skin. *See Part 6: Operational Environment: Chapter 24*

Plan:
Treatment
Primary: <u>Stop ascent!</u> Descend to lower altitude until symptoms resolve. Once symptoms resolve, continue ascent slowly (See Prevention). Treat with **acetazolamide*** 250mg po bid/tid. Oxygen (if available) by mask or nasal cannula or treatment in a portable hyperbaric chamber. (*See Part 8: Procedures: Chapter 30: Portable Pressure Chamber*). **Aspirin, acetaminophen, ibuprofen, indomethacin,** or **naproxen** in usual doses can be used to treat headache pain. Nausea and vomiting can be treated with **prochlorperazine** 10mg po q6h or 25mg by rectal suppository q12h.

Alternative: Stay at higher altitude during day, but sleep at lower altitude (see Prevention). **Dexamethasone*** 4mg po qid (Use for people allergic to **acetazolamide** or other sulfa drugs).

Primitive: Descent is the best treatment for all altitude illnesses (eg, AMS, HACE, HAPE). Native people of the Andes Mountains in South America chew coca leaves or drink coca tea to prevent and treat AMS. Prophylactic: If slow ascent is not possible, acetazolamide* 250mg po bid/tid beginning 12-24 hours before starting ascent and continuing for 48 hours after reach destination altitude. **Dexamethasone*** 4mg po qid is a 2nd line preventive agent for individuals allergic to acetazolamide or other sulfa drugs. *These medications can be stopped 1-2 days after symptoms resolve. AMS symptoms may recur after stopping dexamethasone, but do not recur after stopping acetazolamide. Oxygen or portable pressure chamber treatment can be stopped an hour after symptoms resolve. AMS symptoms are likely to recur within 12 hours if patient remains at same or higher altitude.

Patient Education

General: AMS is caused by ascending too rapidly, before body has chance to adjust to altitude. Symptoms will improve over several days as body adjusts to altitude

Activity: Avoid strenuous activity until acclimatized to altitude

Diet: Stay hydrated. High carbohydrate (starches and sugars) diet to decrease symptoms

Medications: Acetazolamide often causes tingling sensations in lips, nose and fingertips and makes carbonated beverages. These side effects are not harmful. Do not stop taking acetazolamide because of them. Dexamethasone can have serious side effects during treatment and withdrawal. Use should be limited and dexamethasone should be withdrawn slowly (ie, tapered over a week) in patients treated with dexamethasone for more than 3-5 days.

Prevention and Hygiene: Ascend slowly (1,000–2,000 feet/day above 8,000 ft) with a rest day (no ascent) every 3-4 days. Sleep at least 1,000-2,000 ft lower than working altitude. Acetazolamide or dexamethasone* beginning 12-24 hours before ascent and continuing for 48 hours after reaching destination altitude can decrease the risk of AMS. Although no controlled studies exist to prove the recommendation; most climbers drink enough water to keep their urine"gin clear"

No Improvement/Deterioration: Seek medical aid if headache worsens, develop difficulty with walking, coordination, cough, cough up frothy, pink or bloody sputum, "gurgling" sounds in chest when breathing

Follow-up Action

Re-evaluation: No follow up is necessary unless symptoms return.

Evacuation/Consultation Criteria: Evacuate to lower altitude as discussed previously. There is no way to predict which person is more susceptible to AMS. Consider medical profile limiting deployment to altitude for those with recurrent or prolonged AMS.

Chapter 22: High Altitude Illnesses: High Altitude Cerebral Edema
COL Paul Rock, MC, USA (Ret)

Introduction: High altitude cerebral edema (HACE) is a potentially fatal accumulation of fluid (edema) in brain tissue which sometimes occurs in people from low altitude (less than 5,000 feet) that ascend rapidly to high altitude (greater than 8,000 feet; but rare below 11,500 feet) and remain there for several days. It is caused by the decreased amount of oxygen available to the body in the low pressure atmosphere at high altitude. *See Part 6: Operational Environment: Chapter 21: Cerebral Hypoxia*

HACE is a severe form of acute mountain sickness (AMS) (*see Part 6: Operational Environment: Chapter 22: Acute Mountain Sickness*) and most often occurs in people who continue their ascent despite symptoms of AMS. Although relatively rare (1-2% of persons going to high altitude), HACE if left untreated can progress to coma and death in 12 hours or less.

High altitude pulmonary edema (HAPE), which can also be rapidly fatal, often occurs with HACE. *See Part 6: Operational Environment: Chapter 22: High Altitude Pulmonary Edema*

Subjective: **Symptoms**

Early: Symptoms of AMS (severe headache, nausea with vomiting, decreased appetite and fatigue); later: progressive weakness, fatigue and clumsiness; confusion and disorientation; vivid hallucinations (visual and/or auditory)

Focused History: *When did the symptoms begin?* (typically begin 3-10 days after ascent; later than AMS) *Have you had symptoms of AMS?* (risk factor; worsening AMS symptoms after 48-72 hours are likely due to HACE.) *How is your coordination? Have you been stumbling or falling?* (Ataxia and clumsiness are typical.) *Are you seeing or hearing unexpected or unusual things (having hallucinations)? Do you have a cough or difficulty breathing?* (typical of HAPE; accompanies 1/3 of HACE cases) *Have you taken any medications, drugs or alcohol?* (Intoxication could cause similar symptoms.) *Have you been in a tent, cave or vehicle with a stove or motor running?* (Carbon monoxide poisoning could cause similar symptoms.)

Objective: **Signs**

Using Basic Tools: Early: Behavioral changes (agitated or quiet and withdrawn); later: disorientation, confusion, ataxia (cannot do "heel-to-toe-walk"), in coordination and often hallucinations (visual and auditory); abnormal deep tendon reflexes, decreased consciousness, coma and death; may have rales, cough, and frothy, pink or bloody sputum (coexisting HAPE). Blood oxygen levels measured by pulse oximeter will be lower with HACE and other altitude illnesses

Using Advanced Tools: Ophthalmoscope: Retinal hemorrhages and swelling of optic nerve in the back of the eye (papilledema)

Assessment:

Differential Diagnosis

Other causes of headache (eg, migraine, cluster, or tension headache; infection): History of headache at low altitude. Check for stiff neck, fever or increased white cell count. *See Part 4: Organ Systems: Chapter 5: Meningitis*

Head trauma: Check for lacerations, bruising, depressed skull

Intoxication: History of ingesting medications, recreational drugs, alcohol. *See Part 5: Specialty Areas: Chapter 17: Introduction to Poisoning & Chapter 18: Substance Abuse*

Carbon monoxide poisoning: History of exposure to combustion fumes. *See Part 5: Specialty Areas: Chapter 17: Carbon Monoxide Poisoning*

Hypothermia: Lack of headache and nausea. Decreased body temperature. *See Part 6: Operational Environment: Chapter 23: Hypothermia and Cold Water Immersion*

Hyperthermia and/or dehydration: History of decreased fluid intake, elevated body temperature. *See Part 6: Operational Environment: Chapter 24*

AMS: HACE patients have papilledema and/or ataxia, and may have deteriorating mental status. *See Part 6: Operational Environment: Chapter 22: Acute Mountain Sickness*

Plan:

Treatment

Primary:

1. Evacuate to lower altitude immediately (1,000-2,000 feet change may be lifesaving). Do not allow solo descent.
2. Oxygen at 6 L/minute or more by oxygen mask. Insert endotracheal tube if comatose. Portable hyperbaric chamber may be a life saving temporizing measure while descent is being arranged. *See Part 8: Procedures: Chapter 30: Portable Pressure Chamber*
3. **Dexamethasone** 8mg po or IV initially, then 4mg po or IV q6h through medical evacuation and clinical improvement at lower altitude.
4. Evacuate patient to advanced medical care.

Alternative: Oxygen, **dexamethasone**

Primitive: Descent is the best treatment for all altitude illnesses (eg, AMS, HACE, HAPE).

Prophylactic: Two of the drugs used to prevent AMS (ie, **acetazolamide** and **dexamethasone**; *see Part 6: Operational Environment: Chapter 22: Acute Mountain Sickness*) also can be used to prevent HACE.

Patient Education

General: HACE is caused by rapid ascent before the body can adjust to altitude. Symptoms will worsen with further ascent. HACE can be rapidly fatal.

Activity: Bed rest or very limited activity; can descend under own power in emergency, if accompanied

Medications: Dexamethasone can cause psychosis, depression, puffy face, increase appetite and adrenal suppression in patients taking this medication for >3-5 days. Dexamethasone dose should be tapered slowly (ie, over one week) to reduce risk of adrenal insufficiency (eg, hypotension, hypoglycemia, poor response to infection/ trauma).

Prevention and Hygiene: Pre-mission acclimatization. Ascend slowly (less than 1,000 ft/day) with rest day q 3-4 days. Do not continue ascending with symptoms of altitude illness. Sleep at as low an altitude as possible (1,000-2,000 ft lower than working altitude) until body adjusts to altitude (7-10 days). The drugs acetazolamide and dexamethasone may help prevent HACE.

No Improvement/Deterioration: HACE is rapidly fatal if not treated. Seek medical attention if have headache and difficulty with balance or have hallucinations. HACE is often accompanied by HAPE. Seek medical attention for cough or frothy, pink or bloody sputum or gurgling sounds in your chest or throat when breathing.

Follow-up Actions

Return Evaluation: Evaluate survivors for neurological deficits that might affect their performance of military duties. Individuals who have had one episode of HACE are at increased risk of future episodes and should be referred for possible medical profile to restrict exposure to altitudes greater than 8,000 feet.

Evacuation/Consultation Criteria: Evacuate all patients with HACE to higher echelon of medical care, preferably to hospital facility. CT scan or MRI imaging of the brain may show cerebral edema. If not evacuated rapidly, even patients who survive may have prolonged or permanent neurological damage.

Notes: Portable pressure chambers (eg, Gamow bag, CERTEC, Portable Altitude Chamber [PAC]) are not normally available in the US military supply inventory outside of the Special Operations Command, but are available in the civilian sector. A Gamow bag is included in USASOC high altitude medical kits which are available through SOF supply channels. These lightweight, highly portable cloth chambers can be carried in a backpack and are extremely useful in treating HACE and other altitude illnesses. When deploying rapidly to high altitude terrain, strongly consider procuring such a chamber.

Chapter 22: High Altitude Illnesses: High Altitude Pulmonary Edema
COL Paul Rock, MC, USA (Ret)

Introduction: High altitude pulmonary edema (HAPE) is a potentially fatal accumulation of fluid in the lungs (non-cardiogenic pulmonary edema) that occurs when people ascend rapidly (without acclimatization) from a low altitude (less than 5,000 ft) to high altitudes (usually greater than 9,000 ft) and remain there for several days. It is caused by the decreased amount of oxygen available in the low-pressure atmosphere at high altitude (*see Part 6: Operational Environment: Chapter 21: Cerebral Hypoxia*). The symptoms of HAPE often begin after the 1st or 2nd night spent at high altitude and the condition is most common during the 1st week at altitude.

Heavy physical exertion upon arrival at high altitude significantly increases the risk of developing HAPE. Although not common (usually less than 10% of persons going to altitudes above 12,000 ft), once the symptoms of HAPE develop, the condition can be rapidly fatal (in 6-12 hours), if not treated. Children are more susceptible than adults, and individuals with previous diagnosis of HAPE have a significant increased risk of recurrence.

Half of individuals with HAPE will also have additional symptoms of acute mountain sickness (AMS), headache, fatigue, nausea and vomiting (*see Part 6: Operational Environment: Chapter 22: Acute Mountain Sickness*). High altitude cerebral edema (HACE) another potentially fatal complication of altitude may also be present. *See Part 6: Operational Environment: Chapter 22: High Altitude Cerebral Edema*

Subjective: **Symptoms**

Early: Shortness of breath, dry cough, dyspnea on exertion. Later: dyspnea at rest, frequent cough with clear and watery sputum, symptoms of AMS (headache, nausea and vomiting, decreased appetite and fatigue). Still later: frothy, blood-streaked or pink sputum; feel or hear "gurgling" in chest with breathing.

Focused History: *Do you have difficulty breathing or a cough? Are you coughing up frothy, pink or bloody sputum?* (typical symptoms) *When did symptoms begin?* (typically after exercise or after sleeping during 1st week at altitude) *Did you have these symptoms or any illness before going to altitude?* (rule out preexisting condition) *How is your coordination? Have you been stumbling or falling? Are you seeing or hearing unexpected or unusual things (hallucinations)?* (suggest coexisting HACE) *Have you had fever and chills? Have you coughed up thick, greenish or yellow-colored sputum?* (suggests bronchopneumonia) *Do you have any pain or swelling in your legs? Does your chest hurt when you breathe?* (possible blood clot in legs with subsequent blood clot in lungs [pulmonary embolus]) *Have you ever had asthma or hay fever in the past?* (rule out asthma)

Objective: Signs

Using Basic Tools: Early signs: Tachypnea and tachycardia during physical activity (compared to companions at same altitude), dry cough, crackling sounds (rales) in lungs. Progressive signs: Tachypnea and tachycardia at rest (compared to unaffected companions); "gurgling" breath sounds; excessive (compared to companions at same altitude) bluish color of lips, fingernail bed, tip of nose and ears (cyanosis); cough productive of frothy and/or pink, blood streaked sputum; low-grade fever. Late signs: Coma, respiratory failure, death. Pulse ox: Blood oxygen levels will be lower with HAPE or other altitude illnesses.

Using Advanced Tools: CXR: Fluffy infiltrates in mid-lung fields or spreading throughout lungs

Assessment:

Diagnosis is made on basis of clinical presentation during exposure to increased altitude (ie, decreased oxygen).

Differential Diagnosis

AMS or HACE (in addition to HAPE): *See Part 6: Operational Environment: Chapter 22: Acute Mountain Sickness & High Altitude Cerebral Edema*

Pneumonia: Fever greater than 101°F; infected (purulent) sputum; symptoms before traveling to high altitude. *See Part 4: Organ Systems: Chapter 3: Pneumonia*

Pulmonary embolus: Chest pain with breathing, blood clot in leg veins (pain and swelling); *see Part 4: Organ Systems: Chapter 3: Deep Vein Thrombosis and Pulmonary Embolism*

High-altitude cough: Chronic, dry cough can occur at very high altitude (usually greater than 15,000 ft) due to irritation of throat by breathing cold, dry air. Not associated with rales, sputum production, or other signs or symptoms of HAPE.

Asthma: History of asthma; breathing cold air or allergen exposure; wheezing. *See Part 4: Organ Systems: Chapter 3: Asthma*

Plan:

Treatment

Primary:

1. Immediately evacuate by liter to lower altitude. Descent 1,000-2,000 feet lower may be lifesaving. Walking will worsen HAPE; do not allow solo descent

2. Oxygen: 6L/minute or greater by mask. Use of a portable hyperbaric chamber (eg, Gamow Bag) may provide dramatic relief of symptoms during transfer of patient to a lower altitude.

3. **Nifedipine:** Break 10mg capsule and hold under tongue. If BP remains stable, nifedipine 10mg po may be repeated at 30 minute intervals as clinically indicated. **Nifedipine** 20mg sustained release tablet po (swallowed) q6h may be used during evacuation or where evacuation is delayed.

4. If HACE also present, treat it. *See Part 6: Operational Environment: Chapter 22: High Altitude Cerebral Edema*

5. If comatose, endotracheal tube intubation to protect airway. *See Part 8: Procedures: Chapter 30: Intubation*

Alternative:

1. If evacuation to lower altitude not possible, bed rest, high-flow oxygen by mask, **nifedipine**, and treatment in portable hyperbaric ("pressure") chamber*. *See Part 8: Procedures: Chapter 30: Portable Pressure Chamber*

2. If nifedipine not available, use **acetazolamide** 250mg (do not give if allergic to sulfa) po q6-8h or **sildenafil** 25mg po q8h.

3. End-positive-airway-pressure (EPAP) mask may be helpful, if available.

Primitive: Descent is the best treatment for all altitude illnesses (eg, AMS, HACE, HAPE). "Pursed-lip" breathing may help increase oxygenation. Patient in prone, slightly head-down position for brief period (10-20 min) may help drain lung fluid through the mouth temporarily (if patient can tolerate that position).

Prophylactic: If slow ascent is not possible, susceptible individuals (ie, have had HAPE in the past) can take **nifedipine** 20mg sustained release po q8-12h, or **dexamethasone** 8mg po q12h, or **sildenafil** 25mg po q8h, or **salmeterol** 125 micrograms inhaled q12h to try to decrease risk of developing HAPE.

Note: Nifedipine, sildenafil, and salmeterol are not on SOF drug list, but are available through military medical supply channels and civilian sources.

Patient Education

General: HAPE is caused by rapid ascent before the body has a chance to adjust to high altitude. More likely to occur in individuals undergoing strenuous physical activity during first 5 days after ascent, or keep ascending while having symptoms of any altitude illness.

Activity: Bed rest (physical activity makes HAPE worse).

Medications: Nifedipine and sildenafil can lower the BP and cause dizziness when sitting up or standing rapidly from a prone position (**Note:** Patients are often volume depleted). Nifedipine can cause swelling (edema) of the hands, lower legs and feet. Dexamethasone can cause psychosis, depression, puffy face, and increase appetite. Taper dose after taking for more than 3-4 days.

Prevention and Hygiene: Ascend slowly (less than 1,000 ft/day above 8,000) with rest day (no ascent) q 3-4 days. Do not continue ascent with symptoms of altitude illness or difficulty breathing. Sleep at as low an altitude as possible (1,000-2,000 ft lower than working altitude) until body adjusts (7-10 days). Avoid vigorous physical activity for first 5 days after ascent. Individuals with history of developing HAPE have a significantly increased risk of recurrence of HAPE. If operational situation requires ascent, the use of nifedipine, dexamethasone, sildenafil or inhaled salmeterol (at doses listed previously) may decrease risk of recurrence of HAPE in these individuals.

No Improvement/Deterioration: HAPE can be rapidly fatal in individuals not diagnosed and appropriately treated. Individuals with more difficulty than companions breathing during exercise or at rest may deteriorate quickly with onset of cough, (blood or pink colored or frothy sputum), feel "gurgling" in chest or audible breath sounds, symptoms of HACE (eg, severe headache, difficulty keeping balance or hallucinations).

Follow-up Actions

Return Evaluation: If evacuated promptly, patient may recover rapidly (hours to days) and completely. Individuals who have had one episode of HAPE are at increased risk of recurrence and should be referred for possible medical profile or prophylactic treatment when being deployed to high altitude.

Evacuation/Consultation Criteria: Evacuate all patients with more than mild HAPE to a hospital facility. They should be evaluated for possible medical profile to restrict exposure to altitudes above 8,000 ft.

Notes: Portable pressure chambers (eg, Gamow bag, CERTEC, Portable Altitude Chamber [PAC]) are not normally available in the US military supply inventory outside of the Special Operations Command, but are available in the civilian sector. A Gamow bag is included in USASOC high altitude medical kits which are available through SOF supply channels. These lightweight, highly portable cloth chambers can be carried in a backpack and are extremely useful in treating HAPE and other altitude illnesses. When deploying rapidly to high altitude terrain, consider procuring such a chamber.

Chapter 23: Cold Illnesses and Injuries: Hypothermia and Cold Water Immersion
LCDR Steven M. Kriss, MC, USN

Introduction: Hypothermia is a reduction in body temperature below 95°F as measured by a rectal thermometer placed at least 6 inches into the rectum. Risk factors for hypothermia include trauma, wind and wetness, physical and mental exhaustion, psychiatric disorders, alcohol use, inactivity, endocrine disorders, poor nutrition, poor clothing and cold, particularly during rapid changes in weather. Freezing temperatures are not necessary to cause hypothermia. Water immersion can produce extremely rapid cooling. Use core temperature taken via rectum or esophagus. Feeling for patient's body warmth between shoulder blades is a quick field expedient way to get a sense of whether patient is maintaining core temperature.

Subjective: Symptoms *See Table 6-4*

Mild hypothermia (core temperature between 90° and 95°F): Poor coordination, stumbling and shivering.

Moderate hypothermia (82°-90°F): Muscle and joint stiffness, poor coordination, slurred speech, extreme disorientation and confusion.

Severe hypothermia (below 82°F): Asleep or unconscious. Below 77°F: Spontaneous ventricular fibrillation.

Focused History: *How cold, wet and windy is it outside and what were you wearing?* (risk of hypothermia). *Who, what and where?* (Define mental status and the severity of hypothermia.) *How long have you been outside?* (risk of hypothermia) *Any health problems?* (Susceptibility to cold injuries eg, hypothyroidism, slows metabolism and increases the risk of all cold injuries.) *Medications?* (Sedatives and narcotics may impair judgment.) *Alcohol or other substance use?* (Alcohol causes vasodilation which results in a greater loss of body heat) *Have you suffered any trauma?* (Trauma patients are prone to develop hypothermia which can inhibit clotting mechanism worsening the effects of the trauma) *Last meal and hydration?* (People who are poorly nourished and/or poorly hydrated are at greater risk of developing hypothermia.)

Table 6-4. Classification of Level of Hypothermia

Core Temperature 98.6°F	Thermoregulatory Status	Signs and Symptoms	Classification
98.6°F		- Cold Sensation - Shivering	Normal
90–95°F	Control and Responses Fully Active	Physical Impairment Mental Impairment - Fine Motor - Complex - Gross Motor - Simple	Mild
82–90°F	Responses Attenuated/ Extinguished	~ 86°F: - Shivering Stops - Loss of Consciousness	Moderate
<82°F	Responses Absent	- Rigidity - Vital Signs Reduced or Absent - Risk of VF/Cardiac Arrest (Rough Handling)	Severe
<77°F		- Spontaneous Ventricular Fibrillation - Cardiac Arrest	

Objective: **Signs**

Remember the "umbles" of hypothermia: stumbles, fumbles, mumbles and grumbles. This will remind you of some of the signs.

Using Basic Tools: Vital signs: Use rectal thermometer to take core temperature as it has a lower scale. Do not place in stool.

Mild: Lethargic, diminished fine motor control, shuffling, stumbling gait, shivering; **Moderate:** Lack of shivering, slow to react, disoriented, makes major errors in judgment, loses consciousness, paradoxical undressing; **Severe:** Heart and respiration rates slow, difficult to perceive a pulse, muscles become too stiff to move, cardiac arrhythmias often develop. If unconscious, the victim may have spontaneous ventricular fibrillation or cardiac arrest if handled roughly. Below 77°F, spontaneous cardiac arrest is likely. There are often no obvious vital signs and the victim may appear clinically dead, but in fact is not.

Using Advanced Tools: ECGs reveal unusual ST changes called Osborne "J waves." Most ECG machines cannot interpret these J waves, which are usually found in leads V2-V4.

Assessment:

Carefully but thoroughly evaluate to identify other potential injuries or conditions. Some of the following diagnoses both increase risk of hypothermia and may also be considerations in hypothermic patients who do not respond to re-warming.

Differential Diagnosis:

Head trauma: Differentiate by history and clinical exam

Hypoglycemia: History of diabetes (especially with insulin therapy) may be present

Exposure to toxins, drugs or alcohol: May contribute to hypothermia. Identify by history or clinical signs (eg, smell)

Severe infection (sepsis): Impairs thermogenesis and may be a consideration in patients who do not respond to rewarming

Adrenal insufficiency: Suspect in a patient who is ill or injured who previously has been treated for an extended period of time (>1 week) with steroids

Figure 6-6. Hypothermia: EMS Prehospital Care

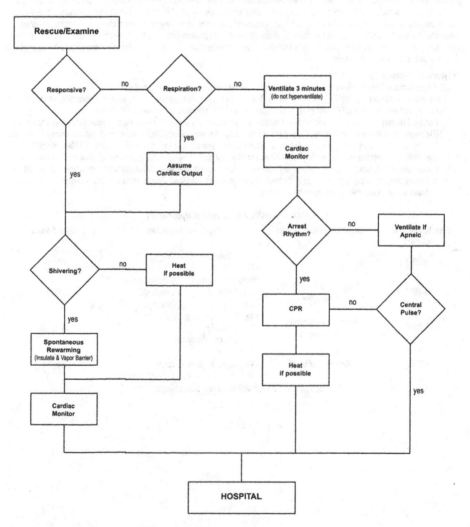

Plan:
Treatment *See Figure 6-6*
   Primary:
1. Handle individuals carefully to prevent ventricular arrhythmias. Patients should be maintained in the horizontal position while being removed from the hypothermic environment and through treatment. Monitor cardiac rhythm (ignore atrial arrhythmias and slow ventricular responses).
2. Ventilate by mouth or by mask, O_2 if available. Ventilation changes the fibrillatory threshold and allows safer transport.
3. If pulse and respiration are absent while in the field (ie, capabilities to analyze rhythm and defibrillator is not available), do not initiate chest compression; merely ventilate. When capability to analyze rhythm and defibrillator is available, use ACLS guidelines for management of hypothermic patient, which differ from normothermic patients. (ie, if patient's temperature is <86°F and a shockable rhythm is identified, defibrillate once at 360 joules, resume CPR and defer cardiac drugs and subsequent defibrillation attempts until core temperature is >86°F.)
4. Remove wet clothes and insulate, particularly the torso, head and neck. Apply a vapor barrier over the insulating layers. Do not delay evacuation to initiate active warming procedures but any warmth applied inside the wrapped insulation layers is useful.
5. If active rewarming therapy is initiated, rewarm the trunk prior to rewarming the extremities to reduce the risk of an "after drop" (additional loss of core temperature that can occur when extremities are warmed returning cold acidic blood to the core). The combination of decreased sensation and reduced blood flow increases the risk of body surface burns in hypothermic patients and care must be taken during any external rewarming to prevent iatrogenic surface body burns.
6. Give sweet fluids orally if awake. Otherwise, give 250-500cc IV bolus of warmed normal saline followed by rapid drip.
7. Patients may appear cold, stiff, blue and may appear to be dead, but this diagnosis cannot be made until they have been rewarmed in a treatment facility.

Patient Education
   General: Follow preventive measures, including proper use of cold weather clothing, staying dry, getting out of the wind, and monitoring buddies.
   Diet: Eat a high calorie, high fat diet to increase heat production and improve performance in the cold.
   Medications: Avoid medications that compromise judgment and shivering, including tranquilizers, alcohol, narcotics and some anti-depressants.
   Prevention and Hygiene: Stay dry, well fed and rested.
   Revaluation: Core temperature may continue to decrease ("after drop") after the patient is removed from the cold. This can be life-threatening if a 2-3 degree drop occurs at a core temperature of 88°F or less.

Follow-up Actions
   Evacuation/Consultant Criteria: Depending on the timeliness of evacuation, patients with severe hypothermia should be transported. Lesser degrees of hypothermia can usually be treated locally.
   Note: Many trauma victims become slowly hypothermic, which may be as life-threatening as the trauma itself as hypothermic trauma patients cannot clot well and lose more blood. While transporting trauma patients, keep them wrapped, insulated and dry and protect them from wind. A short period of successful ventilation oxygenates the patient perceived to be dead, and allows them to be handled, insulated, packaged and transported, while minimizing the likelihood of ventricular fibrillation during this process.
   Note: Cold Water Immersion. The conduction and loss of heat is 24 times greater in water than in air, therefore, patients quickly become profoundly hypothermic in water. Cold water immersion can also decrease the metabolic rate and "preserve" a patient so these patients can sometimes survive longer and require longer resuscitation periods than other typical cold patients. Other problems unique to cold water immersion are the increased risk of drowning due to panic and subsequent aspiration and an increased risk of cardiopulmonary collapse due to vasoconstriction and bradycardia caused by the mammalian "Diving Reflex." Treat these patients gently as any other severely hypothermic patients and be mindful that they may have aspirated water as well. MEDEVAC all severely hypothermic and near-drowning patients, if possible, to an ICU to increase their survival.

Chapter 23: Cold Illnesses and Injuries: Freezing Injury (Frostbite)
LCDR Steven M. Kriss, MC, USN

Introduction: Frostbite occurs at temperatures below freezing (32°F), most often in exhausted, wet, discouraged troops who are poorly dressed and inattentive to prevention. Although there are 4 basic degree categories of frostbite, it is important to differentiate merely superficial from deep or severe frostbite since they are managed differently. Superficial involves just the surface of the skin but no blisters form. Deep or severe frostbite involves partial or full-thickness skin injury, causes blisters and demarcates over a period of days or weeks. Extremities and exposed skin are at an increased risk of injury. Other risk factors include tobacco use and diabetes. **Note:** It is important to check for, rule out and treat hypothermia, if present, as it is often found in frostbite patients. Hypothermia must be treated before frostbite as it can be lethal.

Subjective: **Symptoms**
   Progression from cool, to cold and uncomfortable, to numb and painless tissue; injury is often concealed by mittens, gloves or boots; slow, stiff movements. Injured tissue becomes extremely painful upon rewarming. Deep tissue damage can produce acidosis, rhabdomyolysis, fever and coagulopathies.
   Focused History: *How cold is it outside, how long were you outside and what were you wearing?* (This will determine the person's risk of frostbite.) *What activities were you doing?* (A mountain climber who is exposed to the elements of cold, wind and moisture is at much greater risk of frostbite and develops it faster than others.) *Are you able to move and feel your limbs or affected body parts?*

(This will determine the severity of frostbite.) *Did the affected body part thaw and then re-freeze?* (This leads to a poor outcome because of greater tissue damage.) *Are you a smoker?* (Smoking and tobacco use cause vasoconstriction which will increase the damage from frostbite and impair healing.) *Do you have any health problems?* (Diabetes and other conditions like high cholesterol can worsen the damage of frostbite because of poor blood flow to the tissues.) *Have you been playing with cans of cleaning agents, compressed air or liquid nitrogen?* (These agents can be as cold as -50 to -100°F and can cause frostbite almost instantaneously when in contact with the skin.)

Objective: Signs

Using Basic Tools: Inspection: Frozen tissue is blanched white or pale yellow, completely ischemic and hard to the touch. The skin is immobile over joints. Upon rewarming, the skin becomes red, swollen and may turn gray or deeply red to purple-blue, Large blisters containing either clear or hemorrhagic fluid form in severe frostbite. Dead tissue is known as gangrene, which is identified by a blackened, stiff appearance.

Assessment:

Differential Diagnosis

Gangrene from other sources (ischemia, burns, and severe infections): may present similarly but the history of cold exposure should clarify the diagnosis.

Plan:

Treatment

Primary:

1. Do not thaw tissue if there is any threat of re-freezing during evacuation.
2. Warm superficial frostbite gradually in the axilla, groin or in warm water.
3. Deep frostbite is best managed with:
   a. Moving water immersion (whirlpool) at 104-108°F for 30 minutes. This produces significant pain, but affords the best tissue salvage.
   b. Apply a loose, dry dressing and splint prior to transport.
   c. Low molecular weight **Dextran** (1L of 6% solution IV, followed by 500mL/day for 5 days) or if no increased risk of severe bleeding complications, **heparin** (15 units/kg IV stat, then a total of 70 units/kg in the first 24 hours) can be given to decrease risk of "sludging" of blood and improve perfusion.
   d. Vasodilator **phenoxybenzamine hydrochloride** 10mg po bid. Increase dose 10mg each day to max of 60-80mg po q day.
   e. Surgically débride dead tissue* (*See Part 8: Procedures: Chapter 30: Wound Debridement*)
4. Manage pain: **Aspirin**, NSAIDs or narcotics if indicated. Deep, long standing injury may require **morphine** sedation. *See Part 8: Procedures: Chapter 30: Pain Assessment and Control*
5. All medications have more benefit if given to patient before thawing.
6. Use non-adherent gauze for 1st layer to bandage, pad and then splint affected extremity to avoid further injury during transport.
7. **Tetanus** prophylaxis if required and early use of parenteral antibiotics at 1st signs of any associated infection. *See Part 4: Organ Systems: Chapter 6: Bacterial Infections.* Do not use topical antibiotics which only increase skin maceration. Topical aloe may provide some benefit.

*Note: Debriding frostbitten tissue too early is the most common error in frostbite management. Debriding too early results in retraction, infections, graft failures and removal of viable tissue. Wait to débride mummified tissue for 4-8 weeks unless fever and coagulopathies mandate earlier intervention. There is a 2mm liquefaction line between viable tissue and distal mummifying tissue. Late surgical debridement of indurated tissue should only be to this line.

Patient Education

General: Use personal protective measures to prevent cold injury. Do not walk on frostbitten feet.

Diet: Eat 5% to 10% more calories.

Include more fat and carbohydrates in the diet.

Medications: Give NSAIDs with food. Monitor respiratory status if morphine is used.

Wound Care: Manage wounds with warm water baths bid, pat dry and bandage with a loose, dry dressing.

Follow-up Actions

Evacuation/Consultant Criteria: Minor frostbite can be managed quite successfully in the field, but deep frostbite will require evacuation. Consult a general surgeon as needed for definitive management.

Chapter 23: Cold Illnesses and Injuries: Non-freezing Cold Injury (Immersion Foot/Trench Foot)

LCDR Steven M. Kriss, MC, USN

Introduction: Having cold, wet feet for an extended period (2 days or more) will produce the non-freezing cold injury (NFCI) called immersion or trench foot. Sitting in a life raft with wet extremities produces immersion foot. Tissue death occurs as a result of long-term vasospasm from cold, usually above freezing. The colder it is, the less time it takes to produce damage. This injury is common in POWs, escape and evasion victims, and life raft survivors. It is also common in combat troops exposed to water-filled trenches. Chilblains follow cold, wet exposure of the hands or feet of less than 12 hours. They will be swollen, pink, mildly tender, and pruritic but will recover in 24 hours. A longer exposure (12 hours or more) produces pernio, resulting in thin, partial thickness, necrotic plaques on the dorsum of the hands or feet. These will slough without scarring in a few days, but the area may remain very painful for months or years.

Subjective: **Symptoms**

Initially cold, wet feet progressing to numbness. Upon warming the torso and feet, they become hot and very painful. The patient is unable to wear boots or walk. Those that can walk will have a shuffling gait and describe a feeling of walking on "wooden limbs."
Focused History: *What is the air temperature outside and what is the water temperature?* (This will determine a person's risk of NFCI.) *Which activities were you engaged in outside?* (A person who was doing Ranger training in a swamp or survival training in the jungle or cold weather training is at greater risk of NFCI because of the constant exposure to cold and/or moisture.) *What kind of footwear were you wearing?* (This will influence the patient's risk of NFCI. Footwear that drains readily will lessen the negative effects from moisture whereas footwear like vapor barrier boots stay warm, but keep moisture in and can increase NFCI over a long period if socks are not changed) *Can you feel your affected limb and how does it feel when you walk on it ?* (If someone describes a loss of feeling in a limb and a "woody" feeling while walking they may very well have a NFCI.) *Have you warmed your affected limb rapidly?* (Rapid re-warming of a NFCI is potentially very destructive for the tissue.) *Are you experiencing a lot of pain?* (Painful feet could mean that a person has a significant NFCI.)

Objective: **Signs**

Using Basic Tools: Inspection: Initially pale, pulseless, and numb tissues that have slow capillary refill. Upon warming, they are edematous, bright red or purple, hot and painful. Digital pressure produces pitting and slow rebound. After a number of days, liquefaction necrosis or mummification of distal parts occurs. Fever develops and debridement is necessary.

Assessment: The history of being cold and wet along with visualization of the limbs is diagnostic.

Differential Diagnosis:

Frostbite: Requires below freezing temperatures and produces a dry, mummifying gangrene. *See Part 6: Operational Environment: Chapter 23: Freezing Injury (Frostbite)*
Chilblains: The early stages of trenchfoot and results in just swelling and itching of the extremity, which subsides in 24 hours.
Pernio: Thin, necrotic plaques on the dorsum of the hands or feet. They may be proximal to a more serious distal trenchfoot injury.

Plan:

Treatment

Primary: Pat dry, DO NOT RUB. Elevate the feet, warm the torso and hydrate orally. Urine output (color, frequency) can be used to estimate hydration status. Pain meds help to some degree. NSAIDs may help. Most patients need litters, and may need sleep meds.
Patient Education

General: Keep feet dry. Wounds will have a long, slow healing process. Patients may have residual symptoms for years. Fanning the feet at night might help sleep.
Diet: High calorie diet and adequate hydration
Medications: NSAIDs and sleep meds
Prevention and Hygiene: Change to dry socks daily in cold, wet conditions. Gently massage feet at night to improve blood flow. Treat and/or evacuate those with early symptoms to avoid serious injury.
Wound Care: If necrotic, auto amputation occurs; clean the wound and use loose dry dressings. Evacuate
Follow-up Actions

Evacuation/Consultant Criteria: Patients who are unable to ambulate or perform their mission, have recurrent injury, have auto amputation of digits or develop osteomyelitis should be evacuated.

Chapter 24: Heat-Related Illnesses: Introduction
LTC Ric Ong, MC, USA

Heat injuries fall into a continuum of heat cramps to heat exhaustion to heat stroke. While the mechanism of heat cramps is not understood, there is convincing evidence to suggest it is the result of sodium depletion or over hydration. Heat exhaustion and heat stroke represent a spectrum of disorders, which range in intensity and the severity of tissue damage. The pathophysiology of heat exhaustion and heat stroke are so similar that they may represent a continuum of disease rather then separate, distinct diseases and both are characterized by sodium and water depletion.

Heat cramps, heat exhaustion and heat stroke are all illnesses related to a failure of the body to maintain fluid and electrolyte balance to the challenge of adapting to added heat loads. These conditions may develop over several days, allowing adequate time for effective intervention. The maintenance of adequate diet and fluid intake is essential.

The use of diet supplements such as creatine and amino acids can all lead to dehydration and increased likelihood of heat injury. If sports drinks are used, they should be diluted 1:1 with water to decrease their concentration. Creatine and other diet supplements also increase the requirement for water, while they lack the natural salts and water content of the foods they replace.

When faced with increased heat loads, the body is dependent on sweating to maintain a constant body temperature. The sources of the heat load may be external (a hot day), internal (a road march with 50 pounds of gear) or both (a road march in the desert sun). If the heat load exceeds the body's ability to lose heat, a heat injury will result.

Figure 6-7. Heat Injury: Major Areas of Interaction

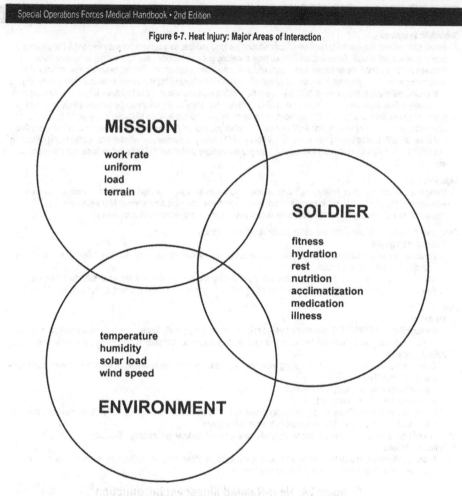

Source: United States Army Research Institute of Environmental Medicine

There are 3 major areas of interaction that determines if a heat injury will occur. These are depicted in *Figure 6-7*. The Soldier represents those personal factors that affect the body's ability to adjust. Physical fitness, hydration, rest, nutrition, acclimatization, the use of medications and illness are factors that influence the body's ability to sweat and therefore, to control its internal temperature. The environment represents those outside conditions that affect the body's ability to lose heat. The mission represents those things that must be modified to allow successful completion of the mission when the heat stress would otherwise overwhelm the body's heat loss mechanisms.

Since the body uses sweat to control temperature, water is essential. There was a myth that the body could adjust to decreased water intake. That has been disproven; being partially dehydrated simply increases the risk of a heat injury. During acclimatization, the body adjusts by beginning to sweat earlier, and the sweat has a lower salt content.

Acclimatization

It takes about 2 weeks to fully acclimatize. During this time the individual should gradually increase heat and activity level. While this reduces the likelihood of becoming a heat casualty, it does not prevent it. Proper caution is always needed. While acclimatization does reduce the salt content of sweat, it does not reduce the water requirement. The rate of sweating and total water requirement actually increases.

Figure 6-8. Wet Bulb Globe Temperature Apparatus

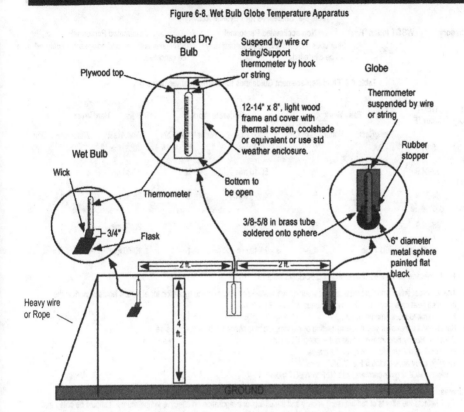

Wet Bulb Globe Temperature

The 4 factors that determine the degree of heat stress exerted by the environment are air wind speed, relative humidity, temperature and heat radiation. These are factored together to a more accurate picture of what the body "feels."

This is called the Wet Bulb Globe Temperature (WBGT). This is calculated using this formula:

WBGT = 0.7 x wet bulb temperature + 0.2 x black globe temperature + 0.1 x dry bulb temperature

Table 6-5. Guidelines for Physical Activity

Category	WBGT Index °F	Non-acclimated Personnel	Acclimated Personnel
I	82-84.9	Use discretion in planning intense physical activity. Limit intensity of work and exposure to sun. Provide constant supervision	Normal duties
II	85-87.9	Strenuous exercises will be cancelled. Outdoor classes in the sun will be cancelled.	Use discretion in planning intense physical Activities. Limit intensity of work and exposure to sun. Provide constant supervision.
III	88-89.9	All physical training, strenuous activities, and parades will be cancelled.	Strenuous outdoor activities will be minimized for all personnel with less than 12 weeks of training in hot weather.

Table 6-5. Guidelines for Physical Activity

Category	WBGT Index °F	Non-acclimated Personnel	Acclimated Personnel
IV	≥90	Strenuous activities and non-essential duty will be cancelled.	Strenuous activities and non-essential duty will be cancelled.

Table 6-6. Fluid Replacement Guidelines for Warm Weather Training

Heat Category	WBGT Index °F	Easy Work		Moderate Work		Hard Work	
		Work/Rest	Water Intake Q/hr	Work/Rest	Water Intake Q/hr	Work/Rest	Water Intake Q/hr
1	78-81.9	NL	½	NL	¾	40/20 min	¾
2 (Green)	82-84.9	NL	½	50/10 min	¾	30/30 min	1
3 (Yellow)	84-87.9	NL	¾	40/20 min	¾	30/30 min	1
4 (Red)	88-89.9	NL	¾	30/30 min	¾	20/40 min	1
5 (Black)	≥90	50/10 min	1	20/40 min	1	10/50 min	1

Note: Applies to average acclimated Soldier wearing BDU; hot weather

- The work/rest times and fluid replacement volumes will sustain performance and hydration for at least 4 hours of work in the specified heat category. Individual water needs will vary ±1/4 qt/hr.
- NL= no limit to work time per hour
- Rest means minimal physical activity (sitting or standing), accomplished in shade, if possible.
- **Caution:** Hourly fluid intake should not exceed 1½ quarts.
- Daily fluid intake should not exceed 12 quarts.
- Wearing body armor adds 5ºF to WBGT Index.
- If wearing MOPP over-garment, add 10ºF to WBGT Index.

Microclimates:
The WBGT reflects the effects of radiant (sun) energy and the effects of evaporation on effective temperatures. It should be noted that anything that changes these factors changes the WBGT. Standing in the shade on a sunny day is cooler, and being below the crest of a hill, protected from the breeze eliminates the cooling effects of the wind, so it is warmer. Being in a narrow valley by a stream (humid) will be hotter then a WBGT taken in a clearing. Local differences can be extremely important. Do not generalize from a single WBGT. Of course, these tables are of no use if a medic does not have a WBGT apparatus. Much of this remains common sense. Without a WBGT reading, most medics should be able to determine reasonable work/rest cycle and fluid intake recommendations given ambient temperature, humidity, local environment, and the mission.

Salt Replacement
The salt contained in the diet is usually sufficient to maintain adequate salt in the body. In high heat stress environments, the body expends more salt in the form of sweat and needs additional salt to replace it. The MRE contains adequate salt to meet the body's needs in a fully acclimated soldier. The use of salt tablets is now discouraged. It is both unneeded and in a form that increases the likelihood of stomach upset. If additional salt is needed, the addition of salt on the food is the preferred method. If the use of oral re-hydration fluids is needed, use the methods in Table 6-7.

Table 6-7. Salt Replacement

Salt	dissolved in	Diluting Water
Oral Hydration Salts		As directed
¼ teaspoon (1 MRE salt packet)		one canteen
1 ⅓ level mess kit spoons		5 gallon can
9 level mess kit spoons		Lyster bag
1 level canteen cup		250 gallon water trailer

Chapter 24: Heat-Related Illnesses: Heat Cramps
LTC Ric Ong, MC, USA

Introduction: The term "heat cramps" is actually a misnomer, as muscle cramping more likely results from sodium depletion during intense activity, not heat. In fact, cooling of a fatigued muscle is often a contributing factor. Heat cramps typically occur in individuals undergoing prolonged, intense activity in a hot and humid environment. Heat cramps are brief, intermittent, and very painful, but can be largely prevented by maintaining an adequate salt and fluid balance prior to and during exertion. **Risk Factors:** More likely to occur in sodium depleted or over-hydrated troops after prolonged strenuous physical activity in a hot, humid environment. Troops that are not fully acclimatized are at increased risk. Heat cramps are a warning and should prompt action to address underlying causes and mitigate risk of more severe heat injury and adverse effect on operational readiness.

Subjective: Symptoms
Painful, tonic contractions of skeletal muscles frequently preceded by palpable or visible fasciculation. Fatigue, giddiness, nausea, vomiting are common.

Focused History: *Which muscles are involved?* (usually all or part of large skeletal muscles currently under exertion) *What does the pain feel like?* (usually severe) *What were you doing at symptom onset?* (strenuous work) *What were the environmental conditions?* (hot, humid) *Have you had similar symptoms previously* (Individuals with multiple previous heat injuries are more susceptible to recurrence.) *Do you have frequent leg cramps at night?* (suggest vascular problems, not heat cramps) *What makes the symptoms worse?* (Manipulation of the muscle may precipitate cramping.) *Have you been ill with any gastrointestinal disorder prior to onset of these symptoms?* (distinguish nausea, vomiting from GI source)

Objective: Signs
Using Basic Tools: Inspection/Palpation: Muscle cramping with possible fasciculations, rapid resolution after oral or IV salt solution. Ill-appearing, fatigued, vomiting.

Assessment:
Differential Diagnosis
Tetany due to alkalosis: Hyperventilation, severe gastroenteritis and cholera more likely cause of generalized muscle tetany v. focal muscle cramping of large voluntary muscles subjected to exertion found in heat cramps.

Tetanus: History of tetanus prone wound in individual with inadequate immunization status. Symptoms generally progress over several days.

Hypocalcemia: Trousseau's sign (eg, carpal spasm when BP cuff is inflated above systolic BP for 3 minutes). Evidence of an underlying condition responsible for hypocalcemia (eg, pancreatitis, sepsis, vitamin D deficiency, rhabdomyolysis)

Strychnine poisoning (rare): Usually occurs within 10-20 minutes of ingestion (eg, history of ingestion of herbal or homeopathic medicine containing strychnine) possibly sooner if source is injection (eg, adulterated street drug). "Awake" spinal shock (tonic clonic seizure with patient awake) is the classic presentation.

Black widow spider envenomation: History of spider bite. *See Part 4: Organ Systems: Chapter 6: Bug Bites and Stings: Spider (Black Widow, Brown Recluse) Bites*

Plan:
Treatment
Primary: Salty foods with oral hydration if thirsty. Re-hydrate with 0.1% salt solution po for mild cases (salt tablets are not recommended) or normal saline solution IV if more rapid treatment needed. If a sports drink is used, dilute it 1:1 with water. Magnesium is used with reported success at Hawaii's Iron Man race and may be helpful.

Secondary: Mild stretching and massage of the contracting muscle will provide some relief to the intense discomfort.

Patient Education
General: Patients with heat cramps usually have sodium deficits or over-hydration. Eating the entire MRE and adding salt to tray pack meals should replenish salt stores over several days. Patients are at risk for developing more severe heat injury which may include irreversible adverse effects (to include significant impact on fitness for duty). Compliance with therapy and mitigation of risk to additional heat injury are critical.

Activity: Allow 2-3 days to replenish salt and water deficits before resuming work in the heat.

Diet: Increase salt application to food and water intake.

Prevention and Hygiene: Consume adequate quantities of salt and water as part of the normal diet and in preparation for planned strenuous activity.

No improvement/Deterioration: If recovery is not rapid (within 1-2 hours with oral fluids, within 15-30 minutes with normal saline), return for reevaluation. Consider heat stroke or hyponatremia.

Follow-up Actions
Consultation Criteria: If recovery is not rapid (within 1-2 hours with oral fluids, within 15-30 minutes with normal saline).

Note: An attempt should be made to determine conditions and circumstances for the episode so that the leadership can be appropriately advised, ie, modify training, mission parameters, or support requirements to prevent more severe casualties.

Chapter 24: Heat-Related Illnesses: Heat Exhaustion
LTC Ric Ong, MC, USA

Introduction: Heat exhaustion is the most common heat illness. Although heat exhaustion in a military setting often manifests after extreme exertion, in reality, it likely develops over several days and is a result of cardiovascular strain as the body tries to maintain normothermia in a hot environment. Heat exhaustion occurs when the demands for blood flow (to the skin for temperature control through convection and sweating, to the muscles for work, and other vital organs) exceed the cardiac output. A body that has developed a state of salt depletion over several days, in combination with extreme exertion, is at risk for heat exhaustion.

Consider the diagnoses of heat exhaustion and heat stroke on the continuum of heat illness. The distinction between heat exhaustion and heat stroke is often unclear, frequently making the diagnosis of heat exhaustion one of exclusion. In general, any end-organ damage, including neurological (especially mental status) changes and laboratory markers for liver, kidney, and muscle damage beyond expected values for exerting individuals leads to a diagnosis of heat stroke, rather than heat exhaustion.

Note that heat exhaustion is not exclusive to hot environments, although it most commonly occurs in this setting. Individuals performing strenuous physical activity in cold weather environments are also susceptible, making the use of appropriate cold-weather gear an important planning factor.

Risk Factors: Dehydrated and sodium-deficient members are at risk after strenuous physical activity in the heat. Operators that are not fully acclimatized are at increased risk. Heat injury can cause permanent damage with potential for long term effects limiting fitness for duty. All steps possible to mitigate risk should be emphasized.

Subjective: Symptoms
Profound fatigue, chills, nausea/vomiting, tingling of the lips, shortness of breath, orthostatic dizziness, headache, syncope, hyperirritability, anxiety, piloerection, heat cramps, heat sensations in head and upper torso. Casualty may or may not feel thirsty.
Focused History: *What have you had to eat and drink in the last 48 hours?* (Water and salt intake may be too low. If they have consumed more than 12L of fluid in the past 24 hours, consider hyponatremia- water intoxication.) *Do you know who you are, where you are and what day it is?* (While heat exhaustion patients may be confused, it is a common sign of heat stroke. A patient with mental status changes should be treated as a heat stroke patient until it is proven otherwise.) *Have you been ill recently?* (Concurrent gastrointestinal illness is not uncommon and may increase risk under appropriate conditions.) *Have you had similar episodes previously?* (Although a single previous episode of heat exhaustion does not increase risk for recurrence, multiple previous episodes certainly does.)

Objective: Signs
Using Basic Tools: Vital signs: Tachypnea, tachycardia, orthostatic hypotension. Temperature may be normal or greater than 104ºF. Inspection: Pale skin; piloerection; profuse diaphoresis; anxiety and agitation; muscle spasms; vomiting; shortness of breath; syncope. If the patient is confused, assume heat stroke until proven otherwise. *IF THE RECTAL TEMPERATURE CONTINUES TO RISE, TREAT AS A HEAT STROKE.* Palpation: Skin cool and moist to touch. It may be dry in desert environments where evaporation is rapid. Neuro Exam: Should be normal; any mental status changes or other neurologic abnormalities suggest heat stroke.

Assessment:
Differential Diagnosis
Heat stroke: Altered mental status, core (rectal) temperature continues to risk. *See Part 6: Operational Environment: Chapter 24: Heat Stroke*
Simple dehydration: Generally milder symptoms (possibly indistinguishable from heat exhaustion), patient will complain of thirst; may include history of diarrhea or other cause of fluid loss. Identify underlying cause and treat dehydration.
Febrile illness: Other history or symptoms of underlying illness may be present

Plan:
Treatment
1. Reduce the load on the heart with rest and cooling. Place casualty in shade and remove heavy clothing. Apply cool water to the skin, if available.
2. Correct water and electrolyte depletion by administering oral or IV fluids. IV fluids replenish the volume and correct symptoms quickly. Patients with resting tachycardia or orthostatic hypotension should initially receive 200-250cc boluses of normal saline (NS) repeatedly until these vital signs are corrected. No more than 2L of NS should be administered without laboratory surveillance. Consider D5/0.5 NS or D5/0.2 NS as subsequent IV fluid replacement if signs of hypoglycemia. Since this is seldom available, alternating D5W with NS or Ringer's lactate may be the best alternative. If patient can tolerate oral fluids, use a 0.1% salt solution or sports drink diluted 1:1.
Note: Giving po fluids creates intravascular volume, which is ideal. D5 can cause an osmotic diuresis, which is counterproductive in dehydration. Use cautiously and only if hypoglycemic

Patient Education
General: Maintain adequate fluid and water intake and work/rest cycles in heat. Avoid direct sunlight and other risk factors.
Activity: Heat exhaustion patients have rapid clinical recovery. However, they all need at least 24 hours of rest and re-hydration under 1st echelon or unit level medical supervision to reverse water-electrolyte depletion.
Diet: Regular diet augmented with salted food and increased water intake.
Prevention and Hygiene: Acclimatize gradually with adequate water and dietary salt. Forced drinking may help to avoid dehydration.
No improvement/Deterioration: Return quickly for reevaluation.

Follow-up Actions
Return Evaluation: If the patient fails to improve rapidly, assume the patient is a heat stroke casualty and treat as such with rapid cooling and evacuation. A single episode of heat exhaustion does not imply a predisposition to heat injury and no continuing follow-up or profile evaluation is required.
Consultation Criteria: Repeated episodes of heat exhaustion require a temporary profile against heat exposure, evacuation and referral for a thorough evaluation.
Recommendations to Leadership: Planning and preparation with awareness of mission requirements and environmental conditions. Acclimatization is best attained by gradual increase in intensity and duration of physical activity over an 8-10 day period.
Notes: A case of heat exhaustion or heat stroke should alert the leadership to reevaluate current environmental conditions and mission requirements, appropriately modify work/rest cycles, and increase water and electrolyte intake accordingly. The difference

between heat exhaustion and heat stroke is often difficult to determine. Soldiers who do not respond dramatically to rest and fluid/electrolyte repletion should be observed for 24 hours for delayed complications of heat stroke. USACHPPM has recommended work/rest/hydration charts available for leaders, providers and troops. *See Tables 6-5 and 6-6*

Chapter 24: Heat-Related Illnesses: Heat Stroke
LTC Ric Ong, MC, USA

Introduction: Heat stroke is a medical emergency, distinguished from heat exhaustion by the presence of end-organ damage, including neurological (especially mental status) changes, and laboratory markers for liver, kidney, and muscle damage beyond expected values for exerting individuals. Heat stroke is the most severe manifestation on the continuum of heat illness. You may see the sudden collapse of an individual under strenuous physical exertion in a hot and humid environment. Loss of consciousness follows and core temperature is often greater than 104ºF. Severity of the condition depends on the degree and duration of temperature elevation. If heat stroke is suspected and body temperature is elevated, start cooling immediately! Do not delay for a diagnostic evaluation. Cooling and evaluation should proceed simultaneously. There are 2 general classifications of heat stroke. Classic Heat Stroke (CHS) occurs when the ambient temperature is very high over several days (heat wave), and affects mainly the elderly with chronic medical conditions and medications that impair the body's natural thermoregulatory mechanisms, and/or with limited access to air conditioning; physical exertion is not the primary cause. Exertional Heat Stroke (EHS) results from strenuous physical activity, typically in hot environments (but may occur in colder environments as well). EHS is the primary concern of our SOF medics, although both CHS and EHS share many pathologic and therapeutic similarities. This section focuses on EHS. **Risk Factors:** Poor physical conditioning and lack of acclimatization, level of exertion mismatched to level of physical fitness, sleep deprivation, dehydration, high work loads in a hottest hours, high humidity, illness with fever, medications that interfere with sweating or contribute to dehydration such as caffeine, alcohol and diuretics. Concurrent gastrointestinal illness with diarrhea. (A history of previous heat stroke was thought to be a predisposing factor, but this is no longer the case. Individuals suffering heat stroke show transient heat-intolerance over the short-term while recovering, but no permanent inability to properly acclimatize and they are able to develop exertional heat tolerance in the long-term. Nevertheless, the military largely considers previous heat injury as a predisposing factor for future heat injury.)

Subjective: Symptoms
Dizziness, exhaustion, weakness, nausea, vomiting, diarrhea, involuntary urination and defecation, difficulty speaking, irritability, aggressiveness, confusion, and other mental status changes.

Focused History (if conscious): *What have you had to eat and drink in the last 48 hours?* (Water and salt intake may be too low. If they have consumed greater than 12L of fluid in the past 24 hours or 8 liters in the past 4-6 hours, consider hyponatremia-water intoxication.) *Do you know who you are, where you are and what day it is?* (Confusion is a common sign of heat stroke but can also be seen in a patient with heat exhaustion. A patient with mental status changes should be treated as a heat stroke patient until it is proven otherwise.) *What were you doing today?* (typical exposure: work in a hot environment) *Have you had similar episodes previously?* (Previous episode of heat exhaustion increases risk for recurrence.) *Have you been able to sleep in a cool or air-conditioned space?* (Sleeping in a cool space decreases the chance getting heat stroke while sleeping in hot conditions increases the risk of heat stroke.)

Objective: Signs
Using Basic Tools: Vital signs: Tachycardia, tachypnea, hypotension, possibly shock. Temperature greater than 104ºF (use core temperature reading from rectum). **Caution:** Heat stroke has occurred with documented normal temperatures. Inspection: Profuse sweating will likely to be present up to the point of collapse (in contrast to earlier beliefs), as almost all exertional heat stroke victims are sweating. In desert environments, dry skin may be seen with rapid evaporation of the sweat. Do not confuse exertional heat stroke sweating as a "good sign" (as in classic heat stroke where lack of sweating is end stage). Diminished urination; urinary and fecal incontinence may be seen. Auscultation: Rapid, deep respirations dropping off to shallow and irregular respirations. Palpation: Hot, red skin; rapid, thready pulse. Neurologic: Convulsions; seizures; ataxia, dysarthria, pin-point pupils, irritability, aggressiveness, irrational behavior, confusion, delirium, coma and other mental status changes.

Using Advanced Tools: Labs: Sodium (high, reflecting severe dehydration, or low), potassium (high or low), calcium (low), phosphate (low), magnesium (low), glucose (low), urine specific gravity (high or low), urine hemoglobin (may be positive from myoglobin present if rhabdomyolysis develops), hemoconcentration

Assessment:
Differential Diagnosis

Infection: Most commonly community acquired pneumonia but consider meningococcemia and *P. falciparum* malaria. *See Part 4: Organ Systems: Chapter 3: Pneumonia; Chapter 6: Bacterial Infections: Meningococcemia & Part 5: Specialty Areas: Chapter 12: Parasitic Infections: Malaria*

Pontine or hypothalamic hemorrhage: Pontine hemorrhage typically leads to deep coma and total paralysis within minutes. If patient is awake may see facial palsy, deafness, dysarthria.

Drug intoxication: Cocaine, amphetamines, phencyclidine, theophylline, tricyclic antidepressants

Alcohol or sedative withdrawal: History of ingestion. *See Part 5: Specialty Areas: Chapter 18: Substance Abuse*

Severe hypertonic dehydration: Typically part of the pathophysiology seen with heat stroke, may be indistinguishable at presentation from heat stroke (ie, only suggested by clinical course and response to therapy)

Neuroleptic malignant syndrome: Typically an idiosyncratic reaction to neuroleptic agents and some anti-emetic drugs (eg, haloperidol, chlorpromazine, promethazine, metoclopramide). Classic sign is described as "lead pipe" muscle rigidity.

Thyroid storm: History of infection or trauma involving the thyroid or long untreated hyperthyroidism. *See Part 4: Organ Systems: Chapter 4: Thyroid Problems*

Hyponatremia and cardiac causes: Consider if the rectal temperature is less than 103ºF

Plan:

Treatment

1. Reduce body temperature rapidly by any means available: Stop physical activity, find shade. Ice water baths are preferred but seldom available in the field. Field expedient baths, which will keep the water cool, can be constructed by digging plastic-lined, shaded pits. Fans (rotor wash from a helicopter), if available, in conjunction with spray bottles to mist water on exposed skin (to maximized evaporative heat loss) is very effective. Ice bags to the large vessels of the femoral and axillary regions if possible. Pouring large amounts of water over the casualty's exposed body with intermittent toweling (renews the evaporative capacity of the skin surface) is also effective. Discontinue active cooling when the rectal temperature reaches 101°F in order to avoid overcooling. Constantly monitor the patient's body temperature and alternate heating and cooling until the temperature stabilizes. Continue monitoring the patient's temperature every 10 minutes for the next 48 hours. CPR is rarely required in heat stroke.
2. Hydrate with 1-2L of NS or LR over the first hour. Titrate IV fluid administration thereafter to hydration status. Over-hydration can increase the likelihood of complications, including pulmonary edema. Consider subsequent D5NS if hypoglycemic, but use with caution as it may cause osmotic diuresis.
3. Control the airway to prevent vomiting. Intubate if patient is unconscious. Consider NG tube.
4. Give **diazepam** 5-10mg IV or IM to control seizures, as seizure activity will increase body temperature.
5. Consider cardiac monitoring with ECG; consider inserting Foley catheter for monitoring urine output.

Note: Epinephrine, sodium amytal and morphine are contraindicated. Atropine and other drugs that interfere with sweating are also contraindicated.

Patient Education

General: Avoid heat exposure until clinical recovery and a thorough medical evaluation are complete. Recovery is primarily a function of the magnitude and duration of the temperature elevation. There is an increased risk for future heat stroke.

Activity: Patient should receive profile restricting heat exposure (a permanent profile may be issued later) until clinical recovery is complete. Consider heat tolerance and other testing. Chronic neurological abnormalities may persist for several months, but even with coma up to 24 hours, most heat stroke casualties will recover completely.

Diet: None during initial symptoms, then as tolerated.

Medications: Avoid alcohol, caffeine and other diuretics during convalescence. Avoid stimulants.

Prevention and Hygiene: Avoid heat exposure for several weeks until the body can thermo-regulate correctly.

No Improvement/Deterioration: Evacuate immediately for additional testing and treatment with continued cooling en route.

Follow-up Actions

Reevaluation: Hypotensive patients who do not respond to saline may benefit from carefully titrated **dopamine**.

Evacuation/Consultation Criteria: All heat stroke patients need mandatory evacuation and referral. Evaluation of the potential complications of heat stroke (encephalopathy, coagulopathy, hepatic injury, cardiac injury renal failure and rhabdomyolysis) requires laboratory tests not available in the basic or advanced management tools.

Follow-on Care: Temporary neurologic impairment may require physical, occupational, and speech therapy until complete resolution of sequelae.

Recommendations to Leadership: Planning and preparation with awareness of mission requirements and environmental conditions. Acclimatization is best attained by gradual increase in intensity and duration of physical activity of 1-4 hours in heat over a 2 week period.

Do:
* treat any heat injury with neurologic or mental status abnormalities as heat stroke
* initiate immediate cooling measures to any heat stroke casualty
* obtain a rectal temperature as soon as possible after collapse (body may cool quickly giving a misleading initial temp if delayed)
* inform the leadership so they may implement appropriate measures to prevent further heat injuries

Do Not:
* delay cooling measures awaiting a definitive diagnosis
* assume that a casualty with or without profuse sweating does not have heat stroke
* give any medications that will increase heart rate or metabolic rate (epinephrine, atropine, creatine, ephedra), decrease blood pressure (morphine), or impede sweating (atropine)
* allow recovering casualty to ingest any diuretic substances (alcohol, caffeine)
* not take this condition lightly, understanding that most will recover completely. Heat stroke can kill!

Chapter 25: Chemical, Biological, and Radiation Injuries: Chemical: Weapons of Mass Destruction

Phillip L. Coule, MD & SSG Chris Pipes, USA

Introduction: There are 4 basic types of chemical weapons: nerve agents, cyanides, vesicants and pulmonary agents, and each type defines its method of action. The time from exposure to onset of signs/symptoms and severity of symptoms varies with the specific agent; duration of exposure, form (liquid, gas, solid); environmental conditions (temperature, humidity, wind); route of absorption (vapor. liquid); personal protective equipment; history of prior exposure or pre and post-exposure treatment. Chemical exposure should be considered whenever there is intelligence or history to suggest agent use, evidence of unknown substance contamination, and incapacitation without obvious mechanism of injury or greater degree of incapacitation than is expected from a specific type of injury. A chemical attack should also be considered with any sudden increase in numbers of unexplained causalities. Toxic industrial chemicals may also cause injury by accidental release (collateral damage) or as agents of "opportunity". The best source of information on toxic materials is the National Institute for Occupational Safety and Health (NIOSH) manual. All suspected chemical exposure should be reported to higher command ASAP.

Focused History for chemical exposure: *Describe the agent. What was the route of exposure? How long ago were you exposed? Were you using protective equipment? What was the time of onset? What are your specific symptoms? What was the type of decontamination used? What was the pre-treatment and initial management?*

Chapter 25: Chemical, Biological, and Radiation Injuries: Chemical: Nerve Agents

Nerve agents are organophosphates specifically designed to inhibit nerve function and can be highly lethal in small quantities. Common nerve agents include Tabun (GA), Sarin (GB), Soman (GD), Cyclosarin (GF) and VX. Cyclosarin (GF) is considered of limited strategic interest but was one of the stockpiled agents discovered in Gulf War 1.

Nerve agents act by preventing acetylcholinesterase (AChE) from breaking down acetylcholine (ACh). This causes the affected nerves to continuously fire, thus giving the overstimulation symptoms. Once the agent remains in contact with the AChE for a period of time, it can become permanently bound. This is known as "aging." The time required to "age" is unique for each different organophosphate.

Treatment strategy for exposure includes removing the patient from further agent contact, competing for receptor sites (Atropine), attempting to unbind the unaged AChE with an oxime (2-PAM) and treating fasciculation or seizures with an anti-convulsant (diazepam). Actual treatment will be casualty dependant based on signs/symptoms NOT suspected exposure. If contact with nerve agent is anticipated, pre-treatment with a non-aging organophosphate is another strategy.

Physostigmine and Pyridostigmine are non-aging cholinesterase inhibitors that "bind" a selected amount of acetylcholine-esterase. Acetycholine-esterase that is bound to the physostigmine and pyridostigmine is then not available to be bound and aged to a nerve agent if exposed and provides a pool of reserve AChE, and increases the survivable dose of nerve agent exposure. Use of pre-treatment agents is a command-level decision.

Casualties are treated according to their level of exposure: Mild, Moderate and Severe. Level of exposure is determined by the signs/symptoms exhibited after exposure.

The most common, Mild, is characterized by Miosis and is caused by vapor exposure only. Moderate exposure is characterized by the parasympathetic overstimulation symptoms: SLUDGE. Severe exposure can be identified by the presence of generalized seizures and/or respiratory arrest.

Casualties are only treated for the actual signs/symptoms they exhibit. Care providers should use caution when making the decision to treat, as over treatment has complications as well. Personnel should also be cautioned against the reflex use of antidote kits unless clearly indicated.

Table 6-8. US DOD Chemical Kits

Kit Name	Contents
Nerve Agent Antidote Kit (NAAK) (aka Mark I)	Atropine 2mg auto-injector Pralidoxime chloride (2-PAM) 600mg auto-injector
Antidote Treatment Nerve Agent Auto-injector (ATNAA) (aka Mark II)	Atropine 2.1mg + pralidoxime chloride (2-PAM) 600mg in a single auto-injector
Convulsive Antidote, Nerve Agent (CANA)	Diazepam 10mg auto-injector

Table 6-9. Nerve Agent Antidotal Therapy

Type of Exposure	Presentation	Antidotal Therapy	Observation/Additional Treatment
Mild Vapor (GA, GB, BD) Exposure	Nasal congestion with mild shortness of breath, miosis	1 Mark Kit*, or 2mg atropine, 1g 2PAMCL	Miosis may not reverse with treatment
Mild Liquid (VX) Exposure	Localized sweating and fasciculations	1 Mark Kit*, or 2mg atropine, 1g 2PAMCL	Observe for return of symptoms or delayed worsening, supportive care
Moderate vapor or liquid exposure	More severe respiratory distress, muscular weakness	1-2 Mark Kits*, or 2-4mg atropine, 1g 2PAMCL IV over 30 min	Observe for return of symptoms or worsening, supportive care. Treat seizures with benzodiazepines or diazepam auto-injector
Severe vapor or liquid exposure	Unconscious, possibly seizing or flaccid, possibly apneic or severe symptoms	3 Mark Kits*, or 6mg atropine and 1g 2PAMCL initially. May require additional doses of atropine	May repeat atropine as needed every 5 mins, and 2PAMCL in 1 hr. Endpoint for atropine administration is drying of secretions and ease of breathing. Treat seizures with benzodiazepines or diazepam auto-injector

*Mark kit refers to Mark I or Mark II kit (Adapted from Soldier Biological and Chemical Command, 2003.)

Vapor Exposure (mild)

Subjective: Symptoms

Complains of: "Can't see" or "It's dark". No parasympathetic symptoms (salivation, lacrimation, urination, defecation, GI distress, and emesis [SLUDGE]).

Objective: Signs

HEENT: Miosis ("pin point" pupils, earliest sign of exposure, may last several days), mild rhinorrhea (runny nose). Other Systems: None

Assessment: Based on clinical signs and symptoms, environment and probability.

Plan:

Treatment of Vapor Exposure (mild)
1. Remove casualty from environment
2. Do NOT give atropine eye drops
3. Administer 1 Mark Kit* or 2mg **atropine** and 1g **2PAMCL** IV
4. Observe and re-evaluate for continued symptoms. Miosis may not reverse with treatment.
5. If symptoms persist after 5 minutes or symptoms worsen, administer additional Mark Kit* or additional 2mg **atropine**.

Vapor/Liquid Contact Exposure (moderate)

Subjective: Symptoms

Complains of: "Can't see" or "It's dark", tightness in chest; runny nose, Parasympathetic symptoms (SLUDGE) are present: Salivation, Lacrimation (uncontrolled tearing), Urination, Defecation, Gastro-Intestinal Motility ("Gurgling" gut –Cramping), Emesis.

Objective: Signs

HEENT: Miosis ("pinpoint" pupils, earliest sign of exposure, may last several days), eye pain, photophobia, uncontrolled lacrimation, nasal congestion, rhinorrhea, hoarseness, drooling
RESP: SOB, dyspnea, tachypnea, wheezing, coughing
CARD: Early tachycardia followed by bradycardia
GI: Nausea, epigastric "gurgling," abdominal cramping, uncontrolled defecation
GU: Uncontrolled urination
CNS: Apprehension, headache, difficulty concentrating, confusion, weakness; localized "sweating"/fasciculation at exposure site is common.

Assessment: Based on clinical signs and symptoms, environment and probability.

Plan:

Treatment of Vapor/Liquid Contact Exposure (moderate)
1. Only treat symptomatic patients*
2. Remove casualty from environment
3. Administer 1-2 Mark Kits* or 2-4mg **atropine** and 1g **2PAMCL** IV
4. Remove contact contamination.
5. Observe and re-evaluate for continued symptoms. Miosis may not reverse with treatment.
6. If symptoms persist after 5 minutes or symptoms worsen, administer additional Mark Kit* or additional 2mg **atropine**.
7. Additional doses of **atropine** may be required and should be administered until secretions dry.
8. Establish vascular access
9. **Atropine** 2mg may be administered every 5 minutes until patient is "dry" or breathing becomes easier
   *DO NOT use heart rate as the end point for atropine administration.
10. Provide airway/respiratory support. MUST have suction to be effective

Vapor/Liquid Contact Exposure (severe)

Subjective: Symptoms

Parasympathetic symptoms (SLUDGE) are present: Salivation, Lacrimation (uncontrolled tearing), Urination, Defecation, Gastro-Intestinal Motility ("Gurgling" gut – Cramping), Emesis. PLUS increased likelihood of seizures/coma

Objective: Signs

HEENT: Miosis ("pinpoint" pupils, earliest sign of exposure, may last several days), eye pain, photophobia, uncontrolled lacrimation, nasal congestion, rhinorrhea, hoarseness, drooling.
RESP: SOB, dyspnea, tachypnea, wheezing, coughing, respiratory arrest.
CARD: Bradycardia.
GI: Nausea, epigastric "gurgling," abdominal cramping, uncontrolled defecation.
GU: Uncontrolled urination.
CNS: Confusion, seizures, coma

Assessment: Diagnosis based on clinical signs and symptoms, environment and probability. *Only treat symptomatic patients*

Plan:

Treatment
1. Remove casualty from environment. Administer 2-3 Mark Kits or 6mg **atropine** and 1g **2PAMCL** IV.
2. Remove contact contamination, Establish vascular access: Give **atropine** 2mg every 5 min. until patient is "dry" or breathing

becomes easier. *DO NOT use heart rate as the end point for atropine administration. Observe and re-evaluate for continued symptoms. Miosis may not reverse with treatment. Additional doses of atropine may be required and should be administered until secretions dry.

3. If seizures/fasciculation are present give (1) CANA **diazepam** Auto-Injector (10mg). If required to control seizures, give **lorazepam** 1mg or **diazepam** 5mg, or **midazolam** 2mg IV/IO titrated to control seizures.

4. Provide airway/respiratory support.

Note: Treatment of atropine overdose/anti-cholinogenic toxidrome ("Hot as a hare, Blind as a Bat, Dry as a Bone, Red as a Beet, Mad as a Hatter")

Mild to Moderate cases: Administer benzodiazepines (**diazepam** 2-5mg IV) and cool the victim.

Severe Atropine Overdose: **Physostigmine** 1.0-2.0mg IM or IV (at NO MORE than 1.0mg/min), repeated every 10 min. until symptoms are controlled.

*CAUTION: Use only for severe atropine (or other anticholinergic) overdose – can have fatal complications including complete heart block. Do not use in setting of use of atropine to treat actual nerve agent exposure.

Chapter 25: Chemical, Biological, and Radiation Injuries: Chemical: Cyanides

Cyanides are naturally occurring chemicals that were one of the first to be "weaponized" by the military. Cyanogen Chloride (CK), Cyanogen Bromide (CB), Bromobenzyl Cyanide (CA) and Hydrogen Cyanide (AC) are all examples of NATO agents. While they have a reputation for rapidly causing unconsciousness and death, these agents still have the same dispersal issues that all chemical weapons posses: a sufficiently high concentration/dose must be absorbed through a susceptible route to have lethal effect. In particular, creating a lethal concentration of cyanide agents on an open battlefield is difficult. In a closed environment such as use in a terrorist attack, cyanide agents are highly lethal.

Military literature often refers to cyanides as "Blood" agents because they prevent cellular respiration: the mitochondria is blocked from using oxygen to metabolize glucose thus creating metabolic acidosis. Cyanides are primarily an inhalation danger but ingestion of sufficient amounts of solid (usually fruit seeds) can also be toxic.

Cyanides are also a contact hazard. Prolonged skin contact with the solid crystals will lead to a skin rash. Contact through broken skin can also lead to toxicity. Detection is primarily by previous intelligence, observed gas formation, fire in a confined space (CO may also be present) or shortness of breath/coma/apnea without other signs or explanation. Odor is a particularly poor indicator.

Treatment is focused on supportive care. Drug therapy is focused on: "Holding" the cyanide in the blood (away from the mitochondria) to gain time for the agent to be detoxified by the liver (Amyl Nitrite, Sodium Nitrite), boosting the natural metabolite excretion pathway (Sodium Thiosulfate, Hydroxocobalamin), and balancing excessive methemoglobin production (Methylene Blue).

Table 6-10. Time Course of Effects for Inhalation Exposure to High Concentration Cyanide Gas

<15 second	Transient increase in rate/depth of respirations
<30 seconds	Seizures
2-4 minutes	Respirations Cease
6-8 minutes	Heartbeat Ceases

*Once removed from environment (evacuation/masking) little risk of delayed onset.
*Cyanides rapidly degrade protective mask filters so "burn through" time should be a major consideration in deliberate planning.

Ingestion/Inhalation Exposure
  Subjective: Symptoms
    Mild: Complaints of: "Can't breathe," "Tightness in chest"
    Severe: none

  Objective: Signs
    RESP: Transient increase in rate/depth of respiration, respiratory arrest. CARD: Arrhythmia, bradycardia, cardiac arrest; GI: Nausea, emesis. CNS: Weakness, dizziness, confusions, seizures, LOC. SKIN: Cyanosis

  Assessment: Cyanide poisoning is a clinical diagnosis based on the likelihood of exposure and signs/symptoms.

  Plan:
    Treatment
    1. Stop exposure and evacuate to "fresh" atmosphere
    2. Inhale crushed **amyl nitrite** ampules (Give even if not appearing to breathe). Cup under nose or in eye pieces of mask. Anticipate side effects of **amyl nitrite** which include sudden vasodilation with drop in BP and rapid heart rate.
    3. Assist ventilation (if required): **amyl nitrite** ampules can be placed inside of BVM mask, if necessary.
    4. Remove contact exposure (skin): soiled clothing, regular shower, may unmask once dust hazard is removed
    5. Establish IV/IO access. If high suspicion of cyanide poisoning and patient is critically ill, or not improved after removal from the environment, give **sodium nitrite** 300-500mg IV (given over 5–15 min) PLUS **sodium thiosulfate** 12.5g IV or **hydroxocobalamin** 5g IV.

Chapter 25: Chemical, Biological, and Radiation Injuries: Chemical: Vesicant (Blister) Agents

Vesicant, or "blister" agents are specifically designed to attack exposed skin and mucous membranes by direct alkylation of the cell proteins. They create large painful blisters that degrade the fighting efficiency and incapacitate the casualty. Often incorrectly called "mustard gas", vesicants are the oldest weapon-specific agent (created in 1820), the easiest to manufacture and therefore are some of the most commonly discovered.

Vesicants are divided into 4 types: sulphur mustard, nitrogen mustard, phosgene oxime and the arsenicals (lewisite). All are oily liquids of varying viscosity and persistence. Rapid decontamination (within minutes) is essential as agent left in contact with the skin or mucosa will not only denature those cellular proteins but cross-link the cell's DNA preventing regeneration.

The mask protects against eye and lung damage but provides only limited protection against systemic effects. Extensive, chemical burns of the eyes, integumentary and respiratory systems slow-healing skin lesions will place a heavy burden not only on the medic but other soldiers as well.

Rapid decontamination (within minutes) is the only method of preventing the skin lesions. No drug is available for the prevention of the effects except for lewisite with the limited benefit of British Anti-Lewisite (BAL). Delayed effects include temporary blindness, intense pain and chemical pneumonia. No drugs are available to prevent the skin and mucous membrane damage that the agents cause, although steroids have been found effective to alleviate symptoms. Contact is typically painless initially; arsenicals being the exception. Masking protects against direct damage to the eye, nose and lung tissue from the liquid and vapor threat but leaves much surface area exposed.

While the burns have a dramatic appearance, the damage is rarely permanent. The vesicant casualty fatality rate for WWI was 2% and for the Iran-Iraq War, 3%. Phosgene oxime was designed to penetrate protective garments more easily than other chemical agents and produces a rapid onset of severe and prolonged effects. When mixed with other chemicals, the rapid skin damage caused by phosgene oxime will make the skin more susceptible to the second agent. It is also the only agent that causes rapid onset of severe pain and urticaria.

Vesicant Contact/Vapor Exposure (mild)
Subjective: Symptoms
Complaints of: Eyes "feel gritty" or "itchy," "can't stop sneezing," Skin is "itchy" or "burns" (delayed)

Objective: Signs
HEENT: Lacrimation, rhinorrhea, hoarseness. RESP: Non-productive cough. SKIN: Erythema

Assessment: Diagnosis based on clinical signs and symptoms, environment and probability.

Plan: Treatment
1. Decontaminate exposed area:
2. Manage eye irritation: Irrigate eyes with water, treat conjunctivitis (**erythromycin** ophthalmic ointment qid until resolution of signs and symptoms)
3. Casualty can return to duty with casual observation.

Vesicant Contact Exposure (moderate to severe)
Subjective: Symptoms (moderate):
Exposed areas are moderately painful (delayed)

Objective: Signs (moderate)
HEENT: Lacrimation, sclera reddening, lid swelling, rhinorrhea, hoarseness. RESP: Non-productive cough. SKIN: Erythema, blisters start to form 2-24 hours post-exposure.

Subjective: Symptoms (severe):
Exposed areas are severely painful (delayed)

Objective: Signs (severe):
HEENT: Lacrimation, sclera reddening, obvious lid swelling, corneal ulceration, miosis, rhinorrhea. RESP: Productive cough, dyspnea, pulmonary edema. CIR: Hypotension from massive plasma leakage. SKIN: Erythema, >25% BSA blisters start to form 2-24 hours post-exposure.

Assessment: Diagnosis based on clinical signs and symptoms, environment and probability. Death is probable in cases demonstrating severe symptoms and signs.

Plan:
Treatment of Moderate and Severe Vesicant Contact Exposure
1. Stop exposure: Remove from environment; mask casualty to prevent further physical contamination; decontaminate; irrigate eyes with water
2. Maintain airway: Suction, cricothyrotomy if severe laryngeal edema
3. Control irritability: **Methylprednisolone**
4. Respiratory support: Positive pressure ventilation (if required), Bronchodilator (if required) **albuterol** inhaler 2 puffs q2-6h. Antitussives (if required): **dextromethorphan** or **benzonatate** pearls. Consider **methylprednisolone** 125mg IV q6h to reduce pulmonary edema. (questionable efficacy)
5. Circulatory support: Establish vascular access. Consider oral fluid resuscitation. Insert NG tube (if required).

6. Treat contact exposure of eyes: Irrigate with saline daily. Apply topical antibiotic like **erythromycin** ophthalmic ointment qid. Apply topical mydriatic. Apply petroleum jelly to lid edges to prevent adherence.
7. Manage pain: *See Part 8: Procedures: Chapter 30: Pain Assessment and Control*
8. Reduce topical swelling: 1% **hydrocortisone** cream qid x 2 days to affected areas.
9. Limit exertion: exertion worsens pulmonary edema with some agents

Note: Dimercaprol (**BAL- British Anti-Lewisite**) is no longer available for topical application. It is available for IM use to reduce the systemic effects of Lewisite exposure. Administer **BAL** 3-5 mg/kg IM q4h x 4 doses. Side effects of BAL include pain at the injection site, nausea, vomiting, headache, burning sensation of lips, mouth and throat and eyes, lacrimation, chest pain, muscle aches and anxiety. BAL is contraindicated in peanut allergy, renal disease, pregnancy (unless life-threatening) and concurrent use of medicinal iron.

Vesicant Ingestion Exposure
Subjective: Symptoms
Moderate to severe abdominal pain, cramping, nausea, vomiting; sore throat

Objective: Signs
HEENT: Drooling, erythema of oral mucosa, hoarseness. Assessment: Diagnosis based on clinical signs and symptoms, environment and probability.

Plan:
Treatment of Vesicant Ingestion Exposure
1. Stop exposure: Decontaminate, drink water/milk.
2. Maintain airway: Suction; cricothyrotomy if laryngeal edema
3. Manage nausea: **Promethazine** 25mg IM
4. Consider oral lavage: NG tube

Chapter 25: Chemical, Biological, and Radiation Injuries: Chemical: Pulmonary Agents

Pulmonary or "choking" agents are the original chemical warfare agent with the first large-scale deployment in 1915. Pulmonary agents cause casualties by either directly damaging respiratory system tissue, causing death by pulmonary edema and eventual respiratory failure or by displacing the ambient atmosphere and creating a low-oxygen environment, causing death by asphyxia. Common agents include chlorine (CL), phosgene (CG), diphosgene (DP), methyl isocyanate, phosphine, bromine (CA), and ammonia.

Warning properties are variable and range from immediate mucous membrane irritation to anxiousness and insidious fatigue that rapidly progresses to unconsciousness and death. Onset of symptoms depends on the agent and can range from immediate (ammonia, methyl isocyanate) to several hours (phosgene, phosphine). Identification of significant pulmonary effects from phosgene exposure may be delayed up to 48-72 hours.

Although the primary effect of these agents is through direct inhalation, eye, skin and mucous membrane irritation occurs with some agents. There is no contact or ingestion danger and thus no need to decontaminate casualties unless significant skin exposure or liquid contact exposure occurs.

Pulmonary Agent Inhalation Exposure
Subjective: Symptoms
Difficulty breathing; tightness, burning, pain in chest; burning eyes, sore throat

Objective: Signs
HEENT: Lacrimation, rhinorrhea, hoarseness, redness/ irritation of throat mucosa. RESP: Tachypnea, wheezing, pulmonary edema, respiratory arrest. CV: Arrhythmia, tachycardia, cardiac arrest. GI: Nausea, emesis. CNS: Anxiety, weakness, dizziness, confusion, seizures, LOC. DERM: Cyanosis, erythema

Assessment: Diagnosis based on clinical signs and symptoms, environment and probability.

Plan:
Treatment of Pulmonary Agent Exposure
1. Stop exposure: Remove from environment; mask casualty to prevent further physical contamination; decontaminate; irrigate eyes with water
2. Maintain airway: Suction; cricothyrotomy if severe laryngeal edema
3. Control irritability: **Methylprednisolone**
4. Respiratory support: Positive pressure ventilation (if required), bronchodilator (if required): **albuterol** inhaler 2 puffs q2-6h. Antitussives (if required): **Dextromethorphan** or **benzonatate** pearls. Consider **methylprednisolone** 125mg IV q6h to reduce pulmonary edema. (questionable efficacy)
5. Limit exertion as it worsens pulmonary edema with some agents

Chapter 25: Chemical, Biological, and Radiation Injuries:
Procedure: Casualty Decontamination Station
Phillip Coule, MD

What: Establish an area in which to decontaminate and treat a casualty. It consists of a <u>decontamination</u> area: triage, emergency treatment (may be co-located with triage) and skin decontamination; a <u>treatment area</u>: clean holding area pending treatment, advanced treatment facility; a clean <u>patient holding</u> area for those pending evacuation (can be located inside the treatment area); and a <u>hot line</u> separating the decontamination and treatment areas.

When: Chemical agents used against your unit, or against personnel you support. Similar procedures can be used to remove nuclear fallout and biological agents.

What You Need: Required: water source, supertropical bleach (STB), shovels, personnel MOPP4 ensemble for decontamination crews, protective shelter (tents, buildings, tree cover, caves, etc.). Optional: medical equipment sets (MES) for patient decontamination and patient treatment (contains many of these items), tentage, plastic sheeting, chemical agent alarms, chemical agent monitors, engineer tape or wire, field radio or telephone, windsock, camouflage netting, brushes and/or sponges, plastic bags, litters, litter stands, and contaminated disposal containers.

What To Do:
1. Select primary and alternate sites.
   a. Select primary and alternate sites in advance of operations. If the prevailing winds change direction, use of the primary site may no longer be possible.
   b. Site selection factors:
      (1) Direction of the prevailing winds
      (2) The location of friendly facilities downwind from the chemical hazard released at the decontamination station
      (3) Availability of protective shelters or buildings to house clean treatment facilities
      (4) Terrain
      (5) Availability of cover and concealment. The protective shelter may have visual, audible and infrared signatures that can compromise concealment
      (6) General tactical situation
      (7) Availability of evacuation routes (contaminated and clean)
      (8) Location of the supported unit's vehicle decontamination point, personnel decontamination point and MOPP exchange point. It is sometimes best to collocate with these unit decontamination sites. The arrangement of the operational areas must be kept flexible and adaptable to both the medical and tactical situations
2. Set up the decontamination area.
   a. Triage area. Do not decontaminate expectant patients. Personal equipment, including weapons, should be returned to the patient's unit if possible, for decontamination and management. Patient equipment can be decontaminated in the decontamination area as an option.
   b. Emergency treatment area. **Note:** Sometimes triage and emergency treatment are conducted in the same area.
   c. Skin decontamination area. Mix the STB with water in buckets and apply to garments and skin with brushes, sponges or rags. Sequentially decontaminate the chemical agent protective ensemble, remove the components as well as any clothing, decontaminate the underlying skin, and pass the clean patient to the shuffle pit.
   d. Overhead cover: erect an overhead cover, at least 20x50 feet, to cover the decontamination, clean waiting and triage/emergency treatment areas. If the protective shelter is used, the overhead cover should overlap the air lock entrance. If plastic sheeting is not available, alternate materials such as trailer covers, ponchos or tarpaulins may be used.
3. Set up the clean side of the decontamination station on the upwind side of the contaminated areas.
4. Set up the shuffle pit on the hot line as the only point of access between the decontamination area and the clean waiting and treatment area.
   a. Turn over the soil in an area that is 1-2 inches deep, and of sufficient length and width to accommodate a litter stand. Can also use mulch, sawdust or similar material if available. The shuffle pit should be wide enough to force the litter bearers to stand in the pit also.
   b. Mix supertropical bleach (STB) with the soil in a ratio of 2 parts STB to 3 parts soil. Transfer newly decontaminated patients into a patient decon bag on a litter in the shuffle pit (if available). If these items are not available, logroll patients from the arms of the decon team to those of the litter team. The patients should then be transported by the litter team to the treatment area.
5. Set up the treatment area on the upwind side of the decontamination area.
   a. Set up a protective shelter over the treatment area attached to the air lock adjoining the clean side of the decontamination station.
   b. When a protective shelter or air lock is not available for use, set up a covered medical treatment facility (use tents, fixed facility, etc.) 30-50 meters upwind from the shuffle pit.
6. Set up the evacuation holding area (can be part of the treatment area).
   a. Set up an overhead cover of plastic sheeting at least 20x25 feet.
   b. Make sure the cover overlaps part of the clean treatment area and part of the protective shelter.
   c. Avoid setting the protective shelter up near the generator.
7. Mark the hot line. Ensure that the entire hot line is clearly marked. Use wire, engineer's tape or other similar material to mark the entire perimeter of the hot line.

8. Establish ambulance points on both the "clean" and "dirty" evacuation routes.
    a. Establish a "dirty" ambulance point downwind from the triage area in the decontamination station.
    b. Establish a "clean" ambulance point upwind from the evacuation holding area on the clean side of the decontamination station.
9. Set up a contaminated (dirty) dump.
    a. Establish the contaminated dump 75-100 meters downwind from the decontamination station.
    b. Clearly mark the dump with NATO chemical warning markers.
10. Emplace chemical agent alarms. Set these alarms around the area, particularly between the decontamination and treatment areas.
11. Camouflage areas IAW tactical directives

What Not To Do:
1. Do not select only one decontamination site. Have an alternate site in case the wind direction or the operational situation changes.
2. Do not fail to determine the prevailing wind direction. It may be different at the primary and alternate sites.

Chapter 25: Chemical, Biological, and Radiation Injuries:
Biological Warfare: Suspected Unspecified Exposure
COL Theodore Cieslak, COL, MC, USA & COL Edward Eitzen, COL, MC, USA (Ret)

Introduction: Dozens of biological organisms and toxins have been mentioned as potential agents of warfare or terrorism. A detailed discussion of each of these agents is beyond the scope of this handbook. Rather than attempting, to discuss each agent, this guide focuses on the 6 agents felt by a panel of military and civilian experts to represent the most significant or problematic threats. Since the motives of terrorists are often difficult to ascertain, and because belligerents may employ weapons of opportunity, these 6 agents are not necessarily those most likely to be employed, but rather those that, IF employed, might pose the greatest threat to health and to operations. Because agents other than the 6 discussed here might be encountered, however, and because patients with virtually any biological agent exposure may present initially (when treatment is likely to be most beneficial) with a nonspecific febrile illness, empiric therapy might often be necessary. Empiric therapy might be offered to casualties with nonspecific symptoms where intentional biological agent exposure is felt to be a distinct possibility. This would be especially true on the battlefield, where sophisticated diagnostic tools and expert consultation are less likely to be available.

Subjective: Symptoms
Biological (and, in fact, chemical) agent casualties may often present with a predominance of pulmonary symptoms. These symptoms may be due to pulmonary pathology per se, or they may be due, in the case of botulism, to neuromuscular impairment and its subsequent effect on the muscles of respiration. Biological casualties may present with little more than a non-specific febrile illness. Subjective signs of a potential biological attack might include fever, headache, myalgias, fatigue, malaise, weakness, cough, and shortness of breath. Obviously, these same signs are seen in a wide variety of endemic diseases. Diagnosis of a biological attack, then, will not depend on the finding of a specific symptom, but on epidemiological clues.

Objective: Signs
Using Basic Tools: Inspection: Fever, tachypnea, dyspnea, cyanosis, diaphoresis, hypotension, and muscular weakness. Obviously, these will vary among diseases and not all findings will be present in the case of a given agent exposure. Auscultation: Rales. Palpation: Tachycardia
Using Advanced Tools: Specific diagnostic tests may often be unavailable in a field setting. Moreover, empiric therapy may be necessary long before confirmatory lab results are available. With this in mind, however, it will likely be beneficial to obtain certain basic lab studies from representative patients when a deliberate biological attack is suspected, even in situations where results will not be readily available and specimens will, of necessity, be sent to reference laboratories. Each of the following might be considered; not all will pertain to a given situation: Complete blood count, nasal swabs for Gram's stain, culture, and Polymerase Chain Reaction (PCR), blood for bacterial culture and PCR, serum for future serologic studies, sputum for Gram's stain, culture, and PCR, blood and/or urine for future toxin analysis, throat swabs for viral culture and PCR, and chest radiographs.

Assessment
A potential biological attack must be differentiated from naturally occurring illnesses and infectious diseases by using epidemiological clues. Potential signs of a deliberate attack might include: tight clusters of casualties, unusually high infection rates, unusual geography (presence of a presumed disease in an area where it does not occur naturally), localized geography, unusual or unexpected clinical presentations, finding of unusual munitions, evidence of a point-source, dead or dying animals and lower attack rates in protected personnel

Plan
Treatment
This section deals with empiric therapy provided when biological attack is suspected, but the identity of the specific agent is unknown. In cases where a specific agent is identified or strongly suspected, the provider should refer to the appropriate section of this manual. Remember that the provision of empiric therapy is not a substitute for the continued pursuit of a definitive diagnosis and the consequent provision of definitive therapy.
Primary: When dealing with casualties exhibiting pulmonary symptoms, or when dealing with large numbers of casualties exhibiting significant but nonspecific febrile illness, empiric antibiotic therapy might be warranted. This would be the case if patients were deteriorating and lives were in jeopardy, and it might also be the case if the tactical situation would be compromised by large numbers of casualties. In this setting, **doxycycline** 100mg po q12h can be prescribed. Supportive care (oxygen, IV fluids, antipyretics) should also be provided as needed.
Alternative: Tetracycline, ciprofloxacin, levofloxacin, ofloxacin, or other fluoroquinolones would be reasonable empiric alternatives.

Chapter 25: Chemical, Biological, and Radiation Injuries:
Biological Warfare: Inhalational Anthrax

Introduction: Anthrax is caused by infection with *Bacillus anthracis*, a gram-positive spore-forming rod. Although cutaneous and gastrointestinal forms are known, it is the inhalational form of the disease that would likely predominate following intentional aerosol delivery. The stability of anthrax spores, the relative ease of their dissemination, and the high lethality of the disease combine to make anthrax one of the most viable of potential biological weapons. *See Part 5: Specialty Areas: Chapter 12: Bacterial Infections: Anthrax*

Subjective: **Symptoms**

Classic inhalational anthrax is said to follow a "biphasic" course. Early in the disease, patients complain of non-specific flu-like symptoms: fever, malaise, fatigue, muscle aches, headaches, mild chest discomfort, and non-productive cough. After a brief period of these symptoms, patients may experience an apparent partial recovery. One or two days later, in the final stage of the disease, patients complain of high fever and significant shortness of breath.

Focused History: *Are you coughing? If so, are you coughing up sputum?* (The cough of anthrax is non-productive.) *Does your chest hurt?* (Chest pain is said to be prominent in cases of anthrax.) *Are you short of breath?* (This is non-specific, but prominent in anthrax.)

Objective: **Sign**

Using Basic Tools: Inspection: Dyspnea, cyanosis, diaphoresis, chest wall edema. Auscultation: Tachycardia, tachypnea. Palpation: Fever, meningismus. Percussion: Increased area of dullness over central chest (due to mediastinal widening) Early: Fever, tachypnea. Late: Fever, tachycardia tachypnea, dyspnea, cyanosis, diaphoresis, hypotension, chest wall edema, meningismus.

Using Advanced Tools: Essential: CXRs will often demonstrate pleural effusions and widening of the mediastinum late in the course of the disease. The lung fields themselves may be relatively clear, allowing differentiation of anthrax from most forms of pneumonia. Early in the disease, CXRs may be normal. Recommended: Blood cultures; Gram's stain of blood may actually demonstrate characteristic gram-positive rods late in the course of disease. *See Appendices: Color Plates: Figure A-23.A*

Assessment

Differential Diagnosis

Pneumonia (both conventional etiologies and other potential biological weapons): Anthrax produces respiratory symptoms but without true pneumonia. Anthrax victims will not likely have rales.

Plague: Will likely have rales and hemoptysis

Tularemia: May have rales

Staphylococcal enterotoxins: May have rales

Gram-negative sepsis: May be very difficult to differentiate from anthrax, but anthrax victims may have a widened mediastinum, which gram-negative sepsis patients will not. Gram's stain of peripheral blood may be useful and is often positive in late-stage anthrax.

Plan:

Treatment

Primary: Ciprofloxacin 400mg IV q12h plus **clindamycin** 900mg IV q12h plus **penicillin G** 4 million units IV q4h; oxygen, IV fluids, antipyretics (eg, **ibuprofen** 400mg po q4-6h prn)

Alternative: IV **doxycycline**, **tetracycline**, **levofloxacin**, **ofloxacin**, or other quinolones may be used if ciprofloxacin is unavailable. **Rifampin** or **clarithromycin** may be substituted if clindamycin is unavailable. **Ampicillin**, **imipenem**, **meropenem**, or **chloramphenicol** may be substituted if penicillin G is unavailable.

Primitive: Ciprofloxacin should be given alone if multi-drug therapy is not feasible. Oral **ciprofloxacin** 500mg q12h may be used if IV therapy is not possible.

Patient Education

General: Anthrax is an extremely serious disease; strict adherence to a regimen of antibiotic therapy is essential to survival; patients should be cared for in an inpatient setting.

Activity: As tolerated

Diet: As tolerated

Medications: Diarrhea is common with antibiotic administration; allergic reactions occasionally occur.

Prevention and Hygiene: Standard precautions are adequate.

No Improvement/Deterioration: Caretakers should watch for worsening respiratory distress, meningeal signs.

Follow-up Actions

Evacuation/Consultation Criteria: Symptomatic patients with presumed inhalational anthrax should be cared for in an inpatient setting, with access to intensive care modalities.

Notes: Immunization is an effective preventive measure against anthrax. Anthrax is not contagious; caregivers need only use standard precautions when dealing with patients. The prognosis for symptomatic anthrax victims is poor; in all likelihood, 50-85% or more of symptomatic victims will succumb, even in the face of appropriate therapy. EARLY treatment, however, may be lifesaving. For this reason, empiric therapy should be considered as soon as anthrax is suspected. These recommendations apply to symptomatic patients. Asymptomatic persons thought to have been exposed to aerosolized anthrax should be started on **ciprofloxacin** 500mg po q12h. **Doxycycline** 100mg po q12h is an acceptable substitute. Other fluoroquinolones, **tetracycline**, or **penicillin V** may be tried if ciprofloxacin or doxycycline is unavailable. In addition, asymptomatic exposed persons who have not received anthrax vaccine should be immunized if possible (with at least 3 doses of vaccine: at "time zero" and at 2 and 4 weeks after the first dose). *See Part 4: Organ Systems: Chapter 12: Bacterial Infections: Anthrax*

Chapter 25: Chemical, Biological, and Radiation Injuries:
Biological Warfare: Botulism

Introduction: Botulism is caused by exposure to one of 7 related neurotoxins produced by *Clostridium botulinum* and related anaerobic bacteria. It is NOT due to infection with the bacteria; antibiotics are thus of no value in its treatment. While botulism might be acquired in a number of ways (by consuming contaminated canned foods, by inhalation, and rarely, by percutaneous inoculation), it is likely to be encountered in aerosol form if weaponized. Botulism would present a similar clinical picture, however, regardless of the route of inoculation. *See Part 4: Organ Systems: Chapter 7: Acute Bacterial Food Poisoning*

Subjective: Symptoms
Botulism causes a descending symmetrical flaccid paralysis. Bulbar findings are prominent early in the course of the disease. Thus, after a latent period of several hours to several days, patients will complain of blurred vision, difficulty swallowing and speaking, dry or sore throat, and dizziness. Weakness and difficulty breathing become significant problems as the paralysis proceeds downward.
Focused History: *Should concentrate on bulbar signs; ask patient to speak* (difficulty articulating [dysarthria] is characteristic of botulism), *and to follow finger movements with their eyes* (extraocular muscle palsies are also characteristic).

Objective: Signs
Using Basic Tools: Inspection: mydriasis, ptosis, extraocular muscle palsies, absent gag reflex, cyanosis
Early: Mydriasis, ptosis, dysarthria, dysphonia,
Late: Postural hypotension, absent gag reflex, extraocular muscle palsies, cyanosis, progressive descending symmetrical muscle weakness. Notably, fever is generally absent.
Using Advanced Tools: There are no routinely positive, clinically relevant laboratory findings available to the clinician in the field.

Assessment: Botulism is a clinical diagnosis.
Differential Diagnosis
Nerve agent exposure: May also cause paralysis on the battlefield, but paralysis in this case is spastic. Moreover, miosis, copious secretions, and immediate onset of symptoms should make nerve agent intoxication readily distinguishable from botulism.
Other causes of flaccid paralysis (myasthenia gravis, Guillain-Barre syndrome, Eaton-Lambert syndrome, poliomyelitis, tick paralysis): May be impossible to differentiate from botulism in a field setting, but multiple patients presenting simultaneously with descending flaccid paralysis should prompt a diagnosis of botulism.

Plan
Patients with symptoms of botulism (or other in the differential diagnosis) cannot be cared for in a field setting and should be evacuated.
Treatment
Primary: Supportive (oxygen, assisted ventilation if necessary, IV fluids). A licensed antitoxin is available through the CDC, but this product is only effective against 2 of the 7 types of botulinum toxin (types A and B). An additional investigational antitoxin, effective against type E toxin, is also available through the CDC. Limited quantities of an investigational antitoxin potentially effective against all 7 types are available through the US Army Medical Research Institute of Infectious Diseases at Ft. Detrick, MD (1-888-USARIID).
Patient Education
General: Recovery from botulism may take several months; patients cannot be cared for in a field environment and evacuation is mandatory.
Activity: Bed rest
Diet: An inability to swallow makes long-term parenteral fluids and nutrition mandatory.
Prevention and Hygiene: Botulism is not contagious; standard precautions suffice.
No Improvement/Deterioration: Continued descent of the level of paralysis signifies a worsening of clinical status; all botulism victims must be evacuated to a facility with intensive care modalities.
Follow-up Actions
Evacuation/Consultation Criteria: Botulism victims will likely require long-term intensive care management and should be evacuated.
Notes: Botulism is not contagious; caregivers need only use standard precautions when dealing with patients. Botulism victims, even those with access to antiserum, may have a very prolonged course, requiring months of recovery. Thus, evacuation is of paramount importance. Adequate ventilatory support throughout this prolonged course is also critical to survival. Asymptomatic persons thought to have been exposed to botulism may be salvaged by prompt administration of antiserum.

Chapter 25: Chemical, Biological, and Radiation Injuries:
Biological Warfare: Pneumonic Plague

Introduction: Plague is caused by infection with *Yersinia pestis*, a gram-negative bacillus. Although bubonic and primary septicemic forms are known, it is the pneumonic form of the disease that would likely predominate after intentional aerosol delivery. *See Part 5: Specialty Areas: Chapter 12: Bacterial Infections: Plague*

Subjective: Symptoms
Patients complain of fever, malaise, fatigue, cough and shortness of breath.
Focused History: *Are you having difficulty breathing? Have you been coughing up blood?* (Most forms of pneumonia do not cause frank hemoptysis.)

Objective: Signs

Using Basic Tools: Inspection: Dyspnea, cyanosis, diaphoresis. Auscultation: tachycardia, tachypnea, rales, diminished breath sounds. Percussion: Dullness over lung fields Early: fever, tachypnea Late: fever, tachycardia, tachypnea, dyspnea, cyanosis, diaphoresis, hypotension, hemoptysis. The classic finding in pneumonic plague is the production of bloody sputum in a previously healthy patient, although this is not present in every case.

Using Advanced Tools: CXRs are consistent with pneumonia. Gram's stain of sputum will demonstrate short bipolar gram-negative rods, often with a "safety-pin" appearance.

Recommended: Blood cultures. 6% of pneumonic plague victims will develop meningitis; patients with meningeal signs should have a lumbar puncture performed for cerebrospinal fluid cell count, glucose, protein, and culture.

Assessment

Differential Diagnosis

Other forms of pneumonia (both conventional etiologies and other potential biological weapons: tularemia, staphylococcal enterotoxins): Most forms of pneumonia do not cause hemoptysis, but these can otherwise be very difficult to differentiate from plague pneumonia in an austere clinical setting.

Pulmonary tuberculosis: TB patients are typically chronically ill, but are not acutely ill and do not generally have high fevers.

Sepsis caused by other gram-negative bacteria: Hemoptysis is not generally a feature of sepsis.

Anthrax: Does not generally cause hemoptysis or true pneumonia.

Plan

Treatment

Primary: Gentamicin 5mg/kg IV q24h, oxygen, IV fluids, antipyretics (eg, **ibuprofen** 400mg po q4-6h prn).

Alternative: Streptomycin 1g IM q12h, **doxycycline** 100mg IV q12h, or **ciprofloxacin** 400mg IV q12h, may be used if gentamicin is unavailable.

Primitive: Doxycycline 100mg po q12h or **ciprofloxacin** 500mg po q12h may be used if IV therapy is not possible.

Patient Education

General: Pneumonic plague is an extremely serious disease; strict adherence to a regimen of antibiotic therapy is essential to survival; patients should be cared for in an inpatient setting.

Activity: As tolerated

Diet: As tolerated

Medications: Diarrhea is common with antibiotic administration; allergic reactions occasionally occur.

Prevention and Hygiene: Droplet precautions are required.

No Improvement/Deterioration: Caretakers should watch for worsening respiratory distress.

Follow-up Actions

Evacuation/Consultation Criteria: Patients with presumed plague should be cared for in an inpatient setting, with access to intensive care modalities, patients should be evacuated.

Notes: There is currently no available vaccine effective at preventing pneumonic plague. Pneumonic plague is contagious; caregivers should employ droplet precautions when dealing with patients. At a minimum, this entails masking of either the casualty or the health-care team and close contacts. Contacts should also be given prophylactic oral **doxycycline** 100mg po q12h x 7 days after the last exposure. The prognosis for symptomatic pneumonic plague victims is very poor; a large percentage of symptomatic victims will succumb, even in the face of appropriate therapy. These recommendations apply to symptomatic patients. Asymptomatic persons thought to have been exposed to aerosolized plague should be started on **doxycycline** 100mg po q12h x 7 days. **Ciprofloxacin** 500mg po q12h x 7 days is an acceptable substitute. Other fluoroquinolones may be tried if doxycycline or ciprofloxacin is unavailable.

Chapter 25: Chemical, Biological, and Radiation Injuries: Biological Warfare: Smallpox

Introduction: Smallpox is caused by infection with *Variola* virus, a member of the Orthopoxvirus family. Naturally occurring smallpox has been globally eradicated, the last case occurring in Somalia in 1977. Authorized stockpiles of virus exist in only two high-security laboratories. The categorization of smallpox virus as a viable weapon stems from the fear that belligerent groups may possess clandestine stocks. Moreover, fear exists that other closely related orthopoxviruses (such as monkeypox or cowpox) might be genetically manipulated to produce *Variola*-like disease.

Subjective: Symptoms

After a relatively lengthy incubation period of 7-17 days, clinical manifestations begin abruptly with malaise, fever, rigors, headache, backache, and vomiting.

Focused History: *Did you receive chickenpox or chickenpox vaccine as a child?* (makes a diagnosis of chickenpox less likely) *Have you been exposed to anyone with chickenpox?* (makes this diagnosis more likely) *Have you had a smallpox vaccination?* (makes smallpox less likely)

Objective: Signs

Using Basic Tools: The hallmark finding in smallpox patients is the characteristic rash, which appears 2-3 days after the onset of symptoms. The rash is synchronous in its progression from macules to papules to pustules to scabs, and is centrifugal in distribution (worse on the hands and face). Patients also exhibit fever and mental status changes. Palpation: Painful, firm "BB"-like pustules on skin. Early: Fever Late: Rash appears within 2-3 days

Using Advanced Tools: No diagnostic tests for smallpox are likely to be available in a field setting. A Tzanck smear prepared from a skin lesion may be helpful in ruling out chickenpox.

Assessment

Differential Diagnosis

Chickenpox: Asynchronous in its progression and centripetal in distribution. *See Part 5: Specialty Areas: Chapter 15: Viral Exanthems*

Monkeypox: Can closely mimic smallpox, but is typically milder. *See Part 5: Specialty Areas: Chapter 12: Viral Infections: Monkeypox*

Enteroviral exanthems: Patients are not typically severely ill.

Plan

Treatment

Primary: Supportive (oxygen, intravenous fluids, antipyretics). Intravenous **cidofovir** may be of some benefit, but is unlikely to be available in a field setting.

Patient Education

General: Recovery from smallpox may take several weeks; patients cannot be cared for in a field environment and evacuation is mandatory.

Activity: Most patients with smallpox will have extreme exhaustion and require bed rest.

Diet: Painful intraoral lesions may render the patient unable to eat and dependent on parenteral fluids.

Prevention and Hygiene: Strict adherence to airborne and contact precautions is required.

No Improvement/Deterioration: Caretakers should guard against dehydration, shock, and organ failure by meticulous attention to fluid status and supportive care.

Wound Care: Lesions should be cared for using contact precautions.

Follow-up Actions

Evacuation/Consultation Criteria: Smallpox victims will likely require a prolonged recovery period and should be evacuated.

Notes: Vaccinia vaccine is effective at preventing smallpox. A single case of smallpox is the gravest of public health emergencies; virtually no one (other than recently vaccinated members of the US military) is immune to the disease and the potential exists for an explosive pandemic to arise from the reintroduction of virus into the world's population. Preventive medicine experts should be consulted at the first suspicion of smallpox. Smallpox is contagious; caregivers should employ airborne and contact precautions when dealing with patients. At a minimum, this entails masking of either the casualty or the health-care team and close contacts, as well as the wearing of gloves when touching the patient. Contacts of smallpox victims should be promptly immunized with *Vaccinia* virus. These recommendations apply to symptomatic patients. Asymptomatic persons believed to have been exposed to smallpox should be promptly vaccinated with *Vaccinia* virus. Those vaccinated within the first several days after exposure may be protected against the development of smallpox. *Vaccinia* Immune Globulin (VIG) is not considered useful in managing smallpox victims.

Chapter 25: Chemical, Biological, and Radiation Injuries: Biological Warfare: Tularemia

Introduction: Tularemia is caused by infection with *Francisella tularensis*, a gram-negative coccobacillary organism. Although several forms are known, it is the pneumonic or typhoidal forms of the disease that would likely predominate following intentional aerosol delivery. *See Part 5: Specialty Areas: Chapter 12: Bacterial Infections: Tularemia*

Subjective: Symptoms

Patients complain of fever, malaise, fatigue, cough, shortness of breath, and abdominal pain.

Focused History: *Are you having difficulty breathing? Have you had contact with rabbits or squirrels?* (Naturally-occurring tularemia arises through contact with these hosts.) *Have you had tick bites?* (Tularemia can be transmitted by ticks.)

Objective: Signs

Using Basic Tools: Inspection: dyspnea, cyanosis, diaphoresis. Auscultation: tachycardia, tachypnea, rales, diminished breath sounds. Percussion: dullness over lung fields. Early: fever, tachypnea. Late: fever, tachycardia, tachypnea, dyspnea, cyanosis, diaphoresis, hypotension, abdominal tenderness.

Using Advanced Tools: CXRs may be consistent with pneumonia. A negative CXR does not rule out typhoidal tularemia. Gram's stain of sputum may demonstrate short gram-negative rods. Blood cultures recommended.

Assessment

Differential Diagnosis

Other forms of pneumonia (both conventional etiologies and other potential biological weapons: plague, staphylococcal enterotoxins): Can be very difficult to differentiate from pneumonic tularemia in an austere clinical setting.

Plague: Typically causes hemoptysis, which tularemia generally does not. *See Part 5: Specialty Areas: Chapter 12: Bacterial Infections: Plague*

Pulmonary tuberculosis: TB patients are typically chronically ill, but are not acutely ill and do not generally have high fevers *See Part 5: Specialty Areas: Chapter 12: Mycobacterial Infections: Tuberculosis*

Sepsis caused by other gram-negative bacteria: Can be very difficult to differentiate from tularemia in an austere clinical setting.

Anthrax: Does not generally cause true pneumonia. *See Part 5: Specialty Areas: Chapter 12: Bacterial Infections: Anthrax*

Plan:

Treatment

Primary: Gentamicin 5mg/kg IV q24h, oxygen, IV fluids, antipyretics (eg, **ibuprofen** 400mg po q4-6h prn). **Chloramphenicol** 25mg kg IV, then 15mg/kg (to a maximum of 4g/day) qid x 14 days should be added to other antibiotic therapy if meningitis is suspected. *See Part 5: Specialty Areas: Chapter 12: Bacterial Infections: Tularemia*

Alternative: Streptomycin 1g IM q12h, or **doxycycline** 100mg IV q12 h, or **ciprofloxacin** 400mg IV q12h may be used if gentamicin is unavailable.

Primitive: Doxycycline 100mg po q12h or **ciprofloxacin** 500mg po q12h may be used if IV therapy is not possible.

Patient Education

General: Pneumonic tularemia is an extremely serious disease; strict adherence to a regimen of antibiotic therapy is essential to survival; patients should be cared for in an inpatient setting.

Activity: As tolerated. This is a debilitating disease and most patients will require a period of bed rest.

Diet: As tolerated.

Medications: Diarrhea is common with antibiotic administration; allergic reactions occasionally occur. Side effects of gentamicin may include kidney and inner ear damage. Report ringing in the ears, hearing loss or dizziness (signs of ear toxicity).

Prevention and Hygiene: Standard precautions are sufficient.

No Improvement/Deterioration: Caretakers should watch for worsening respiratory distress

Follow-up Actions

Evacuation/Consultation Criteria: Patients with presumed pneumonic tularemia will likely require care in an inpatient setting, with access to intensive care modalities, patients should be evacuated.

Notes: Tularemia is not typically contagious; caregivers need only employ standard precautions when dealing with patients These recommendations apply to symptomatic patients. Asymptomatic persons thought to have been exposed to tularemia via aerosol should be started on **doxycycline** 100mg po q12h. **Ciprofloxacin** 500mg po q12h is an acceptable substitute. Other fluoroquinolones or **tetracycline** may be tried if doxycycline or ciprofloxacin is unavailable. Recommended duration of post-exposure prophylaxis is 14 days.

Chapter 25: Chemical, Biological, and Radiation Injuries:
Biological Warfare: Viral Hemorrhagic Fevers

Introduction: The viral hemorrhagic fevers (VHFs) are a diverse group of diseases caused by viruses of at least 4 families. They share a propensity to cause bleeding, but otherwise vary considerably in their clinical manifestations and severity. Included among the VHFs are Ebola and Marburg, certain Hantavirus infections, Argentinian and Bolivian hemorrhagic fevers, Lassa fever, Crimean-Congo hemorrhagic fever, and yellow fever. Most patients will exhibit fever. Bleeding from the gastrointestinal tract is common with some VHFs. Pulmonary hemorrhage occurs in certain of the VHFs. Flushing of the face, conjunctival injection, petechiae, purpura, bleeding from the mucous membranes, and ecchymoses of the skin are typical of many VHFs. Hematuria may be seen. Hypotension, shock, edema, hepatic tenderness, pharyngitis, hyperesthesias, and tremor may also occur.

Subjective: **Symptoms**

Early: fever, malaise, myalgias, headache, photophobia, vomiting, diarrhea, abdominal pain, cough, dizziness

Late: hemorrhage

Focused History: *Have you noticed blood in your stool, urine or are you coughing up blood?* (Bleeding is the hallmark finding of the VHFs.)

Objective: **Signs**

Using Basic Tools: Inspection: bleeding, petechiae, purpura, ecchymoses; Palpation: abdominal tenderness, capillary fragility

Using Advanced Tools: Specific diagnostic tests are unlikely to be available in a field setting. The platelet count, PT, PTT, and serum protein levels are likely to be abnormal in VHF patients, but such findings are not diagnostic. A blood culture is useful for ruling out meningococcemia and typhoid fever. A stool culture may rule out shigellosis. Lumbar punctures may be necessary to rule out meningitis among patients with meningeal signs and/or altered mental status.

Assessment

Differential Diagnosis

Dengue: Can cause hemorrhagic fever but is not transmissible via aerosol. *See Part 5: Specialty Areas: Chapter 12: Viral Infections: Dengue*

Yellow fever: 90% of cases occur in sub-Saharan Africa and the majority of others in S. America (CDC category C biological threat): *See Part 5: Specialty Areas: Chapter 12: Viral Infections: Yellow Fever*

Other causes of bleeding diathesis or disseminated intravascular coagulation (both conventional causes, as well as plague): Malaria, typhoid fever, meningococcemia, rickettsial diseases, leptospirosis, shigellosis, fulminant hepatitis, leukemia, lupus, hemolytic-uremic syndrome, thrombocytopenic purpuras. Many of these topics are specifically addressed in other sections in the handbook.

Plan:

Treatment

Primary: Supportive (oxygen, IV fluids, antipyretics). Aspirin should be avoided, as should intramuscular injections. Intravenous **ribavirin** may be beneficial in certain VHFs (Argentinian & Bolivian hemorrhagic fevers, Lassa fever, Hantavirus infection), but is unlikely to be available in a field setting.

Patient Education

General: The VHFs can be extremely serious diseases; meticulous supportive care and attention to fluid status is essential to survival. patients should be cared for in an inpatient setting.

Activity: As tolerated.

Diet: As tolerated.

Prevention and Hygiene: Contact precautions are required.

No Improvement/Deterioration: Caretakers should pay particular attention to blood pressure and fluid status.

Wound Care: Extreme caution should be used when handling any wounds or secretions.

Follow-up Actions

Evacuation/Consultation Criteria: patients with viral hemorrhagic fevers will likely require care in an inpatient setting, with access to intensive care modalities, patients should be evacuated.

Notes: Many VHFs are contagious; caregivers should employ contact precautions when dealing with patients. At a minimum, this entails the wearing of gloves when touching the patient and the disinfection of medical equipment (such as stethoscopes) between patient encounters. A licensed vaccine is available for one VHF, namely yellow fever. Personnel traveling to areas where yellow fever is endemic (eg, sub-Saharan Africa, tropical South America) should be immunized.

Chapter 25: Chemical, Biological, and Radiation (CBR) Injuries: Radiation: Radiation Injury
COL John Mercier, MS, USA & Col Glen Reeves, USAF, MC (Ret)

Introduction: This chapter focuses on recognizing and managing patients with Acute Radiation Syndrome (ARS) as typically seen following whole body doses above 100 centigray (cGy). Although some signs and symptoms for acute doses have thresholds as low as 50-75cGy, acute whole body doses above 200cGy are usually clinically significant and doses above 700cGy are nearly always fatal regardless of care and treatment. Late effects of whole body radiation exposure are dose dependent and may carry an increased risk of radiogenic cancer(s), leukemia and other somatic effects (eg, cataracts) years after exposure. To date, nearly all ARS patients worldwide received exposures from atomic bombings, nuclear criticality accidents, nuclear reactor accidents and accidents involving highly intense radioactive material sources. Although a nuclear detonation caused by an improvised nuclear device (IND) would certainly lead to ARS casualties, it is very unlikely that a radiation dispersal device (RDD), eg, "dirty bomb", would produce ARS casualties. Cutaneous radiation injury can occur with or without ARS and is more likely in scenarios where the skin receives a much higher dose than the whole body (eg, unsafe handling of a high intensity radioactive source or prolonged nuclear fallout on the exposed skin). More information is available in FM 4-02.283 (Treatment of Nuclear and Radiological Casualties) and via download of the Medical Management of Radiological Casualties Handbook at www.afrri.usuhs.mil. As well, subject matter expertise is available from military health physicists and radiation medicine physicians at major medical centers.

Subjective: Symptoms

Fatigue, listlessness, weakness, and loss of appetite have dose thresholds as low as 50-75cGy. Nausea, vomiting and headache are dose related. Noting the severity and time of onset of symptoms post exposure will aid in estimating dose received.

Focused History: *Do you have a headache?* (Headache can occur at low doses; however, severe headache may indicate a high exposure.) *Do you have diarrhea? Is it bloody? When did it begin? When do you think you were first exposed to radiation?* (If diarrhea is bloody or onset was within first few hours of exposure, the dose was very high. At moderate doses, diarrhea may not begin for several days.) *Have you vomited? When did vomiting start?* (If time of onset of emesis post exposure is more than 4 hours, dose is most likely survivable; if less than 1 hour, probably not survivable [especially in mass casualty situation]).

Objective: Signs

Using Basic Tools: Note areas of skin erythema and record their location and extent. Erythema may appear for a few hours after exposure, then disappear, then recur a few days later (ominous prognostic sign) along with skin erosions, ulcerations, blisters, and pain. Observe for trauma (unrelated to radiation). Dose threshold for hair loss (epilation) is 300cGy. Hair loss generally occurs 2-3 weeks post exposure. Conjunctivitis may occur with beta radiation (dust in eyes) or moderate to high dose external radiation. Patients may present with oropharyngeal lesions within 24-48 hours moderate to high doses.

Using Advanced Tools: Labs: CBC with differential immediately and q6-12h (50% drop in lymphocytes within the first 24 hours, with total lymphocyte count less than $1x10^9$ indicates significant radiation injury). If inhalation suspected, and if less than 1 hour post exposure, collect bilateral nasal swabs. If inhalation of uranium or plutonium is suspected, begin urine sampling 24 hours post exposure. If patient not evacuated and at least 24 hours post-exposure: Collect serum amylase and draw 10cc of peripheral blood in a heparinized tube, refrigerate and forward it with patient for cytogenetic biodosimetry (estimate of dose received) analysis. Radiation Monitoring (if available): Whole-body monitoring with RADIAC meter to ensure proper decontamination or identify significant internal contamination that will require followup.

Assessment: Differential Diagnosis

Radiogenic vomiting may be confused with psychogenic vomiting that often results from stress and fear reactions. Skin damage may be from conventional thermal burns or from high doses of radiation. Diarrhea may be radiogenic or psychogenic (or from other causes); if bloody, not psychogenic and prognosis is very poor.

Clinical Course: ARS is a multi-system injury that presents as a sequence of phased symptoms.

1. Prodromal Phase (within hours of exposure): Nausea, vomiting, diarrhea, fatigue, weakness, fever and headache; time to onset, duration and severity of these symptoms varies with radiation dose received. Transient erythema (skin redness) and an itching or burning sensation may occur for skin doses exceeding 300cGy.
2. Latent Phase (lasting days to weeks depending on dose received): Except for some fatigue and weakness, relatively symptom free.
3. Manifest Illness Phase (follows latent phase): Clinical symptoms are expressed in the affected major organ systems. The organ systems whose injuries are most likely to contribute to death from ARS are the hematopoietic (blood forming), gastrointestinal (GI), skin, and in extremely high doses, cardiovascular and CNS. Infection and sepsis are major causes of severe morbidity and mortality.
4. Recovery Phase (if casualty survives): Slow return of blood counts toward normal; may take months. Skin damage may persist or recur. Other organs (lung, kidney) may express damage months later.

Plan: Treatment
  Primary:
    1. Decontaminate following stabilization. Remove outer layer of clothing and wash exposed skin with soap and water (95% effective). Do not abrade skin. Eyes: Saline rinse. Wounds: saline rinse and/or povidone-iodine scrub. Areas of skin that tend to collect fallout include neck, torso, belt line.
    2. For ARS, supportive care is known to substantially improve survivability for doses below 500cGy (eg, clean environment, fluids to balance electrolytes, administer blood products as needed, broad spectrum antibiotics to control infection/fever, antiemetics and antidiarrheals, etc.). Maintain the gut with oral diet if patient can tolerate it, avoiding raw vegetables and fruits to reduce risk of bacterial ingestion. Control radiogenic emesis with antiemetics: **granisetron** 1mg IV over 30 seconds or **ondansetron** 8mg IM, or IV over 30 seconds is best.
    3. Skin injury: Topical steroids that do not cause atrophy and antihistaminic skin emollients if there are no breaks in the skin.
    4. Wound Care: Definitive surgical management of associated wounds and trauma must be completed (wound closure) within 36 hours in a patient with significant radiological injury so as to avoid infection and increased morbidity associated with poor wound healing.
    5. Fever: If neutropenic but afebrile, consider antibiotic to minimize risk of infection: **Ciprofloxacin** 250-500mg po or IV q12h.
  Patient Education
    General: A patient who receives a low dose (<75cGy) should be reassured and returned to duty, as no symptoms will occur, or be mild and transient. The patient should be informed that any dose suspected of exceeding the peacetime regulatory limit of 5cGy, although clinically insignificant, will be noted in his clinical record should possibly radiogenic illnesses such as solid tissue cancer, leukemia, or certain nonmalignant diseases such as cataracts occur, years later.
    Diet: After discharge from facilities no special diet or medication is required (except for internal contamination from significant quantities of certain isotopes).
    Skin care: Recurrent waves of erythema may occur. Delayed skin injury and hair loss may occur with high skin doses, even if whole body doses are low.
  Follow-up Actions
    Evacuation/Consultation Criteria: Evacuate a patient with suspected significant radiological injury as soon as possible. A patient with lymphocyte depletion within the first 24 hours should be evacuated as quickly as possible for definitive care. At definitive care facilities, access to specialized pharmaceuticals such as **cytokines** may be used, if administered sufficiently early in the treatment cycle, to recover the bone marrow.
    Notes: Although not normally associated with ARS, a variety of antidotes are available for specialized treatment of internal contamination. Common ones include **potassium** or **sodium iodide** (**KI** or **NaI**) to prevent thyroid uptake of radioactive iodine, which occurs after reactor accidents and INDs. Significant internal contamination by plutonium, the primary radioactive contaminant in nuclear weapons accidents, is treated with chelating agents such as **calcium- and zinc- (DTPA)**. Internal contamination with radioactive cesium is treated with **Prussian Blue**.

Chapter 26: Trauma Assessment: Primary and Secondary Survey

COL John Holcomb, MC, USA

Reviewed June 2008 by COL Thomas Deal, MC, USA

Primary Survey

The standard ABC approach as outlined in civilian models provides an excellent methodology for addressing life-threatening injuries in a systematic fashion. The "ABC" mnemonic prioritizes the search for injuries in accordance with their potential to kill the patient; it is simple to remember and it provides an anchor point from which patients can re-assessed if they deteriorate. This system may require some modification in a tactical setting. For example, in a mass casualty situation, the SOF medic may need to address the ABCs of several patients at once. *See Part 1: Operational Issues: Triage in MASCAL*. Simply asking the casualties where they are injured can do this. Those casualties who answer the question appropriately have an intact airway, are breathing and are conscious. The medic should then focus his attention on those casualties who are unconscious or in obvious distress. Meanwhile, the medic can direct the lightly injured casualties or non-medical team members to assist in controlling the bleeding of those patients with active hemorrhage, thus addressing the circulation step. During combat, moving the patient to a safe location takes priority over the Primary and Secondary Survey unless a rapid maneuver can be performed for an obvious life-threatening injury, ie, the application of a tourniquet. Rapid control of hemorrhage is a mainstay of combat casualty care.

Airway: A conscious and spontaneously breathing patient requires no immediate airway intervention. If the patient is able to talk normally then his airway is intact. If the patient is semi-conscious or unconscious, the flaccid tongue is the most common source of airway obstruction. The chin lift or jaw thrust maneuver should be attempted and should readily relieve any obstruction created by the tongue. Once the airway is opened or if further difficulty is encountered, a nasopharyngeal or oropharyngeal airway should be inserted. The nasopharyngeal airway is better tolerated in the semi-conscious patient and the patient with an intact gag reflex. If these measures fail to provide an adequate airway or if the patient is unconscious, unresponsive and apneic, orotracheal intubation should be considered. Orotracheal intubation done on a trauma patient with an intact gag reflex without the use of pharmacological sedation and paralysis will be difficult and may cause additional complications such as vomiting, airway trauma and increased intracranial pressure, and thus should be avoided except as a last resort. If the patient is breathing and definitive airway control if needed, blind nasotracheal intubation (BNTI) may be attempted. Severe facial fractures and basilar skull fractures are relative contraindications to BNTI.

Other adjuncts to airway management can and should be used if available and if the medic is skilled in their use. Other possible adjuncts to airway management include the Laryngeal Mask Airway (LMA), the Intubating LMA, the Combitube, and the Lighted Stylet.

If the patient has obvious maxillofacial trauma with signs of airway compromise or if orotracheal intubation fails, then a surgical cricothyroidotomy may be a necessary and lifesaving maneuver (*see Part 8: Procedures: Chapter 30: Cricothyroidotomy*). The most common mistake when performing a surgical airway is delaying too long before starting the procedure.

Civilian models of trauma care include cervical spine control and immobilization with airway management. Few if any battlefield casualties with penetrating trauma will have associated injury to the cervical spine unless they have combined blunt injuries from vehicle or aircraft crashes, falls or crush injuries, or penetrating injury to the spinal cord. Meticulous attention to presumed cervical spine injury on the battlefield is not warranted if penetrating trauma is the obvious mechanism. Furthermore, the medic or the casualty may sustain additional injury if evacuation from the battlefield, and/or treatment of other injuries such as hemorrhage is delayed while the cervical spine is immobilized.

Breathing: In the conscious patient, who is alert and breathing normally, no interventions are required. If the patient has signs of respiratory distress such as tachypnea, dyspnea, or cyanosis, which may be associated with agitation or decreasing mental status, an aggressive search for an etiology is required. Injuries that may result in significant respiratory compromise include tension pneumothorax, open pneumothorax (sucking chest wound), flail chest, and massive hemothorax. The patient's chest and back should be quickly exposed and inspected for obvious signs of trauma, asymmetrical, or paradoxical movement of the chest wall, accessory muscle use and jugular venous distention. If possible, auscultation should be performed listening for abnormal or decreased breath sounds. The chest wall should be palpated to identify areas of tenderness, crepitus, subcutaneous emphysema or deformity.

Open pneumothorax should be treated with a three-sided occlusive dressing and a tension pneumothorax with needle decompression. *See Part 8: Procedures: Chapter 30: Thoracostomy, Needle and Chest Tube*

The field management of a flail chest centers on controlling the patient's pain and augmentation of the patient's respiratory efforts with bag valve mask (BVM) ventilation. Chest wall splinting with tape, sandbags and the like has been advocated in the past, but should no longer be performed as it decreases the movement of the chest wall and will further compromise the patient's ability to ventilate. These casualties may have significant injury to the underlying lung and may deteriorate rapidly requiring endotracheal intubation and positive pressure ventilation.

Management of a massive hemothorax in the field should be directed at maintaining adequate ventilation with a BVM. If evacuation is delayed and the patient continues to deteriorate, consideration may be given for the placement of a chest tube. If more than 1000cc of blood is immediately drained by the chest tube or if the output is more than 200cc per hour for 4 hours, the patient likely has injury to the great vessels, hilum, heart or vessels in the chest wall that will require surgical repair.

Flail chest and massive hemothorax are difficult injuries to treat in the field and should be evacuated are rapidly as possible.

Circulation: <u>Uncontrolled hemorrhage is the leading cause of preventable battlefield deaths.</u> Rapid identification and effective management of bleeding is perhaps the single most important aspect of the primary survey while caring for the combat casualty.

Obvious external sources of bleeding should be controlled with direct pressure initially followed by a field dressing or pressure dressing. If bleeding is not controlled by the previous measures or if gross arterial bleeding is present, an effective tourniquet should immediately be applied. Clamping of injured vessels is not indicated unless the bleeding vessel can be directly visualized. Blind clamping of vessels may result in additional injury to neurovascular structures and should not be done.

Note: The current ATLS manual discourages the use of tourniquets in the pre-hospital setting because of distal tissue ischemia, tissue crush injury at the tourniquet site, which may necessitate subsequent amputation. This admonition is based on the civilian model of trauma care where most penetrating injuries are low velocity in nature and rapid evacuation to a trauma center is available. Withholding the use of tourniquets on the battlefield for patients with severe extremity hemorrhage may result in additional death or injury that might have otherwise been prevented.

Sources of internal hemorrhage should be identified. A significant amount of blood can be lost into the chest and abdominal cavities, the retroperitoneal space and the soft tissues surrounding fractures of the pelvis and lower extremities. Significant bleeding into the thoracic and abdominal cavities following trauma will require surgical exploration. In the absence of a head injury, hypotensive resuscitation will help prevent more bleeding. Bleeding from injuries to the pelvis and groin or from fractures of the lower extremities not otherwise amenable to treatment with a tourniquet and not associated with thoracic injuries may be controlled with the application of Pneumatic Anti-Shock Garment (PASG), aka Military Anti-Shock Trousers (MAST).

After sources of hemorrhage are identified and controlled, the need for intravenous access should be considered. If the patient has an isolated extremity wound, the bleeding has been controlled and there are no signs of shock, there is no need for immediate intravenous fluid resuscitation. Intravenous access with a saline lock should be considered for all casualties with significant injuries. If there is a truncal injury and if signs of shock are present, or if blood pressure continues to drop, intravenous access should be obtained with a 16 or 18 gauge catheter followed by a 1-2L bolus of normal saline or lactated Ringer's, or 500mL of Hespan. If the patient has improvement of the clinical signs of shock following the initial bolus, subsequent intravenous fluids should be titrated to achieve only a good peripheral pulse and an improvement in sensorium rather than to normalize blood pressure. If there is no clinical improvement following the initial IV fluid bolus, the possibility of severe uncontrolled intra-abdominal or intrathoracic bleeding should be considered. Further fluid resuscitation in uncontrolled hemorrhage is not indicated, may be harmful, and may waste the limited fluids available to the SOF medic.

Cardiopulmonary arrest from hemorrhage has a very high mortality in the hospital setting. Attempting to resuscitate patients who are in cardiac arrest secondary to hemorrhage while in the field will almost certainly be futile.

Disability: A brief neurological assessment should be performed using the AVPU scale:

A - Alert
V - Responds to verbal stimuli
P - Responds to painful stimuli
U - Unresponsive

Exposure: Clothing and protective equipment such as helmets and body armor should only be removed as required to evaluate and treat specific injuries. If the patient is conscious with a single extremity wound, only the area surrounding the injury should be exposed. Unconscious patients may require more extensive exposure in order to discover potentially serious injures but must subsequently be protected from the elements and the environment. Hypothermia is to be avoided in trauma patients.

Vital Signs: Vital signs should be assessed frequently, especially after specific therapeutic interventions, and before and after moving patients. The SOF medic should be sensitive to subtle changes in vital signs in wounded SOF operators. As a group, these patients are in excellent physical condition and may have tremendous physiological reserves. They may not manifest significant changes in vital signs until they are in severe shock. The vital signs include:

Pulse: The rate and character of the pulse should be evaluated. A weak, rapid, barely palpable radial pulse indicates the presence of hemorrhagic shock.

Respiration: Respiratory rate can be an extremely sensitive indicator of physiologic stress. Resting tachypnea should be considered abnormal and should prompt investigation if there is no obvious cause.

Blood Pressure: The SOF medic is not expected to carry a sphygmomanometer during combat operations. Palpation of distal and central pulses provides a rough guide to systolic blood pressure.

Radial - at least 70mmHg
Femoral - at least 60mmHg
Carotid - at least 50mmHg

Temperature: Only if hypo or hyperthermia are suspected. Hypothermia is an often unrecognized and yet significant contributor to traumatic death.

Secondary Survey

During the Secondary Survey, a more methodical search for non life-threatening injuries is conducted. These injuries should be treated as they are encountered. Like the Primary Survey, the Secondary Survey may need to be modified and adapted according to the tactical situation and the number and type of casualties encountered. The vast majority (75%) of casualties who are wounded in action (WIA) will have isolated penetrating trauma to the extremities. These patients do not require a detailed head to toe exam in the Secondary Survey. They will need to have a bandage and/or splint applied with evaluation of their neurovascular status distal to the injury before and after treatment. They then need to be frequently reassessed for signs of deterioration as the tactical situation permits. Patients who are severely injured or unconscious will require a more detailed Secondary Survey. Evacuation should not be delayed to perform a Secondary Survey or for the treatment of non life-threatening injuries. The Secondary Survey should be conducted in a systematic head to toe, front to back fashion using visual Inspection, Auscultation, Palpation and Percussion (IAPP) where applicable.

HEENT: The head and face should be inspected for obvious laceration, burns, contusion, asymmetry or hemorrhage. The bones of the face and head should then be palpated to identify crepitus, bony step-off, depressions or abnormal mobility of the mandible and mid face. The eyes should be opened and examined for signs of trauma, globe rupture, or hyphema. The orbits and zygomatic arches should be palpated for signs of fractures. Pupils should be checked for reactivity and symmetry. If the patient is awake, extra-ocular movements can be assessed along with gross visual acuity. The ears should be inspected for obvious trauma and the ear canals for blood or cerebral spinal fluid (CSF). Battle's sign, indicating possible basilar skull fracture, may be observed over the mastoid processes. The nares should be inspected for blood or CSF. The mouth and oropharynx should be inspected for trauma or bleeding. Loose teeth, dental appliances or other potential airway obstructions should be removed. Any previous airway interventions should be reassessed.

Neck: The neck should be visually inspected searching for obvious trauma or deformity, tracheal deviation, jugular venous distention (JVD), or signs of respiratory accessory muscle use. The cervical spine should be palpated for step-off, tenderness or deformity.

Chest: The chest wall should be observed for penetrating injury or blunt injury, asymmetrical breathing movements or retractions. Auscultation over the anterior lung fields, posterior lung bases and heart should follow. The entire rib cage, sternum and chest wall should be palpated for tenderness, flail segments, subcutaneous emphysema or crepitus. Percussion may be performed looking for hyperresonance or dullness.

Abdomen: The abdomen should be observed for signs of blunt or penetrating injury. The presence or absence of bowel sounds should evaluated. Palpation searching for tenderness, guarding or rigidity should follow. Percussion may elicit subtle rebound tenderness.

Pelvis: The pelvis should be inspected for signs of penetrating trauma or deformity. Pelvic instability and fracture should be suspected with movement of the anterior iliac crests when lateral and anterior pressure is applied. The perineum and genitals are inspected next for signs of injury. Scrotal, vulvar and perineal hematomas or blood at the urethral meatus may indicate pelvic fracture as well as the possibility of a urethral tear that could complicate placement of a urethral catheter. Likewise, the rectal exam will yield information about the location of the prostate, and presence or absence of gross blood in the rectum.

Extremities: The extremities are inspected and palpated proximally to distally. Each bone and joint distal to the pelvis and clavicle should be assessed for crepitus, tenderness, deformity and abnormal joint motion. Distal pulses and capillary refill are then examined. Asking the patient if he can feel the examiner lightly touching his hands and feet tests gross sensation. Gross motor strength is tested by having the patient squeeze the examiner's fingers and by moving his toes up and down against the resistance of the examiner's hands.

Neurological: A field neurological exam should consist of observation of the pupils for reactivity and asymmetry (done during HEENT exam), the level of consciousness, gross sensory and motor function (assessed during examination of the extremities) and calculation of the Glasgow Coma Scale (GCS). The GCS is a useful tool that can be used to monitor the clinical status of seriously injured patients. A declining GCS score over time indicates further neurological deterioration. A GCS less than 9 indicates severe neurological injury (*see Appendices: Table A-5: Glasgow Coma Scale*).

Pain Management: Intravenous **morphine sulfate** is an excellent analgesic for traumatic injuries. **Morphine** has a rapid onset, is easily titratable and can be readily reversed by naloxone if the patient becomes obtunded or experiences respiratory depression. It should be used with caution in patients with injuries that may compromise respiratory function and it is contraindicated in patients with head injuries or altered levels of consciousness. Doses should be given in 5mg increments every 10-15 minutes until adequate levels of analgesia are obtained. The practice of withholding narcotic analgesics or more frequently, giving inadequate doses because of concerns of abuse or respiratory depression in otherwise healthy SOF operators are based on unrealistic concerns and should be avoided. Casualties with combat wounds require treatment for their pain, preferably through the intravenous route. In cases where IV access is not possible, **fentanyl** lollipops may be useful. *See Part 8: Procedures: Chapter 30: Pain Assessment and Control.*

Antibiotics: There are many antibiotic regimens. A reasonable approach is to use **cefotetan** 1-2g IV or IM q12h. It is cheap, readily available, easily stored and rarely causes an allergic reaction. Minor injuries in the field often become infected so pre-hospital antibiotic use should be liberal. Of course all open fractures, abdominal wounds and extensive soft tissue injury should be cleaned, dressed and given antibiotics. For severe injury in patients where medical evacuation is anticipated to be delayed >3 hours, **moxifloxacin** 400mg po or **ertapenem** 1g IV q day through medical evacuation are reasonable choices. *See Appendices: Table A-1. Organism/Antibiotic Chart*

Reassessment: The most valuable diagnostic tool available to the SOF medic while caring for combat casualties is a repeated physical exam. Patients should be frequently reassessed with attention given to potential complications of their particular injuries and treatments. For example, distal pulses and sensation should be re-examined in those patients with extremity injuries, looking for the development of compartment syndrome. Wounds treated with bandages and tourniquets should be reassessed for further bleeding. Patients with head injures should have frequent neurological examinations looking for signs of deterioration. Those with chest wounds will require repeated auscultation to rule out development or re-accumulation of a pneumothorax.

Chapter 26: Trauma Assessment: Primary and Secondary Survey Checklist

Furnished by JSOMTC

Scene Size-Up
    Tactical Situation/Security/Time on Site
    Body Substance Isolation (BSI) Precautions
    Mechanism of Injury (MOI)/History of Events
    Determine # of Patients
    Request Help if needed
    Direct/Provide C-spine Stabilization if indicated (always if multisystem trauma, altered LOC or blunt injury above clavicle)

Primary Survey
    INITIAL ASSESSMENT
        AVPU/GCS (GCS of 8 or less requires intubation)
    Chief Complaint if Conscious
        Determine Apparent Life Threats (Massive Hemorrhage)/Stop Gaps
    ASSESS AIRWAY
        Assess Airway for 5-10 Seconds
        Open Airway/Modified Jaw Thrust/Chin Lift
        Inspect Mouth and Clear (Suction/Heimlich/Laryngoscope)
        Insert Indicated Airway Adjunct (NPA/OPA/ET/CRIC)
        Reassess Airway/BLS as Required
    ASSESS BREATHING
        Inspect Anterior Chest (bilateral rise and fall)

Occlude Chest Wounds
Auscultate Anterior Chest x 1 bilateral
Palpate Anterior Chest
Percuss Anterior Chest x 1 bilateral
Palpate Posterior Chest
Identify/Stop Gap Treat Posterior Wound
Manage Injuries that Could Complicate Breathing

ASSESS CIRCULATION
Identify and Control Major Bleeding Pack, Clamp, Dress prn
Apply Tourniquet prn (Amputation, Major Bleeding)
Assess Pulse (Radial/Femoral/Carotid)
Assess Peripheral Perfusion (Skin Color/Temp)
State General Impression of Patient Based on Injuries/Findings
Log Roll, Identify/Definitively Treat Downside Wounds (tension pneumo after movement if not treated)
Expose as needed
Initiate Movement within 10 minutes

Secondary Survey
Reassess all Previous Treatments Following Movement
Move Patient Safely
Mental Status (AVPU/GCS)
Reassess ABC/TX
Airway (ET if unconscious) (reassess placement prn)
Neck
   Assess for Jugular Vein Distention
   Assess for Tracheal Deviation
   Palpate C-spine
   Treat all Injuries to Neck
Anterior Chest
   Reassess Prior Treatment/Reinforce PRN
   Auscultate x 3 Bilateral
   Auscultate Heart
   Percuss x 3 Bilateral
   Palpate
Abdomen/Pelvis
   Inspect the Abdomen for Obvious Injury
   Assess the Pelvis/Shoulders
Extremities (Hemorrhage/Fracture)
   Inspect & Palpate Arms
   Inspect & Palpate Legs
L-Spine
   Palpate L-spine/Treat Injuries
Log Roll
   Maintain C/L-Spine Control
Assess/TX Posterior
   Head to Foot
Reassess Airway
   Check Placement of ET Tube
Reassess Circulation
   Reinforce Treatments, Apply Stump Dressing prn, etc.
Obtain Baseline Vital Signs
Obtain Patent Percutaneous IV
PERRL
AVPU/GCS
Identify and Treat All Life-Threatening Injuries
Full Set of Vital Signs
Fracture Immobilization
Splint all Long Bone Fractures

Evacuate
Move Patient Safely
Reassess ABCs w/placement Check
Resuscitative Phase
   Vital Signs
   Treat for Hypothermia

Patient Positioning
Perform Detailed Physical Exam
  HEENT
  Thorax/Heart
  Abdomen/GU
  Musculoskeletal
  Neurological
  Identify and Treat all Wounds
  Cricothyroidotomy, Tube Thoracostomy, Venous Cutdown
  Splint Cutdown Site
  9-Line CASEVAC (ASAP)
  Field Medical Card (FMC)

Chapter 26: Trauma Assessment: Mild Traumatic Brain Injury/Concussion: Assessment and Management

Col (S) Michael S. Jaffee, USAF, MC & Katherine M. Helmick, MS, CRNP

Introduction: Traumatic brain injury (TBI) is any structural injury or physiological disruption of brain function due to trauma that includes at least 1 of the following clinical signs immediately following the traumatic event: 1) loss or decreased level of consciousness; 2) loss of memory (ie, for events either before or after the injury); 3) any other decrease in mental function or neurological deficit. The traumatic event can be from an object striking the head or the head striking an object, acceleration or deceleration injury, foreign body penetration, or blast injury. TBI casualties can be some of the most challenging trauma casualties and the primary goal is the initial stabilization of the patient (*see Part 7: Chapter 26: Primary and Secondary Survey; Chapter 27: Hypovolemic Shock & Part 8: Procedures: Chapter 30: Initial Airway Management and Ventilatory Support*). This section will focus on the assessment and management of mild TBI or concussion and patients at increased risk for mild traumatic brain injury (mTBI). Mild TBI and concussion are synonymous terms. Field screening and diagnosis of concussion caused by single or repeated blast or other trauma remains problematic and the SOF medic must remain alert to the possibility of symptoms presenting after the "heat of battle" has passed and through redeployment.

Subjective: Symptoms

Symptoms of mTBI/concussion may present and resolve quickly or be delayed and persist for days to months, with the remote possibility of permanent disability. Typically signs and symptoms will manifest immediately following the event and frequently as:

1. Physical symptoms: headache, nausea, vomiting, dizziness, blurred vision, sleep disturbance, weakness, paresis/plegia, sensory loss, spasticity, aphasia, dysphagia, dysarthria, apraxia, balance disorders, disorders of coordination, seizure disorder
2. Cognitive symptoms of decreased: attention, concentration, memory, speed of processing, new learning, planning, reasoning, judgment, executive control, self-awareness, language or abstract thinking and/or
3. Behavioral symptoms: depression, anxiety, agitation, irritability, impulsivity, aggression.

Focused History: Ask Military Acute Concussion Evaluation (MACE) questions I-VIII (*see Figure 7-3*). *What happened? What do you remember? Were you dazed, confused, "saw stars"? Did you hit your head? What caused your injury? Explosion/blast, blunt object, MVA, fragment, fall, gunshot wound, something else? Were you wearing your helmet? What happened just before your injury? What happened immediately after your injury?* (Evaluate for any gaps in memory. Troop should be able to relay details of the event.) *Did you lose consciousness or "black out"? Who came to your aid? What did you do? Did you smell anything? Were you able to perceive what was going on around you? If blast related, how far away were you from the blast/explosion? How long ago did it happen?* (Suspect mild TBI if an injury event has occurred and there has been an alteration in consciousness; see severity chart below.) Whenever possible, team members or others who witnessed the event should be questioned to add to and validate the accuracy of the patient's answers

Objective: Signs

Using Basic Tools: Neurological exam (include the Glasgow Coma Scale (GCS) in Appendices and the MACE tool sections IX–XIII [*see Figure 7-3*] in this section) **Note:** Consider varying options on MACE section X to mitigate risk that highly motivated individuals may memorize MACE to avoid detection of disability. Specific attention should be given to identify: progressively declining level of consciousness, declining neurological exam, pupillary asymmetry, seizures, repeated vomiting, GCS <15, loss of consciousness (LOC) greater than 5 minutes, double vision, worsening headache, neurologic deficit: motor or sensory, inability to recognize people or disoriented to place, ataxia. *See Appendices: Figure A-32. Neurological Examination Checklist*

Table 7-1. TBI Severity Chart

Severity	Glasgow Coma Score (GCS)	Alteration of Consciousness (AOC)	Loss of Consciousness (LOC)	Post-traumatic Amnesia (PTA)
Mild (Concussion)	13-15	≤24 hrs	0-30 min	≤24 hrs
Moderate	9-12	>24 hrs	>30 min <24 hrs	>24 hrs <7 days
Severe	3-8	>24 hrs	≥24 hrs	≥7 days

Note: The GCS is not a sensitive tool in the evaluation of mTBI or concussion. The GCS score may be 15, but the patient can be impaired enough to threaten unit readiness and mission completion.

Assessment:
Differential Diagnosis
No concussion: No alteration of consciousness or other neurologic symptoms or signs.
Concussion without loss of consciousness
Concussion with loss of consciousness
Operational stress/post-traumatic stress disorder: *See Part 5: Specialty Areas: Chapter 18: Operational Stress*
Hypoglycemia: *See Part 4: Organ Systems: Chapter 4: Hypoglycemia*
Substance abuse: *See Part 5: Specialty Areas: Chapter 18: Substance Abuse*

Figure 7-1. Level 1 mTBI Treatment Algorithm

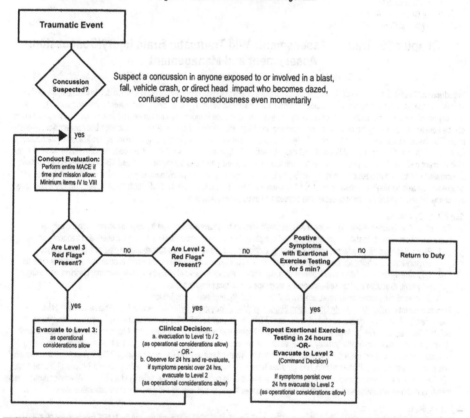

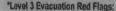

*Level 3 Evacuation Red Flags:	**Level 2 Evacuation Decision:	Treatment:

1. Progressively declining level of consciousness/neurological exam
2. Pupillary asymmetry
3. Seizures
4. Repeated vomiting
	1. MACE (Items IV-VIII)
	2. Red Flags
	  a. Double vision
	  b. Worsening headaches
	  c. Can't recognize people or places, disorientation
	  d. Behaves unusually or seems confused and irritable
	  e. Slurred speech
	  f. Unsteady on feet
	  g. Weakness or numbness in arms/legs
		1. Headache management – use **acetaminophen**
		2. Avoid tramadol, narcotics, NSAIDs, ASA or other platelet inhibitors until CT confirmed negative
		3. Give an educational sheet to all positive mTBI patients.

Plan:

Treatment (*see Figures 7-1 and 7-2*)
1. Protection and prevention of subsequent injury until recovery is completed
2. Management of specific symptoms
3. Do not return to full duty status until asymptomatic, MACE >25 and resting and exertional signs and symptoms are negative.
4. Provide patient support and reassure continuing care through anticipated full recovery.
5. Reevaluate prn for any of these Red Flags:
    a. Progressively declining level of consciousness
    b. Progressively declining neurological exam
    c. Pupillary asymmetry
    d. Seizures
    e. Repeated vomiting
    f. Clinician verified GCS <15
    g. LOC greater than 5 minutes
    h. Double vision
    i. Worsening headache
    j. Neurologic deficit: motor or sensory
    k. Cannot recognize people or disoriented to place
    l. Neurologic ataxia

Note: The following algorithms are a work in progress as the operational situation changes and as more is learned more about concussion sustained in theater.

Figure 7-2. Level 2 mTBI Treatment Algorithm

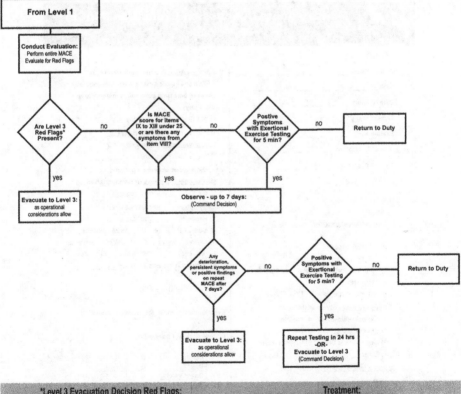

*Level 3 Evacuation Decision Red Flags:	Treatment:
1. Progressively declining level of consciousness/ neurological exam	1. Headache management – use **acetaminophen**
2. Pupillary asymmetry	2. Avoid tramadol, narcotics, NSAIDs, ASA or other platelet inhibitors until CT confirmed negative
3. Seizures	3. Give an educational sheet to all positive mTBI patients
4. Repeated vomiting	

Patient Education:

The most important piece of the education for a concussed patient is the expected course of full recovery. Education should be aimed at identifying symptoms and managing them utilizing the strategies outlined.

Activity: Patient should not return to full duty if any signs of concussion (eg, headache or dizziness) are present. Patients with a very mild concussion and complete resolution of all symptoms may return to duty after 1 day. Patients with any loss of consciousness should not return to full duty for 1-2 weeks following complete resolution of symptoms. Patients who have been diagnosed as having a severe concussion, but who have no neurological deficit may return to full duty in 1 month. Patients with a previous history of concussion should be referred to specialty care for further diagnosis, management and determination of duty status.

Diet: Limit alcohol

No Improvement/Deterioration: Medical care should be sought immediately, at any time of day or night if seizures, double vision, slurred speech or inability to recognize people or places occurs.

Follow-up Actions

Return Evaluation: Follow patients closely on daily basis for signs of improvement or deterioration. **Note:** Medic should be aware of all patients with a history of injury, symptoms or signs that place them at increased risk for mTBI (and other problems, eg, PTSD), and re-evaluate as clinical or operational conditions dictate.

Evacuation/Consultation Criteria: Evacuate patients as indicated in Treatment Algorithms and any patient who does not show improvement within 24-48 hours.

Chapter 26: Trauma Assessment: Mild Traumatic Brain Injury/Concussion: Military Acute Concussion Evaluation

Defense and Veterans Brain Injury Center (DVBIC)

Figure 7-3. MACE, page 1

Military Acute Concussion Evaluation (MACE)

Defense and Veterans Brain Injury Center

Patient Name: _____

SS#: _____-_____-_____ Unit: _____

Date of Injury: ___/___/___

Time of Injury: _____

Examiner: _____

Date of Evaluation: ___/___/___

Time of Evaluation: _____

History: (I – VIII)

I. **Description of Incident**
   Ask:
   a) What happened?
   b) Tell me what you remember.
   c) Were you dazed, confused, "saw stars"?
   ☐ Yes ☐ No
   d) Did you hit your head? ☐ Yes ☐ No

II. **Cause of Injury** (Circle all that apply):
   1) Explosion/Blast   4) Fragment
   2) Blunt object   5) Fall
   3) Motor Vehicle Crash 6) Gunshot wound
   7) Other _____

III. **Was a helmet worn?** ☐ Yes ☐ No
   Type _____

IV. **Amnesia Before:** Are there any events just BEFORE the injury that are not remembered? (Assess for continuous memory prior to injury)
   ☐ Yes ☐ No If yes, how long _____

V. **Amnesia After:** Are there any events just AFTER the injuries that are not remembered? (Assess time until continuous memory after the injury)
   ☐ Yes ☐ No If yes, how long _____

VI. Does the individual report **loss of consciousness** or "blacking out"?
   ☐ Yes ☐ No If yes, how long _____

VII. Did anyone observe a period of **loss of consciousness** or unresponsiveness?
   ☐ Yes ☐ No If yes, how long _____

VIII. **Symptoms** (circle all that apply)
   1) Headache   2) Dizziness
   3) Memory Problems 4) Balance problems
   5) Nausea/Vomiting 6) Difficulty Concentrating
   7) Irritability   8) Visual Disturbances
   9) Ringing in the ears 10) Other _____

Examination: (IX – XIII)

Evaluate each domain. Total possible score is 30.

IX. **Orientation** (1 point each)

Month:	0	1
Date:	0	1
Day of Week:	0	1
Year:	0	1
Time:	0	1

Orientation Total Score ____/5

08/2006   DVBIC.org   800-870-9244
This form may be copied for clinical use.

7-8

Figure 7-4. MACE, page 2

Military Acute Concussion Evaluation (MACE)
Defense and Veterans Brain Injury Center

X. Immediate Memory:

Read all 5 words and ask the patient to recall them in any order. Repeat two more times for a total of three trials.

(1 point for each correct, total over 3 trials)

List	Trial 1		Trial 2		Trial 3	
Elbow	0	1	0	1	0	1
Apple	0	1	0	1	0	1
Carpet	0	1	0	1	0	1
Saddle	0	1	0	1	0	1
Bubble	0	1	0	1	0	1
Trial Score						

Immediate Memory Total Score _____/15

XI. Neurological Screening

As the clinical condition permits, check

Eyes: pupillary response and tracking

Verbal: speech fluency and word finding

Motor: pronator drift, gait/coordination

Record any abnormalities. **No points are given for this.**

XII. Concentration

Reverse Digits: (go to next string length if correct on first trial. Stop if incorrect on both trials.) 1 pt. for each string length.

4-9-3	6-2-9	0	1
3-8-1-4	3-2-7-9	0	1
6-2-9-7-1	1-5-2-8-5	0	1
7-1-8-4-6-2	5-3-9-1-4-8	0	1

Months in reverse order:
(1 pt. for entire sequence correct)
Dec-Nov-Oct-Sep-Aug-Jul
Jun-May-Apr-Mar-Feb-Jan   0   1
Concentration Total Score _____/5

XIII. Delayed Recall (1 pt. each)

Ask the patient to recall the 5 words from the earlier memory test (Do NOT reread the word list.)

Elbow	0	1
Apple	0	1
Carpet	0	1
Saddle	0	1
Bubble	0	1

Delayed Recall Total Score _____/5

TOTAL SCORE _____/30

Notes: _____
_____
_____
_____
_____
_____

Diagnosis: (circle one or write in diagnoses)

No concussion

850.0 Concussion without

Loss of Consciousness (LOC)

850.1 Concussion with

Loss of Consciousness (LOC)

Other diagnoses _____

_____

McCrea, M., Kelly, J. & Randolph, C. (2000). Standardized Assessment of Concussion (SAC): Manual for Administration, Scoring, and Interpretation. (2nd ed.) Waukesa,WI: Authors.

Defense & Veterans Brain Injury Center
1-800-870-9244 or DSN: 662-6345

Trauma: Chapter 27: Shock: Anaphylactic Shock
COL Clifford Cloonan, MC, USA (Ret)

Introduction: Anaphylactic shock is a life-threatening medical emergency that is caused by a generalized allergic reaction affecting the cardiovascular, respiratory, cutaneous, and gastrointestinal systems. It is a severe immune-mediated reaction that occurs when a previously sensitized patient is reexposed to an offending allergen such as: bee/wasp stings, penicillin or other drug allergies (especially when given IM/SC/IV), seafood (especially shrimp/shellfish) and nuts of various types. Allergens may produce an allergic reaction by being ingested, inhaled, injected, or absorbed through the skin/mucous membranes. Shock is produced by the release of histamine that causes "leaky" vessels resulting in hives/edema and hypotension; it also causes bronchospasm/wheezing. This produces both a volume problem and a vascular resistance problem. Anaphylactic shock differs from less severe allergic reactions in that it is characterized by hypotension and obstructed airflow (upper and/or lower) that can be life-threatening. In fatal cases of anaphylaxis, death occurs in less than 60 minutes between exposure to allergen and death. History of allergies is a risk factor. The differential diagnosis for generalized allergic reactions and anaphylaxis should include non-allergic causes of urticaria and angioedema.

Subjective: Symptoms

Malaise, feeling of warmth, anxiety/feeling of impending doom, diffuse itching/"scratchy" sensation in the back of the throat, chest tightness/difficulty breathing, lightheadedness, sudden loss of consciousness. If allergen was ingested, there may be associated nausea/vomiting and diarrhea.

Focused History: *Do you have allergies and any prior history of anaphylaxis? Have you ever had asthma and/or eczema?* (Previous history of allergy and especially anaphylaxis considerably increases likelihood of anaphylactic shock and patients with asthma and or eczema are more likely to have allergic reactions. Family history of allergies, particularly life-threatening allergies, or of the genetic C1-esterase inhibitor deficiency that causes hereditary angioedema [HAE] also increases likelihood of a patient becoming hypotensive as a result of an allergy or allergic-like reaction.) *Have you been recently exposed to likely allergens (foods, drugs, bites, stings, latex) particularly any new medications?* (A recent exposure to common allergen increases likelihood that current symptoms are allergic in origin. Evaluate for common causes of anaphylactic shock.)

Objective: Signs

Using Basic Tools: Vital signs: Pulse: tachycardia; BP: hypotension and orthostatic hypotension; +/- narrowing pulse pressure (systolic-diastolic pressure); Respirations: tachypnea/hyperpnea. **Note:** Children and physically fit young adults may maintain near normal vital signs until significant shock is present and death is imminent. Inspection: Anxious appearance with increased respiratory rate +/- audible stridor, +/- altered mental status, flushed/red skin with urticaria (hives), raised edematous, pruritic, classically pale wheals; may also be red or pink papules that are usually discrete, round/oval in shape ranging from several millimeters to a few centimeters but may coalesce to form very large confluent plaques and may occur anywhere on the body. There may also be edema (especially tongue/periorbital/perioral) with urticarial lesions that form in deep layers of the skin, most commonly in the area of the head and neck but can occur anywhere on the body (angioedema). In angioedema there is much less or no pruritus as compared to urticaria and these deeper lesions tend to be somewhat longer lasting and can be associated with a sense burning, pressure or tightness, or a dull ache. Nasal mucosa may be congested, swollen and inflamed. Profuse watery rhinorrhea, itchy eyes, followed by wheezing are characteristic. Capillary refill: Delayed in shock, longer than 3 seconds. Auscultation: Inspiratory and expiratory wheezing (bronchospasm). Palpation: Warm skin (until severe hypotension develops at which point skin becomes cool/moist). Urticaria. GI: Bowel edema, causing cramps and water diarrhea.

Using Advanced Tools: Pulse oximetry

Assessment: Clinical observation is the only diagnostic test. Use rapidity of onset and constellation of symptoms to suggest the diagnosis. A prior history of similar symptoms may be the only other clue. Observe closely with frequent assessment/reassessment of mental status, vital signs, and pulse oximetry.

Anaphylaxis likely if ANY of the following 3 criteria are met:

1. Acute onset (minutes to several hours) with involvement of skin and or mucosal tissue (hives, pruritus, swollen lips/tongue) plus 1 of the following:
   a. Respiratory compromise (eg, dyspnea, wheezing, stridor or other signs of bronchospasm)
   b. Cardiovascular compromise (eg, decreased blood pressure, syncope)
2. Two or more of the following that occur quickly (minutes to several hours) after exposure to a likely allergen:
   a. Involvement of skin-mucosa (as described previously)
   b. Respiratory compromise
   c. Reduced blood pressure
   d. Persistent GI symptoms (eg, vomiting, abdominal pain)
3. Reduced blood pressure (systolic <90 for adult) after exposure to a known allergen for the patient.

Differential Diagnosis

Allergic reaction without hypotension and/or airway obstruction: Symptoms limited to primarily skin manifestations (eg, itching, rash)

Vasovagal reaction after injection/immunization: Common; quickly resolves when patient is supine.

Cardiogenic shock: Older patient (usually), no evidence of upper airway obstruction (may be in CHF and may have wheezing), no urticaria/erythema.

Acute urticaria: Eg, acute infection (usually viral); cold associated urticaria, and cholinergic (exercise associated) urticaria.

Chronic urticaria: Urticaria associated with rheumatic and other autoimmune conditions (thyroiditis, etc), neoplastic conditions and sometimes associated with parasitic infections such as strongyloidiasis, giardiasis, malaria and amebiasis. Patient is not hypotensive and has history of, or high probability of, parasitic infection or cancer.

Angioedema: Due to hereditary lack of C1 inhibitor or ingestion of an angiotensin converting enzyme inhibitor type BP medication (captopril, enalapril, lisinopril, ramipril, etc.). Patient currently on ACE inhibitor BP medication. No significant hypotension (this is an idiopathic reaction that is not dose dependent and can occur at anytime someone is taking one of these medications). Urticaria is not commonly present -- usually this condition involves significant swelling of the lips.

Plan:

Treatment

REMOVE AND/OR TREAT PRECIPITATING CAUSE:

Epinephrine: Intramuscular (anterolateral thigh) injection of 0.3-0.5mg (0.3-0.5mL of a 1:1000 solution) and repeat in 3-5 minutes if required. If concern for poor perfusion (shock), severe bronchospasm or stridor, or symptoms are not responding to IM epinephrine injections, give IV **epinephrine.**

Warning: Use only the 1:10,000 concentration for IV administration (if only 1:1,000 concentration is available, dilute to 1:10,000 by diluting 1mL of 1:1000 concentration with 10mL of normal saline). Dose: 0.2-0.5mg (1-5mL) of a 1:10,000 solution of **epinephrine** given very slowly IV in 1mL increments every 3-5 minutes (as required by symptoms) for up to 5mL total dose for adults given over 15-20 minutes. Give only as much as needed to control symptoms and monitor closely for recurrence of symptoms. Give **epinephrine** endotracheally if necessary to treat severe hypotension and bronchospasm. If unable to obtain an IV and patient is not intubated, **epinephrine** may be given intraosseously or deep IM (avoid SC administration in hypotensive patients due to poor absorption).

Note: IV administration of **epinephrine** is DANGEROUS if it is given in too large a dose, if given too quickly IV, and/or if given unnecessarily. DO NOT USE IV **epinephrine** to treat a simple allergic reaction without signs of shock and/or severe bronchospasm and/or stridor - give either subcutaneously, or intramuscularly.

Notes: If due to an injected drug or venom, apply loose tourniquet proximal to injection/bite/sting site and place injection site in a dependant position to reduce venous/lymphatic circulation. Apply ice to, and consider injecting small dose of epinephrine (0.1-0.2mL 1:1,000) into the injection site unless contraindicated. If due to bee/wasp sting(s), carefully remove all stingers. Avoid applying pressure to venom sac while stinger is inserted in patient. If due to an ingested food/drug, give **activated charcoal** orally (50g for adults).

Support Airway/Breathing: Immediate intubation if impending airway obstruction from angioedema is suspected. Delay may lead to complete obstruction, difficult intubation and cricothyroidotomy. Give 6-8L oxygen per minute via face mask or up to 100% if intubated. **Albuterol** metered dose inhaler (2-3 puffs) for bronchospasm.

Circulation: Place patient in recumbent position and elevate lower extremities. Crystalloid (saline) fluid bolus IV titrated to restore and maintain blood pressure. Apply PASG (MAST) if available and hypotension is unresponsive to epinephrine and fluids. Adequacy of fluid status (ie, end organ perfusion) should be monitored by urinary output.

Diphenhydramine 50-100mg IV over 3 minutes. Consider adding **cimetidine** 300mg IV q6h if diphenhydramine does not provide rapid relief especially if allergy is due to ingested allergen and continue until symptoms resolve. For certain types of urticaria, other H1 antihistamines have been suggested to be more effective such as **hydroxyzine** 25-50mg po or IM q6h, or **cyproheptadine** 4mg po tid.

Methylprednisolone sodium succinate 125-250mg IV q6h until major symptoms resolve, then convert to tapering course of oral **prednisone** 60mg/day x 2d; 40mg/day x 2d; 20mg/d x 2d

Monitor patient: At least 24 hours following treatment: Recurrence of symptoms may occur in up to 20% of patients (generally within 8 hours but recurrences up to 72 hours following initial resolution of symptoms have been reported).

Patient Education

General: Activity: Following resuscitation, inform patient that he has experienced a life-threatening allergic reaction. If the triggering allergen is known, warn patient to avoid any future exposure.

Diet: Avoidance of allergen.

Medications: Anaphylaxis kit (Epi-Pen autoinjector; Ana-Kit) for use in the event of recurrence. Albuterol (or other beta-agonist) inhaler if bronchospasm was a prominent symptom (be sure to properly teach patient how to use inhaler with spacer).

Prevention and Hygiene: Avoid circumstances in which recurrent exposure is possible/likely

No Improvement/Deterioration: Return immediately for any recurrence of symptoms after first self administering anaphylaxis kit.

Follow-up Actions

Return Evaluation: Return for repeat evaluation/treatment if fainting/near fainting occurs; if difficulty breathing does not resolve with treatment

Consultation Criteria: If cause of allergic reaction is unknown, patient should be advised to seek allergist in an effort to isolate cause.

Chapter 27: Shock: Hypovolemic Shock

COL Clifford Cloonan, MC, USA (Ret)

Introduction: Shock is the state in which perfusion and oxygen delivery to organs is inadequate to maintain organ function. Shock is classified as hypovolemic (insufficient volume), distributive (insufficient vascular tone) or cardiogenic (insufficient pump function of the heart). Hypovolemic shock is the most common type of shock and hemorrhage is the most common cause of hypovolemic shock. Hypovolemic shock may also be caused by burns, severe or prolonged diarrhea (eg, cholera), prolonged vomiting, internal 3rd space loss (as in peritonitis), or crush injury. Tissue injury from trauma may worsen shock by causing microemboli that further activate the inflammatory and coagulation systems. Hemorrhage sufficient to cause shock usually happens in the torso, in the thigh(s) (femur fracture), or externally. Fractures of the femur, pelvis, and/or traumatic amputation are associated with substantial blood loss. From a clinical perspective, attempts to quantify blood loss in order to determine a shock category is of little value because even external blood loss is notoriously difficult to quantify and quite often trauma patients have significant internal as well as external hemorrhage. Treat the patient, not the evident blood loss.

Subjective: Symptoms

Constitutional: Diffuse weakness, anxiety/feelings of impending doom, difficulty concentrating, c/o being chilled to the bone; progressive thirst; shortness of breath. Consider thirst progressing in severity and breathing that becomes progressively deeper and more rapid to be evidence of worsening shock until proven otherwise.

Focused History: *How, where and how long ago were you injured?* (The risk of shock is increased in patients with high energy mechanisms of injury, eg, falls from >15', high speed MVA, penetrating injuries of chest and abdomen or extensive burns.) *Have you lost fluids other than blood?* (severe diarrhea, decreased access to fluids) *Are you thirsty?* (Patients who repeatedly complain of being thirsty are much more likely to be in shock.) *Are there any symptoms to suggest Acute Coronary Syndrome?* (eg, cardiogenic shock) *What is patient's mental status?* (Patients in severe shock will be lethargic/confused. If patient is alert and not complaining of thirst more than an hour after wounding, it is unlikely [but not impossible] that they will develop shock.)

Warning: 1) Patients with low energy mechanism of injury or penetrating wounds not considered likely to have struck major vasculature may still develop hypovolemic shock. 2) Altered mental status may be due to head trauma, not shock.

Objective: Signs

Using Basic Tools: Vital signs: Pulse: Tachycardia is typical. (Unexpected bradycardia may be present with penetrating abdominal trauma, ruptured ectopic pregnancy or other pelvic bleeding.) BP: Progressive hypotension and orthostatic hypotension; narrowing pulse pressure (systolic minus diastolic pressure); Respirations: Tachypnea/hyperpnea; measurement of orthostatic vital signs may be helpful when significant postural hypotension is documented but this test is neither sensitive nor specific for shock. **Warning:** Children and physically fit young adults may maintain near normal vital signs until significant shock is present and death is imminent! Inspection: Pale, diaphoretic, anxious appearing. If degree of shock/hypotension is severe (eg, systolic BP < 60-70mmHg), then there may be evidence of altered mental status (ranges from confusion to unconsciousness). In general, cerebral blood flow is preserved to the last and patient's mental status (MS) may be normal or near normal until right before death (when MS is abnormal look for other causes, especially closed head injury in a traumatized patient). If shock is due to trauma, there is often external evidence of traumatic injury. Auscultation: Lungs sounds are typically normal (unless there is intrathoracic trauma) with deep, rapid respirations. Palpation: Cool, moist skin. In non-hypothermic patients, an ascending palpation of the skin from feet to chest to note the point at which the skin becomes warm is a useful, rapid, method for estimating the degree of shock. The more severe the shock, the more proximal the level of warmth. Capillary refill: Normally prolonged beyond 3 seconds in shock BUT interpretation is difficult in elderly patients (normal is up to 4.5 sec), cold environment or poor lighting. Pulse oximetry may be used to estimate level of tissue perfusion/tissue oxygenation. *See Part 8: Procedures: Chapter 30: Pulse Oximetry Monitoring*

Notes:
1. Most useful of all the vital signs in assessing hypovolemic/hemorrhagic shock is the pulse pressure (systolic - diastolic pressure), which becomes progressively narrowed as shock proceeds. The normal pulse pressure for an adult is between 30-40mmHg. If a BP cuff is not available, estimate the pulse pressure by the strength of the pulse. A weakening pulse implies a narrowing pulse pressure.
2. More important than the absolute value of any of the vital signs at a given point is their trend over time. A falling BP, narrowing pulse pressure, and rising heart rate are signs of severe hemodynamic compromise (shock).

Using Advanced Tools: Placement of Foley catheter with measurement of urinary output as objective measure of the adequacy of intravascular volume.

Assessment:

Differential Diagnosis

Hypovolemic shock:

Plasma loss: History of severe diarrhea or burns that involve extensive body surface area. Body responses intact (narrow pulse pressure). *See Part 3: General Symptoms: Diarrhea, Acute & Part 7: Trauma: Chapter 29: Burns (Thermal, Scald or Chemical)*
Hemorrhagic shock: Intravascular volume depletion through blood loss. Body responses intact (narrow pulse pressure).
Cardiac shock: Loss of sufficient cardiac output to sustain BP. Body responses usually intact (narrow pulse pressure) unless on BP medications. *See Part 4: Organ Systems: Chapter 1: Acute Coronary Syndrome (Acute Myocardial Infarction and Unstable Angina) & Congestive Heart Failure (Pulmonary Edema)*

Distributive (vasogenic) shock:

Septic shock: Loss of vascular tone due to release of infectious toxins in the circulatory system. Body will feel warm to the touch.
Anaphylactic shock: Loss of vascular tone due to an allergic reaction. *See Part 7: Trauma: Chapter 27: Anaphylactic Shock*
Neurogenic shock: Loss of vascular tone due to impaired neural or spinal function.

Psychogenic shock (faint): Transient bradycardia and peripheral vasodilatation caused by parasympathetic stimulation. *See Part 3: General Symptoms: Syncope (Fainting)*
Pulmonary embolus: Massive embolus blocks blood flow through the lungs. *See Part 4: Organ Systems: Chapter 13: Deep Vein Thrombosis and Pulmonary Embolism*
Cardiac tamponade: Mechanical impairment of the pumping action of the heart by increased fluid accumulation between myocardium and pericardium. *See Part 8: Procedures: Chapter 30: Pericardiocentesis*
Tension pneumothorax: Loss of blood return to the thorax and heart due to increased pressure within the chest cavity. *See Part 4: Organ Systems: Chapter 3: Pneumothorax*

Plan:

Procedures

Essential: CONTROL ALL HEMORRHAGE. Eliminate all possible sources of ongoing intravascular volume loss. Once hemorrhage is controlled, initiate blood administration as soon as it can safely be accomplished. If unable to control hemorrhage (eg, intrathoracic/intraabdominal bleeding), urgent evacuation to a medical facility with general surgical capability is indicated ASAP. Do not delay evacuation to initiate procedures (other than to secure the airway). Further efforts at hemorrhage control should be performed en route and should not delay evacuation. Obtain IV access (18 gauge x 2). If hemorrhage has been controlled, administer fluid to insure adequate end-organ perfusion (eg, improving mental status, urine output >50mL/hr). This generally requires a systolic BP >90mmHg (*see Part 7: Trauma: Chapter 27: Resuscitation Fluids*).
Recommended: For lower abdominal/pelvic bleeding and/or large thigh/buttocks wounds or femur fractures, PASG (MAST) application is reasonable and appropriate. In these instances, PASG will tamponade bleeding sites and stabilize the pelvis, thereby reducing/stopping bleeding. Applying PASG when patient has uncontrolled intrathoracic bleeding is contra-indicated. *See Part 8: Procedures: Chapter 30: Pneumatic Anti-Shock Garment*

Treatment

Primary:
1. If hypovolemic shock is due to hemorrhage; measures to control hemorrhage (including evacuation to damage control surgery) take precedence. Fluid resuscitation is a temporizing measure, not a treatment for uncontrolled hemorrhage. Surgery is necessary to treat uncontrolled internal hemorrhage. Attempting to initiate IVs and maintain urinary output (and systolic BP) of patients with on-going, uncontrollable blood loss may temporarily maintain their urinary output at the expense of increasing the rate of red blood cell loss. There is no simple answer to this dilemma and the most appropriate response depends upon a variety of factors, such as prior hydration and health status, anticipated time to surgery,

availability of IV fluids. In cases of profound shock where cerebral perfusion is significantly compromised, fluid resuscitation with Hextend 500mg IV bolus, repeated in 30 minutes if required (no more than 1000mL of Hextend) followed by normal saline or Ringer's lactate as per TCCC is reasonable. Blood is the best resuscitation fluid to replace blood loss. When hemorrhage has been controlled, administer sufficient fluids (po and/or IV) to maintain an hourly urinary output of >50cc/hr. *See Table 7-3*

2. If volume loss is due to other causes (eg, burns, diarrhea, vomiting), attempt to prevent further volume loss or redistribution of fluids (eg, septic, anaphylactic, neurogenic shock). Early aggressive fluid resuscitation is appropriate because the increased BP will improve perfusion (not contribute to further exsanguinating hemorrhage). Monitor clinical signs, measure urine output and fluid loss to guide fluid replacement. For burn patients, use specific published guidelines to direct fluid resuscitation. *See Part 7: Trauma: Chapter 29: Burns (Thermal, Scald or Chemical)*

3. Preserve body heat (ie, attempt to limit hypothermia) by passive rewarming (eg, blanket under and over the patient). External heating (active rewarming) before volume has been restored may cause vasodilation and further decrease BP.

4. Place all badly wounded patients in a position with their feet elevated about 12 inches (Trendelenburg position). Use this head-down position unless it causes obvious distress, labored respiration or cyanosis, even in patients with chest wounds and with head wounds as long as their systolic BP remains below 80mmHg. When the systolic BP has risen above 80mmHg, patient may be gradually returned to a normal supine position.

5. PASG may be useful to control pelvic bleeding (eg, pelvic fracture) and bleeding into the thigh(s).

Note: Do NOT treat bradycardia in hypovolemic patients with atropine. The appropriate treatment is to stop further blood loss and rapidly restore intravascular volume, preferably with blood.

Alternative: If unable to obtain intravascular access, consider the intraosseous (IO) route through either the sternum (use specialized F.A.S.T. IO needle system) or through the tibia (lateral malleolus) using B.I.G. or other similar device. In children, the recommended IO route is the proximal tibial plateau which can be accessed with any strong enough and long enough needle or with a needle specifically designed to enter the bone marrow such as a Jamshidi or Shur-Fast IO needle. Bone marrow can also be accessed through the distal radius. Remember, however, that the administration of fluids (other than blood) via ANY route is not the important issue; control of bleeding, by surgery if necessary, is the key. Focusing on fluid administration rather than hemorrhage control may kill the patient.

Primitive: When IV fluids cannot be administered to restore intravascular volume, rehydrate orally. Start with small volumes and increase as tolerated.

Patient Education

General: Activity: Bedrest

Diet: If surgery is imminent, keep patient NPO, but liquids (except alcohol or caffeine-containing liquids) as tolerated are appropriate in most circumstances.

Prevention and Hygiene: Emphasis on maintaining well hydrated status and importance of use of body armor in combat situations is appropriate.

No Improvement/Deterioration: Stabilize; rule out treatable causes (eg, tension pneumothorax, pericardial tamponade) and evacuate.

Wound Care: Patients in shock are more susceptible to infection than those with normal perfusion. Keep wounds as clean as possible and watch closely for developing infection

Follow-up Actions

Evacuation/Consultation Criteria: Uncontrollable hemorrhage requires rapid evacuation to a general surgeon.

Chapter 27: Shock: Routes of Fluid Administration

CDR Les Fenton, MC, USN (Ret)

Table 7-2. Routes of Fluid Administration

Route	Indication	Potential Benefit	Caution
By mouth	Dehydration, hemorrhage	May use any fluids	Aspiration risk in unconscious Avoid in abdominal wounds if possible
Gastric tube	Unconscious. Avoid in abdominal wounds.	May use any fluids	Aspiration risk, Limit infusion rate to 200mL/hr and check residuals each hour – Stop if more than 200mL
Intravenous	Unable to take oral. Need large volumes	High volumes	Use care in increasing blood pressure for uncontrolled hemorrhage
Intraosseous	Unable to obtain IV	High volumes	Same as IV, watch for leak into tissues
Rectal	No other route available, or no sterile fluids available.	Any fluid	Limit flow rates for 200mL/hr

Chapter 27: Shock: Resuscitation Fluids

COL Cliff Cloonan, MC, USA (Ret)

Table 7-3. Resuscitation Fluids

Fluid	Indication	O$_2$	Potential Benefit	Cautions
Crystalloids Saline Ringer's Lactate	Hypovolemia Dehydration Hemorrhage Shock, Burns	No	Easy to store Inexpensive; no other non-oxygen carrying solution has been proven more effective	Weight ratio requires 3:1 for lost blood Dilution, edema, coagulopathy
Hypertonic Saline 3% 7.5% Hypertonic saline-colloid Combinations HTS Dextran Hetastarch	Hemorrhagic Shock Burns - only one dose initially	No	Lighter weight Small volume = large effect Longer duration of effect than plain HTS?	Hypernatremia Do not use for dehydration from vomiting, diarrhea, or sweating. Do not repeat without addition of other fluids. See Colloids
HTS Colloids Albumin Artificial Colloids Dextran Hetastarch Hextend *Other commercial names depending on country	Hemorrhagic Shock Burns? Third day	No	Longer duration 1:1 replacement for blood More effect for less weight	Hextend standard fluid carried for hemorrhagic shock from wounds. Overuse may lead to "leak" into tissue. Monitor infusion to avoid rapid "spike" in BP, causing rebleeding. Artificial: Coagulopathy Allergic reaction
Oral Rehydration Fluids	Dehydration Controlled hemorrhage Burns	No	Fluids of opportunity. Non-sterile. Ingredients: 4 tsp. sugar 1/2 to 1 tsp. salt 1 liter water	Rehydration in extremity wounds with controlled hemorrhage. Austere option in abdominal wounds and unconscious patients, but use with caution.
Blood; Red Cells	Hemorrhage	Yes	Ideal	Storage, type & cross-match
Artificial blood Hemoglobin based Fluorocarbon based	Hemorrhage	Yes	Easy storage	Experimental only Still not yet available for use Future option?

Notes:
1. End Points of resuscitation:
   a. Controlled hemorrhage (also dehydration and burns): Normal BP, pulse, urine output (0.5-1mL/Kg/Hr), normal capillary refill, good mentation. See specific cases for discussion of fluid requirements (eg diarrhea, burns).
   b. Uncontrolled hemorrhage of the trunk: Accept lower BP (systolic 80–90mmHg or MAP 60–65mmHg). A fluid bolus should not be given. Begin fluids if radial pulse not palpable or pulse is >120. Stop when radial pulse palpable <120. Monitor and restart fluids if indicated. Severe hypotension (SBP <90mmHg) should be avoided whenever possible in patients at risk for Traumatic Brain Injury (TBI). Close clinical monitoring and optimal balance of fluid resuscitation is an additional challenge in these patients.
2. Maintenance rate for IV fluids in patients who are NPO: (Weight in Kg) + 40 = mL per hour. Continue to monitor for adequate volume status (ie, urine output [0.5–1mL/kg/hr], capillary refill, and mental status).

Chapter 28: Bites, Animal and Human: Human and Animal Bites

MAJ Robert Malsby III, MC, USA & CPT Christopher Cole, SP, USA

Introduction: The human ("clenched fist") bite injury poses an especially high risk of infection, but human bites in other areas of the body pose no greater risks than any other animal bites. The 3 most common types of human "bite" wounds that may lead to complications are:
1. Clenched fist injury: This wound results when a clenched fist strikes the mouth/teeth of an adversary and the force of the punch breaks the skin. The hand is flexed when the injury is sustained, inoculating bacteria directly into the wound. When the hand is relaxed, the tendon retracts into its sheath, carrying the inoculum into the tendon sheath, making normal irrigation and cleansing techniques difficult and less effective.
2. Bite to a finger: Fingers are enveloped in only a thin layer of overlying skin that constrains the underlying tendons and their sheaths, only a few millimeters beneath the surface. Hence, when a finger is bitten, even though the wound may appear to be only a superficial abrasion, there is potential for inoculation of the tendon sheaths through an unnoticed skin defect.
3. Puncture wounds about the head: This type of injury is usually sustained during "horseplay" among children of all ages. The tooth impacts the head, producing the wound. Although the wound may appear innocuous on the surface, deep contamination may occur.

Animal Bites: Of the estimated 1-3 million animal bites in the US per year, 80-90% are inflicted by dogs, 5-15% by cats, 2-5% by rodents, and the balance by rabbits, ferrets, farm animals, monkeys, reptiles and other species (see Part 5: Specialty Areas: Chapter 17: Venomous Snake Bites). Dog bites cause a crushing-type wound due to their rounded teeth and strong jaws that may damage deeper structures (bones, vessels, tendons, muscle and nerves). Cats' sharp, pointed teeth cause puncture wounds and lacerations with inoculation of bacteria into deep tissues.

Bites on the hand have a risk of infection due to the relatively poor blood supply, and anatomic considerations that make adequate cleansing of the wound difficult. In general, the better the blood supply, the easier the wound is to clean (eg, laceration vs. puncture), thus lowering the risk of infection. Nearly any group of pathogens (bacteria, viruses, rickettsia, spirochetes, and fungi) may cause infection. Dogs and cats are more likely to host *Pasteurella* and *Staph aureus*, but infected bite wounds are often mixed infections, with any of the organisms ultimately having the potential to produce sepsis, meningitis, osteomyelitis, or septic arthritis.

Subjective: Symptoms

Puncture, laceration, or abrasion possibly with contusions, erythema, edema, pain, throbbing or itching. Because human bite wounds are frequently intentional injuries, always consider the potential for alcohol, child, and spouse abuse.

Focused History: *Who or what bit you? When were you bitten? Where were you bitten?* (This information may help to assess, treat and prevent subsequent injury. The history provided concerning human bites is known to be notoriously unreliable. Animal bites: Determine the kind of animal, general health, rabies vaccination status, behavior, time and location of the incident; circumstances surrounding the bite [ie, defensive vs. unprovoked]; and the whereabouts of the animal [loose in the wild or observable in quarantine]. Animal bites, particularly in developing countries, carry a high risk of rabies infection [*see Part 5: Specialty Areas: Chapter 12: Viral Infections: Rabies*]. Human bite wounds are often infected when patients present because the wound initially appeared innocuous and the patients delayed seeking care. Patient's health status, HIV status of biter, tetanus immunization status, time delay since receipt of the injury, amount of disability can all contribute to the risk of complications.)

Objective: Signs

Using Basic Tools: Superficial surgical extension of the wound may be required to determine involvement of the tendon sheaths. Always maintain a high index of suspicion for infection.

1. Clenched fist injury: Evaluate integrity of extensor tendons; inspect for signs of infection (hot, swollen, red), palpate for crepitus; inspect for loss of knuckle height, or penetration into the joint capsule.
2. Bite to a finger: Carefully inspect and palpate all bite wounds of the fingers for deeper penetration into underlying structures. Evaluate for integrity of the extensor and flexor tendons; inspect for evidence of flexor tenosynovitis.
3. Bites about the head: Ear and nose bites: Inspect for loss of tissue; palpate for cartilage tears and depth of penetration into adjacent structures.
4. Evaluate distal neurovascular status, tendon or tendon sheath involvement, bony injury (particularly in the skull of infants and children), joint space violation, viscera injuries, and foreign bodies (eg, teeth in the wound).
5. Consider possible cervical spine injuries if bite was from a large animal.

Using Advanced Tools: X-Rays: Clenched fist injuries have an associated risk of metacarpal head fracture that may require surgical treatment. "Old" infected bites may reveal cortical erosion; periosteal new bone formation or bone loss seen with osteomyelitis.

Assessment: Diagnose based on history of a bite, wound appearance and captured specimens (teeth).

Differential Diagnosis

Insect bites: History of exposure

Cellulitis or deep hand infections: History of trauma; rule out retained foreign bodies

Plan:

Treatment

1. Assess bite site and appearance:
   a. Superficial human bites (mixture of abrasions and contusions) can be managed adequately with only local cleansing and tetanus immunization.
   b. Bites to the ear and nose: When associated with tissue loss or violation of cartilage, requires consultation with surgery (plastic surgery or ENT if possible). Penetrating bites in cartilage are slow to heal due to the limited blood supply and difficulty in treating chondritis. (*see step 4*)
   c. Consider primary closure in relatively clean wounds or wounds that can be effectively cleansed. Facial wounds, because of the excellent blood supply, are at a low risk for infection even with primary closure.
   d. Deep bite wounds, animal bites, those to the lower extremities, those with a delay in presentation (>8 hours), or those in compromised hosts generally should be left for closure by secondary intention.
2. Irrigate wounds with water or sterile saline (preferred) using a 19 gauge blunt needle and a 35mL syringe to provide adequate pressure (7psi) and volume. Flush individual punctures with approximately 200cc of irrigation solution. Heavily contaminated wounds may require more irrigation. Soaking wounds in a povidone-iodine solution is NOT sufficient.
3. Débride devitalized tissue, particulate matter and clots to provide clean wound edges that will result in smaller scars and promote faster healing.
4. Give antibiotics: Prophylaxis administration is controversial and clinical judgment is indicated. A systematic review was performed in the Annals of Emergency Medicine, 2004. This examined the efficacy of antibiotic prophylaxis in preventing infections following mammalian bites within 24 hours of injury. The authors concluded that insufficient evidence exists to support antibiotic prophylaxis in dog and cat bites, and minimal evidence supports its use for human bites. However, there is evidence that antibiotics significantly reduce the risk of infection in hand bites. Obviously, if signs of clinical infection are present, then antimicrobial therapy is warranted. If antibiotics are used, the duration of therapy should be 7-14 days depending on the severity of the infection and the clinical response. Determine therapy based on species.
   a. Human bites (*Streptococcus viridians; Bacteroides; Corynebacterium; Staphylococcus epidermidis; Staphylococcus aureus; Peptostreptococcus*), Early (not yet clinically infected): **amoxicillin/clavulanate** 875/125mg po bid x 5 days or 500/125mg po tid x 5 days or **clindamycin** 300mg po qid x 5 days or **doxycycline** 100mg po bid x 5 days. Later (signs of infection 3-24

hours): **ertapenem** 1g IV/IM q day x 7-14 days or **ampicillin/sulbactam** 1.5g IV q6h or **cefoxitin** 2.0g IV q8h or **ticarcillin clavulanate** 3.1g IV q6h or **piperacillin/tazobactam** 3.375g IV q6h. If penicillin allergic, use **clindamycin** 300mg po qid (+) either **ciprofloxacin** 500mg po bid or **trimethoprim-sulfamethoxazole DS** po bid x 7-14 days. Consider HIV prophylaxis for all US forces bitten by host nation individuals. If possible, screen biter for HIV. *See Part 5: Specialty Areas: Chapter 12: Viral Infections: Human Immunodeficiency Virus*

   b. Bat, raccoon, and skunk bites (high rabies risks): **Amoxicillin/clavulanate** 875/125mg po bid or 500/125mg po tid po x 7 days or **ertapenem** 1g IV/IM q day x 7-14 days or **ampicillin/sulbactam** 1.5g IV q6h. Alternates: **Doxycycline** 100mg po bid x 7 days. Rabies post-exposure treatment is indicated. *See Part 5: Specialty Areas: Chapter 12: Viral Infections: Rabies*

   c. Cat bites (rabies risk): **Amoxicillin/clavulanate** 875/125mg po bid or 500/125mg po tid x 7 days or **ertapenem** 1g IV/IM qd x 7-14 days or **ampicillin/sulbactam** 1.5g IV q 6h x 24-48h or until the patient makes clinical improvement and can be converted to po antibiotics.
   Alternates: **cefuroxime axetil** 500mg po bid or **doxycycline** 100 mg po bid. Resistant organisms seen; observe for signs of osteomyelitis. *See Part 5: Specialty Areas: Chapter 12: Viral Infections: Rabies*

   d. Dog bites (rabies risk): **Amoxicillin/clavulanate** 875/125mg po bid or 500/125mg po tid x 7 days or **ertapenem** 1g IV/IM qd x 7-14 days or **ampicillin/sulbactam** 1.5g IV q6h. Alternates: **Clindamycin** 300mg po qid (+) **ciprofloxacin** 500mg po bid x 7 days. Do NOT use ciprofloxacin in children. Substitute with **trimethoprim-sulfamethoxazole**.

   e. Cattle and swine: Consider prophylactic treatment for brucellosis and leptospirosis: Brucellosis: **doxycycline** 100mg po bid x 7 days plus **rifampin** 600-900mg po qd x 6 weeks; Leptospirosis: **penicillin** G 1.5 million units IV q6h or **ceftriaxone** 1g IV/IM qd x 7 days or **doxycycline** 100mg IV/po bid or **ampicillin** 0.5-1g IV q6h.

   f. Bites from hospitalized patients: Consider including coverage for aerobic gram-negative bacilli.
   Note: The use of fluoroquinolones in children and adolescents younger than 18 years is contraindicated by the FDA, and tetracycline antibiotics are rarely used in children younger than eight years. Alternatives should be strongly considered.

5. Give **tetanus toxoid, dT, or TDAP** if >5 years since last dose or when tetanus status is unknown. Consider adding immunoglobulin if high suspicion of tetanus.

6. Use narcotics or benzodiazepines judiciously for agitation. *See Part 8: Procedures: Chapter 30: Pain Assessment and Control*

7. Consider anti-rabies therapy, *See Part 5: Specialty Areas: Chapter 12: Viral Infections: Rabies*

8. Monkeys and non-human primates: B virus (*Cercopithecine herpesvirus* 1) is a zoonotic agent that, while rare, can cause fatal encephalomyelitis in humans. The virus naturally infects macaque monkeys including: rhesus macaques, pig-tailed macaques, cynomolgus monkeys, and other macaques, resulting in disease that is similar to herpes simplex virus infection in humans. Although B virus infection generally is asymptomatic or mild in macaques, it can be fatal in humans. Initial symptoms typically begin 5-21 days after exposure (incubation period is 2 days to 5 weeks). After infecting humans, B virus replicates at the site of exposure and may result in the development of a vesicular rash at this site. Additional symptoms can include tingling, itching, pain, or numbness at the site; however, many patients have no symptoms at the site of infection. Some patients develop lymphadenopathy proximal to the site of inoculation. Within the first 3 weeks after exposure, paresthesias may develop and proceed proximally along the affected extremity.
   Associated symptoms can include fever, myalgias, and weakness of the affected extremity, abdominal pain, sinusitis, and conjunctivitis. Other organs, including the lung and liver, may be involved. The virus spreads along the nerves of the peripheral nervous system to the spinal cord and then to the brain. Symptoms of infection can include meningismus, nausea, vomiting, persistent headache, confusion, diplopia, dysphagia, dizziness, dysarthria, cranial nerve palsies, and ataxia. Seizures, hemiplegia, hemiparesis, ascending paralysis, respiratory failure, and coma more commonly occur later in the course of infection. Some patients have presented with symptoms within 48h after exposure to the virus. The overall presentation of late-stage disease is that of brain stem encephalomyelitis that may evolve into diffuse encephalomyelitis during its terminal stages. Among untreated humans, the mortality rate associated with B virus infection is estimated to be 80%. The mortality rate has declined since the advent of antiviral therapy. If the SOF medic is unable to positively identify the primate as a non-macaque species, prompt post-exposure protocol should be initiated:

   a. Irrigate the exposure site with copious saline or water for 15 minutes.

   b. Wash the skin thoroughly with a solution containing detergent such as chlorhexidine or povidone-iodine for 15 minutes. Irrigation with a 0.25% sodium hypochlorite solution is advised for all non-mucous membrane sites.

   c. Treat with prophylactic antibiotics: **Amoxicillin/clavulanate** 875/125mg po bid or 500/125 po tid x 5 days or **doxycycline** 100mg po bid x 5 days. Initiate post-exposure antiviral prophylaxis: **Valacyclovir** 1g po q8h x 2 weeks or **acyclovir** 800mg po 5 x a day x 2 weeks.

   d. Keep close (bid) follow-up with the exposed patient and maintain a high index of clinical suspicion for signs of active disease.

   e. If you suspect an exposed patient may be showing signs of active B-virus, immediately consult with your supervising provider to determine the best disposition of the patient.

   f. Patient isolation is not required, but evacuation to definitive care may be necessary.

   g. Additional informational and reporting resources are listed in the next section.

Patient Education:
   General: Observe for signs/symptoms of infection; close follow-up is needed. Return promptly for fever and hot, red, or swollen wound, particularly if accompanied by swollen nodes or streaks (blood poisoning) traveling away from the wound.

Follow-Up Actions:
   Wound Care/Return Evaluation: Recheck patient in 24-48 hours if not infected at first visit, and followed daily if infected.
   Evacuation/Consultation Criteria: Bites with extensive tissue loss, involvement of complex/deep structures, penetration of the skull, and infection failing to respond to antibiotic regimens should be evacuated ASAP. Consult general surgery or infectious disease specialists in these cases, and others as needed.

Chapter 29: Burns, Blast, Lightning and Electrical Injuries: Burns (Thermal, Scald or Chemical)

COL Leopoldo C. Cancio, MC, USA & Steven J. Thomas, MD

Introduction: Burns can be classified by their cause, as thermal (ie, heat), flame, flash, contact (with a hot radiator, etc.), scald (hot water, oil, or other liquid), chemical, radiation (sunburn, x-rays, nuclear), or electrical (*see Part 7: Trauma: Chapter 29: Lightning and Electrical Injuries*). Inhalation injury may occur with or without skin injury, and may be life-threatening. The depth of burn is often classified as 1st, 2nd, or 3rd degree. "Partial-thickness burns" refers to 1st and 2nd degree burns, whereas "full-thickness burns" refers to 3rd degree burns. A burn of 20% of the total body surface area (20% TBSA) or greater is a life-threatening burn. In the very young, very old, or those with serious medical diseases, 10% TBSA or more can be life-threatening. These patients need IV fluid resuscitation and aeromedical evacuation, if possible. Eschar (a layer of burned skin) will form at the site of injury. With time, the eschar will slough off and be replaced with epithelium (new skin) if the burn is partial thickness, or with granulation tissue if the burn is full thickness. Full-thickness burns may eventually heal, particularly across the joints, by wound contracture. The best definitive treatment for large open wounds is skin grafting.

Subjective: Symptoms

Painful, red skin without (1st degree) or with (2nd degree) blisters; or dry, charred, non-painful skin (3rd degree), or a combination. May complain of hoarseness or coughing

Objective: Signs

Table 7-4. Objective Signs of 1st, 2nd and 3rd Degree Burns

	1st Degree	2nd Degree	3rd Degree
Typical causes	Sun, hot liquids, brief flash burns	Hot liquids, flash or flame, chemical	Flame, prolonged contact with hot liquid or hot object, electricity, chemical
Color	Pink or red	Pink or mottled red	Dark brown, charred, pearly white, translucent with visible, thrombosed veins
Surface	Dry	Moist, weeping, blisters	Dry and inelastic
Sensation	Painful	Very painful	Anesthetic
Depth	Epidermis	Epidermis and portions of the dermis	Epidermis, dermis, and possibly deep structures
Healing	Few days	Few weeks	Skin grafting or slow inward contraction of edges

Warning: Airway obstruction may present suddenly or gradually over a period of hours with: stridor, hoarseness, coughing, carbon in the sputum or in the mouth, rapid or labored breathing, and finally respiratory distress.

Assessment:

Differential Diagnosis

Dermatitis with erythematous or bullous features: Certain skin diseases like Stevens-Johnson Syndrome or Toxic Epidermal Necrolysis Syndrome (TENS) cause extensive blistering and represent life-threatening emergencies. They can be treated similarly to a burn, except that burn creams should not be used.

Abrasions: Combat casualties may have both burns and abrasions (scrapes and cuts). Large surface area abrasions ("road rash") and extensive degloving injuries can be treated like burns.

Blast: Explosions may cause a combination of burns, mechanical trauma, and primary blast injuries. Evaluate patients with burns from an explosion for other injuries, to include tympanic membrane (TM) rupture and traumatic brain injury (TBI).

Plan:

Treatment: Directed toward burns of 20% TBSA or greater, and those with inhalation injury. For small burns, focus on wound care.

Primary:

1. Stop the burning process: Decontaminate chemical burns at the scene. Remove any hot synthetic clothing. For patients with tar burns, immerse the injured areas in cold water until the hot tar has cooled down.
2. Protect the C-spine. Cervical injury is common following high-speed motor vehicle accidents, explosions, high-voltage electrical injury, or falls/jumps.
3. Secure the airway: Prophylactically intubate patients with mild symptoms of airway obstruction (swelling of the face, upper airway or larynx) or smoke inhalation injury, and before a prolonged aeromedical or ground evacuation. See Part 8: Procedures: Chapter 30: Intubation
4. Breathing/Ventilation: Give 100% O_2 by non-rebreather mask for burn, shock or carbon monoxide poisoning. Intubated patients can be bag-ventilated for prolonged periods (up to 12 hours) during evacuation.
5. Circulation: Insert 2 large-bore IV cannulas through unburned skin (preferably) or eschar. Alternatives are an intraosseous cannula or a cut-down. Start lactated Ringer's (LR) at 500cc/hr for adults or 250cc/hr for children age 5-15. Do not give an initial fluid bolus (contraindicated in burn patients) unless the patient has low BP or major mechanical trauma (ie, bleeding). Secure the lines with suture: tape does not stick well to burned skin. This IV fluid rate will need to be adjusted based on burn size and weight. Insert Foley catheter to monitor fluid output. (*See Fluid Resuscitation Notes*)
6. Disability: Do neurological exam and treat neuro injuries. Even patients with massive burn injuries should initially be alert, unless they have received drugs, have sustained a head injury, are in shock, or have ingested a toxic substance (carbon monoxide, drugs, alcohol).

7. Exposure: Keep the patient warm by all available means (aluminum combat casualty blanket, warm IV fluids, sleeping bag, body bags, etc.) Burn patients lose heat through the damaged skin, and severe hypothermia can result if the environment is not kept "hot." Cool only the smallest burns (<10%). Never soak a burn patient in wet linens unless he also has heat stroke (rare). Monitor core temperature as frequently as possible (eg, via a rectal thermometer).

8. Do a careful secondary survey. Remove all the clothing, roll the patient to inspect the back. Remove all jewelry, especially rings, since fingers can swell causing damage beneath rings. Examine the corneas with fluorescein and Wood's lamp, looking for corneal defects in all patients with facial burns and those who complain of eye problems. Treat corneal abrasions with alternating ophthalmic antibiotics such as **erythromycin** and **gentamicin** (1 drop of each, alternating q4h, such that one of the 2 is applied q2h). Look for non-thermal trauma. Burns can make it more difficult to detect spinal or extremity fractures, or intraabdominal injury. Check the TM for rupture in blast injuries.

9. Open fractures in burn patients are at high risk for developing osteomyelitis. Immobilize the fracture with splints. A plaster cast can be used over a burn, but should be immediately bivalved to permit wound care and to allow for post-burn swelling. Definitive care is external fixation.

10. Use frequent, low-dose IV narcotics (eg, **morphine** 2-10mg or **fentanyl** 25-100mcg) for pain control. Depending on response, it may be necessary to re-dose these drugs about q15 min. Avoid IM narcotics during the burn shock period. **Ketamine** 0.25-0.5mg/kg IV repeated q 5-10 min prn is very useful for painful procedures. Consider **promethazine** 25mg IV, IM, or po q8h to potentiate the effects of narcotics and treat nausea.

11. Place a nasogastric tube (NGT) to prevent gastric ileus, vomiting and aspiration. To prevent stress ulceration of the stomach and duodenum, give 30cc of **magnesium** or **aluminum-containing antacids** q2h, preferably via NGT. Clamp the tube for 30 minutes after each dose. Alternatively, give an H2-blocker such as **ranitidine** 50mg IV q8h. Utilize NGT for both feeding and as a route for enteral resuscitation.

12. Immunize against tetanus as needed.

13. If the patient will be evacuated within 24 hrs of injury, then no specific wound care of the burn is needed. Otherwise, clean the burns with an antimicrobial solution (best is **chlorhexidine gluconate**) and daily shower. (Use normal saline or similar to cleanse the face.) In general, do not débride small (<2cm diameter) blisters if they are intact, but unroof them if they rupture, lie across major joints, or are larger. If the burns are in the scalp, shave the hair. An antimicrobial burn cream such as **silver sulfadiazine** or **mafenide acetate** should be applied at least daily (preferably bid). Thorough cleansing with a surgical detergent like chlorhexidine gluconate needs to be done at each such dressing change. Following application, the wounds should be dressed with sterile gauze. Another good choice is a silver dressing such as **Silverseal, Acticoat, Silverlon**, or **SelectSilver**. The silver ions are released slowly and have broad-spectrum antimicrobial activity. Apply silver dressings after wetting with water. Cover with moist gauze dressing. Re-wet q6-8h with water (usually not saline-containing solutions). May leave on for 2-5 days depending on how clean the wounds are. If burn creams or silver dressings are not available, a 0.5% solution of silver nitrate in water is also very effective. Apply this solution to a thick layer of gauze dressings at least once q6h (must be kept moist). Do not put silver nitrate on the face, as it stains the corneas black. **Alternate** topical treatment: Apply **bacitracin** to the face and to burned areas. Other options: any antibiotic ointment, or honey. IV **ketamine** or narcotics are important for pain control during dressing changes. Give an oral benzodiazepine such as **lorazepam** 1-2mg po q8h or **diazepam** 5-10mg po q8h 30-60 minutes before wound care to control anxiety caused by repetitive painful procedures.

14. Do not use prophylactic IV or oral antibiotics. Up to a centimeter of redness surrounding a burn wound is common, and results from local inflammation rather than true infection. If redness spreads (with or without other symptoms of infection), treat as cellulitis. For less severe infection, give **dicloxacillin** 500mg po q6h or **cefazolin** 1g IV q8h x 7–10 days. If more severe infection, give **nafcillin** (or **oxacillin**) 2g IV q4h x 10-14 days. If effective burn creams are not used (especially for burn size of 20% or more), the patient may develop invasive gram-negative burn wound infection. Look for systemic signs of sepsis and changes in the color and odor of the burn wound. This is a life-threatening problem. Monitor vital signs carefully, provide fluid resuscitation and give 2 additional antibiotics that cover *P. aeruginosa* (eg, **piperacillin** 4g IV q4h or **ceftazidime** 2g IV q8h; PLUS **amikacin** 10mg/kg loading dose, then 7.5mg/kg IV q12h or **ciprofloxacin** 400mg IV q12h. (May also inject antibiotics beneath the infected eschar: suspend ½ daily dose **piperacillin** into a sufficient volume of crystalloid solution to treat the entire infected area and inject into the sub-eschar tissues using a 20 spinal needle.) Surgical eschar removal should be done within 12 hours. Evacuate the patient for surgery.

15. Burn patients need more calories and protein. Supplement patients with burns over 30% TBSA with milkshakes or any similar high-calorie, high-protein food source.

16. Burn patients with deep burns across most of the entire anterior and lateral chest may develop a "chest-eschar syndrome" during the first 24hr post-burn. Full-thickness burned skin (leathery, tight, and inelastic) may act like a straightjacket, inhibiting chest movement during inspiration or bag ventilation. Using a scalpel or electrocautery, cut through the eschar on the chest from mid-clavicular line to anterior axillary line down past the costal margin. Then, connect right and left across the epigastrium (*see Figure 7-5*). Do this procedure immediately when it is needed. As a caveat: if you think about doing an escharotomy, then do it!

17. Burn patients with circumferential deep burns of the extremities are at risk for an "extremity eschar syndrome", in which swelling beneath the inelastic eschar causes gradual constriction of the blood vessels. This can result in nerve and muscle damage, and eventually life-threatening infection of dead muscle and/or limb loss. This syndrome is diagnosed by loss of distal pulses in a patient with deep (full-thickness or deep partial thickness) burns of an extremity. Remember that loss of pulses is a late sign. Low BP due to severe shock may also cause loss of peripheral pulses in burn patients.) Treat with escharotomy: incise the tight, inelastic eschar with a scalpel or electrocautery. Place the incision in the mid-lateral and/or mid-medial line of the extremity (*see Figure 7-5*). Cut all the way through the skin, but no deeper into the subcutaneous fat than is necessary to release the tension.

Low-dose IV narcotics or **ketamine** will help control pain. Check distal pulses after the procedure to make sure it was successful. During the first 3 days postburn, keep burned extremities (especially burned forearms/hands) elevated above the heart level on pillows or blankets to prevent worsening of edema.

Figure 7.5 Regions of Escharotomy

Note: Perform escharotomies along the lines shown. Bold lines indicate the importance of the incisions crossing any involved joints.

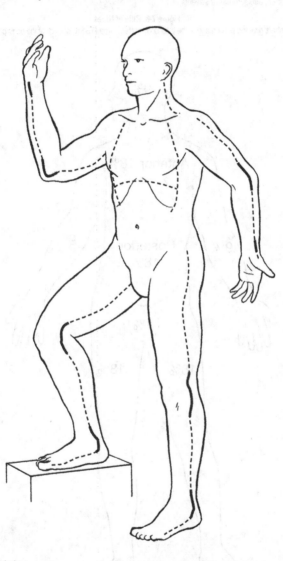

Specific Chemical Injuries:

1. Decontaminate the patient. Decontaminate at the site of injury as thoroughly as possible. Determine exactly what compound caused the injury. Following decontamination, treat in the same manner as thermal injuries.
2. Acids or bases: brush off any solid material, and then flush with copious amounts of water, at least 30 minutes for acids, hours for bases. Test the skin with pH paper to determine when it is safe to stop decontamination. Never attempt to neutralize a chemical by applying a basic compound to an acid burn. Burns of the eyes should be continuously irrigated (can use IV line) at the inner canthus. Alkali burns of the eyes may require irrigation for 8-12 hours.
3. White phosphorus (WP): an incendiary compound that ignites on contact with air at 32°C (89.6°F). To prevent this, wounds containing WP fragments must be continuously immersed in water, saline solution, or similar liquid. Remove the fragments in an operating room and place them in a container of water. A Wood's lamp (UV light) can be used in a dark room to identify these fluorescent fragments.
4. Hydrofluoric acid (HF): HF absorption can cause deep tissue damage and can deplete circulating calcium and magnesium,

resulting in lethal dysrhythmias. Topical application of **calcium gluconate** in a water-soluble lubricating jelly such as **Surgilube** will chelate the fluoride anion and prevent systemic absorption. This mixture can be placed inside a surgical glove for those patients with HF hand burns.

5. Tar and asphalt; Hot tar and asphalt cause a deep thermal injury. Cool the injured areas in water, and then apply white petrolatum (**Vaseline**, etc.), mineral oil, or vegetable oil to the area in order to dissolve and soften the material. Do not apply gasoline or other petroleum-based solvents.

Figure 7-6. Rule of Nines.

The numbers give the percentage of the total body surface area (TBSA) of each of the body parts shown.

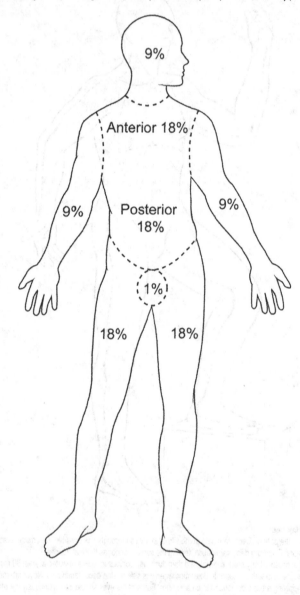

Fluid Resuscitation Notes: After initiating IV fluid therapy, calculate the total body surface area (TBSA) burned using the "Rule of Nines" (see *Figure 7-6*). First-degree burns are not significant and need not be included. The hand, including the 5 fingers, represents approximately 1% of the total body surface. Find out or estimate the patient's pre-burn weight in kilograms (kg). Estimate the total fluid (lactated Ringers) required during the first 24 h after injury by using the modified Brooke formula for adults: 2cc/kg/%TBSA. Plan to give ½ of the estimated fluid in the first 8 hrs. In children weighing less than 30kg, the infusion rate is estimated at 3cc/kg/%TBSA. Plan to give ½ of the estimated fluid over the first 8 hrs. Children will also need maintenance fluids of 5% dextrose in ½ normal saline. This should be given using a rule such as the 4-2-1 rule: 4cc/kg/h for the first 10kg, 2cc/kg/h for the next 10 kg, and 1cc/kg/h for the next 10kg. If a patient's resuscitation is delayed by a few hours, then give fluid more rapidly. Simpler rule for adults ("Ten cc rule"): start infusion at 10cc/TBSA per hour, eg, for a 45% burn, start LR at 10cc/hr x 45 = 450cc/hr. Adjust the initial fluid infusion rate to the urine output. Failure to monitor and record the urine output (catheter or bedpan) and adjust the fluid rate hourly may result in death or in severe complications. Adequate urine output is 30-50cc/h in an adult and 1cc/kg/h in a child who weighs less than 30kg. If the output is greater, or less, than the target for 2 consecutive hours, decrease, or increase, the IV rate by about 20% respectively until the rate is satisfactory. After the first 24 hours, switch resuscitation fluids to albumin (diluted to 5% in normal saline or similar crystalloid) at 0.5cc/kg/%TBSA burned over 24 h at a constant rate. If albumin is unavailable, use fresh frozen plasma or 6% hetastarch, or continue the LR while adjusting the rate as before. At the 24-hour point after injury, also start D5W at 1cc/kg/%TBSA burned each 24 h at a constant rate (subtract any oral water intake from the total needed per day). After 48 hours, patients with large burns continue to need fluid (ie, water or D5W) at 1cc/kg/%TBSA/day, but may be very thirsty, so watch their intake carefully to avoid over-drinking.

Alternate:
1. If LR is not available, you may use normal saline or alternate between normal saline and sodium bicarbonate solution (mix 2 1/2 50meq ampules of sodium bicarbonate per liter of D5W to make a solution of 125meq/L). If you give normal saline alone, you should also start D5W at the rate given below (1cc/kg/TBSA burned/24 h), because of the high sodium concentration in normal saline. You can also use colloid (5% albumin, fresh frozen plasma, or 6% hetastarch) during the first 24 hours post-burn in combination with crystalloid, according to a formula such as colloid (0.5cc/kg/TBSA burned/24 h) plus LR or saline (1.5cc/kg TBSA burned/24 h).
2. If unable to provide IV fluids, start oral (or nasogastric tube) resuscitation using the following oral formula: 1L of water, ¼ tsp of salt, ¼ tsp of sodium bicarbonate (if no bicarbonate, use total of ½ tsp salt), 2 tbsp of sugar or honey and a little orange or lemon juice. May also utilize WHO oral rehydration packets. Salt solutions can also be given by enema (proctoclysis).
3. Intraosseous infusion can be used with burn patients. The infusion rate should be the same as for IV resuscitation.

What Not To Do:
1. Do not over-resuscitate burn patients. IV fluids are usually needed for burn size over 20%, but more is not better. Turn the fluids down whenever the urine output (for adults) is more than 50mL/hr.
2. Do not fail to intubate burn or inhalation injury patients with symptoms of airway obstruction. It is safer to intubate early than to try to rescue a patient with a lost airway.
3. Do not hesitate to do escharotomies on acutely burned, full-thickness circumferential burns of the extremities.
4. Do not fail to elevate acutely burned upper extremities above the level of the heart on blankets or pillows.
5. Do not under medicate burn patients for wound care. Adequate wound care requires adequate analgesia with narcotics or ketamine, as well as prevention of anxiety with benzodiazepines.
6. Do not fail to do aggressive wound care daily or twice daily, to include cleansing with a surgical detergent like chlorhexidine gluconate.
7. Do not miss non-burn injuries (eg, spine fractures, internal bleeding, eye injuries, perforated tympanic membranes [depending on mechanism of injury]).
8. Do not fail to enforce vigorous physical and occupational therapy (basic range-of-motion and out-of-bed mobility).
9. Do not neglect supplemental nutrition especially for those with burns of 20% or more.
10. Do not miss possible child or domestic abuse, which are common worldwide.
11. Do not miss a simple burn-wound cellulitis, but do not use antibiotics unnecessarily.

Patient Education
Wound care: With silver dressings, change dressings every 2-5 days (ie, more often if there is a question about microbial colonization, less often if it is clean). Keep dressings moist. With cream applications, change the dressings at least q day bid, if possible. Soak the dressings off to decrease pain and prevent disruption of the healing process, wash with soap and water, apply topical burn cream and new dressings. Keep the dressings dry and clean. After the burns are healed, apply a moisturizing cream to the burned area bid. Use sunscreen and sun precautions, since burned skin is more susceptible to sunburn.

Activity: Ambulate, and do range of motion exercises 5-10 minutes every hour to prevent edema and contractures.

Diet: Eat a diet high in calories and proteins during the healing process.

Prevention: Avoid burn agents to prevent further accidents. Be careful while cooking and handling fuels.

No Improvement/Deterioration: Return to the clinic for any difficulty breathing, hoarseness, or worsening cough, and for any increased pain in the burn area, increased redness and blanching to the burn area, red streaks from the burn area, or fever.

Follow-up Actions
Return Evaluation: If the patient is reliable, the burn encompasses <10% TBSA partial thickness burn, and there are no associated injuries such as inhalation, the patient may be able to perform wound care at home. See the patient at least twice weekly until healed. If the patient is unreliable or if burns are >10% TBSA, then daily follow-up or hospitalization is recommended.

Evacuation/Consultation Criteria: Evacuate those with >20% TBSA burned or those with serious associated injuries, such as inhalation injury or fractures. Consult a trauma surgeon or emergency medicine specialist for all burn cases other than sunburns.

Chapter 29: Burns, Blast, Lightning and Electrical Injuries: Blast Injuries

Col John M Wightman, USAFR, MC

Introduction: Mechanisms of injury: High-explosive (HE), thermobaric, and nuclear detonations compress air or water molecules creating a devastating blast shock wave that can be transmitted into the human body, causing pressure differentials that can tear tissue. The injury is most extreme where densities change, especially at air-tissue interfaces and the surfaces of solid organs, but damage can occur within the solid organs as well (eg, brain and heart). Damage due to the blast wave itself is termed primary blast injury (PBI), but the most common injuries result from conventional penetrating, blunt, and thermal mechanisms. Ballistic injuries from fragments, shrapnel, and debris are the most common causes of injury and death. Blunt trauma may also occur as the result of the body being blown by the blast wind and striking the ground or other surface (eg, interior parts of or being ejected from a vehicle, or remaining in a vehicle that is then involved in a crash after the explosion). The effects of detonation can range from limited 1st degree flash burns to exposed skin surfaces to severe 2nd and 3rd degree burns from fireballs that completely engulf individuals.

Injuries more common in blast-exposed casualties: PBI may occur in isolation or in combination with conventional injuries. The challenge is to identify and manage internal injuries that may have few symptoms or signs initially but that will have serious adverse consequences if not identified and appropriately managed. The following identify potential consequences of PBI at air-tissue interfaces:

Lung PBI: Hemorrhage into lung tissue (pulmonary contusion); Hemorrhage into pleural cavity (hemothorax); Hemorrhage into airways (hemoptysis [may be massive enough to threaten airway]); Escape of air into pleural cavity (pneumothorax); Escape of air into pulmonary veins (arterial air embolism [AAE]); Escape of air into lung tissue (pulmonary pseudocyst)

Gastrointestinal (GI) tract PBI: Hemorrhage into bowel lumen (upper or lower GI bleeding); Hemorrhage into bowel wall (mass effect leading to obstruction or wall weakening with delayed rupture and escape of contents); Hemorrhage into peritoneal cavity (hemoperitoneum); Escape of stomach or intestinal contents into abdomen – (peritonitis); Escape of esophageal contents into chest (mediastinitis)

Ear PBI: Middle ear (ruptured tympanic membrane [TM], temporary conductive hearing loss); Inner ear (temporary or permanent sensory hearing loss). *See http://emedicine.medscape.com/article/822587* for management of specific penetrating, blunt, and thermal mechanisms of injury.

Blast syndrome: Poorly understood entity that can present as: a brief period of apnea, which the medic is unlikely to see before assessing the casualty; relative bradycardia with mild hypotension and brief syncope; retrograde or antegrade amnesia; and profound apathy. Syncope or lightheadedness can be managed by lying the casualty down, and elevating the lower extremities. Patients should be kept quiet, protected and observed, but further immediate intervention is often not required.

Traumatic brain injury (TBI): TBI following HE detonation is most often due to blunt or penetrating mechanisms. Contributing mechanisms to occult TBI are likely 3-fold: blast waves transmitting stress waves directly through the skull into the brain; high-chest pressures creating something similar to a vasovagal episode; and "water hammer" effects where the blast impulse contacting soft body parts is carried into the rigid skull by pressure pulses up the major arteries and veins. Manifestations of blast syndrome typically resolve on their own within 4 hours, whereas manifestations of TBI may persist for days, weeks, months, or years.

Subjective: **Symptoms**

Focused History:

Pulmonary: *Are you short of breath?* (Dyspnea may indicate pulmonary contusion, tension pneumothorax; hemopneumothorax or shock.) *Do you have chest pain?* (penetrating or blunt trauma, pneumothorax, or myocardial ischemia due to coronary AAE) *What does your pain feel like?* (Pain of pulmonary contusion is often described as dull and diffuse, bronchospasm or difficulty expanding the chest may be described as chest tightness; pain may wax and wane with respirations; pain of pneumothorax will often be sharp and focal, lateral or central, typically aggravated by breathing until the lung is completely collapsed. Chest pain that seems like it would be consistent with ischemic heart attack may be due to AAE.) *How much effort is required to breathe?* (Dyspnea at rest indicates shock due to external or internal hemorrhage, pneumothorax, or serious pulmonary contusion. The less exertion that leads to dyspnea, the more lung injury is likely.)

Abdominal: *Do you have abdominal or testicular pain, nausea, urge to defecate, or blood in your stools?* (PBI of air-containing structures in the GI tract may cause any of these symptoms.) *What does your pain feel like?* (Stretched bowel will feel like a persistent gas bubble with possibly sharp and crampy waves as it is affected by peristalsis. Once the bowel ruptures, pain will decrease until peritonitis begins. The pain of peritonitis is usually diffuse and severe.)

Neurological: *Do you have headache, vertigo, unsteadiness, or nausea?* (Identify patients at risk for mTBI and initiate casualty protection and medical management as early as possible.) Ask questions in sections I–VIII of the Military Acute Concussion Evaluation (MACE). *See Part 7: Trauma: Chapter 26: Mild Traumatic Brain Injury/Concussion: Military Acute Concussion Evaluation; Figure 7-3*

Special senses: *Do you have pain or problems with your eyes or ears?* (Identify penetrating or blunt trauma; any decreased vision is a penetrating foreign body or hyphema until proven otherwise.) Ringing, roaring, or decreased hearing is common and determination of effect on hearing will ultimately be required.) *What does your pain feel like?* (Eye pain is typically severe, and muscle spasms may make thorough examination difficult. Ear pain caused by a ruptured TM is often initially sharp but wanes over time.)

Objective: **Signs**

Using Basic Tools: Vital signs: Tachycardia (hemorrhage, hypoxia); bradycardia (blast syndrome, near-death rhythm); irregular heart rhythm (shock or AAE); hypotension (hemorrhage, other causes of shock, or blast syndrome); tachypnea (hypoxia, shock); bradypnea (blast syndrome, near-arrest respirations). Internal hemorrhage may not manifest obvious external signs, especially when PBI is the primary mechanism. Repeat vital signs as changes over time are much more important than a single set of values. Initial anxiety or pain reactions should improve. Abnormalities associated with internal injuries will more likely be persistent, recurrent, or worsen over time. Inspection: Identify external hemorrhage, apnea or dyspnea, altered mental status, syncope, seizures. Penetrating wounds; traumatic amputations; cyanosis (hypoxia or cyanide); pallor (hemorrhage); mottling of skin, mucous membranes, or tongue (shock if diffuse or AAE if localized); eye injury; drainage or bleeding from ears (TM rupture or basilar skull fracture); drainage or bleeding from nose (blast-induced sinus injury, basilar skull fracture, or exposure to chemical nerve agent); pharyngeal petechiae (predicts higher likelihood of pulmonary contusion); gross rectal bleeding (bowel injury). **Note:** Small wounds from penetrating fragments and debris may be difficult to identify without a complete and careful inspection. The eyes are particularly vulnerable to injury by tiny particles, either accelerated at high velocity to penetrate the globe or circulated in the air to cause a surface conjunctival or corneal foreign body. Although apprehension, sweating, tachycardia, tachypnea, and evidence of peripheral vasoconstriction are all signs of activation of the sympathetic nervous system and may be caused by anxiety, assume these represent response to serious injury until casualty is completely evaluated. Cardiopulmonary and neurological examinations as described in appendix. Auscultation: Unilateral decreased or absent breath sounds (pneumothorax, hemothorax, or extensive pulmonary contusion). Palpation: Subcutaneous emphysema (AAE, pneumothorax); abdominal tenderness (penetrating, blunt, or blast trauma). Pulse Oximeter: S_pO_2 < 95% on room air following blast indicates some degree of pulmonary contusion, inadequate respirations, pneumothorax or hemothorax, shock, or exposure to chemical agent such as cyanide. Persistent S_pO_2 75-95% on room air (mild lung injury) not likely to require assisted ventilation. Persistent S_pO_2 <75% on room air (moderate or severe lung injury) likely to require assisted ventilation immediately or in near future. MACE Sections IX–XIII: *See Part 7: Trauma: Chapter 26: Mild Traumatic Brain Injury/Concussion: Military Acute Concussion Evaluation; Figures 7-3 and 7-4* **Using Advanced Tools:** Ophthalmoscope: Magnification to identify subtle anterior eye trauma (small foreign body, corneal or scleral penetration, hyphema, lens injury); funduscopy to identify posterior eye trauma (lack of red reflex due to hemorrhage, vitreal foreign body). Fluorescein strip: Pooling (corneal abrasion); dilution (corneal penetration with aqueous leak). Otoscope: Ruptured TM. Stool guaiac: Guaiac-positive stool (occult penetrating, blunt, or blast trauma).

Assessment:
Differential Diagnosis
Rapid unconsciousness: Penetrating or blunt brain or cardiac trauma, blast syndrome, cerebral or cardiac AAE, chemical nerve agent or cyanide inhalation.
Airway compromise: Altered mental status, penetrating or blunt face or neck trauma, inhalational injury, massive hemoptysis, foreign body aspiration.
Ventilatory insufficiency: Pulmonary contusion, pneumothorax (all types), hemothorax, rib fractures, bronchopleural fistula, chemical-agent or botulinum-toxin exposure.
Shock: External or internal hemorrhage (more likely due to conventional mechanisms), tension pneumothorax, hypoxia from pulmonary injury, GI bleeding (more often lower), coronary AAE (heart attack with poor pumping and cardiogenic shock), spinal AAE (with generalized vasodilation and neurogenic shock).
Focal neurological deficits: TBI or cerebral AAE (stroke), spinal injury or spinal AAE, peripheral nerve injury.

Plan:
Treatment: Evaluate for necessity of tetanus immunization booster.
1. **External hemorrhage:** Penetrating injury or traumatic amputation
   Primary & Alternative: Standard trauma management
   Evacuation: Category dependent on control of external hemorrhage and shock or not
2. **Massive hemoptysis:** May lead to airway compromise
   Primary: Allow casualty to spit, cough, and find own position for best breathing.
   Alternative: Selective intubation of mainstem bronchus on least injured side (must be done orally, cannot be accomplished nasally) (*See Figure 7-7*). Use lumen of tube to facilitate gas exchange in and out of lung with lighter bleeding. Use cuff to prevent blood from side of heavier bleeding crossing into mainstem bronchus of better lung. Numbers in boxes of algorithm indicate order of preference of interventions listed.
   Evacuation: Administer 100% oxygen. Category usually URGENT-SURGICAL.
3. **Pneumothorax, tension pneumothorax, hemothorax:** May lead to ventilatory insufficiency and hypoxia.
   Primary & Alternative: Standard trauma management
   Evacuation: Category based on relief of respiratory distress and shock or not
4. **Pulmonary contusion:** May lead to hypoxia.
   Primary: Allow casualty to spit, cough, and find own position for best breathing. Do not exert casualty, since this leads to worse outcomes. Predict need for positive-pressure ventilation (PPV) or positive end-expiratory pressure (PEEP) using guidelines. PPV can be accomplished with mouth-to-mask or bag-valve-mask/tube with slower and less forceful deliveries. AAE is one common cause of death in immediate survivors, and often occurs when PPV is initiated because airway pressure is increased.
   Evacuation: Supplemental oxygen as necessary. PEEP will not be available in the field, but may be on evacuation platforms. Category based on improvement in oxygenation or not. Prediction of Respiratory Problems: Insignificant pulmonary injury may be defined as no dyspnea with exertion after 1 hour of post-exposure rest. Significant pulmonary blast injuries may be classified based on pulse oximetry when available. The result may predict likelihood of complications, and requirement for PPV and PEEP. Mild (S_pO_2 >75% on room air): Unlikely to need PPV, normal PEEP if PPV initiated, pneumothoraces occur, bronchopleural fistulae rare. Moderate (S_pO_2 >90% on 100% oxygen): Likely to require conventional PPV, PEEP 5-10cm H_2O usually needed, pneumothoraces common, bronchopleural fistulae occur. Severe (S_pO_2 <90% on 100% oxygen): likely to require unconventional PPV, PEEP >10cm H_2O usually needed, pneumothoraces almost universal, bilateral tension pneumothoraces with bronchopleural fistulae common. Bronchopleural fistulae: Cannot be diagnosed in the field, but are important causes of inability to relieve tension pneumothoraces with one or two needle decompressions, because the volume of air with each breath/ventilation entering the pleural space through the torn trachea or bronchus exceeds the capacity of narrow needles to evacuate it. One or more large-bore chest tubes are required in these situations.

Figure 7-7. Selective Intubation Algorithm

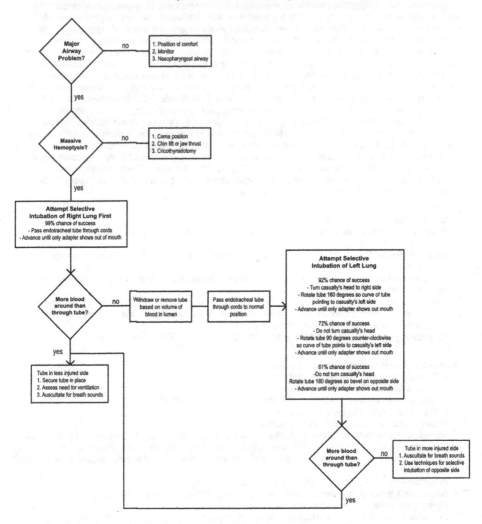

5. **AAE:** Air can lodge in any location creating distal ischemia or infarction.
Primary: Place casualty in recovery position with left side down (halfway between left-lateral decubitus and prone) and head at same level as heart (*see Figure 7-8*).

Figure 7-8. Recovery Position

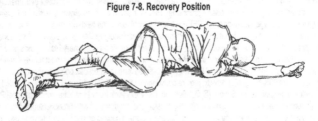

Alternative: Perform in-water recompression as a last resort in divers exposed to blast.
Evacuation: Administer 100% oxygen. Category usually URGENT if symptomatic—ideally to hyperbaric oxygen chamber, if available.

6. **Shock**: Most causes are conventional trauma mechanisms.
   Primary & Alternative: Standard trauma management. Consider smaller fluid boluses with more frequent reevaluation to avoid exacerbating lung or brain injury: normal saline or lactated Ringer's solution 500mL or hetastarch (Hespan) 250mL. Repeat these smaller boluses as necessary to restore mental status, as the indicator of shock reversal.
   Evacuation: Category URGENT or URGENT SURGICAL depending on suspected mechanism. *See Part 7: Trauma: Chapter 27: Hypovolemic Shock*

7. **GI bleeding, GI tract rupture:** May often be difficult to identify unless progressive or severe.
   Primary: NPO and maintenance IV fluid at 125mL/hr. **Ceftriaxone** 2gm IV or IM q day.
   Evacuation: Category PRIORITY for surgical care within 4 hours, unless shock or sepsis is suspected. **Prochlorperazine** 25mg IV or IM up to qid or **promethazine** 25mg IV or IM up to qid, if needed to prevent recurrent vomiting.
   Alternative: Maintenance oral fluids, if no IV and evacuation time >4 hours. **Ciprofloxacin** 500mg po q12h and **metronidazole** 500mg po q8h, if parenteral cephalosporins not carried or casualty is allergic to them. Virtually any broad-spectrum antibiotic coverage is better than nothing when time to definitive care is prolonged.

8. **TBI from blast:** Standard trauma management. Identify, stabilize and evacuate moderate and severe TBI (eg, Glasgow Coma Scale [GCS] score <13, loss of consciousness >30 min, altered mental status >24 hrs, or post-traumatic amnesia >24 hrs). If vital signs and pulse oximetry can be measured, systolic BP <90mmHg and oxygen saturation <90% must be avoided. Even transient decreases can worsen TBI, so effective resuscitation is key to preventing secondary brain injury.

9. **Vertigo:** More often due to TBI than blast effects on the inner ear. May try **meclizine** 25mg po q8h or **diazepam** 5mg po q8h prn to improve symptoms, but these drugs also sedate and impair ability to function and make assessment of mental status more difficult.

10. **TM rupture:** Patient should not dive, swim, or shower until TM heals. Risk of otitis progressing to encephalitis; permanent hearing loss, vertigo, or tinnitus; and other complications.
    Primary: Prevent water and other non-sterile material from entering ear canal. Do not attempt removal of foreign debris. Prophylactic antibiotics not indicated, unless ear canal is grossly contaminated. If infection of external ear canal (otitis externa), TM (myringitis), or middle ear (otitis media) develops, then instill **ofloxacin** otic solution 5-6 drops q12h x 7 days.
    Alternative: Amoxicillin/clavulanate 875mg po q12h (500mg q8h) or **ciprofloxacin** 500mg po q12h, if antibiotic drops not available or ear canal is grossly contaminated.
    Return Evaluation: Inspect area surrounding ear, external ear, ear canal, and TM daily for redness, swelling, or purulent drainage.
    Consultation Criteria: ENT consult within 3 days if significant debris in canal; up to 2 weeks acceptable, if no infection.

11. **Pain control:** Do not use morphine if bradycardic and hypotensive. Do not use anti-inflammatory medications if internal contusion or hemorrhage is possible. *See Part 8: Procedures: Chapter 30: Pain Assessment and Control*
    Primary: Mild pain can be treated with **acetaminophen** 975mg or 1000mg po q4h (do not exceed 4g daily). Moderate-to-severe pain should be treated with an oral opioid such as **hydrocodone/acetaminophen** 5/325mg q4h or 10/650mg q6h; a transmucosal opioid such as **fentanyl lollipop** 400mcg consumed over 15 min; or a parenteral opioid such as **fentanyl** 2mcg/kg IV q half hour or **morphine** 0.05mg IV q half hour or 0.1mg/kg IM q2h up to an initial maximum of 2mg/kg in the first 4 hrs. If respiratory depression occurs, administer **naloxone** 0.4mg IV or IM q20 min and observe the casualty for recurrence as naloxone wears off. If symptomatic bradycardia occurs, **atropine** 0.5mg IV q20 min up to 6 doses. If hypotension occurs as a result of narcotic administration, initiate an IV fluid bolus with normal saline or lactated Ringer's solution 500mL or hetastarch 250mL then administer **diphenhydramine** 25mg IV or IM which may be repeated once a half hour later. *See Part 8: Procedures: Chapter 30: Pain Assessment and Control*
    Alternative: Sedation instead of or in addition to analgesia is an option, but most sedatives carry a risk of respiratory depression in a casualty who may have occult pulmonary injury and relative bradycardia. **Ketamine** 2mg/kg IV or 4mg/kg IM is a good choice for casualties who do not have a head injury or suspected increased intracranial pressure.

12. **Body substance exposure (BSE):** Consider BSE protocols against infectious diseases (hepatitis, HIV, etc.) for penetrating wounds with body parts and mucous-membrane contact with body fluids, particularly following attacks by suicide bombers.

Evacuation through higher altitudes: Pneumothorax, AAE, and bowel-wall stretching injuries are more likely to be initiated or exacerbated by decreased ambient external pressure on the casualty (associated with ascent from dive, travel to altitude in ground vehicle or aircraft, or combination). Reassess frequently! Monitor cardiac rhythm (ECG monitor if available) and pulmonary status (including pulse oximetry) throughout trip. If there is a possibility the patient has a pneumothorax, place a chest tube before any ascent to higher altitudes. Tension pneumoperitoneum affecting respiration is rare, but may require 14 gauge needle decompression in midline just above umbilicus. Remove air from cuffs on Foley catheters and endotracheal tubes and replace with liquid. Notify receiving facility of urgent need for appropriate special services: neurosurgeon, general surgeon, hyperbaric chamber, intensive care, etc.

Chapter 29: Burns, Blast, Lightning and Electrical Injuries: Electrical and Lightning Injuries

Lt Col Jeff Vista, USAF, MC

Introduction: Electrical injuries encompass 3 types of injury (lightning, high-voltage and low-voltage) and span a wide spectrum of direct and secondary injuries. Alternating current (AC) may result in tetanic muscle contractions, preventing the victim from releasing the source. Direct current (DC) tends to cause a single, violent muscle contraction, often throwing the victim from the source. Lightning rarely causes the same injuries associated with generated electricity, due to the extremely brief duration. In mass casualty triage following a lightning strike, avoid use of the expectant category for cardiac arrest patients. Return of spontaneous circulation is not uncommon, and patients may only require airway and other supportive management. Conscious victims of a lightning strike are unlikely to subsequently immediately expire. Victims of electrical injury are not electrically "charged" and may be touched immediately after injury, provided they are no longer in contact with the "live" electrical source.

Subjective: **Symptoms**

Cardiopulmonary arrest, loss of consciousness, entry/exit burns and wounds, disorientation, pain, numbness and tingling.

Focused History: *Were there any witnesses to your injury? If so, what did they see?* (may confirm electrocution and suggest possible associated injuries) *Do you have any pain, numbness, tingling, or other abnormal sensations or feelings?* (directs you to areas of injury for closer evaluation and monitoring on serial exams) *Have you had any change in urine color or frequency?* (Decreased quantity and or frequency of urine, and cola- or tea-colored urine may suggest renal failure due to rhabdomyolysis, which is the pathologic breakdown of muscle tissue, accompanied by the release of potentially toxic cellular contents into the systemic circulation. Clinical sequelae include hypovolemia [due to third-spacing within affected tissues], hyperkalemia, metabolic acidosis, acute renal failure, and, in severe cases, disseminated intravascular coagulation. Evaluation and management tips in this section are aimed at preventing and/or mitigating the effects of these sequelae.)

Objective: **Signs**

Using Basic Tools: Approach patient as any other trauma victim, performing primary and secondary surveys. Assess for evidence of blunt trauma to head, neck and spinal column, chest, abdomen, and musculoskeletal system (fractures, dislocations). Include thorough eye and ear exams (up to two-thirds of lightning strike victims sustain ruptured eardrums). Assess for Compartment Syndrome*. Superficial "fern-like" burns of the skin are indicative of lightning injury. Severe electrical burns may occur with "entrance" and "exit" wounds and extensive tissue damage along the path of the electrical current. Injured muscle releases large amounts of myoglobin that may damage the kidneys. This may be seen clinically as dark tea- or cola-colored urine.

*Compartment syndrome may jeopardize the viability of a limb and results from swelling within tight fascial compartments of the extremities causing compression of nerves and blood vessels. Compartment syndrome may be characterized by the "7 Ps", the last two of which are ominous findings:

1. **P**ain out of proportion to visible injury
2. **P**assive movement-induced pain in the involved muscles
3. **P**ressure palpable over the compartment
4. **P**aralysis or weakness of affected muscles
5. **P**aresthesia in nerve distribution of affected compartment
6. **P**allor
7. **P**ulselessness, a LATE finding (do not wait for this!) *See Part 8: Procedures: Chapter 30: Compartment Syndrome*

Using Advanced Tools: Lab: Presumptively diagnose myoglobinuria if urine dips positive for large amount of blood, and few or no red blood cells visible on microscopic urine exam. Evaluate ECG and cardiovascular status. Monitor hemoglobin/hematocrit and electrolytes as trauma baseline labs; repeat if patient's condition persists or worsens (look for evidence of occult hemorrhage and/or hemolysis). More severely injured patients may need blood typing in anticipation of transfusion.

Assessment: **Differential Diagnosis**

Consider syncope, traumatic head injury, stroke and/or anoxic brain injury (particularly if associated smoke inhalation is suspected) as causes of prolonged altered level of consciousness or coma. Consider internal bleeding (chest, abdomen, GI) as cause of unexplained hypotension.

Plan:

Treatment

Primary:

1. Resuscitate patients based on clinical status as per BLS/ACLS & ATLS protocols. Perform meticulous wound and burn care.
2. Monitor intake and output (I & O): Insert Foley catheter and NG tube in seriously injured patients
3. Treat pain: Nonsteroidal anti-inflammatory drugs (NSAIDs) for the first few days may decrease long-term neurologic damage; although there are no studies on this, they are usually safe and have the added benefit of pain control. Consider **ibuprofen** 400-800mg po tid, or **naproxen** 500mg po bid.
4. Give antibiotics if fever or other signs of infection develop; appropriate choices include **ampicillin/sulbactam** 1.5-3gm IV q6h or **ceftriaxone** 1-2gm IV q24h, or **ciprofloxacin** 200-400mg IV q12h. Ensure up-to-date **tetanus prophylaxis.**
5. Fluids: Due to variable extent and depth of burns, standard fluid resuscitation formulas may underestimate fluid requirements, however overloading with fluids and development of massive edema should be avoided by close monitoring of I & O with titration of IV fluids (normal saline or lactated Ringers) to maintain urine output at 0.5-1mL/kg/hr.
6. Acid suppression for patients at risk for GI ulceration able to take oral medications: **famotidine** 20mg po daily or **omeprazole** 20-40mg po daily. For all patients on prolonged NPO: **famotidine** 20mg per NG tube q6h, or **famotidine** 20mg (10mg/mL) IV over 2 minutes q12h or **esomeprazole** 20-40mg IV injection (evenly distributed over no less than 3 minutes) or infusion (evenly distributed over 30 minutes) daily.

Empiric: If patient develops evidence of myoglobinuria, increase IV fluids to maintain urine output twice normal at 2 mL/kg/hour. Alkalinizing the urine aids in solubility and excretion of myoglobin. Add 1-3 ampules of **sodium bicarbonate** to each liter of IV normal saline or lactated Ringer's. Monitor urine pH with urine dipsticks and adjust amount of bicarb to keep pH greater than 6.5 (add more bicarb to increase urine pH; less to decrease). Monitor lung sounds and jugular veins for evidence of induced pulmonary edema. Consider also giving **furosemide** 20-40mg IV titrated to achieve and maintain diuresis, and/or **mannitol** 1 gm/kg IV bolus. Do not allow patient to become hypotensive from resultant diuresis and hypovolemia; adjust IV fluids accordingly. Monitor blood pressure, urinary output.

Primitive: If sterile IV solutions are not available or are in limited supply, and the patient has bowel sounds present and is not vomiting, consider substituting an oral rehydration solution (ORS). You may use any of the commercially available solutions (eg, Ricelyte, CeraLyte) or make your own ORS**, which can be taken orally or given by NG tube "drip" or "infusion." If the patient develops myoglobinuria, attempt to alkalinize the urine by increasing the amount of baking soda (bicarbonate) to 1-3 tbsp/L and adjusting the drip rate to achieve urine output of 1-2 mL/kg/hour. Adjust the amount of baking soda added to the ORS based on a target urine pH of 6.5 or greater. The solution can be placed into a clean, used IV fluid bag that has been cut open just enough at the top to add the ORS. Then hang the bag with IV tubing attached and the other end of the IV tubing attached to the NG tube. Adjust the flow rate in the same manner as any other IV fluid infusion. The bag and tubing may be used repeatedly in the same patient. Add more ORS solution to the bag as needed. If patient will be going to surgery within 4-6 hours, then discontinue oral/NG tube intake unless told otherwise by the surgical team.

** **ORS Recipe:** 1 tsp of salt, 1 tsp of salt substitute (potassium chloride), 1 tsp baking soda (bicarbonate), 2-3 tbsp of table sugar or 2 tbsp of honey or Karo syrup, all mixed in 1L of clean or disinfected water.

Patient Education

Medications: Furosemide and mannitol are potent diuretic agents. Ibuprofen and naproxen, as mentioned, are common NSAIDs both available over-the-counter.

Prevention and Hygiene: Remember scene safety. Turn off the electrical source before making physical contact with the victim. Rescuers must avoid becoming victims themselves. Remember that lightning does strike twice in the same area. Avoid being the tallest object in an open area, and being near one. If caught in the open, crouch low and/or seek low ground.

Follow-up Actions

Return Evaluation: If myoglobinuria does not clear within 24-36 hours of adequate urine diuresis and alkalinization, then a source of undetected muscle ischemia or necrosis should be sought. Re-examine for areas of swelling and tenderness.

Consultation Criteria: Except for the most trivial of electric shocks, all victims of electrical injury should be evaluated by a physician as soon as tactically and/or operationally feasible. Patients with suspected compartment syndrome might require "limb-saving" fasciotomy. *See Part 8: Procedures: Chapter 30: Compartment Syndrome*

Notes: Fasciotomy is not the same procedure as escharotomy, which is done on third degree (full thickness) burn victims to relieve constricting overlying burn eschar. The escharotomy incision is not as deep, going only to the subcutaneous fat; on the other hand, the fasciotomy incision goes past the subcutaneous fat, down to (and through) the fascia, the thick fibrous tissue enclosing the affected muscle compartment. Victims of electrical injury are not electrically "charged" and may be touched immediately after injury, provided they are no longer in contact with the "live" electrical source.

NOTES:

Chapter 30: Basic Medial Skills: Initial Airway Management and Ventilatory Support

CPT Carl R. Pavel, MC, USA

What: How to assess, establish, and control the patient's airway to achieve adequate oxygenation and ventilation. This guideline does NOT address an entire trauma assessment. *See Part 7: Trauma: Chapter 26: Primary and Secondary Survey*

When: Patient is having respiratory distress. Airway: Establish and maintain a patent airway. Open the casualty's airway and establish the least invasive but most effective airway. Breathing: Determine if the casualty is exchanging air sufficiently to maintain adequate ventilation (ie, oxygen saturation & CO_2 exchange.) Monitor: After checking and correcting the airway and breathing status, monitor to ensure no deterioration. Perform these procedures without causing further injury to the patient.

What You Need: Various sizes of nasal and oropharyngeal airways, laryngeal mask airway (LMA) (if appropriate), gloves, gauze pads, tongue blades, bag-valve-mask (BVM) system, water-soluble lubricant, 10cc syringe to inflate the cuff, stylette, laryngoscope with blades, endotracheal tubes (rough size of little finger diameter; 7-9 for adult, 6-7 for adolescents, 4-6 for children [uncuffed], 3.5-4 for infants [uncuffed]), and oxygen/suction (if available), and emergency drugs.

What To Do:
1. **Assess consciousness: Does casualty respond to shake and shout, or painful stimuli?**
   If patient is conscious, go to **A (Conscious Casualty).**
   If patient is unconscious, go to **B (Unconscious Casualty).**

   A. **Conscious Casualty (Assess airway and respirations)**
      Note: Assessing the airway and respirations are two different steps in the trauma sequence, but every time the airway is assessed, the respiratory effort can also be partially assessed. A clear airway with respiratory effort detected does not fully clear the respiratory system. After assessing the airway, assess respiratory effort bilaterally with a stethoscope to ensure that both lungs are working and air movement is adequate.
      1. Ask casualty simple questions to determine status of airway.
         (a) If casualty can talk to you without difficulty, airway is clear.
         (b) If the patient answers with difficulty, coughing, pain, hoarseness or other difficulty, manage the airway using the same procedure as if the casualty were unconscious (See B. Unconscious Casualty).
      2. Auscultate both lungs to ensure that air is being exchanged equally and bilaterally.
      3. If history does not point to respiratory/airway involvement and there are no signs of respiratory distress present, continue primary assessment.
         (a) Monitor the patient's airway and respirations.
         (b) Monitor for signs and symptoms of hypoxia.
      4. If signs of respiratory distress develop:
         (a) Initiate appropriate treatment immediately.
            Note: Do not attempt to insert oropharyngeal airways or endotracheal tubes in conscious casualties unless they have a history or signs of inhalation burns or injuries.
         (b) Give supplemental oxygen, if available.
            Note: Failure to notice signs and symptoms of hypoxia or respiratory distress early may have a catastrophic effect on the patient.
      5. If casualty becomes unconscious, manage Unconscious Casualty as follows.

   B. **Unconscious Casualty**
      1. **Assess airway and respirations**
         Note: If patient is in a position that makes assessing the airway impossible, move the patient as little as possible to assess the airway. Institute c-spine control and be aware of other possible injuries when moving patient. Remember life has precedent over limb.
         (a) Look, listen and feel for respiratory effort.
            (1) Look for bilateral rise and fall of the chest.
            (2) Listen for air escaping during exhalation.
            (3) On the side of your face, feel for breath exhaling from the casualty's mouth.
         (b) If respiratory effort is detected, assess the respiratory effort for at least 6 seconds.
            (1) Assess the quality of the respiratory effort as strong, moderate, or weak.
            (2) Assess the rhythm of the respiratory effort as regular or irregular.
            (3) Assess the rate of the respiratory effort: <10 respirations per minute or >20 respirations per minute are indicators for assisted ventilations. **Note:** Multiply the number of respirations detected in a 6 second period x 10 to get the number respirations per minute.
         (c) If no respiratory effort is detected, check pulse
            (1) If the casualty is pulseless:
               • In a combat situation, an unresponsive, non-breathing, pulseless casualty is a fatality. End of this task
               • In a noncombat situation, initiate CPR. *See Part 4: Organ Systems: Chapter 1: Cardiac Resuscitation*
            (2) If the casualty has a pulse, establish an airway immediately.
      2. **Open and inspect the airway and provide appropriate airway and ventilatory support based on clinical condition.**
         (a) Inspect head, face, and throat for signs of trauma and inhalation injuries. Signs of inhalation injuries may include reddened face or singed eyebrows and nasal hair.

(b) Open the airway using the appropriate technique.
    (1) If working on a trauma casualty, use the jaw thrust technique:
    (2) Kneel at the top of the casualty's head.
    (3) Grasp the angles of the casualty's lower jaw.
    (4) Rest your elbows on the surface on which the casualty is lying.
    (5) Lift with both hands, displacing the lower jaw forward.

(c) If working on a non-trauma casualty, use the head-tilt/chin-lift method:
    (1) Kneel at the level of the casualty's shoulders.
    (2) Place one hand on the casualty's forehead and apply firm, backward pressure with the palm of the hand to tilt the head back.
    (3) Place the fingertips of the other hand under the bony part of the casualty's lower jaw, bringing the chin forward.
    Cautions:
    • Do not use the thumb to lift the lower jaw.
    • Do not press deeply into the soft tissue under the chin with the fingers.
    • Do not completely close the casualty's mouth.

(d) Inspect the oral cavity for foreign material, blood, vomitus, avulsed teeth, and signs of inhalation injuries. If the casualty has signs of trauma, foreign objects, and/or complications, continue with this step.

    (1) **If airway is clear & casualty is breathing: insert an oropharyngeal airway (J tube). Have suction available before attempting.**
    • The oropharyngeal airway should be approximately the same length as the distance from the corner of the casualty's mouth to tip of his ear lobe.
    • Insert the airway inverted until past the tongue and then rotate 180°.
    Warning: It is more traumatic (and contraindicated in children) to use this "corkscrew" technique. If a tongue depressor is available, it is preferable to use it to depress the tongue and insert the oral airway under direct vision.
    • Check for respiratory effort after J tube is inserted. Respiratory effort should be the same or improved after insertion of J tube. If decreased, remove tube, re-inspect airway, reinsert J tube and reassess.
    • Have assistant provide ventilations if required (*see notes*) and administer oxygen if available.
    • Continue with the survey, remembering that you will eventually need to intubate the unconscious patient.

    (2) **If airway is clear & casualty is not breathing, attempt to give 2 breaths using the rescue breathing technique.**
    • If the breaths go in, intubate and ventilate the casualty. Adequate ventilation requires correct volumes, rates and cadence. Avoid giving excessive tidal volumes, forcing air too quickly or ventilating too rapidly. Squeezing the bag steadily over approximately one full second at a rate of 10-12 breaths per minute will provide adequate ventilation. *See Part 8: Procedures: Chapter 30: Intubation*
    • If the breaths do not go in, attempt to reopen the airway again and give 2 more breaths. Remember C-spine precautions:

    2.1 If the breaths go in, intubate and appropriately ventilate the casualty.
    2.2 If breaths still do not go in, insert laryngoscope and inspect the oropharynx for foreign body, blood, vomitus, swelling or other causes of obstruction.
    2.3 Using forceps, attempt to remove any foreign objects seen.
        2.3.1 If able to clear airway, attempt 2 breaths and assess for return of spontaneous respirations.
        Note: If at any time spontaneous respirations return after clearing an airway, the casualty requires assisted ventilations with an oropharyngeal airway or ET tube. Casualties who were apneic for any length of time will have an elevated CO_2 level. Traumatized casualties who were apneic will have difficulty regaining O_2 saturation. They may start off breathing adequately, but their CO_2 deficit will cause them to destabilize over time. Failure to assist ventilations in a formerly apneic casualty WILL cause harm and possible death.
        2.3.2 If unable to clear airway, perform surgical cricothyroidotomy. *See Part 8: Procedures: Chapter 30: Cricothyroidotomy, Needle and Surgical*
        2.3.3 If the situation makes it impossible to perform an immediate surgical cricothyroidotomy, perform a needle cricothyroidotomy. *See Part 8: Procedures: Chapter 30: Cricothyroidotomy, Needle and Surgical*
    2.4 If no obstruction is seen but vocal cords are visualized, attempt to intubate casualty. *See Part 8: Procedures: Chapter 30: Intubation*
        2.4.1 If successful intubation, ventilate casualty using appropriate techniques.
        2.4.2 If unsuccessful intubation, perform surgical or needle cricothyroidotomy. *See Part 8: Procedures: Chapter 30: Cricothyroidotomy, Needle and Surgical.* If no obstruction of airway is seen but vocal cords are not visualized, perform surgical cricothyroidotomy.
    2.5 **If airway is not clear (obvious bleeding or vomiting), clear the airway:**
        2.5.1 Clear any foreign material or vomitus from the mouth as quickly as possible using forceps or the finger sweep method.
        2.5.2 If casualty is vomiting, turn head to the side or if you suspect C-spine injury, log-roll casualty on side to prevent aspiration
        2.5.3 If casualty is bleeding into the oral cavity, place an ET tube or J tube and then stem bleeding into the oral cavity with packed gauze.

2.5.4 After clearing the obstruction, if you have not yet secured the airway, assess the respirations and determine the type of airway required based on the cause of the obstruction and the situation. If the casualty is breathing on his own with little or no chance of aspiration, insert J tube. If the casualty is not breathing or has minimal respiratory effort, or there is a chance for aspiration, intubation is preferred.

2.5.5 Secure airway with an oropharyngeal airway or an ET tube.

2.5.6 If blockage cannot be removed or injuries make obtaining a secure oral airway improbable, give casualty a cricothyroidotomy immediately. *See Part 8: Procedures: Chapter 30: Cricothyroidotomy, Needle and Surgical*

2.5.7 Assist ventilations with BVM and oxygen if available.

Note: Casualties who are vomiting or bleeding into their naso/oropharynx need a secured airway, ie, ET tube, to protect against aspiration. In a combat situation, the medic may have to settle for a J tube or LMA until time and circumstances permit him to intubate the casualty.

Note: All unconscious casualties will eventually require intubation to further control and protect airway. *See Part 8: Procedures: Chapter 30: Intubation*

Note: If the casualty is in severe respiratory distress or arrest and cannot be intubated, you must perform a cricothyroidotomy. *See Part 8: Procedures: Chapter 30: Cricothyroidotomy, Needle and Surgical*

3. **Monitor airway and respiratory effort at least every 5 minutes while you continue the primary survey.**

4. **After completing the primary survey, periodically reassess the ABCs and immediately address any problems that emerge.** Verify optimal tube placement and confirm adequate oxygenation and ventilation frequently (clinical signs and use of appropriate technique). Whenever possible, continuous pulse oximetry and CO_2 monitoring (capnography) should be used to verify adequate oxygenation and ventilation.

5. **Evacuate casualty to nearest appropriate medical treatment facility. Note:** Providing oxygen allows time to treat the underlying respiratory problem.

   A. The nasal cannula is the simplest method suitable for a spontaneously breathing patient. Each additional L/min of flow adds approximately 4% to the 21% O_2 available normally at sea level.

   B. Facemasks provide higher and more precise levels of inspired oxygen—up to 35%-60%
      (1) Venturi mask delivers 24%-50% fraction of inspired oxygen (FiO_2).
      (2) Non-rebreather delivers 60%-90% FiO_2
      (3) A continuous positive airway pressure (CPAP) device can deliver up to 100%.

   C. Use a BVM device to assist or control ventilation until a more secure airway can be obtained. If used correctly (correct volumes, rates, cadence, with a good seal), 100% oxygen can be delivered this way.

What Not To Do:

1. If it takes 2 additional people to hold down a casualty to intubate them, re-evaluate the need for intubation since they have to be exchanging oxygen to maintain muscle strength and resist.

2. Do not proceed directly to intubation in a patient with respiratory disease without first attempting to improve airway and assisting respiratory effort wherever possible. Ambu or bag-valve mask ventilation, timed with a patient's efforts can help relax and improve their respiratory status, and potentially avoid the risk of intubation.

3. Do not forget to verify optimal tube placement and confirm adequate oxygenation and ventilation frequently (clinical signs and use of appropriate ventilatory technique).

4. Do not give excessive tidal volumes, force air too quickly, or ventilate too rapidly. Squeezing the bag steadily over approximately one full second at a rate of 10-12 breaths per minute will provide adequate ventilation.

Chapter 30: Basic Medical Skills: Intubation

MAJ Leland Bradley Morgans, AN, USA

What: Establish a temporary emergency airway through the mouth or nose, and pharynx.

When: To control the airway during cardiopulmonary resuscitation or respiratory failure, prior to the onset of expected complications (eg, laryngeal edema from inhalation burns), during complications from surgical anesthesia or other complications. Other indications include: disease or trauma to airway, traumatic injuries or musculoskeletal malformations making ventilation difficult, anatomic traits that make mask management difficult or impossible, need for frequent suctioning, prevention of aspiration of gastric contents, type of surgery or position of patient during surgery, need for postoperative ventilatory support. The most experienced airway provider should perform the technique. If failure to intubate and ventilate, one must consider moving quickly to a cricothyrotomy if the provider is trained in the technique. *See Part 8: Procedures: Chapter 30: Initial Airway Management and Ventilatory Support*

What You Need: Oxygen source and tubing if available, suction device, bag-valve-mask (BVM) device with self-inflating reservoir and oxygen coupling, face masks of different sizes, oral and nasopharyngeal airways (different sizes), water-soluble lubricant, straight and curved laryngoscope blades, endotracheal tubes (ETT) of different sizes, a syringe to inflate the cuff, stylets, tongue blades, nasogastric tube, end-tidal CO_2 monitor (if at all possible) and emergency drugs.

What To Do:

Evaluate patient and determine need for intubation and potential for difficulty with airway management. Evaluate the airway during the initial injury assessment, and administer supplemental oxygen during this time if possible. Continual airway assessment is crucial since subtle changes in mental or respiratory status can occur at any time.

Airway characteristics that can make fitting the mask and tracheal intubation difficult include: short, thick, muscular or fat neck with full set of teeth; full beard, facial burns, or facial injuries; receding or malformed jaw; protruding maxillary incisors; poor mandibular (lower jaw) mobility and limited neck extension.

Co-existing injuries such as: known or suspected cervical spine injury, thoracic trauma, skull fractures, scalp lacerations, ocular injuries and airway trauma must be included when planning airway management.

Figure 8-1. Basic Intubation: Initial Blade Position (Macintosh)

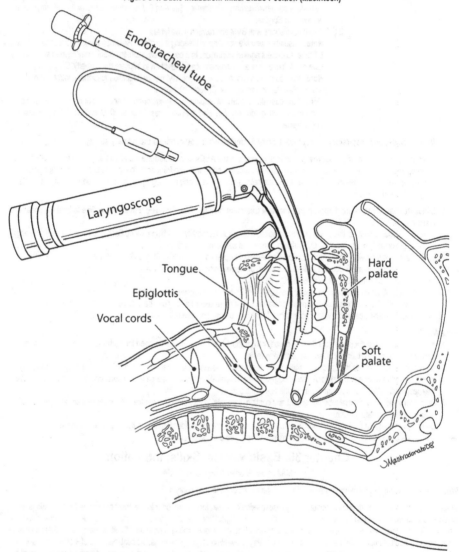

Prepare equipment and patient
1. Gather and check all previously listed equipment for proper function. Check light on laryngoscope, inflate ETT cuff with 5-10cc air and check for leaks, then deflate and leave syringe attached, insert lubricated stylet so that it does not protrude beyond distal end of ETT, bend into hockey stick form, and have suction on.
2. Pre-oxygenate with 100% oxygen for several minutes using BVM.
3. Have assistant hold cricoid pressure if aspiration is a risk.

Intubate the patient and verify adequate oxygenation and ventilation
1. Hold the laryngoscope in left hand and insert the blade on right side of mouth pushing the tongue to the left and avoiding the lips, teeth and tongue. Holding the left wrist rigid (to avoid using the scope as a fulcrum and damaging the teeth), visualize the epiglottis.

2. If a straight (Miller) blade is used, pass the blade tip beneath the laryngeal surface of the epiglottis and lift forward and upward to expose the glottic opening. If a curved (Macintosh) blade is used, advance the tip of the blade into the space between the base of the tongue and the pharyngeal surface of the epiglottis (the vallecula) to expose the glottic opening.

3. Insert the ETT with the right hand through the vocal cords until the cuff disappears. Remove the stylet and slightly advance the tube. Inflate the cuff with air until no leak is heard when ventilated with bag. Adult women need a 7.0mm; men need an 8.0mm ETT.

4. Verify correct placement in 3 breaths: first auscultate the stomach (ruling out esophageal intubation and avoiding insufflation of the stomach), then left lung (ruling out right mainstem intubation – more frequent than a left mainstem), and finally the right lung. You should observe fogging in the ETT on expiration; confirm end-tidal CO_2 present (whenever possible). After appropriate insufflation of the ETT balloon, hold the pilot balloon in one hand and with opposite fingertip, apply repeated pressure to a depth of 1-2cm (ballottement) at the patient's suprasternal notch. This ballottement should be felt in the ETT pilot balloon. This demonstrates location of the balloon past the vocal cords and will minimize a shallow or excessively deep ETT. Note depth of insertion by centimeter markings on the tube at the lips, and tape the tube in place.

5. Ventilate the patient by squeezing the bag steadily over approximately one full second at a rate of 10-12 breaths per minute. This will create a volume of air large enough to cause the chest to rise and provide adequate ventilation. Avoid giving excessive tidal volumes, forcing air too quickly or ventilating too rapidly.

6. Recheck tube placement and confirm adequate oxygenation and ventilation frequently (monitor clinical signs and ventilatory technique). Whenever possible, continuous pulse oximetry and CO_2 monitoring (capnography) should be used to verify adequate oxygenation and ventilation. *See Part 8: Procedures: Chapter 30: Initial Airway Management & Ventilatory Support & Pulse Oximetry Monitoring*

7. For nasotracheal intubation (if no contraindications; see #3 below) when the mouth cannot be opened or the patient cannot be ventilated by another means, or if the patient is conscious and requiring intubation, follow steps 1-3 using a lubricated (water-soluble), size 7-7.5 ET without the stylet. Insert the ETT straight down into the larger nares until it reaches the posterior pharyngeal wall. If doing a blind nasal intubation, listen for the patient to inhale and insert the ETT quickly into the trachea with a single smooth motion. If intubating under direct visualization, insert the blade as previously described and pass the ETT through the cords. Inflate the cuff and verify placement. This technique can be difficult without training. Again, moving to a surgical airway may be the better choice in an emergency.

What Not To Do:

1. Do not mishandle laryngoscope blade and handle. Teeth can be broken and aspirated, or lips or gums lacerated with resultant bleeding. In addition, cardiac arrhythmias can occur with manipulation of the trachea and esophagus.

2. Do not allow the ETT to be moved or removed accidentally. It must be adequately secured after successful placement to avoid compromising respiratory status in order to replace it. Re-verify correct position of tube frequently, especially during and after movement of patient.

3. Do not perform a nasal intubation in a patient with a known or suspected basilar skull fracture or cribriform plate fracture. The ETT can end up in the brain! Never force the ETT against tissue resistance. Bleeding and inflammation can result, making future attempts at intubating difficult or impossible.

4. Be reluctant to intubate a facial trauma patient if they are able to maintain their own airway. They may need to stay seated or lean forward, but lying them flat may cause airway occlusion.

5. Do not forget to adequately ventilate the patient using appropriate technique and available adjuncts (eg, oral airway, nasopharyngeal airway, King LT or ETT). If used correctly (correct volumes, rates, cadence, with a good seal), a BVM can deliver close to 100% oxygen. Constant attention to technique is critical to provide optimal ventilation regardless of the airway used. Avoid giving excessive tidal volumes, forcing air too quickly or ventilating too rapidly. Use pulse oximetry and capnography whenever possible to confirm oxygenation and ventilation.

Chapter 30: Basic Medical Skills: Cricothyroidotomy, Needle and Surgical
Capt Joshua Sill, USAF, MC

What: Two methods to establish a temporary emergency airway through the neck: (1) Needle penetration of the cricothyroid membrane (2) Surgical placement of an airway tube through the cricothyroid membrane when a cricothyroidotomy needle is unavailable or performing a needle cricothyroidotomy is not effective

When: Consider cricothyroidotomy to establish an emergency airway in casualties with a total upper airway obstruction or when inhalation burns or other injuries prevent intubation

What You Need: Gather pre-assembled cricothyroidotomy kit (every medic should have an easily accessible "Cric Kit" that contains all required items) or minimum essential equipment as follows: Cutting instrument: #10 or 11 scalpel, knife blade, 12-14 gauge catheter-over-needle (eg, Angiocath) with 10cc syringe attached for needle cricothyroidotomy. Syringe can also be used to inflate cuff on ET tube (ETT). Airway tube: IV catheter 12-14 gauge, T or Y tube connector (to permit intermittent exhalation), ETT, cannula, or any non-collapsible tube that will allow sufficient airflow to maintain oxygen saturation. In a field setting, an ETT is preferred because it is easy to secure. Use a size 6-7 and ensure that the cuff will hold air. Other instruments: 2 hemostats, needle holder, tissue forceps, scissors. Other supplies: Oxygen source and tubing, Ambu bag, suctioning apparatus, povidone-iodine or chlorhexidine prep, gauze, (sterile) gloves, blanket, silk free ties (for bleeders; size 3-0), 3-0 silk suture material on a cutting needle, and tape.

What To Do: Needle and Surgical Cricothyroidotomy

1. **Preparation**
   a. Place the casualty in the supine position.
   b. Place a blanket or poncho rolled up under the casualty's neck or between the shoulder blades to hyperextend the casualty's neck and straighten the airway. Warning: DO NOT hyperextend the casualty's neck if a cervical injury is suspected.

    c. Assemble needle/syringe set if not already done.

    d. Locate and prep the cricothyroid membrane.

    e. Place a finger of the nondominant hand on the thyroid cartilage (Adam's apple) and slide the finger down to find the cricoid cartilage.

    f. Palpate for the "V" notch of the thyroid cartilage.

    g. Slide the index finger down into the depression between the thyroid and cricoid cartilage, the cricothyroid membrane.

    h. Prep the skin over the membrane with povidone-iodine or chlorhexidine.

    i. Put on gloves (sterile, if available) after assembling equipment and supplies.

2. **Needle Cricothyroidotomy (for percutaneous transtracheal ventilation)** *See Figure 8-2*

    a. Make a small nick in the skin with a #11 blade to open a hole for the IV catheter to slide through the skin

    b. Using the needle/catheter/syringe, penetrate the skin and fascia over the cricothyroid membrane at a 90° angle to the trachea. While applying suction on the syringe, advance the catheter through the cricothyroid membrane.

    c. Once air freely returns into the syringe, STOP advancement, and direct the needle toward the feet at a 45° angle.

    d. Hold the syringe in one hand, and use the other hand to advance the catheter off the needle towards the lower trachea.

    e. Slide the catheter in up to the hub. **Caution:** Do not release the catheter until it is adequately secured into place.

    f. Check for air movement through the catheter by using the syringe to inject air through it and confirm free airflow. If air does not flow freely, straighten the tube and try again or withdraw the catheter and begin again at step 2b.

    g. Use the 3-0 suture to make a stitch through the skin beside the catheter. Secure the catheter to the stitch with several knots.

    h. Connect the catheter (using tubing that has attached to it a T or Y tube connector adequate to provide expiration) to an oxygen source using tube at a flow rate of 15 L/min or 50 psi.

    Note: The passive process of exhalation takes 3-4 times as long as inhalation (with a normal airway). With a smaller opening (as provided here), the process of exhalation takes even longer. Oxygenate the casualty by holding finger over the open T or Y tube and leaving the hole open for exhalation. The appropriate timing for this sequence is approximately 1 second for oxygenation and 4 seconds for exhalation.

        (1) If air flows freely and the patient is breathing on his own, *see Steps 6 and 7* for wound care and on-going management.

        (2) If the patient is NOT breathing on his own, attach the syringe to the catheter, remove the plunger and deliver artificial respirations through the syringe and catheter. If the patient does not recover spontaneous respirations after several minutes, or if oxygen source is not available, proceed to Surgical Cricothyroidotomy.

Figure 8-2. Needle Cricothyroidotomy

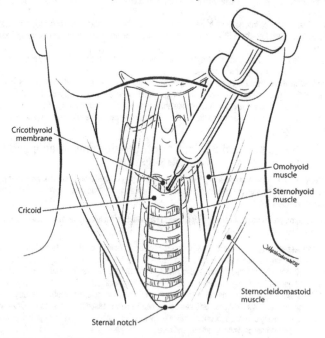

3. **Surgical Cricothyroidotomy** (If needle cricothyroidotomy is not possible or is insufficient) *See Figure 8-3*

    a. Proceed through Step 1 if not already done. Test ETT cuff to ensure it holds air.

    b. Raise the skin to form a tent-like appearance over the cricothyroid space, using the index finger and thumb.

c. With a cutting instrument in the dominant hand, make a 1 inch horizontal incision through the raised skin to the cricothyroid space. **Caution:** Do not cut the cricothyroid membrane with this incision!

d. Relocate the cricothyroid space by touch and sight.

e. Stabilize the larynx with one hand and cut or poke a 1 inch incision through the cricothyroid membrane with the scalpel blade. **Note:** A rush of air may be felt through the opening. Look for bilateral rise and fall of the chest in the spontaneously breathing patient.

f. Insert the ETT or other airway tube through the opening into the trachea at a 90° angle to the trachea. Once in the trachea, direct the tube toward the feet at a 45° angle. Do NOT insert an ETT or other long airway more than 3-4 inches to avoid intubating a single bronchus. Inflate the ETT cuff, if applicable. Do NOT release the airway tube until it is secured (instructions to follow).

g. Connect the Ambu bag to the tube and inflate the lungs, or have someone perform mouth to tube respirations. Auscultate the abdomen and both lung fields. The presence of bilateral breath sounds, bilateral rise and fall of the chest, lack of breath sounds in the stomach, and fog in the ET tube all indicate correct tube placement. If available, attach a colorimetric capnography filter to the ET tube. A change in color from purple to yellow indicates the presence of carbon dioxide, suggesting correct tube placement. If the tube has been placed properly, secure it in place. If not, reposition the tube as follows until adequate placement is obtained:

   (1) Unilateral breath sounds and unilateral rise and fall of the chest indicate that the tube is past the carina. Deflate the cuff on the ETT, retract the tube 1-2 inches, inflate the ETT cuff, and recheck air exchange and placement.

   (2) Air coming out of the casualty's mouth indicates that the tube is pointed away from the lungs. Deflate the cuff on the ETT, remove the tube, reinsert, inflate the cuff and recheck for air exchange and placement.

   (3) Any other problem indicates tube is not in the trachea. Deflate the cuff on the ETT, remove the tube, reinsert, inflate the cuff and recheck for air exchange and placement.

h. If air flows freely, and the patient is breathing on his own, proceed to next step. If the patient is NOT breathing on his own, continue providing respirations via the Ambu bag with oxygen (if available), or via mouth to tube assistance at the rate of 20/min.

i. Secure the airway tube using tape (temporary), or use the 3-0 suture to make a stitch through the skin beside the tube. Secure the tube to the stitch with several knots.

j. Suction the casualty's airway, as necessary. Insert the suction catheter 4-5 inches into the tube. Apply suction only while withdrawing the catheter. Administer 1cc of saline solution into the airway to loosen secretions and help facilitate suctioning. **Note:** Ventilate the casualty several times or allow him to take several breaths between suctioning

4. **Apply a dressing to further protect the tube or catheter and incision using one of these techniques:**
   a. Cut two 4x4s or 4x8s halfway through. Place them on opposite sides of the tube so that the tube comes up through the cut and the gauze overlaps. Tape securely.
   b. Apply a sterile dressing under the casualty's tube by making a V-shaped fold in a 4 x 8 gauze pad and placing it under the edge of the catheter to prevent irritation to the casualty. Tape securely.

5. **Monitor casualty's respirations on a regular basis.**
   a. Reassess air exchange and placement every time the casualty is moved.
   b. Assist respirations if respiratory rate falls below 10 or rises above 20 per minute.

What Not To Do:
   1. Do not remove needle before advancing the catheter into trachea. (NEEDLE Cricothyroidotomy)
   2. Do not forget to ensure that the tube is correctly placed, and secured. (SURGICAL Cricothyroidotomy)
   3. Do not fail to monitor.

Chapter 30: Basic Medical Skills: Thoracostomy, Needle and Chest Tube

MAJ Karin Nicholson, MC, USA

What: Emergency management of tension pneumothorax, simple pneumothorax (if required, eg, prior to aeromedical evacuation) and hemothorax.

When: A needle thoracostomy can be performed faster than a tube thoracostomy in a rapidly deteriorating patient having signs of a tension pneumothorax. This can be life saving and gives enough relief to provide time for the medic to insert a chest tube. Once the chest tube is properly inserted, remove the needle.

What You Need: 10-14 gauge 3.25 inch needle w/catheter, 10-20cc syringe, sterile saline, alcohol pads, povidone-iodine or chlorhexidine, latex sterile gloves, assorted chest tubes (sizes 28-32 French [F] for adult pending air evacuation, 36-40 F for adult with hemothorax, 12-14 F for children), water seal drainage system (eg, Pleur-Evac) and connection tubing for suction (alternate: one-way valve made from finger of latex glove), instruments: scalpel, forceps, gauze (may be in prepared tray), **lidocaine** 1-2 % without epinephrine, petrolatum gauze, external dressing (4x4), adhesive tape, and pulse oximetry.

What To Do: Determine which lung has the pneumothorax! Ensure that the procedure is performed on the side suspected of having a pneumothorax (tension pneumothorax, simple pneumothorax, hemothorax), which will be the lung without breath sounds. Hyper-resonance is also a helpful sign but the lack of breath sounds after penetrating or blunt trauma is a definitive sign.

Figure 8-3. Surgical Cricothyroidotomy

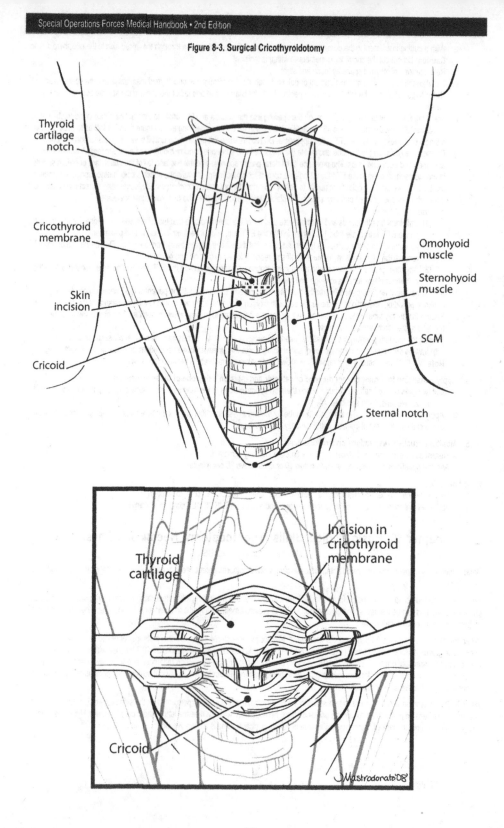

Needle Thoracostomy:
1. Prep the chest wall by pouring povidone-iodine or chlorhexidine over the intended site or swab with povidone-iodine or chlorhexidine wipe.
2. Insert a 10-14 gauge 3.25 inch needle w/catheter into the 2nd intercostal space, along the midclavicular line (an imaginary line from the middle of the collarbone, or clavicle; the interspace immediately below the clavicle is the 1st interspace). Run your finger down the midclavicular line, over the 2nd rib, to the 2nd intercostal space. Insert the IV catheter immediately above the 3rd rib.
3. When the pressure built up in the pleural space is released, there will be a rush of air. Advance the catheter up to the hub, then remove the needle stylette and discard. The patient's ability to spontaneously breathe usually improves immediately. Leave the catheter in place, and attach a 3-way stopcock, which can be used to drain air as it accumulates.
4. This can improve the patient's symptoms and be life saving. Primarily, it is fast and easy to perform, providing enough time for the medic to set up for inserting a chest tube. The life-threatening emergency is the tension pneumothorax, not the simple pneumothorax that remains.
5. Once the chest tube is properly inserted, the catheter can be removed.
Alternative Technique: Remove the plunger from a 10-20cc syringe filled with sterile saline, attach a 10-14 gauge 3.25 inch needle w/catheter and use it to perform the thoracostomy. This allows handling of the needle/IV catheter more precisely and provides visual "bubbles" when the trapped air is released into the syringe. This is helpful in a noisy environment. Once the catheter is placed and the needle removed, setup for chest tube can begin. If the location is not safe for the 2nd procedure, leave the catheter in place, attach a 3-way stopcock to drain air as it accumulates, cover the catheter with gauze and tape, and move to a secure location for the procedure.

Tube Thoracostomy: Setup for a tube thoracostomy is more labor intensive than for a needle thoracostomy. Perform a tube thoracostomy after or in lieu of a needle thoracostomy to treat a simple pneumothorax (required prior to air evacuation).
1. Prep the chest wall by pouring povidone-iodine or chlorhexidine over the intended site.
2. Site of insertion: along the mid-axillary line (a line running straight down from the middle of the armpit); always above the level of nipples in males (5th intercostal space since below this level there is a risk of puncturing the diaphragm).
3. Infiltrate 1% **lidocaine** along the track to be used. Generally, the tube is placed in the 3rd to 5th intercostal space on the mid-axillary line.
4. Cut a 3cm long incision on top of the rib, NOT in the intercostal space. Cut along the axis of the rib, down to the bone, crossing the mid-axillary line.
5. Insert a large curved hemostat (Kelly clamp) with the curve pointed toward the ribs and create a tunnel over the top of the rib. This tunnel helps to stabilize and seal the chest tube after placement. Curve the clamp over the top of the rib. Advance it slowly, opening and closing the jaws of the hemostat to clear a path and then puncture into the thoracic cavity. Do not advance straight in.
6. Digitally explore the pleural space to remove any pleural adhesions and ensure the lung is free to fall away from the chest wall.
7. Have chest tube ready. Use size 28-32 French for adult pending air evacuation, 36-40 F for adult with hemothorax, 12-14 F for children. When in doubt, use a larger size because it will allow drainage of either air or blood from the chest cavity. Grasp the tube between the jaws of the clamp and insert into the pleural space. Direct the clamp tip posterior, towards the apex and the spine. Make sure that the tube is completely inserted so that no holes are left outside the chest.
8. Connect the free end of the chest tube to an underwater seal drainage system (Pleur-Evac), and then suture into place with nylon 2-0. If an underwater seal drainage system is unavailable, make a field expedient version by securing the free end of the tube in a container of water that is lower than the level of the inserted end of the tube. *See Part 8: Procedures: Chapter 31: Chest Tube\Drainage System.* This system prevents the patient drawing air back into the chest cavity. Bubbles coming out of the free end of the tube are a positive sign, indicating that the patient is expelling free air.
9. In emergency conditions, use a 1-way Heimlich valve instead. Cut a finger off of a latex glove. Fasten it as air-tight as possible over the end of the tube: insert the free end of the chest tube inside the open end of the glove finger and tape the glove finger around the tube. Cut a 2cm slit in the closed end of the glove finger. This will allow air to escape, but the glove finger will collapse on inspiration and prevent air from entering the lung. This will also collect blood draining from the chest tube.
10. Place Vaseline-impregnated gauze around the tube at the incision site, cover over that with 4x4 gauze and tape in place. The Vaseline gauze will prevent air leaks.
11. If the patient's condition does not improve, or deteriorates, the placement of the tube is suspect and it should be checked thoroughly for proper placement, or repositioned.
12. Other considerations: Antibiotics: Give **ceftriaxone** 1g IM or IV q12-24h or similar broad-spectrum antibiotic for all chest tubes inserted in the field.

What Not To Do:
1. Do not insert a chest tube if a tension pneumothorax is suspected and the patient is rapidly deteriorating; perform a needle thoracostomy instead for rapid relief.
2. Do not reposition or remove and replace a suspect tube if the patient shows signs of a repeat tension pneumothorax. Perform a 2nd needle thoracentesis, and then insert a 2nd chest tube above or below the original tube.

Chapter 30: Basic Medical Skills: Pulse Oximetry Monitoring
CPT James Woodrow, MC, USA & MAJ Christopher Lettieri, MC, USA

What: Assess oxygen saturation using a pulse oximetry device. Pulse oximeters estimate the percentage of hemoglobin molecules that are carrying oxygen (oxygenated blood – bright red; poorly oxygenated – dark red), by measuring the transmission of red and infrared light through arterial beds. Hemoglobin absorbs red and infrared light waves differently when it is bound with oxygen (oxyhemoglobin) versus when it is not (deoxyhemoglobin). Oxyhemoglobin preferentially absorbs infrared rather than red light and reduced hemoglobin absorbs more red than infrared light. Pulse oximetry reveals arterial saturation by measuring this difference. The pulse oximeter probe contains a sensor and a light source, and is usually packaged in a clip or flat wrap that can be attached to a source of good capillary perfusion. One side (light source) emits wavelengths of light into the arterial bed and the other side (sensor) detects the presence of red or infrared light.

When: There are 3 major reasons to use pulse oximetry:
1. Measure arterial oxygen saturation to determine need for supplemental oxygen
2. Monitor oxygenation saturation in risk of respiratory compromise
3. Monitor pulse rate

What You Need: Commercial pulse oximeters (and extra batteries). Two oximeters and a back-up with additional batteries are recommended.

What to Do:
1. Understand the principles of pulse oximetry
2. Select a site(s): The probe is normally placed on the finger or toe of an uninjured limb in an adult, or on the ear of an infant or small child. A second oximeter may be useful.
3. Understand readings for pulse oximetry:
   a. Normal SaO_2 (oxygen saturation of hemoglobin) is 93% or greater.
   b. SaO_2 below 90% indicates insufficient oxygenation of the blood.
   Note: These patients need supplemental oxygen, evaluation and improvement of ventilation or both.
4. Recognize that certain poisons (eg, carbon monoxide [carboxyhemoglobin] or nitrite [methemoglobin]) can displace oxygen, saturate hemoglobin and produce FALSE normal pulse oximetry readings.
5. Record all findings in the patient's medical record.

What Not To Do:
Do not fail to recognize the following conditions that commonly cause false readings:
Ambient light on the oximeter probe
Presence of specific substances that falsely elevate SaO_2
Carbon monoxide (carboxyhemoglobin)
Nitrites, chloroquine, sulfonamides (methemoglobin)
Conditions that increase vasoconstriction of capillary beds
Hypotension
Hypothermia
Patient's use of vasoconstrictive drugs
Nail polish
Jaundice
Very dark pigmented skin (choose area that has less pigment – finger tips, toes, etc.)

Chapter 30: Basic Medical Skills: Exhaled Carbon Dioxide Detection

MAJ George Lantz, MC, USA

When: You need to determine that the endotracheal tube (ETT) has been placed in the trachea. Look for color change in the end tidal carbon dioxide (CO_2) detector (generally yellow to purple with CO_2 present, but ensure by checking package insert). **Note:** Proper positioning of the distal portion of the ETT for "placement" must still be assessed.

What You Need: An intubated patient, an end tidal carbon dioxide detector, and a controlled bag ventilation apparatus (if the patient requires manual ventilation). This is part of almost all emergency airway kits.

What To Do:
Note: The patient has been intubated.
1. Understand the operation of end tidal carbon dioxide detectors.
   a. The carbon dioxide detector contains a chemical indicator which is sensitive to the exhaled carbon dioxide.
   b. After the detector is attached to the ETT, the color of the indicator changes during exhalation due to an elevated carbon dioxide level.
2. Connect the end tidal carbon dioxide detector to the end of the ETT.
   a. The detector is a flow through device.
   b. One end is designed to attach to the connector of the ETT. Securely attach the device.
   c. The other end of the device is identical to the ETT connector such that all standard oxygen delivery/ventilation equipment can be attached.
   d. It may be left in place without interfering with the flow of oxygen during manual or mechanical ETT ventilation. **Note:** The color change duration will not be infinite.
3. Assess ETT placement with the carbon dioxide detector.
   a. In patients with an ETT in the trachea, you will see a continued color change in the device during exhalation.
   b. In patients with an ETT in the esophagus, you will not see a continued color change in the device during exhalation.
   Note: With very low cardiac output states or during ineffective CPR, there may be no color change in the carbon dioxide detector, even though the ETT is in the trachea (as poor cardiac output means little carbon dioxide carrying blood is returning to the lungs for exhalation).

What Not To Do:
Do not fail to recognize the absence of color change. This means that either the tube is not in the trachea, or that the patient is potentially intubated, but in such a severe medical condition that there is insufficient circulation of blood flow through the lungs to provide carbon dioxide for exhalation and monitoring.

1. Reevaluate and/or re-insert ETT. This should be done by the most experienced medical provider present. Correlate breath sounds, chest rise and fall, or manual/controlled ventilation with color change, or lack thereof in the carbon dioxide detector.
2. Packages not freshly opened or previously exposed to air may not show a color change. Inspect the packaging for damage and ensure that the detector has not expired.

Chapter 30: Basic Medical Skills: ECG: Three-Electrode Rhythm Tracings

BG Joseph Caravalho, Jr., MC, USA

What: Guidelines on preparing for and conducting an electrocardiogram (ECG) using only three electrodes.

When: A 3-electrode tracing is used to monitor the heart solely for dysrhythmia. The following information can be obtained from using Lead II: Rate (how fast the heart is beating electrically; rhythm; and intervals (ie, the pulses' conduction times). The following information cannot be obtained from using Lead II: The presence or location of an infarct; axis deviation or chamber enlargement; right-to-left differences in the conduction impulse formation; or the quality or presence of pumping action. 12-lead ECGs are used for diagnostic purposes. Single-lead rhythm tracings may be used to monitor rhythm disturbances over time. Used to diagnose metabolic and toxic disorders of the heart. (eg, high potassium, low calcium, toxic quinidine or digoxin), chamber enlargement (eg, ventricular and atrial enlargement), acute myocardial infarction (MI) and myocardial ischemia (MI or angina), or dysrhythmias and conduction system abnormalities (eg, bundle branch blocks seen in Chagas' cardiomyopathy). Monitor: Course and effect of therapeutic changes made in any of the conditions mentioned previously.

What You Need: A cardiac monitor/defibrillator, ECG paper, electrodes, heart rate calculator ruler, alcohol prep pads, drapes, and tape

What To Do:
1. Prepare the equipment
   a. Read the manufacturer's instructions for proper use, if not familiar with the equipment
   b. Plug the machine into a grounded wall outlet
   c. Turn the power switch ON and allow the machine to perform its self-check
   d. Check the machine's graph paper supply
   e. Verify that the machine is set on the standard settings: paper speed at 25 mm/sec; amplitude at 10 mm/mV
   f. Verify that all other equipment is on hand: Electrodes, alcohol pads, drapes or towels
2. Ensure the area is:
   a. Free from electrical interference
   b. Comfortable and private for the patient
   c. Free from distractions (noise, traffic)
3. Prepare the patient
   a. Explain the procedure to the patient and answer any questions. Many patients will be apprehensive about being connected to an electrical instrument. Reassure the patient that there is no danger and they will feel no pain.
   b. Ask (or assist) the patient to remove all clothing from the waist up. Provide a chest drape for female patients.
   c. Ask (or assist) the patient to lie supine on the bed or examination table. (Note: Patients with respiratory problems may be unable to tolerate the supine position. If necessary, elevate the head of the bed to 45°.) Caution: When necessary, ensure the patient's IV tubing and/or urinary catheter tubing is handled with care and positioned properly to avoid discomfort to the patient.
   d. Ensure the patient's body is not in contact with the bed frame or any metal objects and that all limbs are firmly supported.
   e. Ask the patient to relax and breathe normally throughout the procedure
4. Apply the electrodes
   a. Clean the sites for electrode placement by rubbing with an alcohol prep pad to remove dead skin, oils, and traces of soap or dirt.
   b. Attach the electrodes, being careful to place them over muscle and not directly over bone
      (1) Attach the white electrode to the right deltoid
      (2) Attach the black electrode to the left deltoid
      (3) Attach the red electrode to the left leg
   c. Obtain a rhythm strip for Lead II
5. Interpret whether the rhythm strip is normal or abnormal
   a. Step 1: Determine whether the rate is normal. Compare to pulse found on patient.
      (1) Six-second method
         (a) Count the number of R-waves in a 6-second interval by noting two 3-second marks at the top of the ECG paper
         (b) Multiply the number of R-waves within the 6-second strip by 10, which will give the heart rate per minute
      (2) Triplicate method
         (a) Locate 2 R-waves that fall on dark lines on the graph paper.
         (b) Assign numbers corresponding to the heart rate to successive dark lines starting with the dark line on which the first R-wave fell.
         (c) The order is 300, 150, 100, 75, 60, 50, and so forth. The assigned numbers are a result of dividing 300 by 1, 2, 3, 4, 5, 6, and so forth.
         (d) The number corresponding to the line where the 2nd R-wave falls is the pulse. Normal rate is considered 60-100 bpm, although some fit individuals will have resting rates down into the 40s.
   b. Step 2: Determine if the rhythm is regular (P-wave and QRS complexes occur at regular intervals). R-waves fall on top of each other when the ECG paper is folded in half and held it up to the light. Not regular is abnormal.
   c. Step 3: Analyze the P-wave. Determine whether there is a P-wave for every QRS complex, the P-waves are upright, and they are regular and similar in appearance. Any "NO" is abnormal. **Note:** 12-lead ECG criteria for ST segment changes cannot be applied to rhythm tracings
   d. Step 4: See Part 4: Organ Systems: Chapter 1: Acute Coronary Syndrome (Acute Myocardial Infarction and Unstable Angina) &

Cardiac Resuscitation and ACLS guidelines, for further discussion of management of selected abnormalities. Stabilize patient based on current ACLS guidelines and evacuate the patient.

What Not To Do:

Do not treat a rhythm tracing. Always treat the patient. Does the information from the tracing correlate to the patient? Example: When a rhythm looks like atrial fibrillation, feel the patient's pulse. If it is regular and full, then the information from the tracing "does not correlate," and is in error.

Chapter 30: Basic Medical Skills: Pericardiocentesis

BG Joseph Caravalho, Jr., MC, USA

What: Mechanism to relieve fluid or air inside the sac surrounding the heart.

When: The patient has sustained a penetrating wound in the chest that may have entered the heart covering (pericardium), and is showing the signs of shock-hypotension, tachycardia, and tachypnea with narrowed pulse pressure, muffled heart sounds, pulsus paradoxus. Pulsus paradoxus is an abnormally large inspiratory decline in systemic arterial pressure (greater than 10mmHg drop in SBP during inspiration) that results in a narrowed pulse pressure (ie, difference between systolic and diastolic pressures). This abnormality occurs during forced respiratory effort, heart failure, pericardial tamponade, severe asthma, hypovolemia, and mechanical ventilation. Pericardiocentesis is dangerous and potentially life-threatening, if not done correctly. The SOF medic should not attempt this procedure without prior training, and then only as a last resort in an attempt to save the patient's life. If vital signs are stable, the SOF medic should continue IV fluids and patient monitoring only. Of note, pericardiocentesis can also be used to treat life-threatening causes of pericardial tamponade (serous fluid in viral pericarditis; air in diving-related pneumopericardium).

What You Need: 18 gauge spinal needle or pericardiocentesis kit with Mansfield catheter, a 60cc syringe, sterile preparation kit (alcohol wipe may be adequate in emergencies), local anesthetic, sterile needles, 3-way stopcock, alligator clips, ECG monitor, gauze pads/bandage. Emergency drugs (**atropine, lidocaine, epinephrine,** oxygen)

What To Do:

Preparation:
1. Have the patient lie supine.
2. Administer oxygen (nasal cannula or face mask) and attach pulse oximeter if available.
3. Start an IV since volume loading may help attenuate the effects of cardiac tamponade.
4. Set up ECG machine to monitor the cardiac rhythm.
5. Clean subxiphoid area with antiseptic

Procedure:

Option A: Emergency Technique to Withdraw Fluid Once
1. Connect 18 gauge spinal needle and 60cc syringe
2. Place your finger 0.5cm below the patient's xiphoid to mark the point of needle insertion. Raise the needle to a 30° angle from parallel to the patient's chest. Aim the needle at the tip of the left scapula.
3. Insert the needle, maintaining slight suction and advance until blood flow is obtained, and then stop advancement.
4. Withdraw as much blood as possible and then remove the needle. Even removing a small amount (5-10cc) can have a marked improvement in vital signs, indicating that the constricting pressure around the heart has been relatively decreased.

Option B: Technique to Withdraw Fluid Multiple Times
1. Attach a central line needle and catheter to a 60cc syringe.
2. Follow the procedure as outlined previously.
3. When fluid is obtained, hold the syringe and needle in one hand, and gently advance (slide) the catheter into the pericardial space. Withdraw the needle from the catheter.
4. Attach the 3-way stopcock (closed position) to the hub of the catheter.
5. Remove the needle from the syringe and discard. Connect one end of IV tubing to one port of the 3-way stopcock, the other end of the IV tubing attach to a 60cc syringe (optional to connect another IV line to the third port of the stopcock for ejecting blood from the syringe).
6. Open the 3-way stopcock to the syringe to withdraw fluid from the pericardial space, and then turn open to ejection port IV line to eject the fluid out.
7. When no further fluid/blood returns, turn the 3-way stopcock to closed or in-between position. The catheter can be left in if the SOF medic has a catheter line that can be switched between the closed and open positions.

Option C: Technique to Monitor Needle Approach with ECG Lead (use with both option A & B) to Withdraw Fluid Multiple Times
1. Connect V1 lead of 12-lead ECG with an alligator clip to the metallic hub of the needle or needle stylet of the catheter, then insert needle as directed previously.
2. During the advancement of the needle, monitor the ECG for ST segment elevation. This indicates that the needle tip is in contact with myocardium and should be withdrawn slightly.
3. This monitoring improves the safety of the procedure, but is not practical in immediate life-and-death field scenarios.

Post-Procedure:
1. Monitor for pneumothorax and dysrhythmias
2. Collect samples of pericardial fluid (in cases not related to penetrating trauma) for later analysis.

What Not To Do:
1. Do not insert the needle more than 1/8 of an inch once blood is obtained.
2. Do not "jiggle" the syringe. Small movements of the syringe can have large effects on movement of the tip of the needle causing lacerations of the myocardium or coronary arteries.

Chapter 30: Basic Medical Skills: Pneumatic Anti-Shock Garment

COL Clifford Cloonan, MC, USA (Ret)

What: Apply pneumatic antishock garments (PASG), also known as Medical or Military Anti-Shock Trousers (MAST)

When: To control otherwise uncontrollable, on-going hemorrhage in the lower abdomen/pelvis and/or buttocks/thigh(s) (used as a device to tamponade bleeding); neurogenic shock (especially when unable to avoid a head-up attitude, eg, during extraction/evacuation) and anaphylactic shock (used as a device to supplement other measures to raise/maintain BP); pelvic fracture, femur/tibia fracture when traction splint not available (used as a pneumatic splint). **Note:** PASG should not to be used for treatment of hemorrhagic shock, particularly when there is on-going, uncontrolled/uncontrollable bleeding.

What You Need: Pneumatic Anti-Shock Garment

What To Do:
1. Apply the garment – there are various methods to do this (follow manufacturer recommendations/ATLS guidelines).
2. Inflate garment, legs first, then abdominal compartment, until Velcro on the suit begins to crackle (indicating that separation is imminent), and/or bleeding is controlled and/or fracture(s) is/are adequately stabilized.
3. If applying a PASG that has a pressure gauge that measures the pressure inside the PASG, it is essential that this pressure not be used as an end-point for inflation. This pressure gauge should only be used to allow the care provider to maintain a constant PASG inflation pressure despite changes in altitude and/or temperature.
4. PASG should only be applied as a temporizing measure and not as a substitute for other interventions.
5. If the patient has on-going bleeding, rapid evacuation for surgical stabilization is indicated.

What Not To Do:

Absolute Contraindication to application of PASG
Pulmonary edema/congestive heart failure/cardiogenic shock: The increased peripheral vascular resistance which PASG produces increases the work of the heart and will worsen these conditions.

Relative Contraindications to application of PASG
Head injury/cerebrovascular accident: Use of PASG will increase intracranial pressure. Severe and uncontrollable bleeding above the diaphragm: The possibility exists of increasing intrathoracic bleeding as the BP increases.
Ruptured diaphragm: Inflation of the abdominal compartment of the PASG will force abdominal contents into the chest cavity.
Third trimester pregnancy: Do not inflate abdominal compartment.
Impaled object in the abdomen: Do not inflate abdominal compartment.
Do not remove PASG until patient is in a location where his underlying problem can be fully addressed (ie, surgery).
Premature removal of the PASG can lead to severe hypotension. When the decision is made to deflate the PASG, slowly deflate the garment, abdominal compartment first, then legs, until the systolic BP drops by 5mmHg. Then discontinue deflation and provide fluid replacement until the pressure is restored. Repeat these steps until deflation is complete. Circumstances may require a more rapid deflation but this should only be done in the OR when the surgeon and the anesthetist/anesthesiologist are fully prepared to deal with the consequences.

Note: Treatment of hypovolemic/hemorrhagic shock by applying PASG has fallen into such disfavor that it is not recommended for this application any more. There are good reasons, however for continuing to recommend its use in combat situations, specifically for use in stabilizing pelvic fractures and to tamponade bleeding in the pelvis, buttocks, and/or groin/upper thigh where a tourniquet cannot be applied to control hemorrhage.

Chapter 30: Basic Medical Skills: Blood Transfusion

COL Richard Tenglin, MC, USA (Ret)

When: You have a trauma patient who may require a transfusion in a medical facility with blood replacement capability. You must correctly assess the trauma patient to determine whether or not he requires blood replacement and if he does, what those requirements are.

What You Need:
1. A thermometer, blood pressure cuff, stethoscope, IV stand, tourniquet, large bore IV catheters, tape, alcohol and povidone-iodine prep pads, Vacutainers, needle and syringe, gloves, crystalloids, and the patient's clinical record.
2. 2 large bore IVs already established and the following materials, blood transfusion recipient set ("Y" type), 500mL or 1000mL bag of 0.9% normal saline, blood, IV stand, needle and syringe.

What To Do:
1. Perform a survey of the casualty to ensure airway stabilization, adequate respirations, and hemorrhage control.
   a. Establish 2 large bore (18 gauge or larger) IV lines.
      (1) Draw blood.
      (2) Request and/or perform labs, H/H with type and crossmatch.
   b. Initiate IV fluids for resuscitation. Give Ringer's lactate as a 1st choice, normal saline as a 2nd choice.
      Note: The usual initial volume for resuscitation is 1-2L in an adult and 20mL/kg in pediatric cases. Other diagnostic decisions are based on the observed response.

     c. Establish a set of baseline vital signs.

     d. Perform other resuscitative procedures as required: ABCs and secondary survey.

2. Monitor patient and determine if patient requires blood transfusion:

     a. Indications that patient does not require a blood transfusion:

         (1) Stable vital signs within normal limits, Class I or Class II shock.

         (2) Patients who have lost less than 20% of their blood volume and are no longer hemorrhaging require no further fluid bolus or immediate blood administration.

         (3) H/H within normal limits.

         Caution: With rapid blood loss, H/H will lag behind actual blood volume. Infusion of crystalloid may further "dilute" the blood, and cause a further drop in hemoglobin/hematocrit.

     b. Indications for blood transfusion:

         (1) Vital signs not stable; patient in Class III shock

         (2) Patients who have lost 20%-40% of their blood volume and are still hemorrhaging will show marked deterioration. Continued fluid therapy and blood replacement are indicated.

         (3) Patients with little or no response to the initial fluid therapy.

         (4) H/H below normal.

         Note: Isovolemic patients can have adequate oxygen carrying capacity with Hb levels as low as 4g/dL, especially if young, healthy and at rest.

3. Determine the type of blood to give to the patient. (Type Specific or Universal Donor - O Negative) **Note:** Response to blood administration should identify patients that are still bleeding and require rapid surgical intervention.

     a. Select the appropriate blood type based on the type and crossmatch and the types of blood available.

     b. Ideally, the patient should receive the same type of blood that they have.

     c. In urgent situations, type O RBCs may be used for patients of other blood types, and either A or B RBCs may be used for AB recipients (but not both together).

     d. Rh-negative patients should always receive Rh-negative blood except in life-threatening emergencies when Rh-negative blood may be unavailable.

     e. Rh-positive patients may receive either Rh-positive or Rh-negative blood.

4. Select the appropriate blood component, if available:

     a. Whole blood: used for rapid massive blood loss. May be necessary if packed red cells are unavailable

     b. Packed RBCs: also used for rapid massive blood loss. Packed RBCs are preferred due to the lower chance of complications.

         (1) Transfused to replace Hb or O_2 carrying capacity, including blood lost at surgery or as a result of trauma.

         (2) Consider the patient's age, cause, degree of anemia, circulatory stability and the condition of heart, lungs, and blood vessels.

         (3) When volume expansion is required, other fluids can be used concurrently or separately.

     c. Fresh frozen plasma is an unconcentrated source of clotting factors except platelets.

         (1) Used to correct a bleeding tendency of unknown cause or one associated with liver failure, or from dilution from large volume transfusion.

     d. Washed RBCs (by continuous-flow washing) are free of almost all traces of plasma, most WBCs, and platelets. Used for patients who are hypersensitive to plasma or who have severe reactions to plasma (eg, severe allergies or IgA immunization).

5. Determine the amount of blood to administer:

     a. Blood is usually replaced until the patient has been stabilized and the reason(s) for transfusion no longer exist.

     b. Stabilization of adequate vital signs is primary indicator of sufficient blood volume.

6. Order type specific or type O blood based on the type and crossmatch.

7. Verify and inspect the blood pack received from the laboratory for abnormalities such as gas bubbles or black or gray colored sediment (indicative of bacterial growth):

     a. Note the time the blood pack was received and record the time.

     b. Check the label for blood components, type, and expiration dates. **Notes:** Two people, if possible, should independently verify the information match of type and crossmatch patient to label. Infusion of a blood pack should be started within 30 minutes of being issued.

8. Establish baseline data:

     a. Reconfirm data from the patient's history regarding allergies or previous reactions to blood or blood products.

     b. Measure and evaluate the vital signs.

     c. Record the vital signs on the chart.

9. Reduce the chances of reactions by applying prophylactic measures:

     a. Meticulous identification and clear labeling at the bedside of casualty's blood samples intended for compatibility testing.

     b. Ensure that blood has been screened for hepatitis, HIV, malaria, and syphilis.

     c. Carefully identify casualty and donor blood at the time of transfusion.

         (1) Identify casualty by ID tags, ID bracelet, or other means.

         (2) Identify the donor blood and have a second person check the blood and the casualty, if possible.

     d. Handle blood products with care to prevent hemolysis or destruction of RBCs.

         (1) Use of microwave ovens to warm blood is contraindicated.

         (2) Use an IV set that includes a heat exchange device, if available, to warm blood gently (but not >37°C) during delivery.

     e. Prevent contact with inappropriate IV solutions such as injections of distilled water or non-isotonic solution.

     f. **Diphenhydramine** 25-50mg po or IV and **acetaminophen** (if no liver disease) 650mg po may decrease the chance of febrile reaction to transfused blood. They will not prevent severe allergic reactions or prevent major hemolytic transfusion reactions.

g. In cases where volume overload is possible, **furosemide**, or another diuretic may need to be given during, or between, transfusions. A rise in venous pressure can be avoided by infusing RBCs at a slow-to-moderate rate. The patient should be observed for signs of increased venous pressure or pulmonary congestion. If possible, direct observation of venous pressure during the infusion is a useful precaution.

h. Administer the first 10-30mL over 15 min, while observing the patient for reactions.

i. Use transfusion sets that include a filter to trap the clots and fibrin shreds present in stored blood units.

j. Use microaggregate filters is available.

k. Guard against the introduction of air into the tubing, though a small amount of air that get infused is unlikely to be of clinical significance and efforts to remove small amounts of air results in manipulation of the IV system that may result in contamination.

Caution: Consult manufacturer's instructions. Microaggregates can be detected in the lungs after massive transfusions and have been implicated as a cause of the syndrome of posttraumatic pulmonary insufficiency, though direct evidence is lacking.

10. Prepare the blood and the blood recipient set:

Note: Use only tubing that is designed for the administration of blood products. It is equipped with a filter designed for the fine filtration required for blood products. If "Y" type recipient tubing is not available, use regular infusion tubing for the normal saline (0.9% normal saline only) and the available blood recipient tubing for the blood pack. Prime each set. Attach a sterile, large bore (16 or 18 gauge) needle to the end of the blood tubing and "piggyback" the blood into the normal saline line below the level of the roller clamp. Hang the blood pack at least 6 inches higher than the normal saline.

a. Close all 3 clamps on the "Y" tubing.

b. Aseptically insert one of the tubing spikes into the container of normal saline. Invert and hang this container about 3 feet above the level of the patient.

c. Open the clamp on the normal saline line and prime the upper line and the blood filter.

d. Open the clamp on the empty line on which you will eventually hang the blood. Normal saline will flow up the empty line to prime that portion of the tubing.

e. Once the blood line is primed with saline, close the clamp on the blood line.

f. Leave the clamp on the normal saline line open.

g. Open the main roller clamp to prime the lower infusion tubing.

h. Close the main roller clamp.

i. Aseptically expose the blood port on the blood pack.

j. Aseptically insert the remaining spike into the blood port and hang the blood at the same level as the normal saline container.

11. Connect the bloodline:

a. Patients receiving blood should have 2 patent IV sites in the event of complications or emergencies. Establish 1-2 new IV sites as needed.

(1) Use a large gauge IV catheter (14, 16, or 18) to enhance the flow of blood and prevent hemolysis of the cells.

b. If the patient already has 2 IV sites, aseptically switch the blood line with one of the existing IV lines or piggyback the blood line into an existing IV line.

12. Begin the infusion of blood:

a. Attach the primed infusion set to the catheter, tape it securely, and open the main roller clamp.

b. Close the roller clamp to the normal saline and open the roller clamp to the blood.

c. Adjust the flow rate with the main roller clamp.

(1) Set the flow rate to deliver approximately 10-30cc of blood over the first 15 minutes.

(2) Monitor the vital signs every 5 minutes for the first 15 minutes and observe for indications of an adverse reaction to the blood.

(3) If after the first 15 minutes, no adverse reaction is suspected and the vital signs are stable, set the main roller clamp to deliver the prescribed flow rate.

Note: Prolonged transfusions pose a hazard of bacterial growth because blood quickly reaches room temperature.

13. Monitor and evaluate the patient throughout the procedure.

a. Monitor vital signs every 15 minutes or IAW local SOP.

b. Compare the vital signs with previous and baseline vital signs.

c. Observe for changes that indicate an adverse reaction to the blood.

d. If a reaction is suspected, stop the blood, infuse normal saline, and identify and treat the reaction *IAW Part 8: Procedure: Chapter 30: Blood Transfusion Reactions.*

Caution: When a transfusion reaction occurs or is suspected, stop the blood immediately and infuse normal saline. The unused blood and recipient tubing must be sent to the laboratory along with a 10mL specimen of the patient's venous blood and a post-transfusion urine specimen.

14. Discontinue the infusion of blood when the patient's vital signs have stabilized or the transfusion is finished.

a. Close the clamp to the blood and open the clamp to the normal saline.

b. Flush the tubing and filter with approximately 50cc of normal saline to deliver the residual blood.

c. After the residual blood has been delivered, run the normal saline at a TKO rate or hang another solution, as needed.

d. Take and record the vital signs at the completion of the transfusion and 1 hour later.

Note: As a rule, a unit of blood should be infused within 2 to 4 hours.

15. Dispose of the used blood pack IAW local SOP.

a. Return it to the laboratory blood bank.

b. Discard it in a container for contaminated waste.

16. Document the procedure and significant observations on the appropriate forms IAW local SOP.

What Not To Do:

1. Do not transfuse blood products when ANY doubt exists as to the crossmatching, or type of blood. Transfusion reactions can convert a critical situation into a "fatal" situation if safe medical procedures are not followed.
2. Do not withhold blood products in a patient that is hypotensive, tachycardic and actively bleeding, with a normal hematocrit. Remember, the hematocrit will take several hours to fall in a bleeding patient, so that a normal percentage is not unusual in acute trauma.

Chapter 30: Basic Medical Skills: Field Blood Transfusion

MAJ Richard A. Angel, MC, USA

Introduction: The transfusion of whole blood from a walking donor can be a lifesaving procedure that has been used successfully in austere environments. However, due to the potential for life-threatening transfusion reactions, this procedure should only be used when a casualty has lost a significant amount of blood, will die without transfusion, and component blood products are not available. Drawing multiple units from a single ABO compatible individual, or units from multiple ABO compatible individuals needs advanced planning and preparation. This includes: identifying the blood types of all team members, (including type O donors on the team/mission), reconfirming their blood type as the recorded blood type may be wrong in up to 10% of the time (use Eldon typing card vs. lab), and carrying single bag transfusion kits.

Packed red blood cell (PRBC) field transfusions are also covered in this section and may be brought on specific missions, where appropriate "cooler" or refrigeration devices are available and monitored.

When: Casualty is dying from hemorrhagic shock as evidenced by worsening mental status (in the absence of traumatic brain injury [TBI]), weak or absent radial pulse, poor response to initial fluid therapy, increasing HR, increasing RR, decreasing BP and decreasing urine output. Remember any IV fluid, including blood, may increase the risk of further bleeding. Blood should be only given in the field to save the life of a casualty dying of hemorrhagic shock when bleeding cannot be stopped, known ABO compatible donors are available, and other therapies (IV fluids) cannot sustain the casualty until definitive care is reached. Evacuation times need to be considered.

What You Need: ABO compatible donor (O Negative is "universal donor"), povidone-iodine swabs, single bag transfusion kits (Fenwal 4R0012MC recommended). Y tubing with 180-micron filter. Casualty with 18 gauge or preferred 16 gauge short IV catheter with NS TKO. IO may be used. **Note:** Do not remove extra bags from triple collection bag set until just before use as system will no longer be sterile and serious contamination may result. Single bag collection kit is strongly recommended. Any sterile collection system may be used in an emergency, however with greater risks.
PRBC transfusion: units of Type O negative PRBCs or type specific, Y tubing, appropriate climate controlled storage.

Note: Do not transfuse PRBCs unless they have been properly transported and maintained in a container with constant internal temperature of 1° to 6°C (34°-39°F). Individual units of PRBCs (in plastic bags) may be transported in an appropriate container (eg, Collins box) with wet ice (in plastic bags) for up to 48 hrs. If ambient temperature is above 32°C (90°F), anticipate and plan for units that will require re-icing every 24 hrs. The temperature in the transporting container should be measured and documented every 4 hours during transport to insure constant internal temperature of 1° to 6°C (34°-39°F).

What To Do:

1. Identify appropriate patient: Consider casualty for possible transfusion if signs of worsening shock present: decreased mental status in absence of TBI, weak or absent radial pulse, HR >120, RR >30, systolic BP <90. Give ABO compatible blood, though, if available, O neg (universal donor) will generally be the safest. In SOF environment, use US Soldier donor who has had regular immunizations and medical care. All attempts must be made to stop any bleeding.

2. Draw blood from donor: Blood types of all team members and accompanying personnel should be identified pre-mission. Additional potential injuries could endanger donor! Consider danger of additional potential combat before drawing blood. In certain situations, non-medic team members may be trained to draw blood to allow medic to attend to dying casualties.
    a. Open and inspect collection bag.
    b. Place collection bag on ground or lower than donor's heart.
    c. Prepare arm with povidone-iodine and apply constriction band.
    d. Remove needle cover and insert needle bevel down.
    e. Monitor for blood flow, moving needle as appropriate to maximize flow. Tape needle in place, remove constriction band.
    f. Allow bag to fill, which should take about 10 minutes. Additional collection bags may be required.
    g. Clamp tube and withdraw needle.
    h. Gently agitate collection bag every few minutes to mix anticoagulant agent present in the bag.
    i. Tie knot 4 inches from collection bag in tube or leave clamp in place.
    j. Blood should be transfused immediately.

3. Give unit of whole blood:
    PRBC transfusion Note: Two people should independently inspect blood units, verify blood type, expiration date and product identification number. Inspect the blood pack for abnormalities such as gas bubbles or black or gray colored sediment (indicative of bacterial growth). Record transfused blood unit number, patient's name, SSN, date and time of transfusion. If possible, warm the PRBCs (should feel as warm as your own face, no greater than 40°C /104°F). Set up the PRBCs in the same manner as whole blood. Hang the blood pack at least 6 inches higher than the normal saline.
    a. Recipient should have NS TKO and large bore IV/IO in place. 16 gauge short IV cath preferred although 18 gauge can be used with greater hemolysis and longer infusion times. Additional IV/IO access preferred to manage complications and as protocol for trauma patient.
    b. Open and inspect Y tubing, ensure all clamps are closed, and spike NS bag. **Note:** Y tubing may be used as the standard IV line tubing in the SOF aid bag.

    c. Open clamp on saline side of Y tubing and fill drip chamber to cover filter with saline.

    d. Open clamp on infusion line to allow saline to fill line, then close clamp.

    e. Open clamp on blood side of Y tubing and allow to fill with saline and drain of air, then clamp both blood and saline sides of Y tubing.

    f. Hang blood bag next to NS and aseptically spike blood bag with blood side of Y tubing.

    g. Check vital signs just prior to the administration of whole blood and pay careful attention to RR and HR. The BP may be difficult to obtain, and can be an unreliable indicator of transfusion reaction in hypotensive dying patient.

    h. Start blood at TKO rate of one drop every 5 seconds. Record time as blood enters recipient.

    i. Take VS again with careful attention to RR and HR. Monitor for transfusion reaction.

    j. Continue TKO rate for 10 minutes, recheck vital signs. If no significantly increased heart rate, respiration rate or other signs of severe hemolytic transfusion reaction, then you may increase rate.

    k. Take vital signs every 5 minutes for the first 15 minutes, then every 15 minutes.

    l. Consider drawing additional units of whole blood as first unit is being given, or warm next unit of PRBCs. **Note:** Transfusion of PRBCs must be completed within 4 hours of removal from "cooler."

    m. Stop transfusion once vital signs have stabilized. Vital signs and mental status should improve. If vital signs are not improving, consider: 1) transfusion reaction, 2) continued bleeding, and/or 3) worsening shock.

    n. Rapid medical evacuation to surgical care is the highest priority at all times and should not be delayed.

    o. Treat hypothermia aggressively.

    p. Label all units given with name and SSN of all donors and send blood samples with casualty for lab testing. Ensure all bags of blood or blood products given are transported with casualty.

4. Monitor for Transfusion Reaction:

There are multiple types and degrees of reaction. The most dangerous and life-threatening hemolytic reaction occurs with type-mismatched blood. Again, recheck and identify all blood types of team members prior to deployment to serve as a walking blood bank. Transfusing females or casualties that have had a previous transfusion may pose a greater risk for immediate and later complications. Signs of severe reaction can be difficult to evaluate in a combat casualty. Feeling of impending doom, pain at injection site, in back, head and neck, increasing heart rate, increasing respirations, and decreasing BP may be indicators of a severe hemolytic transfusion reaction. Stop blood immediately if a severe hemolytic transfusion reaction is suspected and rapidly infuse NS. Pay careful attention to HR and RR, as these should not worsen during procedure and may be the only reliable signs of a severe reaction in the combat casualty. Less severe reactions may be treated and the continuation of the transfusion may be considered. See Part 8: Procedures: Chapter 30: Blood Transfusion Reaction

Note: If donor and recipient blood type are known and transfusion is "compatible", acute hemolytic transfusions reactions are uncommon. In the life-threatening situation that prompts the need for transfusion, the medic may be best advised to "press on" with the transfusion, unless clear and unequivocal signs of an acute hemolytic transfusion reaction are seen.

What Not To Do:

1. Do not give blood to a casualty without physician supervision unless casualty is dying of hemorrhagic shock. Continue to monitor for and control bleeding.

2. Do not fail to monitor carefully for transfusion reactions and stop transfusion if needed.

3. Do not delay evacuation to surgical care.

4. Do not give PRBCs or any blood product that has not been properly stored in an approved "cooler" or refrigeration device. Blood or blood products that have warmed slightly in a poorly controlled environment may appear normal however may cause severe life-threatening infections.

Chapter 30: Basic Medical Skills: Blood Transfusion Reaction

MAJ Richard Angel, MC, USA

When: You have a casualty who has received or is receiving a transfusion of whole blood. The casualty is having a reaction to the transfusion. You must correctly identify a transfusion reaction and manage it without causing further injury to the casualty.

What You Need: Thermometer, blood pressure cuff, stethoscope, IV equipment with 0.9% normal saline, needles and syringes, oxygen and related equipment, **diphenhydramine, epinephrine 1:1000 solution, furosemide, acetaminophen** or **ibuprofen. Note:** Ibuprofen may interfere with blood clotting and may be withheld in the casualty in hemorrhagic hypovolemic shock.

What To Do:

Note: Casualty has received or is receiving transfusions.

1. Monitor the casualty's vital signs during and after transfusion--continuously for the first 5 minutes, then every 15 minutes.

2. Compare baseline vital signs to current vital signs.

3. Monitor the site of the infusion for edema, warmth, and urticaria.

4. Examine the casualty for systemic signs and symptoms of reaction, pay careful attention to respirations and pulse when field transfusing a combat casualty.

5. Important: Identify the type of reaction based on the signs and symptoms.

Note: Hemolytic reaction is the rarest and most severe transfusion reaction. It usually starts within the first 10 minutes of the transfusion. The most severe reaction occurs when donor RBCs are hemolyzed by antibody (Ab) in the recipient's plasma. **STOP THE TRANSFUSION IF A HEMOLYTIC REACTION IS SUSPECTED.**

Observe the patient for the following:

    a. Shortness of breath/increased respiration rate- may be your only sign of severe transfusion reaction in a severely injured patient

b. Chilly sensation; this is more ominous.
c. Shaking chill; stop transfusion
d. Chest or lower back pain
e. Hypotension: decreased blood pressure from initial blood pressure
f. Nausea
g. Urticaria/Itching
h. Hematuria (red urine)
i. Perspiration
j. Arthralgia/Joint pain
k. Headache
l. Pallor
m. Fever, though if low grade and the only sign or symptom, transfusion may be carefully continued.
n. Oozing from wounds or venipuncture sites
o. Pain at venipuncture site.
   Note: Rapid transfusion of cold blood can cause arrhythmia or cardiac arrest.
6. Initiate the appropriate treatment for the transfusion reaction. Give medications through a clear IV line without donor blood.
   a. Treatment for hemolytic reactions.
      (1) Stop the transfusion immediately and change the IV tubing.
      (2) Leave the needle in place and reconnect the new tubing to the needle.
      (3) Send a sample of the patient's fresh blood and urine to the laboratory for analysis, if possible.
      (4) Start Ringer's lactate or normal saline IV to correct hypotension and maintain urine output.
      (5) Monitor vital signs and urine output.
      (6) Administer oxygen.
      (7) Administer medications. To establish diuresis and increase renal blood flow, give **furosemide** 20-40mg IV (IM may be used), increased by 20mg q2h if needed to maintain urine output of 30-100mL/hr.
      (8) Use blankets and warming measures to treat chills and hypothermia.
   b. Treatment for febrile reactions: Febrile transfusion reactions can usually be managed with antipyretics, like **acetaminophen** 500mg po q4-6h (not to exceed 4g/day) or **ibuprofen** 400-600mg po q4-6h (not to exceed 3200mg/day) and gentle patient cooling. Change tubing and keep venous access open with normal saline. Check the patient's temperature every 30 minutes. Document the episode, time, and IV fluid given.
   c. Treatment for circulatory overload. The transfusion should be discontinued immediately. Place the casualty in an upright position. Keep the IV line open with a slow infusion of normal saline. Use diuretic: **furosemide** (dose listed in step 6), if necessary.
   d. Treatment for air embolism: stop the source of the air and bleed or replace the line. Turn the patient on the left side, head down, to allow the air to escape a little at a time from the right atrium. Monitor the patient for pulmonary or cerebral embolisms.
   e. Severe allergic reactions may require **diphenhydramine** 25-50mg IV/IM q6h and **epinephrine** 0.01mL/kg of 1:1000, IM/SC, not to exceed 0.5mL of 1:1000 (5mg) IM/SC if needed. Fluid bolus with NS/LR as above. See Part 7: Trauma: Chapter 27: Anaphylactic Shock
   f. Treatment for arrhythmia or arrest due to infusion of cold blood: Stop the infusion. Manage the arrhythmia or arrest. Warm the blood before resuming infusion.
7. Explain to the patient that there are possible late complications of blood transfusions and that they should notify medical personnel immediately if they develop signs or symptoms of late complications.
   a. Serum hepatitis
   b. HIV virus
   c. Malaria: Can be transmitted by asymptomatic donors. Casualty may develop high fever and headaches weeks after the transfusion.
   d. Syphilis
   Note: All donated blood should be laboratory tested for hepatitis, HIV and other pathogens.
   e. Delayed hemolytic reactions can occur from 1 to 2 weeks after transfusion. Signs are fever, mild jaundice, gradual fall in hemoglobin level, positive Coombs' lab test.
   f. Bacterial infection: A few contaminating bacteria, particularly gram-negative, can grow in refrigerated blood and may cause severe reactions, sepsis and death if transfused. Procedures that allow blood to reach room temperature (prolonged transfusions or warming blood) may accelerate bacterial growth and are potentially hazardous. For these reasons, refrigerated blood should never be stored in a non-approved refrigeration unit without appropriate temperature sensors and monitoring.
8. Record all treatment given.
9. All patients who have received a blood transfusion must be evaluated by a physician.

What Not To Do:
1. Do not continue a transfusion when blood recipient complains of chills, difficulty breathing and/or feeling worse than baseline during a transfusion. Stop the transfusion, continue normal saline and evaluate for possible transfusion reaction.
2. Do not reassure a patient that all transfusions are completely safe and without risk. There is always risk of severe illness or death with transfusion of blood products. In a field environment without physician supervision, give only whole blood to save a dying casualty.

Chapter 30: Basic Medical Skills: Intraosseous Infusion

MAJ John Croushorn, MC, USA

When: Intraosseous (IO) infusion is a reliable option for parenteral drug, fluid or blood administration when IV access is unavailable or difficult or when dealing with chemical warfare or mass casualties. **Indication:** For the infusion of fluids, blood or medications into the proximal or distal tibia, distal femur or proximal humerus of pediatric patients, or the proximal or distal tibia, proximal humerus or sternum of adult patients. IO infusions have been proven to be the medication delivery equivalent of central venous catheters but are somewhat less effective (depending on IO site selected) for fluid resuscitation. IO access has been proven to offer fewer risks than central venous access and is clearly faster than IV access in the emergent setting. Urgency of access, treatment requirements and simplicity should all be taken into consideration when confronted with immediate vascular access needs.

What You Need: Alcohol swabs, IO needle set, IV administration set, and IV solution. **Note:** Package needed supplies together for rapid access.

What To Do:
1. IO infusion should be considered for the adult or pediatric patient when presented with:
    a. Altered level of consciousness
    b. Respiratory compromise
    c. Hemodynamic instability AND when peripheral cannulation is unobtainable or difficult
    Note: IO infusions should be considered for patients in medical or traumatic extremis or in patients who are sedated or unconscious. IO pain medication should be considered to decrease intramedullary pressure for the alert patient.
2. Pediatrics: Of the IO systems currently in use by the DoD, only the EZ-IO PD and the B.I.G product systems are approved by the FDA for use in patients under 39kg. The FAST 1 and EZ-IO are sternal devices approved for use in adult patients only.
3. Apply gloves for personal and patient protection.
4. Clean the site as for an IV infusion.
5. **Site Selection:** There are multiple IO access sites for the pediatric patients.
    a. Proximal tibia, 2 finger widths below the patella, on the medial (flat aspect) of the tibia.
    b. Distal tibia, 2 finger widths above the medial malleolus (ankle) on the medial (flat) aspect of the tibia.
    c. Distal femur, 2 finger widths directly above the patella, mid-line of the anterior aspect of the leg.
    Approved insertion sites for adults are:
    a. The proximal tibia – 1 finger width medial to the tibial tuberosity (large bump directly below the patella)
       Note: The B.I.G. requires that you additionally move 1 finger width proximal (toward the joint).
    b. The proximal humerus – directly in the greater tubercle (lateral, upper aspect of the humerus). Identified by "running" finger proximally (up) the lateral aspect of the humerus to the prominent greater tubercle protrusion
    c. The distal tibia – 2 fingerbreadths proximal to the medial malleolus
    d. The manubrium (top 1/3 of the sternum) on the midline and 1.5cm (5/8 inch) below the sternal notch. (FAST 1 and EZ-IO sternal needle sets only).
       Contraindications to intraosseous infusion:
       (1) Fracture of the bone selected for infusion
       (2) Inability to locate landmarks or excessive tissue over site
       (3) Infection at the infusion site
       (4) Recent use (within 24 hours) of the same bone
       (5) Use of a NON-sternal needle set in the sternum
6. Select an intraosseous (bone marrow) needle set, or commercially available device such as the EZ-IO, FAST-1, B.I.G., or if those are unavailable, a 16 or 18 gauge spinal needle.
7. Put the patient in a supine position. Expose the site and ensure that no fracture is present in the selected bone.
8. Consider anesthetizing the site by raising a subcutaneous **lidocaine** wheal and then injecting down to the surface of the bone. Injecting 1-2mL of 1% **lidocaine** at the surface of the bone will help to anesthetize the periosteum. (Insertion pain has shown to be minimal.)
9. If manually inserting a needle set, use a gentle boring or screwing motion (avoiding excess force) to advance the needle at a 90° angle to the bone until it penetrates into the marrow. There should be a decrease in the resistance once the cortex has been penetrated. Other techniques may be used with the commercially available devices. These techniques are device specific. If you have them, become familiar with them by studying the literature and practicing on a suitable model before deploying – consider website, compact disc or printed material training assistance.
10. To check your catheter placement following insertion consider:
    a. Stability of needle set
    b. Blood at the tip of the stylet upon removal
    c. Flash back in the catheter
    d. Light aspiration of bone marrow into extension set (be aware that it will not always be possible to aspirate marrow.)
    e. Syringe flush (required) with no sign of extravasation
    f. Noted signs of fluids and or medications effects
11. If patient is awake, administer 40mg cardiac **lidocaine** (preservative free) IO to anesthetize the intramedullary space.
12. Rapidly syringe push (bolus) 20mL of NS to establish flow through the intraosseous space.
13. Secure the catheter with tape or supplied dressing.
14. Attach an IV infusion set as with normal IV infusion. Consider using a pressure bag with IO infusions. Failure to syringe push (bolus) 20mL of sterile saline may compromise or limit IO flow. 20mL syringe flush has been shown to dramatically improve flow.
    Note: Crystalloid solutions, blood, and all medications can be administered by the IO route.
15. Record all treatment in the patient's medical record.
16. May be left for up to 24 hours, but each day increases risk of infection, so attempt to change to an IV line when acceptable.

What Not To Do:

1. Do not forget that all medications can be delivered through this route at the same dose that would be given IV.
2. Do not use the sternal technique in small adults or children.
3. Do not use the sternal technique in patients with previous sternotomy (heart by-pass), evidence of sternal skin infection, fracture or vascular injury that could compromise the integrity of the sternum.
4. Do not fail to do syringe flush.

Chapter 30: Basic Medical Skills: Suturing

COL Michael M. Fuenfer, MC, USAR

When: You must stitch a wound closed without contamination. Dirty or contaminated wounds should not be closed primarily (sutures, Steri-Strips, Dermabond, etc) due to the risk of infection. Application of sterile dressings, frequent changing and delayed primary closure at 5-7 days, or allowing the wound to heal by secondary intent should always be considered.

What You Need: Antibiotic ointment (eg, **povidone-iodine, bacitracin, bacitracin/neomycin/polymixin B**), Dermabond, Steri-Strips, Mastisol, sterile dressings (gauze, Xeroform, self-adherent, op-site), tape, a large Kelly clamp, a needle holder, tissue forceps, a mosquito clamp, appropriate sutures and needles or pre-package suture/needle combinations (preferred), four towel clamps, sterile gloves, several 4x8 inch gauze pads, four hand towels, shaving razor, antiseptic solution and sponges, irrigation syringe (may use attached catheter for increased pressure), sterile saline for irrigation and suture wash, surgical bowl(s), a 22-23 gauge needle with 5-10cc syringe, and **lidocaine** anesthesia (with or without epinephrine as appropriate).

What To Do:

1. Gather the appropriate equipment. Inspect for damage or tampering.
2. Prepare the wound site.
   a. Protect the wound with sterile gauze.
   b. Shave carefully the skin 3-5 inches around the wound (avoid creating iatrogenic abrasions).
   c. Perform a surgical scrub.
      (1) Clean the wound area with circular motions, making sure not to let antiseptic solution wash into the wound.
      (2) Clean from the wound edges out.
      (3) Dispose of the sponges.
      (4) Repeat as needed.
   d. Irrigate the wound with sterile solution.
      (1) Irrigate from one end toward the other, usually from the proximal to distal.
      (2) Avoid "suck back" with the syringe.
3. Drape the patient appropriately with hand towels.
4. Check the patient for allergy to medications.
5. Administer the anesthesia.
   a. Inject anesthetic into the subcutaneous layer.
   b. Insert the needle full length.
   c. Aspirate for blood.
   d. Inject anesthesia upon withdrawal of the needle.
   e. Wait for 3 minutes, then test for pain.
   Warning: Do not use **lidocaine** with **epinephrine** to anesthetize the fingers, nose, ears, toes, or penis.
6. Select the proper suture.
   a. Use 5-0 to 6-0 for the face, 3-0 to 4-0 for the arms, legs, and trunk. 2-0 may be used to secure chest tubes and other high-stress applications. Tend to use smaller sizes in children and in lower stress areas.
      (1) Chromic suture: Use for the bowel, muscle, and peritoneum. Resorbs within 14-21 days. Packaged in isopropyl alcohol, which is an irritant. Rinse suture with saline prior to use. Causes less inflammation than plain suture.
      (2) Plain suture (gut): Use for subcutaneous tissue and ligation of small vessels. Resorbs within 7-14 days. Packaged in isopropyl alcohol, which is an irritant. Rinse suture with saline prior to use. Monocryl: monofilament suture that resorbs in 7-10 days.
      (3) Vicryl, Maxon, and Dexon: Strongest absorbable sutures. They are easier to handle and tie than plain suture, have higher tensile strength, and cause less tissue reaction. Resorb in 4-6 weeks. Vicryl comes dyed and undyed - avoid using dyed on the face. PDS suture is a monofilament suture that resorbs in 6-8 weeks.
      (4) Nylon: Most popular skin suture. Not absorbable. Good tensile strength, minimal tissue reaction
      (5) Polyester or Polypropylene: Not absorbable. Easier to tie than nylon. High tensile strength, moderate/ minimal tissue reaction.
      (6) Silk: Not absorbable. Fair tensile strength, excellent handling/knot tying. Moderate tissue reaction.
   b. Use wire sutures on bone. Stainless steel is the strongest suture material, with the most secure knots, and inert resulting in minimal inflammatory tissue reaction. Stiffness of the metal may result in irritation and tissue damage, and when subjected to frequent motion, may break.
   c. Tissue reaction to suture: localized acute, aseptic inflammation. Suture, especially braided suture, can provide a wick through the skin allowing pathogens access to a wound.

Figure 8-4. Suture Techniques

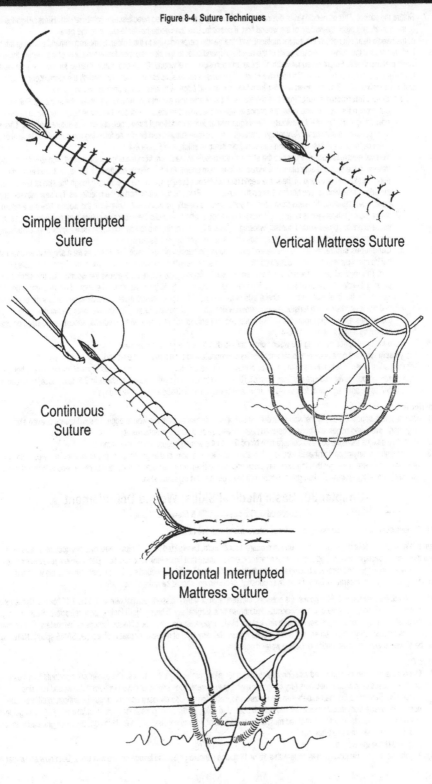

Simple Interrupted
Suture

Vertical Mattress Suture

Continuous
Suture

Horizontal Interrupted
Mattress Suture

7. Suture the patient. Thread needles with desired suture if not using pre-packaged needle/suture combinations. **Hints:** Align the edges of the wound, and stitch the middle of the wound first, if possible. Use the needle holder to clamp on the back of the needle near but not ON the suture material, with the needle perpendicular to the holder. Some recommend grasping the needle half way around the curve. Insert the point of the needle perpendicular to the skin and then follow the curve of the needle through when piercing tissue. Suture an equal width of tissue on each side of the wound. Go deeper rather than wider with the stitches if need to achieve greater wound closure. Do not have stitches too tense - make sure tissue is not blanched by the stitch. Keep stitches uniform approximately 5-10mm apart and 5-10mm from the wound edge, with knots away from the wound edge.

   a. **Simple interrupted suture**: Puncture the skin with the needle and exit into the wound, traversing the skin only. Pull the needle out through the wound, and enter the opposite side of the wound at the same depth. Curve the needle up through the skin, positioning it as described previously. Tie a square knot plus an additional throw, then clip excess suture material. This is the most common suture used. Advantages: strength; successive sutures can be placed following the path of the laceration; distance, depth and tissue eversion can vary from stitch to stitch, see Figure 8-4.

   b. **Vertical mattress suture**: Puncture the skin with the needle at least 1cm from the edge of the wound, and exit into the wound, traversing the skin and subcutaneous tissue (at least 1cm deep). Pull the needle out through the wound, and enter the opposite side of the wound at the same depth (subcutaneous tissue). Curve the needle up through the skin at least 1cm from the edge of the wound, positioning it as on the other side. Reverse the orientation of the needle, as if to sew with the opposite hand. Point the sharp tip away from yourself and insert the needle approximately 5mm from the wound. Make the return suture either subcutaneous or a skin closure. Tie a knot as above and clip the excessive suture material. Advantages: more tissue eversion, broad wound contact, watertight. Useful for preventing broad scar formation (see Figure 8-4). Disadvantage: constricts blood supply at wound edges, possibly causing necrosis and dehiscence.

   c. **Continuous suture**: Insert the needle and exit through the subcutaneous tissue. Tie a knot as for a simple interrupted stitch, but do not clip the suture end. Suture continuously the entire length of the wound without tying any additional knots until the end. This method can be modified to "lock" each stitch by bringing the suture back across the wound after the stitch and passing it under the piece of suture coming from the previous stitch. All the locks should be aligned on the same side of the wound. Tie the final knot on the opposite side of the wound. Clip the excessive material. Advantages: aligns perpendicular to the wound, distributing tension evenly; allows watertight, rapid closure; locking feature prevents continuous tightening of the stitches as suturing progresses. Disadvantages: not able to adjust to tension from edema; should not be used on areas of existing tension, see Figure 8-4.

8. Eliminate the dead space by rolling the wound proximally to distally with a rolled gauze pad.

9. Apply **bacitracin** ointment or other topical antibiotic as appropriate and then bandage the wound.

10. Tell the patient when to return to have the sutures removed or to return earlier if the wound shows signs of infection (red, hot, swollen, wound draining pus; fever; red streaks from wound). Remove stitches from eyelid in 3 days; cheek in 3-5 days; nose, forehead and scalp in 5-7 days; arm, leg, hand, foot in 7-10+ days; and chest, back, and abdomen in 7-10+ days.

What Not To Do:

1. Do not suture opposite sides of the wound at different depths or distances from the wound edge. This will create uneven skin alignment, overriding edges and poor or delayed healing, as well as a poor cosmetic result.

2. Do not tie sutures too tight, so as to compromise blood flow to the wound edges, which need it most.

3. Do not suture a dirty or contaminated wound. If it is still dirty after irrigation, or if irrigation is not possible, allow the wound to heal by granulation. If there is danger that the skin may close prior to the deeper tissues granulating, then pack the wound with iodoform gauze (or **povidone-iodine** soaked gauze) daily until the wound heals up to the skin.

Chapter 30: Basic Medical Skills: Wound Débridement

COL Leopoldo C. Cancio, MC, USA & Steven J. Thomas, MD

What: Remove dead or devitalized tissue to decrease infection and improve healing.

When: It is essential to débride a traumatic wound to prepare it for closure. Devitalized tissue inhibits leukocyte phagocytosis, acts as a culture medium for bacteria growth, and provides an anaerobic environment that limits leukocyte function. Debridement relieves excess tension, provides drainage, and removes bacteria and devitalized tissue that impair the wound's ability to heal. Whether the wound is secondary to an abrasion, laceration, burn, frostbite or gunshot, débridement should be rational, not radical.

What You Need: Recommended: Skin hooks, iris scissors, Metzenbaum or Mayo scissors, scalpel with #10, #11, # 15 blades, tissue forceps, 35cc syringe, 16 or 18 gauge needle or plastic cannula, toothbrush or a surgical scrub brush, NaCl for irrigation, retractors: Sims or Army-Navy. Improvised: Any type of scissors, scalpel with any type of blade or pocketknife, any type of tissue forceps or hemostats, IV with catheter (any type of clean fluid), any type of brush, tap water (boiled if possible), any type of retractor or pliable object (ie, SAMS splint). **Note:** Items should be sterilized with cold sterilization or boiling water if possible.

What To Do:

1. Debridement should be performed as soon as possible after injury, preferably within hours. The exception is patients with frostbite or other causes of avascular necrosis (dry gangrene), who may benefit from a delay of days to weeks if the wound remains uninfected. Determine the margin between devitalized and viable tissue. Use clinical judgment. It may be difficult to differentiate nonviable muscle from muscle that is injured but will heal. Use color, contraction, consistency, and circulation (the 4Cs) as guidelines when excising muscle. Identify devitalized muscle by its dark color, mushy consistency, inability to contract when grasped with forceps and a lack of brisk bleeding when cut.

2. Prep and drape the wound.

3. Irrigate the wound. Historically, a syringe with a 16 or 18 gauge cannula or a pulse lavage device was used. Data now show that high-

pressure irrigation causes tissue damage, drives bacteria into wounds, and increases infection rates. Therefore, use a bulb syringe or gravity flow and normal saline, and irrigate the wound copiously.

Minor wounds not involving muscle

1. Stabilize the skin edges with the skin hooks by retracting the wound at both ends. Use your fingers to pull the skin being débrided perpendicular to the laceration (this will prevent the skin from rolling in, providing an even, clean edge).
2. Using the scalpel with a #11 or #15 blade, hold it angled away from the wound edge and excise the devitalized skin. Holding it at an angle will ensure that eversion is achieved when the edges are approximated.
3. After excising the skin edges, inspect subcutaneous tissue. Excise any devitalized tissue with iris scissors.
4. Irrigate the wound once again with copious amounts of NaCl.
5. Close the wound either as a delayed primary closure or secondarily depending on the location, initial debridement, and the level of contamination. Pearl: A technique that helps distinguish devitalized tissue: apply fluorescein dye to a gauze pack and pack the wound. The fluorescein will stain devitalized tissue, which can then easily be débrided. If unsure, excise the skin until active bleeding starts.

Abrasions

Particular attention should be given to abrasions in order to prevent a traumatic tattoo. These occur when fine particles become embedded and are incorporated into the epithelium.

1. Ensure adequate anesthetic has been administered (either locally or via block).
2. **Lidocaine** gel can be applied to the wound for 5-10 minutes. This may assist in providing adequate anesthesia.
3. Irrigate the abrasion copiously with NaCl.
4. Use a sterile toothbrush or surgical scrub brush soaked with NaCl or surgical soap to help remove the debris.
5. Use the tip of a #11 blade to remove large or deeply embedded particles.
6. Use mineral oil, Vaseline, peanut butter, or mayonnaise (or some other oil-based product) to help remove tar.
7. Leave the wound open and clean it daily.

Penetrating wounds

1. In general, extensive debridement of both low- and high-velocity combat wounds, in the absence of some other indication for surgery (eg, fracture, bleeding, or infection) is no longer recommended. Rather, it is best to treat such wounds conservatively and to treat infections such as abscesses if and when they occur. If debridement of nonviable tissue is necessary, use a scalpel with a #11 or # 15 blade to excise the entry and exit wounds. The incisions should be sufficient to allow optimal surgical exposure and drainage. The excised skin should include the underlying subcutaneous tissue, and be incised oriented parallel to the underlying muscle fiber.
2. Incise the fascia parallel to the muscle fiber with Mayo or Metzenbaum scissors in both directions. Open the muscle surrounding the missile tract in the direction of the fibers to allow adequate exposure for inspecting the tract.
3. Inspect the wound tract. Remove any foreign bodies. Excise any muscle that is nonviable with a scalpel or scissors.
4. Utilize the retractors at this time to help with visualization and debridement. Be careful when using retractors in order to avoid damaging vessels, nerves, and healthy tissue.
5. Perform this procedure at both the entry and exit wounds. Débride the mid-track through extended entry and exit wounds. This prevents cutting across muscle groups to connect the two wounds.
6. Appropriate drainage of the wound may be difficult to achieve. Liberal incisions tend to facilitate drainage from the deep recesses. Remember to excise skin, fascia, vessels, nerves, and bone conservatively, and muscle more liberally. Try to save periosteum and tendons unless severely contaminated or compromised.
7. Irrigate the wound copiously again.
8. Do not tightly pack the wound. The additional pressure can cause tissue necrosis due to its already compromised blood supply. Lightly lay dry sterile gauze in the wound.
9. Leave the wound open with delayed primary closure in 4-10 days.

Pearls:

a. If it does not bleed, it is not "viable" (and will slow, or stop healing).
b. Do not be afraid to put your nose to the wound closely. Much can be learned by smelling it.
c. When in doubt, do not close the wound (an open wound in good biological balance is still a contaminated wound).
d. Always evaluate for a palpable pulse proximal to any extremity wound, as impaired vascular inflow will be problematic for any wound healing.

What Not To Do:

1. Do not débride viable tissue. Wait until the tissue declares itself, or makes it apparent that it is dead.
2. Do not close the débrided wounds, but let them drain. They may be closed later (delayed primary closure) if not infected.
3. Do not pack débrided wounds tightly, but allow them space to expand.
4. Do not fail to use caution with débridement of the hands and feet.

Chapter 30: Basic Medical Skills: Skin Mass Removal

COL Michael M. Fuenfer, MC, USAR

What: Surgical procedures for treating various masses and conditions of the skin including abscess, epidermal inclusion cyst (EIC), lipoma, mole, etc. These masses may be inflamed (abscess) or non-inflamed (lipoma).

When: The patient complains of a mass in the skin that is either infected or a hindrance to activity and mission performance. Manage lesions that do not fit into these categories conservatively until return from the mission. The medic should not remove vascular masses.

Non-inflamed: These are best treated electively with excision (the removal of the entire lesion) and submission for pathologic evaluation. Differential diagnosis includes lipoma, fibroma, neuroma, and fibrohistiocytoma (potentially malignant), hence the need for pathology review.

Inflamed: Although antibiotics can control and sometimes reverse the inflammation of an abscess, those that appear to be infected and unresponsive to conservative therapy should be incised and drained (I&D). This however, creates an open wound that requires dressing changes for 1-2 weeks. An EIC can be excised as opposed to incised as a non-inflamed mass if it is not actively inflamed. An attempt should be made to remove the entire cyst wall. If the wound remains sterile (the cyst is not accidentally opened during the procedure), it can be closed at the end of the procedure. If the EIC is actively infected, treat it as an abscess.

What You Need: Sterile prep and drape, povidone-iodine, needles: 18 and 24-27 gauge, 10cc syringe, alcohol prep pads, local anesthetic, preferably with **epinephrine**, scalpel: #15 blade, irrigation: sterile NS/LR/water or hydrogen peroxide, sterile gloves, sterile 4x4s, sterile hemostat, Adson pickups, Metzenbaum or iris scissors, Allis clamp (if available), specimen container and label (store/send in a watertight container [eg, urine cup] filled with formaldehyde), saline, IV fluid or sterile water, tape and dressings. Excision: 3-0 dissolvable suture (taper needle), back lesion: 2-0 nylon (cutting needle), extremity or scalp lesion: 3-0 nylon (cutting needle) I&D: 2x2 or 4x4 gauze (or iodoform) for packing, tape

What To Do: Prep: For inflamed and non-inflamed lesions, scrub and prep the area around the lesion with povidone-iodine and drape with sterile towels. Infiltrate local anesthetic in a field block at 2-4 sites around the area of the lesion. This is a much more tolerable approach to anesthetizing the inflamed lesion but works well in providing pain control for either lesion. Try not to inject the EIC, as the distention of the capsule can cause increased pain or spray the contents of the lesion out through the EIC orifice back at the surgeon. Allow several minutes for the anesthesia to take effect. Subcutaneous lesions (lipomas, etc.) require deeper anesthesia but they should likewise NOT be injected. Plan an incision along the lines of Langer (natural lines of tension) to minimize the scar formation and promote efficient healing. Make the incision: using an elliptical incision for excision of an epidermal mass or EIC, but use a straight incision for an abscess or subepidermal lesion. Include the entire epidermal lesion, as well as the EIC (skin overlying cyst plus punctate, follicular orifice), in the excised tissue to prevent recurrence. Similarly, remove deeper masses in their entirety.

Non-inflamed superficial mass: Do not remove these lesions unless they fit the criteria. Make an elliptical incision around any superficial mass. Grasp the tissue to be excised with a clamp to allow retraction and demonstration of the lines of tension of the surrounding tissue. Dissect under the mass, remaining in the dermis if the mass is indeed superficial. Remove the tissue plug. Control hemostasis by gentle pressure. Irrigate the wound then close it in one layer with nylon suture. Standard guidelines: The specimen should be sent to the pathologist for evaluation. Use mattress suture technique rather than simple interrupted technique in areas of higher tension (ie, back, joints) to prevent dehiscence of the wound. A dry bandage should be kept in place for 36-48 hours to allow re-epithelialization of the wound. Sutures should be left in 5 days on the face, 7-10 days elsewhere, and 10-14 days on high-tension areas. No antibiotics are needed. Profile of the Soldier/patient should include limited movement of the surgical wound for 2-3 weeks.

Non-inflamed subcutaneous mass: Do not remove these lesions unless they fit the criteria. Unless the lesion is an EIC, make a single incision through the skin over the mass, large enough to allow visualization and dissection in the wound. If it is an EIC that is not actively inflamed, make an elliptical incision for a superficial mass. Be certain the ellipse will include both the EIC and its epidermal opening. Gently spread the subcutaneous tissue to locate the mass, and use scissors when needed to dissect the mass out of the wound intact. The capsule of the EIC is usually adjacent to the dermis. Dissection should proceed carefully in order to prevent rupture of the EIC capsule and spillage of the foul smelling contents. If the mass has a capsule that ruptures, attempt to remove the mass and capsule "piecemeal." Inspect the wound for retained fragments of wall. If the rupture was large, or the capsule cannot be entirely removed, manage the mass as an inflamed subcutaneous mass. Otherwise, send the specimen to the pathologist for evaluation. Control hemostasis by gentle pressure. Irrigate the wound, and then close it in 1-2 layers. Close the dermal layer using inverted, interrupted stitches with dissolvable suture. Include some fat in the stitch if the dissection extended into the fat tissue. Follow the standard guidance. Use this surgical approach for the removal of all non-infected, subcutaneous masses such as lipomas or fibromas. It is important to send lesions for pathologic evaluation, as further radical surgery may be necessary for the rare malignancy.

Inflamed superficial or subcutaneous mass: Treat with appropriate antibiotics (*see Part 4: Organ Systems: Chapter 6: Bacterial Infections*). If the lesion is an EIC that responded to therapy, treat as in the previous paragraph. If the lesion is an abscess or unresponsive EIC (or similar lesion, such as furuncle), interferes with the mission performance and cannot be safely managed until the end of the mission, perform the following surgery. Mark any sinus tract by placing a needle or other object into the tract. Incise the abscess/cyst (avoid spraying the contents on any person) and evacuate its contents. Explore the cavity with a hemostat and spread the jaws to break down walls and adhesions in the abscess. If the abscess had a sinus tract communicating with the epidermis, open the tract and expose it to therapy. Obtain hemostasis with pressure. Irrigate with hydrogen peroxide or saline and pack with damp (sterile saline) 2x2s or 4x4s (or iodoform), and apply a dry dressing. Do not close this infected wound. Do not continue antibiotics unless cellulitis is severe, the infection does not resolve with I&D or the patient is immunosuppressed (ie, diabetic, HIV, malnourished, on chemotherapy). Then continue antibiotics only until the wound demonstrates that it is healing. Start wet-to-dry dressings.

Wet-to-dry dressings: This requires moist packing that "dries" during the interim between dressing changes. Removing the packing débrides the wound by removing the dead cells that stick to it. Do not allow the packing to dry completely. If it does, then change the dressing more frequently. Remove the packing daily with non-sterile gloves, irrigate the wound, and replace the packing until the wound closes (1-3 weeks). The irrigation does not need to be "sterile" as potable water can be used (the wound is already colonized with skin flora and is by definition not sterile). **Note:** Only the wound should be in contact with the moist dressing, because exposure of the surrounding skin to the continuous moisture can denude the skin and lead to further infection. The patient can even remove the packing, take a shower and wash the wound with soap and water, before repacking the wound.

What Not To Do:
1. Do not leave obvious cyst wall behind in the wound.
2. Do not close grossly infected wounds.
3. Do not forget to send the lesion to a pathologist.
4. Do not attempt to remove a lump over a joint at the wrist or fingers; this is often a ganglion cyst and connects directly to a tendon sheath and the joint space.
5. Do not electively remove lesions involving the face or hands.
6. Do not attempt to remove potentially malignant lesions (eg, melanomas, sarcomas).
7. Do not attempt to remove masses adjacent to large peripheral vascular structures or nerves.

Chapter 30: Basic Medical Skills: Joint Aspiration

COL Frank Anders, MC, USA

When: To analyze joint fluid for suspected infection or for therapeutic reasons; relieve pain by draining an effusion from a swollen synovial space; infuse medications.

What You Need: Alcohol swabs, iodine prep solution, sterile gloves and towels, gauze, forceps, local anesthesia (**lidocaine** 1 or 2%), appropriate syringes, needles, and chocolate (Thayer-Martin) agar if gonococcal arthritis is suspected. If instilling anti-inflammatory drug, will need **betamethasone** or **triamcinolone**.

What To Do:
General Procedure
1. Identify landmarks and mark the entry point with a scratch or indentation on the skin.
2. Sterilize the skin in a wide field around the puncture site.
3. If you intend to inject the joint to facilitate a better physical exam after aspiration, draw up the medication in a smaller separate syringe and put it aside on the sterile field.
4. Anesthetize the skin with 1 or 2% lidocaine with a 10mL syringe and 25 to 27 gauge needle; continue down to the joint capsule.
5. Select an appropriate needle (usually 20 gauge for knee, shoulder, elbow, or ankle; 25 gauge for small hand joints).
6. Stabilize the joint to be aspirated. Advance the needle into the joint space while continually applying suction. Generally, a sudden "give" will be felt on the plunger when the needle passes through the synovium into the joint space.
7. Withdraw as much fluid as possible.
8. If infusion (medicine) is desired, remove the aspiration syringe with the needle in place and apply infusion syringe then inject. **Betamethasone** (Celestone Soluspan) is desirable, but equivalent dose of other steroid injectables (eg, **triamcinolone**) is acceptable at about a 1 to 2 ratio of steroid to local anesthetic (1% **lidocaine without epinephrine**). Reasonable rule of thumb is: 40mg steroid (1mL) for a large joint (eg, shoulder or knee), 30mg steroid for a medium sized joint (eg, wrist, ankle, elbow) and 10mg steroid for smaller spaces (eg, metacarpal, interphalangeal, tendon sheath).
9. Withdraw the needle and apply firm pressure over the site for 1-2 minutes.
10. Cover the site with an adhesive dressing.

Specific Joint Techniques
Shoulder: Have patient sit with forearm in lap (this positions the shoulder in mild internal rotation and adduction). Identify insertion site inferior and slightly lateral to tip of coracoid. Direct the needle (20-22 gauge 1½ inch needle) into joint space medial to the head of the humerus and just lateral to the palpable tip of the coracoid process.
Wrist: Place the patient's forearm on a flat surface with a folded towel under the wrist. Position the wrist in the pronated position with about 40° of flexion. Identify insertion site by marking the distal ends of the ulna and radius. Enter the bulging joint capsule at the wrist dorsally at prominent areas of swelling between the two marks. Avoid inserting needles into the palmar aspect of the wrist to prevent damaging nerves or blood vessels crossing the joint. Use a 20-22 gauge ½ or 1 inch needle.
Elbow: Have patient sit with the arm supported horizontal to the ground and the elbow flexed at about 30°. Identify insertion site on the lateral aspect of the elbow in the shallow depression immediately anterior and inferior to the lateral epicondyle of the humerus. Advance the needle medially into the joint space. With significant effusion, the bulging synovium should be evident laterally. Use a 20 or 22 gauge ½ inch needle. **Caution:** Confirm correct diagnosis (ie, diagnosis is fluid within the joint and not an olecranon bursitis, which would not require a joint procedure).
Knee: Place patient supine with quadriceps muscle relaxed (patella should be freely movable). Identify the insertion site immediately beneath the lateral or medial edge of the superior pole of the patella. Enter the joint space either medially or laterally. Pressure on the opposite side of the joint will make the synovium bulge more prominently toward the needle. Direct the needle parallel to the plane of the underside of the patella aiming for the suprapatellar pouch. From the lateral aspect, the entrance site is at the intersection of lines extended from the upper and lateral margins of the patella. Fluid should be obtained before the needle tip reaches midline. Use a 20-22 gauge 1½ inch needle. If a traumatic hemarthrosis (bloody effusion) is suspected, a larger bore needle is recommended.
Ankle: Seat the patient with lower leg and foot suspended. This joint is most safely entered through anterior and lateral aspect. A 1/2 or 1 inch needle should suffice. Palpate the distal tibial border and insert the needle perpendicular to the long axis of the tibia immediately distal to the border aiming toward the center of the joint.

Synovial Fluid Analysis: Record the physical characteristics of the fluid:
1. Total volume
2. Color and clarity
3. Viscosity (joint fluid usually will stretch 1-2 inches)
4. Presence or absence of visible fat globules if bloody

Laboratory Studies: (if available)
1. Cell count and differential
2. All fluids should have a Gram's stain.
3. Examine for crystals: Examine the specimen immediately under the microscope.
4. Culture: Blood agar (GC requires special agar)
5. Fluid glucose: Low fluid glucose suggests infection (<20mg/dL).
6. Fat stain: Sudan stain (a few drops of glacial acetic acid and Sudan III in ethanol). Positive indicates the presence of free fat that suggests intra-articular fracture.

What Not To Do:
Do not perform under the following circumstances:
1. Local infection along the proposed needle tract (eg, overlying cellulitis, periarticular infection)
2. Uncooperative patient, especially if unable to keep the joint immobile throughout procedure.
3. Difficulty in identifying bony landmarks
4. A poorly accessible joint space, as in hip aspiration in the obese patient
5. Inability to demonstrate a joint effusion on physical examination, except when septic arthritis is strongly suspected.

Chapter 30: Basic Medical Skills: Compartment Syndrome

COL Martha Lenhart, MC, USA

What: Diagnosis and management of compartment syndrome

When: Compression of muscle, nerves and blood vessels within a confined fascial compartment can result in the condition known as compartment syndrome (CS). Sustained, pressure elevation within a defined anatomic space causes decreased tissue perfusion and ultimately cell death (necrosis). Internal factors leading to CS include intra-compartmental bleeding from penetrating injuries, fractures, vascular injuries and swelling from contusions. External conditions leading to CS include skin constriction from burns and compartment compression from restrictive splints/casts/bandages. The most common site of CS is the leg, followed by the forearm. Early evaluation includes direct manual compression of the extremity to assess compartment tenseness in comparison to the contralateral extremity. Additionally, pain within the compartment of concern with passive motion of distal joints is indicative of CS. Outcomes of undiagnosed/untreated CS includes limited extremity function and limb loss.

What You Need: IV fluids/IV infusion set, bandages/splinting material, pain medication, antibiotics, tetanus prophylaxis, minor surgical set (scalpel, forceps, retractors, scissors), +/- urinary catheter

What To Do:
1. **Establish diagnosis**
   a. Fracture: Open or closed. Despite an impression that open fractures/open wounds have decompressed compartments, these may indeed be associated with development of CS.
   b. Contusion: Following low or high-energy trauma. Low energy injury as in a direct blow to leg during soccer or low speed MVA may result in the development of CS but is more likely to occur in higher energy traumas.
   c. Vascular injury: Penetrating injury to a major vessel or partial vascular occlusion from compression or spasm may result in direct intra-compartmental bleeding or compartment ischemia.
   d. Burn: Swelling and eschar formation may result in significant compartment compromise.
   e. Bites: Less common in the US; most US snakes have fangs that are generally too short to penetrate fascial compartments.

2. **Perform exam for CS using the Ps:** Pain/Pressure/Passive stretch/Paresis/Paresthesia/Pallor-Pulses
   a. Subjective complaint of increasing extremity pain.
   b. Pain out of proportion to the primary injury
   c. Pain with passive stretch of muscles by passive movement of digits distal to injury (toes/fingers)
   d. Palpation/manual compression of affected area – may feel tense, rock hard compartment and significantly different from contralateral, uninjured extremity
   e. Paresis: muscle weakness in injured extremity due to nerve involvement, muscle ischemia or guarding. **Note:** Isolated nerve injuries are associated with little pain.
   f. Paresthesia (anesthesia) in conscious/cooperative patient evaluate sensory deficit in distribution of potential nerve involvement
   g. Pulses: palpable in most patients/cases of CS. **Note:** Isolated arterial injuries are usually associated with absent pulses.
   h. Pallor: capillary refill routinely present.

3. **Monitor patient**
   a. Monitor (and maintain) vital signs and urinary output to maintain tissue perfusion.
   b. Perform repeated extremity evaluations to assess for CS.

4. **Manage non-surgically**
   a. Administer pain medication. Be aware that need for increased dosing of pain medication associated with decreased pain relief may signal the development of CS. *See Part 8: Procedures: Chapter 30: Pain Assessment and Control*
   b. Administer antibiotic if indicated (eg, GSW, shrapnel, other penetrating or open trauma). Give **cephazolin** 1g IV q8h or **clindamycin** 900mg IV q8h or **moxifloxacin** 400mg po daily through medical evacuation, and tetanus as indicated based on nature of the wound and immunization status.

  c. Loosen/release casts, circular dressings, constricting splints/bandages. Remove completely if symptoms do not improve within 1 hour.

  d. Maintain extremity at heart level as elevation above this height may decrease extremity perfusion.

  e. Re-examine the extremity regularly for evidence of improvement or deterioration. If deteriorating, proceed to manage surgically.

5. **Manage surgically:** Surgical decompression is the primary method of relieving compartment pressure.

  a. Evacuate all cases of suspected CS. (8 hours is the limit of tissue tolerance to severe, sustained elevation in compartment pressure)

  b. If evacuation is not possible, proceed as follows: (This procedure should NOT be performed without prior instruction.)

Figure 8-5. Lower Leg Compartments
Source: Emergency War Surgery, 3rd Revision, Borden Institute, 2004 p. 22-13

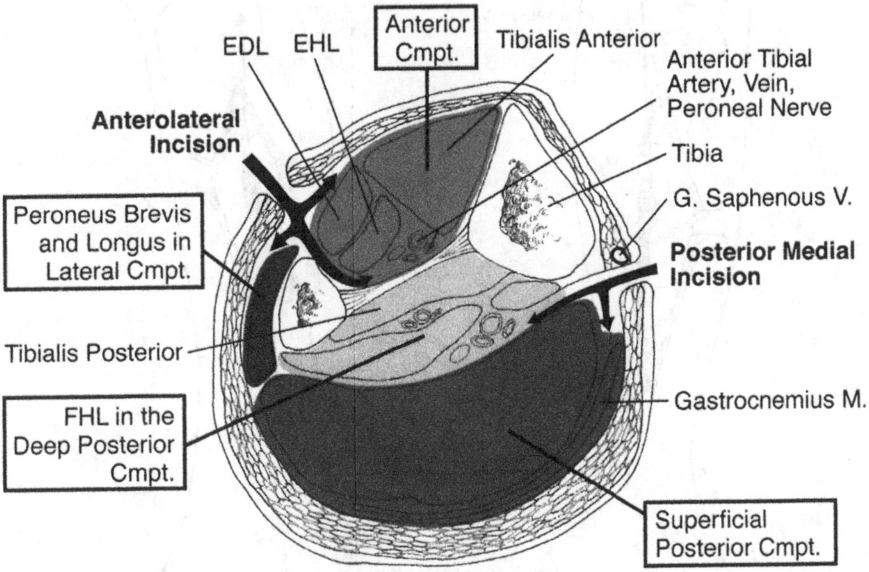

  c. Review leg anatomy.

   (1) Leg Compartments: The calf has 4 compartments: **(1) Lateral** containing peroneal brevis and longus; **(2) Anterior** containing extensor hallucis longus, extensor digitorum communis, tibialis anterior, and peroneus tertius; **(3) Superficial posterior** containing gastrocnemius and soleus; **(4) Deep posterior** containing the flexor hallucis longus, flexor digitorum longus, and the tibialis posterior.

    (a) Using the following surgical technique, release all involved leg compartments to relieve pressure.

     1.1 Use 2-incision technique (lateral and medial) to release the 4 leg compartments

     1.2 Incisions must extend the entire length of the calf to release all compressing skin.

     1.3 Place a lateral incision centered between the fibula and anterior tibial crest.

     1.4 Identify the lateral intermuscular septum and superficial peroneal nerve and release the anterior compartment with scissors in line with tibialis anterior muscle, proximally toward the tibial tubercle, and distally toward anterior ankle.

     1.5 Release the lateral compartment through this same incision

     1.6 Release the fascia with scissors in line with the fibular shaft, proximally toward the fibular head, distally toward the lateral malleolus.

     1.7 Make a 2nd incision medially at least 2cm medial to the medial-posterior palpable edge of the tibia.

     1.8 Avoid placing incisions over the surface of the tibia to prevent exposure of the tibia when tissues retract.

     1.9 The saphenous vein and nerve are identified/protected/retracted anteriorly.

     1.10 Using scissors, release the superficial compartment along its length.

     1.11 Release the deep posterior compartment over the FDL.

     1.12 Last, identify the tibialis posterior and release its fascia.

Figure 8-6. Compartment Syndrome: Lower Limb 2-Incision Technique
Source: Emergency War Surgery, 3rd Revision, Borden Institute, 2004 p. 22-12

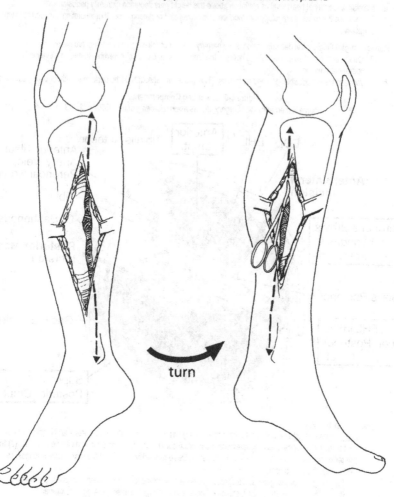

turn

(2) <u>Forearm Compartments:</u> The forearm has 3 compartments: **(1) mobile wad** proximally; **(2) volar** compartment;
 (3) dorsal compartment.
    (a) Using the following surgical technique, release all involved forearm compartments to relieve pressure.
        1.1   Use 2 incisions to release the 3 forearm compartments.
        1.2   Place a palmar incision between the thenar and hypothenar musculature in the palm, releasing the carpal
                  tunnel as needed.
        1.3   Curve this incision across the wrist flexion crease then extended up the volar forearm. At the elbow, just
                  radial to the medial epicondyle, curve this incision across the elbow flexion crease. Use of a curved skin
                  incision allows for soft-tissue coverage of the neurovascular structures at the wrist and elbows, and
                  prevents contractures from developing later at the flexion creases.
        1.4   Release the deep fascia with scissors.
        1.5   At the antecubital fossa, the fibrous band of the lacertus fibrosus overlying the brachial artery and median
                  nerve should be carefully released.
        1.6   Make a 2nd straight dorsal incision to allow release of the dorsal forearm compartment and reaching
                  proximally to release the mobile wad if necessary.

Figure 8-7. Forearm Compartments
Source: *Emergency War Surgery, 3rd Revision, Borden Institute, 2004 p. 22-11*

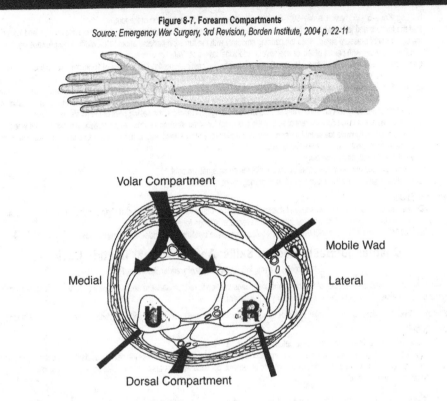

6. **Post-Op Care:**
   a. After fasciotomy, leave leg and forearm incisions open.
   b. Apply saline moistened gauze on exposed muscle (and neurovascular structures) and a clean, dry, bulky, nonconstricting bandage for coverage. Reinforce dressing as needed.
   c. Splint extremity in functional position following compartment release. Position ankle in neutral at 90° as tolerated, hand in "beer can holding" position.
   d. Observe for reduced pain (incisional pain now present but overall pain level and pain with passive stretch decrease) and resolving paresthesia
   e. Keep surgical site covered until evacuation/transfer to higher level care accomplished.
   f. Additional surgery for debridement of devitalized tissue and skin closure is performed at higher level of care.

What Not To Do:
1. Do not delay diagnosis/management of compartment syndrome: This is a limb-threatening emergency.
2. Do not perform compartment releases without prior instruction.
3. Do not close incisions immediately after fasciotomy.

Chapter 30: Basic Medical Skills: Splint Application
COL Winston J. Warme, MC, USA (Ret) & Alexander Bertelsen, PA-C

When: A casualty has a fractured or dislocated bone that requires stabilization. Apply a splint to relieve pain and prevent further harm by immobilizing the underlying bone, the joint above the injury and the joint below the injury.

What You Need: Water (NOT HOT), padding material (rolled cotton or Webril), a knife, scissors or cast saw, plaster or fiberglass casting material. Alternatives for splints: thin boards, sticks, or adjacent body parts for fingers/toes/legs or to splint an arm against the body. Alternatives for padding: cut sections of clothing/uniform.

What To Do:
1. Before applying a splint, inspect skin carefully to ensure that there are no sores or breaks in the skin that should be cleaned and dressed with Telfa before application of casting material. Small puncture wounds might actually be open fractures and should be treated emergently to decrease the incidence of infection. Patients with open fractures should receive tetanus prophylaxis and antibiotics if available (eg, **ceftriaxone** 1g IM or IV) before being evacuated.
2. Immobilize the injury in a position of function while immobilizing the joint above and below the fracture. Position the patient and encourage them to relax.
   a. Arm: Wrist–in a natural position, 15° extension (as if holding a can). Elbow–at a 90° angle

b. Leg: Knee–5°-15° flexion; Ankle–90°. There should be no inversion or eversion of the foot.

3. Pad the fracture and joint area with sheet cotton or Webril in acute injuries and postoperative cases to provide comfort and lessen the possibility of pressure sores. Wrap the padding smoothly with the turns overlapping about ½ the width of the previous layer. Pad bony prominences with pieces of felt, or use several additional layers of Webril or cotton.

4. Use 5x30 inch splints or rolls torn/cut to size. Dip and squeeze the casting material. Use a splint of 10 thicknesses (plies) of casting material on the posterior lower leg and continuing onto the plantar surface of the foot for ankle injuries. Extend out beyond the toes on the foot. Similarly, use 5-ply casting material to make medial and lateral splints for the arm. Extend just to the proximal palmar crease on the hand. Rub the plaster/fiberglass smooth as it is applied so that the layers blend. Rub and mold the splint with your hands over the contour of the body part until it is firmly set. Continue molding until reaching the setting point of the plaster/fiberglass.

5. Make sure the splint is not circumferential so that there is room for some swelling to occur. Avoid creating a pressure spot when holding the extremity while the splint hardens. Elevate the extremity above heart level to minimize the swelling and maximize comfort. Encourage the patient to wiggle toes and fingers.

6. Cover the splint with an Ace bandage.

7. Check peripheral neurovascular status to ensure that the splint is not too tight.

8. Evacuate the patient to orthopedics for definitive management.

What Not To Do:

1. Do not forget to reassess neurovascular status later. Remember that inflammation and swelling can continue and result in loss of neurovascular function 8-12 hours later. Inform the patient and arrange for re-examination.

2. DO NOT CAST AN ACUTELY INJURED PATIENT. Allow for tissue swelling with a non-circumferential splint.

Chapter 30: Basic Medical Skills: Apply External Traction Devices

COL Winston J. Warme, MC, USA (Ret) & Alexander Bertelsen, PA-C

When: When a casualty has a fracture of the lower limb that needs traction to reduce, stabilize and align a fracture. Apply the correct amount of traction to the extremity without causing further injury to the patient.

What You Need: Moleskin, elastic bandage, felt pads or cotton, stockinette, rope or cord, a spreader bar, soap, water, a razor and blades.

What To Do:

1. Inspect the skin of the lower extremity to determine the scope of injury.

2. Check the pulse in the lower extremity to ensure blood circulation. **Note:** If none, assess the neurovascular status before, after, and at intervals during the procedure. If pulses continue to be absent, continue with this task and evacuate as soon as possible.

3. Wash the lower extremity.

4. Shave the leg.

5. Pad the bony prominences of the leg (medial/lateral malleoli and fibular head) to prevent injury.

6. Apply moleskin to the medial and lateral aspects of the leg to protect the skin from breakdown.

7. Apply a long piece of stockinette from the medial proximal tibia to the lateral proximal tibia, leaving a loop below the foot. Attach the spreader bar to the stockinette, in line with the long axis of the extremity. Secure the stockinette to the limb with an elastic bandage.

   a. If stockinette is not available, improvise with rope, torn clothing or belts.

   b. The spreader bar can be a stiff branch, a canteen cup with a hole drilled in the center, or an unopened abdominal bandage taped to the device.

8. Align the rope over a pulley or pivot point with tension in line with the long axis of the extremity.

9. Attach 5 pounds of weight to the construct. More may be needed.
   Caution: The device used to attach the weight to the extremity must not be so tight that it restricts blood flow. The force applied by the weight must NOT exert uneven pressure that would cause skin necrosis.
   Note: Add additional weight until the patient experiences relief of pain. The relief will often be dramatic by adding as little as 2-3 pounds. Reduce the weight over the following days as the muscle spasm (that the traction device is designed to overcome) diminishes.

10. Perform a postreduction examination of the extremity to evaluate the following:

    a. Reduction efficacy.

    b. Neurovascular status. **Caution:** Pain may indicate the possibility of compartment syndrome. Re-examine the patient frequently for this complication. *See Part 8: Procedures: Chapter 30: Compartment Syndrome*

11. Check the pulses in the extremity hourly by palpation or if available, Doppler.

12. Record the procedure.

What Not To Do:

1. Do not add too much weight.

2. Do not constrict the limb, which restricts blood flow and causes necrosis.

Chapter 30: Basic Medical Skills: Urinary Bladder Catheterization

LTC Steve Waxman, MC USA, & LTC Douglas Soderdahl, MC, USA

What: Drain urinary bladder by passing a catheter through the urethra.

When: Monitor urinary output in critically ill patient; confirm adequate fluid resuscitation. In patient unable to void or who has distended urinary bladder due to poor emptying of the bladder (suggested by physical exam and [q15-20 minutes] voiding).

What You Need:

1. Catheter (options):
   a. Foley catheter: Has balloon at end of straight tip. Sizes generally used are 16 or 18 Fr. Balloon sizes are 5 and 30cc. 5cc balloon is most commonly used.
   b. Red rubber Robinson: Red colored straight catheters without balloons.
   c. Short female straight catheters: 14 or 16 Fr.
   d. Coudé catheter: Has curved tip with or without balloon. If balloon is attached, check to see if the balloon port is on the same or opposite side as the curved tip. If no balloon, there is usually a small raised bump or ridge at the opposite end to orient to the tip.
2. Antiseptic solution. If none is available, use soap and water.
3. (Sterile) Water soluble lubricant or **lidocaine** gel. **Lidocaine** gel can be made by mixing 10cc of 1% **lidocaine** solution with 10cc of lubricant to make a viscous solution.
4. 5-30cc syringe to inflate Foley balloon.

When You Do Not Have Everything (options):

1. If no Foley or Coudé, use feeding tube, nasogastric tube, small diameter chest tube or IV tubing (try to round the edges). Standard catheter size is about 3/8 inch diameter.
2. If no sterile tube, can boil tube. A clean non-sterile tube can be safely used as long as the bladder is emptied regularly and there is no evidence of break in the mucosal lining (gross bleeding). Risk of infection is low with clean intermittent catheterization.
3. If no sterile lubricant, try to find water-soluble lubricant or petroleum jelly. If nothing available: either use water, passing the catheter very slowly; or use saliva (preferably patient's).

What To Do:

1. Using sterile technique, wash the urethral meatus with antiseptic soap. In females, do not allow the labia to close over the washed urinary meatus. Lubricate the catheter with water soluble lubricant and gently pass the catheter into the bladder. In males, it is necessary to pass the catheter until the hub or flange is in contact with the urethra.
2. In young males, the pain caused by the catheter may cause the patient to clamp down with his sphincter preventing passage of the catheter. In such cases, use 10-20cc of **lidocaine** gel (1-2%). Squirt the **lidocaine** gel into the urethra and squeeze the meatus shut and hold for 1-2 minutes.
3. In older males, the prostate may make it difficult to pass a catheter. A Coudé catheter with the tip pointing up toward the patient's head may be easier to pass. A larger, stiffer Coudé in the 20-22 Fr size may be easier to pass. If only a small catheter can be passed, a urethral stricture may be present.
4. In females, the meatus may be tucked under a fold in the vaginal opening or obscured by the labia. "Frog leg" the patient as much as possible and elevate the buttocks. This is best accomplished with the patient in stirrups at the end of an exam table. An assistant may be required to spread the labia apart. A strong light is also very useful.
5. Have patient empty the bladder. Measure the residual, dipstick the urine and send for a culture if possible. Record the amount emptied from the bladder and the results of the testing. Normal post-void residuals should be generally under 100mL. In patients with large bladder capacities, a residual representing 20-25% of the total initial bladder volume is considered normal. Example: patient voids 450cc and has 150cc left. The initial bladder volume was 600cc with 25% remaining. This is acceptable.
6. If the bladder is palpable, place a Foley catheter. Empty the bladder as much as possible. Patients that have very large volumes (>1000mL) when suddenly emptied may experience a profound vasovagal reaction. To avoid a vasovagal reaction, with patient in the supine position, empty the bladder by letting out 400mL every few minutes. Extremely large bladders, when drained often will cause rupture of bladder mucosal veins that had been compressed by the bladder. Do not be surprised if the urine turns bloody. Irrigate to remove blood clots, as needed using sterile saline or water using a catheter tip syringe.
7. If the catheter is to be left in more than a day, daily cleaning of the meatus with antiseptic soap will decrease incidence of infection. Prophylactic antibiotics are not necessary. If there is a concern for recurrence of urinary retention, perform a "fill and pull" at the time of catheter removal by priming the bladder with 300-400mL in order to rapidly assess emptying and determine the need for re-catheterization.

What Not To Do:

1. Do not inflate the balloon unless urine flows through the catheter, and the catheter flange is at the meatus. If this is not done, the balloon may be inflated in the prostatic urethra.
2. Do not make more than 2 attempts to pass the catheter if there is injury to the urethra. Allow the patient to try to void. Consider a suprapubic catheter and evacuation.
3. Do not use saline to inflate the balloon if the catheter is to be left more than a day; use sterile water. (Saline may crystallize in the balloon port resulting in inability to deflate the balloon.)
4. Do not leave catheters in for more than 1 month without changing them.
5. Do not forget to always pull the foreskin of an uncircumcised male back down over the glans to prevent development of paraphimosis.

Chapter 30: Basic Medical Skills:
Suprapubic Bladder Aspiration (Tap) or Catheter Placement

LTC Steve Waxman, MC, USA & LTC Douglas Soderdahl, MC, USA

What: Insert a needle or catheter through the supra-pubic skin and abdominal wall into the urinary bladder and aspirate urine.

When: Bladder is palpable above pubic bone, patient cannot void and the urethra is unable to be successfully catheterized.

What You Need: Long spinal needle, if available (if not, use a 2 inch or longer needle for adults; 1½ inch for children), antiseptic skin prep, 10cc syringe , 60cc syringe, stopcock and IV tubing (desirable), 10cc of 1% **lidocaine** local anesthetic (optional), Kelly clamp (optional). Suprapubic "punch" kits specifically made for this purpose.

What To Do:
1. Confirm bladder is full:
   a. Palpate abdomen above pubic bone. If there is a midline mass above the pubic bone, confirm that this is the bladder by pressing on the mass. If there is increased urge to void, this suggests that the mass is the bladder. Then percuss abdomen above pubis. If the mass is dull and firm, this also suggests the mass is the bladder. Visualize the bladder by ultrasound if available (sono-cite) or other modality if present (CT scan).
   b. Do a bimanual rectal or vaginal exam to feel for an enlarged bladder.
      Warning: IF YOU CANNOT PALPATE THE BLADDER, DO NOT ATTEMPT A TAP. IF THE BLADDER IS NOT FULL, YOU MAY INJURE THE BOWEL OR MAJOR PELVIC BLOOD VESSELS. If the patient has a surgical scar in the lower middle abdomen, beware of underlying bowel even with a distended bladder and consider immediate referral to urologist, if practical.
2. Prep the skin, an area about the size of your hand, centered on a spot in the midline 1-2 finger-widths above the pubic bone with alcohol prep pads or povidone-iodine.
3. If you have **lidocaine**, fill the 10cc syringe and anesthetize the skin as described. This is about as painful as the tap will be, but the patient will be less likely to move during the procedure.
4. Attach the spinal needle (or appropriate length needle) to the lidocaine syringe and infiltrate the skin in the midline about 1-2 finger-widths above the pubic bone. Infiltrate the tough fascia below the skin and subcutaneous fat. Direct the needle straight down, perpendicular to the long axis of the body. Do not angle up toward the head or down toward the feet. You may infiltrate below the fascia.
5. If you are using a large 18 gauge needle, now insert the supplied obturator (wire that goes inside the needle) with the needle. If the needle is smaller, you may use a syringe to aspirate in place of the obturator. Attach the stopcock, tubing and 60cc syringe (if available) to siphon out the urine.
6. Pass the needle in the area that was anesthetized. Again, direct the needle straight down.
7. The bladder should be encountered within 1 inch below after going through the fascia (tough layer below the skin). If you do not get urine back, slowly withdraw the needle while aspirating.
8. Once urine is encountered, advance the needle about ½ inch. A Kelly clamp or other large clamp may be used to stabilize the needle. Use the 60cc (or the 10cc) syringe to aspirate urine.
9. Withdraw the needle once urine aspiration stops.
10. For suprapubic catheter placement, follow instructions on the specific catheter package insert. Do not attempt suprapubic catheter placement if you have not previously been instructed in the technique as misplacement can result in serious bowel or vascular injury.

What Not To Do:
1. Do not make repeated passes in different directions.
2. Do not insert the needle far from the pubic bone.
3. Do not advance the needle too deep. In most average size adults, it is difficult to go too deep. However, do not press the hub of the needle into the skin. In children, the bladder is higher (more superior) and much closer to the skin.

What to look for when emptying the bladder:
1. Suddenly emptying a large bladder (volumes >1000mL) may precipitate a profound vasovagal reaction, so empty the bladder with the patient lying down. To avoid a vasovagal reaction, empty the bladder by letting out 400mL every few minutes. Drainage of extremely large bladders can cause rupture of bladder mucosal veins that had been compressed by the urine, so do not be surprised if the urine turns bloody.
2. Some patients will have a marked increase in urine output after the bladder is decompressed. This signifies a significant obstruction to the bladder and kidneys that results in a post-obstructive diuresis. The urine output can be very high (eg, over 500mL/hour). In most cases, the patient's thirst mechanism may allow for adequate hydration. If urine output is very high (>200cc/hr), monitor the vital signs every hour and ask the patient if they feel lightheaded. If the pulse rate becomes elevated (>100) or there are orthostatic symptoms (lightheadedness) or decreased BP and increased pulse from supine to standing position, insert an IV catheter and give D5 ½ NS. Infuse the crystalloid over the next 2 hours at a rate to replace half the urine volume of the previous 2 hours.

Chapter 30: Basic Medical Skills: Portable Pressure Chamber
COL Paul Rock, MC, USA (Ret)

What: Portable hyperbaric ("pressure") chambers are fabric bags that can be internally pressurized to create a hyperbaric (higher pressure) condition inside the bag. The higher pressure inside is generated and maintained by a small hand, foot or battery powered air pump. Hyperbaric environments are useful for treating altitude illnesses because high pressure increases the oxygen available to the body. For a patient inside the pressure chamber bag, increased air pressure simulates descent to lower altitude. The difference between the air pressure outside and inside the chamber bag at high altitude determines the amount of simulated descent that can be achieved for the patient; the higher the actual altitude, the greater the pressure difference and the greater the simulated descent. For most chamber bags, the difference in pressure at 15,000 feet is the equivalent of a descent to an elevation of about 8,000 feet. Because the pressure difference between the inside of the bag and the atmosphere is less at lower elevations, the degree of simulated descent is less there. However, because descent of even a few thousand feet can be a life saving treatment for some altitude illnesses, pressure bags are still useful at altitudes as low as 9,000 feet.

Portable pressure chambers are relatively lightweight (generally less than 15 lbs) and can be folded for easy carrying in backpacks. They are commercially available in the civilian sector in several countries and can be purchased or rented through outdoor/travel medical suppliers. Available chambers include the Gamow Bag (USA), the CERTEC (France), the PAC (Portable Altitude Chamber, Australia). Portable pressure chambers are not normally available in the US military supply inventory outside of the Special Operations Command, but are available in the civilian sector. A Gamow bag is included in USASOC high altitude medical kits which are available through SOF supply channels. These lightweight, highly portable cloth chambers can be carried in a backpack and are extremely useful in treating high altitude illnesses when evacuation or descent to lower altitude is not possible. When deploying rapidly to high altitude terrain, strongly consider procuring such a chamber.

When: For temporary treatment of altitude illnesses (acute mountain sickness [AMS], high altitude cerebral edema [HACE], and high altitude pulmonary edema [HAPE]) when descent or evacuation is not available, or while waiting for evacuation. The light weight of portable pressure chambers allows the patient to be transported in the chamber by litter and aircraft.

What You Need: Required: Portable hyperbaric chamber (fabric "pressure chamber" bag) with pressure gauge, ventilation pump (hand-, foot- or battery powered), and connection hoses. Useful/Optional: Carbon dioxide absorption device ("CO_2 scrubber"; placed inside chamber), mat or blanket for patient to lie upon (for increased comfort), supplemental oxygen (can be placed inside fabric chamber).

What To Do:
Note: Follow specific instructions for the type/brand of pressure chamber being used.
Begin Treatment
1. Attach ventilation pump to chamber using hose.
2. Place patient in chamber (Be sure patient's head is visible in viewing window.)
3. Close chamber (If patient is alert, instruct them to hold the fabric away from their face.)
4. **IMMEDIATELY** begin pressurizing/ventilating the chamber with ventilation pump.
5. Watch pressure gauge. When chamber is pressurized enough, ventilation valve will open automatically to exhaust CO_2 and prevent over-pressurization. Listen for sound of air exhaust from ventilation/dump valve to confirm ventilation.
6. Continue pumping at slower rate to maintain pressure and ventilation. Do not stop pumping while patient is inside chamber.

Length of Treatment
1. Treatment in hyperbaric chamber can be life-saving and should be continued while awaiting and throughout descent to lower altitude. If medical evacuation is not possible, treat until symptoms have completely resolved (usually takes more than 2-3 hours). Altitude illness will most likely return in 12 hours if the patient does not descend.
2. Continuously observe patient through chamber window. Talk to patient to reassure; chambers transmit voices easily.

End Treatment
1. Instruct patient to equalize ears as necessary during chamber decompression by swallowing or Valsalva maneuver.
2. Open exhaust ("dump") valve. Continue pumping at low rate to maintain ventilation.
3. Watch pressure gauge. When pressure inside chamber is equal to pressure outside (gauge reads "0"), open chamber and remove patient. Opening chamber before pressures are equal causes sudden decompression and can damage patient's ears or sinuses. Theoretically, sudden decompression could also cause DCS ("bends").

What Not To Do:
1. Do not stop ventilation pump while patient is inside chamber. (Constant pumping is required to insure continued oxygen supply and to exhaust carbon dioxide.)
2. Do not decompress chamber at rapid rate or open it before pressure inside is equal to pressure outside. (necessary to avoid sudden decompression problems)

Chapter 30: Basic Medical Skills: Pain Assessment and Control
COL Chester 'Trip' Buckenmaier III, MC, USA

What: Pain control is an integral part of the overall management of the sick or injured patient and often the most neglected aspect of trauma care. Many studies have shown that health care providers are poor at recognizing and treating pain and that untreated acute pain can lead to chronic pain syndromes. The medic should not allow his own feelings or bias toward pain influence how he perceives his patient's reaction to injury, but simply recognize that each person handles pain in their own way and try to alleviate the pain to the maximum extent possible given the circumstances. In the austere medical condition of war or disaster medicine, effective pain control can reduce the burden of a casualty on mission completion. Casualties relieved of pain can better assist with mission objectives or be active participants in their own evacuations. The SOF medic should teach the patient that it is easier to prevent pain than to "chase" or treat it once it has become established, and that communication of unrelieved pain is essential to its relief.

When: Pain should be assessed at its onset and reassessed frequently.

What You Need: Assessment of pain (based on history [see mnemonic] and exam), reference list of medications and related information (including side effects), availability of medications and delivery mechanisms (needle, syringe, etc.). A general understanding of new pain technologies available in the continuum of care is vital, even if these technologies are not presently available to the SOF medic.

What To Do:
1. Assess patient's pain using history and exam. This mnemonic will be helpful.
   OPQRST Mnemonic for Pain Assessment
   <u>O</u> = Onset: What caused the pain? Was it sudden or gradual?
   <u>P</u> = Palliate/Provoke: What palliates or provokes the pain? What makes it better or worse?
   <u>Q</u> = Quality: What does the pain feel like? (sharp, dull, tearing, etc.)
   <u>R</u> = Radiate: Where is the pain most intense on the body? Does the pain radiate? If so, from where to where?
   <u>S</u> = Severity: How bad is the pain on a scale of 0 to 10? (with 0 being no pain, and 10 being the worst imaginable) This number is used to guide pain treatment. Usually a pain level of 4 or less is the goal of treatment.
   <u>T</u> = Time: How long have you been in pain? Is it continuous or intermittent? Has it gotten worse, better, or stayed the same?
2. Consult reference material and use a stepped approach for the control of pain:
   a. **Mild to Moderate Pain:** Begin, unless there is a contraindication, with a non-steroidal anti-inflammatory drug (NSAID) or **acetaminophen.** NSAIDs or single injections of local anesthetics alone may control mild to moderate pain after relatively minor surgical procedures. NSAIDs decrease levels of inflammatory mediators generated at the site of tissue injury. At

present, one NSAID (**ketorolac**) is approved by the FDA for parenteral use. All but two NSAIDs (**salsalate** and **choline magnesium trisalicylate**) appear to produce a risk of platelet dysfunction that may result in clinically significant bleeding and carry a small risk of GI bleeding. (Chronic use of NSAIDS can lead to a substantial increase of this risk.) **Acetaminophen** does not affect platelet aggregation, but neither does it provide peripheral anti-inflammatory activity. Agonist-antagonist medications such as **butorphanol** or **nalbuphine** bind to various opioid receptors producing agonist and antagonist effects and are useful in managing moderate pain. These potent analgesics, while possibly less easily titrated (and possibly less effective in men) to reduce pain compared to pure opioid agonists, tend to be associated with a reduced incidence of respiratory depression. Benzodiazepines (anti-anxiety drugs) such as **midazolam** are often used to reduce agitation and anxiety associated with painful injuries, but this class of medications cannot be used alone to manage pain since they possess no analgesic effect.

b. **Moderately Severe to Severe Pain:** Normally treated initially with an opioid analgesic, especially for more extensive surgical procedures that cause moderate to severe pain. The concurrent use of opioids, NSAIDs, regional anesthetics, among other pain medications (multimodal therapy) often provides more effective analgesia with fewer drug side-effects than any one drug class used alone. Multimodal therapy has the added benefit of reducing opioid requirements, minimizing the potentially devastating side effect of respiratory depression associated with this class of drugs. In contrast to opioids, NSAIDs and local anesthetics do not cause sedation or respiratory depression, nor do they interfere with bowel or bladder function. For these reasons, special emphasis on the use of NSAIDS and regional anesthetic blocks (*see Part 5: Specialty Areas: Chapter 19: Local/Regional Anesthesia*) with local anesthetics for managing pain in extreme environments is recommended to keep the wounded Soldier "in the fight" if possible.

c. **Opioid Tolerance or Physiological Dependence:** Patients should be reassured that these complications are very unusual in short-term use by opioid naive patients. Likewise, psychological dependence and addiction are extremely unlikely to develop when patients without prior drug abuse histories use opioids for acute pain. Proper use of opioids involves selecting: 1) appropriate drug, initial dose, and frequency of administration; 2) consideration of non-opioid analgesics (multimodal therapy), 3) a clear understanding of incidence and severity of side effects. Titrate opioids to achieve the desired therapeutic effect and to maintain that effect over time.

d. **Other Pain:** When increasing doses of opioids are ineffective in controlling postoperative pain, search for another source of pain, and consider other non-opioid analgesics in a multimodal pain plan. Unusual diagnoses such as neuropathic pain (ie, burning, tingling or electrical shock sensation triggered by very light touch, and accompanied by a sensory deficit in the area innervated by the damaged nerve) may complicate pain management in patients with previous injury.

e. **Other Therapies:** Remember that interventions such as relaxation, distraction, and massage can reduce pain, anxiety, and the amount of drugs needed for pain control. Stabilization and splinting of fractures along with protective padding around wounds can significantly reduce the pain of injury. A confident and compassionate treatment approach to the patient's pain will enhance the effectiveness of any pain management plan.

Table 8-1. Suggested Dosages of Opioids for Acute Pain Control in the 70 kg Opioid-Naive Military Casualty

Some of the medications and devices are not presently available to the SOF medic (in white italics) but in the rapid evacuation environment of modern warfare it is likely these medications and devices will be encountered now and in the near future. The SOF medic should be familiar with these recent medication and technology additions to the battlefield.

Opioid	Intravenous/ Intramuscular[1]	PCA[2]	Oral	Plasma half-life	Comments[3]
Morphine	5-15mg q3-4 hours	1-2mg q6-12 minutes	10-30mg q2-3 hours	3 hours (1-5 hours)	Principal medical alkaloid of opium, active metabolites, respiratory depression, increased intracranial pressure
Hydromorphone	2-3mg q3-4 hours	0.2-0.8mg q8-12 minutes	2-3mg q 4-6 hours	2-3 hours	Semi-synthetic opioid, approximately 5 times more potent then morphine and a useful alternative
Fentanyl	25-100µg q5 minutes titrated to effect at bedside	25-50µg q8-12 minutes, rare applications	Sublingual preparation available	7 hours (3-12 hours)	Synthetic, usually not available far forward. Novel delivery technologies are in development that will increase use in the near future.
Oral transmucosal fentanyl citrate (fentanyl lollypop)	N/A	N/A	400-800µg unit consumed over 15 minutes	7 hours (3-12 hours)	Use with caution. Patients should be monitored at all times.
Fentanyl iontophoretic transdermal system (PCA transdermal patch)	N/A	40µg/activation Patient-activated	N/A	7 hours (3-12 hours)	Currently under development.

Table 8-1. Suggested Dosages of Opioids for Acute Pain control in the 70 kg Opioid-naive Military Casualty, continued

Opioid	Intravenous/ Intramuscular[1]	PCA[2]	Oral	Plasma half-life	Comments[3]
Meperidine	75-150mg q2-3 hours	10mg q6-12 minutes, rare applications	100-300mg q3 hours	3-5 hours	Toxic metabolite normeperidine can lead to seizures, increased risk of abuse due to rapid onset and associated "rush"
Codeine	15-60mg q4 hours IM only	N/A	30-60mg q4 hours	2-4 hours	Antitussive, combined with acetaminophen as Tylenol-3; ineffective in 10% of Caucasians
Oxycodone	N/A	N/A	10-20mg q4-6 hours	3-4.5 hours	Combined with aspirin as Percodan and acetaminophen as Percocet; high abuse potential
Tramadol	50-100mg q4-6 hours	N/A	50-150mg q4-6 hours	5-7 hours	Respiratory depression is not a common side effect; can decrease the seizure threshold
Nalbuphine	10-20mg q3-6 hours, 160mg maximum daily	N/A	10mg q3-6 hours	5 hours	Acute withdrawal in persons addicted to opiates synthetic agonist-antagonist; tends to be more effective in women
Butorphanol	0.5-2mg q3-4 hours	N/A	N/A	4-7 hours	May cause dysphoria; nasal spray 1mg q 4 hours for migraine

[1]Generally, the intramuscular administration of opioids should be avoided in favor of intravenous administration.
[2]Patient controlled analgesia (PCA) is a preferred method for opioid pain control when equipment is available and the patient is able to operate the PCA device. This Level 3 medical device may be available further forward in the near future.
[3]Naloxone is an opioid antagonist that will reverse systemic opioid effects (analgesia, sedation, respiratory depression, etc.) and should be available when opioids are used. Naloxone 0.2-0.04mg doses are titrated to desired effect every 2-3 minutes; the effect is dose dependent lasting 20-60 minutes.

Table 8-2. Equianalgesic Opioid Conversion (mg)

Opioid	Intravenous	Oral
Morphine	1	3
Hydromorphone	0.2	0.6
Meperidine	10	30
Fentanyl	0.01	0.03

Table 8-3. Suggested Dosages of Nonsteroidal Anti-inflammatory Drugs (NSAIDs) for Acute Pain Management in the Military Casualty

NSAID	Intravenous/ Intramuscular	Oral	Plasma half-life	Comments
Acetaminophen	N/A	325-1000mg q 4-6 hours up to 3000 mg/day	1-4 hours	Does not produce gastric irritation or alter platelet aggregation; weak antiinflammatory; hepatotoxic in large doses
Ketorolac	30mg then 15-30mg q6 hours	10mg q 4-6 hours	5 hours	30mg IV is equivalent to 10mg of morphine; moderate antiinflammatory activity; may cause life-threatening bronchospasm in asthma patients

Table 8-3. Suggested Dosages of Nonsteroidal Anti-inflammatory Drugs (NSAIDs)
for Acute Pain Management in the Military Casualty, continued

NSAID	Intravenous/ Intramuscular	Oral	Plasma half-life	Comments
Acetylsalicylic acid (Aspirin)	N/A	325-650mg q4-6 hours	2-3 hours	Antipyretic, low intensity pain, effective platelet activation inhibitor; useful for acute angina or myocardial infarction, can induce asthma in up to 20% of asthmatics
Ibuprofen	N/A	400-800mg q8 hours	2 hours	Low incidence of GI side effects
Naproxen	N/A	250-500mg q12 hours	12-15 hours	Longer half-life allows twice daily dosing
Indomethacin	N/A	25-50mg q8 hours	4.5 hours	Potent anti-inflammatory
Celecoxib	N/A	400mg loading dose followed by 100-200mg daily	11 hours	Highly selective COX-2 inhibitor, greater cardiovascular risk than other NSAIDs

(1) **Benzodiazepines: Diazepam:** Indications: Muscle relaxation, sedation. Contraindications: Respiratory depression. Routes: Oral, IV, IM, Rectal. Dose: Oral: 5-10mg every 8 hours for sedation, IV: 5-10mg, IM: 10mg, Rectal: 10mg (1 day only). Side Effects: Respiratory depression, cardiovascular collapse, paradoxic excitation. **Midazolam:** Indications: Same as diazepam. Contraindications: Same as diazepam. Routes: IV, IM. Dose: IV: 1-2mg; IM: 5-10mg, Side Effects: Respiratory depression. **Lorazepam:** Indications: Sedation in acute psychotic agitation. Contraindications: Same as diazepam. Routes: IV, IM. Dose: 0.05-0.1mg/kg over 2-4 minutes. Maximum dose 8mg in 12 hours. Usually mixed with **haloperidol** 10mg IM for the treatment of acute psychotic agitation. Side Effects: Same as diazepam.

(2) **Local Anesthetics:** Indications: Local or regional anesthesia (*see Part 5: Specialty Areas: Chapter 19: Local/Regional Anesthesia*). Contraindications: Allergy. Routes: Local infiltration subcutaneously. Dose: short acting local anesthetics - **lidocaine:** 3mg/kg, mepivacaine: 8mg/kg. Dose: long acting local anesthetics – **ropivacaine:** 1.5mg/kg, **bupivacaine:** 1.5mg/kg. Side Effects: CNS and cardiovascular toxicity if injected intravascularly (especially bupivacaine).

(3) **Other Agents:**
   a. **Ketamine:** Indications: Painful invasive procedures. Contraindications: Hypertension. Head or eye injury. Chest or abdominal surgery. Routes: IV, IM. Dose: IV 1-2mg/kg. IM 4mg/kg. IV infusion of 0.5-1mg/kg per hour approved for adult use only for prolonged procedures. **Atropine** at 0.1mg/kg for children to 1-2mg for adults should be added to control secretions. Side Effects: Emergence hallucinations (mostly in adults, benzodiazepines can mitigate this effect) Hypertension, respiratory depression if given rapidly IV.
   b. Reversing Agents: **Naloxone** - Indications: Reversal of side effects of opiates. Contraindications: No absolute. Will trigger opiate withdrawal. Routes: IV, IM, SC. Dose: 0.1-2.0mg q 2-3 min to max of 10mg. Side effects: Acute withdrawal may exhibit combativeness. **Flumazenil** - Indications: Reversal of benzodiazepine overdose resulting in airway compromise or significant hypotension. Contraindications: Benzodiazepine dependence or if used for seizure control as it will trigger intractable seizures, concomitant ingestion of tricyclic antidepressants (TCAs), presence of increased intracranial pressure such as in head injury. Routes: IV. Dose: 0.2mg IV every minute until desired response to a maximum dose of 3mg. Side effects: *see contraindications.*

What Not To Do:
1. **Do not** give insufficient pain medication to achieve relief.
2. **Do not** give pain medication only after the pain has returned. Anticipate the onset of pain, and give the medication 30 minutes BEFORE the pain returns to provide effective relief.
3. **Do not** fail to consider all classes of pain medications and their few side effects before prescribing. A patient that gets good pain control from morphine, but starts to vomit repeatedly as a side effect, might have benefited from a non-opioid medication. Favor the use of NSAID and local anesthetic medications in the pain management plan.
Note: Do use multimodal pain therapies selecting drugs from each class thus improving overall pain control while minimizing the dose related side-effects of any one drug. Continuously reassess the patient for pain and medication related side effects.

Chapter 30: Basic Medical Skills: Length of Use for Compressed Oxygen Cylinders

COL Jackie A. Hayes, MC, USA

Introduction: Gas cylinders containing oxygen are frequently used to provide supplemental oxygen for patient care. It is beneficial to maintain awareness of the supply of gas remaining in the cylinder. This will help ensure that adequate supplies are available and allow planning for replacement of cylinders. In general, a full E cylinder with a flow rate of 10 liters/minute will last approximately 60 minutes. A full H cylinder with a flow rate of 10L/minute will last 10 times as long or approximately 10 hours. These figures are approximate and only to be used as a general guide:

Table 8-4. Length of Use for Compressed Oxygen Cylinders: An Approximate Guide

Cylinder	D	E	G	H
Liters	356	622	5260	6900
Flow (LPM)	Length of Use (minutes)	Length of Use (minutes)	Length of Use (minutes)	Length of Use (minutes)
2	178	311	2630	3450
4	89	155	1315	1725
6	59	104	876	1150
8	44	78	658	862
10	35	62	526	690
12	30	52	438	575
15	23	41	350	460

To Estimate Duration of Use for Oxygen Cylinders

The duration of gas flow can be estimated if the cylinder size, gas flow rate and cylinder pressure are known. This information outlines a method of calculating the duration of gas flow in cylinders of varying sizes and flow rates. The duration of flow is proportionate to the amount of gas in the cylinder and the size of the cylinder. The duration of flow is inversely related to the flow rate.

Duration of Flow = Contents of cylinder/Flow rate

The contents of the cylinder are usually measured in cubic feet or gallons and the flow rate is usually measured in liters/minute. Because of the difference in units of measurement, a conversion has to be made. Rather than converting units of measurement for each size of cylinder, a cylinder factor can be used. The assigned cylinder factors for oxygen are in Table 8-5:

Table 8-5. Cylinder Factors for Calculation of Duration of Oxygen Flow

Cylinder Size	D	E	G	H and K
Factor	0.16	0.28	2.41	3.14

Once you have the cylinder factor and the amount of pressure remaining in the cylinder, the duration of flow can be calculated with the following equation:

Duration of Flow (minutes) = Pressure (psig) x Cylinder Factor/Flow (L/min)

For example, if an E cylinder with a current psi of 1400 was being used at a flow rate of 2L/min, the duration of flow could be calculated as follows:

Duration of Flow (minutes) = 1400 x 0.28/2 L/min = 196 minutes

An H cylinder with a current PSI of 1500 and flow rate of 10L/min would have the following duration of flow:

Duration of Flow (minutes) = 1500 x 3.14/10 L/min = 471 minutes

This will allow for estimation of duration of flow for oxygen cylinders of varying sizes and varying flow rates.

Chapter 30: Basic Medical Skills: Teleconsultation

LTC Charles Lappan, MSC, USA (Ret) & COL Ronald Poropatich, MC, USA

When: Medical specialists may not be readily available at all locations, so a multispecialty teleconsultation service available is to all deployed providers and to Independent Duty Medical Technicians. Consultations are answered 7 days a week within 24 hours by a medical technician working under the authority of a provider. Consultations are provided by specialists from all branches of the military. The teleconsultation system is accessible on the Army Knowledge Online (AKO) portal.

What You Need: Specialties organized into email groups – send teleconsultation to appropriate email

Table 8-6. Existing Teleconsultation Specialties

Medical Specialty	Email Address
Burn-trauma	burntrauma.consult@us.army.mil
Cardiology	cards.consult@us.army.mil
Dermatology	derm.consult@us.army.mil
Ophthalmology	eye.consult@us.army.mil
Infectious Diseases	id.consult@us.army.mil
Internal Medicine	im.consult@us.army.mil
Nephrology	nephrology.consult@us.army.mil
Neurology	neuron.consult@us.army.mil
Orthopedics and Podiatry	ortho.consult@us.army.mil
Traumatic Brain Injury	tbi.consult@us.army.mil
Pediatric Intensive Care	picu.consult@us.army.mil
Preventive Medicine	pmom.consult@us.army.mil
Rheumatology	rheum.consult@us.army.mil
Toxicology	toxicology.consult@us.army.mil
Urology	urology.consult@us.army.mil

Table 8-7. "As Requested" Teleconsultation Specialties

Other specialties "as requested" – send teleconsultation to chuck.lappan@us.army.mil

Medical Specialty	Email Address
Allergy	chuck.lappan@us.army.mil
Endocrinology	chuck.lappan@us.army.mil
EENT	chuck.lappan@us.army.mil
Flight Medicine	chuck.lappan@us.army.mil
Gastroenterology	chuck.lappan@us.army.mil
General Surgery	chuck.lappan@us.army.mil
Hematology	chuck.lappan@us.army.mil
Legal	chuck.lappan@us.army.mil
Neurosurgery	chuck.lappan@us.army.mil
Nutrition	chuck.lappan@us.army.mil
OB-GYN	chuck.lappan@us.army.mil
Oncology	chuck.lappan@us.army.mil
Oral & Maxillofacial Pathology	chuck.lappan@us.army.mil
Pharmacy	chuck.lappan@us.army.mil
Plastic Surgery	chuck.lappan@us.army.mil
Pulmonary Diseases	chuck.lappan@us.army.mil
Psychiatry	chuck.lappan@us.army.mil
Radiology	chuck.lappan@us.army.mil
Speech Pathology	chuck.lappan@us.army.mil
Vascular Surgery	chuck.lappan@us.army.mil

What To Do: **How To Send A Consult**

Gather patient history, images and other attachments and email them to the specialty emails listed in the specialties organized into email groups or to chuck.lappan@us.army.mil for other specialties "as requested" that are not included in the specialties generic emails.

Patient History

1. When did it start? Days? Weeks? Months? Years?
2. Patient symptoms now?
3. Chronicity: Getting better? Worse? Staying the same? Spreading?
4. What was used to previously treat the patient?
5. Effectiveness of previous treatments?
6. Laboratory and test results if any?
7. Your diagnosis and/or differential diagnosis
8. Limitations you have in treating the patient such as medications, procedures, lab tests?

Include patient demographics: branch of service, age, and gender. If not US military, state their nationality. Identify if contractor, detainee, foreign military, etc

Include digital images if appropriate

1. Use the JPEG format for images
2. Check images before transmitting to ensure they are in focus and accurately portray the problem as you see it
   a. Usually 3 to 5 images is all we need
   b. When in doubt, overload us with images
3. Other attachments:
   a. PDFs of ECGs
   b. JPEGs of radiographs
   c. Copies of laboratory and pathology reports

What Not To Do:

1. Do not include any patient identifying information especially patient's name or SSN.
2. Do not resend additional request to the consultant who answered your consult; consultants work on a call-roster and look for consults only for the period they are on-call. They usually delete all consults after they have answered them. A new consult file is made by the Project Manager for each file that is sent to the generic email address and that re-consult will be sent only to the current on-call consultant.
3. Do not include "archive" attachments as certain file types such files are automatically blocked.
4. Do not send images or other attachments in any other format other than PDF or JPEG.
5. Do not include more than one patient per teleconsultation.

Chapter 31: Nursing Procedures: Nursing Assessment

Gay D. Thompson, RN, MPH

When: You have a sick and/or injured patient that you have stabilized medically, but he will need your prolonged nursing care in an austere environment. Your patient may not be able to perform even the most minimal of his acts of daily living; breathing, swallowing, coughing, drinking, eating, re-positioning (turning, moving extremities), toileting, and hygiene. The patient needs regular physical assessments to monitor his condition, as well as multiple nursing interventions to prevent him from developing complications from his injuries/illness and from the risks of invasive tubes and the hazards of immobility, such as DVT, pneumonia, pressure sores, fecal impactions, and urinary tract infections. You must assess your patient's overall needs to see what kind of nursing care he will need while he is in your hands. All nursing care must be individualized according to your patient's age, gender, mental status, and clinical condition. You must adapt the priorities of your care plan as your patients condition changes from hour to hour, and you must "triage" the needs for your nursing care if you have multiple patients. This section includes some basic questions you must ask yourself as you do your initial and periodic nursing assessments on your medically stable patients.

What To Do:

1. Vital signs: *How often do I need to check VS on this patient? What would be the norms for this patient? Should I measure oral, rectal, or axillary temperature? Is his temperature a reflection of a hot or cold environment, or is it because of a physiological change in his condition? Do I have the correct size BP cuff for this patient? If I cannot take the BP on the arm because of injury, can I measure it on his leg? What are the signs of deterioration in this patient? Does this patient need repeated neuro exams? How will this patient express pain? What pain meds are most appropriate for this patient and his condition?*
2. Tubes: *What tubes does the patient have? ET, NG, chest tube, IV, Foley? How often will I need to check them for patency? Are they well secured if the patient pulls at them or is turned, or if I have to move him quickly? How do the insertion sites appear?*
3. Pulmonary status: *Is the patient positioned so his airway is patent? How is his pulse ox? Does he exhibit signs of hypoxia? Are his lungs clear to auscultation? Does he need suctioning? Can he turn over on his own? Do I need to do postural drainage?*
4. Hydration/nutrition status: *How do I monitor his hydration status? How long can I sustain him with just IV fluids? Will he be able to eat or drink? What do I have on hand that could be crushed to feed him? Do I need to insert a NG tube to keep him hydrated and fed? How often do I need to tally up the intake and output?*

5. Wounds and dressings: *How often do I need to check for drainage or bleeding? How often do I need to irrigate the wounds and change the dressings? Are there signs of wound infection? How can I prevent him from getting infections, or from infecting others? Does he have any rashes or lesions?*

6. Splints: *Are they too tight or too loose?*

7. Bowel care: *When was his last BM? Is he impacted? Is he having diarrhea?*

8. Bladder care: *When was his last voiding? Is his bladder distended? Is he dribbling urine? Should I do and in and out catheterization or does he need an indwelling catheter?*

9. Eye care: *Was he wearing contact lens at the time of his injury? Do I need to tape his eyes shut for protection? How often do I need to instill lubricating drops or ointment?*

10. Mouth care: *Does he have any loose teeth? Are his mucous membranes dry or cracked? How can I clean his mouth?*

11. Mobility: *Can he move at all? Will his condition permit sitting up? How often do I need to reposition him or do range of motion on his extremities?*

12. Skin care: *Does he have any signs of pressure sores? Is he continent? If not, what is the skin condition of around his buttocks/genitals/groin?*

13. Communication: *Can he hear me? Can he see me without his glasses? How can I best communicate with this patient?*

Chapter 31: Nursing Procedures: Nursing Interventions

LTC Prospero C. Donan, Jr., AN, USA

Introduction: The principles of the nursing process outlined in this section can be applied to austere conditions in which SOF medics work. It is written in a holistic manner so that it will apply to as many patient conditions that might be encountered in austere environments. The care is cyclical and recurs as often as the need arises. For the sake of succinctness and space limitations, detailed explanations of rationales are not discussed. This is to be used in conjunction with medical, surgical, and pharmacologic treatment modalities prescribed in other chapters, and in the detailed nursing care described in the rest of this chapter, and on the electronic version. Each of the system interventions provided addresses the issue of prolonged bed rest, limited neuromuscular activity, and maintenance in a fixed position. Document every patient condition, nursing intervention, and patient outcome.

What You Need: BP cuff, stethoscope, body and oral hygiene equipment, basin (helmet), watch with 2nd hand, gloves, thermometer, liquid measuring device (for urine, watery stools, vomitus), pillows, tubing, blankets, heat/cold packs, marker (for dressings), flashlight, water-soluble lubricant, suction catheters, hot water, syringes of various sizes, padding, gauze pads.

Respiratory Care:
1. For patients with artificial airways: monitor ventilatory status, assess breath sounds every 2 hours, and assess for secretions.
2. Suction mouth and throat using clean technique. Use sterile technique if suctioning tracheostomy or ET tube.
3. Humidify the air using a humidifier, moist gauze, or a boiling pot of water (keep away from patient).
4. Provide mouth care using mouthwash or diluted hydrogen peroxide.
5. Keep the head of the bed elevated.
6. Change position every two hours.
7. Perform chest physical therapy:
   a. Diaphragmatic breathing
      (1) 2 count inhalation through nose
      (2) 4 count exhalation through mouth
      (3) Focus on movement of abdomen, not chest
      (4) Perform for 1 minute, rest for 2 minutes
      (5) Work up to 10 minutes 4x per day.
   b. Pursed-lip breathing
      (1) 2 count inhalation through nose
      (2) 4 count exhalation through pursed lips
      (3) Tighten the abdomen.

8. Perform postural drainage: Percuss using cupped hands for 1-2 minutes. Repeat according to patient's tolerance. Avoid percussing over spine, kidneys, spleen, clavicle, scapula, or sternum.
   a. To drain lower lobes, superior segment, place patient in prone position with pillow under hips.
   b. To drain upper lobes, anterior segment, place patient in supine position with pillow under hips.
   c. To drain lower lobes, anterior basal segment, place patient right side down with pillow under hips, and elevate the foot of bed.
   d. To drain lower lobes, lateral basal segments, place patient left side down with pillow under hips, and elevate the foot of bed.
9. Decrease the risk of pulmonary embolism using non-pharmacologic care:
   a. Promote early mobilization
   b. Do passive and active range of motion exercises.

Cardiovascular Care:

1. Place the patient is a semi-Fowler's position (elevated head and back); provide O_2; monitor VS and dysrhythmias. Assess pain level, UO, and bleeding. Encourage deep breathing. Decrease anxiety.
2. Goals: saturation >92%, decrease PVCs, ↓ pain, ↓ anxiety. Talk to the patient. Explain what you are doing at every step, even if you are not sure he can hear you.
3. Hypervolemia: ↑ BP and ↑ pulse, venous distention, headache, anxiety, SOB, tachypnea, coughing, pulmonary crackles. Monitor: I/O, infusion at KVO, observe for bladder distention, elevate head of bed
4. Hypovolemia: ↓ BP, ↓ UO, and ↑ pulse. Monitor I/O, ↑ fluids.
5. Decrease the risk of deep vein thrombosis:
   a. Use thigh-high graduated compression elastic stockings
   b. Elevate the legs
   c. Use pneumatic calf compression, if available
   d. Isometric exercises of the lower extremity
6. Monitor BP before attempting to mobilize a patient that has been at bed rest for 3-5 days. Have him sit for brief periods of time before trying to stand up.

Neurologic/Sensory/Skin Care:

1. Bed rest.
2. Elevate head of bed.
3. Monitor neurologic status, temperature, VS, bowel, and bladder control frequently.
4. Insert urinary catheter if not already done.
5. Always talk to the patient and keep him oriented to time and place. Touch the patient and speak slowly. Keep him involved in his care.
6. Bathing and toileting needs: give patient a bed bath every 24 hours. Provide clean clothes. Clean groin and perineal area with soap and warm water. Urine and feces will break down skin quickly.
7. Fever: Cold compresses to head, forehead, in armpits, and groin.
8. Perform range of motion exercises. Massage and pad pressure points. Turn every 2 hours. Avoid creases underneath the patient's sheet. Keep skin clean and moisturized.
9. Parts of the body that are at risk for ulcerations in the supine position are: occiput, spine, sacrum, elbows, and heels. In the sitting position, it is the ischial tuberosities.
10. Promote early ambulation to maintain balance and gait.

Endocrine and Metabolic Care:

1. Endocrine disorders affect metabolic functions.
2. If a laboratory is available, monitor the patient's electrolytes and serum glucose.
3. VS, ECGs, I/O, weight changes, and edema.
4. Explain care slowly and repeatedly because the patient might be confused, mentally slow, or lethargic.

Musculoskeletal Care:

1. Elevate injured extremity above the level of the heart.
2. Pad pressure points. Improvise with boot pads, helmet liners, foam.
3. Inspect and clean wounds, change dressings, and assess neurovascular status. Do not over-constrict dressing.
4. Monitor for shock and hemorrhage.
5. If possible, let the patient ambulate.
6. Use anti-embolism stockings.
7. Observe for pulmonary emboli (restlessness, confusion, irritability, and disorientation are the first signs), and compartment syndrome.
8. Change position every 2 hours, apply lotion, massage dependent areas, avoid creases in linen, and perform ROM exercises.
9. There is a 3% strength loss per day of bed rest and 50% strength loss in 3 weeks of bed rest. To prevent this:
   a. Only immobilize what is absolutely required
   b. Perform 30% maximum voluntary isometric contraction for 5 seconds, with 10 second rest. Repeat x3. Do this every 2x/day. Do not exercise patients with unstable spine.
   c. Help patient move his joints through its full range of motion passively or actively 3-5 times, 2x/day.
   d. Use the foot board to maintain the ankle in a neutral position.
   e. Use trochanteric rolls to prevent external rotation of the hips. Lying prone for 30 minutes a day also prevents hip flexion contractures.
   f. Three basic extremity positions you can use when changing positions:
      (1) Shoulder abducted and externally rotated with elbow flexed and forearm pronated
      (2) Shoulder abducted and internally rotated with elbow flexed and forearm pronated
      (3) Shoulder abducted with elbow extended and forearm supinated.

Post-operative Nursing Care:

1. Place in lateral position unless contraindicated. Turn every 1-2 hours. This position promotes lung expansion.
2. Teach deep breathing exercises or use incentive spirometer if available, to prevent hypostatic pneumonia.
3. Monitor VS every 5 minutes x 3, then every 15 minutes, then every 4 hours. Adjust VS monitoring interval depending on patient's condition. Monitor I/O.
4. Early symptoms of shock and hemorrhage: cool extremities, U/O <30mL/hr, capillary refill >3 sec, lower BP, pulse. Nursing intervention: O$_2$, ↑ fluids, elevate feet. If elevating the feet is contraindicated, then prop up the foot of the bed.
5. Maintain normothermia. Avoid shivering.
6. Nausea and Vomiting: Head to side to prevent aspiration. Offer mouthwash. Offer small sips of clear carbonated drinks.
7. Thirst: ↑ fluids via IV or mouth if tolerated; sips of hot tea with lemon juice; moist gauze over lips to humidify the air; rinse mouth with mouthwash; or offer sugarless hard candy or chewing gum.
8. Constipation/gas: Ambulate if capable; ↑ fluids; use non-opioids for pain; assess bowel sounds; with lubricated gloves, break up impaction if necessary; administer oil, soapy, or saline enema; administer laxatives, suppositories, or stool softeners.

Wound Care:

1. Wear personal protective equipment to protect you and the patient. Use sterile technique.
2. Have all supplies close to you. Use alcohol wipes to remove stuck tape. Carefully remove old dressing by layers to avoid wound trauma. Use sterile saline to remove stuck dressing.
3. With sterile saline moistened gauze, start cleaning along the edge using small circular motions. Repeat pattern as necessary using new sterile saline moistened gauze. Do not scrub. Only use topical antiseptics on intact skin around the wound. Do not use it within the wound.
4. Apply new dressing. If there is excessive drainage, use more gauze to decrease dressing changes. Use minimal tape to avoid skin irritation.
5. Keep surrounding tissue clean.
6. Monitor for local and systemic infections.

Chapter 31: Nursing Procedures: Measuring Intake and Output

LT Susan Schmidt, NC, USNR

When: Intake and output (I & O) measurements are used to determine if a patient is retaining fluid or diuresing (putting out more fluid than is being taken in). The patient retaining fluid is at risk for respiratory failure due to pulmonary edema, cardiac compromise due to congestive heart failure and increased risk of skin breakdown due to increased fluid in the tissue. I & O also gives the medic a quick snapshot of renal function and perfusion. Urinary output that averages less than 30cc/hour is marginal and may be an indicator of decreased renal perfusion and/or function. Increased urinary output may indicate a hormonal imbalance (diabetes insipidus), or be the expected result of a medication (eg, furosemide, hydrochlorothiazide, mannitol). Diabetes insipidus is the loss of free water caused by an imbalance of ADH (anti-diuretic hormone) secreted by the pituitary gland and controlling renal function. I & O should be calculated at least every 24 hours. Intake should be recorded as it is given and output as it occurs. When the caregivers are working in shifts, it is beneficial to subtotal at the end of each shift.

What You Need: Pencil, paper, and various sizes of liquid measuring devices are all that are needed. Most urine collection (Foley) bags have some markings on them for measuring output. Extra canteen cups, approximate volume of 500mL, would be easy to use. Other measuring devices include syringes (50 and 30), water bottles, empty IV bags, urine specimen cups from lab tac set, and items from kitchen.

What To Do:

1. Measure and record all input, which is any fluid that goes into the patient; IV fluids, fluids by mouth, fluids via NG tube, IV medications. Input would also include irrigation fluids not returned at the time of irrigation (nasogastric and bladder).
2. Measure and record all output, which is urine, emesis, liquid stool, and anything coming out of a drainage tube (nasogastric tube; chest tube; or wound drain; ie, Hemovac, Jackson-Pratt or Penrose).
3. Subtract the larger number is subtracted from the smaller. If input is larger the patient is positive, and if output is larger, the patient is negative in balance.

What Not To Do: Do not over or underestimate the volumes of intake and output. This can give a false picture to the providers at the next stop for the patient and be a factor in choice of treatment.

Chapter 31: Nursing Procedures: Bowel Assessment and Care

LT Susan Schmidt, NC, USNR

When: Sick and/or injured bedbound patient comes under your care.

What You Need: Stethoscope, gloves, water-soluble lubricant. (If gloves are not available, proper hand hygiene with soap and water both before and after checking is required. Using a scrub brush would be advantageous.) If a water soluble lubricant is not available, a petroleum based product could be substituted.

What To Do: Upon arrival to your care and stabilized, the patient (if awake and not confused) should be asked when their last bowel movement (BM) was and what their normal bowel patterns are. If the patient is unconsciousness and/or intubated, a rectal check should be performed to check for an impaction (unless contraindicated) but only after a thorough, non-invasive abdominal exam to include auscultation and palpation has been performed. Contraindications would include abdominal surgery, open abdominal wounds or the presence of a colostomy.

1. Gather supplies
2. Wash hands
3. Explain procedure to patient. Inspect abdomen for visible peristalsis.
4. Listen for bowel sounds in all 4 quadrants.
5. Palpate abdomen for regions of tenderness and solid masses. It should be non-tender and supple.
6. Put on gloves
7. Apply generous amount of lubricant to index finger of gloved hand
8. Placed finger with lubricant on rectal sphincter and apply gentle pressure.
9. As applied pressure allows finger to enter rectum, feel cavity for presence of stool as far up as digit can reach. If hard stool is felt, break up with finger and remove as much of impaction as possible. Be sure to maintain adequate amounts of lubricant while removing impaction.
10. Slowly remove finger from rectum, remove gloves and wash hands.

What Not To Do: Do not do a rectal exam in a patient with a soft, non-tender abdomen, but continue to assess for pattern of BMs and bowel sounds. Invasive procedures should be avoided when possible.

Chapter 31: Nursing Procedures: Nasogastric Tube Placement
LT Douglas Tratchel, NC, USNR

When: To decompress the stomach through removal of air or gastric contents, to lavage the stomach and analyze stomach contents, or to instill medications or feedings.

Complications of NG Tube Insertion. Hypoxia, cyanosis, or respiratory arrest can result from inadvertent passage into the trachea. Cardiac compromise as a result of vagal response secondary to gagging. Nasal irritation, rhinorrhea, epistaxis from trauma during insertion. Sinusitis, esophagitis from the tube irritation. Vomiting and aspiration resulting in aspiration pneumonia secondary to gagging during tube placement.

What You Need: 60cc catheter tip syringe, water-soluble lubricating jelly, tape, stethoscope, a nasogastric (NG) tube. The double lumen Salem sump tube allows for suction through tube and keeps tube from sucking against the stomach wall. Meds and feedings can also be instilled through this tube. The single lumen Levin tube can be used for feeding and decompression.

What To Do:
1. Position conscious patient in a high Fowler's position.
2. Position unconscious patients head down, preferably lying on the left side.
3. Measure tube from the tip of the nose to the ear, then down to the epigastric area.
4. Mark the tube with a piece of tape.
5. Lubricate the tip of the tube; choose the nostril that is the largest and not obstructed, thread the tube through the nostril, aiming back to the posterior of the nostril.
6. When the tube gets to the pharynx, the patient should flex their neck forward with chin to chest. Flexing forward allows for passage of the tube past the epiglottis and down the esophagus into the stomach.
7. While you are passing the tube down the posterior pharynx and down the esophagus, have the patient sip on water through a straw forcing the patient to swallow.
8. Pass the tube to your pre-marked depth.
9. When the tube is in place, check placement by instilling 60cc of air with the 60cc syringe through the tube while listening over the epigastric region with the stethoscope. When you hear the air bubble pass into the stomach, you can then tape the tube in place. Ask the patient to say their name and listen for proper phonation.
10. Use a split-tape method to secure the tube. Tear off about 4 inches of tape and split lengthwise to about halfway. Tape the unsplit end to the end of the nose and crisscross the split ends around the tube.
11. Secure the tube to your patient's clothes to reduce discomfort from its weight and protect it from becoming dislodged. Loop a rubber band around the tube by making a slipknot, or create a tab with tape. Then run the pin through a rubber band loop or tab and into the fabric of the patient's clothes, about 10-12 inches from the nose. For a sump tube, position the pigtail above the level of the stomach to prevent backflow of gastric secretions.

What Not To Do:
1. Do not force the tube in. Reposition and try again.
2. Do not suture the tube to the nose. Use tape or commercially prepared device only.

Chapter 31: Nursing Procedures: Nasogastric Tube Feeding
LT Douglas Tratchel, NC, USN

When: Enteral nutrition (EN) is indicated when patients with a functional GI tract cannot eat. It is for patients who are or may become malnourished and to maintain structural and functional integrity of GI tract and enhance utilization of nutrients.

What You Need: 60cc catheter tip syringe, Disposable gavage bag and tubing, pH paper, liquid supplement

What To Do:
1. Bolus Feed:
   a. Place patient on right side in high Fowler's to reduce risk of pulmonary aspiration should patient regurgitate supplement.
   b. Check for abdominal distention and auscultate for bowel sounds.

    c. Aspirate gastric content to determine residual; if greater than 50-100mL hold until residual diminishes. This is also a good time to double-check placement with pH paper to ensure tube has not migrated. The pH of normal stomach contents is acid, from 0 to 4.

    d. Push gastric content back into tube

    e. Clamp tube

    f. Remove plunger from barrel of syringe and attach adapter.

    g. Fill syringe with supplement

    h. Allow supplement to infuse slowly; continue adding until desired amount administered

    i. Flush tubing with 30-60mL of water

2. Intermittent/Continuous Gavage Feeding:

    a. Hang supplement bag on IV pole above patient head

    b. Remove air from bag

    c. Attach distal end of tubing to feeding tube adapter and adjust drip.

    d. When supplement finished add 30-60mL of water, then clamp.

    e. Check placement of tube q4h.

    f. Check residual q8h. If greater than 100mL, hold until residual diminishes.

    g. Turn patient q2h to promote digestion.

    h. Administer water with and between feedings as directed.

    i. Ensure documentation of I & O

Complications:

1. Gastric retention: signs and symptoms; nausea, vomiting, and cramping.
2. Aspirate exceeds 100mL in 4 hours or absent bowel sounds may indicate ileus.
3. Assess patient for pulmonary aspiration by checking gag reflex, if absent suction, discontinue feeding and remove tube if signs of respiratory distress.
4. Keep patient in high Fowler's to prevent aspiration if vomiting occurs, if vomiting; suction.
5. It may become necessary to dilute some supplements to prevent diarrhea.

What Not To Do:

1. Do not infuse feeding by pressure on plunger. Allow it to drip in with gravity.
2. Do not fail to check position of tube before feeding.
3. Do not infuse anything through small vent lumen of Salem sump tube.

Chapter 31: Nursing Procedures: Bladder Catheter Care

LT Traci Johnson, NC, USN

Bladder Catheterization: *See Part 8: Procedures: Chapter 30: Urinary Bladder Catheterization*

What: A patient with an indwelling urinary catheter is in your care.

What You Need: Soap and water, rubber band, safety pin, gloves, tape, drainage collection container with measurement marks

What To Do:

1. Make sure that urine is flowing out of the catheter into the drainage bag.
2. Keep the urinary drainage bag below the level of the bladder. Coil the drainage tube on the bed so the urine does not collect in the loops hanging below the patient.
3. Clean around the urethral meatus bid and prn with soap and water. Check the area around the urethral meatus for inflammation or signs of infection, such as irritated, swollen, red or tender skin at the insertion site or drainage around the catheter.
4. Make sure that the urinary drainage bag does not drag and pull on the catheter. Tape the catheter to the thigh in women. In men, tape the catheter to the thigh or the anterior abdominal wall.
5. When turning the patient from side to side, crimp the tubing before raising the bag above the left of the patient's bladder. Hang the bag on the side that the patient is facing.
6. Empty the drainage bag q8h. Always wash your hands with soap and water or an available hand sanitizer and wear disposable gloves before touching the bag or catheter.
7. Unfasten the tube from the drainage bag.
8. Fasten the tubing clamp and remove the drainage cap.
9. Drain the urine into another container and then empty it in designated area. Avoid touching the tubing or drainage cap on the collection container or the floor.
10. Measure the amount of urine before you have emptied the urine.
11. Replace the drainage cap, close the clamp, and refasten the collection tube to the drainage bag. Wash your hands again with soap and water or an available hand sanitizer.
12. Remember the signs and symptoms of complications of an indwelling catheter.

    a. No urine or very little urine is flowing into the collection bag for 4 or more hours.

    b. No urine or very little urine is flowing into the collection bag and the patient feels like his bladder is full.

    c. Urine is leaking around the catheter at the urethral meatus.

    d. Patient has a new pain in abdomen, pelvis, legs, flank, or back.

e. A fever of 100°F or higher.

f. Urine has a foul odor, has changed color, is very cloudy, looks bloody, or has large blood clots in it.

g. The urethral meatus becomes very irritated, swollen, red, or tender, or pus draining from the around the catheter insertion site.

h. Patient develops nausea, vomiting, or shaking chills.

What Not To Do:

1. Do not place the drainage bag on the floor or the ground. If the patient is on a litter on the ground, place a clean towel or drape underneath the drainage bag.
2. Do not disconnect the catheter from the drainage tube unless the catheter must be irrigated.

Chapter 31: Nursing Procedures: Peripheral Intravenous Access and Maintenance

Maj Ricky Sexton, USAF, NC

What: Start and maintain peripheral intravenous access

When: You have a patient requiring resuscitation and/or emergency medications associated with a cardiac arrest or pain control.

What You Need: Gloves and protective equipment, appropriate size catheter 14-18 gauge IV catheter, non-latex tourniquet, alcohol swab/other cleaning instrument , non-sterile 2x2 gauze, Tegaderm or any other transparent dressing, tape to secure IV after insertion, IV bag with solution set (tubing) (flushed and ready) or saline lock, sharps container

What To Do: Assemble and prime the fluid bag and IV tubing prior to starting the procedure:

1. Check IV bag for expiration date and clarity
2. Open IV line and tighten clamp
3. Remove protective covers on the spike and the long outlet on the fluid bag
4. Insert spike into IV bag using a twisting motion to ensure there are no leaks
5. Elevate bag and line 18-24 inches in order to prime the line
6. Squeeze the drip chamber several times to fill chamber half way with solution
7. Open clamp and loosen the cap on the distal end of the line to allow the IV line to prime
8. Tighten clamp and secure protective cover over distal end after priming
9. Keep primed IV line in close proximity to be attached after the IV catheter has been inserted.

Starting the IV:

1. Choose the most distal site available, avoiding injured extremities if possible.
2. While the ante-cubical (AC) space is probably the most desirable site, do not neglect the forearm or hand. These sites are easier to maintain flow because the catheter can get kinked when inserted into the AC simply by the patient bending his arm. When the patient is "packaged" and ready for transport on a NATO litter, the most distal sites are the easiest to access and maintain.
3. Apply the constricting band approximately 2 inches above the desired venipuncture site
4. Vein selection is accomplished by visualization and palpation of the potential site and can be done without gloves. Methods to increase vein dilation: gently tap; apply warm wrap; have patient make a fist, or dangle his arm below his heart.
5. Cleanse the site using alcohol swabs or povidone-iodine swab. Clean in a circular motion, moving outward from intended puncture.
6. Hold the catheter with your dominant hand, and remove protective cover.
7. Hold the flash chamber with thumb and index finger; align catheter parallel to the selected vein.
8. Stabilize the vein and apply counter tension to the skin
9. With the needle bevel facing up, and parallel to the selected vein, insert it approximately ½ inch below the selected site puncturing the skin at a 20-30° angle. Decrease the angle as you continue advancing the needle and catheter through the wall of the vein.
10. Observe for a "flashback" as the blood fills the chamber near the thumb and index finger indicating the needle has penetrated the vein wall.
11. Advance the needle approximately 1cm into the vein.
12. Continuing to hold the end of the catheter with your thumb and index finger, pull the needle (only) back 1 cm with your middle finger and slowly advance the catheter.
13. Pay careful attention to the catheter to ensure the needle does not advance, potentially puncturing the vein completely
14. Remove the tourniquet
15. Occlude the distal end of the catheter with the 3rd, 4th and 5th fingers of your non-dominant hand.
16. Secure the catheter hub with your thumb and index finger and carefully remove the needle.
17. Attach the tubing to the catheter and begin the flow of fluids. Observe for signs of infiltration.
18. Cover and secure site with Tegaderm or other transparent dressing and anchor IV tubing using tape.
19. Document IV location, catheter size, fluid, and time

Maintaining an IV:

There is evidence that infections occur related to IV procedures. However, they can be minimized by cleaning the site prior to the procedure and removing the IV as soon as feasible (48 hours or less). Infections related to IVs increase drastically when left in place for more than 72 hours. In a care under fire scenario, it might not be practical to thoroughly clean the site prior to insertion. If this is the case, another IV needs to be started when conditions improve and the first IV needs to be removed. If IV fluids are infusing, the line should stay patent. However, if the IV has a saline lock in place, you need to flush it at least q8h with 3-5cc of normal saline or sterile water. If during this time frame you are pushing medications and flushing the saline lock before and after, there is no need to duplicate this procedure again.

Complications of Intravenous Infusions:

Infiltration occurs when the IV fluids escape from the vein into the surrounding tissues due to the catheter becoming displaced. Signs and symptoms of Infiltration can include: IV site is cool to the touch; unable to establish a flow rate; swelling of the IV site or the entire limb. If a patient's IV is suspected to have infiltrated, discontinue the IV. Apply warm packs to increase fluid absorption.

Positional IV is detected when the IV fluid does not flow because the vein containing the catheter is compressed or the catheter tip is up against the vein's wall. When the limb is repositioned, the infusion should flow without difficulty. If the infusion does not flow despite repositioning and flushing, it may be infiltrated.

Circulatory overload results from excessive fluid being introduced into the circulatory system. Signs and symptoms can include: shortness of breath; increased respiratory rate; jugular vein distention, excessive cough; increased BP. If you think your patient is in circulatory overload, reduce the flow rate to keep vein open (30mL/hr), give high flow oxygen, and place patient in position that most comfortable for breathing.

Blood in the IV line is one sign of that you have a patent line. However, if that blood is not flushed back into the veins it could easily clot the IV. First, raise the IV bag higher and determine if the fluid flushes the blood back into the vein. If this process keeps the blood out of the line, keep the IV bag elevated. If the bag needs to be lowered for transport, you may need to utilize a pressure bag in order to keep the blood out of the line and into the vein.

Air in the IV line can be introduced into an IV line if the bag is allowed to run completely dry, during changing of an IV bag, or by motion. The procedure to remove air from an IV line is:

1. Close slide or roller clamp
2. Clamp off or kink IV tubing distal to port
3. Wipe injection port with alcohol swab distal to air bubbles
4. Insert assembled 21 gauge needle and 10cc syringe into port
5. Gently aspirate air and fluid by pulling back on plunger of syringe
6. Close slide or roller clamp
7. Remove needle and syringe, dispose appropriately without recapping
8. Release tubing and reset roller clamp for desired drip rate

Calculate Flow Rates:

Intravenous solutions are delivered through administration sets

1. Microdrip (60 drops/mL) set
2. Macrodrip (10 or 15 drops/mL) set

To calculate a flow rate in gtt (drops) per minute, use the following equation:

$$gtt/min = \frac{volume \ to \ be \ infused \ x \ gtt/mL \ of \ administration \ set}{Time \ of \ infusion \ in \ minutes}$$

For example, if you were to deliver 100 mL per hour using a macrodrip set:

$$gtt/min = (100 \ x \ 10) \ / \ 60$$

Result: Approximately 17gtt/min

Note: Also refer to *Appendices: Table A-4: IV Drip Rates* to cross reference your calculations

What Not To Do:

Reasons NOT to Start IVs on All Casualties:

1. Minimize interference with combatants who can continue to participate in the engagement
2. Conserve limited IV fluid supplies
3. Attend to casualties with more severe wound.
4. Avoid delaying tactical movement

Working in Austere Environments:

When working in austere environments, common sense needs to be applied. First, there is little to no substitution for the IV catheters. So, you have what you carry. They are small on weight and cube so you might want to carry a few more than you think you will really need. If you run out of alcohol swabs or povidone-iodine swabs, wash the site with water and soap if available prior to starting the IV. The goal, of course, is to get the site as clean as possible to prevent infection. After starting the IV, the site needs to be covered to help prevent dislodgement and to prevent the further possibility of infection. If Tegaderm or other transparent dressing is not available, you have a couple of options. If povidone-iodine is available, thoroughly clean the site and let it dry. Take a small piece of gauze and put it over the hub and entrance site and cover with tape. Remember, the goal is to keep the dirt out. Another option is to use an empty IV bag and cut it into a square and use in the place of a Tegaderm and tape into place. The clear IV bag will allow you to see if the site is leaking or bleeding. Of course, it will not adhere to the skin but it will provide ample protection from dirt entering the insertion site. Consider adding 550 cord and shower hooks to your bags. When IV poles are not available, the cord can be dropped from trees, rafters, d-rings and attached to a shower hook to allow the ability to hang IV bags.

Chapter 31: Nursing Procedures: Intramuscular Injection Sites

Maj Ricky Sexton, USAF, NC

Figure 8-8. IM Injection Sites

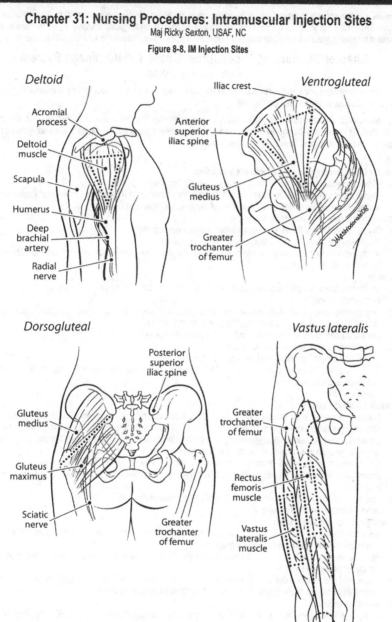

Deltoid

- Acromial process
- Deltoid muscle
- Scapula
- Humerus
- Deep brachial artery
- Radial nerve

Ventrogluteal

- Iliac crest
- Anterior superior iliac spine
- Gluteus medius
- Greater trochanter of femur

Dorsogluteal

- Posterior superior iliac spine
- Gluteus medius
- Gluteus maximus
- Sciatic nerve
- Greater trochanter of femur

Vastus lateralis

- Greater trochanter of femur
- Rectus femoris muscle
- Vastus lateralis muscle

Deltoid. Feel the edge of the acromial process that is in line with (lateral arm) the axilla. Drop down 1.5-2 inches from this intersection point (2-3 fingerbreadths). Inject at this site with the needle at right angles to the skin. A typical injection volume is 0.5-2.0mL. You can bunch the muscle with your thumb and forefinger before needle insertion with any IM injection.

Dorsogluteal. Draw an imaginary line from the posterior superior iliac spine to the greater trochanter of the femur. Inject above and outside this line. Alternatively, divide the buttock into four quadrants. Inject 2-3 inches below the iliac crest in the upper outer quadrant. A typical injection volume is 1-5mL. Inject 90° to the skin.

Ventrogluteal. Feel the greater trochanter of the femur with the heel of your hand (lateral leg). Point and spread your index and middle fingers superiorly with the tip of the anteriorly positioned finger at the anterior superior iliac spine. The spread between your fingertips will be about 3 inches. Inject in the middle of this V 90° to the skin. The typical injection volume is 1-5mL.

Vastus lateralis. Use the central and/or lateral area of the quadriceps muscles (rectus femoris/vastus lateralis) on the anterior part of the leg above the knee. The injection site should be in an area one handbreadth (5 inches) below the greater trochanter to one handbreadth above the superior border of the knee. A typical adult injection volume is 1-5mL, and a typical infant/child injection volume is 1-3mL. Inject 90° to the skin.

Chapter 31: Nursing Procedures: Chest Tube/Drainage System

Maj Ricky Sexton, USAF, NC

When: A casualty requires chest tube insertion to remove air and/or fluid in the pleural cavity. It allows for lung re-expansion and adequate gas exchange, and prevents air and/or fluid from returning.

What You Need: A traditional chest drainage unit (CDU) that consists of a collection chamber, a water seal which allows air or fluids to drain from the chest but not return, and a suction control chamber which regulates the uncontrolled suction to levels acceptable for thoracic drainage; Sterile water, Heimlich valve, hemostats, tape, and suction

What To Do:
1. **Set up the CDU according to the manufacturer's instructions**
   a. Fill water seal chamber per manufacturer instruction (usually 2cm sterile H_2O)
   b. Prepare suction and attach to drainage system if available (the level of sterile H_2O controls the amount of suction being applied, not the suction control valve). High levels of suction can damage lung tissue!
   c. If patient is aware and time allows, explain procedure
   d. Oxygen should be provided as required to maintain oxygen saturation >95%.
   e. Provide analgesia to patient if time and hemodynamic status allow
   f. Monitor patient throughout procedure. Pay particular close attention to the patient's vital signs, skin color, and breath sounds before and after the procedure.

2. **Procedure**
   a. Attach chest tube to the collection chamber. If a Heimlich valve is available, place it into the chest tube first and then attach to the collection device
   b. Once the chest tube is inserted, place an airtight occlusive dressing around tube/insertion site. The ideal dressing would be Vaseline gauze wrapped around the base of the tube at the insertion site.
   c. Cover at the base of the tube with a 4x4 gauze and secured with tape (ideally foam tape).
   d. Attach suction control chamber if suction available
   e. Tape all connections and ensure no air leakage in system.
   f. Secure the tube to the patient; tube will dislocate if not properly anchored. Secure entire length of tube to patient using multiple strips of tape down torso.
   g. X-ray if available

3. **Maintaining Drainage System**
   a. Monitor system for air leaks, bubbles noted in water seal chamber. When using a water-seal chamber, the fluid level rises when the patient inhales and drops when the patient exhales. (The opposite occurs if the patient is mechanically ventilated.) These fluctuations (tidaling) indicate the patency of the chest tube. Constant bubbling indicates an air leak. To determine the origin of an air leak, momentarily occlude the chest tube close to the insertion site. If the bubbling in the water-seal chamber stops, the air leak originates from the patient, either at the insertion site or in the pleural cavity. If the bubbling does not stop, the leak is in the drainage system. Check to ensure tight connections. The drainage system may need to be replaced.
   b. Keep system below the chest to allow fluids to flow into the connection chamber.
   c. Avoid dependent loops in the tubing

4. **Monitoring Patients with Chest Tubes**
   a. Auscultate chest at least every 2 hours and listen for breath sounds on the affected side to ensure lung expansion.
   b. Assess the insertion site for subcutaneous emphysema
   c. Perform pulmonary toilet to include chest percussion, coughing/deep breathing and postural drainage to prevent atelectasis (collapse of part or all of a lung)
   d. Assess color and amount of drainage; document amount characteristics in medical record. Surgical intervention usually is required if blood loss is 1000-1500mL immediately or 200-300mL/hr in the adult patient.
   e. **Activity permitted:**
      (1) Can have regular diet if no particulate matter out of chest tube (suggests esophageal injury) and if patient is not too sedated.
      (2) Can walk with system on water seal. If a one-way valve is not used, be sure to keep the collection system lower than the insertion site to prevent fluid from returning back into the pleural space

5. **Improvise a Drainage System:** Drainage system can be constructed from materials on hand
   a. Field expedient chest tube drainage system
      (1) Attach chest tube to Heimlich valve. This allows air to flow out, and prevents air from re-entering chest.
      (2) Provide some system to collect fluid.
      (3) Connect Heimlich valve to collection container
         (a) Air must be able to escape the container
         (b) Container must be kept lower that chest for drainage

b. System can be constructed using one, two, or three bottles. If possible, use the same size bottles for all three. If different sizes are used, the larger of the three needs to be the collection bottle. While both glass and plastic bottles will work, there are a couple of concerns with each; glass breaks and plastic will collapse. If plastic is used, a more rigid composite would work best to prevent the collapse in the event the water seal is lost. First bottle will collect drainage fluid. Second bottle will act as water seal. Third bottle will act as suction control.

c. Setting up the system
    (1) Use surgical tubing to connect the chest tube to the first bottle
    (2) Tubing will be used to connect the three bottles together
    (3) In the second bottle, fill approximately ¼ of the bottle with water for seal. Tubing going from first to second bottle must go beneath water in second bottle to produce the seal .
    (4) Third bottle must be vented and then connected to suction

6. Removal of chest tube
a. Criteria for removing the chest tube
    (1) There is no air leak on the underwater seal.
    (2) <100cc drainage in 24 hours
    (3) CXR
        (a) No pneumothorax
        (b) None or slight residual fluid. Even if the criteria are met, DO NOT REMOVE before air evacuation or mechanical ventilation.

b. Technique for removing the tube
    (1) Have dressings, tape, and scissors available
    (2) Remove dressings and suture securing the tube.
    (3) Have patient inhale and exhale slowly
    (4) Pull the tube in one continuous motion at start of exhalation
    (5) Appy occlusive dressing
    (6) Monitor patient for S&S pneumothorax

What Not To Do:
1. Do not apply rapid suction to a patient with pulmonary edema; this can result in unilateral edema.
2. Do not allow dependent loops that can cause fluids and air to drain improperly.
3. Do not routinely strip tubing to help with drainage. This practice increases pain and intrathoracic pressure, and may damage lung tissue. OK to strip tubing if chest tube stops functioning or has an obvious clot in it.
4. Do not remove the tube if patient will be flying within 24 hours. Removing a chest tube will delay aeromedical evacuation.
5. Do not forget to remove the suture securing the chest tube before pulling from the chest.

Chapter 31: Nursing Procedures: Heat Therapy
LT Douglas Tratchel, NC, USN

When: Apply heat for pain associated with muscle spasm; leg cramps; superficial thrombophlebitis; chronic pain relief for musculoskeletal injury or injuries with no inflammation. Heat can also reduce muscle spasm after back injury, and can also aide in finding peripheral IV site by elevating blood flow.

What You Need: Hot water bottle, warm bag of saline or sterile water used as warm compress, moist warm towel/cloth, warming blanket, Bair Hugger warmer system if available, heating pad if available.

What To Do:
1. Apply heat source to affected area, being cautious of heat intensity.
2. When utilizing compresses it may be necessary to first wrap heat source in a towel/cloth to avoid burning the affected area.
3. When utilizing a warming blanket it may be necessary to first cover patient with a sheet to avoid direct skin contact.
4. Treatment should last no longer than approximately 20 minutes.
5. Affected area should be checked q5min to ensure patient is not receiving a burn secondary to treatment.

Complications:
1. Local burn injury
2. Orthostatic symptoms (warm bath, shower)
3. Precipitation of coronary ischemia (warm bath, shower)

What Not To Do: Contraindications for heat therapy:
1. Acute inflammation or hemorrhage
2. Bleeding disorder
3. Decreased sensation poor circulation, ie, diabetic
4. Do not use on open wound or over suture site
5. Avoid treatment on eyes or genitalia

Chapter 31: Nursing Procedures: Cold Therapy

LT Douglas Tratchel, NC, USN

When:
1. Acute injuries to prevent swelling, inflammation, and treat pain.
2. Low back pain; research suggests that cold works better for individuals who have had back pain for more than 14 days.
3. To reduce muscle spasm by making them less sensitive to stretching.
4. Nose bleeds, by wrapping ice in a cloth and placing over nose while elevating head.
5. Minor burn Tx; immediate application of ice or cold packs for superficial burns and burns of less than 20% total body surface area decreases pain, edema, erythema, and blistering. For optimal results in cases of trauma, cold should be applied before significant edema and hemorrhage occur.
6. To reduce limb metabolism (prior to amputation).

What You Need: Ice packs, (bag of frozen vegetables can be used as an alternative), ice in Dixie cups, towels/rags/whatever is available that can be soaked in cold/cool water and used as cold wraps, canteens/Camelback to cool/immerse as needed.

What To Do:
1. Utilize cold packs, commercial or field expedient.
2. Apply to area of injury for approximately 15-20min per application.
3. RICE principle can be utilized for extremity injuries.
    a. Relative rest
    b. Ice
    c. Compression, apply Ace wrap
    d. Elevate
4. Remove ice if skin becomes numb
5. Observe skin frequently
6. Use caution with fingers and toes

Complications:
1. Frost Bite
2. Superficial nerve injury

What Not To Do: Contraindications for cold therapy:
1. Hypertension (due to secondary vasoconstriction)
2. Raynaud disease
3. Local limb ischemia
4. History of vascular impairment, such as frostbite or arteriosclerosis
5. Cold allergy (cold urticaria)
6. Paroxysmal cold hemoglobinuria

Chapter 31: Nursing Procedures: Eye Irrigation

LT Traci Johnson, NC, USN

What: Eye irrigation is a widely accepted therapeutic must in first aid treatment. The burning agent is removed, diluted, and if possible neutralized.

When:
1. To avoid removal of corrosive substance from the eye.
2. To remove secretions from conjunctival sac.
3. To treat infection.
4. To relieve itching.
5. To provide moisture of the eyes of the eyes of an unconscious patient.
6. To irrigate chemicals or foreign bodies from the eye.

What You Need: Irrigation fluids. Usually water, NaCl 0.9%, Ringer's lactate or phosphate buffer are the most accepted rinsing solutions; bottle IV tubing or oxygen tubing

What To Do:
1. Help patient into either sitting or lying position with head and neck well supported
2. Wash and dry your hands with soap and water or an available hand sanitizer.
3. If the patient is able, have him pull down his lower lid. Hold the eyelid open during this process.
4. Hold the irrigating tip 1-1½ inches away from the patient's eye.
5. Direct a steady flow of irrigation from the inner portion of the eye to the outer portion to minimize contamination of the lacrimal duct.
6. Instruct the patient to look up to expose the conjunctival sac and lower surface of the eye.
7. Instruct the patient to look down to expose the upper surface of the eye.

Duration of Irrigation: For harmless substances, irrigation only needs to be carried out for 2-3 minutes. For stronger chemicals that cause more irritation and stinging, flush the eye for 15-20 minutes.

What Not To Do:
1. Do not exert pressure on the eye globe.
2. Do not touch the irrigation tip to the eye.

Chapter 31: Nursing Procedures: Hygiene

LT Susan Schmidt, NC, USNR

When: Patients need daily skin care to help prevent skin breakdown. Body hygiene should be performed daily. Perineal care should be performed bid at a minimum, and whenever else it may be needed. Oral care should be performed bid, morning and evening for a patient that is not intubated. Oral care should be performed q2h with repositioning for the patient that is intubated.

What You Need: Soap, water, clean cloths to wash with and a towel to dry the patient off are all that is necessary. Toothbrush, or improvise toothbrush with a tongue blade wrapped with a 4x4 gauze.

What To Do: Beginning with the patient's face and working toward the feet, wash the front then back. The perianal area should be washed last. When washing female genitalia, remember to wash front to back to assist in the prevention of urinary tract infections.

What Not To Do: Do not let a patient that is incontinent lie in urine or stool. This contributes to skin breakdown and infection of wounds.

Chapter 31: Nursing Procedures: Positioning

LT Susan Schmidt, NC, USAR

When: Re-positioning should be done q2h for anyone unable to reposition their torso or an extremity. Repositioning is necessary to prevent skin breakdown and pressure ulcers.

What You Need: Pillows, rolled towels, rolled sheets, rolled clothing, any soft items may be used to prop patients on their side or elevate an extremity.

What To Do: There are 3 main positions when positioning a patient; right side, left side and back. It may simplify things to post a turning schedule so a patient on his/her back does not go back to the previous side with the next turn. Pillows should be placed behind the patient's back and hips to keep off the sacrum and coccyx. Padding should also be placed between knees and ankles while lying on either side to prevent the bony prominences from causing pressure areas. Support should be placed under the patient's head when lying on either side. Patients positioned on their backs will benefit from having pillows or rolled blankets placed under the knees and ankles. Elevation of the knees is helpful for alignment of the spine and low back comfort, and elevating the ankles allows the heels to be "floated" keeping pressure off the area.

What Not To Do: Patients should not be left in any single position for more than 2 hours. The circulation of a patient lying down and unable to make position changes unassisted is compromised and the continued weight on the bony prominences makes them more susceptible to skin breakdown and pressure ulcers. Pressure ulcers are more difficult to heal than they are to prevent.

Chapter 32: Lab Procedures: Wet Mount and KOH Prep

MAJ Timothy M. Pellini, MC, USA

When: To assess sample (discharge, scraping, biopsy) for presence of Candida or Tinea.

What You Need: Sample, slide, coverslip, normal saline in dropper or vial, 10% KOH (potassium hydroxide), small cotton swab, and a microscope.

What To Do:
1. Obtain specimen. Collect fluid or discharge on cotton swab. Put a scraping sample or biopsy directly on slide.
2. For fluid or discharge, place 1 drop of discharge on right and left end of slide.
3. Place one small drop of KOH on one drop of sample. Perform whiff test by smelling for amine odor. A strong amine or fishy odor is suggestive of bacterial vaginosis.
4. Place one small drop of normal saline on other spot.
5. Cover each sample with glass cover slip. The slides usually dry quickly and can still be interpreted before they dry.
6. Observe under microscope. Examine the KOH portion for hyphae and spores under the 10X objective. Examine the saline portion for trichomonads and clue cells under the 40X objective.
7. For dry specimens of skin scrapings or biopsies, place a drop of KOH over the specimen already on the slide, cover with a coverslip (probably not practical with biopsy), and observe under microscope.
8. Look for:
   a. **Candida (Yeast) and Fungi (Tinea)**: KOH causes the epithelial cells to swell and break open which will allow a clear view of any filamentous or branching yeast or fungi.
   b. **Clue Cells**: Vaginal epithelial cells to which bacteria are attached, obscuring the cell border. The edges of vaginal epithelial cells are normally sharp and clear. The attached bacteria make the edges of the cell appear fuzzy on low power. Small bacteria will be visible on higher power.
   c. **Trichomonas**: Motile flagellated protozoa; look like sperm with balloon-shaped heads and are about the size of a normal epithelial cell.

What Not To Do:
1. Do not add too much KOH or saline allowing the fluids to mix or run off the slide. Alternatively the collected specimen/discharge may be placed on 2 separate slides.
2. Normal saline can be placed on one slide and 10% KOH added to other. Follow the remaining instructions as above.
3. Do not forget to perform the whiff test (strong amine or fishy odor).

NOTES:

Anatomical Plates: Skeletal System, Anterior View
Figure A-1

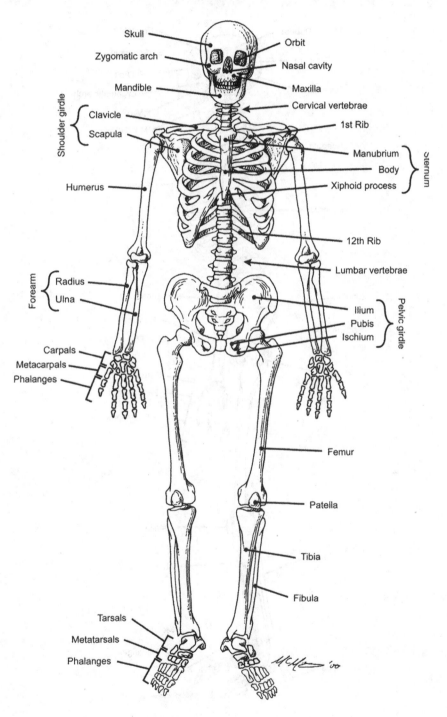

Anatomical Plates: Skeletal System, Lateral View
Figure A-2

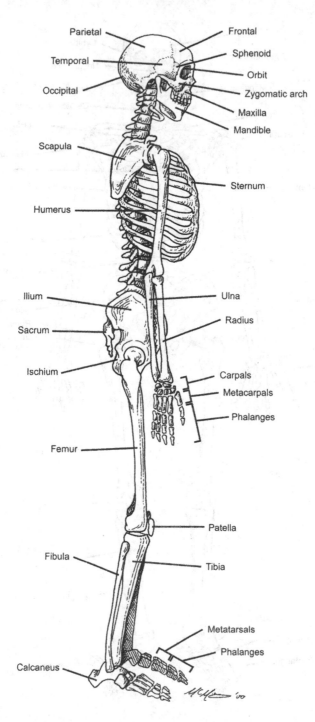

Anatomical Plates: Vertebral Column
Figure A-3

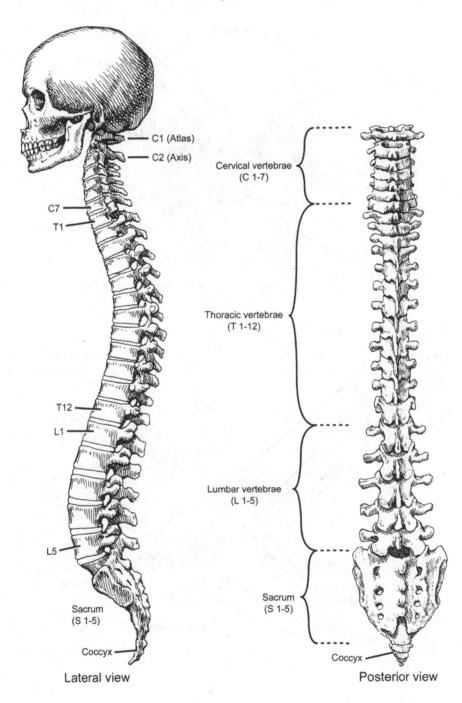

C1 (Atlas)
C2 (Axis)

Cervical vertebrae
(C 1-7)

C7
T1

Thoracic vertebrae
(T 1-12)

T12
L1

Lumbar vertebrae
(L 1-5)

L5

Sacrum
(S 1-5)

Sacrum
(S 1-5)

Coccyx

Coccyx

Lateral view

Posterior view

Anatomical Plates: External Anatomy of the Skull
Figure A-4

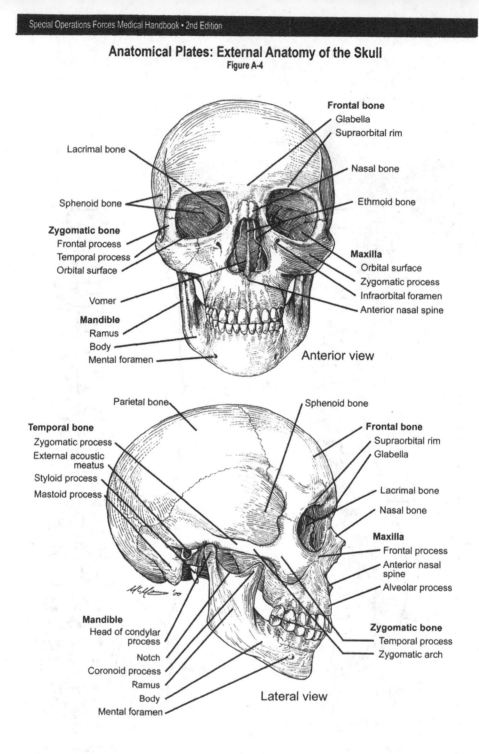

Frontal bone
Glabella
Supraorbital rim

Nasal bone

Ethmoid bone

Lacrimal bone

Sphenoid bone

Zygomatic bone
Frontal process
Temporal process
Orbital surface

Maxilla
Orbital surface
Zygomatic process
Infraorbital foramen
Anterior nasal spine

Vomer

Mandible
Ramus
Body
Mental foramen

Anterior view

Parietal bone

Sphenoid bone

Temporal bone
Zygomatic process
External acoustic
meatus
Styloid process
Mastoid process

Frontal bone
Supraorbital rim
Glabella

Lacrimal bone

Nasal bone

Maxilla
Frontal process
Anterior nasal
spine
Alveolar process

Mandible
Head of condylar
process
Notch
Coronoid process
Ramus
Body
Mental foramen

Zygomatic bone
Temporal process
Zygomatic arch

Lateral view

Anatomical Plates: Cervical Vertebrae and Related Structures
Figure A-5.A

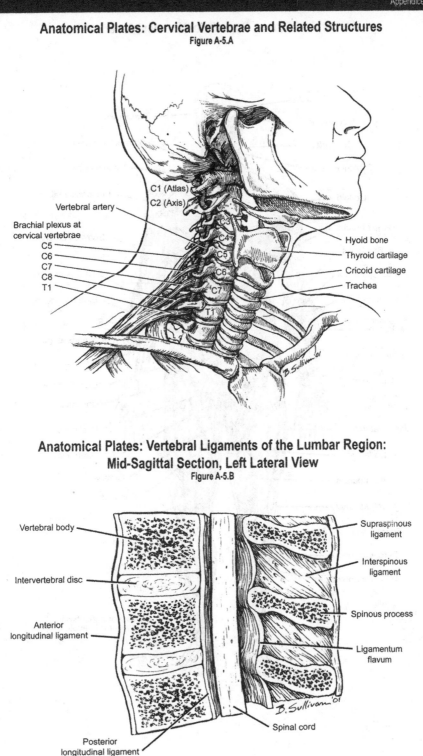

Vertebral artery

C1 (Atlas)
C2 (Axis)

Brachial plexus at
cervical vertebrae
C5
C6
C7
C8
T1

C3
C4
C5
C6
C7
T1

Hyoid bone

Thyroid cartilage

Cricoid cartilage

Trachea

B. Sullivan '01

Anatomical Plates: Vertebral Ligaments of the Lumbar Region:
Mid-Sagittal Section, Left Lateral View
Figure A-5.B

Vertebral body

Intervertebral disc

Anterior
longitudinal ligament

Posterior
longitudinal ligament

Supraspinous
ligament

Interspinous
ligament

Spinous process

Ligamentum
flavum

Spinal cord

B. Sullivan '01

Anatomical Plates: Superficial Muscles, Anterior View
Figure A-6

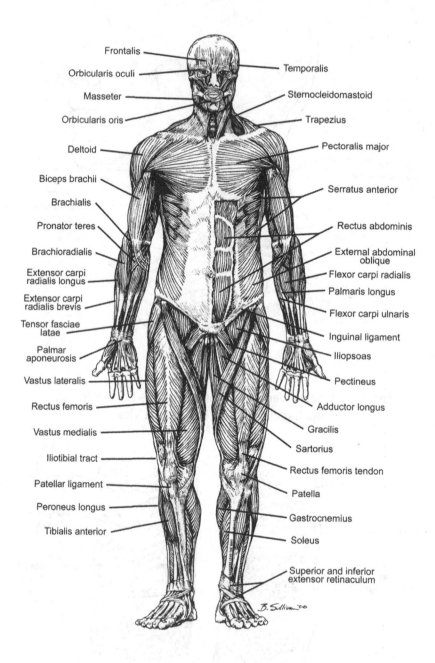

Frontalis
Orbicularis oculi
Masseter
Orbicularis oris
Deltoid
Biceps brachii
Brachialis
Pronator teres
Brachioradialis
Extensor carpi radialis longus
Extensor carpi radialis brevis
Tensor fasciae latae
Palmar aponeurosis
Vastus lateralis
Rectus femoris
Vastus medialis
Iliotibial tract
Patellar ligament
Peroneus longus
Tibialis anterior

Temporalis
Sternocleidomastoid
Trapezius
Pectoralis major
Serratus anterior
Rectus abdominis
External abdominal oblique
Flexor carpi radialis
Palmaris longus
Flexor carpi ulnaris
Inguinal ligament
Iliopsoas
Pectineus
Adductor longus
Gracilis
Sartorius
Rectus femoris tendon
Patella
Gastrocnemius
Soleus
Superior and inferior extensor retinaculum

B. Sullivan '00

Anatomical Plates: Superficial Muscles, Posterior View
Figure A-7

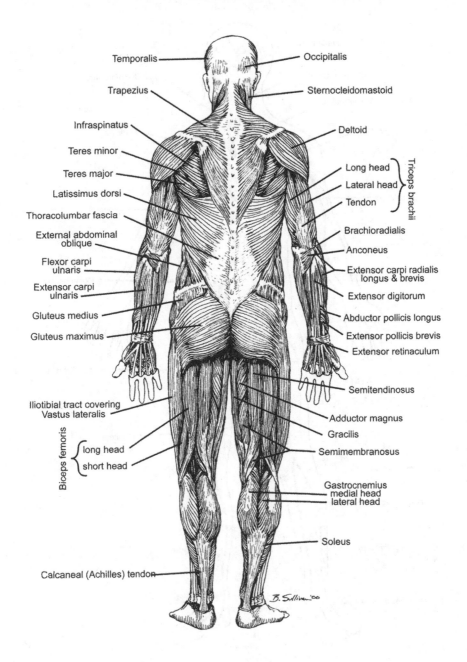

Temporalis

Trapezius

Infraspinatus

Teres minor

Teres major

Latissimus dorsi

Thoracolumbar fascia

External abdominal
oblique

Flexor carpi
ulnaris

Extensor carpi
ulnaris

Gluteus medius

Gluteus maximus

Iliotibial tract covering
Vastus lateralis

Biceps femoris
{ long head
short head

Calcaneal (Achilles) tendon

Occipitalis

Sternocleidomastoid

Deltoid

Long head
Lateral head   Triceps brachii
Tendon

Brachioradialis

Anconeus

Extensor carpi radialis
longus & brevis

Extensor digitorum

Abductor pollicis longus

Extensor pollicis brevis

Extensor retinaculum

Semitendinosus

Adductor magnus

Gracilis

Semimembranosus

Gastrocnemius
medial head
lateral head

Soleus

B. Sullivan '00

A-7

Anatomical Plates: Arterial System
Figure A-8

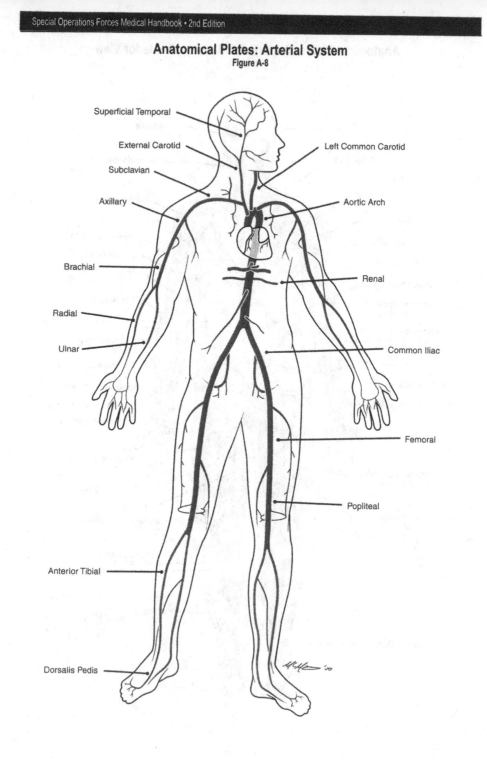

Anatomical Plates: Venous System
Figure A-9

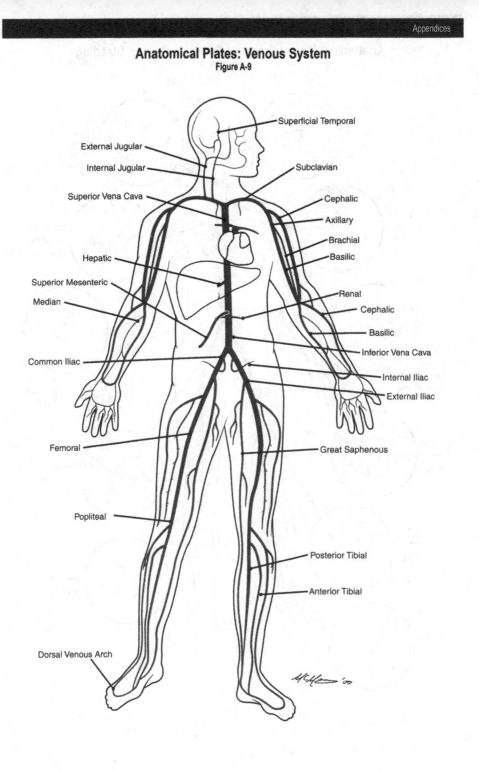

Anatomical Plates: Pressure Points to Control Bleeding
Figure A-10

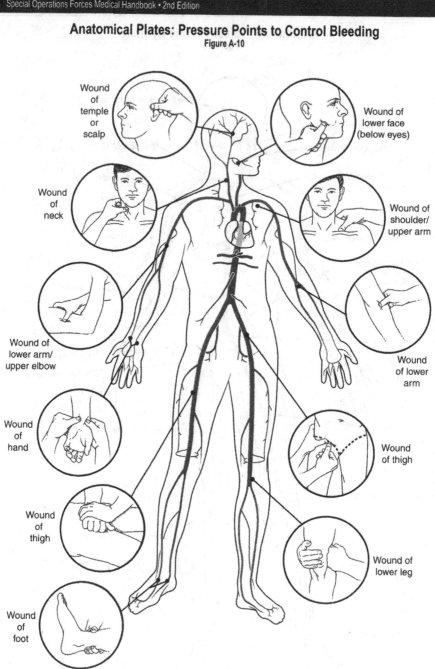

Anatomical Plates: Lymphatic System (major components)
Figure A-11

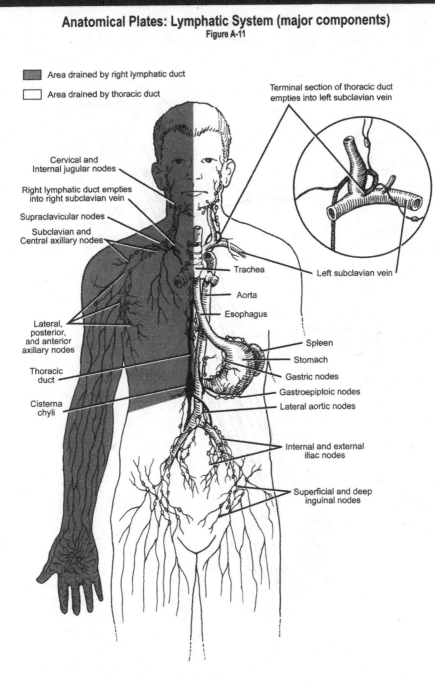

Area drained by right lymphatic duct

Area drained by thoracic duct

Terminal section of thoracic duct empties into left subclavian vein

Cervical and Internal jugular nodes

Right lymphatic duct empties into right subclavian vein

Supraclavicular nodes

Subclavian and Central axillary nodes

Trachea

Left subclavian vein

Aorta

Esophagus

Lateral, posterior, and anterior axillary nodes

Spleen

Stomach

Gastric nodes

Gastroepiploic nodes

Thoracic duct

Lateral aortic nodes

Cisterna chyli

Internal and external iliac nodes

Superficial and deep inguinal nodes

Anatomical Plates: Nerves of the Arm
Figure A-12

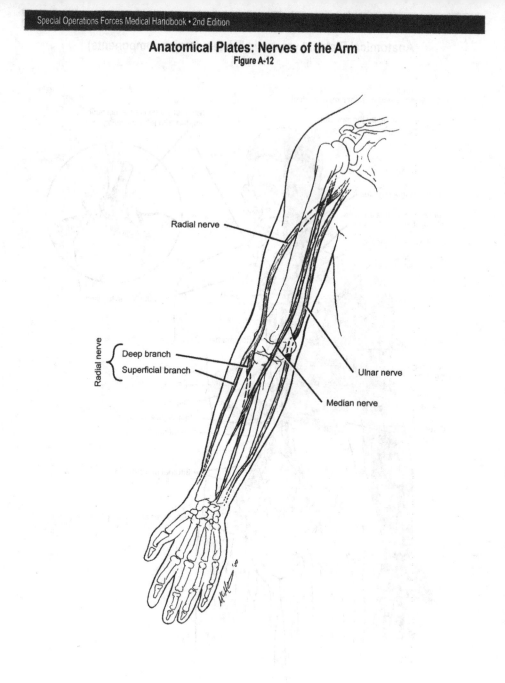

Anatomical Plates: Nerves of the Leg
Figure A-13

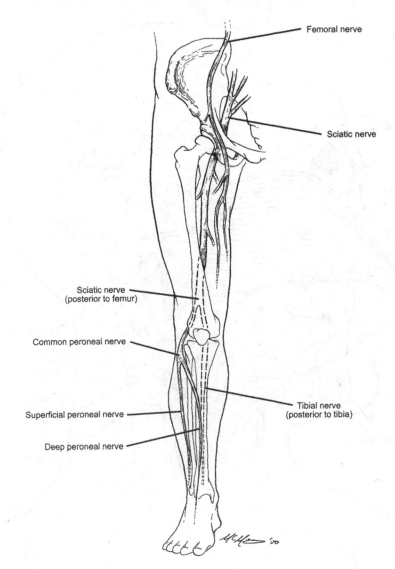

Femoral nerve

Sciatic nerve

Sciatic nerve
(posterior to femur)

Common peroneal nerve

Superficial peroneal nerve

Deep peroneal nerve

Tibial nerve
(posterior to tibia)

Anatomical Plates: Key Structures of the Head and Neck, Sagittal View
Figure A-14

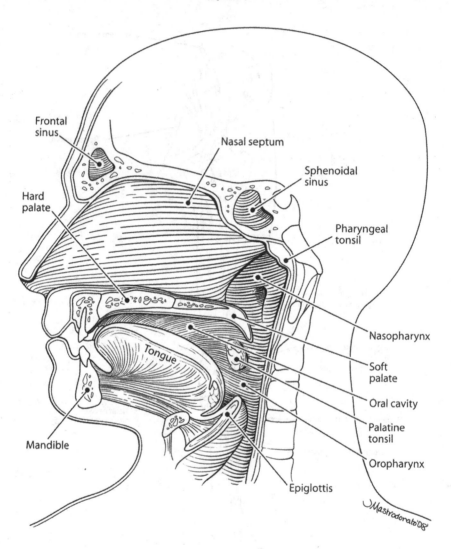

Frontal sinus

Nasal septum

Sphenoidal sinus

Hard palate

Pharyngeal tonsil

Nasopharynx

Tongue

Soft palate

Oral cavity

Palatine tonsil

Mandible

Oropharynx

Epiglottis

Anatomical Plates: Eye Anatomy
Figure A-15

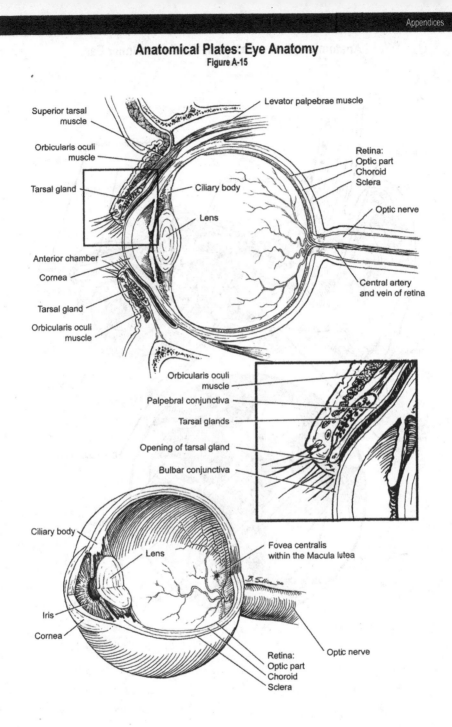

Superior tarsal muscle

Orbicularis oculi muscle

Tarsal gland

Anterior chamber

Cornea

Tarsal gland

Orbicularis oculi muscle

Levator palpebrae muscle

Ciliary body

Lens

Retina:
Optic part
Choroid
Sclera

Optic nerve

Central artery and vein of retina

Orbicularis oculi muscle

Palpebral conjunctiva

Tarsal glands

Opening of tarsal gland

Bulbar conjunctiva

Ciliary body

Lens

Iris

Cornea

Fovea centralis within the Macula lutea

Retina:
Optic part
Choroid
Sclera

Optic nerve

Anatomical Plates: External, Middle and Inner Ear
Figure A-16

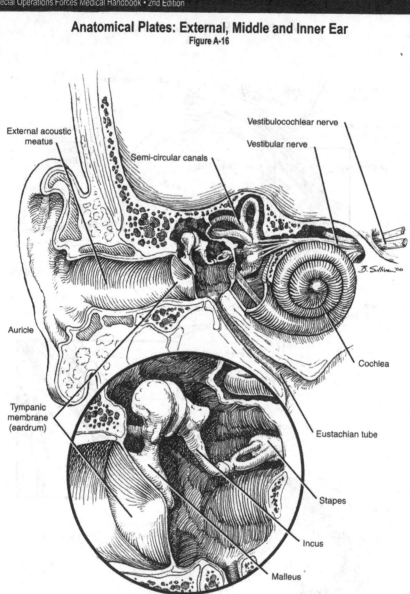

Anatomical Plates: Respiratory System
Figure A-17

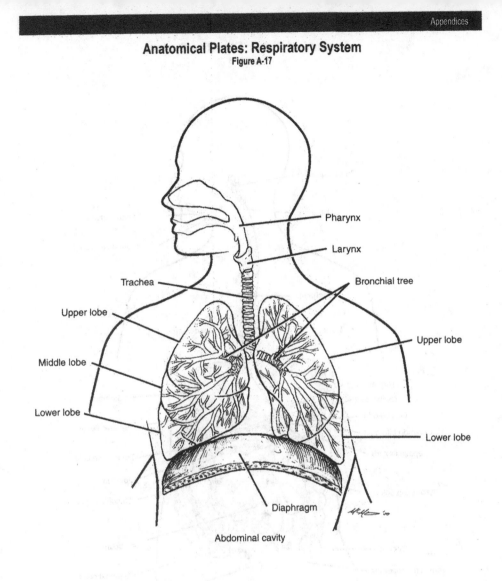

Pharynx

Larynx

Trachea

Bronchial tree

Upper lobe

Upper lobe

Middle lobe

Lower lobe

Lower lobe

Diaphragm

Abdominal cavity

Anatomical Plates: Digestive System
Figure A-18

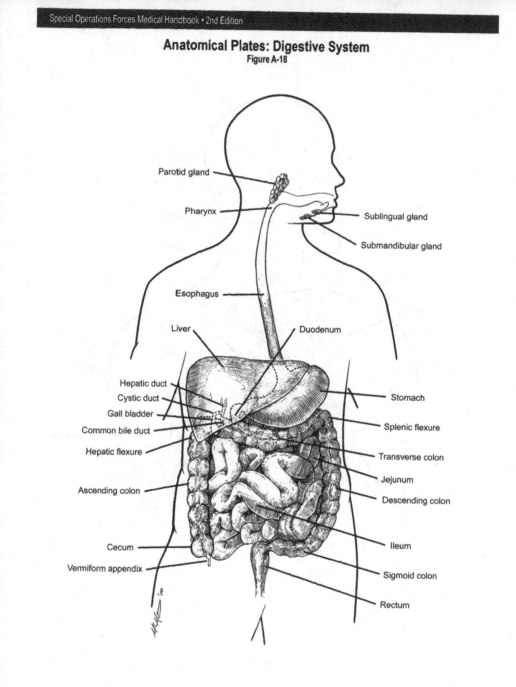

Anatomical Plates: Endocrine System
Figure A-19

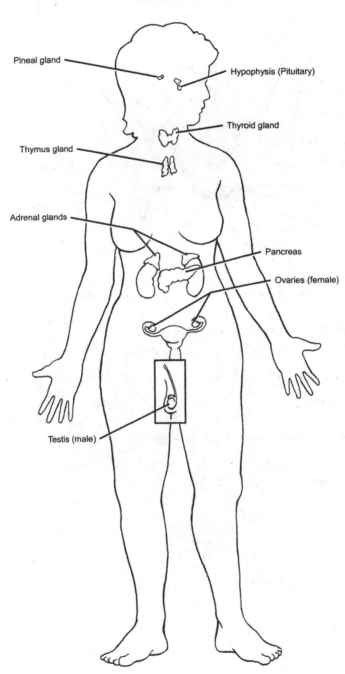

Pineal gland

Hypophysis (Pituitary)

Thyroid gland

Thymus gland

Adrenal glands

Pancreas

Ovaries (female)

Testis (male)

Anatomical Plates: Male and Female Reproductive Systems
Figure A-20

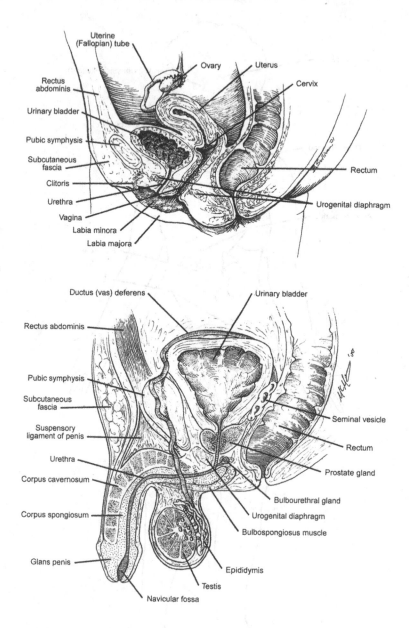

Color Plates

Figure A-21.A. Dermatophyte Onchomycosis

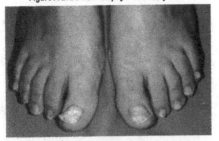

(courtesy of MAJ Dan Schissel)

Figure A-21.B. Dermatophyte Ringworm

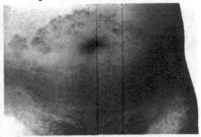

(courtesy of MAJ Dan Schissel)

Figure A-21.C. Dermatophyte KOH

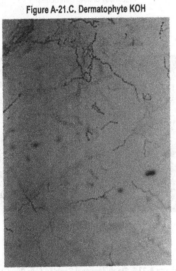

(courtesy of MAJ Dan Schissel)

Figure A-21.D. Disseminated Gonococcal Infection

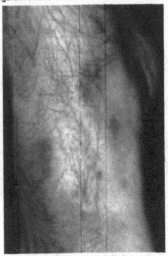

(courtesy of MAJ Dan Schissel)

Figure A-21.E. Erysipelas

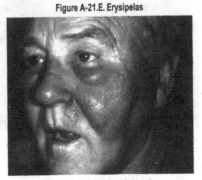

(courtesy of MAJ Dan Schissel)

Figure A-21.F. Tache Noire Lesion of Scrub Typhus

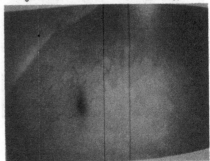

(courtesy of the Textbook of Military Medicine)

Color Plates

Figure A-22.A. Enlarged Lymph Node of Cat-Scratch Disease

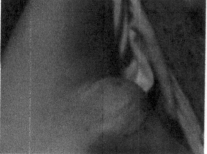

(courtesy of COL Naomi Aronson)

Figure A-22.B. Impetigo Contagiosa

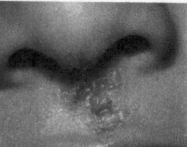

(courtesy of MAJ Dan Schissel)

Figure A-22.C. Herpes Zoster: Back Close-up

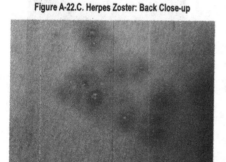

(courtesy of MAJ Dan Schissel)

Figure A-22.D. Herpes Simplex

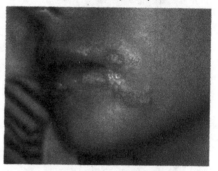

(courtesy of MAJ Dan Schissel)

Figure A-22.E. Molluscum Contagiosum

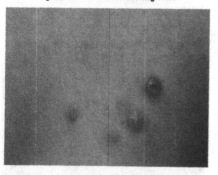

(courtesy of MAJ Dan Schissel)

Figure A-22.F. Staphylococcal Scalded Skin Syndrome

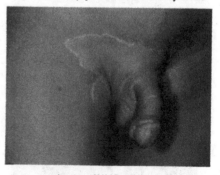

(courtesy of MAJ Dan Schissel)

Color Plates

Figure A-23.A. *Bacilus anthracis* Gram's Stain

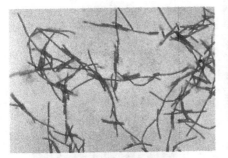

(courtesy of CDC/Dr. William A. Clark)

Figure A-23.B. *Strongyloides stercoralis* First-Stage Larva Preserved in 10% Formalin

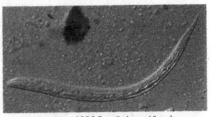

(courtesy of CDC Parasite Image Library)

Figure A-23.C. *Haemophilus ducreyi*

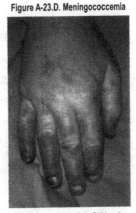

(courtesy of COL Naomi Aronson)

Figure A-23.D. Meningococcemia

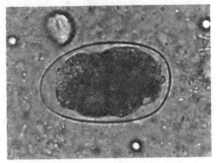

(courtesy of MAJ Dan Schissel)

Figure A-23.E. Erythema Migrans of Lyme Disease

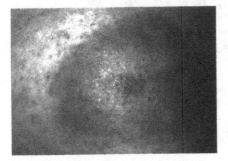

(courtesy of MAJ Joseph Wilde)

Figure A-23.F. Hookworm eggs examined on wet mount

(courtesy of CDC Parasite Image Library)

Color Plates

Figure A-24.A. Leishmaniasis Skin Ulcer

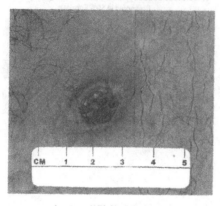

(courtesy of LTC Glenn Wortmann)

Figure A-24.B. Monkeypox

(Courtesy of USAMRIID & LTC Kathleen Dunn Farr)

Figure A-24.D. Lesions of the Skin

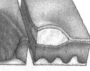

Epidermis
Dermis

Stratum corneum
Stratum lucidum
Stratum granulosum
Stratum spinosum
Stratum basale

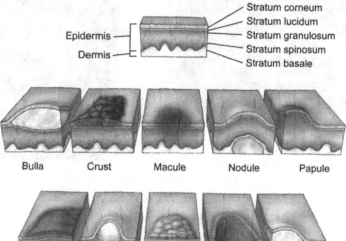

Bulla   Crust   Macule   Nodule   Papule

Plaque   Pustule   Scale   Ulcer   Vesicle

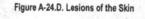

Color Plates
Figure A-25. *Plasmodium falciparum*

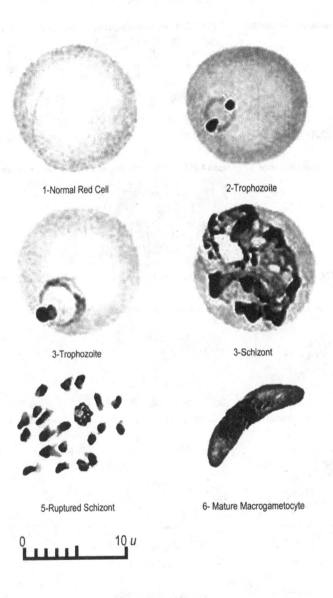

1-Normal Red Cell   2-Trophozoite

3-Trophozoite   3-Schizont

5-Ruptured Schizont   6- Mature Macrogametocyte

0   10 *u*

(courtesy of CDC Parasite Image Library)

Color Plates

Figure A-26.A. *Aeromonas shigelloides*

Courtesy of CDC/Dr. William Clark

Figure A-26.B. *Enterococcus species*

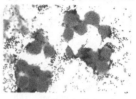

Courtesy of CDC/Dr. Richard Facklam

Figure A-26.C. *Staphylococcus aureus*

Courtesy of www.bact.wisc.edu

Figure A-26.D. *Clostridium novyi*

Courtesy of CDC/Dr. William Clark

Figure A-26.E. *Streptococcus pyogenes*

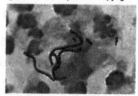

Courtesy of www.bact.wisc.edu

Figure A-26.F. *Streptococcus mutans*

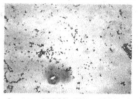

Courtesy of CDC/Dr. Richard Facklam

Figure A-26.G. *E. coli*

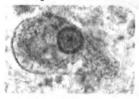

Courtesy of COL Naomi Aronson

Figure A-26.H. *Trichuris* species

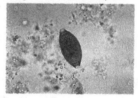

Courtesy of CDC/Dr. Mae Melvin

Figure A-26.I. *Plasmodium falciparum*

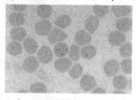

Courtesy of CDC/Dr. Mae Melvin

Figure A-26.J. *Filaria*

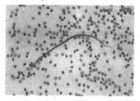

Courtesy of CDC/Dr. Lee Moore

Figure A-26.K. *Trypanosoma* forms

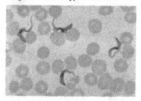

Courtesy of CDC/Dr. Myron Schultz

Figure A-26.L. *Plasmodium ovale*

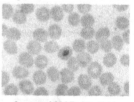

Courtesy of CDC/Dr. Mae Melvin

Figure A-26.M. *Schistosoma haematobium*

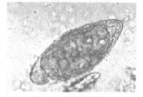

Courtesy of CDC-PHIL

Figure A-26.N. *Vibrio cholerae*

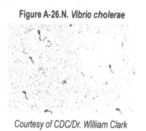

Courtesy of CDC/Dr. William Clark

Figure A-26.O. *Plasmodium vivax*

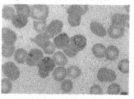

Courtesy of CDC-PHIL

Table A-1. Organism/Antimicrobial Chart

COL Glenn Wortmann, MC, USA & COL Duane Hospenthal, MC, USA

Infecting Organism	Medication of Choice	Alternatives
I. AEROBIC BACTERIA		
A. Gram-positive Cocci		
1. Staphylococci		
a. *S. aureus* (methicillin-sensitive)	PRP, Cephalosporin (1st generation)	Vancomycin, clindamycin, TMP-SMX
b. *S. aureus* (methicillin-sensitive)	Vancomycin	Clindamycin, TMP-SMX, linezolid, or daptomycin
c. *S. epidermidis*	Vancomycin	Linezolid, daptomycin
2. Streptococci		
a. *Streptococcus*, Group A, B, C, G, *S. viridans* and *penicillin-sensitive S. pneumoniae*	Penicillin G or V	1st gen vancomycin, clindamycin, erythromycin, azithromycin*
b. *S. pneumoniae* with high level penicillin-resistance	Vancomycin	ASF
c. Enterococci	Ampicillin + gentamicin	Vancomycin + gentamicin
B. Gram-positive Bacilli		
1. *Bacillus anthracis*	Penicillin or APF	Doxycycline
2. *Corynebacterium diphtheriae*	Erythromycin + Antitoxin	Clindamycin or penicillin G
3. *Listeria monocytogenes*	Ampicillin or penicillin	TMP-SMX
C. Gram-negative Cocci		
1. *Neisseria gonorrhoeae*	Ceftriaxone or Fluoroquinolone	Cefixime
2. *Neisseria meningitidis*	Penicillin G or V	Ceftriaxone
3. *Moraxella catarrhalis*	TMP-SMX or amox-clav	Azithromycin* or doxycycline
D. Gram-negative Bacilli		
1. *Escherichia coli*	TMP-SMX	3rd gen cephalosporin or APF
2. *Enterobacter species*	Imipenem**	APF or 3rd gen cephalosporin
3. *Klebsiella species*	Imipenem**	APF or 3rd gen cephalosporin
4. *Pseudomonas aeruginosa*	APP	Cefepime, ceftazidime, or imipenem**
5. *Proteus species*	APP	3rd gen cephalosporin or APF
6. *Serratia marcescens*	3rd gen cephalosporin	Imipenem** or APF
7. *Salmonella typhi*	Ceftriaxone or APF	TMP-SMX
8. *Haemophilus influenzae*	Ceftriaxone or APF	Azithromycin, doxycycline, or amox-clav
9. *Haemophilus ducreyi*	Ceftriaxone or APF	Amox-clav, azithromycin,* or erythromycin
10. *Brucella species*	Doxycycline + rifampin	Doxycycline + gentamicin
11. *Francisella tularensis*	Streptomycin or gentamicin	Doxycycline
12. *Yersinia pestis*	Streptomycin	Gentamicin
II. ANAEROBIC BACTERIA		
1. *Clostridium tetani*	Penicillin + tetanus toxoid + tetanus immune globulin	Imipenem,** clindamycin, or metronidazole
2. *Bacteroides species*	Metronidazole	Imipenem,** clindamycin, or BL-BLI
III. ACID FAST BACILLI		
1. *Mycobacterium tuberculosis* (TB)	Isoniazid + rifampin + pyrazinamide + ethambutol	Isoniazid + rifampin + pyrazinamide + streptomycin
2. *M. kansasii*	Isoniazid + rifampin+ ethambutol	
3. *M. avium intracellulare complex*	Clarithromycin + ethambutol + rifabutin	Azithromycin + ethambutol + rifabutin
4. *M. leprae*	Rifampin + dapsone (paucibacillary disease)	Rifampin + dapsone + clofazimine (multibacillary disease)

Table A-1. Organism/Antimicrobial Chart, continued

Infecting Organism	Medication of Choice	Alternatives
IV. ACTINOMYCETES		
1. *Nocardia* species	TMP-SMX	Sulfadiazine
2. *Actinomyces* species	Penicillin	Clindamycin
V. MISCELLANEOUS BACTERIA		
1. *Chlamydia* species	Doxycycline	Erythromycin or azithromycin*
2. *Rickettsia* species	Doxycycline	Chloramphenicol
3. *Treponema pallidum* (syphilis)	Penicillin	Ceftriaxone or doxycycline
4. *Mycoplasma pneumoniae*	Azithromycin*	Doxycycline or ASF
VI. FUNGAL		
1. *Aspergillus* species	Voriconazole	Amphotericin B or itraconazole
2. *Blastomyces dermatitidis*	Amphotericin B	Itraconazole
3. *Candida* species	Amphotericin B	Fluconazole or Echinocandin***
4. *Coccidioides*	Amphotericin B	Fluconazole or Itraconazole
5. *Cryptococcus neoformans*	Amphotericin B	Fluconazole
6. *Histoplasma capsulatum*	Amphotericin B	Itraconazole
7. *Pneumocystis*	TMP-SMX	Pentamidine
8. *Sporothrix schenckii*	Itraconazole	Saturated solution of potassium iodide
9. Tinea versicolor	Topical selenium sulfide	Ketoconazole
VII. VIRUSES		
1. Herpes simplex	Acyclovir	Valacyclovir or famciclovir
2. Herpes zoster	Acyclovir	Valacyclovir or famciclovir
3. Influenza	Oseltamivir or zanamivir	Amantadine or rimantadine****

Abbreviations/Classifications:

1st gen cephalosporin, 1st generation cephalosporin: Cefazolin, cephalexin

3rd gen cephalosporin, 3rd generation cephalosporin: Ceftriaxone, cefotaxime, ceftazidime, cefixime

APF, antipseudomonal fluoroquinolone: Ciprofloxacin, levofloxacin

APP, antipseudomonal penicillin: Piperacillin, mezlocillin, ticarcillin

ASF, antistreptococcal fluoroquinolone: Levofloxacin, gatifloxacin, moxifloxacin

BL-BLI, ß-lactam- ß-lactamase inhibitor combination: Ampicillin-sulbactam; amox-clav, amoxicillin-clavulanic acid; piperacillin tazobactam; ticarcillin-clavulanate

PRP, penicillinase-resistant (antistaphylococcal) penicillin: Nafcillin, oxacillin, dicloxacillin, cloxacillin

TMP-SMX, trimethoprim-sulfamethoxazole

*Clarithromycin can be substituted based on availability.

**Meropenem can be substituted for imipenem in most cases. Ertapenem may be substituted except for use against Pseudomonas or Acinetobacter

***Echinocandin: Anidulafungin, caspofungin, micafungin

****Widespread resistance to amantadine and rimantadine has been documented in the US.

DISCLAIMER: This chart does not account for the fact that these organisms may cause a range of diseases from UTI or mild skin infections to life-threatening sepsis and meningitis. It also does not account for local resistance patterns, cost-effectiveness, or what drugs may be available. Microbiology support to identify organisms and produce susceptibility results greatly increases the success of antimicrobial therapy.

MEDICAL EDITOR'S NOTE: The use of broad spectrum antibiotics is without a doubt adding to the increase of resistant organisms and EVERY reasonable effort to limit the use of broad spectrum antibiotics should be made. It must be emphasized that broad spectrum antibiotics are NOT required for every instance of injury (eg, limited extremity trauma where imminent medical evacuation is available). It is strongly recommended to obtain cultures to prove the identification of the infecting bacteria and use antibiotics based on those results whenever possible.

Table A-2. Common Photosensitizing Medications
LTC Gwendolyn Thompson, MS, USA

Class	Medication	Phototoxic Reaction	Photoallergic Reaction
Antibiotics	Tetracyclines: doxycycline, tetracycline	Yes	No
	Fluoroquinolones: ciprofloxacin (Cipro), ofloxacin (Floxin), levofloxacin (Levaquin)	Yes	No
	Sulfonamides (Septra)	Yes	No
Nonsteroidal anti-inflammatory drugs (NSAIDs)	Ibuprofen (Motrin)	Yes	No
	Ketoprofen (Orudis)	Yes	Yes
	Naproxen (Naprosyn)	Yes	No
	Celecoxib (Celebrex)	No	Yes
Diuretics	Furosemide (Lasix)	Yes	No
	Bumetanide (Bumex)	No	No
	Hydrochlorothiazide	Yes	Yes
Retinoid	Isotretinoin (Accutane)	Yes	No
	Acitretin	Yes	No
Hypoglycemics	Sulfonylureas: glipizide (Glucotrol), glyburide (Micronase)	No	Yes
Neuroleptic drugs	Phenothiazines: chlorpromazine (Thorazine), fluphenazine (Stelazine), perphenazine (Tofranil), thioridazine (Mellaril)	Yes	Yes
	Thioxanthenes: thiothixene (Navane)	Yes	No
Anti-fungal drugs	Terbinafine (Lamisil)	No	No
	Itraconazole (Sporanox)	Yes	Yes
	Voriconazole (Vfend)	Yes	No
	Fluorouracil (5-FU)	Yes	Yes
	Amiodarone (Cordarone)	Yes	No
	Diltiazem (Cardizem)	Yes	No
	Quinidine	Yes	Yes
	Hydroxychloroquine (Plaquenil)	No	No
	Coal tar	Yes	No
	Dapsone	No	Yes
	Oral Contraceptives	No	Yes

Phototoxic reactions occur because of the damaging effects of light-activated compounds on cell membranes and, in some instances, DNA. By contrast, photoallergic reactions are cell-mediated immune responses to a light-activated compound. Phototoxic reactions develop in most individuals if they are exposed to sufficient amounts of light and drug. Typically, they appear as an exaggerated sunburn response. Photoallergic reactions resemble allergic contact dermatitis, with a distribution limited to sun exposed areas of the body. However, when the reactions are severe or prolonged, they may extend into covered areas of skin.

Table A-3. Distinguishing Characteristics of Phototoxic and Photoallergic Reactions

Feature	Phototoxic Reaction	Photoallergic Reaction
Incidence	High	Low
Amount of agent required for photosensitivity	Large	Small
Onset of reaction after exposure to agent and light	Minutes to hours	24-72 hours
More than one exposure to agent required	No	Yes
Distribution	Sun-exposed skin only	Sun-exposed skin, may spread to unexposed areas
Clinical characteristics	Exaggerated sunburn	Dermatitis
Immunologically mediated	No	Yes; Type IV

Table A-4. IV Drip Rates
CPT Joseph Fansano, AN, USA

Drip Chamber Drop Sizes (Select Your Drip Chamber Size)

* Hours to Deliver 1000mL	mL per hour	10 Drops per mL Drops Per Minute (DPM)	15 Drops per mL Drops Per Minute (DPM)	20 Drops per mL Drops Per Minute (DPM)	60 Drops per mL Drops Per Minute (DPM)
Fractions are rounded to closest number, except where shown.	10	1.7 DPM	2.5 DPM	3 DPM	10 DPM
	30	5 DPM	7.5 DPM	10 DPM	30 DPM
	50	8 DPM	12.5 DPM	17 DPM	50 DPM
	70	12 DPM	17.5 DPM	23 DPM	70 DPM
	90	15 DPM	22.5 DPM	30 DPM	90 DPM
* 8 Hours	125	20.8 DPM	31 DPM	42 DPM	
	175	29 DPM	43.8 DPM	58 DPM	
	250	41.6 DPM	62.5 DPM	83 DPM	

Table A-5. Glasgow Coma Scale

Eye Opening Response	Spontaneous	4
	To Verbal Command	3
	With Painful Stimulus	2
	No Response	1
Best Verbal Response	Oriented	5
	Confused	4
	Inappropriate Words	3
	Incomprehensible Sounds	2
	None	1
Best Motor Response	Obeys Command	6
	Localizes Pain	5
	Withdraws (pain)	4
	Flexion (pain)	3
	Extension (pain)	2
	None	1
Total		**3 to 15**

Any patient with a GCS of 8 or less is considered to have a severe head injury. Those in the 9 to 12 range are considered moderate, but may require airway control. Any GCS of 13 to 15 is considered indicative of mild head injury, but even these patients can deteriorate and should be observed or evacuated per the guidelines in *Part 7: Trauma: Chapter 28: Mild Traumatic Brain Injury/Concussion*

Table A-6. Mini-Mental Status Exam

The Mini-Mental Status Exam (MMSE) is the most useful tool for assessing brain function in the field. Once a baseline score is established with an initial MMSE, improvement or worsening mental status can be observed with repeated testing.

Specific Test Function	Brain Area Tested	Points
What is the year/season/month/date/day of the week? (1 for each correct answer)	Orientation (Frontal)	5
What state/country/hospital/floor are you in? (Use other cues, such as military unit, etc., when appropriate)	Orientation (Frontal)	5
List three items. Have the patient repeat the list.	Registration (Frontal)	3
Serial sevens – ask the patient to count backwards by 7 from 100, or have them spell "WORLD" backwards.	Concentration (Frontal)	5
Name an object you point to, such as wristwatch or pen.	Naming (Dominant Temporoparietal)	2
Have patient report, "No ifs, ands, or buts"	Expressive Speech (Dominant Frontal)	1
3-part command: Take this paper in your right hand, fold it in half & put it on the table.	Command (Frontal)	3
Read "close your eyes," on the paper and do it.	Reading (Dominant Temporoparietal)	1
Recall the three items listed earlier.	Short-term Memory (Hippocampal)	3
Write a sentence.	Writing (Dominant Temporoparietal)	1
Copy intersecting pentagons	Construction (Nondominant Parietal)	1
Total		30

Figure A-32. Neurological Examination Checklist (Sheet 1 of 2)

Patient's Name: _____ Date/Time: _____

Describe pain/numbness: _____
_____

HISTORY

Type of dive last performed: _____ Depth: _____ How long: _____

Number of dives in last 24 hours: _____

Was symptom noticed before, during, or after the dive?_____

If during, was it while descending, on the bottom, or ascending? _____

Has symptom increased or decreased since it was first noticed? _____

Have any other symptoms occurred since the first one was noticed? _____

Describe: _____

Has patient ever had a similar symptom before? _____ When: _____

Has patient ever had decompression sickness or an air embolism before?____ When: _____

MENTAL STATUS/STATE OF CONSCIOUSNESS

COORDINATION

Walk: _____
Heel-to-Toe: _____
Romberg: _____
Finger-to-Nose: _____
Heel-Shin Slide: _____
Rapid Movement: _____

CRANIAL NERVES

Sense of Smell: (I): _____
Vision/Visual Fld (II): _____
Eye Movements, Pupils (III, IV, VI): _____
Facial Sensation, Chewing (V): _____
Facial Expression Muscles (VII): _____
Hearing (VIII): _____
Upper Mouth, Throat Sensation (IX): _____
Gag & Voice (X): _____
Shoulder Shrug (XI): _____
Tongue (XII): _____

STRENGTH (Grade 0 to 5)

Upper Body

Deltoids	L _____	R _____
Latissimus	L _____	R _____
Biceps	L _____	R _____
Triceps	L _____	R _____
Forearms	L _____	R _____
Hands	L _____	R _____

Lower Body

Hips

Flexion	L _____	R _____
Extension	L _____	R _____
Abduction	L _____	R _____
Adduction	L _____	R _____

Knees

Flexion	L _____	R _____
Extension	L _____	R _____

Figure A-33. Neurological Examination Checklist (Sheet 2 of 2)

REFLEXES

(Grade: Normal, Hypoactive, Hyperactive, Absent

Biceps	L ___ R ___	**Ankles**	
Triceps	L ___ R ___	Dorsiflexion	L ___ R ___
Knees	L ___ R ___	Plantarflexion	L ___ R ___
Ankles	L ___ R ___	**Toes**	L ___ R ___

Sensory Examination for Skin Sensation
(Use diagram to record location of sensory abnormalities – numbness, tingling, etc.)

LOCATION

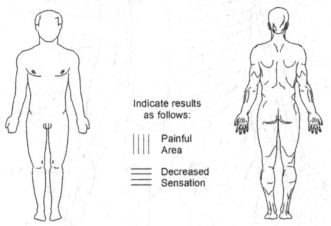

Indicate results
as follows:

|||| Painful
Area

= Decreased
= Sensation

COMMENTS

_____
_____
_____
_____
_____
_____
_____
_____

Examination Performed by: _____

Figure A-34. Dermatomes of Cutaneous Innervation, Anterior View
United States Navy Diving Manual, Revision 6

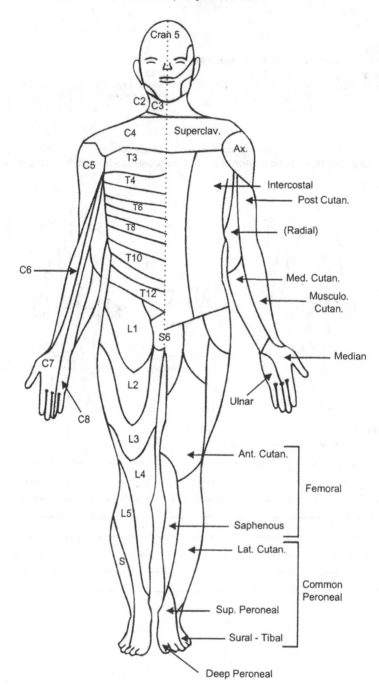

Figure A-35. Dermatomes of Cutaneous Innervation, Posterior View
United States Navy Diving Manual, Revision 6

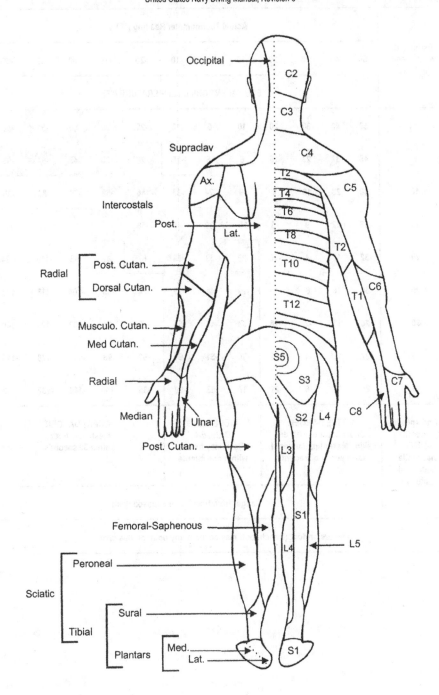

Figure A-36. Wind Chill Chart

Estimated wind speed (in MPH)	Actual Thermometer Reading (°F)											
	50	40	30	20	10	0	-10	-20	-30	-40	-50	-60
	EQUIVALENT CHILL TEMPERATURE (°F)											
Calm	50	40	30	20	10	0	-10	-20	-30	-40	-50	-60
5	48	37	27	16	6	-5	-15	-26	-36	-47	-57	-68
10	40	28	16	4	-9	-24	-33	-46	-58	-70	-83	-95
15	36	22	9	-5	-18	-32	-45	-58	-72	-85	-99	-112
20	32	18	4	-10	-25	-39	-53	-67	-82	-96	-110	-124
25	30	16	0	-15	-29	-44	-59	-74	-88	-104	-118	-133
30	28	13	-2	-18	-33	-48	-63	-79	-94	-109	-125	-140
35	27	11	-4	-21	-35	-51	-67	-82	-98	-113	-129	-145
40	26	10	-6	-21	-37	-53	-69	-85	-100	-116	-132	-148
Wind speeds greater than 40 MPH have little additional effect	LITTLE DANGER Under 5 hours with dry skin. Maximum danger of false sense of security			INCREASING DANGER Flesh may freeze within one minute			GREAT DANGER Flesh may freeze within 30 seconds.					
	Danger from freezing of exposed flesh											
	Immersion foot (trench foot) may occur at any point on this chart											

SOF Medical Handbook Abbreviations

AAE - arterial air embolism
A/B ratio - acid/base ratio
ABC - airway, breathing, circulation; atomic, biological, chemical
ABE - acute bacterial endocarditis
ABG - arterial blood gas
ac - *ante cibum* [L] - before meals
AC - acromioclavicular; alternating current
ACD - allergic contact dermatitis
AChE - acetylcholinesterase
ACIP - Advisory Committee on Immunization Practices
ACL - anterior cruciate ligament
ACLS - advanced cardiac life support
ACS - acute coronary syndrome
ACTH - adrenocorticotropic hormone
ACVD - acute cardiovascular disease
ad lib - *ad libitum* [L] - as desired
ADH - antidiuretic hormone (vasopressin)
ADL - activities of daily living
AE - above elbow
A/E - air evacuation
AED - automatic external defibrillator
AFB - acid-fast bacilli
AFib/AFlut - atrial fibrillation/atrial flutter
AFIP - Armed Forces Institute of Pathology
AFMIC - Armed Forces Medical Intelligence Center
AFP - acute flaccid paralysis
AFRCC - Air Force Recovery Coordination Center
A/G ratio - albumin/globin ratio
AGA - appropriate for gestational age
AGE - arterial gas embolism
AGL - above ground level
AHA - American Heart Association
AHD - atherosclerotic heart disease
AIDS - acquired immune deficiency syndrome
AJ - ankle jerk
AK - above knee
AKA - above-the-knee amputation; also known as
ALL - acute lymphoblastic or lymphocytic leukemia
ALS - amyotrophic lateral sclerosis
AM - *ante meridiem* [L] - before noon
AMI - acute myocardial infarction
AML - acute myelocytic/myeloblastic leukemia
AMPLE - allergies, medications, previous injury, last meal, events
AMS - altered mental status; acute mountain sickness
AN - Army Nurse
ant - anterior
ante - before
ANUG - acute necrotizing ulcerative gingivitis
AO - area of operations
AOM - acute otitis media
AP - anterior-posterior
AP & Lat - anteroposterior and lateral
ARDS - acute respiratory distress syndrome
AROM - active range of motion
ARS - acute radiation syndrome
ASA - acetylsalicylic acid (aspirin)
ASAP - as soon as possible
ASD - atrial septal defect
ASHD - arteriosclerotic heart disease
ARF - acute rheumatic fever

ATA - atmosphere absolute
ATLS - advanced trauma life support
ATP - advanced tactical provider
AUB - abnormal uterine bleeding
AV, A-V - arteriovenous; atrioventricular
AVIP - Anthrax Vaccine Immunization Program
AVMA - American Veterinary Medical Association
AVPU - alert, verbal stimulus response, painful stimulus response, unresponsive
BAC - blood alcohol concentration
BAT - blood alcohol test
BBB - bundle branch block
BCC - basal cell carcinoma
BCG - bacillus Calmette-Guerin (vaccine)
BCL - bandage contact lens
BCP - birth control pills
BE - barium enema
BF - battle fatigue
bicarb - bicarbonate
bid - *bis in die* [L] - twice a day
bil or bilat - bilateral
bili - bilirubin
BK - below knee
BKA - below-knee amputation
BLS - basic life support
BM - bowel movement
BMR - basal metabolic rate
BNTI - blind naso-tracheal intubation
BP - blood pressure
BPH - benign prostatic hypertrophy
BPM - beats per minute
BPV - benign positional vertigo
BR - bed rest
BSA - body surface area
BSE - body substance exposure
BSI - blood stream infection; body substance isolation
BSR - blood sedimentation rate
BUN - blood urea nitrogen
BVM - bag-valve-mask
BW - biological warfare
Bx - biopsy
c - *cum* [L] - with
C - Celsius or centigrade
C1 to C7 - cervical nerves or vertebrae 1 to 7
Ca - calcium; cancer; carcinoma
CA - Civil Affairs
CABG - coronary artery bypass graft
CAD - coronary artery disease
CAGE - cut down, annoyed, guilty, eye-opener
CAM - chemical agent monitor; complementary and alternative medicine
CANA - convulsant antidote for nerve agents
CASEVAC - casualty evacuation
CAT - computerized axial tomography
cath - catheter
CBC - complete blood count
CBR - chemical, biological, radiological
CBRNE - chemical, biological, radiological, nuclear, explosive
cc - cubic centimeter
CC - chief or current complaint

SOF Medical Handbook Abbreviations

CD - Cesarean delivery
CD - contact dermatitis
CDC - Centers for Disease Control
CDU - chest drainage unit
CERP - Commander's Emergency Response Program
CF - cystic fibrosis
cGy - centigray
CHF - congestive heart failure
CHPPM - Center for Health Promotion and Preventive Medicine
CHS - classic heat stroke
Cl - chloride
CLC - cutaneous larva currens
CLM - cutaneous larva migrans
cm - centimeter
CMV - cytomegalovirus
CN - cranial nerve
CNS - central nervous system
CO - carbon monoxide
CO_2 - carbon dioxide
c/o - complains of
COHb - carboxyhemoglobin
COIN - counter-insurgency
COPD - chronic obstructive pulmonary disease
CPAP - continuous positive airway pressure
CPD - cephalopelvic disproportion
CPK - creatinine phosphokinase
CPP - chronic pelvic pain
CPR - cardiopulmonary resuscitation
CRAO - central retinal artery occlusion
CRF - chronic renal failure
CRNA - certified registered nurse anesthetist
CRVO - central retinal vein occlusion
CS - compartment syndrome
C & S - culture and sensitivity
C-section - Cesarean section
CSF - cerebral spinal fluid
CSH - combat support hospital
CT - clotting time; computed tomography
CVA - cerebrovascular accident; costovertebral angle
CVD - cardiovascular disease
CVP - central venous pressure
CXR - chest x-ray
d - day
D5W - dextrose 5% in water
DAN - Divers Alert Network
DBP - diastolic blood pressure
DC - duty cycle; Dental Corps; direct current
D/C - discharge or discontinue
D & C - dilatation and curettage or curettement
DCS - decompression sickness
DEC – diethylcarbamazine citrate
DGI - disseminated gonococcal infection
DHF - dengue hemorrhagic fever
DIC - diffuse intravascular coagulation
DIP - distal interphalangeal
DJD - degenerative joint disease
DKA - diabetic ketoacidosis
DM - diabetes mellitus
DMAC - disseminated Mycobacterium avian complex
DMARD - disease modifying antirheumatic drug

DMO - Diving Medical Officer
DNA - deoxyribonucleic acid
DNBI - disease/non-battle injuries
DNR - do not resuscitate
DO - Doctor of Osteopathy
DOA - dead on arrival
DOB - date of birth
DOE - dyspnea on exertion
DOT - directly observed therapy
DPN - drops per minute
DRE - digital rectal exam
DRI - dietary reference intake
DS - double strength
DSS - dengue shock syndrome
DT - diphtheria toxoid and tetanus toxoid; delirium tremens
DTP - diphtheria toxoid, tetanus toxoid, pertussis vaccine
DTR - deep tendon reflexes
DTs - delirium tremens
DVBIC - Defense and Veterans Brain Injury Center
DVT - deep vein thrombosis
Dx - diagnosis
EAC - external auditory canal
EBA - emergency breathing apparatus
EBL - estimated blood loss
EBV - Epstein-Barr virus
EC - enemy combatant
ECG - electrocardiogram
EDC - estimated date of confinement
EEE - eastern equine encephalitis
EEG - electroencephalogram
eg - *exempli gratia* [L] - for example
EGA - estimated gestational age
EHEC - entero-hemorrhagic *Escherichia coli*
EHS - exertional heat stroke
EIC - epidermal inclusion cyst
EKG - electrocardiogram
ELISA - enzyme-linked immunoassay
EM - erythema migrans
EMD - electromechanical disassociation
EMG - electromyogram
EMS - emergency medical service
ENT - ear, nose, and throat
EOM - extraocular movement
EPW - enemy prisoners of war
ER - emergency room; external rotation
ESR - erythrocyte sedimentation rate
ESRD - end-stage renal disease
ET - endotracheal; Eustachian tube
etc - *et cetera* [L] - and so forth
ETOH - ethyl alcohol
ETT- endotracheal tube
F - Fahrenheit
F Hx - family history
FABER – flexion, abduction, external rotation
FB - foreign body
FBS - fasting blood sugar
FDA - Food and Drug Administration
FDI - Fédération Dentaire Internationale
Fe - iron
FEV - forced expiratory volume

SOF Medical Handbook Abbreviations

FEV1 - forced expiratory volume in 1 second
FFP - fresh frozen plasma
FHR - fetal heart rate
FHT - fetal heart tone
fib - fibrillation
FiO_2 - fraction of inspired oxygen
FITT - frequency, intensity, time, type
FM - field manual, frequency modulation
FMC - field medical card
FP - family practice
Fr - French (catheter size)
FST - forward surgical team
fsw - feet of salt water
ft - foot; feet
FT - full term
FTA - fluorescent treponemal antibody
F/U - follow-up
FUO - fever of unknown or undetermined origin
FVC - forced vital capacity
Fx - fracture
g - gram(s)
ga - gauge
GABHS - group A beta-hemolytic streptococci
GB - gallbladder
GBS - group B streptococcus
GC - gonococcus; gonococcal
GCA - giant cell arteritis
GCS - Glasgow coma scale
GDV - gastric dilatation/volvulus
GERD - gastroesophageal reflux disease\
GI - gastrointestinal
gm - gram
GPMRC - Global Patient Movement Requirements Center
GPS - global positioning system
G6PD - glucose 6-phosphate dehydrogenase
GSW - gunshot wound
Gt or gtt - *gutta* [L] - drop; drops
GTT - glucose tolerance test
GU - genitourinary
GYN; Gyn - gynecology
h - hour
H - hydrogen
H_2O - water
H_2O_2 - hydrogen peroxide
HA or H/A - headache
HAA - hepatitis-associated antigen
HACE - high altitude cerebral edema
HAHO - high altitude, high opening (parachute)
HALO - high altitude, low opening (parachute)
HAPE - high altitude pulmonary edema
HAV - hepatitis A virus
Hb or hgb - hemoglobin
HBO - hyperbaric oxygen
HBP - high blood pressure
HBV - hepatitis B virus
HC - head circumference
HCC - hepatocellular carcinoma
HCG - human chorionic gonadotropin
HCl - hydrochloric acid
HCPS - hantavirus cardiopulmonary syndrome

Hct or HCT - hematocrit
HCV - hepatitis C virus
HDCV - human diploid cell vaccine
HDL - high-density lipoprotein
HDV - hepatitis D virus
HE - high explosive
HEENT - head, eyes, ears, nose, throat
HEV - hepatitis E virus
HF - hydrofluoric
HFRS - hemorrhagic fever with renal syndrome
Hg – mercury
H/H - hematocrit/hemoglobin
Hib – *Haemophilus influenza* type B
HIV - human immunodeficiency virus
HLZ - helicopter landing zone
HN - host nation
HNP - herniated nucleus pulposus
H/O - history of
H & P - history and physical
HPF - high power field
HPI - history of present illness
HPS - hantavirus pulmonary syndrome
HPV - human papillomavirus
hr - hour
HR - heart rate
HRIG - human rabies immune globulin
HRO - human relief organization
hs - *hora somni* [L] - at bedtime
HSV - herpes simplex virus
ht - height
HTN - hypertension
HTS - hypertonic saline
Hx - history
Hz - hertz
IAI - intraamniotic infection
IAPP - inspection, auscultation, palpation and percussion
IAW - in accordance with
IBS - irritable bowel syndrome
ICD - irritant contact dermatitis
ICP - intracranial pressure
ICRC - International Committee of the Red Cross
ID - infectious disease; identification
ID-MED - immediate, delayed – minimal, expectant, dead
I & D - incision and drainage
ie - *id est* [L] - that is
IED - improvised explosive device
IM - intramuscular; infectious mononucleosis
IMCI - Integrated Management of Childhood Illness
in - inch
IND - improvised nuclear device
inf - inferior
INH - isonicotinic acid hydrazide; isoniazid; isonicotinoyl hydrazine
IO - intraosseous
I & O - intake and output
IOP - intraocular pressure
IPPB - intermittent positive pressure breathing
IPV - inactivated polio vaccine
IR - internal rotation
IRM - intermediate restoration material
ITBS - iliotibial band syndrome

SOF Medical Handbook Abbreviations

IU - international unit
IUCD; IUD - intrauterine contraceptive device
IV - intravenous
IVF - intravenous fluids
IVIG - intravenous immunoglobulin
IVH - intraventricular hemorrhage
IVP - intravenous pyelogram
JBAIDS - Joint Biological Agent Identification and Diagnostic System
JE - Japanese encephalitis
JOMAC - judgment, orientation, mentation, abstraction, calculation
JVD - jugular vein distention
K - potassium
kg - kilogram
KIA - killed in action
KJ - knee jerk
kL - kiloliter
km - kilometer
KOH - potassium hydroxide
KS - Kaposi's sarcoma
KUB - kidney, ureter, and bladder
KVO - keep vein open
L - liter
LA – long acting
lac - laceration
LAIV - live attenuated influenza vaccine
lap - laparotomy
laser or LASER - light amplification by stimulated emission of radiation
lat - lateral
lb - pound
L/B - live birth
LBBB - left bundle branch block
LBP - low back pain
LBRF - louse-borne relapsing fever
LBW - low birth weight
L & D - labor and delivery
LCP disease - Legg-Calves-Perthes disease
LDL - low-density lipoprotein
LE - lower extremity
LGV - lymphogranuloma venereum
lig - ligament
LLE - left lower extremity
LLL - left lower lobe (of lung)
LLQ - left lower quadrant
L/M - liters per minute
LMA - laryngeal mask airway
LMP - left mentoposterior (position of fetus); last menstrual period
LMWH - low molecular weight heparin
LOC - loss of consciousness; level of consciousness
LOD - line of duty
LOM - limitation of motion
LP - lumbar puncture
LPF - low power field
LQ - lower quadrant
LR - lactated Ringer's
L-S - lumbosacral
LSD - lysergic acid diethylamide
LTBI - latent tuberculosis infection
LUL - left upper lobe (of lung)

LUQ - left upper quadrant
LV - left ventricular
LZ - landing zone
lymphs - lymphocytes
m - meter
ma - milliampere
MA - mortuary affairs
MAC - minimum alveolar concentration
MACE - Military Acute Concussion Evaluation
maint - maintenance
MAP - mean arterial pressure
mAs - milliamps
MASCAL - mass casualties
max - maximum
MC - Medical Corps
mc; mCi - millicurie
mcg - microgram
MCHC - mean corpuscular hemoglobin concentration or count
MCL - mid clavicular line
MCP - metacarpal phalangeal
MDAD - major depression adjustment disorder
MDI - multidirectional instability
MEA/DMSO - monoethylamine/dimethylsulfocxide
MEB - medical evaluation board
med - medicine or medication
MEDCAP - medical civic action program
MEDEVAC - medical evacuation
mEq - milli equivalent
MES - medical equipment set
MET - meteorological; mission essential task
mg - milligram
Mg - magnesium
MG - myasthenia gravis
MHz - megahertz
MI - myocardial infarction
MIA - missing in action
min - minute
misc - miscellaneous
MK1 - MARK 1
mL - milliliter
MMR – measles-mumps-rubella
MMSE - mini mental status exam
mm - millimeter
mm Hg - millimeters of mercury
MOI - mechanism of injury
Mono - mononucleosis
monos - monocytes
MOPP - mission oriented protection posture
MOTT - mycobacteria other than tuberculosis
MRE – meal, ready to eat
MRI - magnetic resonance imaging
MRSA - methicillin-resistant *Staphylococcus aureus*
MS - multiple sclerosis
MSDS - material safety data sheet
MSL - mean sea level
mTBI – mild traumatic brain injury
MTF - medical treatment facility
MU – million units
MVA – motor vehicle accident
MVE - Murray Valley encephalitis

SOF Medical Handbook Abbreviations

MWD - military working dog
Na - sodium
NA - not applicable
NAAK - Nerve Agent Antidote Kit
NAD - no acute distress
NAEPP - National Asthma Education and Prevention Program
NAIAD - nerve agent immobilized enzyme alarm and detector
NaPent - sodium Pentothal
NBC - nuclear, biological, chemical
NC - Nurse Corps
NCI - National Cancer Institute
ND - not determined
NEC - necrotizing enterocolitis
neg - negative
NEI - National Eye Institute
NFCI - non-freezing cold injury
NG - nasogastric
NGO - non-government organization
NGT- nasogastric tube
NGU - non-gonococcal urethritis
NKA - no known allergies
NKDA - no known drug allergies
nl; norm - normal limits
NLDO - nasolacrimal duct obstruction
NLT - no later than
No - number
NP - neuropsychiatric
NPA - nasopharyngeal airway
NPH insulin - neutral protamine Hagedorn insulin
NPO - *non per os* [L] - nothing by mouth
NS - nervous system; normal saline
NSAID - non-steroidal anti-inflammatory drug
NSN - national stock number; nonstandard number
NTG - nitroglycerin
NTM - non-tuberculous mycobacterial
N & V - nausea and vomiting
NWB - non-weight bearing
NSS - normal saline solution
O₂ - oxygen
OB - obstetrics
OB-GYN - obstetrics and gynecology
OBS - organic brain syndrome
OC - oral contraceptive
OCOKA - Observation and fire, Concealment and cover, Obstacles, Key terrain, and Avenues of approach
OD - overdose; *oculus dexter* [L] - right eye
OM - otitis media
OME - otitis media with effusion
O & P - ova and parasites
OPA - oropharyngeal airway
OPV - oral poliomyelitis vaccine
OPQRST - onset, provokes, quality, radiates, severity, time
OR - operating room
ORS - oral rehydration solution
ORT - oral rehydration therapy
os - *os* [L] - mouth
OS - *oculus sinister* [L] - left eye
OSA - obstructive sleep apnea
OTC - over the counter (drugs)
OU - oculus uterque [L] - each eye

oz - ounce
PA & Lat - posterior-anterior and lateral
PAC - premature atrial contractions; portable altitude chamber
PA-C - physician assistant-certified
PAD - peripheral artery disease
PALS - pediatric advanced life support
PAM Cl - pralidoxime chloride
Pap test - Papanicolaou's test
PASG - pneumatic anti shock garment
PBI - primary blast injury
pc - *post cibum* [L] - after meals
PCA - patient controlled analgesia
PCP - phenyl cyclohexyl piperidine
PCR - polymerase chain reaction
PDL - periodontal ligament
PFB - pseudofolliculitis barbae
PE - physical examination; pulmonary embolus
PEA - pulseless electrical activity
PEEP - positive end-expiratory pressure
PEP - postexposure prophylaxis
PERRLA - pupils equal, round, and react to light and accommodation
PE tubes - pressure-equalizing tubes
PFB - pseudofolliculitis barbae
PFS - patellofemoral syndrome
PFSH - past, family, social history
PFT - pulmonary function test
PH - past history
PHF - potentially hazardous foods
PHTLS - pre-hospital trauma life support
PI - present illness
PID - pelvic inflammatory disease
PIES - proximity, immediacy, expectancy, simplicity
PIP - proximal interphalangeal
Pit - Pitocin
PKU - phenylketonuria
PM - preventive medicine; *post meridiem* [L] - after midday or noon
PMCC - Patient Movement Control Center
PMH - past medical history
PMI - point of maximum impulse
PNM - polymorphonuclear neutrophil leukocytes
PND - paroxysmal nocturnal dyspnea
PNS - peripheral nerve stimulator
PO - post-operative
po - *per os* [L] - by mouth; orally
p0₂ - partial pressure oxygen
POD - post-operative day
POIS - pulmonary over inflation syndrome
pos - positive
postop - postoperative
POW - prisoner of war
PP - post partum; pulsus paradoxicus
PPB - positive pressure breathing
PPD - purified protein derivative
PPH - postpartum hemorrhage
PPI - proton pump inhibitor
ppm - parts per million
pPROM – preterm premature rupture of membranes
PPV - positive-pressure ventilation
Pre med - premedication

SOF Medical Handbook Abbreviations

pre-op - preoperative

PRBC - packed red blood cells

PRICEMM - Protection, Relative Rest, Ice, Compression, Elevate, Medication, Modalities

prn - *pro re nata* [L] - as needed

PROM - premature rupture of membranes; passive range of motion

PROMED - Program for Monitoring Emerging Diseases

PSA - prostate-specific antigen

PSI - pounds per square inch

PSVT - paroxysmal supraventricular tachycardia

Pt - patient

PT - physical therapy; prothrombin time

PTA - peritonsillar abscess

PTB - preterm birth

PTL - preterm labor

PTSD - post-traumatic stress disorder

PTT - partial thromboplastin time

PTB - primary tuberculosis

PUD - peptic ulcer disease

PULHES - physical profile factors: P--physical capacity or stamina; U--upper extremities; L--lower extremities; H--hearing and ears; E--eyes; S--psychiatric

PVC - premature ventricular contractions

q - *quaque* [L] - every

QC - quality control

qd - *quaque die* [L] - every day

qh - *quaque hora* [L] - every hour

q2h - *quaque 2 hora* [L] - every 2 hours

q3h - *quaque 3 hora* [L] - every 3 hours

qid - *quater in die* [L] - four times a day

qt - quart

qty - quantity

r - roentgen

R - right

Ra - radium

RA - rheumatoid arthritis

RADIAC - radiation detection, indication and computations

RBC - red blood cells or corpuscles

RDA - recommended dietary allowance

RDD - radiation dispersal device

RDS - respiratory distress syndrome

RE - relative effectiveness

REM - rapid eye movement

REF - reference

Ret - retired

RHS - radial head subluxation

RMW - regulated medical waste

RNA - ribonucleic acid

ROWPU - reverse osmosis water purification unit

RPM - revolutions per minute

RPR - rapid plasma reagin

Rh factor - Rhesus blood factor

RHS - radial head subluxation

RICE - rest, ice, compression, elevation

RLL - right lower lobe (of lung)

RLQ - right lower quadrant

RML - right middle lobe (of lung)

RMSF - Rocky Mountain spotted fever

R/O - rule out

ROM - range of motion

ROS - review of systems

RPR - Reiter protein reagin

RR - respiratory rate

RRRR - rest, reassurance, replenishment, restoration

RTD - return to duty

RUL - right upper lobe (of lung)

RUQ - right upper quadrant

RVA - rabies vaccine adsorbed

Rx - prescription; treatment; take

SA - Staphylococcus aureus

S-A; SA node - sinoatrial node

SALT - Sort, Assess, Life Saving Interventions, Transport/Treatment

SBE - subacute bacterial endocarditis

SBP - systolic blood pressure

SC - subcutaneous

SCC - squamous cell carcinoma

SCI - spinal cord injury

SCFE - slipped capital femoral epiphysis

SCUBA or scuba - self contained underwater breathing apparatus

Sed rate - erythrocyte sedimentation rate

SEV - surface equivalent

SF - Special Forces; standard form

SG - specific gravity; Surgeon General

SGA - small for gestational age

SH - social history

SIPE - submersion induced pulmonary edema

SLE - systemic lupus erythematosus; St. Louis encephalitis

SLR - short leg raise

SO - special operations

SOAP - subjective, objective, assessment, plan

SOB - shortness of breath

SODARS - special operations debrief and retrieval system

SOF - special operations forces

SOP - standing operating procedures

SP - Specialist (Army Corps for physician assistants, dieticians, occupational therapists, physical therapists)

S/P - status post

sp. gr. - specific gravity

SPK - superficial punctate keratitis

spp. - species

SQ - subcutaneous

SSRI - selective serotonin reuptake inhibitor

S & S - signs and symptoms

SSSS - staphylococcal scalded skin syndrome

staph - staphylococcus

STAT - *statim* [L] - immediately

STB - super tropical bleach

STD - sexually transmitted disease

strep - streptococcus

STS - serologic test for syphilis

SVP - Smallpox Vaccination Program

Sx - signs; symptoms

T - temperature

T & A - tonsillectomy and adenoidectomy

tab - tablet

TAH - total abdominal hysterectomy

TB - tuberculosis

TBD - to be determined; to be developed

TBE - tick-borne encephalitis

SOF Medical Handbook Abbreviations

TBRF – tick-borne relapsing fever
TBI - traumatic brain injury
Tbs or tbsp - tablespoon
TBSA - total body surface area
TCCC - tactical combat casualty care
Td - tetanus toxoid and diphtheria toxoid
TEH - thrombosed external hemorrhoid
temp - temperature
TENS - toxic epidermal necrolysis syndrome
TIA - transient ischemic attack
tid - *ter in die* [L] - three times a day
TIG - tetanus immune globulin
TIVA - total intravenous anesthesia
TKO - to keep open
TM - tympanic membrane
TMJ - temporomandibular joint
TNTC - too numerous to count
TPMRC - Theater Patient Movement Requirements Center
TPR - temperature, pulse, respiration
TSE - testicular self exam
TSH - thyroid-stimulating hormone
tsp - teaspoon
TURP - transurethral resection, prostate
TVH - total vaginal hysterectomy
Tx - treatment
U - unit
UA - urinalysis
UE - upper extremity
UGI - upper gastrointestinal
UNHCR - United Nations High Commissioner for Refugees
UPAC - Universal Portable Anesthesia Complete
UQ - upper quadrant
URI - upper respiratory infection
URQ - upper right quadrant
URTI - upper respiratory tract infection
US - ultrasound
USACHPPM - US Army Center for Health Promotion and Preventive Medicine

USAID - United States Agency for International Development
UTI - urinary tract infection
UV - ultraviolet
UW - unconventional warfare
VPP - vaccine-associated paralytic poliomyelitis
VC - Veterinary Corps
VDRL - venereal disease research laboratory test
V-Fib - ventricular fibrillation
VHC - Vaccine Healthcare Centers
VHF - viral hemorrhagic fevers
VIG - vaccinia immune globulin
vit - vitamin
Vol - volume
VPB - ventricular premature beats
vs - against
VS - vital sign(s)
VT - ventricular tachycardia
V-Tach - ventricular tachycardia
VZV - varicella-zoster virus
WBC - white blood cell
WBGT - wet bulb globe temperature
WEE - Western equine encephalitis
WHO - World Health Organization
WIA - wounded in action
wk - week
WMD - weapons of mass destruction
WN - west Nile
WNL - within normal limits
w/o - without
WP - white phosphorus
WPW - Wolff-Parkinson-White
wt - weight
W/U - workup
X - times
y/o - year old
yr -year
xr - x-ray

Trade Names of Generic Drugs

Generic Name	Trade Name(s)
acetaminophen	Tylenol
acetaminophen/butalbital/caffeine	Fioricet
acetaminophen/codeine #3	Tylenol with codeine
acetaminophen/dichloralphenazone/isomeheptene	Midrin, Duradrin
acetaminophen/oxycodone	Percocet, Endocet
acetazolamide	Diamox
activated charcoal	Actidose-Aqua
acyclovir	Zovirax
albendazole	Albenza
albuterol	Proventil, Ventolin
alfuzosin	Uroxatral
aluminium hydroxide gel	Amphojel
amantadine	Symmetrel
amikacin	Amikin
ammonium lactate lotion	Lac-Hydrin
amoxicillin	Amoxil, Trimox, Wymox
amoxicillin/clavulanate	Augmentin
amphotericin B	Fungizone
amphotericin B liposome	AmBisome
ampicillin	Omnipen, Polycillin, Principen
ampicillin/sulbactam	Unasyn
amyl nitrite	Aspirol, Vaporole
antipyrine/benzocaine ear drops	Aurodex
artesunate	Artenex
aspirin, non-enteric	Ecotrin, Empirin
aspirin/butalbital/caffeine	Fiorinal
atenolol	Tenormin
atovaquone	Mepron
atovaquone/proguanil hydrochloride	Malarone
atropine eye drops	Atropisol, Isopto Atropine
atropine sulfate injection	AtroPen
azithromycin	Zithromax
bacitracin eye ointment	Ak-Tracin, Bacticin, Ocu-Tracin
bacitracin topical	Baciguent
bacitracin/neomycin/polymyxin B eye ointment	Ak-Spore Ointment, Neosporin Ophthalmic Ointment, Ocutricin
bacitracin/neomycin/polymyxin B topical	Neosporin, Triple Antibiotic Ointment
baclofen	Lioresal
beclomethasone inhalant	Beclovent, Vanceril
beclomethasone nasal spray	Beconase AQ Nasal Spray
benzene hexachloride (lindane)	Kwell
benznidazole	Radanil, Rochagan
benzocaine/menthol spray	Dermoplast
benzonatate	Tessalon
betamethasone inject	Celestone
betamethasone topical	Alphatrex, Beta-Val, Betaderm, Betatrex, Diprolene, Diprosone, Luxiq, Maxivate, Uticort, Valisone
bisacodyl	Dulcolax
budesonide	Entocort EC, Pulmicort
bupivacaine	Marcaine
bupivacaine with epinephrine	Marcaine with epinephrine
butorphanol	Stadol
calcium carbonate	Tums, Caltrate
calcium gluconate	Kalcinate
calcipotriene topical	Dovonex

Trade Names of Generic Drugs

Generic Name	Trade Name(s)
cantharidin topical	Canthacur
carbamazepine	Tegretol
cefaclor	Ceclor, Raniclor
cefazolin	Ancef, Kefzol, Zolicef
cefixime	Suprax
cefotaxime	Claforan
cefotetan	Cefotan
cefoxitin	Mefoxin
ceftazidime inject	Tazicef, Fortaz
ceftriaxone inject	Rocephin
cefuroxime inject	Zinacef
cefuroxime axetil po	Ceftin
celecoxib	Celebrex
cephalexin po	Keflex
cephalothin inject	Keflin
cephazolin inject	Kefzol
chloral hydrate	Noctec
chloramphenicol	Chloromycetin
chlorhexidine oral rinse	Peridex, PerioGard
chloroprocaine	Nesacaine
chloroquine	Aralen
chlorpheniramine maleate	Chlor-Trimeton, Chlorphen
chlorpheniramine maleate/pseudoephedrine	Chlor-Trimeton D
chlorpromazine	Thorazine
clarithromycin	Biaxin
clobetasol topical	Temovate, Clobex
ciclopirox nail lacquer	Penlac
cimetidine	Tagamet
ciprofloxacin	Cipro
ciprofloxacin HCl/ hydrocortisone otic	Cipro HC Otic
citalopram	Celexa
clindamycin	Cleocin
clofazimine	Lamprene
clonidine	Catapres
clopidogrel	Plavix
clotrimazole	Mycelex (mouth), Lotrimin (skin), Gyne-Lotrimin (vaginal)
codeine	Generic only. No brands available.
colchicine	Generic only. No brands available.
cromolyn inhaled	Intal- inhaler
crotamiton topical	Eurax
cyclobenzaprine	Flexeril
cyclopentolate eye drops	Ak-Pentolate, Cyclogyl
dapsone	Avlosulfon
dexamethasone	Decadron
dextroamphetamine po	Dexedrine, Dextrostat
dextromethorphan	Benylin
diazepam	Valium
diclofenac sodium	Voltaren
dicloxacillin	Dynapen, Pathocil
diethylcarbamazine	Hetrazan
dimercaprol	British Anti-Lewisite (BAL)
dihydrostreptomycin (vet use)	Pfizer-Strep
dimenhydrinate	Dramamine
diphenhydramine	Benadryl

Trade Names of Generic Drugs

Generic Name	Trade Name(s)
docusate	Colace, Surfak
doxepin	Sinequan
doxycycline po	Vibramycin, Oracea, Adoxa, Atridox
enalapril	Vasotec
enoxaparin	Lovenox
epinephrine	Adrenalin
ertapenem	Invanz
erythromycin inject	E-Mycin, Erythrocin
erythromycin eye ointment	AK-Mycin
erythromycin po	E-Mycin, Eryc, Ery-Tab, PCE, Pediazole, Ilosone
esomeprazole	Nexium
ethambutol	Myambutol
famciclovir	Famvir
famotidine	Pepcid
fentanyl oral transmucosal lozenge	Actiq
fentanyl inject	Sublimaze
fentanyl transdermal	Duragesic
fluconazole	Diflucan
flumazenil	Romazicon
flunixin meglumine (animal use only)	Banamine
fluocinonide topical	Fluonex, Lidex
fluocinolone topical	Synalar, Derma-Smoothe/FS
fluoxetine	Prozac
fluticasone propionate spray	Flonase Nasal Spray
fluticasone/salmeterol	Advair HFA Inhaler
folinic acid	Folinic acid
furosemide	Lasix
gabapentin	Neurontin
gatifloxacin eye drops	Zymar
gentamicin inject	Garamycin, G-Mycin
gentamicin ophthalmic	Gentak, Gentasol, Garamycin Ophth
glipizide	Glucotrol
glyburide	Micronase
glycerin supp	Fleet
granisetron	Kytril
glucagon IV	GlucaGen
griseofulvin po	Fulvicin-U/F, Grifulvin V
guaifenesin	Fenesin, Guaifenex , Robitussin
haloperidol	Haldol
heparin	Calciparine, Liquaemin
heparin, low molecular weight (enoxaparin)	Lovenox
hetastarch	Hespan
homatropine eye drops	Isopto Homatropine
hydralazine	Apresoline
hydrocortisone po	Hydrocortone, Cortef
hydrocortisone injectable	A-Hydrocort, Solu-Cortef
hydrocortisone topical	Ala-Cort, CaldeCort, Cortaid
hydrocortisone/neomycin/polymyxin b otic	Cortisporin
hydromorphine	Dilaudid
hydroxyzine po	Atarax, Vistaril
hyoscyamine	Levsin
human diploid cell vaccine	Imovax
human rabies immune globulin	Hyperab S/D, Imogam Rabies HT
ibuprofen	Advil, Motrin

Trade Names of Generic Drugs

Generic Name	Trade Name(s)
imipenem and cilastatin	Primaxin
imipramine	Tofranil
imiquimod topical	Aldara
indomethacin po	Indocin
insulin, NPH	Humulin-N
insulin, regular	Humulin-R
ipecac syrup	Generic only. No brands available.
ipratropium bromide nasal spray	Atrovent HFA
isoniazid	INH, Laniazid, Nydrazid
itraconazole	Sporanox
ivermectin	Mectizan, Stromectol
ketamine	Ketalar
ketoconazole po	Nizoral
ketorolac eye drops	Acular
ketorolac	Toradol
labetalol	Normodyne, Trandate
lactulose	Cephulac, Chronulac, Constilac, Duphalac
lansoprazole	Prevacid
levalbuterol	Xopenex
levofloxacin inject	Levaquin
levofloxacin eye drops	Quixin
lidocaine gel	Xylocaine Viscous
lidocaine with epinephrine inject	Xylocaine with Epinephrine
lidocaine without epinephrine inject	Xylocaine for Injection
lindane topical	Kwell, Scabene
lisinopril	Prinivil, Zestril
loperamide	Imodium
loratidine	Alavert, Claritin
lorazepam	Ativan
mafenide acetate	Sulfamylon
magnesium citrate po	Citroma
magnesium sulfate IM	Generic only. No brands available.
mannitol	Osmitrol
mebendazole	Vermox
meclizine	Antivert, Antrizine
mefloquine	Lariam
melatonin	Generic only. No brands available.
meperidine	Demerol, Pethidine
mepivacaine HCL inject	Carbocaine, Polocaine
meropenem	Merrem IV
methenamine/methylene blue/phenyl salicylate/benzoic acid/atropine sulfate/hyoscyamine	Urised
methimazole	Tapazole
methylprednisolone	Solu-Medrol
metoclopramide	Reglan
metoprolol	Lopressor
metronidazole po	Flagyl
miconazole vaginal cream	Monistat
midazolam	Versed
minocycline	Arestin, Minocin, Dynacin
misoprostol	Cytotec
modafinil	Provigil
monochloroacetic acid topical	Generic only. No brands available.
montelukast	Singulair

Trade Names of Generic Drugs

Generic Name	Trade Name(s)
morphine inject	Roxanol, Astramorph
moxifloxacin eye drops	Vigamox
moxifloxacin	Avelox
mupirocin ointment	Bactroban
naproxen	Naprosyn
nalbuphine	Nubain
nafcillin	Nafcil, Unipen
naloxone	Narcan
naratriptan	Amerge
n-acetylcysteine po	Mucomyst
neomycin/polymyxin B/gramicidin	Neosporin
neosporin eye ointment	Neosporin Ophthalmic
nifedipine	Adalat, Procardia
nifurtimox	Lampit
nitazoxanide	Alinia
nitrofurantoin	Furadantin, Microbid
nitrogen, liquid	Generic only. No brands available.
nitroglycerin sublingual	Nitrostat, NitroQuick
nortriptyline	Aventyl, Pamelor
nystatin cream	Mycostatin
nystatin/triamcinolone acetonide cream	Mycolog
ofloxacin eye drops	Ocuflox
ofloxacin otic	Floxin Otic
ofloxacin po	Floxin
oseltamivir	Tamiflu
omeprazole	Prilosec
ondansetron	Zofran
oxybutynin chloride	Ditropan
oxycodone	Oxy-Contin
oxycodone/acetaminophen	Tylox
oxycodone/aspirin	Percodan, Roxiprin
oxacillin	Bactocill, Prostaphlin
oxybutynin	Ditropan
oxymetazoline nasal spray	Afrin
oxytocin	Pitocin
pantoprazole	Protonix
paromomycin	Humatin
paroxetine	Paxil
penicillin	Penicillin
penicillin G	Pfizerpen
penicillin G benzathine suspension	Bicillin LA, Permapen
Penicillin G potassium	Pfizerpen
penicillin G procaine	Wycillin
penicillin V	Pen-Vee K, pen-v.
penicillin V potassium	Beepen-VK,
pentavalent antimony	Glucantime
permethrin topical	Acticin, Elimite, Nix
petrolatum gel	Vaseline
phenoxybenzamine hydrochloride	Dibenzyline
phenobarbital	Luminal, Solfoton
phenylbutazone (for animal use)	Butazolidine, Butatron
phenytoin	Dilantin
piperacillin	Pipracil
piperacillin/tazobactam	Zosyn

Trade Names of Generic Drugs

Generic Name	Trade Name(s)
piroxicam	Feldene
podofilox topical	Condylox
polymixin B sulfate	Aerosporin
potassium chloride IV	Generic only. No brands available.
potassium chloride po	Cena K, K-Dur, K-Lor, K-Tab, Kaon-Cl, Kaon-CL, Kay Ciel, Klor-Con, Micro-K, Rum-K
podophyllin topical	Podocon-25; Podofin
pralidoxime chloride	Protopam
pramoxine/menthol/benzyl alcohol gel	PrameGel
praziquantel	Biltricide
prednisone po	Sterapred
prednisolone acetate eye drops	Econopred Plus, Pred Forte
prilocaine	Citanest 4% Plain Dental
primaquine phosphate	Generic only. No brands available.
prochlorperazine	Compazine
promethazine	Phenergan
propofol	Diprivan, Disoprofol
proparacaine eye drops	Alcaine, Ophthetic
propranolol po	Inderal
propylthiouracil	Propyl-Thyracil, PTU
protriptyline	Vivactil
pseudoephedrine	Sudafed
psyllium	Metamucil, Fiberall
pyrantel pamoate	Pin-Rid, Pin-X
pyrazinamide	Generic only. No brands available.
pyrethrin topical	Nix (1%), Elimite (5%)
pyrimethamine	Daraprim
quinidine	Quinalan (gluconate); Quinora (sulfate)
quinine	Qualaquin
rabies immune globulin	HyperRAB S/D, Imogam Rabies-HT
rabies vaccine adsorbed	Generic only. No brands available.
racemic epinephrine	AsthmaNefrin; MicroNefrin
ranitidine	Zantac
ribavirin	Rebetol
rifampin	Rifadin, Rimactane
rimantadine	Flumadine
rizatriptan	Maxalt
ropivacaine	Naropin
salmeterol inhaled	Serevent
salicylic acid topical	Compound W, Hydrisalic, Keralyt
scopolamine eye drops	Isopto-Hyoscine
selenium sulfide topical	Selsun Blue
senna fruit extract	Senokot, Gentlax
sertraline	Zoloft
sildenafil	Viagra
silver nitrate	Generic only. No brands available.
silver sulfadiazine cream	Silvadene
sodium nitrite IV	Part of Cyanide Antidote Kit
sodium thiosulfate IV	Part of Cyanide Antidote Kit
streptomycin inject	Generic only. No brands available.
succinylcholine	Anectine, Quelicin
sulfadiazine	Microsulfon
sumatriptan	Imitrex
syrup of ipecac	Generic only. No brands available.

Trade Names of Generic Drugs

Generic Name	Trade Name(s)
tamsulosin	Flomax
terbutaline sq	Terbutaline for injection
tetanus antitoxoid	Decavac
tetanus, diphtheria and pertussis vaccine	Adacel (age 11-64yr)
tetanus (human) immune globulin	Hyper-TET S/D
tetracaine eye drops	AK-T-Caine PF, Pontocaine
tetracycline po	Sumycin, Achromycin V
thiabendazole	Mintezol
thiamine inject	Generic only. No brands available.
ticarcillin	Ticar
ticarcillin/clavulanate	Timentin
tinidazole	Tindamax
tramadol	Ultram
triamcinolone inject	Kenalog, Aristospan
triclabendazole	Fasinex
triamcinolone topical	Kenalog
trichloroacetic acid topical	Tri-Chlor
trimethoprim-sulfamethoxazole DS	Septra DS, Bactrim DS
trimethoprim sulfate	Primsol, Proloprim
tobramycin	Nebcin
tolmetin po	Tolectin
tolterodine LA	Detrol LA
topiramate	Topamax
valacyclovir	Valtrex
valproic acid	Depakene, Depakote
vancomycin	Vancocin
vecuronium	Norcuron
verapamil po	Calan
vitamin K	Generic only. No brands available.
xylazine (for animal use)	Rompun
zaleplon	Sonata
zanamivir nasal spray	Relenza
zinc oxide topical	Generic only. No brands available.
zolmitriptan	Zomig
zolpidem	Ambien

Index of Figures

Index of Tables

Index of Terms

NOTES:

NOTES:

NOTES:

NOTES:

NOTES:

NOTES:

NOTES:

NOTES:

NOTES:

NOTES:

NOTES:

NOTES:

NOTES:

NOTES:

NOTES:

NOTES:

NOTES:

NOTES:

NOTES:

NOTES: